INTRODUCTION TO
Health Science

SECOND EDITION

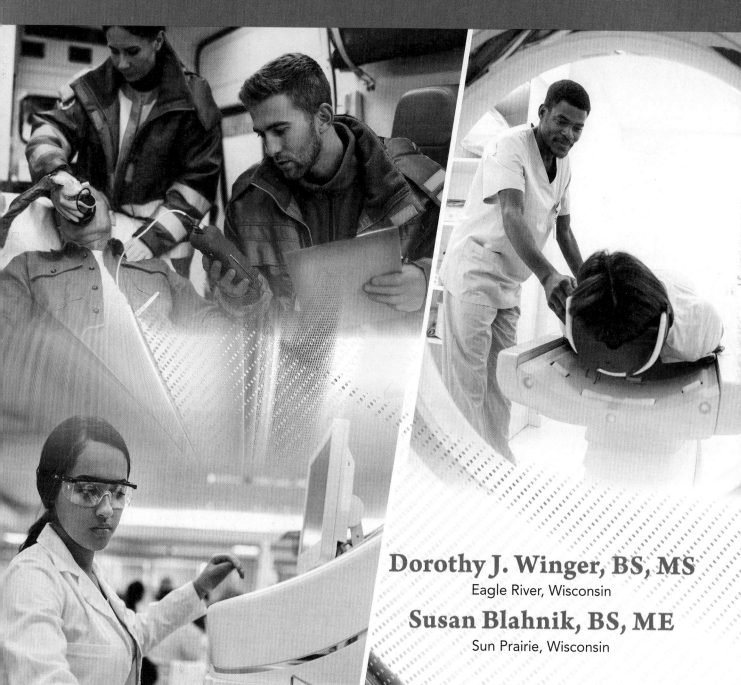

Dorothy J. Winger, BS, MS
Eagle River, Wisconsin

Susan Blahnik, BS, ME
Sun Prairie, Wisconsin

Publisher
The Goodheart-Willcox Company, Inc.
Tinley Park, IL
www.g-w.com

About the Authors

Dorothy Winger has more than 25 years of experience as a teacher and leader in health science and curriculum development. She taught Introduction to Health Occupations, Body Structure and Function, Medical Terminology, and Health Information Office Assistant at Madison East High School, in addition to dual-credit Medical Terminology for Madison Area Technical College. She was also the program coordinator for Nursing Assisting and led Madison Metropolitan School District's health science curriculum writing team. She served as a HOSA advisor, Red Cross blood drive coordinator, and Youth Health Service Corp advisor. She has coauthored multiple curriculum and standards projects at state and local levels and presented at the state and national levels. She served as president of Wisconsin Health Occupations Professional Educators, was Wisconsin HOSA advisor of the year, and served on the Wisconsin Governor's Task Force on the Health Care Worker Shortage and Wisconsin's Disciplinary Literacy Standards Leadership Team. She was a Continuing Professional Development Specialist for the University of Wisconsin School of Medicine and Public Health Pediatric Department, setting up educational events for American Medical Association continuing education credits. She continues to serve as an education consultant.

Sue Blahnik is a dedicated educator whose teaching career spans 40 years. Focusing on secondary education, she has taught career and technical coursework in health science, as well as family and consumer education. She developed a health science career pathway program for her local high school, established and managed the nursing assisting program, supervised youth apprentices, and advised the local HOSA chapter. Sue has written statewide curriculums and served on the statewide team to develop health science standards. She has presented at both national and state conferences and served as the president of the Wisconsin Health Occupations Professional Educators. An avid supporter of service learning, Sue mentored students and fellow educators and has been awarded several grants to support health science instruction and service-learning projects. Sue continues her commitment to students and learning as an educational consultant and author.

Acknowledgments and Reviewers

Goodheart-Willcox Publisher would like to thank HOSA—Future Health Professionals for reviewing and contributing to the development of this program.

Goodheart-Willcox Publisher would also like to thank Mary Kennedy, who helped write the review sections in this book. Mary Kennedy is a national presenter, educational consultant, STEM/STEAM trainer, and veteran teacher of 34 years. She coauthored the *Goals for Living* textbook with Goodheart-Willcox.

Thanks also to Jane Heibel, who carefully reviewed the manuscript before publication. Special thanks to those who completed interviews and posed for pictures that appear in the Healthcare Insider features.

Thanks to Starla Ewan at Starla's Creative Teaching Tips for the many years of sharing teaching techniques and successful ways of delivering difficult body system content.

The author and publisher wish to thank the following industry and teaching professionals for their valuable input into the development of *Introduction to Health Science*.

Chante Ford
Red Oak High School
Red Oak, Texas

Zachary Green
Pharmacy Technician Certification Board (PTCB)
Washington, DC

Charleen Handzel
Lewisville ISD- Technology Exploration Career
    Center West
Lewisville, Texas

Sarah Hansen
Atascocita High School
Humble, Texas

Deborah Hunt
William B Travis High School, Fort Bend ISD
Richmond, Texas

John Ko
Wayne State University College of Pharmacy and
    Health Sciences Clinical Laboratory Science
    Program
Detroit, Michigan

Lovett Lowery
Alabama State University
Montgomery, Alabama

Cyndi Sandusky
Sandusky Editorial Services
Walhalla, South Carolina

Katherine Sawyer
The Austin Center for Radiation Oncology
Austin, Texas

Ellen Shorosky
Hackensack Meridian Health
Edison, New Jersey

Alisha Smith
Summer Creek High School
Houston, Texas

New to This Edition

The second edition of *Introduction to Health Science* has been reorganized to better support instruction that follows the National Health Science Standards. For example, content about teamwork is now contained within one lesson to support instruction that follows the sequence of these standards. This new edition has also been updated to reflect the ever-changing advances in medical understanding and technology. New HOSA Event Prep activities in each chapter support connections to HOSA events.

HOSA—Future Health Professionals

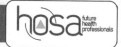

HOSA—Future Health Professionals is a global, student-led organization empowering future health professionals through collaboration, education, and experience. This organization introduces students to health careers and provides opportunities to build key leadership, communication, interpersonal, and healthcare skills.

Available at the middle school, secondary, and postsecondary levels, HOSA is a powerful instructional tool for equipping and educating future health professionals. If there is a HOSA chapter at your school, this course and text can help prepare you to participate, demonstrate your knowledge, and earn recognition through competitive events. If there is not a HOSA chapter at your school, you can talk with your instructor about starting one.

Throughout *Introduction to Health Science*, HOSA Event Prep icons identify activities specifically crafted to help you practice for competitive events. Some examples of how this program supports HOSA events follow:

- HOSA Event Prep features at the beginning of every chapter suggest HOSA events related to chapter content. Examples include *Family Medicine Physician* in Chapter 3: Health Science Career Preparation, *Healthy Lifestyle* in Chapter 9: Health Maintenance for Health Professionals and Patients, and *Medical Terminology* in Chapter 17: Medical Terminology and Body Organization.
- Activities at the end of each chapter help prepare you for competitive events such as *Prepared Speaking* and *Health Informatics*.

Precision Exams by YouScience Certification

Goodheart-Willcox is pleased to partner with You-Science to correlate *Introduction to Health Science* with their National Health Science Certification (NCHSE National Exam), Foundations of Healthcare Professions, and Essential Healthcare Practices certification standards. Students who pass the exam and performance portion of the exam can earn a Career Skills certification. Precision Exams by YouScience and Career Skills Exams were created in partnership with industry and subject matter experts to align real-world job skills with marketplace demands. Students can showcase their skills and knowledge with industry-recognized certifications—and build outstanding resumes to stand out from the crowd!

And for teachers, Precision Exams by YouScience provides:

- Access to a library of Career Skills Exams, including pre- and post-assessments for all 16 National Career Clusters
- Suite of on-demand reporting to measure program and student academic growth
- Easy-to-use, 100% online administration

To see how *Introduction to Health Science* correlates to Precision Exams by YouScience standards, visit the Correlations tab at www.g-w.com/introduction-health-science-2024. For more information about Precision Exams by YouScience, visit www.youscience.com/certifications/career-clusters/.

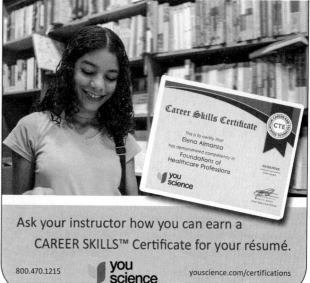

I earned a CAREER SKILLS™ Certificate in FOUNDATIONS OF HEALTHCARE PROFESSIONS. You can earn one too!

Ask your instructor how you can earn a CAREER SKILLS™ Certificate for your résumé.

800.470.1215   youscience.com/certifications

MesquitaFMS/E+ via Getty Images

Guided Tour

The instructional design includes student-focused learning tools to help students succeed. This visual guide highlights the features designed for the textbook.

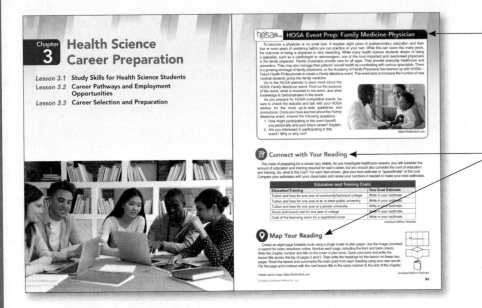

HOSA Event Prep activity introduces HOSA events related to the chapter.

Connect with Your Reading and **Map Your Reading** activities help you organize your notes and think about the chapter's topics before reading, a proven strategy for strengthening comprehension.

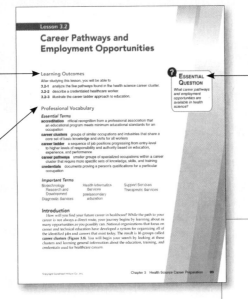

Learning Outcomes clearly identify the knowledge and skills to be obtained when the lesson is completed.

Professional Vocabulary lists the key terms to be learned in the lesson. You will need to learn the essential terms listed before you begin your reading. These terms, highlighted in yellow within the text, will help you understand the main concepts of the lesson. In addition, you will see bold terms explained where they first appear. These terms will deepen your understanding of the topics presented. Both will become part of your professional vocabulary.

Essential Question provides a starting point for thinking about the material in the lesson.

Healthcare Professions connect health science content to real-world experiences in a true introduction to healthcare careers.

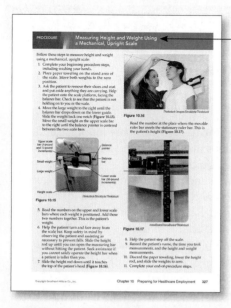

Step-by-Step Procedures are highlighted throughout the text to provide clear instructions for healthcare tasks. You can refer back to these procedures easily.

Lesson Review questions at the end of each lesson provide opportunities to extend your learning and help you apply knowledge.

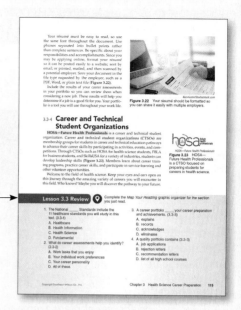

Chapter Summary provides an additional review tool for you and reinforces key learning outcomes.

Maximize Your Professional Vocabulary and **Reflect on Your Reading** activities help you remember and use key vocabulary and reflect on what you have read.

Build Core Skills activities help you apply and use what you have learned in connection with key skills such as math, reading, speaking, and critical thinking.

Review and Recall questions allow you to demonstrate knowledge, identification, and comprehension of chapter material.

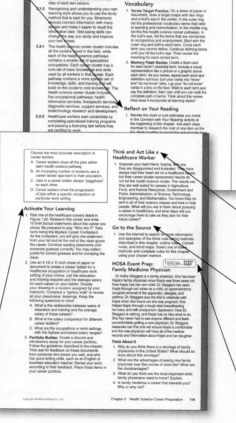

Think and Act Like a Healthcare Worker activities help you practice performing key career skills.

Go to the Source provides practice reading primary source documents and demonstrating other realistic reading tasks of a healthcare worker.

HOSA Event Prep activity helps prepare you to participate in HOSA events related to the chapter.

Activate Your Learning activities give you opportunities to physically use the information from the chapter.

TOOLS FOR STUDENT AND INSTRUCTOR SUCCESS

Student Tools

Student Text

Introduction to Health Science is an introductory health science textbook for high school students, written by health science instructors. *Introduction to Health Science* delivers essential content in an accessible, inviting, lesson-based format that strengthens students' literacy skills and healthcare vocabulary.

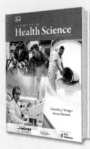

Companion Website

- E-flash cards and vocabulary exercises allow interaction with content to create opportunities to increase achievement.
- Interactive activities reinforce key concepts from the text with engaging and informational graphics.

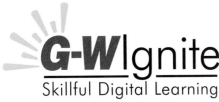

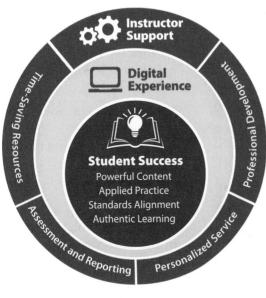

Instructor Support

Digital Experience

Student Success
Powerful Content
Applied Practice
Standards Alignment
Authentic Learning

Time-Saving Resources

Professional Development

Assessment and Reporting

Personalized Service

Instructor Tools

G-W Ignite

G-W Ignite provides a seamless user experience for both you and your students. The easy-to-navigate interface and class rostering capabilities make setting up a course easy and intuitive. Instructors can quickly and easily share assignments with students. Autograded activities and assessments make grading easier than ever, and rubrics are provided for ease of grading when required. Extensive reporting capabilities allow instructors to view students' progress and evaluate performance against learning outcomes and key standards. Students have their own My Progress dashboard where they can view grades and comments from their instructor.

G-W Ignite provides a complete learning package for you and your students. The included digital resources help your students remain engaged and learn effectively:

- The **Online Textbook** is a reflowable digital textbook that works well on all devices. It also works well with screen readers and accessibility tools.

- **Digital Activities** provide opportunities for students to reinforce understanding of learning outcomes in the text. Instructors can easily assign activities for each lesson, while easy grading tools, such as autograding, integrated answer keys, and rubrics, save time.

- **Videos** demonstrate important procedures or dive deeper into key concepts from the text. These videos clarify steps and aid students in visualizing important skills. Guided worksheets are provided to help students take notes as they watch each video. Video quiz questions help assess student comprehension in real time.

- **Drill and Practice Vocabulary Activities**, which are provided for all professional vocabulary terms in every lesson, provide an active, engaging, and effective way for students to learn the required terminology.

- Use the **Pretests**, **Posttests**, and **Exams** to assess students' knowledge of learning outcomes and key standards. These prebuilt assessments help you measure student knowledge and track progress in achieving learning outcomes.

- The **Instructor Resources** provide instructors with time-saving preparation tools such as answer keys, editable lesson plans, and other teaching aids.

- **Instructor's Presentations for PowerPoint**® are fully customizable, richly illustrated slides that help you teach and visually reinforce the key concepts from each chapter.

See www.g-w.com/introduction-health-science-2024 for a list of all available resources.

Professional Development

- Expert content specialists
- Research-based pedagogy and instructional practices
- Options for virtual and in-person Professional Development

Brief Contents

Contents

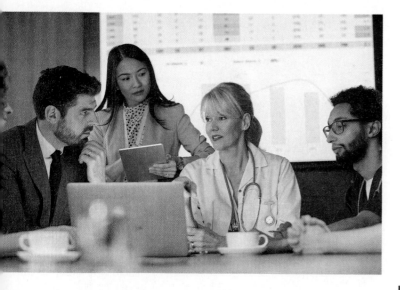

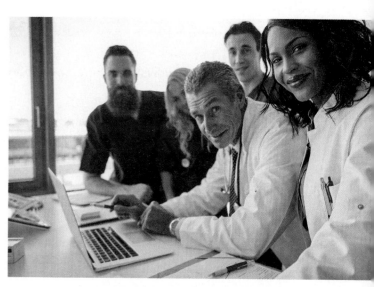

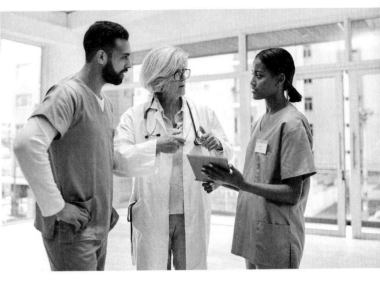

Feature Contents

HOSA Event Prep

Healthcare Professions

PROCEDURES

Welcome to the field of health science!

We hope you will enjoy learning from the experiences and insights of health-care workers as you read about the wide variety of careers in healthcare. You will study the five health science career pathways and will learn professional skills and standards of behavior used by workers in each pathway.

As you use the reading supports provided in this text, including professional vocabulary, mapping your reading, and connecting with and reflecting on your reading, you will improve your understanding of health science content. At the same time, you will strengthen your reading and comprehension skills.

Whether you have a specific career in mind or are just beginning your search, you will be excited to know that there are literally hundreds of healthcare occupations from which to choose. When you read about work personalities, leadership styles, and preferences for data, people, things, or ideas, take time to consider your own personal preferences, and you will discover satisfying career options for your future. Practicing the technical skills associated with each pathway will provide additional clues to your preferred career pathway.

Prepare for challenging health science coursework by sharpening your study skills. Use the memory techniques for learning vocabulary, try different methods for taking notes, and assess your personal learning style to improve your study habits. If you develop a plan for managing your time and learn skills for taking exams now, you will see the benefits throughout your school and work life.

Above all, we hope you will be excited to learn about the amazing variety of healthcare careers and will feel prepared to discover the pathway to your future career!

Dottie Winger

Sue Blahnik

Unit 1
Welcome to the Field of Health Science

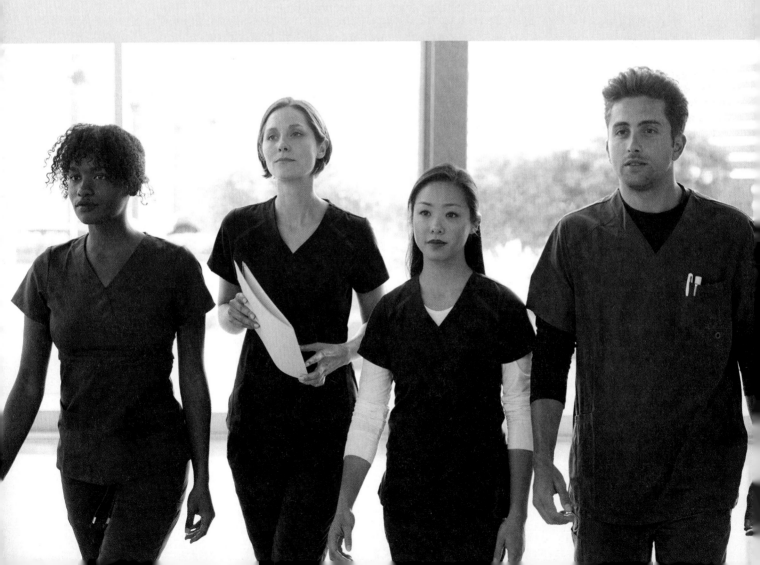

Healthcare Insider

Lauren, BS Marketing, Director of Public and Community Relations

I like my job because I have the opportunity to share success stories from the patients treated at Shriners Hospitals for Children. I work directly with news reporters and photographers to capture footage for stories, which has also allowed me to learn about pediatric orthopedics. My job duties include managing the Shriners Hospitals for Children brand, which means I have a hand in all advertising and marketing material.

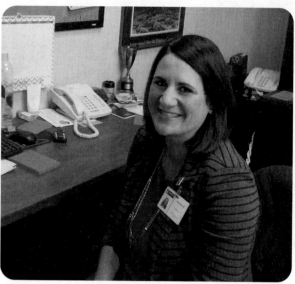

Courtesy of Lauren Elm, Director of Public and Community Relations, Shriners Hospitals for Children—Twin Cities

I have to make sure all of our brand requirements are met. It's fun to find new ways of sharing the amazing work that is done with pediatric orthopedics at Shriners Hospitals for Children. I feel lucky to be able to share that information every day.

Discussion Activity

Lauren says that she feels lucky in her job because she gets to share the amazing work done at Shriners Hospitals.

1. What would make you feel lucky to have a job in healthcare?
2. What daily tasks or work opportunities are exciting for you to consider?
3. If you have a particular career in mind, what tasks of that job do you think you will enjoy?

Chapter 1 The Evolution of Healthcare

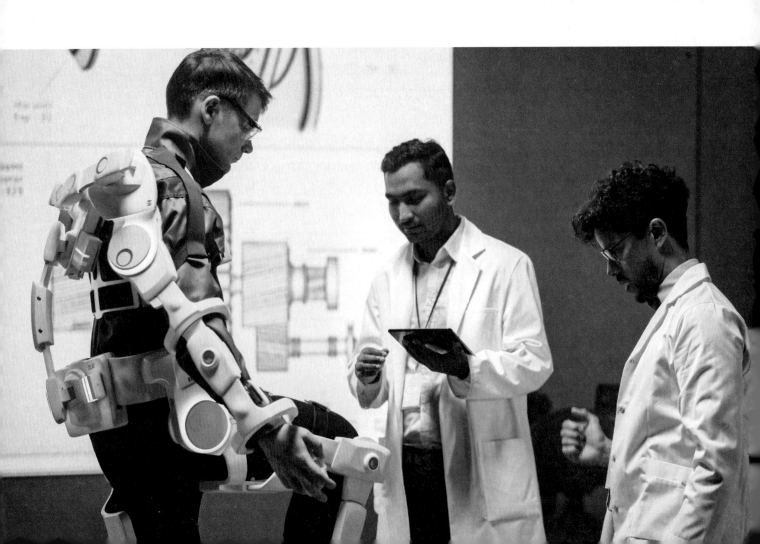

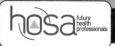

Healthcare professionals use reading to stay informed about the latest practices and advances in the field of health science. They read research papers and professional journal articles about their medical specialties. As you continue your education, reading skills will be important in your studies. Learning to read for content and remembering that information will help in any subject you are studying. You may find that you enjoy reading more when you are learning about a career field that interests you. Perhaps you will enjoy reading about diseases or cures. HOSA has a health science event called *Medical Reading*. Each year HOSA selects health science books to read for this competition. Some are leadership books, while others are biographies about physicians or true medical stories. This is a great event for expanding your knowledge about the field of health science.

Go to the HOSA website to learn more about the HOSA *Medical Reading* event. Find out the purpose of the event, what is involved in the event, and what knowledge is demonstrated in the event.

As you prepare for HOSA competitive events, be sure to check the website and talk with your HOSA advisor for the most up-to-date guidelines and procedures. Once you have learned about the *Medical Reading* event, answer the following questions:

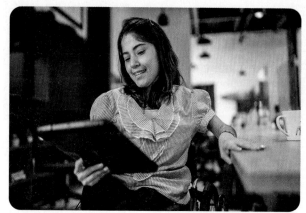

1. How might participating in this event benefit you personally and your future career? Explain.
2. Are you interested in participating in this event? Why or why not?

FG Trade Latin/E+ via Getty Images

 ## Connect with Your Reading

Consider a medical condition or disease, perhaps one that affects members of your own family. What treatment would your grandparents have received for this illness? What treatment would you receive for this disease today? What treatment do you predict your grandchildren will receive if they are affected by this disease? Pair with another class member and share your thoughts.

 ## Map Your Reading

Create a chart like the one shown. Skim through this chapter and list the three lessons in the chapter. Next, read the opening paragraph of each lesson and create a question about the content that you will read. Record each question in your chart. Finally, after reading each lesson, write an answer for each question using your own words rather than repeating the text.

The Evolution of Healthcare		
Lesson	**Possible Question**	**Answer the Question**
Write the name of the lesson.	*Write a possible question.*	*Answer the question.*
Write the name of the lesson.	*Write a possible question.*	*Answer the question.*
Write the name of the lesson.	*Write a possible question.*	*Answer the question.*

Goodheart-Willcox Publisher

Chapter opener image: Gorodenkoff/Shutterstock.com

Historical Changes in Healthcare

Learning Outcomes

After studying this lesson, you will be able to

1.1-1 describe historical changes in healthcare pioneered through the contributions of countless individuals.

1.1-2 relate the influences that change attitudes and beliefs about healthcare.

1.1-3 analyze the importance of accepting new research in healthcare.

Professional Vocabulary

Essential Terms

alternative, complementary, or integrative therapies   healthcare practices and treatments that minimize or avoid the use of surgery and drugs

holistic care   therapies that treat the patient as a whole person after assessing the individual's physical, social, mental, and spiritual well-being

Western medicine   the most common form of medical care in the United States; uses medication and surgery to treat the signs and symptoms of illness

Important Terms

antioxidant

infusion

Introduction

People have used medical treatments throughout the course of history, and countless individuals have contributed to advancements in the world of medicine. Within the last century, dramatic changes have occurred in the practice of medicine. Only a hundred years ago, a physician had a small home office and made frequent visits to the homes of patients. There were not many treatments available, so a physician was able to carry all the necessary medical care supplies in a single bag. Today, diagnostic and treatment options have multiplied, and medical research and development guide the acceptance of new attitudes and beliefs about healthcare.

1.1-1 Medical Advancements

A century ago, a physician studied the symptoms and courses of many diseases in medical school. A physician could diagnose an illness and tell patients the likely outcome of their disease. The physician might have been able to treat the pain involved with a disease, but could not cure the disease itself. Physicians provided personal care and support, as well as advice to family members regarding care for the patient.

Top 10 Lifesaving Medical Advances		
Scientist	**Medical Advance**	**Lives Saved**
Karl Landsteiner	Blood transfusions	1,100,000,000 lives
John Enders	Modern vaccines	340,000,000 lives
Howard Florey	Penicillin for bacterial diseases	203,000,000 lives
Frederick Banting	Insulin for diabetes	200,000,000 lives
Piero Sensi	Tuberculosis-curing drugs	75,000,000 lives
David Nalin	Oral rehydration therapy for cholera and diarrhea	57,500,000 lives
David Cushman	Blood pressure drugs	55,000,000 lives
Andreas Gruentzig	Angioplasty to widen arteries	52,000,000 lives
Akira Endo	Statins for heart attacks and strokes	26,000,000 lives
James Jude	Cardiopulmonary resuscitation (CPR)	25,000,000 lives

Goodheart-Willcox Publisher

Figure 1.1 These valuable scientists worked with others to develop healthcare treatments. Though their names may not be well-known, their work has saved millions of lives.

Patients sometimes recovered if they received good care at home. Physicians wished that more hospitals were available because they knew that good nursing care could improve patient outcomes. Often their job was to prepare patients for death from a disease that could not be treated.

Fifty years later, it was far more likely that physicians could treat the illnesses they diagnosed. Medical research and scientific discoveries changed medical care. Newly developed antibiotics such as sulfa drugs and penicillin shortened the course of infections. They even cured some diseases, such as meningitis, that were previously fatal. Insulin became available to treat diabetes, and X-rays could check for broken bones. Smallpox and tetanus vaccinations greatly reduced the incidence of illness (**Figure 1.1**).

During the past 50 years, technological advances have continued to change the methods and outcomes of medical treatment (**Figure 1.2**).

Healthcare Advances

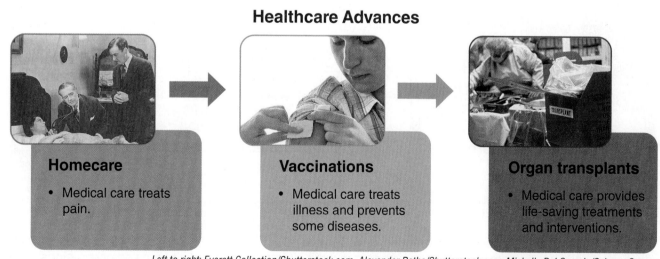

Homecare
- Medical care treats pain.

Vaccinations
- Medical care treats illness and prevents some diseases.

Organ transplants
- Medical care provides life-saving treatments and interventions.

Left to right: Everett Collection/Shutterstock.com, Alexander Raths/Shutterstock.com, Michelle Del Guercio/Science Source

Figure 1.2 Healthcare has rapidly evolved in the past 50 years alone. *What evolutions in healthcare do you predict for the next 50 years?*

Today, hospital patients receive life-saving treatments, such as heart bypass operations, heart valve replacements, and kidney transplants. An **infusion** (injection directly into a vein) of clot-busting drugs can reverse paralysis caused by a stroke. Some cancers that were previously fatal are now treatable.

In the fast-changing field of healthcare, doctors are not the only ones who have seen the demands and capabilities of their profession grow. For example, many students today plan to pursue a career in nursing because it provides the opportunity to work in a wide variety of healthcare environments. Nursing as a profession has only existed for about 150 years. Florence Nightingale felt compelled to care for people who were sick or injured. Her early efforts to establish good nursing standards and practices in the 1800s have evolved into programs that train nurses in many specialty areas. Nursing informatics, organ transplantation, midwifery (mid-WIF-eh-ree), advanced practice nursing, and anesthesia are some of the specialties within the nursing profession (**Figure 1.3**).

Nursing Professions

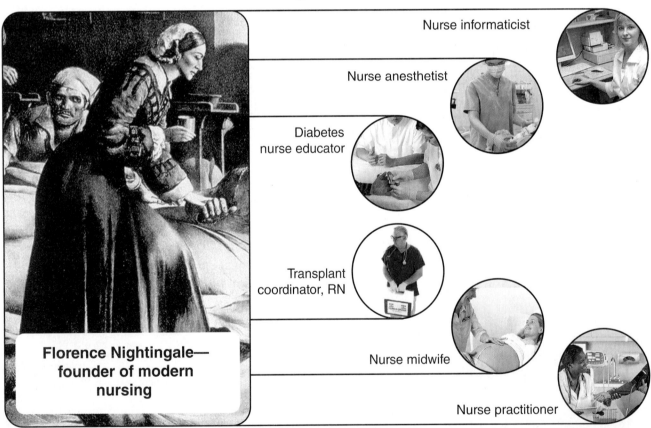

Left: Everett Collection/Shutterstock.com; Right, top to bottom: Univega/Shutterstock.com, Anettta/Shutterstock.com, Ian Hooton/Science Source, Catherine Yeulet/iStock/Thinkstock, Jeffery B. Banke/Shutterstock.com, Tyler Olson/Shutterstock.com

Figure 1.3 The role of nurses has expanded since Florence Nightingale, the founder of modern nursing, developed early nursing practices. Today, nurses can work in a variety of specialty nursing occupations. *Can you name additional specialty nursing roles?*

Healthcare Professions: Student Choices

Gerry's long stay in the hospital led him to appreciate the care he received from all types of healthcare professionals. June noticed the thoughtfulness shown to her dad by hospice personnel during his terminal illness. Fatou wants to return to her home country and work to improve healthcare there. Ron's dad, an athletic trainer, encouraged Ron to explore healthcare occupations in his career search. These students each have different situations and different experiences, but all of them are being led toward the same goal—a career in healthcare.

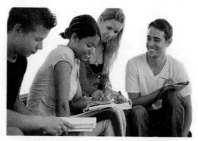

Diego Cerva/Shutterstock.com

Think about your own life experiences. Can you identify the influences that have led you to consider a career in healthcare? Whether you have a specific career in mind or are just beginning your search, you will be excited to know that there are literally hundreds of healthcare occupations from which to choose. As you identify your personal skills and connect them to the job opportunities in this field, you will discover satisfying career options for your future.

1.1-2 New Attitudes and Beliefs

The evolution of healthcare is not limited to changes in patient care and treatment. It also includes changes in the current attitudes and beliefs of people who will (or will not) benefit from those treatments. The discoveries of archeologists show that ancient cultures practiced medicine based on their spiritual beliefs and the use of herbal remedies. For example, scientists reject the ancient practice of removing "impure" blood from a patient, called *bloodletting*, to treat appendicitis. Today, appendicitis is treated surgically. However, not all spiritual and herbal treatments should be rejected in the practice of healthcare.

Alternative, Complementary, or Integrative Therapies

The neurosurgeon Benjamin Carson used prayer in his practice of medicine. Research shows that prayer and other practices such as meditation and yoga can improve a patient's mental health by reducing anxiety and stress. As a result, blood pressure may be lower, and the body's immune system may be stronger.

Research also shows benefits for some herbal treatments. Modern science has begun to validate some traditional uses for herbal teas. Peppermint and ginger teas really do improve nausea. Sage tea can improve memory, and chamomile tea really is calming. Green tea has many **antioxidant** (an-tee-AHK-suh-duhnt) benefits. Antioxidants promote health by reducing cell deterioration and may contribute to disease prevention. History is a valuable tool for advancing medical care when helpful information is accepted and information proven to be harmful is rejected (**Figure 1.4**).

Highlights in the History of Medicine

Location and Period in History	Medical Practice	Beneficial/Not Beneficial		Related Medical Practice Today
Many parts of the world (6000–3000 BC)	Trepanning—removing part of skull to release bad spirits; some patients actually survived	👎	👍	Craniotomy, the temporary removal of part of the skull, is used to prevent brain damage due to brain swelling.
Many parts of the world (6000–3000 BC)	Use of plants and herbs, such as foxglove and opium poppy	👍	👍	Digitalis, which regulates heartbeat, is made from foxglove. Morphine, which is used for pain relief, is made from the opium poppy.
Egypt (3000–300 BC)	Accurate health records	👍	👍	Accurate records are a legal requirement of medical care.
Egypt (3000–300 BC)	Bloodletting using leeches	👎	👍	Leeches are used to restore blood circulation to skin grafts.
China (1700 BC–220 AD)	Acupuncture	👍	👍	Acupuncture successfully treats osteoarthritis, migraine headaches, and more.
Greece (1200–200 BC)	Research into physical causes of disease	👍	👍	Research results form the basis for medical treatments.
Rome (700 BC–300 AD)	Building of aqueducts and sewers to improve sanitation and prevent disease	👍	👍	There is a renewed focus on handwashing and hygiene practices to reduce infections.
Arabic/Islamic civilization (700–1500 AD)	Universal healthcare and licensing for doctors and pharmacists	👍	👎	Many citizens have no health insurance and cannot access regular medical care.
Europe (400–1400 AD)	No medical advancements; millions of deaths caused by epidemics	👎	👍	Rapid medical advancements are made. Vaccines prevent > 20 life-threatening diseases.
Europe (1400–1700 AD)	Medical schools established	👍	👍	Educational training is established for more than 300 healthcare occupations.
Europe/America, 17th and 18th centuries (1600–1800 AD)	Study of anatomy and physiology through human dissection	👍	👍	3D imaging allows for anatomy study without using cadavers.
Europe/America, 17th and 18th centuries (1600–1800 AD)	Microscope invented; pathogens seen for the first time	👍	👍	Nanotechnology will develop targeted treatments that use devices and particles too small to be seen by a microscope.
Europe/America, 17th and 18th centuries (1600–1800 AD)	Many deaths caused by uncontrolled infections	👎	👎	"Superbug" infections remain a health issue.

Goodheart-Willcox Publisher

Figure 1.4 These medical practices used throughout history have influenced modern medical practices used today. Understanding how these treatments worked or did not work has shaped modern-day healthcare. (continued)

Highlights in the History of Medicine (continued)			
Location and Period in History	**Medical Practice**	**Beneficial/ Not Beneficial**	**Related Medical Practice Today**
Europe/America, 17th and 18th centuries (1600–1800 AD)	Bifocals invented	👍 👍	Bifocals are still used, but surgery can correct many vision conditions.
Europe/America (1800–2000 AD)	First female physician	👍 👍	Females equal or outnumber males in medical school.
Europe/America (1800–2000 AD)	First use of antiseptics and anesthetics	👍 👍	The use of aseptic and clean techniques and of general and local anesthetics is standard practice.
Europe/America (1800–2000 AD)	Discovery of penicillin	👍 👎	Overuse of antibiotics results in antibiotic-resistant bacteria.
Europe/America (1800–2000 AD)	Study of psychology and psychiatry	👍 👍	Therapies and medications treat "diseases of the mind."
Europe/America (1800–2000 AD)	Molecular structure of DNA modeled	👍 👍	The human genome is mapped.

Traditionally, **Western medicine**, which is practiced in the United States, has rejected forms of healthcare that do not focus on physical signs of illness. Some ancient practices are considered **alternative, complementary, or integrative therapies** because they do not focus mainly on treating symptoms with medication or surgery.

Holistic Care

Today there is a greater acceptance of the idea that wellness and the treatment of disease require a holistic approach. This means that healthcare focuses not only on the physical needs of an individual, but also on social, mental, and spiritual needs.

This kind of healthcare, called **holistic care**, works to maintain or restore wellness by promoting a balanced relationship between the mind, body, and spirit (**Figure 1.5**). People are most familiar with the components of physical wellness, which include a healthy diet, physical activity, and routine medical care. Other important components include the following:

- Mental/intellectual wellness—intellectual curiosity, lifelong learning, creativity, and problem solving
- Social wellness—communicating and interacting well with others and maintaining positive personal relationships
- Spiritual wellness—living according to personal values, ethics, and morals; may incorporate religious practices

People's personal history and culture also affect healthcare beliefs and practices. Your cultural heritage may determine whether you say a prayer, visit a shaman (SHA-muhn), or shop at a health food store in times of illness. Think about any home remedies you have used. Gargling with salt water for a sore

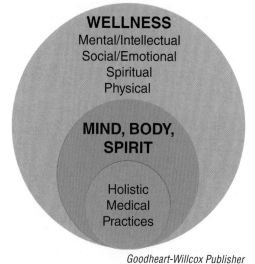

Goodheart-Willcox Publisher

Figure 1.5 Holistic medical practices can be found at the heart of preserving wellness by treating the mind, body, and spirit.

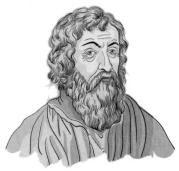

madjembe/Shutterstock.com

Figure 1.6 Hippocrates, known as the *Father of Medicine*, was a Greek physician who practiced medicine in 400 BC. His oath of medical ethics is still taken by physicians today. He believed in holistic care and promoted the wellness aspects of diet, rest, and cleanliness as part of the natural healing process.

throat is a home remedy that has stood the test of time. On the other hand, research has shown both positive and negative results for using zinc lozenges (LAH-zuhnj-ez) to shorten the duration of a cold. When evaluating treatments for illness, medical care providers still use Hippocrates's advice to "do no harm" (**Figure 1.6**).

1.1-3 Accepting New Research

Although medical research may show the need for changes in healthcare practices, both healthcare workers and healthcare consumers must understand and accept research before changes can be made. Over the course of history, many "healthcare heroes" contributed to medical advancements (**Figure 1.7**). Surprisingly, their discoveries and practices were often rejected by their peers.

Healthcare Workers

To understand the importance of healthcare workers accepting research, consider Ignaz Semmelweis. Ignaz Semmelweis advocated for handwashing. At the time, physicians were performing autopsies and then delivering babies without ever washing their hands. As a result, many people who had given birth died from puerperal (pyoo-UR-pur-uhl) fever caused by a bacterial infection. Semmelweis directed doctors to wash their hands and instruments in a chlorine solution. When they did, infections and deaths dramatically decreased. Sadly, Semmelweis' fellow physicians resented him. They did not like the idea that they were responsible for spreading disease. Eventually they gave up handwashing and fired Semmelweis.

Today people know that handwashing and using hand sanitizer are some of the most important tools in public health. They can prevent the spread of disease. Convincing healthcare providers to practice hand hygiene diligently is still a challenge. Every year, thousands of patients get hospital infections that are difficult to treat. The Centers for Disease Control and Prevention (CDC) says hand hygiene is one of the most important ways to prevent these infections.

Famous Healthcare Heroes	
Healthcare Hero	**Description**
Hippocrates	Father of medicine; recorded signs and symptoms of diseases
Leonardo da Vinci	Used dissection to sketch realistic human figures
William Harvey	Described the circulation of blood to and from the heart
Rene Laennec	Invented the stethoscope
Clara Barton	Founded American Red Cross
Joseph Lister	First doctor to use antiseptic during surgery
Florence Nightingale	Developed modern nursing practices
Louis Pasteur	Father of microbiology; pasteurized milk to kill bacteria
Alexander Fleming	Discovered penicillin
Jonas Salk	Developed the polio vaccine

Goodheart-Willcox Publisher

Figure 1.7 These top 10 well-known individuals advanced the practice of healthcare throughout history. *Whom would you include in your top 10 healthcare heroes?*

Healthcare Consumers

Healthcare consumers must learn about and accept new research in order to experience health benefits. For example, when they became new parents in the 1960s or 1970s, today's grandparents were taught to place an infant facedown or on the side for sleeping. They were warned that placing an infant on their back for sleeping could result in possible death due to choking.

In contrast, today's parents are taught to place an infant on their back for sleeping. They are warned that placing an infant facedown for sleeping greatly increases the risk for sudden infant death syndrome (SIDS). The basis for this turnaround was medical research that showed sleeping facedown significantly increased the risk of SIDS.

In 1994, a Back to Sleep® campaign from the American Academy of Pediatrics (AAP) began to educate parents, caregivers, and healthcare providers about ways to reduce the risk of SIDS. Since the start of this campaign, the percentage of infants placed on their backs to sleep has increased dramatically. Overall SIDS rates have declined by 50 percent. Today, the Safe to Sleep® campaign continues to educate parents and caregivers to reduce sudden and unexpected infant deaths (**Figure 1.8**).

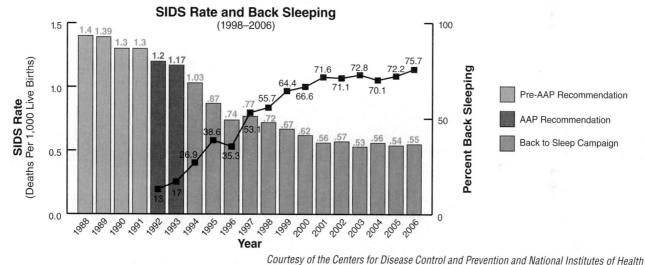

Courtesy of the Centers for Disease Control and Prevention and National Institutes of Health

Figure 1.8 In the graph shown here, the bars represent deaths due to SIDS during different time periods. The black line represents the percentage of babies being put to sleep on their backs.

Lesson 1.1 Review

 Complete the *Map Your Reading* graphic organizer for the section you just read.

1. As recently as 100 years ago, a doctor could often (1.1-1)
   A. treat an illness, but not diagnose it
   B. cure an illness, but not treat it
   C. cure an illness, but not diagnose it
   D. diagnose an illness, but not treat it

2. Examples of advancements in healthcare include (1.1-1)
   A. Landsteiner's work with blood typing
   B. Landsteiner's work with blood transfusions
   C. Salk's work on the polio vaccine
   D. Salk's work on the meningitis vaccine

3. Many healthcare professionals today are embracing a(n) _____ approach that considers more than the physical needs of a patient. (1.1-2)
   A. surgical   C. conventional
   B. holistic   D. targeted

4. Healthcare practices change not only when research verifies the benefits, but also when healthcare _____ understand and accept the research findings. Choose all that apply. (1.1-3)
   A. consumers   C. politicians
   B. broadcasters   D. workers

Future Trends in Healthcare

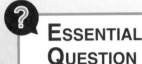

ESSENTIAL QUESTION

What trends will shape healthcare in the future?

Learning Outcomes

After studying this lesson, you will be able to

1.2-1 explain how genomic medicine could personalize healthcare.

1.2-2 explain trends and advancements in regenerative medicine.

1.2-3 give examples of how technology is advancing healthcare.

Professional Vocabulary

Essential Terms

genomic medicine   personalized medical care that uses a patient's unique combination of genes and chromosomes to prevent illness and maintain health

nanotechnology   a field of science that manipulates individual atoms and molecules to create devices that are thousands of times smaller than current technologies allow

regenerative medicine   a form of medical care that creates living tissue to replace tissue or organ functions lost due to age, disease, injury, or birth disorder

telesurgery   surgery performed by robotic equipment that is monitored and controlled from a remote site

Important Terms

3D printing	in vitro	stem cells
artificial intelligence (AI)	mammogram	stents
chronic	pacemakers	virtual reality
gene therapy	prosthetics	

Introduction

As you prepare for a career in healthcare, know that constant change is normal. It is entirely possible that someday you will work in a position that does not even exist today. In 1950, doctors in practice could expect the total amount of medical knowledge to double every 50 years. Now it doubles in just 73 days. The healthcare and scientific communities are learning more every day. This makes teamwork and the sharing of medical knowledge more important than ever before. For a technically savvy generation of healthcare workers, global sharing of information will lead to even more rapid advances in healthcare.

Today, advances in deep brain stimulation can treat patients with obsessive-compulsive disorder. This treatment is also being tested to help patients with Alzheimer's disease improve memory and judgment. It shows promise in helping patients recover from a stroke.

What advances in medical care will you see? What issues will affect your practice and delivery of care? These are important questions for future healthcare workers. While the future cannot be predicted, current research can provide insight into how medical care may change. In this lesson, you will learn about the areas of genomic medicine, regenerative medicine, and medical technology.

1.2-1 Genomic Medicine

Genomic (jih-NOH-mihk) **medicine** identifies and studies sequences in deoxyribonucleic acid (DNA), which carries the genetic information of organisms (**Figure 1.9**). A *genome* is the complete sequence of DNA for every chromosome in an organism—in this case, a human being. When scientists compare the genomes of human beings, they look at the genes on DNA. While 99 percent of genes are identical between people, a few are different. Those differences explain why one person will develop a disease or respond to a drug and another will not.

Future medical care will focus on predicting whether a specific person will develop a particular disease. Treatments will include methods for preventing a disease, as well as improved methods for treating it. Medical care will also become more personalized. Healthcare workers will be able to determine which drug will be most effective for a particular patient based on that patient's unique combination of genes and chromosomes. Genomic medicine will allow doctors to make accurate predictions about how a patient's disease will progress and which medications will produce the best response with the fewest side effects. Drugs will be personalized to be effective and safe for a specific individual.

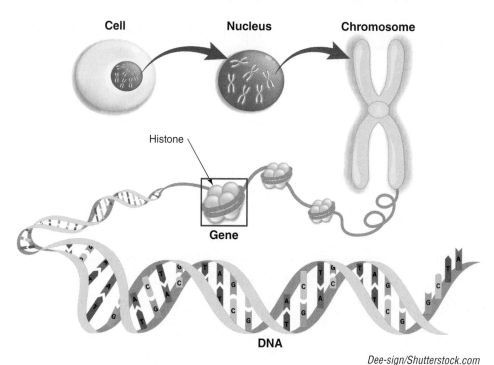

Dee-sign/Shutterstock.com

Figure 1.9 Genomic medicine studies the sequences in DNA, which carries the genetic information of organisms. Eventually, treatments will be tailored to a patient's particular genomic makeup.

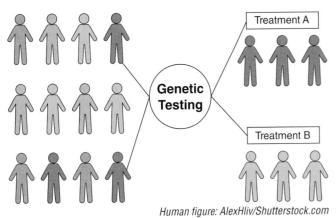

Human figure: AlexHliv/Shutterstock.com

Figure 1.10 Individual genetic information will help physicians select the type of treatment that will be most effective for a specific patient. *What types of illnesses might genomic medicine help treat?*

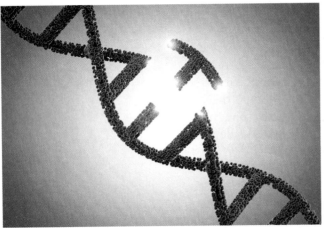

Phonlamai Photo/Shutterstock.com

Figure 1.11 Scientists use a technique called CRISPR to modify DNA to prevent or cure genetic diseases. A gene therapy to treat sickle-cell anemia is being tested in clinical trials at the NIH.

Another use of genomic medicine is genetic testing. Genetic tests are already being developed today to predict the potential onset of a disease later in life. For example, some people carry a gene that greatly increases their risk for developing breast cancer. For these people, earlier and more frequent **mammogram** screenings may detect any developing cancer to treat in its earliest stages. Mammograms are X-rays used to test for breast cancer. As another example, prostate cancer research shows that patients with a testosterone-based genetic variation have different responses to certain drugs. In the future, this could lead to personalized treatments to fight prostate cancer.

In the future, designer vaccines may be developed for a specific person (**Figure 1.10**). Scientists could use fragments of a person's DNA to create a vaccine that would prevent or treat an illness in only that person. Genomic medicine will help scientists develop vaccines to treat many diseases that are not yet preventable. This includes long-lasting, or **chronic** (KRAH-nihk), illnesses such as heart disease or cancer. For example, consider the benefits of the hepatitis B vaccine. Because chronic hepatitis B can lead to a form of liver cancer, this vaccine prevents both hepatitis B and the development of this specific type of cancer. In the future, many vaccines will be given in new ways, such as by mouth, inhalation through the nose, or skin patches. In addition, often only one dose of each vaccine will be needed.

Eventually, genomic medicine may include **gene therapy**, which involves the insertion of a new gene to replace an abnormal gene (**Figure 1.11**). For example, *CRISPR* is a genome-editing method that could revolutionize genomic medicine. It may allow scientists to edit immune system cells to help them fight off cancer cells. Research into gene therapy is ongoing with the goal of developing treatments for genetic diseases and disorders, such as sickle cell disease or hemophilia.

1.2-2 Regenerative Medicine

The goal of **regenerative** (rih-JEH-nuh-ray-tiv) **medicine** is to use a patient's stem cells to develop tissues and organs that replace damaged ones. **Stem cells** are basic cells that can develop into specific types of cells. Organs created using stem cells are developed from a patient's DNA. This should eliminate the current problem of organ rejection experienced by transplant patients today. With advances in regenerative medicine, organ donation would become a thing of the past.

There are two types of stem cells—embryonic and adult. Embryonic (ehm-bree-AH-nihk) stem cells can become all types of cells found in the body. These stem cells come from discarded embryos created as part of *in vitro*, or *test tube*, fertilization. The use of embryonic stem cells is controversial.

Adult stem cells are found in tissues and are more limited in their ability to generate the various cells of the body. While researchers once believed adult stem cells could only produce similar types of cells, newer evidence indicates they may be more adaptable than previously thought. Despite some limitations, adult stem cells do appear to help repair damage caused by illness or injury (**Figure 1.12**).

Today, adult stem cells are used for bone marrow transplants to treat severe forms of blood cancer and anemia. In the future, stem cells could be developed to help heal heart tissue after a heart attack or create pancreatic cells for patients with type 1 diabetes. Stem cell injections could repair worn-out knee cartilage, removing the need for surgical joint replacement.

Clinics across the United States already offer stem cell therapies, but not all therapies are approved by the Food and Drug Administration (FDA). The FDA is increasing its enforcement of regulations in stem cell clinics that use unapproved stem cell products. Unproven stem cell treatments have produced severe adverse, or harmful, reactions.

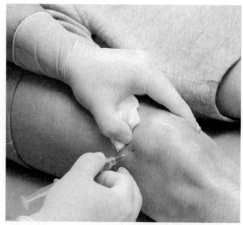

photoshoot2015/Shutterstock.com

Figure 1.12 While stem cell therapies show great promise for new treatments, the FDA has issued a warning to consumers to avoid stem cell clinics that use experimental procedures. Treatments without FDA approval have resulted in tumor growth and other negative effects.

1.2-3 Technology and Medicine

Just as technology is bringing major changes in our everyday lives, it is also fueling important advances in medicine. Virtual reality, artificial intelligence, data mining, digital devices, and biomechanical technologies will all influence medical care.

Healthcare Professions: The Evolving Nature of Healthcare

Consider the experience of Addison, a surgical technologist at a major university hospital. She was hired before she graduated from her training program. During the first year of her job, Addison assisted surgeons as they performed brain surgeries and observed the deep brain stimulation procedures for treating patients with Parkinson's disease. The following year, she was part of a medical team researching the installation of a magnetic resonance (REHZ-uh-nuhnts) imaging (MRI) scanner within the surgical suite. This new technology improved the surgical experience for patients with Parkinson's disease. Now, just three years out of school, Addison is a *preceptor* (prih-SEHP-tuhr), or teacher, who trains future technologists in the use of magnetic resonance imaging during surgery.

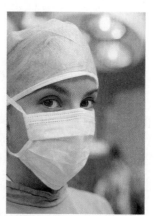

wavebreakmedia/Shutterstock.com

Virtual Reality

Virtual reality technology shuts out all parts of the environment and provides an entire simulation. This can be used in psychiatry to treat irrational fears, called phobias. Virtual reality helps patients manage pain by focusing attention away from the sensation of pain. Many fitness apps use it to make physical activity more entertaining.

Mixed reality, a combination of virtual and physical environments, enhances medical education. An instructor can project the human body in its full size in front of students. Students can examine organs, veins, or bones accurately in 3D. This can replace the use of cadavers and make 3D anatomy more accessible for students (**Figure 1.13**).

One concern with new technologies is that excessive use will produce new illnesses and conditions. For example, video games can provoke seizures in people with photosensitive epilepsy. Could virtual reality gaming produce a form of post-traumatic stress disorder (PTSD)? Could virtual battles produce the same symptoms as actual warfare? Therapists are already treating patients with "text neck," the neck pain and damage caused by looking down at your cell phone, tablet, or other wireless devices too often and for too long.

Data Mining and Artificial Intelligence

Examining data from many different research studies already offers insight into answering current health questions. Researchers today can access repositories (collections) of scientific data from a wide variety of scientific fields.

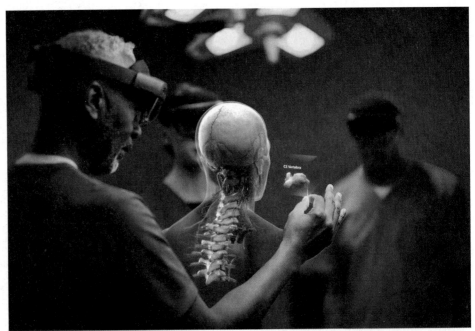

Used with permission from Microsoft

Figure 1.13 Medical students find virtual/mixed reality anatomy instruction appealing and efficient when they access the images. *What other medical applications for virtual reality are suggested in this image?*

Advances in data mining and artificial intelligence include microdevices, machine learning, and voice technologies.

- **Microdevices.** In the future, researchers may be able to conduct clinical trials without animals or people. Instead, they will use human organs on chips. These *microdevices* lined with living human cells could imitate the functions of human organs (**Figure 1.14**). This makes them ideal for replacing clinical testing. In the future, a computer simulation may be able to develop or evaluate a medication or medical device with no risk to animals or people.

- **Machine learning.** Correctly identifying cancer cells in a tissue sample is vital to successful treatment. Using **artificial intelligence (AI)** to produce *machine learning*, computers can be trained to detect cancerous cells in a tissue sample. They can find the cells as accurately as a human, but in a matter of seconds. AI could also calculate the precise dosage of a cancer drug that will shrink tumors with the fewest toxic side effects.

- **Voice technologies.** Voice technologies can help physicians diagnose diseases and disorders. Researchers have found that characteristics of patients' voices, called *vocal biomarkers*, reveal a lot about their health. So far, vocal biomarkers have helped diagnose mental health conditions and coronary artery disease, and more options are expected in the future.

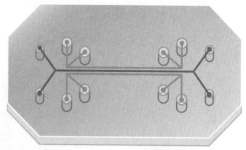

XOHDY/Shutterstock.com

Figure 1.14 Microdevices lined with living human cells can imitate the functions of human organs. This makes them ideal for use in clinical testing and eliminates the risk to human subjects.

Voice technology can also help healthcare providers with administrative tasks. Using artificial intelligence combined with voice technologies could allow physicians and patients to talk during appointments while a voice assistant listens and records interpreted text in a patient's electronic health record.

Digital Devices

Healthcare applications (apps) for digital devices are expanding rapidly. For example, a smartphone app may be able to help detect pancreatic cancer by checking the whites of a person's eyes for signs of jaundice. Take a selfie, and the app checks for elevated bilirubin levels, a sign of the disease.

People already track their steps, calories, and sleep quality using digital devices. Newer devices can also measure electrical impulses of the heart and detect atrial fibrillation. Some measure blood pressure and blood oxygen levels, while others measure heart and lung sounds like a digital stethoscope.

In the future, digital tattoos may be available. These flexible skin patches could be worn for days or weeks. They would provide continuous monitoring and transmit data to smartphones or other devices. Healthcare professionals could monitor and diagnose critical health conditions such as heart arrhythmias, heart activities of premature babies, and sleep disorders.

Biomechanical Technologies

Biomechanical technologies are another changing area of healthcare. Some applications of these technologies could include 3D printing, brain implants, and telesurgery.

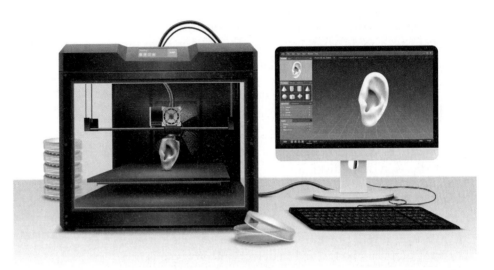

Figure 1.15 3D printed prosthetics can easily be reproduced in multiple sizes to adjust for a child's growth, for example. *Would you consider a prosthetic that enhances your skills rather than replacing your natural abilities?*

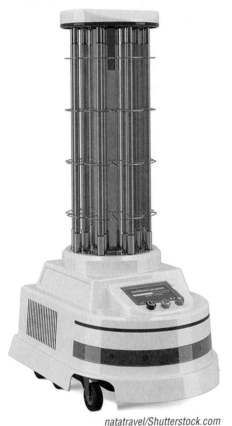

Figure 1.16 This robot disinfects a hospital room in 10 minutes. *Can you name other uses for robots in healthcare?*

3D printing is already producing **prosthetics** (artificial body parts) for people who have had a limb amputated. Prosthetics can be created for a specific individual using measurements scanned by a mobile phone. After printing, prosthetics can be shipped anywhere in the world. 3D printing creates a three-dimensional solid object from a digital file (**Figure 1.15**). This process can also produce medications in layers that dissolve more easily or shapes that appeal to young patients. Commercially produced printed medications may be available in a few years.

3D bioprinting technology could create liver or skin tissues or even a cancerous tumor for use in testing new treatments. Eventually replacement organs might be printed to address organ donor shortages.

Brain implants could someday provide perfect vision and hearing. Could a brain implant combined with an exoskeleton for support allow a person with paralysis to move? That technology is already being developed. How about a contact lens that monitors blood sugar? Would you consider an implant even if you did not have a medical condition? Would you wear earbuds that make you multilingual?

Robots already assist in surgery, but newer technologies could allow physicians to perform robotic surgery remotely using wireless 5G networks. In this way, **telesurgery** could bring the expertise of specialists to less populated areas. Robots will become more common in healthcare as they are used to disinfect hospital environments, assist with lifting and moving patients, and administer medication (**Figure 1.16**).

Nanotechnology

The combined efforts of engineering and medicine are producing smaller and more powerful medical devices. Healthcare already uses tubes called **stents** that keep arteries open and tiny devices called **pacemakers** that regulate heartbeats.

The science of **nanotechnology** (na-noh-tehk-NAH-luh-jee) is expected to develop devices so small they cannot be seen by a microscope. These tiny devices will be able to swim through the bloodstream or lymphatic fluid. They could enter a cell to deliver a targeted medication or kill cancer cells before a tumor can form. If these devices could deliver insulin directly to the blood, people with diabetes would not need multiple daily shots, and oral tablets would replace insulin injections.

Micro-robots are another advance in nanotechnology. Tiny micro-robots can be folded into a medication capsule that makes them easy to swallow. A micro-robot might contain a magnet, so that when the capsule opens in your digestive system, the micro-robot can grab a battery that has been swallowed and carry it out of the body—no surgery required (**Figure 1.17**). In the future, specialized nanobots could perform surgeries inside the body while surgeons use a magnetic field to guide the bots. These nanobots are even smaller than micro-robots. They could drill through blocked arteries to restore blood flow or collect tissue samples for biopsy.

Which of these trends will prove beneficial to medical care? Which of these new treatments will be a part of your future career? Some new treatments will become a part of routine medical care, while others will not fulfill their promise. They will be abandoned as new research moves forward.

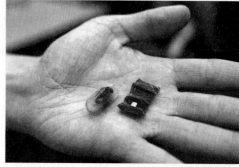

Melanie Gonick/MIT

Figure 1.17 This tiny "origami" robot unfolds from a swallowed capsule. Steered by outside magnetic fields, it moves across the stomach wall to remove a swallowed button battery or patch a wound.

Lesson 1.2 Review

 Complete the *Map Your Reading* graphic organizer for the section you just read.

1. Which of the following is a genome-editing method that could be used to develop treatments for genetic diseases and disorders? (1.2-1)
   A. Telesurgery
   B. Gene therapy
   C. CRISPR
   D. CABG

2. Organ rejection could be eliminated if new organ tissue is generated using a patient's own (1.2-2)
   A. assimilation
   B. basal cells
   C. stem cells
   D. adaptation

3. Extreme miniaturization produced by scientists in which field could one day deliver medicine to individual cells, allowing doctors to treat a disease without damaging healthy tissue? (1.2-3)
   A. Biotechnology
   B. Immunotechnology
   C. Nanotechnology
   D. Prosthetics

4. In which practice can a physician use a robot to perform surgery on a patient in another city or possibly even another country? (1.2-3)
   A. Digital surgery
   B. Telesurgery
   C. Online surgery
   D. Deep brain stimulation

5. Which of the following techniques may be used to create prosthetic devices or medications? (1.2-3)
   A. Modern teleprinting
   B. 3D printing
   C. Artificial intelligence
   D. Machine learning

Healthcare Challenges

? ESSENTIAL QUESTION

What challenges are influencing healthcare today?

Learning Outcomes

After studying this lesson, you will be able to

1.3-1 provide reasons for the increased use of complementary and alternative medical practices.

1.3-2 explain how the affordability of healthcare services influences patient health.

1.3-3 explain how the accessibility of healthcare services influences patient health.

1.3-4 identify how current issues in healthcare are being addressed.

Professional Vocabulary

Essential Terms

integrative medicine   care that combines practices and treatments from alternative medicine with conventional medicine

Patient Protection and Affordable Care Act (ACA)   a healthcare reform law that increased access to and coverage by health insurance plans

Introduction

As medical care becomes more specialized, patients are missing the personal connection with their healthcare provider. They are using a variety of options for seeking personal wellness. Affordability and access are also big issues challenging healthcare today. People in the United States are finding it increasingly difficult to pay for their healthcare costs, and lack of primary care in rural areas is rising. This means that more people are at risk of dying earlier due to lack of medical care. People are making efforts, however, to address these important healthcare issues.

1.3-1 Back to the Basics of Care

Many patients are frustrated by a lack of personal attention in their medical care. As they move from one doctor to another, patients feel as though they are a set of symptoms or a disease rather than a valued person who is seeking relief. Patients are looking for medical care that is more holistic, paying attention not only to their physical needs, but also to their emotional, social, and even spiritual wellness.

A growing number of patients are turning back to ancient healthcare practices, such as acupuncture (AK-yu-puhnk-cher) and homeopathy (hoh-mee-AH-puh-thee). These patients are finding relief from pain while using fewer medications and surgeries. Many alternative healthcare practices are not covered by insurance, so patients must be finding them effective. If these techniques were not providing relief, patients would not be willing to pay for the treatment.

Western medical providers are taking note of this trend. Many US hospitals, universities, and medical schools have established centers for **integrative medicine**. These centers offer conventional Western medical care combined with alternative and complementary therapies (**Figure 1.18**).

The National Institutes of Health (NIH) has created a National Center of Complementary and Integrative Health (NCCIH). This organization conducts scientific studies to determine which alternative therapies are effective. As research confirms the benefits of therapies, medical doctors will begin to include or integrate these therapies into patient care plans. In many cases, research has shown that a particular therapy is effective, but the reason why is still unknown. As with any other kind of treatment, doctors must know both the pros and cons of alternative therapies before fully adopting them (**Figure 1.19**).

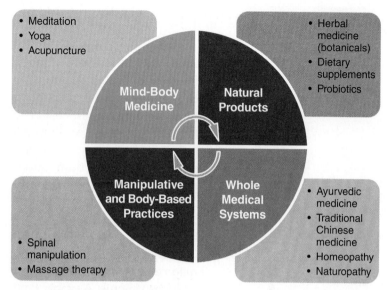

Data courtesy of the NCCIH

Figure 1.18 Other Complementary and Alternative Medicine (CAM) practices include movement therapies such as Pilates and the Feldenkrais method. Traditional healers, including the Native American medicine man, are considered CAM practitioners. The energy practices of magnet therapy, light therapy, qi gong, and Reiki are also considered CAM therapies.

Alternative Therapies	
Benefits of Select Alternative Therapies	**Precautions for Select Alternative Therapies**
Acupuncture has proven beneficial in treating pain caused by osteoarthritis, dental surgery, migraine headaches, and other causes.	Choose a reputable and experienced practitioner who can provide credentials. Be aware that insurance may not cover treatment costs.
A combination of glucosamine and chondroitin sulfate has proven beneficial for some patients with severe osteoarthritis pain. Omega-3 supplements can reduce the risk factors for heart disease.	Herbal remedies are regulated for safety but not for effectiveness. Natural products may interfere with other medications. Not all natural compounds are safe for use.
Massage benefits the development of premature infants and can provide relief from stress, anxiety, and the pain of migraine headaches.	Select a therapist who is trained and licensed. Avoid massage therapy if you take blood thinners or have a history of blood clots.
Meditation can reduce anxiety, depression, and chronic pain symptoms.	People with physical limitations may not be able to participate in meditative practices involving physical movement. Research is needed to determine if meditation can worsen symptoms in people who have certain psychiatric conditions.

Goodheart-Willcox Publisher

Figure 1.19 When looking into alternative therapies, it is important to think of the precautions as well as the benefits. *After studying the pros and cons of these alternative therapies, would you be willing to try any of them? Why or why not?*

1.3-2 Affordable Healthcare

Healthcare costs in the United States have been rising for several years. As a result, the United States surpasses most other industrialized countries in terms of dollars spent on healthcare per resident (**Figure 1.20**). Healthcare costs have been rising faster than the rate of inflation. An increase in the inflation rate could push costs even higher. As a result, employers and workers are finding it more and more difficult to afford health insurance. The average premium for family coverage has increased 54 percent over the last 10 years, significantly more than workers' wages. Healthcare spending is projected to grow faster than the economy over the next decade. Cost control, therefore, is a critical consideration for healthcare reform efforts.

Why are healthcare costs rising so rapidly? There is no simple answer because many factors are influencing this trend. One factor is the cost of newly developed healthcare technologies. The research and development costs of medications and new medical technologies increase the costs of newly developed treatments. As more consumers require or demand newer, more expensive treatments and procedures, overall spending increases.

In addition, people in the United States are living longer because of better treatments for chronic illnesses. This means that people receive more medical care for more years of life, which increases their total healthcare costs. As the baby boomer generation (people born between 1946 and 1964) ages, a larger number of people will need increased healthcare services.

Some researchers also cite poor lifestyle choices as a factor in rising healthcare costs. For example, poor diet and lack of physical activity have led to increasing obesity rates, most notably in children and teens. As a result, the number of diagnosed diabetes cases has increased. Because a higher number of newly diagnosed people with diabetes are young, they will require many years of healthcare treatment.

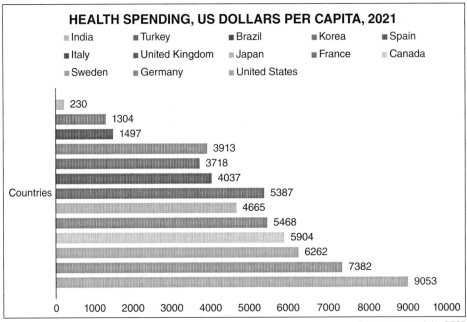

Data courtesy of the OECD

Figure 1.20 This chart shows how much money different countries spend on healthcare per person. *Why do you think the US spends so much money on healthcare?*

1.3-3 Accessible Healthcare

The cost of health insurance and out-of-pocket costs not paid by insurance create a barrier to accessing healthcare. As the cost of health insurance increases, some employers increase the amount that employees must pay to receive insurance or simply stop offering health insurance.

In the United States, healthcare costs for an average family of four are more than $28,000 per year. A family's out-of-pocket costs for healthcare are often greater than the amount spent on food, clothing, or transportation. In some cases, these costs are almost as much as a family spends on housing (**Figure 1.21**). When insurance is offered through an employer, the average worker pays $400 to $500 per month for insurance premiums. In addition, people must pay other healthcare costs, such as insurance deductibles and co-pays for prescriptions.

While low-income families can qualify for Medicaid insurance and older individuals can sign up for Medicare, a growing number of middle-class individuals and families are unable to afford health insurance. In 2013, about 50 million people in the United States lacked basic health insurance and accessed care only in an emergency. This emergency care is expensive, and most people cannot pay for it without help. As a result, hospitals and taxpayers are spending about $43 billion dollars each year to cover the costs of those who were treated but could not pay.

A shortage of primary care physicians, especially in rural areas, creates another healthcare accessibility challenge. Many US physicians choose to specialize in a specific area of medicine. As a result, there is a shortage of primary care physicians. Individuals must travel many miles to access medical care. It may take an hour or more to reach the nearest hospital.

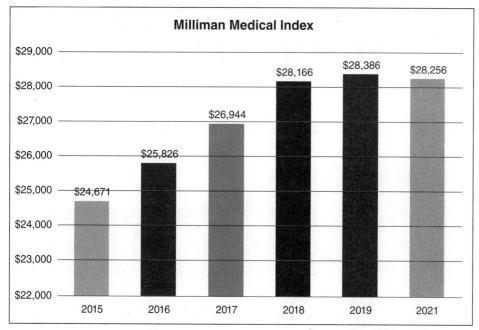

Data courtesy of Milliman Medical Index

Figure 1.21 This chart from Milliman, a statistical consulting firm, shows how much the average family spent on healthcare in recent years.

1.3-4 Addressing the Issues

Many cost-containment measures have already been tried in the healthcare industry. For example, diagnostic-related groups (DRGs) classify treatments in a way that limits the amount paid to a hospital for a patient with a specific diagnosis. Health maintenance organizations (HMOs), which aim to provide lower-cost healthcare through contracts between insurance companies and healthcare providers, often provide preventive care for free or at little cost. This system is based on the belief that prevention of illness reduces potential treatment costs. Preferred provider organizations (PPOs) require members to choose from a select group of medical providers who have agreed to provide services for a specific cost. The use of home healthcare services and outpatient surgical centers also reduces hospital costs. None of these measures, however, has been able to control the rising cost of healthcare.

On March 23, 2010, a national healthcare reform bill called the **Patient Protection and Affordable Care Act (ACA)**, or the Affordable Care Act, was signed into law. The law called for major changes to the healthcare system to provide insurance for a larger number of people in the United States. Major provisions of this law included:

- requiring most people in the United States to have health insurance by 2014
- creating a healthcare exchange or marketplace in each state where individuals and families can compare health insurance plans and enroll in coverage
- expanding Medicaid to cover a larger number of low-income individuals
- requiring employers with more than 50 employees to offer health insurance
- requiring health insurance plans to cover all individuals, regardless of their health status
- increasing payments for primary care services
- eliminating co-payments for specific preventive care services
- increasing support for prevention, wellness, and public health services

Since the law was implemented, the number of individuals without health insurance has decreased from 46.5 million to 27 million. Today, however, the number of uninsured individuals is rising once again (**Figure 1.22**).

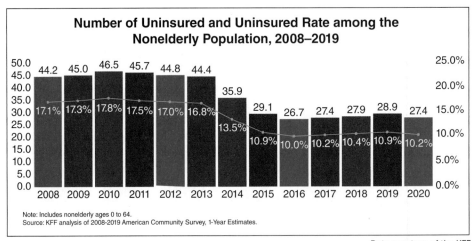

Number of Uninsured and Uninsured Rate among the Nonelderly Population, 2008–2019

Note: Includes nonelderly ages 0 to 64.
Source: KFF analysis of 2008-2019 American Community Survey, 1-Year Estimates.

Data courtesy of the KFF

Figure 1.22 Provisions of the Affordable Care Act require most people in the United States to have health insurance. *What are some other provisions of this law?*

While everyone agrees on the need to control healthcare costs and make healthcare affordable for all, not everyone agrees with the requirements of this law. The changes required by the Affordable Care Act have faced strong political and policy challenges. Since its implementation, some states have rejected the Medicaid expansion, leaving more residents uninsured. In addition, the requirement for all people in the United States to have health insurance has been rendered ineffective. Continuing challenges to the law will impact the affordability and accessibility of healthcare for the foreseeable future.

Today, physician assistants and nurse practitioners provide an increasing percentage of primary care. As a result, these two professions are high-growth healthcare occupations. Legislation to increase federal support for medical education seeks to increase the number of future physicians, and telemedicine plays an expanding role in the delivery of care.

Lesson 1.3 Review

 Complete the *Map Your Reading* graphic organizer for the section you just read.

1. Which of the following organizations studies the effectiveness of alternative medical treatments? (1.3-1)
   A. NCCIH
   B. PERRLA
   C. FDA
   D. WHO

2. Which of the following factors may contribute to increasing healthcare costs? (1.3-2)
   A. Increasing age of people in the United States
   B. New technologies
   C. Increase in number of diagnosed diabetes cases
   D. All of these.

3. A shortage of _____ restricts access to healthcare, especially in rural areas of the United States. (1.3-3)
   A. medical specialists
   B. people
   C. healthcare workers
   D. primary care physicians

4. The Patient Protection and Affordable Care Act has brought changes to healthcare such as reducing the number of (1.3-4)
   A. people with insurance
   B. people without insurance
   C. employers that provide insurance
   D. insurance claims

Chapter 1 Review and Assessment

Chapter Summary

1.1-1 Both the practice of and attitudes toward healthcare have evolved over the centuries. Multiple individuals, some well-known and some not, have made life-saving contributions to the advancement of healthcare.

1.1-2 New attitudes and beliefs are shaping healthcare. New attitudes value a holistic medical approach, which works to maintain or restore mental, spiritual, and social wellness in addition to physical wellness.

1.1-3 New healthcare research reveals new treatments, technologies, and advancements. Change requires that healthcare workers and consumers accept new research.

1.2-1 Genomic medicine will use a patient's DNA to select the best methods to diagnose, treat, or even prevent illness for a specific patient.

1.2-2 Regenerative medicine will use stem cells to heal and repair tissue damaged by illness or injury.

1.2-3 Healthcare is rapidly changing due to technological advances. For example, telesurgery will bring the expertise of specialists to less populated areas. Nanotechnology will allow treatments to happen inside the body at the exact location needed to avoid damage to healthy surrounding tissue.

1.3-1 Because patients want more holistic care, healthcare systems are providing options for integrative medicine. The National Center of Complementary and Integrative Health oversees scientific research studies to determine the effectiveness of alternative therapies.

1.3-2 The cost of medical care in the United States has been rising faster than the rate of inflation. Increased inflation may lead to even higher healthcare costs.

1.3-3 Access to healthcare is a problem for many people in the United States, either because they cannot afford health insurance or because there is no physician practicing in their community.

1.3-4 Many people and organizations are trying to address current issues in healthcare. The Patient Protection and Affordable Care Act calls for major changes to the US healthcare system to provide care to a larger number of citizens.

Maximize Your Professional Vocabulary

1. **Stand Up/Sit Down Terms Review.** Form two rows of chairs and stand in front of them with one student per chair, facing each other to form two teams. A leader, chosen by the class, will walk between the rows asking students for either a term or a definition. A correct answer allows the student to sit down. The first team with all students sitting wins.

2. **Terms Sort Review.** Make three columns in a document or a sheet of paper. In the first column, list all the professional terms that describe new healthcare technologies. In the second column, list any remaining terms that relate to medical treatments. Finally, record any unused terms in the third column. Compare your lists with a classmate. Define any terms that you listed in different columns and share the reasons for your placement. Then take turns stating the definitions for any remaining terms.

Reflect on Your Reading

1. Review the disease treatment predictions you made in the *Connect with Your Reading* activity at the beginning of this chapter. How have your predictions changed now that you have finished reading the chapter? Select one healthcare trend that interests you. Why do you think this trend is significant? Reconnect with your class partner and share your thoughts.

Review and Recall

1. Which of the following statements best describes the change in the role of physicians during the last century? (1.1-1)
   A. Physicians can diagnose illness, but treatment options are very limited.
   B. Physicians focus mainly on the prevention of illness by employing a holistic model of wellness.
   C. Physicians use more life-saving treatments due to advances in technology.
   D. None of these.

Match these individuals with their contributions to advancing healthcare. (2–5) (1.1-1)

A. Clara Barton
B. Joseph Lister
C. Jonas Salk
D. Alexander Fleming

2. Discovery of penicillin
3. Use of antiseptic during surgery
4. Founder of Red Cross
5. Developed polio vaccine

6. Which of the following historical medical practices are still used today? Choose all that apply. (1.1-2)
   A. Handwashing
   B. Leeches
   C. Acupuncture
   D. Trepanning/craniotomy

7. During a medical appointment, Dr. Jones asks what symptoms her patient is having. She is careful to seek the correct diagnosis and treatment. Sometimes she recommends massage therapy or yoga to improve the patient's outcome. Which term best describes her model of care? (1.1-2)
   A. Integrative medicine
   B. Western medicine
   C. Alternative medicine
   D. Complementary medicine

8. Before new research results can change patient care practices, (1.1-3)
   A. healthcare workers must accept the research
   B. healthcare agencies must set new policies
   C. healthcare workers and consumers must understand and accept the research
   D. healthcare consumers must understand the research

9. Personalized drugs and vaccines are an advancement in (1.2-1)
   A. genomic medicine
   B. regenerative medicine
   C. holistic care
   D. electronic health records

10. Which of the following are part of regenerative medicine? Choose all that apply. (1.2-2)
    A. Organ donation elimination
    B. Lab-grown tissue
    C. Gene therapy
    D. Stem cell therapies

Match each medical advance with its corresponding example. (11–14) (1.2-3)

A. Nanotechnology
B. Virtual reality
C. Artificial intelligence
D. Robotics

11. Telesurgery
12. Computers that identify cancer cells
13. Micro-robots
14. Treatment for phobias

15. One example of nanotechnology is the (1.2-3)
    A. dental implant
    B. fitness app
    C. heart pacemaker
    D. 3D printing

16. Today, patients want medical care that is _____ and pays attention to more than just physical symptoms. (1.3-1)
    A. segmented
    B. advanced
    C. intuitive
    D. holistic

17. This graph shows the percentage of adults 18–64 years old who skipped or delayed medical care because of cost. It tells a story about the reasons people skip or delay needed medical care. Choose the most complete version of the story. (1.3-2)

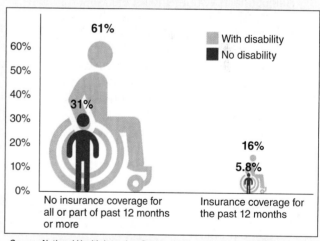

Source: National Health Interview Survey, 2009. Icons: Ecelop/Shutterstock.com

A. Lack of health insurance makes healthcare more expensive and keeps people from seeking needed medical care.
B. Individuals with disabilities who have no health insurance are most likely not to receive regular medical care.
C. Having a disability makes it difficult to access healthcare and keeps people from seeking needed medical care.
D. Individuals with rising healthcare costs are likely not to seek needed medical care.

18. Which of the following contributes to the shortage of primary care physicians in the United States? (1.3-3)
    A. Lack of interest in healthcare
    B. Specializations among physicians trained in the United States
    C. Lower healthcare costs
    D. Artificial intelligence

19. The _____ Act brought major changes to the US healthcare system and increased the number of citizens covered by health insurance. (1.3-4)
    A. Insurance Portability and Accountability
    B. National Health Defense
    C. Patient Self-Determination
    D. Patient Protection and Affordable Care

Build Core Skills

1. **Writing.** Review the section titled *Medical Advancements* in Lesson 1.1. Write a paragraph summarizing the major changes in healthcare in the past century.

2. **Critical Thinking.** Scan Figure 1.4 and note the discoveries that are still important in today's delivery of healthcare. Use online resources to search for important people in the history of medicine who helped to make these discoveries. Select one individual and list the person's main accomplishment, when it occurred, and its importance to healthcare today. Form groups based on the periods in history identified in Figure 1.4. As you share your findings with the class, note the number of students in each group. Can you use this information to draw a conclusion about the rate of medical advances made throughout history?

3. **Math.** Refer to Figure 1.8 to answer the following questions.
   A. Read the title of the graph. What is the AAP (American Academy of Pediatrics) recommending and why?
   B. Why are some bars green, some blue, and some purple?
   C. What do the numbers at the top of each bar tell you?
   D. What is the purpose of the black line in the graph?
   E. The largest decline in SIDS rates occurred between 1992 and which year?
   F. Between 1994 (the year the Back to Sleep® campaign began) and 1999, the overall SIDS rate in the US dropped by more than what percentage? Did rates for back sleeping more than double or triple?

G. Even though the percentages of infants sleeping on their backs has continued to increase, what has happened to the number of deaths?

The rest of the story: Researchers observed that other sleep-related causes of infant death were rising, so they expanded the focus of their program. Today the Safe to Sleep® campaign works to reduce not only SIDS, but also accidental suffocation and other causes of infant death.

4. **Critical Thinking.** Review the description of holistic care. For each of the four components of wellness, provide an illustration of a patient issue that needs to be addressed. For example, physical wellness could be represented by a patient who does not get regular physical activity. Review your list when you have finished. Are the patient issues connected? What conclusions can you draw about the value of holistic care?

5. **Speaking and Listening.** Choose one individual from the following list of lesser-known healthcare heroes. Research this person's contribution to improved healthcare. Decide whether this person should be in the "Top 10" list of healthcare heroes and be ready to explain your decision using the information you learned.
   A. Karl Landsteiner
   B. John Enders
   C. Howard Florey
   D. Frederick Banting
   E. Piero Sensi
   F. David Nalin
   G. David Cushman
   H. Andreas Gruentzig
   I. Akira Endo
   J. James Jude

6. **Problem Solving.** Research the number of primary care physicians per resident in your community. Do you have a shortage? Across the United States, the average number of primary physicians per 1,000 residents ranges from 0.9 to 2.8. According to the chapter, what is one factor contributing to the shortage of primary care physicians in the United States? Suggest ways to solve this problem.

7. **Critical Thinking.** In your own words, explain the differences between genomic medicine and regenerative medicine.

8. **Math.** Healthcare costs are increasing, and so is the cost of health insurance. Just how much does medical care cost? Research the following healthcare treatments and list the average costs without insurance.

A. Dental checkup with X-rays

B. Sore throat visit to an urgent care clinic

C. Sports physical exam

D. X-ray of an injured leg

E. Appendectomy

You can buy dental insurance for $50.00 per month. You see the dentist twice each year for a cleaning, exams, and X-rays. Should you buy insurance? Explain your answer.

Activate Your Learning

1. Connect with one or two healthcare workers you know. Ask what changes they have seen in healthcare during their careers. Note both positive and negative changes.

2. Next, talk with one or two older family members. Ask what changes they have experienced as patients. Again, note both positive and negative changes. Be prepared to discuss your notes.

Think and Act Like a Healthcare Worker

1. Pretend that you are a physician. Like Ignaz Semmelweis, you have discovered a simple change in practice that will improve patient health. Your research shows that, like handwashing, this change could revolutionize healthcare. Semmelweis was unsuccessful at convincing his fellow physicians to wash their hands. They were offended midwives, who commonly washed their hands when delivering babies, were providing better care, so they chose not to believe that their habits could cause patient death. They ignored Semmelweis' advice and fired him as a physician. How will you convince your fellow physicians that your discovery is worth making a change in the way they practice medicine?

Go to the Source

1. Use the NCCIH website to research an alternative therapy of your choice. Write a one-paragraph case study about the experiences of a patient who uses that therapy. In your account, include one result that is factual and one result that is a myth or untrue. Review your case studies as a class to see if your fellow students can recognize the myths.

2. Locate an article about a future healthcare trend. Two possible sources are the "NIH MedlinePlus" magazine or the "Findings" magazine published by the National Institute of General Medical Sciences. Both can be accessed online. Use any of the topics in this chapter or research a future healthcare trend that interests you. Print the article and write a two-paragraph summary. In the first paragraph, summarize the main points of the article. In the second paragraph, include your personal thoughts and reactions to what you have read. Be prepared to discuss your summary with your fellow students.

HOSA Event Prep: Medical Reading

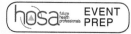

The Radium Girls, the newest novel release from author Kate Moore, is the story of the women who worked in radium-dial factories in the United States. The radium they use to paint the numbers on the faces of watch-dials covered the women from head to toe. Many women even ingested the chemical as they licked the tips of their paintbrushes to paint fine lines. The radium caused these women to glow. Slowly, the women began to fall ill with mysterious symptoms, such as wounds that would not heal and bones that deteriorated. There seemed to be no one on their side as they sued the companies for their illnesses. Eventually, the women moved forward to set the standards for the rights of workers in the United States in the 20th century.

Think About It

1. What does this story illustrate about working conditions in radium-dial factories?

2. Explain the main idea supported by this story about the "radium girls."

Chapter 2

Safety—A Priority for Health Science Workers

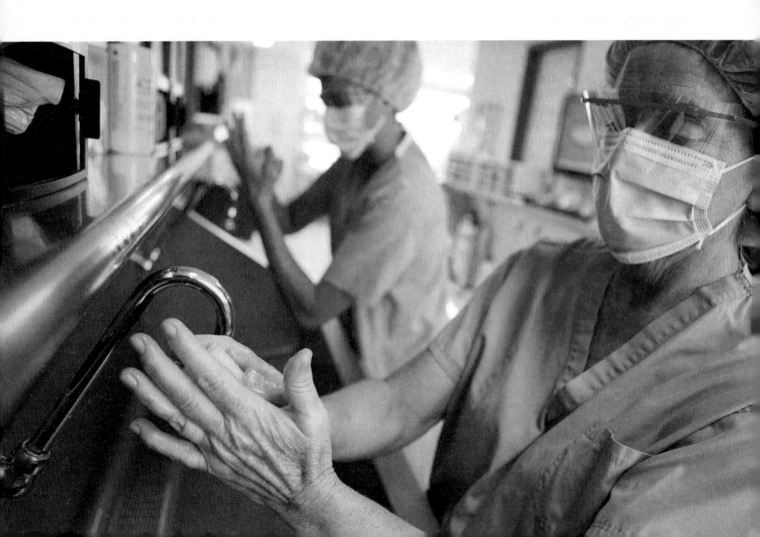

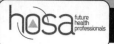
On the evening of December 25, 2015, a tornado hit the town of Rowlett, Texas. This disaster required the activation of the community volunteers who had completed CERT training. *CERT* stands for Community Emergency Response Team. These teams are trained to respond to emergencies, including disasters and accidents. One of the HOSA Emergency Preparedness Events showcases CERT skills.

Go to the HOSA website to learn more about the HOSA *CERT Skills* event. Find out the purpose of the event, what is involved in the event, and what knowledge is demonstrated in the event.

As you prepare for HOSA competitive events, be sure to check the website and talk with your HOSA advisor for the most up-to-date guidelines and procedures. Once you have learned about the *CERT Skills* event, answer the following questions:

1. How might participating in this event benefit you personally and your future career? Explain.
2. Are you interested in participating in this event? Why or why not?

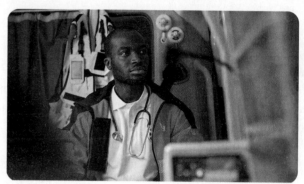

Gorodenkoff/Shutterstock.com

Connect with Your Reading

Have you ever been in a dangerous situation? Were you able to stay calm and remember what to do to keep yourself and others safe? Learning and practicing safety skills before you need them will help you feel more confident when an emergency arises. Whether you provide direct patient care or not; whether you are in a small office, a lab, a large hospital, or someone's home; you will encounter safety hazards. Everyone has a role in creating a safe healthcare environment.

Map Your Reading

Can you describe the broad reach of safety issues in healthcare? Make a visual summary to record your ideas. Begin with a square sheet of paper—an 8½-inch square works well. Fold each of the four points of the square to the center. Label each of the four resulting flaps with one of these topics: *Patient rooms, Public areas, Office areas,* and *Laboratories.* Label the center square inside with *All Areas.* When you finish reading each lesson in the chapter, open the appropriate flaps and add pictures, symbols, or words to illustrate your understanding of how the safety topic presented impacts different areas of the healthcare environment.

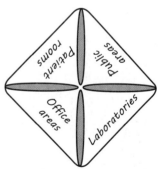

Goodheart-Willcox Publisher

Chapter opener image: Tyler Olson/Shutterstock.com

Personal and Patient Safety

ESSENTIAL QUESTION

How can you promote personal and patient safety in the healthcare environment?

Learning Outcomes

After studying this lesson, you will be able to

2.1-1 identify procedures and equipment used for personal and patient safety in the healthcare environment.

2.1-2 identify ways to respond to common safety hazards.

2.1-3 describe physical safety procedures to protect workers and patients from injury.

Professional Vocabulary

Essential Terms

body mechanics   correct position of the body to help a person avoid injury during a physical task

Safety Data Sheet (SDS)   an OSHA-required document that explains the risks of a chemical product

safety precaution   information about the safe operation of a piece of equipment, which is usually found in the instruction manual or on equipment labels

Important Terms

ergonomics	Occupational Safety and Health Administration (OSHA)	pesticides
		posture
		workplace violence

Introduction

Looking around a hospital will quickly show you that healthcare can be a dangerous environment. There are many people moving about and lots of complex pieces of equipment. In this noisy, busy environment, many things can go wrong. Despite the distractions and complexity, healthcare workers must perform their work in ways that protect their own safety and the safety of others, including patients, visitors, and coworkers. Safety is a priority for all healthcare workers.

As you think about your future career, are you worried about safety? Fortunately, many laws make healthcare safer. The **Occupational Safety and Health Administration (OSHA)** is a federal agency responsible for ensuring safe and healthy work environments. You will need to be trained and follow OSHA and Centers for Disease Control and Prevention (CDC) guidelines to prevent accidents and injury (**Figure 2.1**). Your first day on the job should include an orientation to the specific safety guidelines and procedures for your facility. Knowing what is expected and practicing these skills in advance will help keep you and your patients safe.

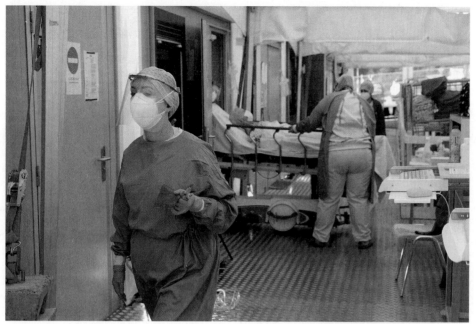

Alexandros Michalidis/Shutterstock.com

Figure 2.1 Healthcare settings have many safety issues. *What hazards are you most concerned about in a future healthcare career?*

2.1-1 Environmental Safety

Safety begins with creating a safer environment. As you look around your home and school, you can identify protections put in place for your safety. Key areas of concern in healthcare are using equipment and chemicals safely, preventing falls, and reducing workplace violence. Safety hazards need to be identified and corrected as quickly as possible.

Equipment Safety

You will likely work with a variety of equipment if you provide direct patient care. Correct use of equipment can protect both you and your patients from injury. For example, using lift equipment can make physical tasks such as lifting or moving your patients easier and safer. The type of lift you should use depends on the task, the patient's need for assistance, weight-bearing ability, body weight, and ability to follow instructions. You should use full-body lifts for patients who cannot support their own weight (**Figure 2.2**). Choose a stand-up lift for patients who can stand with support. Using the wrong piece of equipment or using it the wrong way can cause serious injury.

It is important to be trained on new equipment before you use it. Each piece of equipment has its own set of **safety precautions**. You can refresh your memory on the steps for safe operation of equipment by reading the manual or equipment labels (**Figure 2.3**). If you are unsure how to use a piece of equipment, stop and ask for help. Always follow safety signs, symbols, and labels provided.

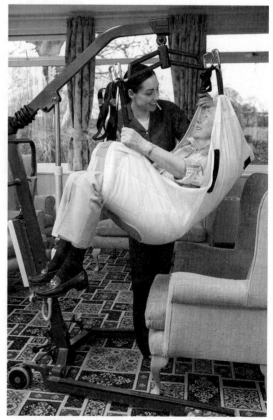

iStock.com/SolStock

Figure 2.2 Full-body lifts are often used in hospitals, long-term care facilities, and physical therapy departments. *How do workers know safety precautions for its use?*

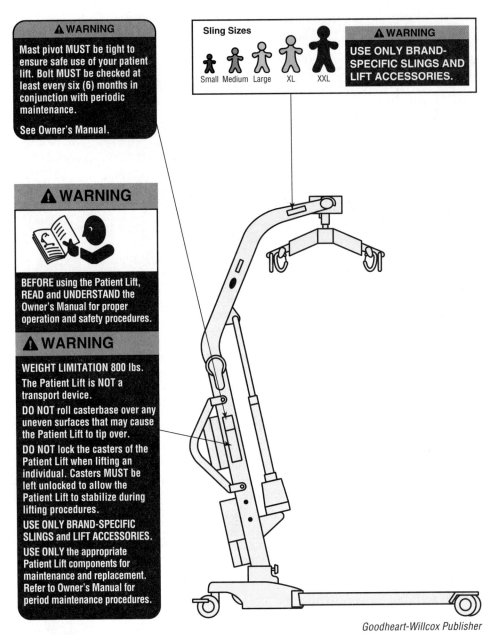

WARNING

Mast pivot MUST be tight to ensure safe use of your patient lift. Bolt MUST be checked at least every six (6) months in conjunction with periodic maintenance.

See Owner's Manual.

Sling Sizes

Small Medium Large XL XXL

WARNING

USE ONLY BRAND-SPECIFIC SLINGS AND LIFT ACCESSORIES.

WARNING

BEFORE using the Patient Lift, READ and UNDERSTAND the Owner's Manual for proper operation and safety procedures.

WARNING

WEIGHT LIMITATION 800 lbs. The Patient Lift is NOT a transport device.

DO NOT roll casterbase over any uneven surfaces that may cause the Patient Lift to tip over.

DO NOT lock the casters of the Patient Lift when lifting an individual. Casters MUST be left unlocked to allow the Patient Lift to stabilize during lifting procedures.

USE ONLY BRAND-SPECIFIC SLINGS and LIFT ACCESSORIES.

USE ONLY the appropriate Patient Lift components for maintenance and replacement. Refer to Owner's Manual for period maintenance procedures.

Goodheart-Willcox Publisher

Figure 2.3 Healthcare workers must follow the operating instructions on equipment such as this patient lift.

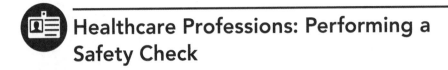

Healthcare Professions: Performing a Safety Check

Antonio is a patient care assistant in a nursing home. Many of his residents need help getting out of bed, dressing, and bathing. When Antonio enters a patient's room, the first thing he does is perform a *safety check*. He wants to find and remove potential hazards before they become a problem. He greets his resident and scans the room for any issues that need to be addressed.

After assessing the situation, Antonio plans ahead. He thinks about where he will be moving the resident and how the equipment will fit. He determines whether he will need a helper for the task. He clears a path for the equipment and prepares a chair to transfer the resident into.

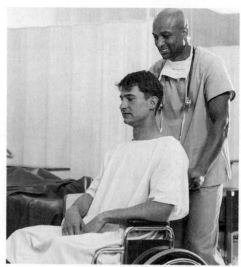

kali9/E+ via Getty Images

Antonio knows to check that equipment is clean and working properly before he uses it. He checks for frayed electric cords before he plugs in equipment. When he finds equipment that is damaged or not working correctly, he reports it immediately and does not use it. He also makes sure any protective pads or safety straps are in place before he begins.

He lets the resident know what is going on so the resident can help during the procedure. He makes sure each person understands what is expected of them, including the resident. Clear instructions avoid confusion and reduce fear. He uses an agreed-upon signal, such as "One, two, three, lift," so everyone's actions are coordinated.

After the procedure, Antonio performs a final safety check before he leaves the room. He returns the patient's bed to its lowest position, returns furniture to its place, and locks the bed wheels, if required. He checks that the resident has everything needed within reach. Finally, he removes the equipment to clean and recharge it for the next use. He knows equipment should not be left in hallways or obstructing traffic. Antonio's residents and coworkers feel safe and comfortable with him because of his organized approach to tasks.

Ergonomics

Healthcare workplace safety is important for all healthcare workers. Even office workers can experience injuries in the workplace. Digital eye strain and repetitive motion injuries (RMIs) are increasingly common workplace problems and account for a large percentage of worker absences. These injuries are caused by the overuse or poor positioning of a body part while it is under stress. Health informatics workers commonly have RMIs in the hands, wrists, elbows, and shoulders.

Computer use is a common cause of injury. Have you experienced pain from poor wrist position when typing or using a mouse? pain in your neck from looking down at your phone or tablet? lower back pain after sitting, standing, or lifting with your back in a poor position? Did the problem get worse the longer you remained in that position? Attention to ergonomics can reduce many of these injuries. **Ergonomics** is the study of designing and arranging a workplace to increase productivity and safety.

To reduce your risk of developing RMIs, you can arrange your workspace to limit unnecessary movement from one place to another. You can set furniture and equipment at heights that allow freedom of movement, reduce strain, and position your body to work at its best (**Figure 2.4**). Use the following guidelines for good alignment:

- Your hips and knees should form 90-degree angles while seated.
- Your back should be upright and supported.
- The screen should be below eye level to prevent hyperextension of the neck.
- Your feet should be flat on the floor or supported on a footrest.
- Your lower arms should be supported and form a 90-degree angle to your upper arms.
- Your wrists should be supported at a natural angle where the thumb is in line with the lower arm.

You should also stretch frequently to increase your comfort and reduce RMIs. Take a short break or change your position every 20 to 30 minutes. Some employers may provide an adjustable desk height so you can stand for a period of time. Stretch and flex your muscles to encourage circulation and range of motion. Try this now:

1. Make a fist, then spread your fingers wide.
2. Arch your back and move your shoulders in circles.
3. Shift your weight from side to side.
4. Tighten your abdominal muscles to straighten your back.
5. Stretch your arms above your head and out to the sides.
6. Let your head hang down, then straighten up and rotate it from side to side.

Taking a few moments to stretch on a regular basis will make you more productive and can help prevent pain.

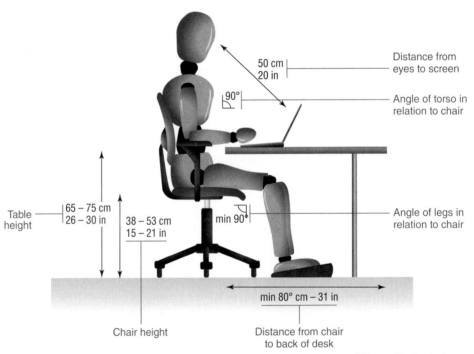

Maluson/Shutterstock.com

Figure 2.4 Paying attention to ergonomics and body alignment can help prevent repetitive motion injuries. *When typing, how should your wrists be positioned?*

You can also arrange your workspace to prevent injury from electronic screens. A link has been shown between exposure to electronic screens and several health conditions. Studies suggest that short-wave, high-energy blue light from LED lights, computers, and digital screens disrupts sleep cycles. Extended screen time can also cause digital eye strain and computer vision syndrome. Symptoms include headaches, burning or red eyes, blurred vision, eye twitching, and double vision. You can increase eye comfort by positioning the screen an arm's length from the eyes, turning on blue light filters, adjusting screen contrast, reducing screen time at night, and taking regular screen breaks. Remember 20-20-20: every 20 minutes, shift your focus to an object 20 feet away for 20 seconds to rest the eyes.

If you notice signs of RMI or eye strain, speak with your supervisor about possible changes to your workstation that may help prevent or relieve the strain. Federal regulations require your employer to take actions to reduce these injuries. If you help transport heavy materials, ask for a wheeled cart or other assistance. Consider ways to break your tasks down into smaller loads to protect yourself from injury.

General Guidelines to Prevent Falls

Falls are among the most common accidents that cause occupational injuries. Your fall may cause another accident, such as a patient's fall or a hazardous material spill. Following these general precautions will make your work environment safer:

- **Always walk.** Hallways are full of workers, patients, visitors, and equipment. Running increases your risk of colliding with people or objects and causing a fall.
- **Stay to the right.** Walk on the right side of hallways, stairwells, and double doors. Leave the other side for people moving in the opposite direction.
- **Use corner mirrors to look ahead where corridors meet.** Healthcare facilities typically mount mirrors high on the walls where corridors intersect. This allows you to see oncoming traffic and avoid potential collisions. This is especially important when you cannot see over the load you are pushing or cannot stop quickly.
- **Clean hallways by halves.** Wet floors are slippery. Clean one half of a hallway at a time to leave space for others to use the opposite side where it is dry.
- **Post a sign and clean up spills as soon as possible.** Place a caution sign on wet floors to warn people of the danger of slipping. Clean up spills as quickly as possible (**Figure 2.5**).
- **Keep walkways clear.** Avoid throw rugs, which are a tripping hazard. Remove excess equipment, push in chairs, and do not clutter hallways. Monitor fire exits and remove anything that prevents easy access to exits during an emergency.

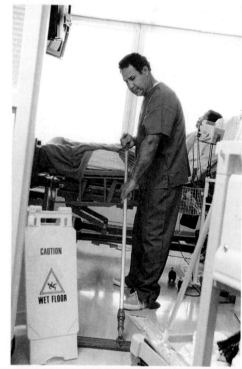
©iStock.com/monkeybusinessimages

Figure 2.5 Yellow caution signs are used to warn against potential hazards. *Where else might you see a caution sign?*

2.1-2 Common Safety Hazards

Following safety policies and procedures can prevent illness and injury. Labels provide important safety information. Some chemical, drug, and radioactive materials can be hazardous with even low levels of exposure. If an accident occurs, additional safety procedures may help prevent future problems.

Working with Hazardous Chemicals

Did you read the label the last time you sprayed disinfectant in your bathroom or glass cleaner on your kitchen window? People tend to assume that the products available in the store are safe to use, but safety depends on products being used correctly.

Using Safety Data Sheets

OSHA's Hazard Communication Standard aims to increase awareness and safe handling of hazardous substances. This includes blood and other body fluids, disinfectant sprays, and chemicals used in diagnostic tests. Your employers must make you aware of any hazardous substances in your work environment and their risks. The law requires employers to provide a document called a **Safety Data Sheet (SDS)**, formerly known as a *material safety data sheet (MSDS)*, from the manufacturer for each hazardous substance. The SDS explains the risks of the chemical and what to do if you are exposed to it. These documents must be readily accessible in the work area where the substances are used (**Figure 2.6**). In addition, the packaging of the hazardous substance must have a label with condensed SDS information.

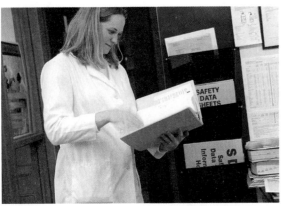

Huntstock/Thinkstock

Figure 2.6 Safety Data Sheets (SDS) must always be accessible to healthcare workers. *What information does an SDS contain?*

Many of the cleaning products you will use in healthcare contain **pesticides** regulated by the Environmental Protection Agency (EPA). A pesticide is any substance or device used to repel, kill, or prevent the growth of any insect, rodent, fungus, weed, or other pest or plant. Pesticides can also be carcinogenic (cancer-causing) or toxic (poisonous) to humans. Antimicrobial pesticides are commonly used against germs. The EPA maintains a list of chemicals appropriate for killing germs while minimizing risks to the environment.

 ## Healthcare Professions: Working with Cleaning Products

As a hospital food service worker, Bryan completed ServSafe® training. In addition to safe food preparation, he learned how to handle chemicals in the kitchen. When he sprays down the kitchen counters before food preparation, he needs a cleaner that can kill common disease-causing organisms. He only chooses products approved for use around food.

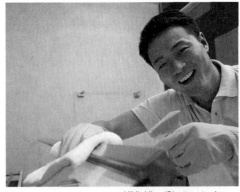

XiXinXing/Shutterstock.com

Although he has used the products before, he rechecks the label for instructions each time. He needs to be sure the cleaner is left on long enough and at the proper strength to kill all of the disease-causing organisms. The label tells him whether he needs to rinse the product off after sanitizing or if it can air-dry. He knows that a harmful residue might remain when some products are left on too long.

Bryan is also careful to change cleaning cloths when he changes cleaning products. He knows that mixing different types of chemicals together can produce toxic gases or even an explosion.

It is important to use the correct solutions when working with chemicals. Lab workers should read the label three times: when gathering chemicals, before using them, and after using them. Never use solutions stored in unlabeled bottles. Do not mix solutions from different containers unless directed by your supervisor. If an error is made, report it immediately so it can be corrected. Some chemicals and biohazardous materials require special safety precautions and treatment that you can find on the SDS.

Handling Exposures and Accidents

If chemicals, hazardous materials, blood, or body fluids touch your skin, eyes, or a mucous membrane, flush the area with water. Eyewash stations provide a stream of water to rinse your eye. Never rub the affected eye because this can lead to serious complications.

When a spill occurs, you should notify nearby workers of the hazard. Check the SDS for instructions on cleaning up hazardous materials and never pick up broken glass with your hands. Using tongs, forceps, or a dustpan and brush is much safer (**Figure 2.7**). You can remove fine fragments that remain by wiping with several layers of wet paper towel. Be sure to wear gloves while cleaning to protect yourself. After the spill is cleaned, disinfect anything that requires it and clean or dispose of the contaminated material.

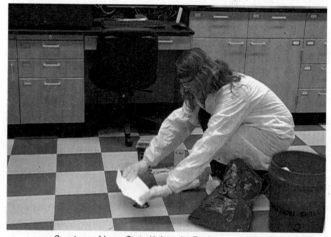

Courtesy of Iowa State University Environmental Health and Safety

Figure 2.7 Spills in the lab must be handled and reported properly. *What should you do if a spill occurs in the lab?*

You must report any accident, cut, spill, malfunctioning equipment, or other problems to your supervisor. OSHA requires an incident report to be filled out for any injury or illness. Records of all accidents must be kept for five years in case problems arise. If you are poked by a sharp object or exposed to a hazardous material in the lab, you may need to have a blood test to determine if it caused any disease. After an incident, follow-up should include an evaluation of why it happened and how to avoid similar incidents in the future. Annual incidence rates should be reviewed to identify problems or progress in preventing work-related illnesses and injuries.

As an extra precaution, some institutions require medical clearance and follow medical surveillance procedures if you will be working with hazardous substances. Medical clearance may include vaccination or health tests prior to beginning your work. Surveillance procedures include taking baseline measures of your health through blood tests and tissue samples. This allows for later identification of any changes if you suspect you have been infected or exposed to hazardous materials.

Medical Imaging Safety

You may have had X-rays of your teeth at the dentist even if you have not had other types of medical imaging done. Your reproductive organs and other sensitive tissues should have been covered with a heavy lead apron to shield them from radiation. Although the risk during each exposure is low, medical imaging procedures can put both patients and technicians at risk.

Radiation from X-rays, computed tomography (CT) scans, and nuclear imaging can cause cell mutations that may be passed on to future generations and can lead to cancer and other health conditions. Technicians must set radiation to the prescribed levels and stop exposure after the planned amount of time. If proper safety steps are used and the number of exposures is minimized, the risk for patients is low.

Radiologic technicians are at a higher risk for radiation exposure because of the number of imaging exams they perform. If you work as a radiologic technician, the federal government will require you to wear protective gear, including lead aprons and gloves, to guard against overexposure (**Figure 2.8**). Technicians must also wear a badge that shows the amount of radiation they are receiving and tracks their lifetime exposure to radiation.

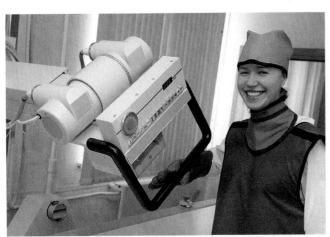

Dmitry Kalinovsky/Shutterstock.com

Figure 2.8 Radiologic technicians must wear protective gear to prevent overexposure to radiation. *What protection is provided for patients receiving X-rays?*

Some imaging techniques avoid the use of harmful radiation. Magnetic resonance imaging (MRI) scans use a strong magnet instead of radiation. You would screen patients receiving an MRI scan for metal implants and remove all jewelry and clothing containing metal. The magnetic field heats up metal fibers in accessories or clothing, which can cause second-degree burns. You would also remove or secure any metal objects in the room, such as an oxygen tank or IV pole, so they are not drawn to the center of the machine where the patient is lying. This could cause serious or fatal injury.

Ultrasound is the safest form of medical imaging. It uses sound waves to create images from inside the body. This can be used for mammograms, prenatal exams, and many other procedures. Transillumination is a radiation-free technology that allows a dentist to capture digital images of your teeth with near-infrared light. New technology is constantly developing to make the healthcare environment safer.

Reducing Workplace Violence

Healthcare is very emotional work. This can bring out both the best and the worst in people. Threats or acts of physical violence, harassment, and intimidation are a major concern for both employers and workers. The risk for these types of **workplace violence** is five times greater in healthcare than any other profession. It may come from patients, their families, or coworkers.

Healthcare Professions: Managing Stress

Jada works as a nurse in a hospice care facility. She provides end-of-life care for patients and their families. Although she finds the work rewarding, it can be very stressful. Her patients and their families often become emotional and sometimes look for someone to blame. Jada finds it helpful to take walks outside on her lunch break. She is glad that her facility provides a free employee assistance program to help with

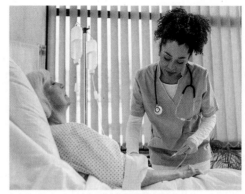

LightField Studios/Shutterstock.com

situations that are causing emotional distress. The hospice staff also have weekly check-ins to discuss their emotional struggles and honor the patients who have passed away that week. These tools help her keep stress in check. Jada uses her calm demeanor to help ease the fears of her patients and their families.

Patient Violence

Working with people who may have unpredictable behavior, such as those with a history of substance abuse or behavioral challenges, increases your chances of being hurt on the job. Workers in direct contact with the public or in high-crime areas are at the greatest risk. Healthcare and social services workers also commonly deliver bad news, which can trigger violent behavior.

About 80 percent of all healthcare worker injuries involve direct patient care. Creating a prevention program can avoid many of these incidents. This should include an evaluation of the work setting, preventive measures, and employee training.

Your employers should identify risks for violence in your work environment. For example, emergency room staff may be at risk when treating wounded members of a gang or people experiencing intimate partner violence. Home health aides may assist clients in violent neighborhoods or households with abuse. Once identified, the risks can be addressed.

Your employers should tell you about potential issues and train you on what to do. Caregivers should learn to identify warning signs and calm down tense situations. Think first about the safety of yourself and those around you, then try to de-escalate the conflict and call for assistance.

There should be clear procedures for how you handle potentially violent situations. For instance, if a floor nurse is preparing to give an injection to a patient who reacts violently to being touched, hospital rules may require the nurse to have one or two other staff members present before approaching the patient. All staff should know their facility's code words for emergency situations and how to respond.

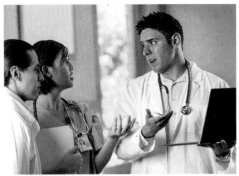

©iStock.com/Steve Debenport

Figure 2.9 The stress involved in a healthcare job may cause tempers to flare among coworkers. *How can you avoid conflicts with fellow healthcare workers?*

Workplace Harassment

Personal problems can add to on-the-job worries and cause some workers to lash out or react inappropriately toward patients or fellow workers (**Figure 2.9**). Many organizations require workers to receive training on cultural sensitivity and sexual harassment issues. Simply stated, if a person finds your behavior offensive and asks you to stop, then you should stop. All healthcare workers and patients should be treated with respect.

You may be embarrassed or feel uncomfortable reporting a coworker who threatens or harasses you, but it is important to address the problem so it can be resolved. This is a situation in which a strong administration is important. A zero-tolerance policy sets consequences for inappropriate behavior, regardless of the circumstances or the person's position in the organization. This sends a message to everyone that no one will be allowed to harass or intimidate another employee. When a patient, coworker, or supervisor treats others inappropriately, the behavior should be corrected. You should not go to work each day dreading harassment.

2.1-3 **Physical Safety**

This text focuses on safety first for a good reason. According to the CDC and Bureau of Labor Statistics (BLS), healthcare workers are more likely to be injured than workers in any other occupation. More than 500,000 healthcare workers are injured on the job each year, with the highest rates occurring in long-term care facilities. Nurses, nursing assistants, and physical therapists are the most frequently injured. Many nurses leave their jobs due to back injuries. You can avoid workplace injuries by following some basic physical safety guidelines for body mechanics, patient handling, and food safety.

 ## Healthcare Professions: Back Pain

Malaika took a class to become a nursing assistant while she was in high school. Now, she is in nursing school and works in home care in the evening and on weekends. She was trained to use lifts for getting her residents out of bed, but that equipment is not always available in her clients' homes. She sometimes works in awkward positions because one of her clients uses a low bed to reduce injuries from falling out of

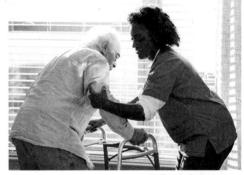

kali9/E+ via Getty Images

bed. Some of her clients are often confused and change positions suddenly. Malaika does not have anyone else to help her with clients who are very overweight, or *bariatric*. She has noticed that her lower back often hurts by the end of her shift. She realizes she needs to change the way she is lifting or she will not be able to continue her work as a nurse when she graduates next year.

Using Good Body Mechanics

Body mechanics describes the correct way to position and move your body to complete tasks more safely and efficiently. Body mechanics alone does not make manual lifting safe. It does, however, reduce muscle fatigue and make lifting, pulling, or pushing safer and easier.

When possible, raise your patient's bed to working height: hip-level for moving a patient and waist-level for patient care. Good **posture**, or body position, is an important part of body mechanics. When lifting, keep your head, back, and hips in a straight line, or *alignment*. Tighten your abdominal muscles to protect your back. A broad base of support gives you the most stability, so place your feet shoulder-width apart. Keep the patient close to your body and directly in front of you to avoid leaning down or twisting sideways. If you need to turn, pivot on the balls of your feet and turn your whole body.

When lifting heavy objects, use the large muscles in your legs rather than the small back muscles. Bend at the knees and hips to lift the object rather than curling your spine to reach down. Bring the object close to your body before lifting. Keep your chin up during the lift to help maintain a straight back (**Figure 2.10**).

It may be easier to push a heavy object instead of lifting it. This allows you to use the weight of your whole body. Avoid pulling a heavy object to prevent injury to your wrist, arm, or shoulder muscles and joints. If an object weighs more than 50 pounds, get help from a coworker or a lift device. OSHA recommends reducing manual lifting of patients when possible. Do not manually lift a patient who requires more than 35 pounds of support and do fewer than 20 lifts per shift. When combined with good decision-making about manual lifting, body mechanics can help prevent strains or injury to both you and your patient.

Transfer and Ambulation Safety

Moving and walking, or *ambulation*, protects patients from health complications. It is important for patients to be up and moving soon after surgery, but this creates safety risks for both you and your patients.

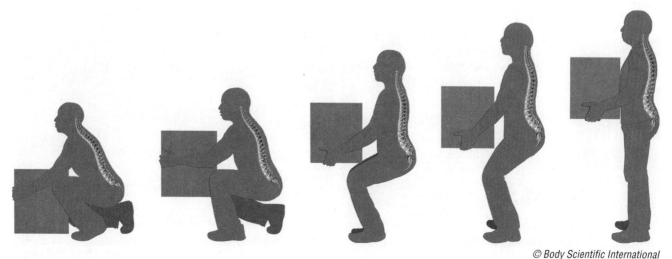

© *Body Scientific International*

Figure 2.10 When lifting heavy objects, always bend at the knees and keep your chin up to maintain a straight back.

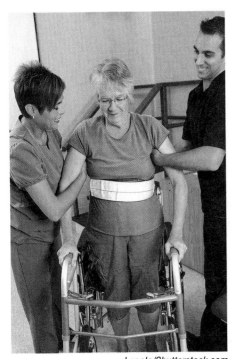

Lopolo/Shutterstock.com

Figure 2.11 Some patients require two people to safely assist them to stand or walk.

Accidents often occur when people are tired, distracted, or rushed. You should be properly trained and approved to perform transfer and ambulation procedures. Falls during patient care can injure both the patient and the healthcare worker. Following these precautions can help prevent falls from occurring:

- **Know the patient's orders and level of assistance needed.** Check for any recent changes in the patient's condition. Verify if they can stand and walk independently, or what assistance from people or equipment they require (**Figure 2.11**). Plan how far they will be walking and where you will have them sit when they are done.
- **Prepare equipment before you begin.** Will you need a lift, walker, cane, or transfer (gait) belt to help the patient stand or walk? Is the wheelchair or lift in place? Is the bed in its lowest position? Did you lock the wheels? Do not leave your patient at the edge of a bed if you forgot something!
- **Non-slip footwear is required.** Some facilities use socks with rubber grips on the bottom, but footwear with a solid sole and secure fit is better. Make sure you tie any laces.
- **Use proper body mechanics.** Protect your back by keeping your back straight, keeping your chin up, and using your larger arm and leg muscles. Do not twist or use jerking motions.
- **Dangle before standing.** Help your patient sit up and swing their legs over the side of the bed, then sit for a few minutes before standing (**Figure 2.12**). This allows their blood pressure to adjust and reduces dizziness.
- **Use a transfer belt and your body's position to support the patient.** Hold on to your patient's transfer belt, if they have one, using an underhand grasp. When transferring from sitting to standing, brace your patient's feet or legs with yours to prevent them from slipping.

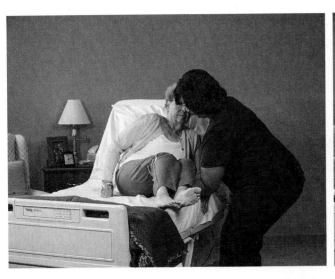
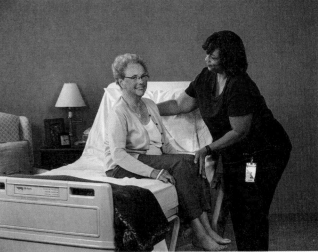

© Tori Soper Photography

Figure 2.12 Before getting them out of bed, help your patient adjust to being upright by dangling at the edge of the bed.

Allow your patient to hold on to your arms or waist, but not around your neck (**Figure 2.13**).

- **Provide instructions for the patient before you begin.** Let them know what you are doing and how they can help. Check that they understand before you begin. Arrange a signal, such as "1, 2, 3, stand."
- **Watch for signs of tiring.** Walk at your patient's pace and offer encouragement (**Figure 2.14**). Watch for slowing pace, unsteadiness, increasing difficulty in moving feet, heavy breathing, sweating, or pale skin color. Your patient may even say they feel weak. Lower them safely to a chair or the floor instead of rushing them back to their room.
- **Control a fall.** Further injury can result from trying to keep a falling person upright. Stand a little behind and to the weaker side of your patient while they walk, keeping your hands ready or on the transfer belt if they have one. If your patient becomes weak, grasp the sides of their transfer belt or wrap your arms under their armpits and around their chest from behind. Bring them close to your body, lower them safely to the floor, and protect their head. Step back with one leg as you lower them down and use your other leg as a slide to help support their weight (**Figure 2.15**). Call for help so your patient's condition and the cause of the incident can be assessed before getting them up.

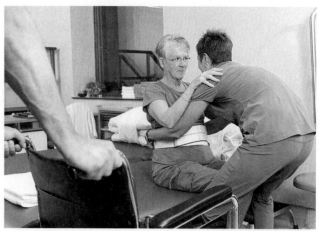

Lopolo/Shutterstock.com

Figure 2.13 Proper body position and use of body mechanics reduces falls and back injuries. *What body mechanics techniques can you identify in this image?*

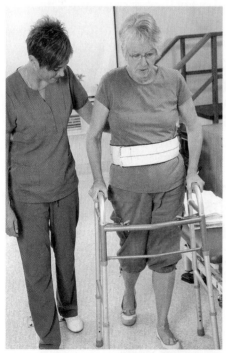

Lopolo/Shutterstock.com

Figure 2.14 Stand slightly behind and to the side of the patient while supporting them to walk.

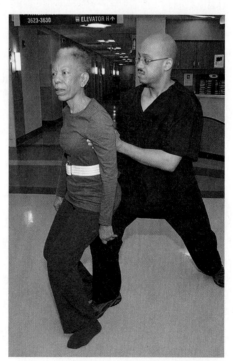

Wards Forest Media, LLC

Figure 2.15 If your patient begins to fall, pull them close to your body and support them as they slide down your leg to the floor. *How was this CNA able to create a wide base of support?*

- **Leave the patient in a safe and comfortable position.** After a transfer, remove the sling and smooth your patient's clothing and bedding. Their body should be left in good alignment. Ask if they are comfortable and can reach everything they need, such as the call button. Is their bed in the lowest position? Are the wheels locked?

Wheelchair and Transport Safety

Wheelchair transport is a common task. You should learn to move your patients through a facility safely. Pay special attention to these safety guidelines when transporting your patients in wheelchairs or on gurneys:

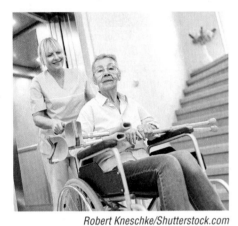

Robert Kneschke/Shutterstock.com

Figure 2.16 When moving patients over the gap at an elevator door, transport technicians should always move backward.

- **Lock all wheels before transferring.** Wheelchairs and gurneys have brakes or lockable wheels to prevent accidental rolling that can lead to a dangerous fall. After a transfer is complete, wheelchair locks are considered a restraint if your patient cannot unlock them independently.
- **Be sure the patient is secure.** After placing your patient on a gurney, secure the straps over their legs, waist, and upper torso. Leave their arms free, but remind the patient to keep their arms and hands close to their body. Raise the side rails on the gurney or place their feet on the wheelchair's footrests before moving. Use any seatbelt and shoulder harnesses provided in a wheelchair transport vehicle.
- **Recognize situations that require backward movement.** Always warn your patient before moving backward, as it can be disorienting. When moving up stairs, down ramps, or over gaps such as an elevator door, backward movement will prevent your patient from tipping forward out of the device (**Figure 2.16**).

Food Safety

Improper food handling can result in *foodborne illness,* meaning any illness caused by eating contaminated food. Foodborne illnesses can happen when germs grow during food storage and are transferred or not killed during food preparation. Because patients in a healthcare facility already have compromised health, an outbreak of foodborne illness may have even more serious outcomes than it would in a healthy population.

 ## Healthcare Professions: Improper Food Handling

Surya thought she had the flu. She had stomach cramps, a headache, and a mild fever. The next day, the diarrhea started, and her fever spiked. She became dehydrated and was admitted to the hospital. Lab tests showed she had *Salmonella,* a type of foodborne illness. She was one of a small group of people who had become ill from something they ate.

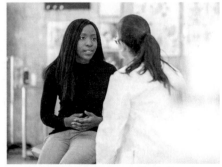

FatCamera/E+ via Getty Images

Health officials investigated the cluster of illnesses and traced it to contaminated food in a restaurant salad bar. Undercooked chicken and failure to keep foods at the proper temperature were the cause of the illnesses. Surya was a vegetarian and did not eat the chicken, but the sprouts on her salad were likely contaminated by someone using one salad tongs for multiple food items. Surya's illness responded to antibiotics, but she now avoids public salad bars!

The mnemonic *FAT TOM* can help you understand how to limit the growth of germs in food, an important part of preventing foodborne illness (**Figure 2.17**).

FAT TOM: Facts for Limiting Pathogens in Food		
Letter	**Example**	**Description**
F is for food	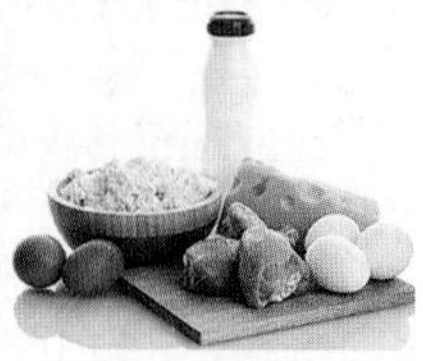	Protein-rich foods are most likely to cause foodborne illnesses.
A is for acid	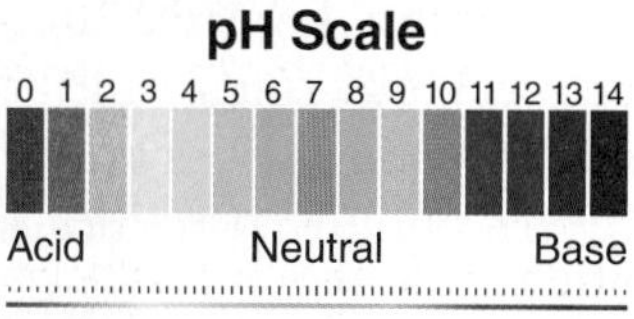	Bacteria grow best in an environment that is neutral or slightly acidic. Bacteria can multiply quickly in low-acid foods like meat, beans, peas, carrots, potatoes, and lettuce.
T is for time	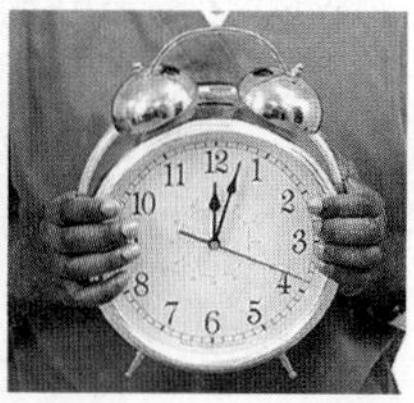	Microorganisms reproduce by cell division: more time = more microorganisms. Limit serving times to less than two hours, and discard leftovers after two hours.
T is for temperature	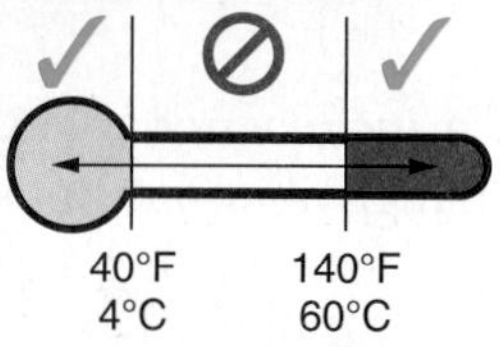	Microorganisms grow quickly in the *danger zone* between 40°F and 140°F. Keep hot foods hot (over 165°F). Keep cold foods cold (under 40°F).
O is for oxygen	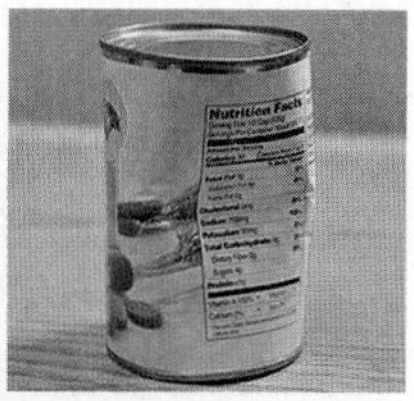	Avoid dented or bulging cans. Oxygen has caused food to spoil. Improper canning may allow the growth of botulism spores, which are toxic and deadly. When in doubt, throw it out!
M is for moisture	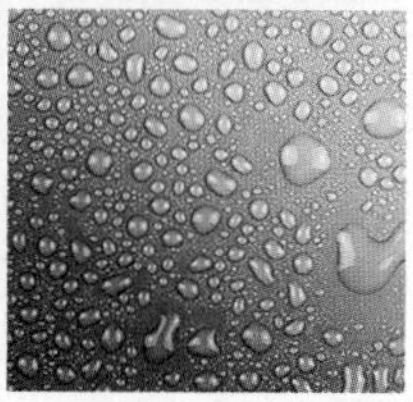	Bacteria, yeast, and mold multiply rapidly in moist foods like meat, produce, and soft cheeses. Bacteria have difficulty growing in dry foods or those preserved with salt or sugar, such as jams and jellies.

Top to bottom: Africa Studio/Shutterstock.com, Svetolk/Shutterstock.com, val lawless/Shutterstock.com, Goodheart-Willcox Publisher, Wards Forest Media, LLC, Mario7/Shutterstock.com

Figure 2.17   The mnemonic FAT TOM can help you understand how to limit the growth of pathogens in food as a first step in preventing foodborne illness.

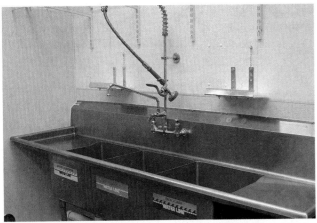

Courtesy of Chef's Shared Kitchen

Figure 2.18 Three-compartment sinks are essential for a hospital kitchen. *Explain how this equipment helps dietary workers clean dishes and instruments.*

You also need to handle food and equipment correctly during preparation and serving. Anyone who handles food must follow safety procedures prescribed by OSHA and the Food and Drug Administration (FDA).

- **Wash your hands before handling food.** This is especially important after you go to the bathroom; cough, sneeze, or blow your nose; and touch uncooked meat or produce. If you touch your face or hair, answer the phone, or pick up something from the floor, then you will need to wash your hands again.
- **Clean and sanitize all utensils, equipment, and food preparation surfaces.** You should do this before and after each food preparation task. The heat of a dish machine and special sanitizing solutions help kill bacteria. You must sanitize larger equipment by hand. Use a sink with three compartments to separate the tasks of food scraping, washing, and sanitizing (**Figure 2.18**).
- **Wash fresh produce before serving.** You should wash away the bacteria on fresh fruits and vegetables under running water if bacteria will not be killed by cooking. Scrub firm produce, such as apples, with a produce brush while washing.
- **Keep raw foods separate to avoid cross-contamination.** Use different-colored cutting boards and knives for uncooked meat, cooked meat, unwashed vegetables, salads, and bakery items. This will prevent the transfer of any harmful bacteria in raw foods onto foods that will not be cooked or washed.
- **Use gloves, utensils, or tissues to handle ready-to-eat foods.** Do not touch food with your bare hands, which may carry germs or allergens picked up from other surfaces.
- **Avoid foods that can trigger allergic reactions.** Change your gloves after handling foods with nuts and change utensils after serving seafood. This can prevent a patient with allergies from having a severe reaction.
- **Do not touch the parts of dishes and utensils that patients eat from.** Touch only the handles of silverware. Hold cups and plates from the bottom rather than the rim.
- **Sick employees may not work with food.** Do not work with food if you have a fever, sore throat, or runny nose. Notify your supervisor of any symptoms of illness that could be transmitted through food. Do not handle food if you have any cuts, scrapes, or open sores that cannot be bandaged and covered with gloves (**Figure 2.19**).
- **Make sure food supplies are fresh.** Follow the *first in, first out* (FIFO) rule, placing new stock behind older items. Check expiration dates and discard expired products.

Contaminated food may not look, smell, or taste spoiled. If you are uncertain about the safety of any food, follow the guideline that states, *when in doubt, throw it out.* It is better to be overly cautious than to risk illness due to contaminated food. Dietary workers also need to look for signs of aspiration or choking as a patient eats.

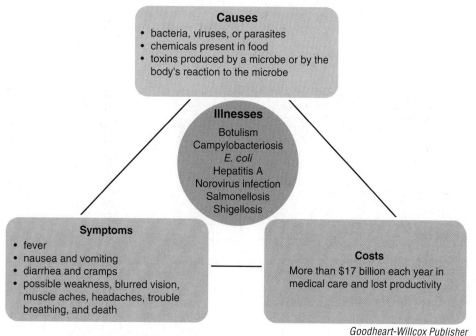

Causes
- bacteria, viruses, or parasites
- chemicals present in food
- toxins produced by a microbe or by the body's reaction to the microbe

Illnesses
Botulism
Campylobacteriosis
E. coli
Hepatitis A
Norovirus infection
Salmonellosis
Shigellosis

Symptoms
- fever
- nausea and vomiting
- diarrhea and cramps
- possible weakness, blurred vision, muscle aches, headaches, trouble breathing, and death

Costs
More than $17 billion each year in medical care and lost productivity

Goodheart-Willcox Publisher

Figure 2.19 Infectious diseases that spread through food or beverages are a common and sometimes life-threatening issue for millions of people in the United States.

Lesson 2.1 Review

 Complete the *Map Your Reading* graphic organizer for the section you just read.

1. Which of the following is *not* a patient safety procedure? (2.1-1)
   A. Perform an equipment safety check
   B. Plan ahead
   C. Lock wheels before transferring
   D. Hold up a falling patient

2. Which of the following is ergonomically correct positioning? (2.1-1)
   A. Allow feet to dangle from the chair
   B. Place screens above eye level
   C. Keep back upright and supported
   D. Support wrists at a 90-degree angle to the arm

3. Which of the following are safety precautions for lab workers? Choose all that apply. (2.1-2)
   A. Check the SDS for handling chemicals
   B. Follow medical clearance and surveillance procedures
   C. Wear gloves to clean up spills
   D. Put on gloves if chemicals have touched your skin

4. Which of the following can reduce workplace violence? Choose all that apply. (2.1-2)
   A. Identifying risks
   B. Training employees to fight back
   C. Providing employee assistance programs
   D. Using zero-tolerance policies

5. Which of the following should you do when lifting? (2.1-3)
   A. Bend at the hip and use your leg muscles
   B. Keep your chin down
   C. Tighten the back muscles
   D. Hold the object away from yourself

6. How do you keep food out of the "danger zone"? (2.1-3)
   A. Keep cold food below 40 degrees
   B. Refrigerate leftovers within three hours
   C. Defrost frozen foods at room temperature
   D. Keep hot food above 100 degrees

Protecting Against Infectious Diseases and Epidemics

ESSENTIAL QUESTION

How can you help prevent the spread of diseases?

Learning Outcomes

After studying this lesson, you will be able to

2.2-1 describe types of pathogens.

2.2-2 explain the links in the chain of infection and how each can be broken to prevent spread.

2.2-3 explain the use of standard precautions to prevent the spread of infection.

2.2-4 explain how transmission-based precautions prevent the spread of infection.

2.2-5 describe how exposure to bloodborne pathogens is controlled in healthcare facilities.

2.2-6 differentiate between sanitization, disinfection, antisepsis, and sterilization in their use to control the growth of pathogens.

Professional Vocabulary

Essential Terms

aseptic techniques   practices used by healthcare professionals to keep an environment free of pathogens and prevent the spread of infections

chain of infection   the elements required for an infection to spread from one source to another

pathogen   a disease-causing microorganism

personal protective equipment (PPE)   equipment such as gloves, masks, gowns, respirators, and eyewear worn to protect skin, clothing, and the respiratory tract from infectious agents

standard precautions   steps that a healthcare worker takes with all patients to prevent the spread of infection

transmission-based precautions   special steps used in addition to standard precautions, chosen based on how the patient's infection is spread

Important Terms

bacteria	infectious	reservoir
clean technique	infectious agent	respiratory hygiene
epidemic	isolation	sharps
fungi	mode of transmission	sterile technique
hand hygiene	parasite	susceptible host
healthcare-associated infections (HAIs)	portal of entry	terminal cleaning
	portal of exit	virus

Introduction

When you begin your career in healthcare, you will want to protect your own health as much as that of your patients. This lesson will help you understand and avoid the spread of infection.

The World Health Organization (WHO) and Centers for Disease Control and Prevention (CDC) want to protect everyone's health. They track patterns of **infectious** diseases, meaning those that spread. They are most concerned about highly *contagious* diseases that spread easily from one person to another. The more widespread a disease becomes, the more concerning it is. An *outbreak* is a small but visible increase in the number of cases. You may hear of an outbreak of children with diarrhea at a daycare. A disease that has spread over a larger area and is growing is called an **epidemic**. A germ that is both contagious and difficult to kill can cause an epidemic, in which many people become ill from the same disease.

The focus during an outbreak or epidemic is on stopping the spread of disease. More crowded areas usually have more epidemics, and disease spreads faster due to closer contact. Regular handwashing, good respiratory hygiene, and vaccines are important protective measures to reduce the spread of disease. Isolating those who are sick and avoiding close contact will also help. These were the initial steps taken when the novel coronavirus disease (COVID-19) was discovered in 2019.

When an infection has spread across many countries and is growing out of control, it is called a *pandemic*. At this point, the focus shifts to reducing the severity of the effects. During the COVID-19 pandemic, people were asked to self-quarantine, use social-distancing, and wear masks to "flatten the curve." Pandemic diseases can cause secondary infections and other complications that require hospitalization. Quarantines helped spread the rate of infection over a longer period of time to avoid overwhelming hospitals with more cases than they could handle at once. The focus was on saving lives, once people realized they could not contain the spread of the infection.

2.2-1 Infectious Agents

Infection control is a key area of concern for healthcare worker safety. Many different healthcare careers have the potential for exposure to infectious blood and body fluids. Phlebotomists who take blood samples for evaluation, lab workers who handle these samples, and pathologists who evaluate them are at high risk. So are surgeons, emergency room workers, nurses, nursing assistants, dental hygienists, and many others who provide direct patient care. Infectious waste, which is any item or product with the potential to transmit disease, must be handled carefully. That means housekeepers, maintenance workers, and other nonpatient contact careers may also be exposed. Even office workers who only share common hallways can be exposed if germs are accidentally transferred to other surfaces. Whatever healthcare career you choose, you will need to have some understanding about infection control.

Types of Pathogens

When you feel ill and tell your friend, "I have a 'bug,'" what are you really talking about? Understanding what you are fighting and how it can be eliminated is the first step in your ability to control the spread of infections. Infections are caused by pathogens. **Pathogens** are disease-causing organisms, such as bacteria and viruses.

Figure 2.20 shows the six major types: bacteria, viruses, fungi, protozoa, helminths, and rickettsiae. These are the *infectious agents* that cause disease. Each has unique characteristics and methods for controlling it.

Bacteria are one-celled microorganisms, so small you can only see them under a microscope. Names of bacteria often describe their shape and arrangement. For example, *cocci* (KAHK-sI) are round, *bacilli* (buh-SIHL-I) are rod-shaped, and *spirochetes* (SPI-roh-kehts) are corkscrew-shaped. *Streptococci* (strehp-toh-KAHK-sI) are twisted chains of round bacteria responsible for strep throat, pneumonia, and a variety of other bacterial infections. Bacteria can be classified by their need for oxygen. Aerobic bacteria require oxygen to live and are common in many environments. Anaerobic bacteria do not need oxygen. *Antibiotics* are medications used to treat bacterial infections. Alternative treatments that destroy the DNA of bacteria are also being developed.

A **virus** is a very small pathogen that takes over and reproduces inside other cells. Viruses usually spread through contact with body fluids. Chicken pox, herpes, hepatitis, mononucleosis (mono), influenza, HIV, and the common cold are all caused by viruses. *Latent viruses*, such as herpes, may lie dormant in your body for a long time and flare up later during times of stress. Immunizations, or *vaccines*, can help prevent viral infections, and antiviral medicines can help reduce the effect of viruses if taken within 48 hours of becoming sick.

Most **fungi** are parasitic microbes that live in the soil and on plants. A one-celled fungus called *yeast* commonly causes infections in the vagina or mouth. Mold spores can cause lung infections. You can use antifungal medications and creams to control infections caused by these microbes.

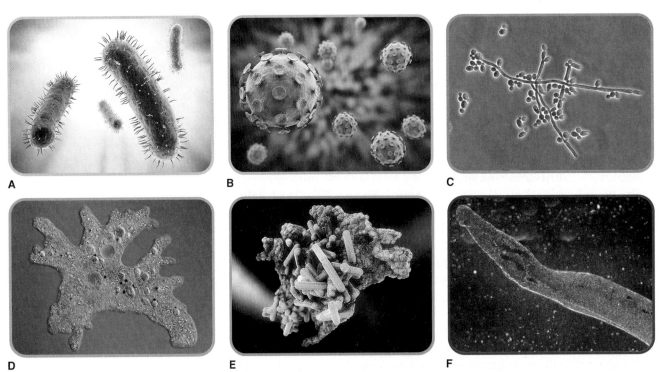

Left to right, top to bottom: iStackphotons/iStock/Thinkstock, Peeradach Rattanakoses/Shutterstock.com, Andre Nantel/Shutterstock.com, micro_photo/iStock/Thinkstock, MichaelTaylor3d/Shutterstock.com, defun/iStock/Thinkstock

Figure 2.20 Types of pathogens include bacteria (A), viruses (B), fungi (C), protozoa (D), rickettsiae (E), and helminths (F). *Can you name one disease caused by each of these types of pathogens?*

A **parasite** is an organism that lives on or inside a host that provides its food. Some are more common in less developed countries, where the conditions are right for them to grow and spread. *Protozoa* are one-celled microorganisms often found in dirty water and decaying material. Drinking water that contains these microorganisms can cause malaria, dysentery, and trichomoniasis. *Helminths* are worms, such as roundworms, thorny-headed worms, and tapeworms. They can spread from the feces of an infected animal to a food source or water supply. *Ecto-parasites* include blood-sucking insects, such as mosquitoes, fleas, or ticks. When an ectoparasite bites another animal or a human, it can act as a transmitter, or *vector*, to pass pathogens from one host to another. Lyme disease, spread by blacklegged ticks, is the most common vector-borne disease in the US. *Rickettsiae* (rih-KEHT-see-ee) are very small bacteria commonly passed through ectoparasite bites. They cause infections such as Rocky Mountain spotted fever and typhus. Antiparasitic drugs are available to prevent and treat many of these infections.

Drug-Resistant Bacteria

While antibiotics can be used to treat many infections, the rise of *drug-resistant bacteria* has become a growing concern. These are strains of a treatable bacterium that have developed the ability to resist normal antibiotic treatment. Drug-resistant bacteria are created when you use antibiotics inappropriately.

 ## Healthcare Professions: Drug-Resistant Bacteria in Pediatrics

Dr. Williams was seeing a young boy, Ethan, and his mother for the second time this week. Ethan was not feeling well. He had flu-like symptoms: coughing, a runny nose, and sore throat. Dr. Williams had told the mother it was probably a virus and Ethan should feel better in a week or two. His strep test came back negative, but Ethan's mother was insistent he needed a prescription. Ethan had a soccer game and he wanted to play. If he could have some antibiotics, his mother was sure it would help.

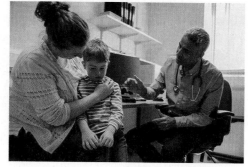

SolStock/E+ via Getty Images

Against his better judgment, Dr. Williams gave in and wrote the prescription. He knew it would not make Ethan's virus go away any sooner, but it would make the mother feel better.

Ethan did not like swallowing pills. He was upset to learn he would be taking two pills with each meal for the next 10 days. He gave in for several days, but did not see any reason to continue taking them after his game on Saturday. He was feeling a bit better, and the pills gave him diarrhea. His mother finally threw away the remainder of the prescription.

A few weeks later, Ethan and his mother were seen in the emergency room. Ethan had abdominal pain and a high fever. Lab tests showed he had a drug-resistant bacterial infection. Unfortunately, the pills would not work this time. He was admitted to the hospital for IV antibiotics. He survived and learned an important lesson about the appropriate use of antibiotics.

A patient helps with the development of resistant strains by not taking all of the pills in a prescribed antibiotic treatment. By not taking the full dose of medicine, the patient allows the strongest bacteria to survive and build resistance to the drug. Antibiotics may also kill bacteria in the intestines that support digestive health. When antibiotics are overprescribed or overused on animals in the food supply, drug resistance increases.

Drug-resistant bacteria cause many **healthcare-associated infections (HAIs)**, which develop as a result of medical care and were formerly known as *nosocomial infections*. Antimicrobial stewardship programs can help you use antibiotics more effectively for patient health and more carefully to prevent further resistance. If a resistant bacterial strain is identified, you can use lab tests to determine which antibiotic will have the best results against it. Remember that antibiotics work against bacteria, not viruses.

Methicillin-resistant *Staphylococcus aureus* (MRSA), vancomycin-resistant *Enterococcus* (VRE), and tuberculosis (TB) are examples of multidrug-resistant organisms (MDROs) listed as serious threats by the CDC. MRSA is a type of bacterial, or *staph*, infection that lives in the skin. It is most common in healthcare settings but is increasingly found in other settings. Increasingly stronger courses of antibiotics may treat MRSA infections. VRE is another bacterial infection that is most often contracted in healthcare settings. While the VRE bacterium has developed immunity to vancomycin (van-kuh-MI-suhn)—the usual treatment for *Enterococcus* (en-ter-oh-KAHK-uhs)—other antibiotics can be effective against it. Regular use of antibacterial hand sanitizers is most effective against these bacteria.

You will probably be asked to take a TB test before you can work in a healthcare setting. Tuberculosis (too-ber-kyuh-LOH-suhs) is a very serious infection that most commonly affects the lungs. Before the development of antibiotics, TB was generally fatal. With the development of multidrug-resistant forms of TB, there are fewer treatments, and it is again difficult to cure.

MDROs are difficult to control and cause serious infections that kill thousands of people each year. *Clostridium difficile* is a strain of bacteria found in human and animal feces. It is the most common cause of healthcare-associated diarrhea, affecting thousands of patients per year. New MDROs are rising in numbers. You will need to use specific disinfectants recommended by the CDC when MDROs are present. The CDC creates guidelines for disinfection during an epidemic or pandemic, such as the highly contagious norovirus (NOR-oh-vI-ruhs) known as the *cruise ship virus* or the novel coronavirus that caused the COVID-19 pandemic.

2.2-2 The Chain of Infection

The chain of infection will help you think about how to protect yourself and your patients from pathogens. The **chain of infection** describes all of the elements that must be present for infectious diseases to spread (**Figure 2.21**). Because all the elements must be present, each link in the chain is an opportunity to prevent the spread of infection.

The first link in the chain is the **infectious agent**, or pathogen causing the infection. Bacteria, viruses, and other pathogens spread differently and are killed by different types of medications. Rapid diagnosis and identification through diagnostic testing will help you know the best way to control the pathogen.

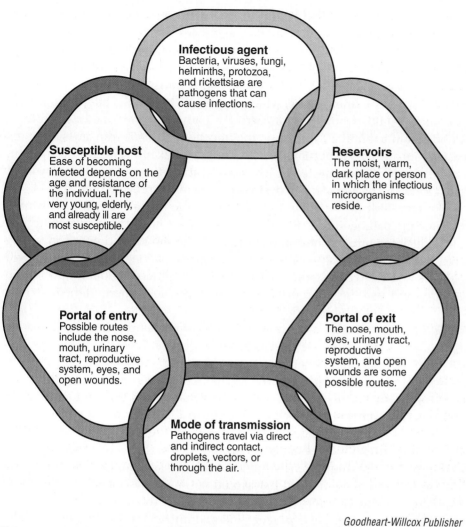

Goodheart-Willcox Publisher

Figure 2.21 All of the elements in this chain must be present for an infection to occur. *How can healthcare workers break this chain to prevent infection?*

The next step is the **reservoir**, which is a place where the pathogen can live, such as the human body, animals, food, or water. Microorganisms like to live in places that are moist, warm, dark, and have a food source. Using good personal hygiene such as handwashing helps remove pathogens from the skin, while heat and chemicals kill pathogens in food or on surfaces. It is important to keep skin, equipment, and the environment clean and dry so pathogens do not have a place to live.

A pathogen leaves its reservoir through a **portal of exit**, the next link in the chain of infection. Both natural body openings and breaks in the skin are ways for pathogens to leave the body. You can cover wounds with a bandage, cover the mouth when coughing or sneezing, and control fluids leaving the body. Covering portals of exit protects you, your patient, and everyone around you from pathogens.

The **mode of transmission** describes how a pathogen moves from its reservoir to a new host. There are several different modes of transmission. *Direct contact* by touching infected body fluid is a common way to spread pathogens such as the cold virus and hepatitis B virus (HBV). *Oral transmission* occurs when a pathogen is ingested. Common vehicles for oral transmission are food and water, such as *Salmonella* in undercooked chicken or *Cryptosporidium* in contaminated water.

Indirect contact through a dirty object, or *fomite*, can also transfer pathogens. Droplet transmissions from a cough, sneeze, or spray of body fluids can travel several feet. Small airborne pathogens can hang in the air for some time before they are inhaled by others. Some pathogens are also transferred by the bite of an infected *vector*, or host. Malaria, which is transmitted by mosquito bites, is one example. Lyme disease, which is transmitted by the bite of a deer tick, is another. Fluids from a vector carry the pathogen from one infected host's bloodstream to another, spreading the infection. *Zoonotic* transmission of diseases from animals to humans is increasing. One example is bird flu. You cannot tell if someone is infected by just looking at them, so all healthcare workers must learn the proper steps to destroy pathogens or prevent their spread.

The next link in the chain of infection is the **portal of entry**, which is a way for the pathogen to enter a new reservoir or host. Protective equipment can reduce the number of portals available. The mouth and nose can be covered with a face mask. Breaks in the skin can be bandaged. If you work with patients who have contagious conditions, you will need to follow special procedures and use the appropriate equipment to block these pathogens from entering the body.

Finally, a **susceptible host** completes the chain of infection. A susceptible host is anyone who can contract a disease. The immune systems of the very young and very old are less prepared to fight off an infection. Those who are already ill may be overwhelmed by an infection that would not be a problem for someone who is healthy (**Figure 2.22**). Hormonal changes, poor nutrition, and stress can also lower the immune system's ability to fight disease. *Opportunistic infections* take advantage of a weak immune system. A person with a weak immune system can die from a pathogen that would not make most people seriously ill. You can support your patients' natural defenses by ensuring good hygiene, proper fluid and nutritional intake, and efforts to reduce stress.

Vaccination exposes your body to a weakened or inactive pathogen or substance to help your body's immune system build an immune response to that disease. It is important to follow immunization schedules to keep up your protection against common pathogens. Vaccinations, natural body defenses, and good health all reduce your chance of contracting an infection.

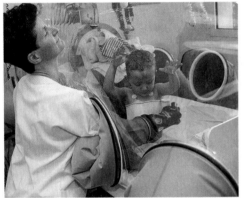

Laurent/Science Source

Figure 2.22 A condition known as severe combined immune deficiency (SCID) often requires those affected to be quarantined from others. A relatively minor infection could be fatal for a person with SCID.

2.2-3 Standard Precautions

This section introduces skills you should practice until you are comfortable and can remember the steps without prompting. Infection control is an essential skill for all healthcare workers in all environments. You will use these skills every day.

The Centers for Disease Control and Prevention developed **standard precautions** to prevent the spread of infections in healthcare settings (**Figure 2.23**). Standard precautions are the basic level of infection control you should use in the care of *all* patients, *all* the time, in *all* settings. You may not know if someone has an infection, and these procedures reduce the risk of transferring pathogens from one person to another. Proper use of standard precautions protects you from infections carried by your patients. It also protects your patients from infections present in the healthcare facility.

Standard Precautions Recommended by the CDC	
Precaution	**Recommendation**
Handwashing	Perform after touching blood, body fluids, secretions, excretions, and contaminated items; immediately after removing gloves; and between patient contacts.
PPE: gloves	Use when touching blood, body fluids, secretions, excretions, and contaminated items; also when touching mucous membranes and non-intact skin.
PPE: gown	Use during procedures and patient-care activities when contact of clothing/exposed skin with blood/body fluids, secretions, and excretions is anticipated.
PPE: mask, eye protection (goggles), face shield	Use during procedures and patient-care activities likely to generate splashes or sprays of blood, body fluids, and secretions, especially suctioning and endotracheal intubation.
Removal of soiled patient-care equipment	Handle in a manner that prevents the transfer of microorganisms to others and to the environment; wear gloves if visibly contaminated; perform hand hygiene.
Environmental control	Develop procedures for routine care, cleaning, and disinfection of environmental surfaces, especially frequently touched surfaces in patient-care areas.
Textiles and laundry	Handle in a manner that prevents the transfer of microorganisms to others and to the environment.
Needles and other sharps	Do not recap, bend, break, or handle used needles; if recapping is required, use a one-handed scoop technique only; use safety features when available; place used sharps in a puncture-resistant container.
Patient resuscitation	Use a mouthpiece, a resuscitation bag, or other ventilation devices to prevent contact with the patient's mouth and oral secretions.
Isolation	Prioritize patient for a single-patient room if the patient is at increased risk of transmission, is likely to contaminate the environment, does not maintain appropriate hygiene, or is at increased risk of acquiring infection or developing an adverse outcome following infection.
Respiratory hygiene/cough etiquette	Instruct anyone with symptoms to cover their nose and mouth when sneezing/coughing; use tissues and dispose of them in a no-touch receptacle; use hand hygiene after contact with nose, mouth, secretions, or used tissues; wear a surgical mask if tolerated or stay at least 3 feet away from the person with symptoms, if possible.

Goodheart-Willcox Publisher

Figure 2.23 Standard precautions break the chain of infection by interrupting the mode of transmission and blocking portals of exit and entry.

Using standard precautions prevents the transmission of diseases spread through blood, body fluids, and mucous membranes. The term *body fluids* refers to all types of fluid coming out of the body except sweat, even if they do not contain visible blood. *Mucous membranes* are the moist linings of body cavities that open to the outside, such as inside the mouth, nose, and vagina. Mucous membranes and broken, or *non-intact*, skin must be protected as both portals of exit and entry for pathogens. The standard precautions you should take to prevent the spread of infection include:

- hand hygiene
- personal protective equipment (**Figure 2.24**)
- respiratory hygiene (cough etiquette)
- appropriate patient placement
- needle and sharps safety
- safe injection practices
- proper handling, cleaning, and disinfecting or sterilizing of the environment, equipment, instruments, and laundry

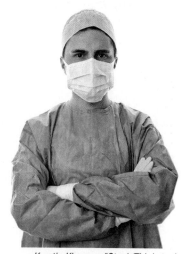

Kerstin Klaassen/iStock/Thinkstock

Figure 2.24 Personal protective equipment (PPE) is part of standard precautions. *What does PPE include?*

Hand Hygiene

Since you cannot disinfect or sterilize skin, frequent handwashing removes pathogens that cause disease. That makes **hand hygiene** one of the most important ways to reduce the spread of infection. Hand hygiene includes regular handwashing using plain or antibacterial soap and the use of alcohol-based gels. Alcohol-based hand gels are the preferred method of hand hygiene when hands are not visibly dirty. You should practice hand hygiene before and after giving care in all situations (**Figure 2.25**). Your patients and visitors also have an important part in preventing infections. When patients practice hand hygiene and remind others to wash their hands, they are reducing their own and others' risk.

The goal of handwashing is to clean your hands without recontaminating them in the process. You do not want to touch a dirty or contaminated surface, such as the sink or faucet. Pay close attention to how long you are supposed to wash and what you should *not* touch with your clean hands. **Figure 2.26** shows the steps to follow when washing your hands.

Alcohol-based hand gels act quickly to kill many types of microorganisms on your hands. You need a coin-sized amount of gel to cover all surfaces. Remember to rub until the hands are dry. Alcohol-based sanitizers do not work well on hands that are greasy, visibly dirty, or exposed to chemicals. **Figure 2.27** shows steps to follow when using alcohol-based hand gels.

Personal Protective Equipment (PPE)

During COVID-19, people got used to wearing masks but why did they do it? At first, scientists thought avoiding contact could stop spread of the disease, but then research showed it was mainly spread through the air. Masks help filter the air and prevent small droplets of body fluid from entering or leaving your nose and mouth. They are a form of personal protective equipment.

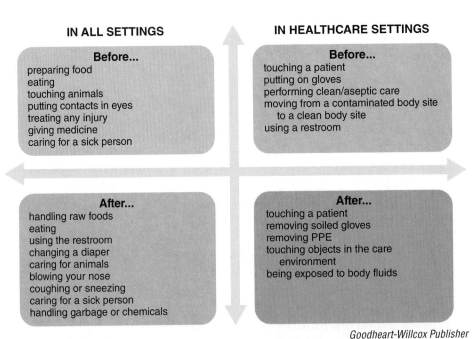

Goodheart-Willcox Publisher

Figure 2.25 Hand hygiene controls the spread of infection in daily life as well as in healthcare settings. *Always* wash hands that are visibly dirty or contaminated with body fluids. *If your hands are not visibly soiled, what other hand hygiene method can you use?*

Personal protective equipment (PPE) creates a barrier to protect your skin, clothing, mucous membranes, and respiratory tract from infectious agents. You should use PPE whenever the possibility of exposure exists. Here are a few guidelines for when you will use PPE in your healthcare career:

- Wear *gloves* when touching blood, body fluids, nonintact skin, mucous membranes, and dirty objects.
- Wear a *mask*, *face shield*, or *goggles* when there is a risk of body fluid or blood splashing or spraying into your nose, mouth, or eyes.
- Wear a *gown* to cover your skin or clothing that will be exposed to blood or body fluids.

How to Handwash?

WASH HANDS WHEN VISIBLY SOILED! OTHERWISE, USE HANDRUB

Duration of the entire procedure: 40-60 seconds

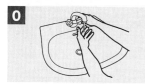

Wet hands with water;

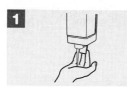

Apply enough soap to cover all hand surfaces;

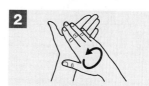

Rub hands palm to palm;

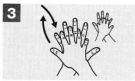

Right palm over left dorsum with interlaced fingers and vice versa;

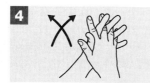

Palm to palm with fingers interlaced;

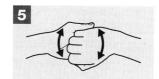

Backs of fingers to opposing palms with fingers interlocked;

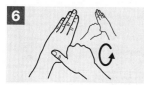

Rotational rubbing of left thumb clasped in right palm and vice versa;

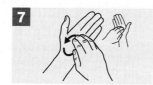

Rotational rubbing, backwards and forwards with clasped fingers of right hand in left palm and vice versa;

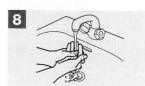

Rinse hands with water;

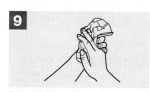

Dry hands thoroughly with a single use towel;

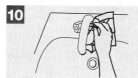

Use towel to turn off faucet;

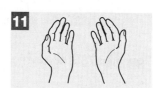

Your hands are now safe.

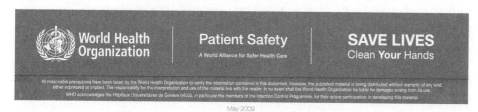

World Health Organization | Patient Safety — A World Alliance for Safer Health Care | SAVE LIVES — Clean **Your** Hands

Courtesy of the World Health Organization

Figure 2.26 This instructional poster shows how to properly wash your hands.

How to Handrub?

RUB HANDS FOR HAND HYGIENE! WASH HANDS WHEN VISIBLY SOILED

🕐 **Duration of the entire procedure: 20-30 seconds**

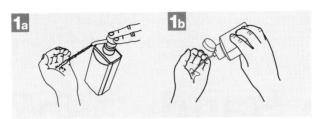
Apply a palmful of the product in a cupped hand, covering all surfaces;

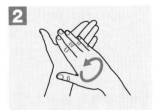
Rub hands palm to palm;

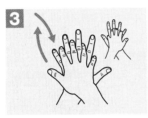
Right palm over left dorsum with interlaced fingers and vice versa;

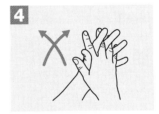
Palm to palm with fingers interlaced;

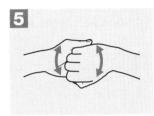
Backs of fingers to opposing palms with fingers interlocked;

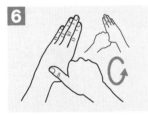
Rotational rubbing of left thumb clasped in right palm and vice versa;

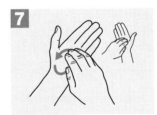
Rotational rubbing, backwards and forwards with clasped fingers of right hand in left palm and vice versa;

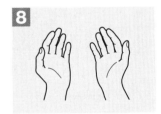
Once dry, your hands are safe.

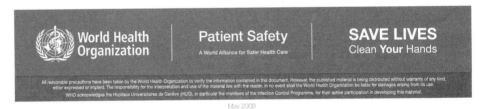

World Health Organization | **Patient Safety** A World Alliance for Safer Health Care | **SAVE LIVES** Clean **Your** Hands

All reasonable precautions have been taken by the World Health Organization to verify the information contained in this document. However, the published material is being distributed without warranty of any kind, either expressed or implied. The responsibility for the interpretation and use of the material lies with the reader. In no event shall the World Health Organization be liable for damages arising from its use. WHO acknowledges the Hôpitaux Universitaires de Genève (HUG), in particular the members of the Infection Control Programme, for their active participation in developing this material.

May 2009

Courtesy of the World Health Organization

Figure 2.27 The correct method of using alcohol-based hand gel is shown here.

If you work with acids or other hazardous materials, you may also need a rubber apron or special gloves. You might wear a hazardous material suit for full-body coverage in a research lab. This suit will keep you from bringing hazardous biological materials from the lab into public areas. It can also prevent you from contaminating your experiments.

You should remove PPE immediately after use. Following the correct steps for removing PPE helps you avoid spreading pathogens to your skin or clothing (**Figure 2.28**). Follow your facility's guidelines for disposing of PPE and remember to wash your hands. In some instances, when PPE is saturated with blood or body fluid, a special biohazard bag is required for safe disposal.

SEQUENCE FOR PUTTING ON PERSONAL PROTECTIVE EQUIPMENT (PPE)

The type of PPE used will vary based on the level of precautions required, such as standard and contact, droplet or airborne infection isolation precautions. The procedure for putting on and removing PPE should be tailored to the specific type of PPE.

1. GOWN

- Fully cover torso from neck to knees, arms to end of wrists, and wrap around the back
- Fasten in back of neck and waist

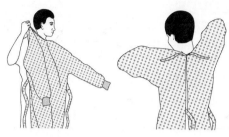

2. MASK OR RESPIRATOR

- Secure ties or elastic bands at middle of head and neck
- Fit flexible band to nose bridge
- Fit snug to face and below chin
- Fit-check respirator

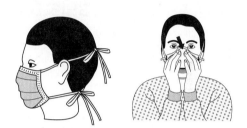

3. GOGGLES OR FACE SHIELD

- Place over face and eyes and adjust to fit

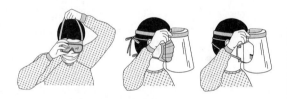

4. GLOVES

- Extend to cover wrist of isolation gown

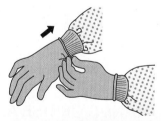

USE SAFE WORK PRACTICES TO PROTECT YOURSELF AND LIMIT THE SPREAD OF CONTAMINATION

- Keep hands away from face
- Limit surfaces touched
- Change gloves when torn or heavily contaminated
- Perform hand hygiene

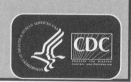

Courtesy of the Centers for Disease Control and Prevention

Figure 2.28 It is important to carefully follow the steps for putting on and taking off personal protective equipment.

(Continued)

HOW TO SAFELY REMOVE PERSONAL PROTECTIVE EQUIPMENT (PPE) EXAMPLE 1

There are a variety of ways to safely remove PPE without contaminating your clothing, skin, or mucous membranes with potentially infectious materials. Here is one example. **Remove all PPE before exiting the patient room** except a respirator, if worn. Remove the respirator **after** leaving the patient room and closing the door. Remove PPE in the following sequence:

1. GLOVES

- Outside of gloves are contaminated!
- If your hands get contaminated during glove removal, immediately wash your hands or use an alcohol-based hand sanitizer
- Using a gloved hand, grasp the palm area of the other gloved hand and peel off first glove
- Hold removed glove in gloved hand
- Slide fingers of ungloved hand under remaining glove at wrist and peel off second glove over first glove
- Discard gloves in a waste container

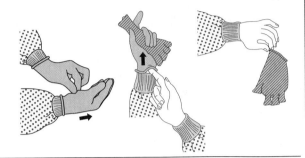

2. GOGGLES OR FACE SHIELD

- Outside of goggles or face shield are contaminated!
- If your hands get contaminated during goggle or face shield removal, immediately wash your hands or use an alcohol-based hand sanitizer
- Remove goggles or face shield from the back by lifting head band or ear pieces
- If the item is reusable, place in designated receptacle for reprocessing. Otherwise, discard in a waste container

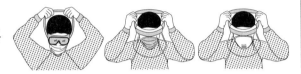

3. GOWN

- Gown front and sleeves are contaminated!
- If your hands get contaminated during gown removal, immediately wash your hands or use an alcohol-based hand sanitizer
- Unfasten gown ties, taking care that sleeves don't contact your body when reaching for ties
- Pull gown away from neck and shoulders, touching inside of gown only
- Turn gown inside out
- Fold or roll into a bundle and discard in a waste container

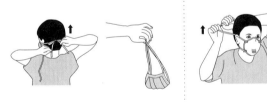

4. MASK OR RESPIRATOR

- Front of mask/respirator is contaminated — DO NOT TOUCH!
- If your hands get contaminated during mask/respirator removal, immediately wash your hands or use an alcohol-based hand sanitizer
- Grasp bottom ties or elastics of the mask/respirator, then the ones at the top, and remove without touching the front
- Discard in a waste container

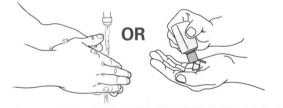

5. WASH HANDS OR USE AN ALCOHOL-BASED HAND SANITIZER IMMEDIATELY AFTER REMOVING ALL PPE

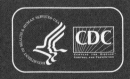

OR

PERFORM HAND HYGIENE BETWEEN STEPS IF HANDS BECOME CONTAMINATED AND IMMEDIATELY AFTER REMOVING ALL PPE

CDC

Figure 2.28 (Continued)

Respiratory Hygiene

COVID-19 made people very conscious of germs spread by coughing and sneezing. You will need to practice and teach your patients about **respiratory hygiene**, or *cough etiquette*, to reduce the spread of respiratory secretions. The tiny spray of droplets can quickly spread infections to others in common areas, such as waiting rooms and cafeterias. The following are basic elements of respiratory hygiene:

- Cover your nose and mouth with a tissue or the inside of your elbow when coughing or sneezing.
- Provide tissues, hand gel, masks, and waste containers in waiting areas.
- Discard tissues after one use and perform hand hygiene.
- Post respiratory hygiene guidelines in common areas.
- Ask patients with signs of respiratory illness to wear a mask in common areas or provide them with a private waiting area.
- Place seats in waiting areas 3 to 6 feet apart to reduce close contact.

Healthcare Professions: Standard Precautions in the Dental Office

Suzanne has her own dental practice. She is training a new dental assistant, Calysta, to support her during dental procedures. Today, they are filling a cavity in a patient's tooth.

The patient checks in and sits down to wait. She had a cold and blows her nose so it will not bother her during the procedure. She puts the tissue in her pocket, then takes out her phone.

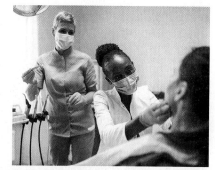

NoSsystem images/E+ via Getty Images

Calysta goes to the waiting room to call the patient. She introduces herself and shakes the patient's hand, then escorts the patient from the waiting room to the dental chair. She washes her hands and puts on gloves, then adjusts the chair, turns on the operating light, and gathers her tools. She opens the door to let Suzanne know they are ready for her, then chats with the patient for a few minutes.

When Suzanne arrives, she puts on gloves and her face shield before giving the injection to numb the patient's tooth. Then she removes her PPE, uses hand gel, and asks Calysta to let her know when the numbing takes effect. The patient has never had a filling before, so Calysta shows her the tools on the tray and answers her questions.

In about 10 minutes, Calysta calls Suzanne in. Suzanne puts on her gloves and a face shield to protect herself from the fine mist of water created during drilling. Calysta rubs her itchy eyes before putting on her face shield. She has been working hard and is very tired and run down. When the patient asks her to stop and change her gloves, Calysta is embarrassed, but complies. After she has washed her hands and put on clean gloves, Calysta holds the suction and hands tools to Suzanne as they are needed.

At the end of the procedure, Calysta provides water for the patient to rinse, then suctions her mouth. Suzanne gives the patient a few last instructions, then removes her gloves, sanitizes her hands, and removes her face shield.

Calysta removes her face shield and washes her hands, then shows the patient out. Whom do you think may become ill after this procedure? What corrections would make this a safer healthcare environment?

Preventing Sharps Injuries

According to the CDC, healthcare workers suffer more than 380,000 sharps injuries each year. **Sharps** are needles, scalpels, or other sharp-edged objects that can puncture the skin. Not all healthcare workers have a high risk, but you should know how to avoid this type of injury. Disposable syringes and suture needles cause more than one-half of all sharps injuries. Most injuries occur while the sharp is being used, but there is still a high risk for injury after use or during disposal. The risk of serious infection from hollow-bore needles used for drawing blood and giving injections is high because these needles can hold blood from the patient. This raises the risk of spreading infections such as human immunodeficiency virus (HIV) and hepatitis.

One way to reduce your chance of injury is to reduce your use of sharps. Needleless intravenous connection systems have greatly reduced the use of needles. Similarly, the use of safer hinged needles and winged-steel needles reduces sharps injuries for phlebotomists (**Figure 2.29**). You should never recap needles because this increases your chances of sticking yourself.

Carefully disposing of sharps after you use them can also prevent injuries. To fit with federal regulations, you must use a durable, puncture-proof container that can be closed. It must be easily available, positioned away from doors, and attached so it cannot tip over. You should be able to put sharps inside with just one hand (**Figure 2.30**). Never fill the container past the level specified on the outside.

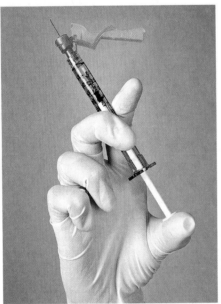

Elena Elisseeva/Shutterstock.com

Figure 2.29 Hinged needles have a cap that can be removed and replaced easily, preventing accidental needlesticks.

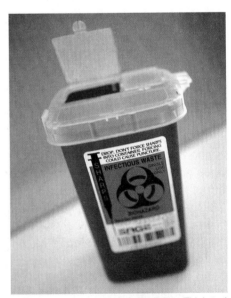

Ingram Publishing/Thinkstock

Figure 2.30 Sharps containers must be easily available so healthcare workers can dispose of needles and other sharps quickly and safely.

Biohazard signs should be posted in areas where there is medical waste containing sharps, chemicals, or blood products. Red biohazard bags and puncture-proof containers are commonly used. This alerts you to use the necessary precautions to prevent injury (**Figure 2.31**). In addition, your facility must work with a disposal company specially equipped to handle biohazardous materials.

2.2-4 Transmission-Based Precautions

In addition to the standard precautions listed in Figure 2.25, the CDC recommends you take extra care with patients who are or may be infected with certain serious pathogens. These **transmission-based precautions** focus on how the identified infection spreads. The goal is to anticipate and prevent the spread of infection before it even begins.

Healthcare workers use transmission-based precautions when standard precautions are not enough to prevent the possible spread of a pathogen. Based on how a pathogen is spread, transmission-based precautions are divided into three categories:

- **Contact precautions.** These are used when the infection can spread by direct contact with a patient or indirect contact through the environment. These precautions are used for infections such as *Staphylococcus aureus* or diarrhea, when contact with body waste can result in infection. When contact precautions are needed, the patient should be placed in **isolation** in a single-person room or have a bed at least 3 feet from the bed of another patient. Use of dedicated or disposable equipment also reduces transmission between patients. You should put on PPE before entering the room when your patient needs contact precautions. You should also take off and dispose of that PPE before leaving the room and wash your hands. This can be time consuming, but it is important to maintain regular contact with your patient so their needs are not ignored and they do not become depressed during isolation.
- **Droplet precautions.** When a pathogen can spread by close contact with respiratory secretions or mucous membranes, droplet precautions are needed. Place your patients with a respiratory infection, such as influenza or pertussis, in a single-person room or in a bed at least 3 feet away from other patients. In addition, draw the curtains around their bed to help contain any droplets. Wear a mask while with the patient. If your patient must travel out of the room and move through the facility, have them wear a mask as a form of reverse-isolation. If the patient cannot wear a mask due to age or respiratory status, instruct them on cough etiquette and hand hygiene.
- **Airborne precautions.** These steps are needed for infections that float through the air for a great distance, such as the viruses that cause measles, chickenpox, and tuberculosis. Place these patients in a single-patient isolation room with negative air pressure and special equipment to filter and vent the air. You will need to wear a mask or respirator while caring for these patients, depending on the pathogen present. TB pathogens are so small they require a special N95 respirator mask to filter them (**Figure 2.32**).

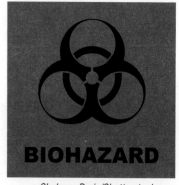

ChekmanDaria/Shutterstock.com

Figure 2.31 This red biohazard symbol with interlocking rings tells healthcare workers to take precautions to avoid contamination or infection.

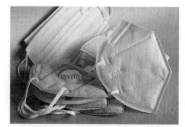

Mau47/Shutterstock.com

Figure 2.32 Different types of masks have different purposes. *What type of mask is required for very small pathogens, such as TB?*

Transmission-based precautions can be put in place before a pathogen is identified, based on the symptoms of a disease. When a symptom can indicate more than one possible pathogen, more than one transmission-based precaution may be needed. For instance, if your patient has a rash of unknown origin and has traveled to a country with outbreaks of very high fever in the past 10 days, you should use both airborne and contact precautions. This is because the possible viruses causing the symptoms spread in different ways.

Transmission-based precautions are used in addition to standard precautions when the risk of transmitting a disease is high. When your patient has symptoms of coughing or diarrhea, for example, you should follow transmission-based precautions as long as those symptoms last. If your patient has a drug-resistant infection, you should continue transmission-based precautions for at least several weeks after they have been treated or no longer have symptoms. This allows time to make sure the drug-resistant infection has not returned. You can return to standard precautions after the increased risk of infection has passed.

2.2-5 Bloodborne Pathogen Exposure Control

The Occupational Safety and Health Administration (OSHA) requires specific safeguards when there is a potential for *occupational exposure* to bloodborne pathogens. This means an employee is likely to encounter this hazard while doing their job. This is common for anyone who obtains or handles specimens. It creates a higher risk of exposure to infections such as human immunodeficiency virus (HIV), which causes acquired immunodeficiency syndrome (AIDS); the hepatitis B virus (HBV); and the hepatitis C virus (HCV).

Your employer must have a written exposure control plan of steps to take if a situation poses a hazard to workers or the public at large. Employers must train anyone at risk for occupational exposure to bloodborne pathogens. They also must offer HBV vaccination to employees with potential exposure, provide you with PPE such as gloves and gowns, and use devices to decrease your exposure to needlesticks and other sharps.

2.2-6 Aseptic Practices

Aseptic techniques maintain a clean environment to prevent HAIs during the process of caring for patients. According to the CDC, on any given day, approximately one in 31 patients has an HAI. Preventing infection is a matter of breaking the chain of infection at any step in the process. Proper handwashing and wearing the appropriate PPE are standard precautions to prevent most transmissions of infection. Other measures include limiting the number of surfaces you touch, planning your procedures to move from the cleanest to the dirtiest areas, and keeping your environment clean.

Your movements should follow the principle of "clean to dirty." This means starting in a clean area with clean materials and equipment and only moving toward dirty surfaces. Never bring contaminants back into the clean area. Of course, you then need to change equipment or gloves before you can go back to touching clean materials.

Most healthcare settings require some level of *asepsis*, or elimination of pathogens, through **clean technique** to limit the spread of infection.

Sanitization uses cleaning to lower the number of bacteria on a surface, but it does not kill viruses. You will usually sanitize areas less likely to have pathogens. *Disinfection* uses powerful chemicals, such as bleach, to kill pathogens. You will want to disinfect high-contact surfaces such as counters, doorknobs, and some equipment. Medical asepsis uses clean techniques, handwashing, standard precautions, and PPE to reduce the number of pathogens and their ability to transfer to new surfaces. This helps to prevent the spread of infection.

Surgical asepsis, or *antisepsis,* is achieved through **sterile technique.** This technique uses sterilization and a sterile field to prevent the introduction of pathogens during invasive procedures. *Sterilization* means using heat or chemicals to destroy all microorganisms on an object or surface. Covering the area with sterilized barriers creates what is called a *sterile field.* You will use this process for surgery, caring for open wounds, inserting tubes in the body, and any procedure that breaks the patient's skin. An autoclave sterilizes surgical tools, and operating rooms are kept dry, cool, and well lit to deter pathogens. How else can you prevent a healthcare facility from providing a reservoir for pathogens?

Cleaning and Disinfecting the Healthcare Environment

The CDC ranks healthcare environments as *noncritical, semicritical,* or *critical* based on classifications developed by Dr. Earle Spaulding (**Figure 2.33**). These classifications rank the potential for infectious disease to spread via equipment, instruments, and furniture. They also consider the level of sterility normally required for the part of the body that will touch the surface.

Typically, waiting areas need only general cleaning. This involves removing dirt and dust and using detergents, scouring powders, and toilet bowl and glass cleaners. This is similar to cleaning an office building or hotel. Patient rooms, however, need both general cleaning and low-level disinfecting. Surgical suites require high-level disinfecting as well as sterilization of instruments. Cleaning and disinfecting in an appropriate and organized manner will protect you and your patient from infections and exposure to toxic chemicals.

OSHA regulates the safe disposal of dangerous, or *hazardous,* medical waste. An entry-level housekeeping employee must be trained in these safety procedures to avoid exposure to infectious organisms, as well as in the steps for cleaning a patient hospital room.

Spaulding's Classifications				
Level	**Definition**	**Procedure**	**Goal**	**Example**
Critical	Objects that enter sterile tissue or vascular system	Sterilization	Kill all organisms, including spores	Sterilization of surgical instruments
Semicritical	Objects that touch mucous membranes or non-intact skin	High-level disinfection	Kill all vegetative organisms; spores not killed	High-level disinfection of endoscopes
Noncritical	Objects that touch only intact skin	Low-level disinfection or cleaning	Removal of pathogenic organisms	Cleaning patient room

Goodheart-Willcox Publisher

Figure 2.33 Dr. Spaulding created a system for identifying the level of cleanliness required for different objects in the healthcare environment.

Specific steps are used to clean and disinfect a patient hospital room in preparation for a newly admitted patient. This **terminal cleaning** procedure is especially important in preventing the infection of a new patient with an HAI.

When a patient room needs to be cleaned for a new patient, follow these steps:

1. Wash your hands and put on gloves.
2. Strip all linens, including pillows, by folding them in on themselves. Some facilities use disposable pillows.
3. Hold linens away from your uniform as you deposit them directly into the linen hamper or laundry bag.
4. Use your facility-approved disinfectant to wash the mattress, making sure you thoroughly disinfect all areas on the mattress slide handles.
5. Discard all items left in the room. This may include cards, flowers, magazines, newspapers, and more.
6. Disinfect all surfaces that are likely to be touched (**Figure 2.34**). This includes tabletops, faceplates of medical equipment, countertops, bed controls, and side rails. Remember that door handles, computer keyboards and screens, and television controls are frequently touched. While less common now because of cell phones, some rooms still have telephones that need disinfection as well.

7. Mop the floor using a disinfectant solution.
8. Clean, disinfect, and store the commode (portable toilet).
9. Clean the bathroom's toilet, sink, and shower. Mop the floor.
10. Discard your gloves and wash your hands.
11. Make the bed, wearing gloves if required by your facility.
12. Remove and properly store all cleaning equipment. Remove gloves, if worn. Wash your hands.

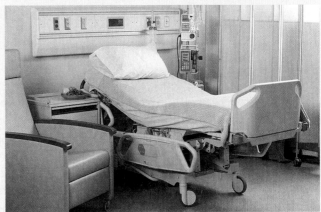

Monkey Business Images/Shutterstock.com

Figure 2.34 Disinfect all surfaces that are likely to be touched. *What surfaces would you disinfect in a hospital room?*

Guidelines for infection control change as new chemicals and treatment procedures are developed. New ultraviolet light systems disinfect without the use of harmful chemicals. They use UV-C waves to penetrate the cell wall of microorganisms and alter their DNA. Just 15 minutes of exposure can kill even the most challenging pathogens that cause HAIs. They can also be used in heating and cooling systems to treat the air people breathe. UV-C lights are beginning to replace the use of disinfectants in the terminal cleaning process.

Cleaning and Sterilizing Equipment

Contamination is the unwanted presence of harmful substances or microorganisms. Cleaning is the first step in removing bloodborne pathogens or other potentially infectious material (OPIM), such as other body fluids or tissues, from equipment. If visible debris is not removed before equipment enters an autoclave, contaminants stuck to the item will be baked on, and pathogens may not be destroyed.

When you are cleaning and sterilizing equipment, the goals are the same for both large hospitals with employees who maintain a central supply of ready-to-use equipment and for small medical offices where one assistant maintains equipment for one doctor. Whether a lab runs clinical tests or research experiments, effective protocols for preventing contamination are required.

Ultrasonic Cleaners

Ultrasonic cleaning is preferred over manual scrubbing and soaking because it is safer for workers. *Ultrasonic cleaners* use sound waves to create millions of water jets that gently remove debris (**Figure 2.35**). Keep in mind that ultrasonic cleaning does not sterilize equipment. Viruses and spores remain on items even after this process.

Autoclaves

Once equipment is cleaned, it is ready to be sterilized. All materials need to be wrapped or packaged in a specific way before you place them in the *autoclave*. Then, this device uses pressurized steam at temperatures high enough and time periods long enough to kill most microorganisms.

Autoclaves sterilize items in both clinical and research facilities. Many items can be autoclaved, including surgical instruments, glassware, plastic tubes, pipette tips, solutions, water, animal food and bedding, and hazardous waste materials. These items should be cleaned and sterilized immediately after a clinical procedure. In a laboratory setting, autoclaves are typically used at both ends of a research project. Initially, glassware and lab instruments are sterilized to ensure experiments are free of biological contaminants. At the end of a project, the autoclave inactivates any microorganisms found in the waste products from an experiment.

Several types of wraps are available for this procedure, including autoclave paper, plastic or paper bags designed for autoclaving, and autoclave containers. Steam will penetrate these wraps during the autoclaving process. Autoclave indicators, which include special tape or sensitive marks on bags or containers, are placed at the center of a group of items and on the outside of the wrap. The indicators change color during the autoclaving process. This color change does not guarantee the equipment is sterile. The tape can change color without being exposed for the full time or to the required level of pressure.

Autoclaves must be properly maintained to remain effective, and employees must know how to operate the autoclave correctly to prevent injury. Manufacturers sell many types and sizes of autoclaves. You must learn the guidelines for using your own facility's machine to sterilize the specific products used at your facility. Maintaining the autoclave's proper function and using it correctly provide the best assurance that items are properly sterilized.

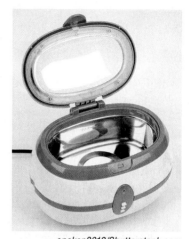

anaken2012/Shutterstock.com

Figure 2.35 Ultrasonic cleaning is preferable to manual scrubbing and soaking because it is safer for workers. *How do ultrasonic cleaners work?*

 Healthcare Professions: Sterilizing

One of Calysta's duties as a dental assistant is to sterilize dental tools after a procedure. She has been trained to use the autoclave in her office but is nervous after her last patient interaction. She knows she needs to brush up on her infection control practices before she makes another mistake. Calysta's dental office uses autoclave paper to wrap dental instruments for autoclaving. She wants to ensure all the edges of the wrap are sealed to keep out pathogens. She checks her notes on how to wrap the equipment and follows the steps carefully to avoid any further mistakes.

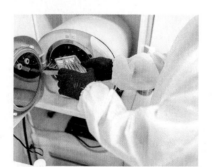

Kosamtu/E+ via Getty Images

Follow these steps to wrap equipment for an autoclave correctly.

1. Wash your hands and put on a gown or lab coat, a mask, and gloves.
2. Clean the items to be sterilized using an ultrasonic cleaner.
3. Select the correct type of wrap, making sure it is large enough to enclose the equipment completely. Use a single or double thickness according to your facility's policy.
4. Position the wrap diagonally with one corner pointing toward you.
5. Open hinged items so that steam can sterilize all surfaces.
6. Place the equipment and an indicator strip in the center of the wrap (**Figure 2.36A**).
7. Fold the bottom corner of the wrap in toward the center and fold a small corner back, forming a tab (**Figure 2.36B and C**).
8. Fold the left edge over to the center and fold the corner back (**Figure 2.36D**).
9. Repeat with the right side (**Figure 2.36E**).
10. Close the package by folding the remaining corner over the top of the package and tucking it in or by folding the package up from the bottom (**Figure 2.36F and G**).
11. Check to see that items are wrapped securely for handling but loose enough that steam can circulate during the autoclaving process.
12. Seal the wrap with indicator tape, leaving a tape tab at one end to allow for easy opening (**Figure 2.36H**).
13. Label the tape with the date, package contents, and your initials (**Figure 2.36I**).
14. Remove and discard your PPE according to your facility's policy. Wash hands.

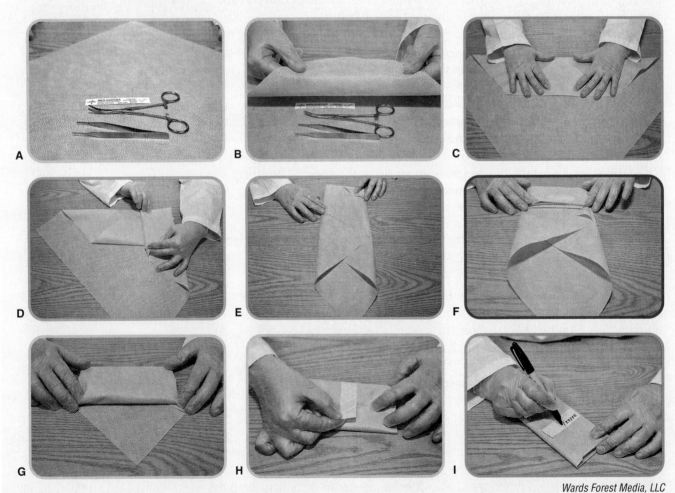

Wards Forest Media, LLC

Figure 2.36 Study these images and the steps listed in the text to learn how to wrap instruments for autoclaving.

As new techniques are developed, safety procedures will continue to adapt. It is important to stay up-to-date with the latest safety and health risks in all healthcare careers. That is why you will review safety and infection control annually as part of your required continuing education for healthcare workers.

Lesson 2.2 Review

 Complete the *Map Your Reading* graphic organizer for the section you just read.

1. Microorganisms known to cause disease are called (2.2-1)
   A. normal body flora
   B. pathogens
   C. HAIs
   D. resistant

2. All of the following are ways to break the chain of infection, *except* (2.2-2)
   A. full vaccination
   B. frequent handwashing
   C. wearing PPE all the time
   D. terminal cleaning

3. Which of the following are examples of standard precautions? Choose all that apply. (2.2-3)
   A. Hand hygiene
   B. PPE
   C. Cough etiquette
   D. Sharps safety
   E. Environmental cleaning

4. The symbol used to identify biohazards is (2.2-3)
   A. four intersecting circles on a red background
   B. a fire within a yellow triangle
   C. a skull and bones within a diamond
   D. All of these.

5. Transmission-based precautions are used for (2.2-4)
   A. all patients, all the time
   B. only susceptible hosts
   C. patients with symptoms of infections that can easily spread
   D. only airborne infections

6. In transmission-based precautions, used PPE should be removed (2.2-4)
   A. wherever you are standing for the procedure
   B. at the doorway before you exit the room
   C. in the hallway outside the room
   D. in the locker room

7. Occupational exposure to blood increases risk for (2.2-5)
   A. HIV
   B. asthma
   C. tuberculosis
   D. psoriasis

8. Which of the following destroys all microorganisms, including bacteria and viruses? (2.2-6)
   A. Disinfection
   B. Sanitization
   C. Sterilization
   D. Clean technique

Responding to Emergency Situations

ESSENTIAL QUESTION

What steps should you use to respond in emergency situations?

Learning Outcomes

After studying this lesson, you will be able to

2.3-1 discuss appropriate emergency response for different situations.

2.3-2 identify the steps for handling a fire emergency, including use of a fire extinguisher.

2.3-3 identify safety hazards around oxygen equipment.

2.3-4 identify safety hazards in the use of electrical equipment.

2.3-5 discuss measures used to prevent bioterrorism.

Professional Vocabulary

Essential Terms

electrical shock   a physical reaction to electricity passing through the body

Pull, Aim, Squeeze, Sweep (PASS)   an acronym for remembering the steps to use a fire extinguisher

Rescue, Alarm, Contain, Extinguish/Evacuate (RACE)   an acronym used to remember the steps to take in response to a fire emergency

Important Terms

fire triangle
grounding
select agents

Introduction

You have probably taken part in fire drills, tornado drills, code reds, and other emergency drills since kindergarten. These practice drills are recommended for all businesses and homes so that you feel prepared when an actual emergency occurs. Healthcare facilities must have well-developed plans for responding to emergency situations. These plans should include prevention, preparedness, response, and recovery stages. They should also cover a broad range of possibilities, such as a natural disaster, pandemic, fire, terrorist attack, threat to safety, or sudden influx of patients. As a healthcare worker, your role in these situations will go beyond evacuating or taking cover for yourself. You will also need to help your patients protect themselves.

2.3-1 Basic Emergency Preparation and Response

Some emergencies can be prevented. Safety officers look for possible safety threats and ways to avoid them. Following safety guidelines, adding guard railings, updating electrical wiring, installing surveillance cameras, and training staff to de-escalate tense situations can all prevent problems before they occur. You may be able to prevent a potentially violent situation by recognizing and reporting warning signs. Alert your human resources department if you notice signs of withdrawal and paranoid behavior or hear comments about dangerous weapons and getting revenge.

Some problems cannot be avoided, but it is possible to be prepared. Severe weather can cause power outages with serious consequences for those who depend on electrical equipment. For preparedness, healthcare facilities have backup generators to provide electricity during a power outage (**Figure 2.37**). Healthcare facilities also maintain an emergency water supply for handwashing, providing drinking water, laundering dirty linens, and other needs. Pandemics, such as COVID-19, reinforce the need to have backup PPE and emergency supplies available.

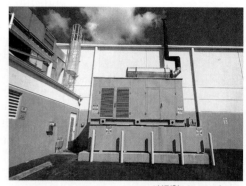

arnet117/Shutterstock.com

Figure 2.37 A backup generator is one important component of a healthcare facility's disaster plan. *What are some other components of a typical disaster plan?*

Facilities must have a plan for responding to a variety of different emergencies. Managers should make sure that staff members are well trained and practice emergency procedures so they go smoothly when the time arises. In the event of an emergency, healthcare workers should follow these basic rules:

- **Remain calm for your own sake and project a sense of calm.** Your calm manner will help reassure patients, prevent them from panicking, and make them easier to manage.
- **If safe, move anyone who is in danger out of the threatening situation.** Keep yourself out of danger so you can help others.
- **Sound the alarm and contact emergency personnel.** If not already called, use an outside phone line to dial 911. Provide the address and your location within the building, type of emergency, and a status report.
- **Mentally review your emergency training and where emergency equipment is located.** You should know the location of fire extinguishers, fire doors, first aid kits, and AEDs.
- **Follow your facility's evacuation procedure and your assigned role during emergencies.** Use the assigned escape and shelter locations for your area. Follow posted exit signs and evacuation maps if you are not in a familiar place. These are generally found near the main entrances.
- **Use stairways rather than elevators and make use of emergency exits.** Some patients may require assistance for evacuation. Those who cannot exit should be taken to a designated area of refuge.

Active shooter threats require different action steps. According to the Department of Homeland Security, your first response to an active shooter should be to evacuate if you can get to an exit. If you cannot leave the area, then look for a protected place to hide out of the shooter's view. Lock or barricade yourself in, if possible. Silence phones and devices that might draw attention and stay as quiet as possible. Text someone to call 911 or alert police, if possible. Only take direct action against the shooter if someone's life is in immediate danger and they cannot escape.

The recovery phase after an emergency involves restoring normal function, evaluating the events, and learning from them. When Hurricane Harvey hit Texas and Louisiana in 2017, facilities had only two days to prepare. Twenty hospitals were evacuated due to flooding. Communication problems sent patients into facilities that were evacuating. Nearby hospitals filled beyond capacity and ran out of food and clean water. Emergency shelters were not equipped to care for people with medical needs such as quadriplegia and dialysis. Morgues reached maximum capacity. There were licensure challenges that delayed healthcare professionals offering support from other states. Gaps and barriers in emergency plans were apparent.

When the COVID-19 pandemic began, some of these problems were avoided. Daily communication between healthcare services and local governments helped distribute equipment and get information out to the public to slow the spread of infection and avoid overwhelming emergency rooms. States created emergency licensing rules to allow support from medical students, providers in other states, and similarly trained professionals. Refrigeration trucks served as emergency morgues. Manufacturers reconfigured production lines to make more masks, sanitizers, and ventilators. Labs began immediate research into treatments and vaccinations. Learning from past mistakes and fast response rates helped reduce the total number of fatalities.

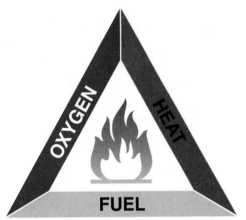

Goodheart-Willcox Publisher

Figure 2.38 The fire triangle shows the three elements needed for a fire to occur—fuel, heat, and oxygen.

2.3-2 Fire Safety in a Healthcare Setting

In a healthcare setting, carelessness while smoking or electrical sparks resulting from frayed wires or overloaded circuits may cause fires. A fire must have oxygen, fuel, and a heat source. These three elements are called the **fire triangle** (**Figure 2.38**). Removing any of these three components will prevent a fire or stop a fire in progress.

Every healthcare facility has a fire plan, and every employee is responsible for knowing that plan. Employees should practice once a month so that everything goes smoothly when there is a real fire.

Handling a Fire Emergency

Your first impulse when you hear fire alarms is probably to get out of the burning building. Healthcare facilities such as hospitals and nursing homes do not evacuate immediately. They defend in place. This is because of the large number of people who would need assistance to evacuate. Healthcare facilities require many fire protection features, but your safety and that of your patients will still rely on you knowing what to do in the event of a fire.

The acronym **RACE** will help you remember the steps to take when there is a fire. RACE stands for **r**escue, **a**larm, **c**ontain, and **e**xtinguish/**e**vacuate:

- Remove or **rescue** patients who are in the same room as the fire and in immediate danger from it.
- As you remove patients from the room, alert others to the fire by pulling the safety **alarm** and calling for help.

- **Contain** the fire by closing all the doors and windows. This limits the amount of oxygen available. Fire doors may close when the fire alarm is pulled. Shut off electrical equipment and oxygen tanks that may fuel the fire.
- If the fire is small, **extinguish** it using a fire extinguisher, a fire blanket, or another means of smothering the flame. In a kitchen, put the lid on a burning pan. Begin **evacuating** the rooms directly above, below, and next door to the area if the fire cannot be contained or is too large to be extinguished. If a full evacuation is required, patients who cannot walk or be transferred to a wheelchair may need extra help. An entire bed may be wheeled out of the facility. A mattress can also be dragged to transport a patient. Never use the elevators during a fire.

Types of Fire Extinguishers

Fire extinguishers eject substances to smother a fire. By cutting the oxygen supply to the flames, they eliminate one corner of the fire triangle and thus stop the fire. Different types of fires require specific types of fire extinguishers (**Figure 2.39**). Using the wrong type of extinguisher can cause injury to the user and increase the fire rather than put it out.

Fire Classifications				
Class	**Description**	**Type**	**Picture Symbol**	**Letter Symbol**
A	**Ordinary Combustibles** (Materials such as wood, paper, or textiles)	Pressurized water	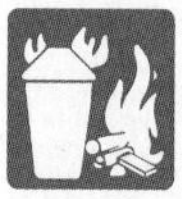	A
B	**Flammable Liquids** (Liquids such as grease, gasoline, oils, and paints)	Carbon dioxide (CO_2)	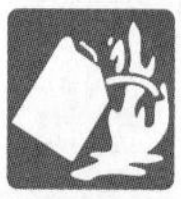	B
C	**Electrical Equipment** (Wiring, computers, switches, and any other energized electrical equipment)	Dry chemical	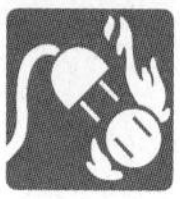	C
D	**Combustible Metals** (Flammable metals such as magnesium and lithium)	Dry chemical	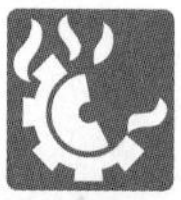	D
K	**Kitchen Fires** (Grease, fat, and oil fires in commercial kitchens)	Dry chemical or wet chemical	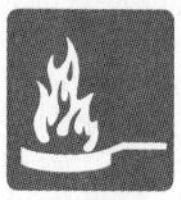	K
Multipurpose ABC	Labeled for use on ordinary combustibles, flammable liquids, and electrical equipment fires	Multipurpose or wet chemical	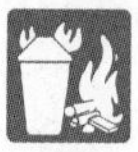 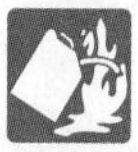 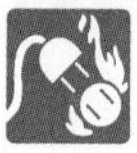	A B C

Figure 2.39 Choose the correct type of fire extinguisher to avoid increasing the fire and risk to the user.

Operating a Fire Extinguisher

In the event of a fire, you will need to make a quick decision about whether to try to extinguish the fire or evacuate. Before you try to use a fire extinguisher, be sure the fire is small, you have the right type of extinguisher, and you know how to use it.

You can remember the steps for operating any fire extinguisher by using the acronym **PASS** (**Figure 2.40**). This stands for **p**ull the pin, **a**im the extinguisher, **s**queeze the handle, and **s**weep the nozzle:

- *Pull* the pin at the bottom of the trigger. Removing this safety pin allows you to operate the trigger.
- *Aim* the nozzle at the base of the fire from about 6 to 10 feet away. Be sure to aim at the base of the flames. If you aim too high or too low, the fire will not be extinguished and may be blown around to start more fires.
- *Squeeze* the trigger with your fingers to discharge the extinguisher solution while holding the extinguisher firmly.
- *Sweep* the fire extinguisher from side to side to smother all the flames.

Fire extinguishers must be kept in good working order. The Occupational Safety and Health Administration (OSHA) requires a monthly visual inspection, annual maintenance by a qualified individual, and testing every 5 to 12 years, depending on the type of extinguisher. Once a fire extinguisher has been used, it must be recharged or replaced.

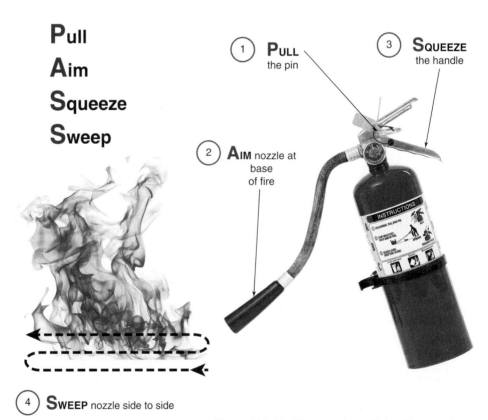

Pull
Aim
Squeeze
Sweep

① **P**ULL the pin

③ **S**QUEEZE the handle

② **A**IM nozzle at base of fire

④ **S**WEEP nozzle side to side

Thomas M Perkins/Shutterstock.com, Valeev/Shutterstock.com

Figure 2.40 The PASS acronym can help you learn how to use a fire extinguisher properly and effectively.

2.3-3 **Oxygen Safety**

Some patients with respiratory conditions require constant delivery of oxygen so they can breathe and function (**Figure 2.41**). You have probably seen oxygen masks on patients in a hospital or ambulance, but they are also found in patients' homes. The oxygen may be delivered from a large metal tank or a concentrator that pulls oxygen from the air. As you know, oxygen is one of the components of the fire triangle. As a result, fire is a very serious threat when an oxygen tank is present. To prevent hazards associated with oxygen use, follow these rules:

- **Secure the oxygen tank.** Make sure the tank is stable and unlikely to fall or tip over.
- **Post warning signs when oxygen is in use.** Signs that read "No Smoking—Oxygen in Use" should be placed near patients who are receiving oxygen.
- **Keep sparks and flames away from oxygen.** Oxygen helps fires burn, so you should take extra precautions to keep any heat source, such as cigarettes and electrical equipment that can spark, away from oxygen supplies or tubing.
- **Use cotton clothing and blankets for patients receiving oxygen.** Avoid wool and synthetics that may create static electricity, which could spark a fire.

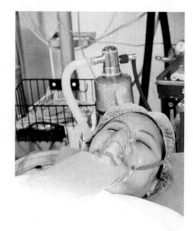

Apples Eyes Studio/Shutterstock.com

Figure 2.41 Because oxygen is one element in the fire triangle, you should take extra precautions around patients using oxygen equipment.

2.3-4 **Electrical Safety**

You have probably felt the light shock of static electricity on a dry winter day and found it annoying. **Electrical shock** is the physical reaction to electricity passing through the body. This can range from almost unnoticeable static electricity to a fatal electrocution. In a hospital setting, patients may be connected to multiple electronic devices, increasing the chances something could go wrong (**Figure 2.42**).

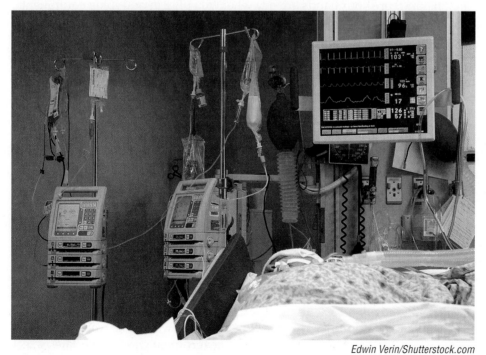

Edwin Verin/Shutterstock.com

Figure 2.42 Electronic equipment in a patient's room can pose a threat of electrical shock. *How can you ensure electrical safety?*

This equipment can cause electrical shock, fires, and explosions if used improperly or not maintained. You will want to avoid all types of electrical hazards for yourself and your patients.

Electrical current is very dangerous. Three to 5 milliamperes (mA) of current can produce a shock that forces a person to pull away. Six or more mA of current cause painful shocks, and 9 to 15 mA can cause muscle contractions that make it impossible for a person to let go. One hundred to 300 mA interrupt heart rhythm, and if contact lasts for three minutes or more, can cause death. Electrical hazards generally have a red "Danger" sign and a lightning bolt symbol to alert people.

The chief causes of electrical hazards are faulty equipment or wiring, damage to receptacles or connectors, and unsafe work practices. OSHA recommends several practices to ensure electrical safety:

- Install and use equipment according to the instructions provided. Make sure that electrical equipment is kept free from hazards noted on the label.
- Provide sufficient working space around electrical equipment to allow for safe access, operation, and maintenance.
- Make sure all electrical equipment near water is properly grounded. **Grounding** carries current safely away from an electrical circuit to prevent shocks or electrical fires when there is a problem with the circuit. A *ground-fault circuit interrupter (GFCI)* will break the circuit at the outlet when unexpected grounding causes an imbalance. Circuit breakers and fuses cut the flow of electricity at the power box.
- Inspect electrical cords, plugs, and equipment regularly. Remove from service and report any receptacles or equipment that show signs of damage.
- Do not overload circuits by plugging in too many devices at once and avoid the use of extension cords.
- Follow safe procedures when using electrical equipment, including making sure your hands are dry when you plug in or unplug equipment.

If electrical shock does occur, treatment will depend on the severity of the incident. Burns and other health conditions caused by electrical shock may require first aid or more extensive medical treatment.

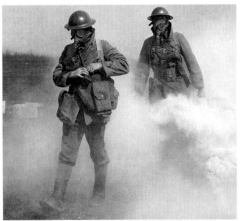

Everett Historical/Shutterstock.com

Figure 2.43 Chemical warfare was frequently used in World War I and World War II.

2.3-5 **Bioterrorism**

The potential for world war involving chemical and biological weapons may sound like a scene from an old movie, but these deadly weapons remain a threat (**Figure 2.43**). Educating healthcare workers to recognize the signs of a bioterrorist attack allows a faster response and minimizes the impact.

The federal government has identified some 30 substances as **select agents**, which are highly dangerous because they can be used to develop biological or chemical weapons. These agents include the Ebola and Marburg viruses, which cause deadly diseases; *Botulinum* toxins, which are also potentially fatal; ricin, which can make a highly deadly gas; and *Yersinia pestis*, the bacterium that causes what was known in the Middle Ages as the *Black Plague*. The federal government strictly regulates select agents to limit the possibility of accidental release or a deliberate terrorist attack.

Despite agreements signed by many countries to ban chemical and biological weapons, a nerve gas released in the Tokyo subway in 1995 killed 13 people and injured thousands. An anthrax attack in the US killed five people in 2001. The Assad regime in Syria killed as many as 1,800 people with sarin gas in 2013–2014. Nanotechnology has made new biological weapons possible, and the FBI has expressed concerns that databases for precision medicine will make it easier to target specific populations. Government intelligence agencies believe that more terrorist groups are working to weaponize select agents.

Simulations of major disasters and bioterrorism events are useful in preparing for these uncommon but critical emergencies. Scenario-based interactive training allows you to identify potential problems, improve performance, increase efficiency, and reduce anxiety surrounding these events.

Lesson 2.3 Review

 Complete the *Map Your Reading* graphic organizer for the section you just read.

1. You hear the emergency code for an active shooter. You are in a patient's room. What should you do? (2.3-1)
   A. Check the hall and call for help.
   B. Lock the door, cover the window, and text for help.
   C. Find a weapon to attack the shooter.
   D. Put your patient in a wheelchair and run for the nearest exit.

2. What is the correct order of steps for using a fire extinguisher? (2.3-2)
   A. Aim at the flame, squeeze, pull the pin, and sweep
   B. Squeeze, sweep, aim at the flame, and pull the pin
   C. Pull the pin, aim at the flame, squeeze, and sweep
   D. Sweep, pull the pin, aim at the flame, and squeeze

3. Which of the following is safe for use around oxygen equipment? (2.3-3)
   A. Polyester blankets
   B. Electric razors
   C. Lighters
   D. Cotton clothing

4. GFCI outlets (2.3-4)
   A. should not be used in patient rooms
   B. allow additional devices to be plugged in safely beyond the capacity of the circuit
   C. provides grounding to prevent electrical shock
   D. require special training

5. Which of the following is true of select agents? (2.3-5)
   A. They are strictly regulated.
   B. They are biological weapons.
   C. They have readily available treatments.
   D. They cannot be managed safely.

Chapter 2 Review and Assessment

Chapter Summary

2.1-1 Environmental safety is a priority for healthcare workers. Ergonomics can help reduce repetitive motion injuries and eyestrain. Following safety guidelines can help prevent falls and injuries.

2.1-2 Safety Data Sheets (SDS) must be readily available to provide information about hazardous chemicals. Radiologic technicians must monitor the amount of radiation they and their patients receive. Procedures for handling potentially violent situations can also prevent injuries.

2.1-3 Good body mechanics and posture can help healthcare workers avoid injuries during lifting and moving. Follow safety precautions when transferring and ambulating patients. Safe food handling and hygiene procedures reduce foodborne illness.

2.2-1 Microorganisms can be aerobic or anaerobic, pathogenic or not. Six broad types of pathogens are bacteria, viruses, fungi, protozoa, helminths, and rickettsiae. Some healthcare-associated infections have developed resistance to standard antibiotics.

2.2-2 The chain of infection outlines the steps by which pathogens spread to cause infection. Breaking any one link can stop the pathogen.

2.2-3 Standard precautions, including handwashing and wearing required personal protective equipment (PPE), are used with all patients at all times and in all settings to prevent or interrupt the chain of infection.

2.2-4 Transmission-based precautions are used depending on how an infection is transmitted: through contact, droplets, or airborne.

2.2-5 Occupational exposure to bloodborne pathogens is a risk in healthcare. Your employer must have an exposure control plan for situations that could endanger workers or the public.

2.2-6 Aseptic techniques maintain a clean environment to prevent healthcare-associated infections. Sanitization lowers the number of bacteria; disinfection kills pathogens. Antisepsis creates a sterile environment for procedures such as surgery.

2.3-1 Healthcare institutions need to be prepared for emergencies, which includes having an emergency action plan, assigned escape and shelter locations, and regular practice with emergency scenarios.

2.3-2 Removing one of the three elements of the fire triangle—fuel, heat source, or oxygen—can put out a fire. It is important to use the correct type of fire extinguisher for the type of fire.

2.3-3 Safety around oxygen equipment is important because of the potential fire hazard. Avoid any source of static, sparks, or flames. Post "No Smoking" signs.

2.3-4 Proper grounding, maintenance, and use of electrical equipment can help prevent electrical fires.

2.3-5 The federal government tries to prevent bioterrorism by carefully controlling access to and use of select agents.

Maximize Your Professional Vocabulary

1. **Connecting Terms.** Write terms on a sheet of paper or in a document. Draw lines between terms you think are connected or closely related to each other. Explain to a partner or the class why or how you think the terms are connected.

Reflect on Your Reading

1. Review your visual summary from the *Map Your Reading* activity at the beginning of this chapter. Can you describe the broad reach of safety issues in healthcare? What types of issues affect different work environments? Who is responsible for creating a safe healthcare environment? Try to use your new professional vocabulary as you support your points.

Review and Recall

1. Which of the following is an appropriate way to ensure the safety of patients who cannot walk independently? (2.1-1)
   A. Hide their shoes so they must have you help
   B. Leave their cane ready by the door
   C. Make sure they can reach their call bell without getting up
   D. Leave a lift device in their room

2. After drawing a blood sample, a lab worker breaks the tube. They should (2.1-2)
   A. post a "wet floor" sign, call housekeeping, and continue working
   B. alert others to avoid the area, put on gloves, wipe up the spill, disinfect the area, and complete an incident report
   C. evacuate the area, wait until the liquid has dried, pick up the glass, then use a bleach solution to clean the floor
   D. report the incident to a supervisor and ask them to take care of it.

3. Which of the following will *not* protect you from injury? (2.1-3)
   A. Sitting upright with your arms supported when typing
   B. Taking frequent breaks to rest your eyes and stretch
   C. Pulling heavy loads rather than lifting
   D. Limiting unnecessary movement in your workspace

Match the types of pathogens with the illnesses they cause (4–7). (2.2-1)

A. bacteria   4. Malaria
B. virus   5. Vaginal yeast infection
C. fungi   6. Strep throat
D. parasite   7. Hepatitis

Match the links in the chain of infection with their definitions. (8–12) (2.2-2)

A. Mode of transmission   8. The pathogen that causes infection
B. Reservoir   9. Place where the pathogen lives
C. Infectious agent   10. How the pathogen leaves the place it lives
D. Portal of entry   11. How the pathogen travels
E. Portal of exit   12. How the pathogen enters a susceptible host

13. What is the correct order for removing PPE? (2.2-3)
    A. Gloves, goggles, gown, mask
    B. Gown, gloves, goggles, mask
    C. Mask, gloves, gown, goggles
    D. Goggles, mask, gown, gloves

14. A patient in your care is sneezing and has a runny nose. Which precautions are most appropriate? Choose all that apply. (2.2-4)
    A. Standard precautions
    B. Contact precautions, including a gown
    C. Droplet precautions, including a surgical mask
    D. Airborne precautions, including an N95 respirator mask

15. To reduce the risk of exposure to bloodborne pathogens, employers must (2.2-5)
    A. instruct employees to purchase PPE
    B. use devices to increase risk for needlesticks
    C. offer HBV vaccination
    D. not allow employees to handle specimens

16. What level of asepsis can be achieved with a bleach solution? (2.2-6)
    A. Sanitization
    B. Disinfection
    C. Sterilization

17. How do active shooter and natural disaster responses differ? (2.3-1)
    A. You may need to lock yourself in, rather than evacuating, for an active shooter.
    B. You are more able to prepare for a natural disaster.
    C. You have a more active role helping patients with an active shooter.
    D. You can do more to prevent a natural disaster.

18. Which of the following is an appropriate response to an electrical fire? (2.3-2)
    A. First, pull the fire alarm.
    B. Select a type K fire extinguisher.
    C. Let the sprinkler system put out the flames.
    D. Shut off power to the electrical equipment fueling the fire.

19. Which of the following is a fire hazard when your patient is on oxygen? (2.3-3)
    A. An open window
    B. Cigarette butts in the waste basket
    C. Cotton blankets on the bed
    D. A longer oxygen tube to allow more movement

20. Which of the following are electrical safety hazards? Choose all that apply. (2.3-4)
    A. Equipment blocking access to the electrical breaker box
    B. Frayed cord on electrical equipment
    C. Five-mA device plugged in a 15-mA circuit
    D. GFCI outlet next to a sink

21. Which of the following helps prevent bioterrorism? (2.3-5)
    A. Select agents
    B. Nanotechnology
    C. OBA regulations
    D. EPA regulations

Build Core Skills

1. **Writing.** Refer to the section titled *Types of Pathogens* in Lesson 2.2. Select one and research a disease caused by this type of pathogen. Create a chart with the headings *Pathogen type*, *Name of pathogen*, *Signs/Symptoms of infection*, and *Treatment*. Share your results with the class to build a table of infectious diseases.

2. **Problem Solving.** How can healthcare workers help interrupt the chain of infection? In your own words, describe the chain of infection and the steps that can be taken at each point to prevent the occurrence of infection.

3. **Math.** The CDC's HAI prevalence survey in 2018 found that approximately 1 in 25 hospital patients in any given day had an HAI. If a hospital was the size of your school, how many patients would have an HAI today?

4. **Critical Thinking.** Create a Venn diagram to compare and contrast standard precautions and transmission-based precautions. When are transmission-based precautions necessary?

What can they achieve that standard precautions cannot?

5. **Reading.** Find an SDS sheet at school, work, or online. Take notes on the risks and safety measures listed. Compare your findings with the class. Which was the most hazardous substance?

6. **Speaking and Listening.** Work with a partner. Take turns listing and explaining lab safety rules. How many can you describe?

7. **Problem Solving.** Imagine that you work in a hospital kitchen. While moving a pot of boiling soup off the gas stove, you drop a towel on the burner, and it catches fire. By the time you can set down the soup without scalding yourself, the blaze is a foot high. What should you do?

8. **Critical Thinking.** Identify a healthcare-related need for each of the different types of fire extinguishers.

9. **Writing.** You work in occupational therapy. You were asked to do a brief demonstration on proper body mechanics for lifting and transporting patients. Create an outline for key points to include in your slide presentation.

Activate Your Learning

1. You will be most prepared to help a person who becomes weak and is falling if you have practiced the procedure. Ask a nurse or physical therapist to demonstrate, then practice the procedure in a safe location, such as a gym with wrestling mats on the floor.

2. Pair with another student to practice the handwashing skill in Figure 2.26. Watch your partner's washing procedure and provide feedback, and vice versa. You can spread glitter glue on your hands as the "dirt" before you begin washing. You will be able to see the glitter in areas that are not cleaned well enough.

3. Review the steps for completing terminal cleaning of the patient environment. Assemble the necessary supplies and practice this procedure.

4. Watch a demonstration or video of cleaning and sterilizing lab equipment. Assemble the necessary supplies and practice wrapping equipment for autoclaving.

5. Search for biohazard symbols in the school setting. What biohazards exist? Where are they located? What precautions are used to prevent exposure?

6. Place a small candle on a fire-proof surface, such as a glass plate. Light the candle. Which leg of the fire triangle is removed in each of these tests? 1) Place a glass cup over the candle: What happens? Why? 2) Use a square of tinfoil with a slit to the center. Place the candle wick through the slit and move it up and down: What happens? Why? 3) Sprinkle water over the flame: What happens? Why?

7. Ask your local fire department to demonstrate proper use of a fire extinguisher. If allowed, practice the PASS procedure so you can experience using a fire extinguisher.

Think and Act Like a Healthcare Worker

1. Suppose you work as a radiologic technician in an emergency room. A trauma patient is brought in after a car accident and requires X-rays before going into surgery. You can see a broken rib protruding from the chest, and the patient is coughing up blood. What special precautions will you take for both your safety and the patient's?

2. Imagine you work in a busy emergency room. A patient's husband is frustrated that his wife has not yet been seen for an injury to her arm. He is agitated and aggressive. What should you do? Role-play with a partner or small group.

3. A supervisor is training staff on new oxygen and electrical equipment. What precautions should be included? What are the risks to health and safety if they are not followed?

Go to the Source

1. Locate the safety stickers for a piece of equipment that would be used for patient care. List three key points from the sticker in your own words and tell why they are important.

2. Visit the CDC website to read about the differences between surgical masks and respirator masks. Search the CDC website for relevant articles and other information on this topic. Then write a brief essay explaining the differences between masks and respirators and why respirator masks are required in some healthcare settings.

3. Watch the "STOP STICKS" video on the CDC website or interview a healthcare worker who handles sharps as part of the job. What are the potential consequences for a healthcare worker who is stuck by sharps on the job?

4. Check your nurse's office or search online for one of the CDC's "Get Smart" posters. Summarize the main message of the poster. Explain how the poster's topic relates to the information in this chapter.

HOSA Event Prep: CERT Skills

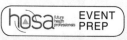

Dan and his friend took the free CERT training his town offered last spring. During training, they learned basic first aid and CPR, fire safety, search-and-rescue techniques, and teamwork. Those who successfully completed the training were placed on a call list if they chose and had quarterly drills. One night in the summer, the phone rang, calling all CERT team members to Main Street, where there had been an Amtrak passenger train derailment. Dan and his friend quickly got to the scene. As they performed search and rescue, they found and safely rescued a mom and her child. Because the community had a CERT team of volunteers, many lives were saved that night.

Test Your Knowledge

1. Which of the following are CERT team members *not* trained for?
   A. Basic first aid
   B. CPR
   C. Rescue from a burning building
   D. Search and rescue

2. Which of the following factors could be safety risks for this train derailment?
   A. They could freeze to death.
   B. The train was carrying hazardous materials.
   C. They could trip on uneven terrain along the tracks at night.
   D. The people they are rescuing could be armed and dangerous.

3. What information would be useful for this CERT team? Choose all that apply.
   A. How many people they are looking for
   B. What resources or tools they have available to help
   C. What the search plan is
   D. What hazards are present

Unit 2 Career Knowledge and Skills for Health Science

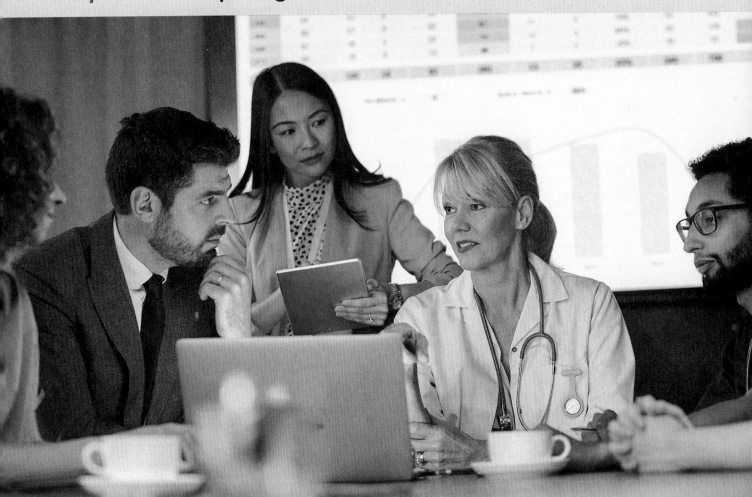

Healthcare Insider

Nathan Drendel, M.S., R.D., L.D., ProMedica's Wellness Dietitian

When people hear I'm a dietitian, they always think I'm in the hospital telling people what to eat. In reality, I have such an amazingly unique job that it's hard to explain. Being a Wellness Dietitian means I get to test recipes and try to improve them, but also film cooking and educational videos and provide educational lectures. I'm able to counsel individuals to help them

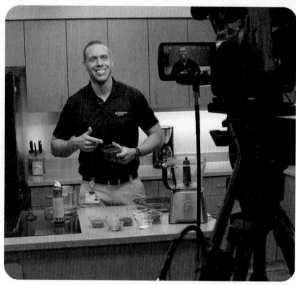

Courtesy of ProMedica

achieve their nutritional and wellness goals. My workdays are never the same, which is just another perk of my job. Being in the role of a "proactive dietitian" rather than a "reactive dietitian" means I get to help people prevent nutritional issues before they progress to serious health issues.

Discussion Activity

Nathan is excited to have a unique job. He films videos, gives lectures, and counsels patients. It is the variety in his job that makes it interesting for him. Discuss the following questions:

1. What will make your future career interesting?
2. Do you prefer to have a fixed schedule and know what your workday will bring, or does facing something new each day appeal to you?

Chapter 3
Health Science Career Preparation

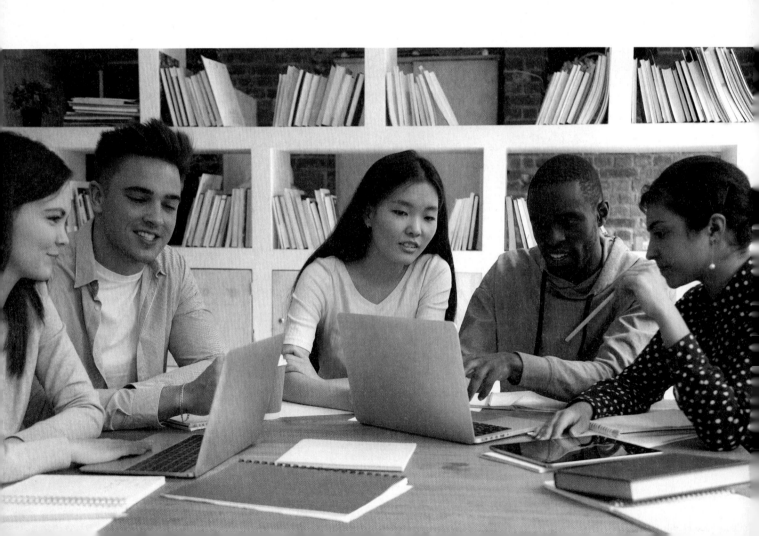

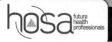

HOSA Event Prep: Family Medicine Physician

To become a physician is no small task. It requires eight years of postsecondary education and then four or more years of residency before you can practice on your own. While this can seem like many years, the outcome of being a physician is very rewarding. While many health science students dream of being a specialist, such as a cardiologist or neurosurgeon, one of the most important and overlooked physicians is the family physician. Family physicians provide care for all ages. They provide everyday healthcare and prevention. They may also manage their patients' overall health by coordinating with various specialists. There is a growing shortage of family physicians, so the American Academy of Family Physicians has teamed up with HOSA—Future Health Professionals to create a *Family Medicine Physician* event. This event aims to increase the number of new medical students going into family medicine.

Go to the HOSA website to learn more about the HOSA *Family Medicine Physician* event. Find out the purpose of the event, what is involved in the event, and what knowledge is demonstrated in the event.

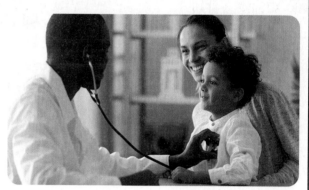

As you prepare for HOSA competitive events, be sure to check the website and talk with your HOSA advisor for the most up-to-date guidelines and procedures. Once you have learned about the *Family Medicine Physician* event, answer the following questions:

1. How might participating in this event benefit you personally and your future career? Explain.
2. Are you interested in participating in this event? Why or why not?

fizkes/Shutterstock.com

 ## Connect with Your Reading

The costs of preparing for a career vary widely. As you investigate healthcare careers, you will consider the amount of education and training required for each career, but you should also consider the cost of education and training. So, what is the cost? For each item shown, give your best estimate or "guesstimate" of the cost. Compare your estimates with your classmates and revise your numbers if needed to make your best estimates.

Education and Training Costs	
Education/Training	**Your Cost Estimate**
Tuition and fees for one year of community/technical college	*Write in your estimate.*
Tuition and fees for one year at an in-state public university	*Write in your estimate.*
Tuition and fees for one year at a private university	*Write in your estimate.*
Room and board cost for one year of college	*Write in your estimate.*
Cost of the licensing exam for a registered nurse	*Write in your estimate.*

Goodheart-Willcox Publisher

 ## Map Your Reading

Create an eight-page foldable book using a single sheet of plain paper. Use the image provided or search for video directions online. Number each page, including the front and back covers. Write the chapter number and title on the cover of your book. Open your book and write the lesson title across the top of pages 2 and 3. Then write the headings for this lesson on these two pages. Read the lesson and summarize the main point from each heading using your own words. Flip the page and continue with the next lesson title in the same manner to the end of the chapter.

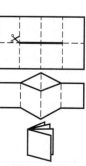

Chapter opener image: fizkes/Shutterstock.com

Goodheart-Willcox Publisher

Study Skills for Health Science Students

Learning Outcomes

After studying this lesson, you will be able to

3.1-1 explain strategies for improving reading comprehension.

3.1-2 describe how to use note-taking to organize and review information.

3.1-3 apply study strategies to learn and remember academic information.

Professional Vocabulary

Essential Terms

learning style   an individual's preferred way of gaining or processing new information

mnemonic device   a learning tool that helps students memorize information

Important Terms

auditory learners	kinesthetic learners	outline notes
Cornell style notes	mind maps	visual learners

Introduction

When studying health science, you may feel overwhelmed by the amount of reading required and the large amount of information you must learn. You can avoid this feeling by using specific strategies to improve your learning. These strategies will help you comprehend or understand the material and remember it. You will identify your learning style and practice a variety of study methods to better remember the information you are learning. Just as your body sorts the materials coming in and decides how to use them, your brain needs to sort information to digest everything you will learn in your health science courses.

3.1-1 Reading Strategies

Reading for information is different from reading for enjoyment. You must learn and recall important concepts and details. Use these steps to make your reading more meaningful.

Survey

Begin by surveying the reading material. What is its source, and why are you reading it? Skim the chapter title, headings, and subtitles. What is the main topic? How is the text organized? How much time will you need to read and understand this information? Are there natural divisions so you can break the reading into manageable segments?

Preview

Next, preview the introduction and summary sections for a shortened version of what you will be reading. What do you already know about this topic? What do you expect to read about in each of the sections? What questions do you have? How will the figures and vocabulary terms be important to understanding this topic? Your preview will help you organize your thoughts before you read and take notes (**Figure 3.1**).

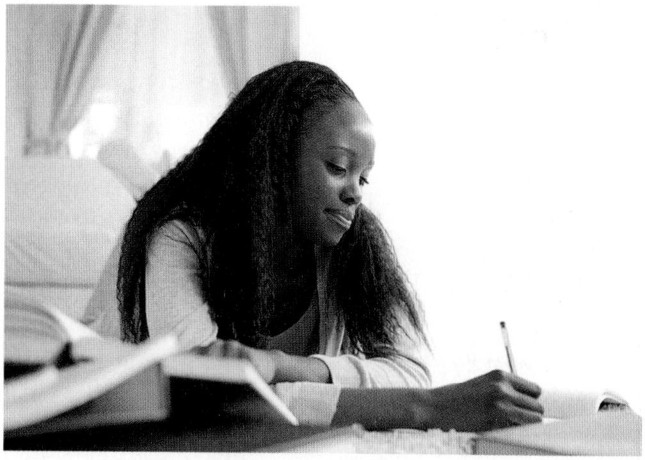

Identify Main Ideas

After your preview, set your brain up to look for information as you read. Turn the title of each section of material into a question. As you read, look for information to help you answer that question. This process sets a purpose for your reading. It helps you find the main ideas. For example, this section is titled *Reading Strategies*. You might ask yourself, "What skills will help me read more efficiently?" The details that answer this question are what you should highlight or include in your notes. Ask yourself who, what, when, where, why, or how for each heading before you begin to read. Once you have set the purpose by developing a question, you are ready to begin reading the text content. Pay special attention to the topics that appear in both the text and your teacher's lecture. Listen for the ideas your teacher emphasizes or spends the most time on in class. Note what they write on the board or hand out in class. These are the main ideas to highlight or write in your notes.

Highlight Important Information as You Read

It will be helpful to mark your text as you read (**Figure 3.2**). Write in the margins of the book (if allowed) or use sticky notes that can be removed. Ebooks generally have a note-taking feature that allows you to virtually mark up the text. Write down the question you created as you set your purpose for reading. Check the pictures and figures for more information that explains the topic. As you read, allow yourself to ask more questions about the material and look for connections to things you already know. Make short notes of these questions and connections. Highlight or bookmark text passages that you find helpful or important.

Your highlighting will be more effective if you use a contrasting color to mark the main idea and key terms. Use a different-colored highlighter or underlining for supporting details. If you stay focused on the most important points, less than one-third of your page should be marked up when you are done.

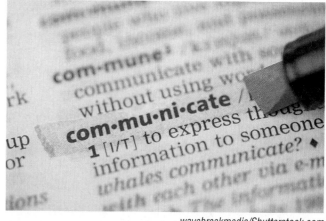

©iStock/MBI

Figure 3.1 Surveying and previewing the material you are about to read can help you prepare to take notes on the reading.

wavebreakmedia/Shutterstock.com

Figure 3.2 If it is allowed, highlighting important terms in your text can help you better remember them. Use sticky notes if you are not supposed to write in your text.

3.1-2 Note-Taking

Next, you should organize your information in a meaningful way. There are many styles for organizing your thoughts. Be sure to write all information in your own words rather than copying straight from the text. Converting the information into your own words will help you develop your understanding of the new information and remember it (**Figure 3.3**).

OUTLINE NOTES

1. Organized
   A. Hierarchy
      i. Big ideas to left
      ii. Smaller ideas indented
         a. dash/bullet
         b. number/letter
   B. Follows textbook format well
      i. Use heading size as clue
      ii. Follows in order
      iii. Details from reading
   C. Teacher may provide outline format for lecture
      i. Copy format from board or overhead
      ii. Add details by listening
         a. Word signals—"there are two ways..."
         b. Examples
      iii. Need to keep up
   D. Easy to share/Get notes from a friend
2. Use
   A. Phrases—not complete sentences
   B. Own words
   C. Key words and facts
3. Leave space between topics
   A. Review in text/lecture/study time and add more info
   B. May come back to ideas again in lecture

Outline Style Notes

Class Notes/Textbook Notes

Name: _____
Class: _____
Period/Block: _____
Date: _____

Topic: _____

Questions/Main Ideas	Notes

Summary, Reflection, Analysis

Cornell Style Notes

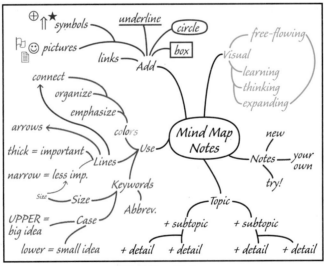

Mind Map Notes

Goodheart-Willcox Publisher

Figure 3.3 Depending on how you learn best, one of these styles of note-taking might help you learn and study. *Which of these styles would you be most likely to use?*

Note-Taking Styles

Following are some note-taking styles you can use.

- **Outline notes**. Notes taken in an outline format are easy if you use the headings from the chapter. However, you may end up with a list of details you do not understand if you are not reading the information as you outline. Stop after reading each section and restate the main idea aloud before adding it to your notes.
- **Cornell style notes**. The two-column, or *Cornell*, style is good for merging notes from more than one source and reviewing information. In this style, you list the main ideas and supporting details from the lecture or text on the right side of a page and use the left side to note prior knowledge, additional information from the lecture, remaining questions, or memory cues. Leave a blank line between topics.
- **Mind maps**. Mind maps, or *web notes*, use color, symbols, arrows, size, and other visual connections to show how ideas are related. They do not use many words. If a visual image for your mind map does not exist, create one! Your mind map should group information into manageable chunks and relate the categories of information to each other. This style of note-taking helps organize information so you can make meaningful connections.

Using Your Notes

No matter what style of note-taking you use, your brain needs review time to process and absorb the new information. If you took notes during a lecture, go back to your text and compare the information. If you took notes from your text, notice how the teacher's lecture and activities organize and connect the same ideas in a new way. It may be helpful to guess potential test questions from the main headings of your text, then attempt to answer the questions from memory and check against your notes. Put the information into your own words or explain it to someone else. This will help you sort through it and build your own understanding. Add notes about connections you see between this topic and other classes, your personal life, the news, and other reading material. New information is easier to remember when you make it personal.

Review your notes in small chunks on a regular basis. A few short review sessions are better for learning than one long cram session. Walking into a test (or doing a medical procedure) when you are tired and your brain is overloaded will not lead to long-term memory or success. Review notes or practice with flash cards or a smartphone app for a few minutes several times a day—on the bus, waiting in line, or during commercials. The more times you reread the information, the more easily you will recall it later. Put the information in your own words and repeat it aloud before you put the notes away. These short practice sessions will build both understanding and memory.

Digesting your reading in this manner is the most efficient way to absorb new information. Stopping to process information in small segments prevents your mind from straying or becoming overwhelmed. Previewing and questioning will help you pay attention to the most important information. Taking notes in your own words will help you actively process the information. Summarizing and reviewing that information will make sure it remains in your memory. Try these techniques as you read the remainder of this chapter.

3.1-3 Learning and Assessment of New Information

There is a lot of information to remember when you are learning health science content. Paying attention to the way you learn can help you better understand this new information.

Adapting to Your Learning Style

Your **learning style** guides the way you take in, store, and recall information. Recognizing and understanding your own learning style helps you use the study method that is best for you.

The way you prefer to take in information determines your learning style. **Visual learners** prefer pictures and have a good understanding of direction, spacing, and location. A visual-linguistic learner likes to see written words through reading and writing tasks. A visual-spatial learner may have a hard time with written activities but does better with charts, demonstrations, and videos. **Auditory learners** use sounds, rhythm, and music to store and recall information. They usually remember spoken words the best. **Kinesthetic learners** use their body, hands, and sense of touch to learn. Movement and touch help them pay attention (**Figure 3.4**).

Do you recognize your preferred learning style from these descriptions? Check your school's online guidance program and look for a learning style assessment to give you more information about your preferences. Although you will naturally use your preferred method of learning most often, you can practice using and building the skills for all these styles. The more tools you have for learning and recalling information, the better off you are.

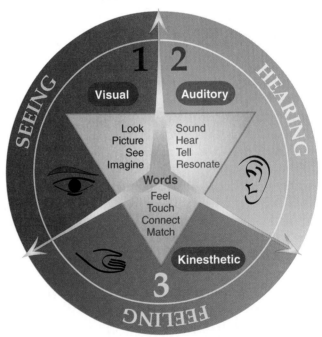

artellia/Shutterstock.com

Figure 3.4 Learning style identifies the ways you prefer to take in information. *Do you recognize your preferred learning style from these descriptions?*

Some classes do not appeal to all types of learners. What should you do when your learning style does not match the instructor's teaching style? You can make some changes to tailor information to your learning style:

- **Map a lecture.** If it is hard for you to pay attention to a lecture, try taking outline notes or creating a mind map of the information (**Figure 3.5**). Use symbols and pictures to represent the details. Visual learners benefit from seeing the words or pictures in this method, while kinesthetic learners benefit from the hands-on activity of doing the writing.

- **Request an outline.** If you get lost in the details of a lecture, ask for a brief outline before the lecture begins. If you are an auditory learner, you might record the lecture to review with your notes after class.

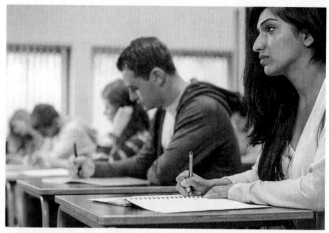

Figure 3.5 Creating visual notes such as an outline or a mental map can help visual learners better recall information presented in class. *What are some study tips for auditory or kinesthetic learners?*

- **Find a picture or a video.** When wordy descriptions do not create a mental image for you, ask for a picture. Try searching for related video or image files on the internet as part of your review.

- **Create a model or diagram.** Building a model or drawing diagrams helps kinesthetic learners understand or remember new ideas.

- **Ask yourself questions.** Auditory learners can ask questions out loud to clarify or confirm their ideas.

- **Use a study group.** Form a study group as a fun support system. The practice of recalling and explaining new information to others is a great way to build your own memory and understanding.

Take the time to adapt your study habits to reflect your learning style. You may be surprised by the results. As you read this chapter, look for ways to connect with the content through your preferred style.

Studying New Vocabulary

It is nearly impossible to memorize all the medical terms you will hear in class or the workplace, but learning some common word parts will make it easier to understand the spoken and written terms used in patient care. It will also help you figure out the general meanings of body structures, diseases, and procedures.

People use a variety of methods to study and remember new terms. One common technique is to make and use flash cards. The time spent creating and reviewing the cards is what makes this technique work, so develop games or a schedule to use them often.

Some people play with the way a word looks to remember its meaning. For example, *parallel* means *equal,* and the *ll* in the middle of the word looks like a sideways equal sign. When studying a term, try drawing or reshaping the letters creatively.

Another technique is to look for familiar words that share the same word part, such as *ortho*dontists who straighten teeth and *ortho*pedists who straighten bones. You can use this strategy with everyday English words too.

Some students like to investigate the origins of a new word. For example, *hypochondriac* [*hypo* = below, *chondr* = cartilage, *ac* = pertaining to] literally means "pertaining to the area below the cartilage." However, in medical usage, it means "below the ribs" because some ribs are attached by cartilage. The term *hypochondriac* may also describe people who always think they are ill. Interestingly, many people hold the area under the ribs when complaining they do not feel well.

This text breaks medical terms down into their Latin and Greek origins to help you understand their meanings. You will study these word parts in the anatomy chapters. In addition, use the other techniques described in this lesson to expand your medical vocabulary.

Using Mnemonic Devices

Mnemonic (nih-MAH-nihk) **devices** often seem silly, but they create powerful connections in our memories. Different areas of the brain store sounds, colors, smells, tastes, touch, and emotions. Vividly connecting information with many senses makes it easier to recall the information later. Use these suggestions for creating your own mnemonic devices:

- Make up acronyms to remember the parts of a concept or procedure. For example, the acronym *SOMBER* can remind you of the symptoms of depression: *S*adness, *O*verwhelmed, *M*emory issues, *B*ehavioral changes, *E*ating changes, and *R*estlessness.
- Use the spelling sequence of a word to remember the order of items in a list. For instance, *SOAP* describes the steps for recording narrative progress notes: *S*urvey/Subjective, *O*bservation/Objective, *A*ssessment, and *P*lanning.
- Use rhythm and rhyming to recall information. For example, "*i* before *e* except after *c*" reminds you of a basic spelling rule. You can also create lyrics from information and set them to a familiar tune or make up one of your own.
- Play the sound of the word you are learning off the sound of a word you already know. For instance, the word part *later*, which means *side*, sounds like *ladder*. To remember this term, you can imagine climbing up the side of a ladder.
- Use vivid or unusual images to recall new terms. Try imagining a deck of playing cards for the term *cardi*. This means "heart," so you might see yourself holding a handful of pulsing, bloody hearts during your card game. The more vivid and unusual the image, the better.
- Exaggerate the size of important parts of an image. For example, a motor homunculus (hoh-MUHN-kyuh-luhs) [*homin* = human, *ule* = small, *us* = structure] is an exaggerated drawing used to help you recall how much area in the brain is required for muscle control of the different parts of the body (**Figure 3.6**). The motor homunculus has a very large tongue, lips, eyes, and hands to show that these parts use a larger area of the brain for motor control than the legs or nose. You can create an exaggerated image like the homunculus for whichever term you are trying to learn.

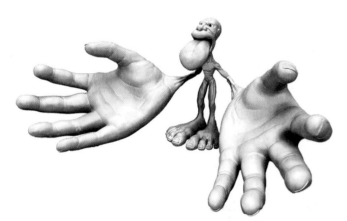

Courtesy of Bandha Yoga Publications

Figure 3.6 You can exaggerate important aspects of a term or image to better remember it. *Which term in this chapter could you memorize by creating an exaggerated visual representation?*

- Create a short scene with dramatic voices and actions for the information you are trying to remember, then practice acting it out. You will remember that the "brachial region" is on your arm if you hold your arm and say in a childish voice, "I breaky my arm!"
- Use humor, especially if it is shocking. This can make things very hard to forget. For example, you might think of the interesting contrast between *cleave*, which means "to cut or split apart," and *cleavage*, which is created by pressing the breasts together.

The more strongly you can picture what you are trying to learn and associate it with something you already know, the more easily you will recall it later. Make your learning more memorable by using all of your senses as you study.

Preparing for Tests

Focus on test-taking skills to change the way you study and improve your test scores. When you get a test back, keep a log of the errors you have made. Study your incorrect answers to find your most common errors. Then practice your test-taking skills. Ask your teacher for a practice test or use your notes to create test questions.

In addition to relearning the concepts you missed, look for problems with your test-taking skills. Watch for these common errors:

- misreading the question
- focusing on the wrong information in the question
- failing to study the correct information

Most tests have several multiple-choice questions. The answers contain distractors that try to take your attention away from the correct answer. Try to answer a multiple-choice question in your head before looking at the answer options. However, read the entire question and all the choices before marking your answer. Use the process of elimination to narrow your options. Begin by looking for the answer that is least correct. It will often be the opposite of the correct response. Next, look for the answer that sounds correct, but does not actually answer the question being asked. Finally, look for the answer that is partially correct, but is either incorrect for this situation or not true in every situation. The remaining answer should be the correct response (**Figure 3.7**).

1. Which statement gives the best description of learning styles?
   A. Learning styles teach everyone the same methods for acquiring information.
   B. Many teachers use learning-style theory to design classroom activities.
   C. Learning styles can be grouped according to the way you prefer to take in information.
   D. Auditory learners always use their sense of hearing to take in and recall information.

Goodheart-Willcox Publisher

Figure 3.7 Use the process of elimination to select the correct multiple-choice answer. *Can you identify the least correct and partially correct answers, as well as the one that does not answer the question?*

When you take a test, start by previewing the entire test to decide how much time to spend on each section. Make notes about formulas or information you will need to use. Start with the easiest or most familiar questions. Then work on the more difficult questions. Use all of the test time your teacher allows, rechecking difficult questions after you have completed the test.

If you have chosen the right career path, you should enjoy the content of most of your classes. That does not mean your classes will all be easy, but the effort you put into them will be worthwhile. Use your reading and note-taking strategies, learning style study methods, mnemonic memory devices, and test-taking skills to help you through the challenging times.

Lesson 3.1 Review

 Complete the *Map Your Reading* graphic organizer for the section you just read.

1. When reading, you should (3.1-1)
   A. diagram the material, then organize the introduction and summary sections
   B. survey the material, then preview the introduction and summary sections
   C. organize the material, then survey the introduction and summary sections
   D. preview the material, then diagram the introduction and summary sections

2. Before you take notes, identify the main idea by (3.1-2)
   A. turning the title of each section into a question
   B. guessing what you think the idea is
   C. highlighting key terms and their definitions
   D. None of these.

3. Taking notes using _____ helps you understand and remember the information. (3.1-2)
   A. text language
   B. your own words
   C. words you do not know
   D. other people's words

4. Identifying your _____ helps you understand how you take in, process, and store new information. (3.1-3)
   A. reading style
   B. learning style
   C. reacting style
   D. mind style

5. _____ devices can help students remember and organize new information. (3.1-3)
   A. Mechanical
   B. Pneumonic
   C. Mnemonic
   D. Abbreviation

6. Vividly connecting information with unusual _____ makes it easier to recall information later. (3.1-3)
   A. images
   B. people
   C. objects
   D. ideas

Career Pathways and Employment Opportunities

Learning Outcomes

After studying this lesson, you will be able to

3.2-1 analyze the five pathways found in the health science career cluster.

3.2-2 describe a credentialed healthcare worker.

3.2-3 illustrate the career ladder approach to education.

Professional Vocabulary

Essential Terms

accreditation official recognition from a professional association that an educational program meets minimum educational standards for an occupation

career clusters groups of similar occupations and industries that share a core set of basic knowledge and skills for all workers

career ladder a sequence of job positions progressing from entry-level to higher levels of responsibility and authority based on education, experience, and performance

career pathways smaller groups of specialized occupations within a career cluster that require more specific sets of knowledge, skills, and training

credentials documents proving a person's qualifications for a particular occupation

Important Terms

Biotechnology Research and Development

Diagnostic Services

Health Informatics Services

postsecondary education

Support Services

Therapeutic Services

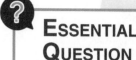

ESSENTIAL QUESTION

What career pathways and employment opportunities are available in health science?

Introduction

How will you find your future career in healthcare? While the path to your career is not always a direct route, your journey begins by learning about as many opportunities as you possibly can. National organizations that focus on career and technical education have developed a system for organizing all of the identified jobs and careers that exist today. The result is 16 groups called **career clusters** (**Figure 3.8**). You will begin your search by looking at these clusters and learning general information about the education, training, and credentials used for healthcare careers.

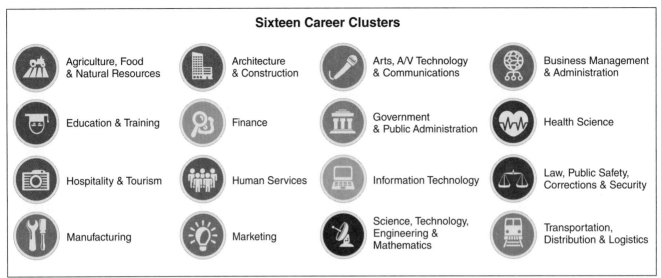

Sixteen Career Clusters

Agriculture, Food & Natural Resources

Architecture & Construction

Arts, A/V Technology & Communications

Business Management & Administration

Education & Training

Finance

Government & Public Administration

Health Science

Hospitality & Tourism

Human Services

Information Technology

Law, Public Safety, Corrections & Security

Manufacturing

Marketing

Science, Technology, Engineering & Mathematics

Transportation, Distribution & Logistics

Icons: Lisses/Shutterstock.com

Figure 3.8 All occupations in the US workforce are addressed within these 16 career clusters. This text will discuss many possible careers within the health science cluster. *How many occupations can you name that are part of the health science career cluster?*

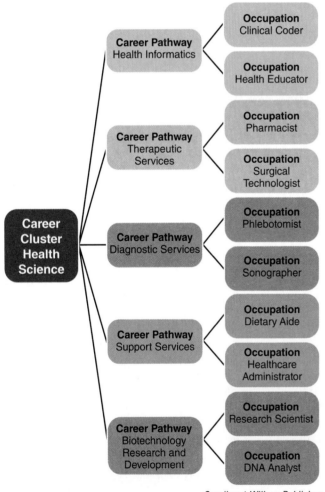

Goodheart-Willcox Publisher

Figure 3.9 This flowchart shows different healthcare occupations organized by cluster and pathway.

3.2-1 Career Clusters and Pathways

Each career cluster contains a specific group of occupations and industries based on the similar knowledge and skills they require. High schools and colleges use the clusters to develop courses that will prepare students for career success. You will use the career clusters to discover your personal interests and preferences. The clusters can help you choose an occupational area that will lead you toward a satisfying career.

Within each career cluster, you will find individual pathways (**Figure 3.9**). A **career pathway** includes a smaller set of specialized occupations. Each career cluster has a core set of basic knowledge and skills used by all workers in that cluster. Each pathway contains a more specific set of knowledge, skills, and training that will build on the cluster's core knowledge.

Understanding Health Science Career Pathways

To understand the wide variety of available healthcare careers, you will want to explore the entire health science cluster.

The health science career cluster includes five distinct career pathways:

- **Health Informatics Services**—occupations focused on documenting patient care, as well as managing healthcare data and information.
- **Therapeutic** (thair-uh-PYU-tihk) **Services**—occupations that change the health status of a patient over time. These careers provide direct care for people.
- **Diagnostic Services**—occupations that create a picture of a patient's health status at a single point in time. These careers provide diagnostic imaging and testing.
- **Support Services**—occupations that create a therapeutic environment for providing patient care. These careers support healthcare and wellness.
- **Biotechnology Research and Development**—occupations involved in bioscience research and the development of treatments and devices that improve human health.

More than 300 different occupations are spread out over these five pathways. Sometimes the tasks of a particular occupation fall into more than one pathway. Consider the physician who both diagnoses (diagnostic pathway) and treats (therapeutic pathway) an illness.

As you study health science careers and learn core health science content, consider how workers across the five health science career pathways use the information (**Figure 3.10**).

Employment Opportunities

The Bureau of Labor Statistics (BLS) is a national agency that tracks statistical data about occupations and industries in the United States. The BLS predicts that healthcare occupations will grow 16 percent from 2020 to 2030, adding about 2.6 million new jobs. In fact, healthcare and social assistance occupations are projected to add more jobs than any other occupational group. Home health aides and personal care attendants will have more job openings from growth than any other occupation.

Two factors that affect healthcare costs—an aging population and longer life expectancy—also drive the growth in healthcare employment. As the baby boomer generation ages, this large segment of the population will need additional healthcare services. The result is an increased need for healthcare workers.

Due to improved nutrition and healthcare, life expectancy for people in the United States has increased dramatically in the past century. People born in 1900 could expect to live an average of 49 years. People born just a hundred years later, in 2000, can expect to live an average of 77 years, and a person born in 2020 can expect to live 78.9 years. Longer lives mean a longer time to maintain health. Again, the result is an increased need for healthcare workers.

Career Education and Training

Jobs in healthcare require different levels of education and training. Some entry-level workers receive on-the-job training, but most jobs require education beyond a high school diploma. Education past high school is called **postsecondary education**. Community colleges, vocational or technical colleges, public and private universities, institutes of technology, and career colleges deliver this education.

Examples of Healthcare Occupations by Pathway

Career Pathway	Sample Career Specialties			
Therapeutic Services	Acupuncturist Art/Music/Dance Therapist(s) Athletic Trainer Audiologist Certified Nursing Assistant Chiropractor Dental Hygienist Dental Lab Technician Dentist	Dialysis Technician Dietitian/Nutritionist Dosimetrist Home Health Aide Licensed Practical Nurse Massage Therapist Medical Assistant Nurse Practitioner Occupational Therapist	Occupational Therapy Assistant Ophthalmic Technician Orthotist/Prosthetist Paramedic Pharmacist Pharmacy Technician Physical Therapist Physical Therapy Assistant Physician (MD/DO)	Physician Assistant Psychologist Psychiatrist Radiation Therapist Registered Nurse Respiratory Therapist Social Worker Speech Language Pathologist Surgical Technologist Veterinarian
Diagnostic Services	Audiologist Blood Bank Technician Cardiovascular Technologist Clinical Laboratory Technician Computed Tomography (CT) Technologist Cytogenetic Technologist Cytotechnologists	Diagnostic Medical Sonographer Electrocardiographic (ECG) Technician Neurodiagnostic Technologist Exercise Physiologist Genetic Counselor Histotechnician Histotechnologist Magnetic Resonance (MR) Technologist	Mammographer Medical Technologist/ Clinical Laboratory Scientist Nuclear Medicine Technologist Nurse Practitioner Nutritionist/Dietitian Occupational Therapist Ophthalmic Technician/ Technologist	Ophthalmic Dispensing Optician Optometrist Phlebotomist Physical Therapist Polysomnographic Technologist Positron Emission Tomography (PET) Technologist Radiologic Technician Respiratory Therapist
Health Informatics	Admitting Clerk Applied Researcher Cancer Registrar Certified Compliance Technician Clinical Account Manager Clinical Coder Clinical Data Miner Clinical Data Manager Clinical Data Specialist Data Quality Manager	Decision Support Analyst Epidemiologist Ethicist Health Educator Health Information Administrator Health Information Technician Healthcare Administrator Healthcare Finance Professional	Information Security Officer Managed Care Contract Analyst Medical Assistant Medical Illustrator Medical Librarian Medical Records Technician Patient Account Manager Patient Account Technician	Patient Advocate Patient Information Coordinator Quality Data Analyst Reimbursement Specialist Risk Manager Transcriptionist Unit Coordinator Utilization Review Manager
Support Services	Behavioral Disorder Counselor Biomedical/Clinical Engineer Biomedical/Clinical Technician Clinical Simulator Technician	Central Service Manager Central Service Technician Community Health Worker Dietary Manager Dietary Aide	Environmental Services Facilities Manager Healthcare Administrator Healthcare Economist Maintenance Engineer Industrial Hygienist Interpreter	Materials Manager Patient Navigator Telehealth Presenter Transport Technician Substance Abuse Counselor
Biotechnology Research and Development	Biochemist Bioinformatics Associate Bioinformatics Scientist Biomedical Chemist Biomedical/Clinical Engineer Biostatistician Cell Biologist Clinical Pharmacologist	Clinical Trials Monitor Clinical Trials Research Coordinator Geneticist Laboratory Assistant Laboratory Technician Medical Editor/Writer Microbiologist	Molecular Biologist Pharmaceutical/Clinical Project Manager Medical Sales Representative Pharmaceutical Scientist Pharmacologist Product Safety Associate/Scientist	Process Development Associate/Scientist Processing Technician Quality Control Technician Regulatory Affairs Specialist Research Assistant Research Scientist Toxicologist

Courtesy of NCHSE

Figure 3.10 Each health science career pathway contains many different career specialties.

When you enter a postsecondary training program, you will earn college credit for the courses you complete (**Figure 3.11**). A class that meets for three hours each week usually earns you three credits. While that sounds easy compared to high school, college programs expect students to complete about two hours of homework for every hour of class time. So, a full-time student taking 15 credits is expected to attend 15 hours of class time and complete 30 hours of homework, for a total of 45 hours per week. Clearly, knowing how to read efficiently and study independently is important for college success.

When choosing your college program, look for one that is accredited. **Accreditation** means the program has been approved by an agency that makes sure the program has quality standards and truly prepares its students for employment.

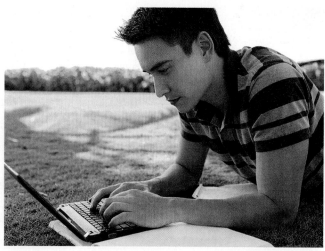

Figure 3.11 College students are expected to complete many hours of independent study.

Healthcare Professions: The Importance of Accreditation

Liam learned about the importance of accredited programs the hard way. He happily enrolled in the new nursing program at a local career college when he learned there was no waiting list. While the school cost more than the local technical college, Liam figured finishing faster would make the higher cost worthwhile.

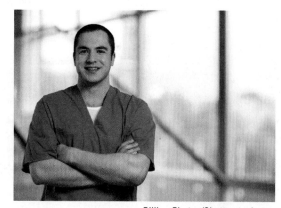

Billion Photos/Shutterstock.com

Everything went well until graduation, when Liam learned the school had applied for accreditation, but had not yet been approved by the accrediting agency. This meant that Liam and his fellow graduates were not eligible to take the national certification test and could not legally work as registered nurses.

Fortunately, this story has a happy ending. The school did receive accreditation within a few months. Liam passed the certification test and now works at a local hospital. Nevertheless, he had many anxious moments during those months after graduation. He wondered if he would ever be able to work as a registered nurse. Be sure to check that your chosen school or training program is accredited.

Postsecondary programs award different types of degrees based on the number of credits earned. The occupation you choose will determine the type of degree you need. For example, an occupational therapy assistant needs an associate's degree, but an occupational therapist must have a master's degree. Different schools offer different degrees. **Figure 3.12** shows the types of degrees healthcare workers can earn. **Figure 3.13** shows three medical professions and the level of education needed for each.

Postsecondary Program Degrees		
Length of Program	**Degree Awarded**	**Educational Institution**
Four or more additional years	Doctor of Philosophy (PhD)	University/graduate school
Two or more additional years	Master's degree (MS or MA)	University/graduate school
Four-year academic program	Bachelor's degree (BS or BA)	University/undergraduate school
Two-year technical program	Associate's degree	Community or technical college
One-year technical program	Diploma	Community or technical college
Less than one-year technical program	Certificate	Community or technical college
On-the-job training	None	None

Goodheart-Willcox Publisher

Figure 3.12 Postsecondary degrees vary in the lengths of programs, degrees awarded, and educational institutions offering them.

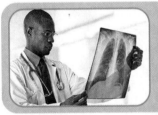

Medical Doctor—MD
Training Needed
- Completion of a bachelor's degree followed by four years of medical school
- Completion of three or more years of residency after medical school

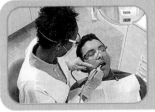

Dentist—DDS or DMD
Training Needed
- Completion of a bachelor's degree followed by four years of dental school
- Completion of an additional two to four years for a specialty

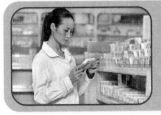

Pharmacist—PharmD
Training Needed
- Completion of an associate's degree or more commonly a bachelor's degree
- Completion of four years of pharmacy school

Top to bottom: Minerva Studio/Shutterstock.com, bikeriderlondon/Shutterstock.com, DmitryKalinovsky/Shutterstock.com

Figure 3.13 Medical doctors, dentists, and pharmacists all require different levels of training.

3.2-2 Job Titles and Credentials

Healthcare organizations want to hire credentialed workers. This means that, in addition to earning a degree, workers need to pass a special test that further proves they are skilled in performing the duties of a specific healthcare occupation. After passing such a test, workers have the credentials to perform the job for which they have been trained.

The terms *certification, licensure,* and *registration* all refer to a healthcare worker's **credentials**. While these terms have slightly different meanings, they all tell a future employer that a worker is qualified (**Figure 3.14**). Certification is awarded after a person has completed a course of study. Licensure is given after people pass a licensure exam that proves they meet the qualifications for a particular occupation. Registration refers to the official record of individuals who have passed an examination and are qualified to perform the tasks of a specific occupation.

The titles of healthcare jobs can often tell you the level of education and training required (**Figure 3.15**). Entry-level titles such as *aide* or *assistant* indicate occupations that require fewer years of training and education. Advanced titles such as *technologist* or *therapist* indicate the need for several years of training and education. As you determine how many years of training and education you want to pursue, you may want to compare the duties of an aide, technician, and therapist within an occupation such as physical therapy or medical lab careers.

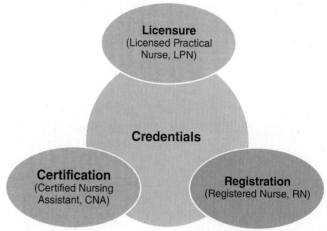

Goodheart-Willcox Publisher

Figure 3.14 These are the different types of credentials available and examples of healthcare occupations that require credentials. *Why are credentials important?*

Education and Training Requirements			
Job Title	**Education and Training**	**Examples**	**Exceptions**
Technologist or therapist	Bachelor's degree; often master's degree	Occupational therapist, medical lab technologist	Respiratory therapist, surgical technologist (both can be associate's-degree programs)
Technician	Associate's degree	Dental lab technician, biomedical technician	Pharmacy technician, healthcare technician (both require one year or less of education and training)
Aide or assistant	Diploma or certificate program requiring one year or less of education and training	Medical assistant, dental assistant, therapy aide	Occupational therapy assistant, physical therapy assistant (both are associate's-degree programs)

Goodheart-Willcox Publisher

Figure 3.15 A job title can tell you what level of education and training is needed for that job.

3.2-3 Career Ladders

Due to the rising cost of college, students are looking for ways to make postsecondary education more affordable. Many choose to use a **career ladder** approach to their education (**Figure 3.16**). A career ladder represents the progression of jobs within a specific occupation or particular work setting. The bottom of the ladder is the entry-level position that requires the least amount of training. As you move up the ladder, the job titles indicate increased education and training, as well as increased responsibility. Most jobs within the same occupation "piggyback" on each other. However, some jobs within the same work setting may have completely different education and training requirements.

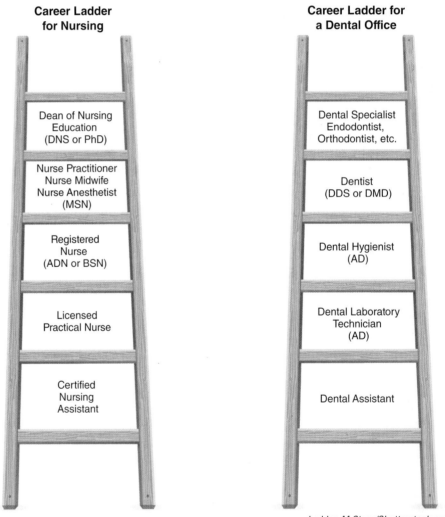

Ladder: M.Stasy/Shutterstock.com

Figure 3.16 Entry-level jobs appear at the bottom of the career ladder. As you "climb the ladder," additional education and training are required. Jobs within the same occupation "piggyback" on each other. For example, you need to have an RN license before training to become a nurse anesthetist. However, jobs within the same work setting may have completely different education and training requirements. For example, you do not have to train as a dental hygienist before studying to become a dentist.

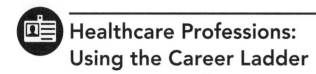

Healthcare Professions: Using the Career Ladder

Lamar used a career ladder approach to his education by taking health science classes in high school. While he wanted to become an X-ray technician, he took a nursing assistant course so he could get an entry-level job in healthcare. After high school, Lamar enrolled in the local community college and lived at home to save money. He continued to work at a local nursing home and learned that he enjoyed the tasks involved in the nursing profession.

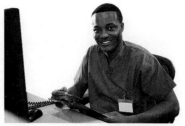

MBI/iStock/Thinkstock

The next year, Lamar transferred to the state university in a nearby city and continued to live at home. He found a nursing assistant job in a hospital close to his new school and continued to work while studying for his bachelor's degree in nursing. Lamar's employer helped pay some of the tuition costs of his classes. Employers often support the education of employees who are seeking advanced degrees or certification. Since they want to maintain a skilled workforce, employers may repay student loans or reimburse tuition for employees.

After completing his bachelor's degree in nursing, Lamar passed the national examination for nurses and became a registered nurse. The hospital was happy to hire him because they already knew he was an energetic and compassionate worker with strong communication skills for interacting with patients. Taking an entry-level position while studying and working his way up the career ladder was a good strategy for Lamar.

Lesson 3.2 Review

 Complete the *Map Your Reading* graphic organizer for the section you just read.

1. The smaller groups of occupations within a career cluster are called (3.2-1)
   A. techniques
   B. skills
   C. pathways
   D. mini-clusters

2. Make sure to attend an _____ educational program, so that you will be eligible to work in your chosen healthcare career. (3.2-1)
   A. associated
   B. adjudicated
   C. accredited
   D. applied

3. Most healthcare jobs require further _____ after you finish high school. (3.2-2)
   A. postsecondary education
   B. university education
   C. technical college education
   D. four-year education

4. In addition to completing a specialized training program, healthcare workers often need to obtain _____, which are documents proving a worker is qualified for a specific occupation. (3.2-2)
   A. registration
   B. recognition
   C. credentials
   D. certification

5. As individuals gain experience or complete additional education, they can move up the _____ in their occupation. (3.2-3)
   A. scale
   B. wall
   C. chain
   D. ladder

Career Selection and Preparation

Learning Outcomes

After studying this lesson, you will be able to

3.3-1 explain the purpose for the National Health Science Standards.

3.3-2 describe the role of career assessments in choosing a healthcare career path.

3.3-3 summarize the purpose for and elements of a quality career portfolio.

Professional Vocabulary

Essential Terms

career portfolio   a written record of career planning and preparation

HOSA—Future Health Professionals   a career and technical student organization for future health professionals

National Health Science Standards   statements developed by the National Consortium for Health Science Education that describe the knowledge and skills workers need to succeed in healthcare careers

résumé   a short, one-page document that contains your accomplishments and experiences and explains how these relate to a job in which you are interested

Important Terms

career and technical student organizations (CTSOs)

career assessments

Introduction

How do you begin to prepare for one of the 300 different healthcare occupations? High school health science courses introduce the core knowledge and skills you need for a healthcare career. Career assessments will help to narrow your career choices. Developing a career portfolio prepares you for entering the job market, and participating in a career and technical student organization builds your professional job skills.

3.3-1 National Health Science Standards

The National Consortium for Health Science Education (NCHSE) took on the overwhelming task of organizing the knowledge and skills that healthcare workers need. This group developed the **National Health Science Standards**.

In this text, you will study these 11 standards. They provide the essential knowledge common across health professions to prepare students for college and future health careers.

The standards teach students how to contribute to the delivery of safe and effective healthcare (**Figure 3.17**). They represent the core set of skills most workers need to succeed in healthcare careers. More than 1,000 healthcare employers, as well as college and high school health science teachers, contributed to the development of the standards.

This text guides you through the content of each foundation standard. Reading about the experiences of workers in the five health science career pathways will enhance your understanding. By noting the differences among the pathways and the experiences of workers within each pathway, you will be able to refine your career search and learn the core skills you will need for a successful healthcare career.

3.3-2 Selecting a Career

The first step in finding a satisfying and rewarding career is to learn about your job preferences. Once you know your preferences, you can analyze career opportunities and find those that fit you personally. Friends, teachers, counselors, and family members may give you career advice with the best intentions, but it will only be good advice if the suggested occupation matches your personality and work preferences.

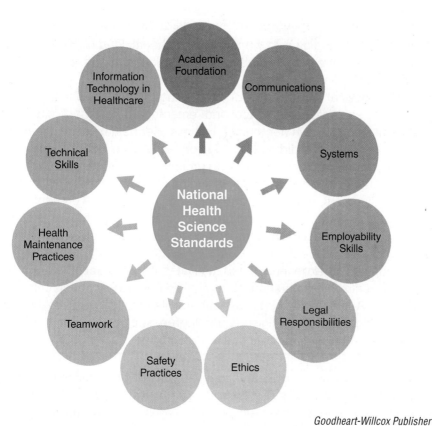

Goodheart-Willcox Publisher

Figure 3.17 Studying these content standards develops core skills for healthcare workers.

Identifying Your Interests and Strengths

Taking a career cluster survey will identify your top occupational interest areas. Sometimes students with a strong interest in health science are surprised when the health science cluster is not their top choice in the survey results. Career interests often come from life experiences, which are powerful motivators. It is important to examine many careers. When you look at the daily tasks of your chosen career, you may find they do not fit your personal preferences or strengths.

 ## Healthcare Professions: Career Choice

When Angie was in elementary school, her beloved grandmother became ill with cancer. Through many months of treatment, Angie observed several different nurses who provided care for her grandmother. She was impressed and moved by their compassionate care. As a result of this experience, she decided to become a nurse. As a high school student, she took every available health science class. The science and math courses were not her favorites, but she worked hard to learn the skills needed for a nursing career. When it came time to take a nursing assistant course, Angie found the clinical practice agonizing. Her stomach clenched each time she thought about going back to work with the patients. One night she broke down in tears in the employee lounge. It was time to reconsider her choice.

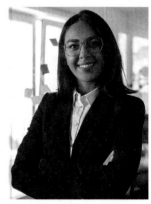

Mangostar/Shutterstock.com

Angie still had a strong desire to help people, but found she did not enjoy the close physical care aspects of the nursing profession. She thought about the classes she enjoyed in school and remembered how much she liked the business projects in her marketing class. Her health science teacher reminded her that she did an excellent job leading the HOSA—Future Health Professionals service-learning project. The teacher also identified some of Angie's natural strengths, including recruiting and training fellow student volunteers, developing and delivering a healthcare presentation to 300 students, and designing and producing hands-on activities for students. Angie also had a positive attitude and could always get fellow students excited about HOSA activities.

Though her life experiences had motivated Angie to become a nurse, she soon realized her personal strengths did not fit that chosen career. Eventually, Angie decided she was better suited to a career in marketing than one in nursing. When she finishes her degree, she hopes to do marketing or public relations work for a healthcare organization.

Knowing the career cluster and pathway you are interested in pursuing helps you create a program of study for high school and college. As a health science student, for example, a program of study based on your chosen career pathway can help you understand why math and science courses are important to your future. Knowing your program of study may also offer opportunities to earn college credit while you are still in high school. Many high schools offer dual-credit and advanced-placement college coursework that is relevant to a student's career goals. In some cases, students attend courses at a college located near their high school. Following the sequence of courses outlined in your program of study will prepare you for employment in your chosen career.

As you research your healthcare career, include career clusters other than health science in your search. You may be surprised to learn that many occupations found in other career clusters are part of the healthcare industry (**Figure 3.18**). **Career assessments** are tools such as questionnaires and surveys that you can use to find careers that will match your individual needs. If you have completed a career cluster survey, you know your top career clusters. Even if health science was not one of your top clusters, you can find ways to use your chosen career in the healthcare field. For example, computer scientists, public relations personnel, and accountants all come from different career clusters. Yet, all of these people can work in healthcare facilities.

Career Personality

Career clusters are organized according to different jobs within an industry. Since the clusters are not organized according to work interests, you will want to narrow your career search based on your own interests. By identifying your work interests, you can determine your career personality.

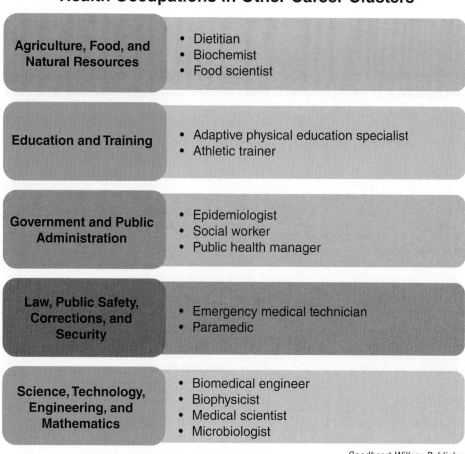

Health Occupations in Other Career Clusters

Agriculture, Food, and Natural Resources	• Dietitian • Biochemist • Food scientist
Education and Training	• Adaptive physical education specialist • Athletic trainer
Government and Public Administration	• Epidemiologist • Social worker • Public health manager
Law, Public Safety, Corrections, and Security	• Emergency medical technician • Paramedic
Science, Technology, Engineering, and Mathematics	• Biomedical engineer • Biophysicist • Medical scientist • Microbiologist

Goodheart-Willcox Publisher

Figure 3.18 Other career clusters also contain many different health-related occupations.

Career psychologist John Holland identified six basic personality types through many years of work and research in the field of psychology. Review the chart in **Figure 3.19** to identify your top three personality types. Then, consider careers that match those personality types. Matching your personality to your career can lead to job satisfaction and success.

As you investigate careers that interest you, look for those that match your work preferences and personality type. Do you prefer to work indoors or outdoors? Are you willing to work only on weekdays and only during the daytime? How long do you want to attend school? How much income do you want to earn? These preferences regarding the practical parts of a career are important to your job satisfaction. Compare each career you are interested in with your list of personal preferences as you develop your career plan.

Primary Work Tasks

As you continue to search for a satisfying health science career, consider the primary tasks of an occupation. Look for jobs that include tasks you enjoy performing. Knowing your likes and dislikes in your hobbies and activities will help you plan for a career that is a good match for you. All job tasks focus primarily on people, data, things, or ideas:

- People-oriented jobs provide care and services to people. They lead or guide people or sell products to people. These jobs may be a good choice if you enjoy helping someone who is sick, running for an elected office, listening to a friend's problems, or showing a child how to do a new task.

Health Science Careers by Personality Type		
John Holland Personality Type	**Characteristic**	**Health Science Career Examples**
Realistic/doer	Likes mechanical hands-on activities	• Central supply worker • Electrocardiograph technician • Surgeon
Investigative/thinker	Is an analytical problem solver	• Medical laboratory technician • Nurse practitioner • Psychologist
Social/helper	Is cooperative and people-oriented	• Certified nursing assistant • Health science educator • Physical therapist
Enterprising/persuader	Is a competitive leader	• Pharmaceutical sales representative • Healthcare administrator • Dean of nursing at a college or university
Conventional/organizer	Pays attention to detail	• Dental assistant • Medical coding specialist • Operating room nurse
Artistic/creator	Likes creative activities	• Medical photographer • Music therapist • Community health nurse

Goodheart-Willcox Publisher

Figure 3.19 Career personality types identify personal interests that match well with different health science careers.

- Data-oriented jobs deal with facts, numbers, and files of information. They involve business procedures. Do you like to complete science experiments? serve as a club treasurer? write a computer program? research an interesting topic?
- Ideas-oriented jobs work with knowledge, insights, theories, and new ways of doing or saying something. Are you interested in decorating a room? writing stories or music? performing in a play or a concert? inventing a new product?
- Things-oriented jobs involve working with equipment and machines; living things; or materials such as food, metal, or plastic. Do you find satisfaction in repairing a car? building something out of wood? gardening and lawn care? making craft projects? preparing food? operating computers, cameras, and other electronic equipment?

All jobs involve a combination of people-, data-, ideas-, and things-related tasks. You will be most satisfied when your preference for one or two of these areas matches the primary tasks of your job (**Figure 3.20**).

For example, Brittany knew that she was a people person. She studied nursing because she wanted to work with people but learned through a career assessment that she has a strong enterprising personality. She realized she enjoys the tasks of influencing people and helping them choose appropriate products more than tasks of caring for them directly. So she switched to studying business and became a medical sales representative.

When you research specific careers, read about the nature of the work to learn about the actual tasks performed by workers in your chosen career. Ask yourself if a job's tasks match your own preferences for working with people, data, ideas, or things.

DATA	PEOPLE
Medical Coder	Nurse
Biostatistician	Paramedic
Admitting Clerk	Pharmaceutical Sales
Clinical Data Specialist	Representative
Unit Coordinator	Rehabilitation Counselor
Patient Account Technician	Dietary Manager
Quality Control Technician	Healthcare Administrator
	Social Worker

THINGS	IDEAS
Central Service Technician	Radiologist
Hospital Maintenance Engineer	Geneticist
Medical Lab Technologist	Epidemiologist
Product Safety Scientist	Forensic Scientist
Dental Lab Technician	Speech-Language Pathologist
Optician	Molecular Biologist
Nurse Anesthetist	Exercise Physiologist

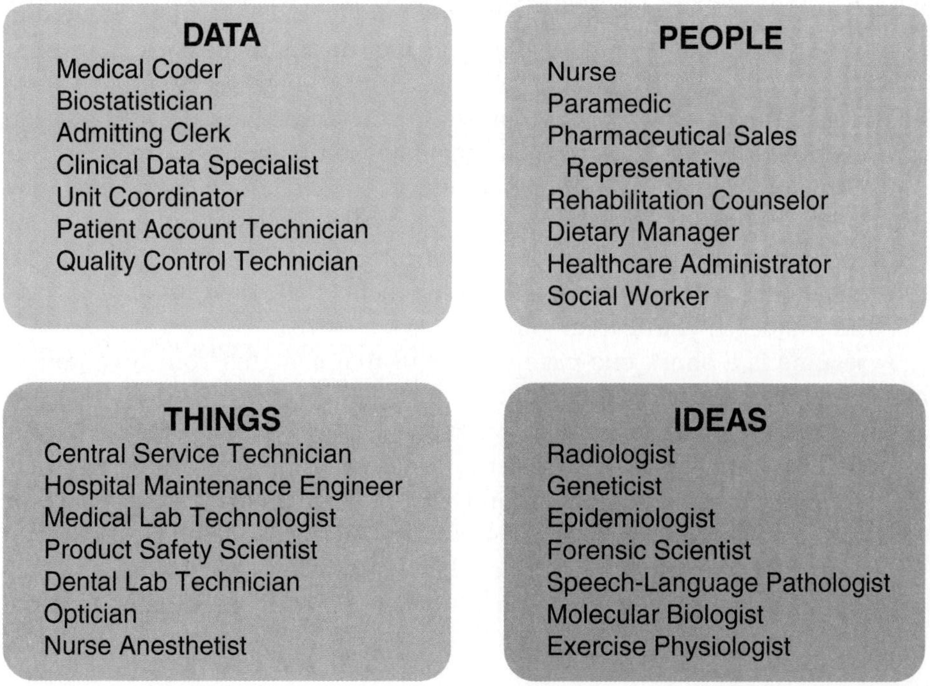

Goodheart-Willcox Publisher

Figure 3.20 Based on your interests, you may want to pursue jobs that specifically include people-, data-, ideas-, or things-related tasks. *Choose the category that best fits with your interests and investigate jobs that include that type of task.*

3.3-3 Career Portfolios

Your **career portfolio** records the work you have done to prepare for a career or get a specific job. You can use the contents of your portfolio to plan your high school course schedule, apply to college programs, complete scholarship applications, or apply for a specific job. Preserving your portfolio and keeping it up-to-date makes these tasks easier because you have all the information you need in one organized location.

A quality portfolio highlights your knowledge, experiences, skills, and abilities (**Figure 3.21**). It contains:

- a personal statement
- your résumé (REH-zuh-may)
- letters of recommendation
- records of paid and volunteer work experiences
- samples of projects and presentations that illustrate your skills
- health certifications you have earned
- a list of school and community activities in which you have participated
- scholastic and professional awards you have received

As you learn health science skills, you will develop your own career portfolio. Store your portfolio digitally for easier updates as you acquire more job skills and experiences.

A personal statement reflects your personality, passions, and goals for your career and your life. It should answer some basic questions. What experiences and interests have led you to this career? Why is this work important to you, and what do you think you can contribute to this career? What goals have you set for yourself in this career? Include an example of one of your positive characteristics. You may use information from this document as you write a college application essay or fill out job applications and prepare for interviews. Do not send your personal statement out to potential employers. Instead, use it to guide your decisions as you begin your career journey.

A **résumé** is a short, one-page document that contains your accomplishments and experiences and explains how these relate to a job in which you are interested. An online template can make it easy to create and revise your résumé. List your name and contact information at the top of your résumé. Include your educational background, employment history, extracurricular activities, employment certifications, and special awards or honors. Keep a separate list of references to include when specifically requested. Each time you apply for a job, adjust your résumé to fit the specific requirements of the position.

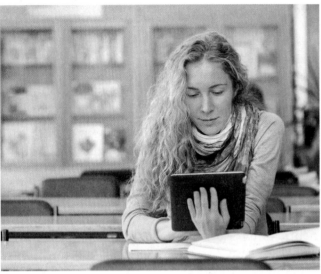

Ermolaev Alexander/Shutterstock.com

Figure 3.21 Keep your career portfolio on hand when applying for jobs. Your portfolio should contain all the information you might need for a job application.

Your résumé must be easy to read, so use the same font throughout the document. Use phrases separated into bullet points rather than complete sentences. Be specific about your responsibilities and accomplishments. Since you may be applying online, format your résumé so it can be posted easily to a website; sent by email; or printed, mailed, and then scanned by a potential employer. Save your document in the file type requested by the employer, such as a PDF, Word, or plain text file (**Figure 3.22**).

Include the results of your career assessments in your portfolio so you can review them when considering a new job. These results will help you determine if a job is a good fit for you. Your portfolio is a tool you will use throughout your work life.

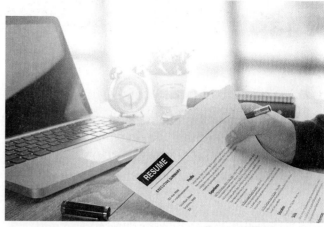
Neomaster/Shutterstock.com

Figure 3.22 Your résumé should be formatted so you can share it easily with multiple employers.

3.3-4 Career and Technical Student Organizations

HOSA—Future Health Professionals is a career and technical student organization. **Career and technical student organizations (CTSOs)** are membership groups for students in career and technical education pathways to advance their career skills by participating in activities, events, and competitions. Through CTSOs such as HOSA for health science students, FBLA for business students, and SkillsUSA for a variety of industries, students can develop leadership skills (**Figure 3.23**). Members learn about career training programs, practice career skills, and participate in service-learning and other volunteer opportunities.

Welcome to the field of health science. Keep your eyes and ears open on this journey through the amazing variety of careers you will encounter in this field. Who knows? Maybe you will discover the pathway to your future.

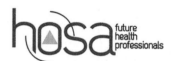
HOSA—Future Health Professionals

Figure 3.23 HOSA— Future Health Professionals is a CTSO focused on preparing students for careers in health science.

Lesson 3.3 Review

 Complete the *Map Your Reading* graphic organizer for the section you just read.

1. The National _____ Standards include the 11 healthcare standards you will study in this text. (3.3-1)
   A. Healthcare
   B. Health Information
   C. Health Science
   D. Fundamental

2. What do career assessments help you identify? (3.3-2)
   A. Work tasks that you enjoy
   B. Your individual work preferences
   C. Your career personality
   D. All of these.

3. A career portfolio _____ your career preparation and achievements. (3.3-3)
   A. explains
   B. records
   C. acknowledges
   D. eliminates

4. A quality portfolio contains (3.3-3)
   A. job applications
   B. rejection letters
   C. recommendation letters
   D. list of all high school courses

Chapter 3 Review and Assessment

Chapter Summary

3.1-1 Using specific reading strategies helps you comprehend the reading material and remember more information.

3.1-2 To develop your understanding of new information, use your own words as you take notes. Short and frequent review sessions build both understanding and memory. Turning chapter headings into questions will help you to find the main idea of each text section.

3.1-3 Recognizing and understanding your own learning style allows you to use the study method that is best for you. Mnemonic devices connect information with many senses and make it easier to recall the information later. Test-taking skills can change the way you study and improve your test scores.

3.2-1 The health science career cluster includes all the careers found in the field, while each of the health science pathways contains a smaller set of specialized occupations. Each career cluster has a core set of basic knowledge and skills used by all workers in that cluster. Each pathway contains a more specific set of knowledge, skills, and training that will build on the cluster's core knowledge. The health science career cluster includes five occupational pathways: health informatics services, therapeutic services, diagnostic services, support services, and biotechnology research and development.

3.2-2 Healthcare workers earn credentials by completing specialized training programs and passing a licensing test before they are certified to work.

3.2-3 Healthcare workers often progress to more advanced positions by seeking additional education and training.

3.3-1 Students learn how to contribute to the delivery of safe and effective healthcare by studying course content that is based on the National Health Science Standards.

3.3-2 Career assessments help to identify potential careers that will lead to job satisfaction.

3.3-3 A quality career portfolio highlights your knowledge, experiences, skills, and abilities. At a minimum it contains your résumé, letters of recommendation, your current references, and a list of your professional certifications.

Maximize Your Professional Vocabulary

1. **Terms Target Practice.** On a sheet of paper or document, draw a target shape with two rings and a bull's-eye in the center. In the outer ring, list the professional vocabulary terms that refer to learning and memorization. In the middle ring, list the five health science career pathways. In the bull's-eye, list the terms that are connected to occupations and employment. Start with the outer ring and define each term. Circle each term you cannot define. Continue defining terms until you hit the bull's-eye. Then review the meaning for each circled term.

2. **Memory Flash Review.** Create a flash card for each level-1 essential term. Include a visual representation like a picture or a graphic above each term. As you review, repeat each word and definition out loud. Sort your cards into "know" and "do not know" piles. Lay your "do not know" cards in a line on the floor. Walk to each term and say the definition. Start over until you can walk the complete path of terms. Think about this review. How does it incorporate all learning styles?

Reflect on Your Reading

1. Review the chart of cost estimates you made in the *Connect with Your Reading* activity at the beginning of this chapter. Ask each class member to research the cost of one item on the list. Work together to record the actual costs from your research. Add tuition and room and board fees and consider these questions: How much does a four-year bachelor's degree cost? How do you think students pay for college education expenses? Discuss your findings with class members. Think about your own experiences regarding the costs of education and training. List some options that can help to cover the costs.

Review and Recall

1. Which of the following is *not* a reading strategy? (3.1-1)
   A. Survey the material
   B. Preview the introduction and summary
   C. Identify the main idea
   D. Reclaim the information

2. Which steps will help you determine the main idea of a text section? Choose all that apply. (3.1-2)
   A. Turn the section title into a question.
   B. Set a purpose for your reading.
   C. Ask who, what, when, where, or how.
   D. List all your text information in your notes.

3. What is likely to be the most effective study technique for a kinesthetic learner? (3.1-3)
   A. Ask for an outline of the lecture.
   B. Ask yourself questions about the lecture.
   C. Create a diagram of the lecture.
   D. Join a study group to review the lecture.

4. You need to remember the names of all the Great Lakes: Huron, Ontario, Michigan, Erie, and Superior. Look closely at the name of each lake. What mnemonic device works well for this task? (3.1-3)
   A. Create an acronym.
   B. Use rhythm and rhyming.
   C. Create vivid images.
   D. Create a short scene with dramatic voices.

5. Which of these is *not* a health science career pathway? (3.2-1)
   A. Health Informatics Services
   B. Therapeutic Services
   C. Pediatric Services
   D. Biotechnology Research and Development

6. Ruth plans to become a speech and language pathologist. Which career cluster and pathway represent the knowledge and skills required for this occupation? (3.2-1)
   A. Human Services/Community Services
   B. Human Services/Early Childhood Services
   C. Health Science/Therapeutic Services
   D. Health Science/Support Services

7. Healthcare workers earn credentials by completing specific _____ and passing a test before they are certified to work in their profession. (3.2-2)
   A. college coursework
   B. career assessments
   C. high school coursework
   D. training programs

8. Which of the following best illustrates a career ladder approach to education? (3.2-3)
   A. Pharmacy technician to surgical technician
   B. Respiratory therapist to physician's assistant
   C. Dental assistant to dental hygienist
   D. Medical laboratory technician to registered nurse

9. Which statement best describes the purpose for the National Health Science Standards? (3.3-1)
   A. They organize the knowledge and skills needed by all healthcare workers.
   B. They contain 11 standards.
   C. They prepare students for college and future health careers.
   D. They strengthen communication and teamwork skills.

10. Jasmine just heard a presentation by a polysomnographer (sleep specialist) who spoke to her health science class. She is excited to pursue this career. What steps should she take next? Choose all that apply. (3.3-2)
    A. Complete a career cluster assessment.
    B. Complete a career personality assessment.
    C. Decide whether she likes working nights.
    D. Apply for a position in this career.

11. Choose the best description of a career portfolio. (3.3-3)
    A. It is a record of your work history.
    B. You use this document to get a work reference.
    C. You give it to the person who interviews you for a job.
    D. You use this document to apply for educational programs and job openings.

Nursing Degree	Certified Nursing Assistant	Licensed Practical Nurse	Bachelor's of Science–Nurse	Master's of Science–Nurse
Cost of education for tuition and fees (Costs are for public colleges and universities)	$600 (one course)	$5,500 (one year)	$40,000 (four years)	$64,000 (six years)
Beginning yearly salary	$28,000	$36,000	$65,000	$90,000
Total 10-year income assuming annual 4% raises	*Write answer here.*	*Write answer here.*	*Write answer here.*	*Write answer here.*
Total income minus the cost of education	*Write answer here.*	*Write answer here.*	*Write answer here.*	*Write answer here.*

Build Core Skills

1. **Math.** The table above shows the education costs and beginning yearly salaries of several nursing degrees. For this activity, find the total dollar amount earned in a 10-year period minus the cost of education for each of the nursing credentials shown. Calculate total dollar amount using compounded 4-percent increases for salary each year and round totals to the nearest dollar amount. Does more education equal more income? Is further education worth the cost? Discuss with your classmates.

2. **Critical Thinking.** Complete a career clusters interest survey. Search the internet for "career clusters interest survey" and select an online or printable version. After completing the survey, identify your three top clusters of career interest. What factors will you consider as you choose a healthcare career if health science is not your first choice in the cluster quiz?

3. **Critical Thinking.** Select two of your own healthcare experiences from the following list. For each experience, identify a healthcare worker who played a role in that experience. Identify that worker's health science pathway and describe the credentials required for that healthcare career.

    Healthcare experiences: eating hospital food, having hearing checked, having a blood test, having vision checked, receiving oxygen, having teeth cleaned, reading a medical bill, taking a sick pet to a doctor, taking a prescription medication, seeing a baby on a sonogram, riding in an ambulance, receiving physical therapy

4. **Critical Thinking.** Review the five health science career pathways. For each job task, write the health science career pathway of the worker who would perform the task.
    A. Determine the cause of a disease outbreak.
    B. Repair an ultrasound imaging machine.
    C. Take an X-ray.
    D. Give a vaccination.
    E. Fill a prescription.
    F. Register a new patient.
    G. Inspect a new medical device for defects.
    H. Print a physician's appointment schedule.
    I. Run a urine test (urinalysis).
    J. Disinfect a hospital room.

5. **Problem Solving.** Review the chapter section about identifying main ideas. Create a question for each of the section titles listed. Then read each section and respond to your question using the chapter information.
    A. Career Clusters and Pathways
    B. Employment Opportunities
    C. Career Education and Training
    D. Job Titles and Credentials
    E. Career Ladders
    F. National Health Science Standards

6. **Writing.** Take a learning style survey. Access a survey online through your school's career program or use a handout from your teacher. Write a one-page summary describing five study techniques that match your preferred learning style.

7. **Problem Solving.** Review the section titled *Using Mnemonic Devices.* Develop a device for recalling the five pathways in the health science cluster.

8. **Critical Thinking.** Review the figure that explains how to complete multiple-choice questions. Can you identify the least correct, and partially correct responses, as well as the response that does not answer the question? Use the same techniques to answer the following question. Identify the least correct, correct, partially correct, and "does not answer the question" responses.

Choose the most accurate description of career ladders.
A. Career ladders show all the jobs within each health science pathway.
B. An increasing number of students use a career ladder approach to their education.
C. Jobs in a career ladder always "piggyback" on each other.
D. Career ladders show the progression of jobs within a specific occupation or particular work setting.

Activate Your Learning

1. Pick one of the healthcare careers listed in Figure 1.20. Research this career and write 10 brief factual statements about the career you chose. Be prepared to play "Who Am I?" Take turns being the Mystery Career Contestant. As the contestant, you will give one statement from your list and let the rest of the class guess the career. Continue reading statements until someone guesses correctly. You may collect points for correct guesses and for stumping the class.

2. Use an 8 1/2 x 11-inch sheet of paper or document to create a career ladder for a healthcare occupation or healthcare work setting of your choice. List the education and training required and the average salary for each career on your ladder. Display your drawing in a location assigned by your instructor. Complete a "gallery walk" to review all your classmates' drawings. Keep the following questions in mind:
   A. What is the relationship between years of education and training and the average salary of these careers?
   B. What is the salary comparison for different career ladders?
   C. What are the occupations or work settings with the highest and lowest salary ranges?

3. **Portfolio Builder.** Create a résumé and personal statement for your career portfolio. Follow the guidelines described in the chapter. Then ask for feedback on these documents from someone who knows you well, and who has good writing skills, such as an English or business education teacher. Revise your work according to their feedback. Place these items in your career portfolio.

Think and Act Like a Healthcare Worker

1. Suppose your best friend, Sophia, tells you they are disappointed and frustrated. They have always had their heart set on a healthcare career, but their career cluster assessment results do not list the health science cluster. The results say they are well suited for careers in Agriculture, Food, and Natural Resources; Government and Public Administration; or Science, Technology, Engineering, and Mathematics. You know they do well in all of their science classes and love to help people. What will you say to them about pursuing a career in healthcare, and what steps will you encourage them to take as they plan for their future career?

Go to the Source

1. Use the internet to search for more information and examples of the three note-taking methods described in this chapter: outline notes, Cornell notes, and mind maps. Select one of these methods and complete notes for this chapter using your chosen method.

HOSA Event Prep: Family Medicine Physician

HOSA future health professionals **EVENT PREP**

Dr. Kathy Steggers is a family physician. She has been Kayla's family physician since Kayla was three years old. Now Kayla has her own child. Dr. Steggers has seen Kayla through ear tubes as a child, an appendectomy (surgical removal of the appendix), allergies, and asthma. Dr. Steggers was the first to celebrate with Kayla when she found out she was pregnant. She helped Kayla through a tough start breastfeeding her baby and with postpartum depression. Now Dr. Steggers is retiring, and Kayla has no idea what to do. She has never had to see anyone different and feels uncomfortable getting a new physician. Dr. Steggers reassures her that she will ensure Kayla is comfortable and the new physician will have all of the medical records and information about Kayla and her daughter.

Think About It

1. Why do you think there is a shortage of family physicians in the United States? What should be done about this shortage?

2. What are the advantages of seeing one family physician over the course of one's life? What are the disadvantages?

3. What do you think are the most important skills family physicians need to know? Explain.

4. Is family medicine a career that interests you? Why or why not?

Chapter 4 Career Skills in Health Informatics Services

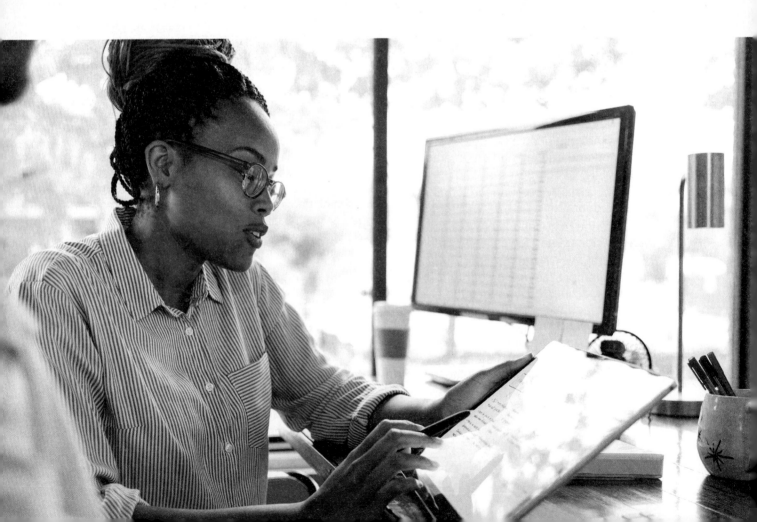

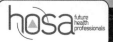

HOSA Event Prep: Health Informatics

We live in a technological world. In the world of healthcare, technology allows medical records to be shared quickly, decreases the need for paper and physical storage of records, and has even helped deliver healthcare. Health informatics is a thriving branch of healthcare. If you are torn between a career in technology and a career in healthcare, then health informatics may be the right fit for you. One of HOSA—Future Health Professionals' newer competitions is *Health Informatics*. By competing in this event, you can dive deeper into careers in health informatics.

Go to the HOSA website to learn more about the HOSA *Health Informatics* event. Find out the purpose of the event, what is involved in the event, and what knowledge is demonstrated in the event.

As you prepare for HOSA competitive events, be sure to check the website and talk with your HOSA advisor for the most up-to-date guidelines and procedures. Once you have learned about the *Health Informatics* event, answer the following questions:

1. How might participating in this event benefit you personally and your future career? Explain.
2. Are you interested in participating in this event? Why or why not?

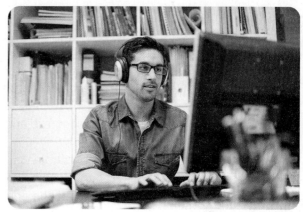

alvarez/E+ via Getty Images

Connect with Your Reading

Before you read this chapter, take time to think about a past experience you have had with healthcare. Create a bubble diagram in which the center bubble represents you. In each surrounding bubble, list a healthcare worker you saw or talked to during that healthcare experience. What seemed to be the main job of each person? Did each person work mostly with people, equipment, or information? Write your answer to this question in each person's bubble. Share and compare your diagram with a classmate.

Map Your Reading

Create a radial diagram of this chapter using the figure shown as a guide. Fill in the chapter title and main headings. As you read each section, answer the accompanying questions. Then answer the questions that follow.

1. Consider your own personal traits. Which of the traits described in this chapter do you possess?
2. Select any career discussed in this chapter. Describe how it suits your aptitudes and interests.

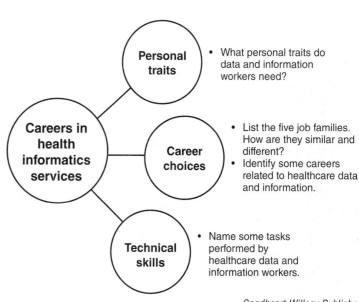

Careers in health informatics services

Personal traits
- What personal traits do data and information workers need?

Career choices
- List the five job families. How are they similar and different?
- Identify some careers related to healthcare data and information.

Technical skills
- Name some tasks performed by healthcare data and information workers.

Goodheart-Willcox Publisher

Chapter opener image: SDI Production/E+ via Getty Images

Lesson 4.1

Personal Traits and Career Choices in Health Informatics Services

ESSENTIAL QUESTION

What jobs are found in the health informatics services pathway, and how do personal traits benefit this work?

Learning Outcomes

After studying this lesson, you will be able to

4.1-1 identify personal traits of healthcare workers and explain how health informatics workers apply them.

4.1-2 compare and contrast occupations within each of the five health informatics services job families.

4.1-3 illustrate ways that advancing technology is changing health informatics services.

4.1-4 describe education, training, and the career outlook for health informatics services jobs.

4.1-5 identify health informatics jobs that include more interaction with people.

Professional Vocabulary

Essential Terms

health informatics services   career pathway that involves methods, devices, and resources used to acquire, store, retrieve, and work with healthcare and biomedical information

internship   practical work or training experience that allows students to apply what they have learned in class

medical coding   the act of assigning numbers to descriptions of a patient's diseases, injuries, and treatments according to established codes

personal traits   an individual's unique combination of qualities and characteristics

Important Terms

Coding and Revenue Cycle

Compliance and Risk Assessment

confidential

dictation

Informatics and Data Analytics

Information Technology Infrastructure

medical history

Operations and Medical Record Administration

personal identifying information

transcriptionist

Introduction

When considering healthcare careers, most people think of becoming doctors or nurses, yet there are hundreds of different healthcare jobs. Some fall into the career pathway of health informatics services. If you have a desire to help others and enjoy learning about the latest technology, you should consider a career in health informatics services. In this lesson, you will learn about job opportunities in **health informatics services** and begin to assess your personal traits.

For example, when asked about her job, Myesha always says she loves what she does. Myesha is a puzzle solver. As a health informatics employee, she works with patient data every day, doing the **medical coding** for every patient visit in the medical office where she works. Medical coding assigns numbers to each patient diagnosis and treatment. Myesha has a strong background in anatomy. She understands the origins, symptoms and signs, diagnostic tests, treatments, and outcomes of diseases.

The information Myesha provides allows the physician she works for to receive payment for treatment services. Correctly coded information also allows the patient to receive health insurance benefits for those services. One of Myesha's favorite parts of her job is working with Medicare patients to arrange treatment plans that meet complex insurance requirements. Patients with serious illnesses feel a great sense of relief when they find out their medical costs will be reimbursed.

Myesha likes to help people, but she does not provide direct, hands-on care. Instead, she helps patients by ensuring their medical records contain accurate information.

4.1-1 Personal Traits

Are you well organized? Are you thorough and attentive to detail when you work? Is correct spelling important to you? If you possess these **personal traits**, then you might enjoy a career in the health informatics services pathway.

As you might guess from the name, information is the focus of the health informatics worker. Because a patient's health can depend on the accuracy of medical records, health informatics workers must be thorough, reliable, and trustworthy.

Workers use self-control to protect the privacy of patient information. Keeping information **confidential**, or private, requires more than just not talking about a patient's condition in public. Health informatics workers do not share their computer passwords. They close any computer screen that shows patient information before leaving their work area and do not leave medical documents in a fax machine where other people can see them. They know who is allowed to receive a patient's medical information and what parts can be shared. They share only facts and do not make judgments or assumptions about the patient.

Do you enjoy working with computers? Do you like learning new things? Medical records are almost completely electronic, so the computer is a constant companion of the health informatics worker. As a result, willingness to learn new skills is a trait of successful health informatics workers.

Adjusting to new equipment, updated technologies, and revised software is common for health informatics workers. Workers must interpret rules and detailed instructions and keep up with constantly changing guidelines for coding and recording information. Health informatics workers welcome the challenge of adjusting to these changes because they want to improve the process for keeping accurate medical records.

Healthcare Professions: Professionalism

When you visit your local medical clinic, Kia's bright smile welcomes you. She is the medical assistant who greets you at the reception desk. As a health informatics worker, Kia accesses your account to update your personal information and checks information about your insurance coverage. She schedules your appointments

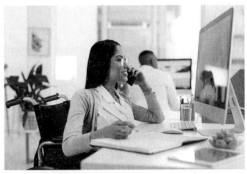

PeopleImages/iStock/Getty Images Plus via Getty Images

and forwards your phone call to the correct worker when you call the clinic.

Kia's appearance and attitude must leave patients with a positive impression of the clinic. Without a good first experience, patients may assume the clinic's medical care is poor and choose to find a different medical provider. A medical office is like any other business: it cannot stay open if it does not make money.

Kia loves fashionable clothes, but strives for a professional appearance at work. For her position, professional clothing includes suits, dress pants and shirts, sweaters, and sport coats. Short dresses, jeans, and leggings are not permitted. Her clothing must fit well and be neat and clean. She was surprised to learn she should not wear strong-smelling cologne and scented lotions, but this made sense when she thought about the sick patients arriving at the clinic. Her facility has specific guidelines for tattoos and piercings. Kia is careful to follow her clinic's dress code. She realizes she needs to look mature and competent, or capable, to patients of all ages. As the first person patients meet, she understands her appearance is just as important as her behavior.

Kia conveys a positive attitude naturally. She admits it was a challenge, however, to learn the practical steps for maintaining confidentiality in a medical clinic. She reminds herself to speak quietly so others cannot hear patient information. She is careful not to use a patient's name when calling coworkers over the intercom for a phone call. She has learned to avoid conversations about patients when she is in the elevator or cafeteria.

4.1-2 Job Families in Health Informatics Services

Jobs in health informatics services do not focus on hands-on patient care. Instead, they combine a knowledge of healthcare and technology. These jobs appeal to people who are interested in the data and information involved in healthcare.

This area of healthcare is changing rapidly. Originally, health informatics workers simply documented patient care. However, technology is increasing the amount of data and information collected in healthcare. Today, health informatics workers use skills in information science and computer science along with their knowledge of healthcare (**Figure 4.1**). Health informatics services jobs are organized into five groups, or families, based on their primary tasks (**Figure 4.2**).

Operations and Medical Record Administration

The **Operations and Medical Record Administration** job family focuses on complete and accurate patient medical records. Workers in this family assemble and organize a patient's health information to create a medical record. This document includes a **medical history** that lists

- all of the diseases and surgeries a patient has had;
- current symptoms;
- results of examinations and diagnostic tests;
- treatments; and
- other health services.

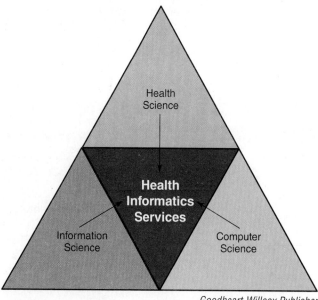

Goodheart-Willcox Publisher

Figure 4.1 Health informatics services combines knowledge and skills from the fields of health science, information science, and computer science. *How many of these fields appeal to you?*

The record also lists the patient's family medical history because some health concerns are genetic. The presence of a genetic marker for cancer or heart disease can shed light on a patient's illness or set of symptoms. Finally, the medical record contains **personal identifying information**, such as a Social Security number, to connect a patient to the correct record.

Medical record employees work with electronic health records, which are stored in a computer database instead of paper files. They understand the flow of information within healthcare facilities, from large hospital systems to a physician's private practice. These workers are vital to the daily collection, management, and protection of health information. Examples of job titles in this family include health information technician, patient or cancer registrar, medical office administrator, health information manager, and meaningful use specialist.

Coding and Revenue Cycle

The **Coding and Revenue Cycle** job family processes patient financial and health information for the purpose of receiving payment for medical services. For example, Myesha from earlier in this lesson codes diagnoses and procedures using a numbering system. Each numerical code determines the payment the healthcare provider receives from Medicare, Medicaid, or other insurance programs. Workers in this area complete insurance claims and bill patients for medical services. Other job titles in this family include benefits coordinator, collections clerk, medical biller, and clinical documentation improvement specialist.

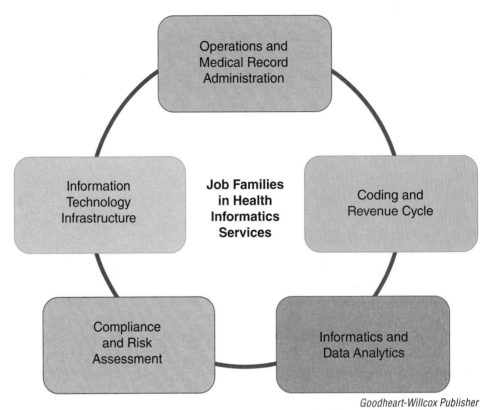

Goodheart-Willcox Publisher

Figure 4.2 Shown here are the job families in health informatics services. *Can you identify the job family that requires the highest level of computer knowledge?*

Informatics and Data Analytics

The **Informatics and Data Analytics** family studies electronic data to further medical research and education. Examining data sets can improve patient outcomes. For example, identifying the number of patients who return to the hospital after surgery can lead to more follow-up care for discharged patients. Avoiding a return to the hospital saves money and enhances patient recovery. Biomedical scientists can use large databases of patient information to research a wide range of health issues such as risk factors for heart disease or reasons certain groups are at higher risk of cancer. Some of the job titles in this family include data analyst, clinical informatics coordinator, and research and development scientist.

Compliance and Risk Assessment

The **Compliance and Risk Assessment** family manages patient information to satisfy the legal requirements for storage and security. These workers make sure the correct information is collected. They develop and monitor security systems to maintain the privacy of patient information. In addition, compliance workers ensure that all employees meet governmental credential standards. They confirm that employees are properly trained and certified according to state and federal regulations. They also verify that all the services provided by the facility meet industry standards set by federal and state regulations. Jobs titles in this family include credentialing specialist, compliance auditor, privacy officer, and information security manager.

Information Technology Infrastructure

The last health informatics job family is **Information Technology Infrastructure**. These workers focus on computer science. Some develop the computer programs that collect, share, and store patient information. Others update programs, repair glitches in software, or install computer hardware. Some job titles are system analyst, implementation support specialist, and data quality manager.

Health informatics services workers are found in all types of medical facilities, from dental offices to medical clinics to hospitals. Day shifts are common, and evening and night shifts are available in 24-hour facilities. As you might expect, health informatics and data analytics professionals work in hospitals with research programs and large healthcare provider organizations. They are also employed by government agencies, insurance companies, and software development and production organizations. Because many health informatics workers have limited contact with patients, their workspaces may be out of the way. It is common to find medical records departments in the basements of healthcare facilities. The COVID-19 pandemic increased opportunities for remote health informatics positions. A variety of healthcare businesses have improved their technology infrastructure to allow remote health informatics specialists to work securely with patient data.

4.1-3 Changing Technology in Health Informatics Services

Because health informatics services uses ever-changing technology, job descriptions continue to change as well. For example, the medical **transcriptionist** used to type medical record information from a physician's recorded **dictation**, or verbal recording describing a patient's symptoms and the treatment given. This was a special skill that involved listening, pausing the recording, and accurately typing what was said. Recent improvements in speech-recognition software have made typing almost unnecessary.

Transcriptionists may now be called *medical editors* or *medical proofreaders* (**Figure 4.3**). Their job is to correct errors made by speech-recognition software. They often do this work at home, sometimes far away from the facility. These workers may live in a different state or even a different country from the facility where they work.

Medical coders are learning to work with computer-assisted coding software that analyzes healthcare documents and assigns medical codes for specific phrases and terms in the document. Coding is becoming a hybrid system in which the computer-assisted coding program performs many routine medical coding tasks. Medical coders work on more complex patient scenarios and review the work of the software program to check for errors.

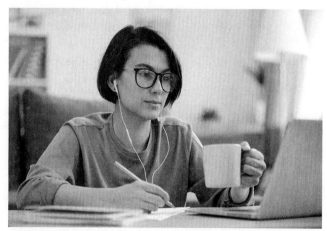

Media_Photos/Shutterstock.com

Figure 4.3 Transcriptionists, or *medical editors*, utilize technology in their job every day. Many work from home and provide an important service to a healthcare facility.

When correctly programmed, this combined system speeds up the coding process and saves money for the facility. As technology advances, fewer transcription and coding employees will be needed.

4.1-4 Education, Training, and Career Outlook

A high school diploma may qualify you for an entry-level health informatics services position. Technical diplomas and associate's degrees, however, are common educational requirements at the entry level. Employers prefer to hire credentialed technicians and professionals. To become credentialed, a worker must pass a test to become certified. The worker will continue to take classes each year to keep that certification up to date. Health information technicians, for example, have several certification options (**Figure 4.4**).

Advancing in a health informatics services career usually means getting more education and experience. With a bachelor's or master's degree, experienced technicians can become compliance or privacy officers, medical records managers, or revenue cycle managers. Those who advance typically have strong business and management skills. Work in more advanced positions can involve long hours. Managers may have to respond to problems at all hours of the day. They must adapt to changing technology, interpret complex regulations, and work to improve efficiency while maintaining quality care.

Health informatics services jobs for computer science workers are increasing rapidly, so there should be many opportunities in this job family. Workers with healthcare knowledge and experience in addition to computer science skills will be in highest demand. As a result, this job family receives the highest salary among informatics workers. A bachelor's degree or higher is required for these positions.

Unlike many healthcare workers, health informatics and data analytics professionals are experts in more than one field. Most of these jobs require a combination of computer and information science knowledge, as well as a healthcare or business background. Employment often requires a bachelor's or master's degree in medical informatics, computer science, public health, or another field related to health science. Many workers have specialized healthcare degrees in medicine or nursing as well.

Certifications for Health Information Technicians	
Certification	**Description**
Certified Professional in Electronic Health Records (CPEHR)	Beginning certification for working in electronic health records
Registered Health Information Administrator (RHIA®)	Manages patient health information and medical records
Registered Health Information Technician (RHIT®)	Ensures that medical records are complete, accurate, and entered in the correct format
Certified Professional Coder (CPC®)	Qualified to code in both hospitals and physician practices

Goodheart-Willcox Publisher

Figure 4.4 There are different types of certifications for health information technicians.

As this area of health informatics services evolves, workers have a growing number of specialty areas from which to choose. Current specialty areas include clinical research, consumer health, public health, and clinical services (**Figure 4.5**).

4.1-5 Related Careers with Patient Interaction

If you want more contact with patients than traditional health informatics workers do, consider becoming a medical assistant, health educator, or medical scribe. These jobs work with health information, but also involve interaction with patients.

Medical Assistants

Medical assisting is one of the fastest-growing occupations, which means many jobs are available. Medical assistants work in a medical office for physicians, chiropractors, or other healthcare professionals. They keep the office running smoothly by performing many different tasks. If you are looking for variety, you will find it as a medical assistant (**Figure 4.6**).

Medical assistants usually complete a one- or two-year training program that includes an **internship**. Interns spend time at a healthcare facility performing skills they learned in school. This work is part of their training and is usually unpaid. They are supervised by a healthcare employee and a school instructor. Graduates of medical assistant programs can become certified and choose a specialty area. Examples of specialties include podiatry (puh-DI-uh-tree), which is a medical practice concerning the feet, or ophthalmology (ahf-thal-MAH-luh-jee), a medical practice concerned with the eyes. Experienced assistants can advance to other occupations, such as office management, nursing, or laboratory technology, through additional training or education.

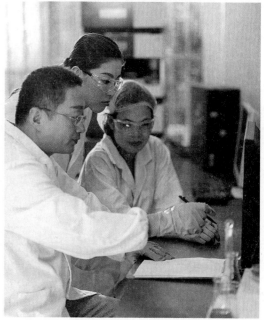

zhudifeng/iStock/Thinkstock

Figure 4.5 People working in public health informatics—a specific focus within health informatics—track disease patterns that might threaten humans. *Would you be interested in this type of work?*

Tasks of a Medical Assistant	
Administrative/Clerical	**Clinical**
Scheduling • Hospital admissions • Clinic appointments • Laboratory services Filing insurance forms Answering the telephone Greeting patients Writing letters and memos Updating patient records Processing billing	Taking medical histories Recording vital signs Assisting with examinations Performing basic lab tests Collecting and preparing laboratory specimens Instructing patients about medication and special diets Authorizing prescription refills as directed Drawing blood

Goodheart-Willcox Publisher

Figure 4.6 Tasks of a medical assistant vary between administrative duties and clinical duties. *Do any of these tasks sound like job duties you would find interesting?*

Health Educators

Helping patients use information to prevent illness and manage chronic conditions is becoming more important as healthcare costs increase. Health educators have at least a bachelor's degree and work with individual patients and groups of people in a variety of locations. In medical offices, they educate patients about their diagnoses. On college campuses, they teach students about healthy lifestyle choices. As public health workers, they provide information to the media and public during an emergency. Think about a past outbreak of an illness like influenza (the flu) or COVID-19 in your community. Did you see signs about vaccination clinics or hear advice about handwashing to reduce infections? These were produced by a public health worker.

 ## Healthcare Professions: Health Educators and Serving People

Health educators help people by providing health-related, scientific information. Adam loves science and chose biology as his major in college. He became a biotechnology (bI-oh-tehk-NAH-luh-jee) research scientist and worked to develop new products to prevent and treat disease.

Over the years, Adam noticed how much he enjoyed explaining new processes to his fellow employees. He often volunteered to develop training programs for other workers. Eventually, he realized he had a strong interest in working with people. Since that was missing from his research job, Adam transferred to an institute

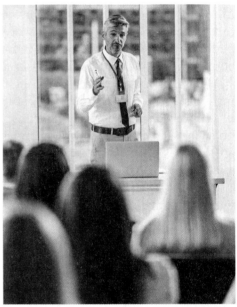

skyneshar/E+ via Getty Images

for biotechnology education and became an education specialist. Now he trains science teachers and educates students about biotechnology and its research methods.

Medical Scribes

Medical scribes are becoming more common as physician workloads and electronic health record documentation increase. These fast-paced workers complete medical data entry in real time. They accompany physicians to the exam room to document patient care. Their work allows the physician to focus on the patient exam and treatment. Medical scribes also gather information for patient visits and monitor the progress of lab tests. They serve as personal assistants to physicians and increase physicians' abilities to see more patients, perform medical procedures, and communicate with nursing staff.

Medical scribes need to understand medical terminology and have computer and typing skills. They must be responsible and mature and have a passion for medicine. Their role is very fast paced as they listen to encounters and record the relevant information in real time. Health science students are good candidates and can use this work experience to enhance acceptance into medical, nursing, and physician assistant training programs.

Other health informatics services career paths include medical librarians, illustrators, and historians. Health informatics workers can also be found in the finance or accounting departments of healthcare facilities. These workers, like all the professions described in this lesson, focus on information. If you love medical language and want to work in healthcare, but touching patients and handling body fluids are not for you, search the health informatics services pathway for your future career.

Lesson 4.1 Review

 Complete the *Map Your Reading* graphic organizer for the section you just read.

1. Healthcare workers must use self-control to keep patient information (4.1-1)
   A. public
   B. accurate
   C. confidential
   D. concise

2. Which of the following are personal traits of health informatics workers? Choose all that apply. (4.1-1)
   A. Extremely friendly
   B. Well-organized
   C. Pay attention to details
   D. Focus attention on the supervisor

3. Unlike doctors and nurses, health informatics workers focus on _____ rather than on direct patient care. (4.1-2)
   A. data
   B. people
   C. things
   D. creations

4. What is the focus of coding and revenue cycle workers? (4.1-2)
   A. Medical payments
   B. Research and education
   C. Medical records
   D. Information security

5. Health informatics workers frequently use computers and must adapt to ongoing changes in (4.1-3)
   A. regulations
   B. office organization
   C. technology
   D. patient symptoms

6. Which of the following will you need to get more of to advance in a health informatics career? Choose all that apply. (4.1-4)
   A. Patients
   B. Information
   C. Education
   D. Experience

7. Which job offers more patient contact than traditional health informatics jobs? (4.1-5)
   A. Health information technician
   B. Medical coder
   C. Data analyst
   D. Medical assistant

Technical Skills in Health Informatics Services

Learning Outcomes

After studying this lesson, you will be able to

4.2-1 describe the forms completed for the medical record of a new patient and the steps taken to protect the privacy of patient information

4.2-2 demonstrate filing records using the alphabetical system.

4.2-3 list the steps needed to build an effective patient schedule.

4.2-4 explain how HOSA participation can build your health science skills and which competitive events can improve your health informatics skills.

Professional Vocabulary

Essential Terms

competitive events   HOSA program that recognizes competencies developed by members through health science education and training

technical skills   practical tasks performed in a specific healthcare discipline or department

Important Terms

family history
medical history form
patient registration form

Introduction

Technical skills are the practical functions and tasks a worker performs on the job. In each of the five health science pathways, you will practice a few entry-level technical skills. This experience will help you determine your future career direction.

In this lesson, you will learn guidelines for maintaining a patient's medical record and scheduling patient appointments. These are important technical skills for a job in health informatics services. You will also learn how to improve your professional skills by participating in activities sponsored by HOSA—Future Health Professionals.

4.2-1 Patient Records

Health information technicians work with several forms to create a complete patient medical record or chart. All written forms become part of this record. It communicates information about the patient's medical status to healthcare workers. It is a legal document that provides evidence of the care the patient has received.

Healthcare workers also use the information in medical records for research, public health initiatives, and patient education. Because they are critical to patient care, these records must be accurate and complete, but also brief.

How Forms Are Completed and Used

When a new patient makes an appointment, a medical clinic or office may send forms for the patient to complete and bring to the appointment. This is more efficient than having the patient fill out forms while waiting to see the doctor. The patient has time to gather information and think carefully about the questions while at home. As a result, the medical office receives a more accurate and complete medical history.

Many medical offices have a website where patients can download and print these forms or set up a private account and complete them online. Occasionally, a technician will contact the patient by phone to obtain the information. If the office uses electronic health records, all handwritten forms are scanned into the patient's chart. Some facilities shred paper forms to protect patient privacy. Others archive the paper records by filing and storing them as a backup to the electronic record.

When a new patient arrives for an appointment, identify the patient before proceeding with the details of the visit. Name, address, and date of birth are common patient identifiers. Protect personal information by speaking privately with the patient to clarify information given on a medical form. Reception areas are arranged so others waiting in line cannot hear conversations that may include private health information. All protected health information (PHI), such as the patient's name, birth date, Social Security number, and more, must remain confidential. You can only share PHI with people who are authorized to receive it.

You should never share patient information outside the patient care team. This is both illegal and unethical. Patient forms, electronic health records, emails, documents, conversations with the patient, phone calls, and messages about the patient are all confidential. Written forms must be protected from unauthorized access. You should not leave forms where others may see them. Make sure your screen is not visible to unauthorized people and log off when leaving your computer.

Healthcare Professions: Maintaining Accuracy

Deepika is a health information technician. She makes sure patient information is complete and clarifies any handwriting that is difficult to read. Using a private area to consult with patients or making sure others cannot hear the discussion is a legal requirement. Deepika double-checks the forms for all required signatures so that claims for service can be sent to the insurance company. Accurate registration avoids future problems.

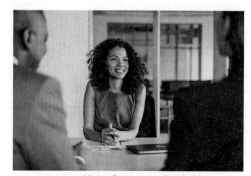

VioletaStoimenova/E+ via Getty Images

Common Types of Forms

In this section, you will learn about some common types of forms health information technicians use.

- **Patient registration forms.** The **patient registration form** tells you how to contact the patient and includes insurance information. **Figure 4.7** shows a complete registration form ready for the patient signature. In this case, the patient is a minor child, so a parent or guardian must sign the form. The *responsible party* is the person in charge of payment for healthcare services the patient receives. Ask the patient about any blank spaces on this document. If items do not apply to the patient, you can indicate this by writing Ø, *N/A*, or *None*. Typically, you will scan the patient's insurance card and enter the patient's information into the electronic record.

SUN VIEW MEDICAL — ***NEW PATIENT REGISTRATION FORM***

PATIENT INFORMATION

PATIENT'S LAST NAME: Wolf	FIRST NAME: Bryan	M.I.: J.	DATE OF BIRTH: 01-10-1999	PRIMARY CARE PHYSICIAN: Dr. Nolan
MAIDEN NAME: N/A	NAME YOU GO BY: BJ			MARITAL STATUS: ☒ S ☐ M ☐ D ☐ W
STREET ADDRESS: 1025 Sun City Dr.				APT. NO.: Ø
CITY: Star Prairie	STATE: TX	ZIP: 74260	HOME PHONE: 123 - 701 - 6529	
SOCIAL SECURITY NUMBER: 000 - 00 - 0000	AGE: 13	GENDER: ☒ Male ☐ Female	CELL PHONE: 123 - 217 - 2220	
EMPLOYER: N/A	OCCUPATION: Student		WORK PHONE: N/A	
EMERGENCY CONTACT (NOT LIVING WITH YOU) / RELATION TO PATIENT: Charmayne Prue - Grandmother			EMERGENCY CONTACT PHONE: 123 - 701 - 3507	

SPOUSE OR PARENT / RESPONSIBLE PARTY INFORMATION

LAST NAME: Ohman	FIRST NAME: Melissa	M.I.: K	RELATIONSHIP TO PATIENT: ☒ Parent ☐ Legal guardian ☐ Other	
STREET ADDRESS: 1025 Sun City Dr.		APT. NO.: Ø	HOME PHONE: 123 - 701 - 6529	
CITY: Star Prairie	STATE: TX	ZIP: 74260	CELL PHONE: 123 - 217 - 0472	
SOCIAL SECURITY NO.: 000 - 00 - 0000			DATE OF BIRTH: 02 - 15 - 1977	
RESPONSIBLE PARTY EMPLOYER: RNK Associates	OCCUPATION: Accountant		RESPONSIBLE PARTY WORK PHONE/EXT.: 123 - 701 - 6000	

SECOND PARENT INFORMATION

LAST NAME: Wolf	FIRST NAME: Marvin	M.I.: J	RELATIONSHIP TO PATIENT: ☒ Parent ☐ Legal guardian ☐ Other	
STREET ADDRESS: 425 Monroe St.		APT. NO.: 2	HOME PHONE: 123 - 701 - 5490	
CITY: Star Prairie	STATE: TX	ZIP: 74260	CELL PHONE: 123 - 217 - 3320	
SOCIAL SECURITY NO.: 000 - 00 - 0000			DATE OF BIRTH: 06 - 22 - 1970	
RESPONSIBLE PARTY EMPLOYER: MJW Electric	OCCUPATION: Electrician		RESPONSIBLE PARTY WORK PHONE/EXT.: 123 - 701 - 2000	

INSURANCE INFORMATION

PRIMARY INSURANCE COMPANY: Whole Health Care		COPAY: $25.00	EFFECTIVE DATE: 01-01-2011
ID (POLICY NO.): 000100623	GROUP NO.: 67018X		
SUBSCRIBER: Melissa Ohman	RELATIONSHIP TO SUBSCRIBER: Child		SUBSCRIBER'S DATE OF BIRTH: 02-15-1977
SUBSCRIBER'S EMPLOYER: RNK Associates		SUBSCRIBER'S SOCIAL SECURITY NO.: 000-00-0000	
SECONDARY INSURANCE COMPANY: N/A		COPAY:	EFFECTIVE DATE:
ID (POLICY NO.):	GROUP NO.:		
SUBSCRIBER:	RELATIONSHIP TO SUBSCRIBER:		SUBSCRIBER'S DATE OF BIRTH:
SUBSCRIBER'S EMPLOYER:		SUBSCRIBER'S SOCIAL SECURITY NO.:	

Insurance payment and records release authorization: *I authorize my insurance benefits to be paid directly to Sun View Medical. I am financially responsible for any unpaid balance. I authorize the release of any information requested by my insurance company.*

Signature of Patient or Responsible Party ______________________ ***Date*** __________

PLEASE BRING INSURANCE CARD(S) TO YOUR APPOINTMENT. THANK YOU!

Goodheart-Willcox Publisher

Figure 4.7 A registration form contains a patient's personal information, such as contact details, age, and full name. *Who would need to sign this form?*

- **Medical history form.** The **medical history form** contains all the information about the patient's health, medical conditions, and treatments (**Figure 4.8**). **Family history** is the current health status and past conditions or diseases of the patient's biological family, including parents, grandparents, and siblings. Again, you will enter the information provided into the patient chart or record.
- **Privacy notice.** A clinic must give every patient a notice of privacy practices. This notice should explain how protected health information is kept confidential and under what circumstances the information can be released to others. You will collect the patient's signature on this form. Depending on your facility, you might scan this into the record or send it to the scanning section of the medical records department.

SUN VIEW MEDICAL

MEDICAL HISTORY FORM
(please print/type)

Last Name	First Name	Middle Name
Date of Birth	Age	Date of Last Physical Exam
Occupation		
Chief Complaint		

HAVE YOU HAD:

	YES	NO		YES	NO		YES	NO
Head Injury with Unconsciousness			Sexually Transmitted Disease			Counseling/Mental Health Treatment		
Asthma			Malaria			Recreational Drug Use		
Recurrent Headaches			Chicken Pox			Tobacco Use		
Seizure Disorder			Scarlet Fever			Alcohol Use		
Hearing Loss			Hay Fever			# times per week		
Recurrent Ear Infections			Rheumatic Fever			amount per session		
Visual Problems (other than glasses)			High Cholesterol			Exercise: # times per week		
Thyroid Problem			Hepatitis A, B, or C			Surgeries / Dates:		
Heart Problem/Murmur			Diabetes					
Kidney/Urinary Tract Problem			High Blood Pressure			Chronic Health Problems:		
Gynecology Problem(s)			Digestive Tract Problem					
Recent Weight Change			Cancer/Tumor/Cyst					
Bleeding/Blood Disorder			Spinal Cord Disruption			Alternative Medicine Practices:		
Tuberculosis			Eating Disorder					

Medications (List all medications you are currently taking)	Allergies (List all allergies.)

Family Health History

Family Member	Age	Serious Illness/Cause of Death
Father		
Mother		
Brother		
Sister		
I am adopted.		

HAS ANY FAMILY MEMBER EVER HAD:

(parent, sibling, or grandparent)	YES	NO	Relationship		YES	NO	Relationship
Tubercolosis				Asthma			
Drug/Alchohol Use				Thyroid Disease			
Diabetes				Seizure Disorder			
Kidney Disease				Blood Disorder			
Heart Disease				Cancer			
High Blood Pressure				Stroke			
Arthritis				Obesity			

OTHER CONCERNS/INFORMATION:

Goodheart-Willcox Publisher

Figure 4.8 A medical history form contains clinical information, such as a patient's past diagnoses and treatments, as well as health information about close family members.

- **Insurance and information-sharing forms.** Additional signed forms give a facility permission to bill an insurance company or to share confidential information with any other individual chosen by the patient.

PROCEDURE — **Complete a New Patient Registration Form**

Mrs. Thomas is a new patient visiting your clinic for the first time. When she scheduled her appointment, she received a registration form to complete and bring to her appointment. Today you will enter this information into her new electronic health record.

1. Log in to your computer using your own password credentials.
2. Greet Mrs. Thomas using her full name. Make eye contact and smile as you greet her.
3. Ask if she has brought the registration form with her. Also ask for her insurance cards.
4. Scan the insurance cards into the electronic record and return the cards to Mrs. Thomas.
5. Open a patient registration form in the new chart for Mrs. Thomas and enter the information from her handwritten form.
6. Fill in all required information. Include dashes and letters when entering insurance policy numbers. Check all spelling and numbers for accuracy.

7. Do not leave blank spaces. Enter Ø, *N/A*, or *None* in any space that does not apply to the patient.
8. Politely ask for clarification of any information that is missing or unclear. Remember to use a quiet voice so others cannot hear you. Use a private room if necessary to maintain confidentiality.
9. Obtain electronic signatures for the notice of privacy and the authorization to bill the insurance company. Save those documents in the patient's electronic record. If you cannot use electronic signatures, complete signatures on paper copies and scan those into the electronic record. Archive or shred paper copies according to facility policies.
10. Verify that the insurance policy is active, and the patient has coverage for provider services. Collect required copays.
11. Ask Mrs. Thomas to be seated and wait for the nurse to take her to an exam room.

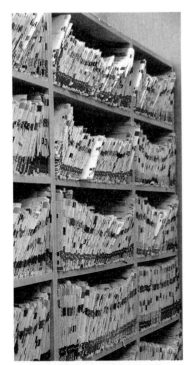

Elena Elisseeva/Shutterstock.com

Figure 4.9 Color-coding is one effective method for organizing paper files.

4.2-2 Filing

While most medical records are stored electronically, workers may still need to access paper records maintained as a backup storage system. Depending on federal and state requirements, healthcare facilities may keep records for as long as 10 years. Proper filing of records helps avoid potential lawsuits by keeping all necessary information available for review. Medical records are stored either alphabetically or by number (numerically).

- **Alphabetic filing.** The alphabetic system files records in order of the patient's last name. File tabs or folders with a different color for each letter group—for example, green for A to F and yellow for G to L—make it easy to spot files that are out of order (**Figure 4.9**). In this system, you will alphabetize files by the patient's last name and then by the first name when two patients have the same last name. Electronic systems save a great deal of time by automatically alphabetizing charts for digital storage. The alphabetic system can cause confusion when two patients have the same name. When this happens, check the patient's name and date of birth to select the correct file (**Figure 4.10**).
- **Numeric filing.** Numeric filing systems give each patient a unique number. Most systems use six digits, and charts are filed in numeric order. This avoids the problem of name duplication and helps protect patient privacy. It is important to write numbers clearly so charts are not misfiled. A poorly written 7 can easily look like a 1. This system also requires a master index of patient names and numbers so you can find the correct chart for a specific patient.

Alphabetic Filing Tips		
Tip	**Patient Name**	**File As**
File by last name, then first name, then middle initial.	Jon C. Byers	Byers, Jon C.
Hyphenated names should be treated as one word.	Gabriel Garcia-Marquez	GarciaMarquez, Gabriel
Abbreviated parts of names are filed as if spelled out.	Susan St. Cyr	Saint Cyr, Susan
Put professional titles and initials at the end of the name. They are not part of the system.	Dr. Mai Vang, MD	Vang, Mai, MD
Use birth dates for patients with identical names. Usually, the most recent date is first.	1. Nicole M. Grimm; DOB: 10/22/1951 2. Nicole M. Grimm; DOB: 03/15/1979	1. Grimm, Nicole M. 03/15/1979 2. Grimm, Nicole M. 10/22/1951

Goodheart-Willcox Publisher

Figure 4.10 Following these filing tips for keeping patient files in order makes records easier to retrieve.

Systems other than alphabetic or numeric include geographic, chronologic, and by subject. A geographic system organizes files by location, such as state or city. This works well for a mobile clinic where patients live in several different areas. Chronologic (krah-nuh-LAH-jik) filing uses dates, such as years or months. Research studies often use this system to record their progress. Filing by subject, such as personnel files, inventory records, or accounts payable, may be used for storing information other than patient charts.

4.2-3 Scheduling

Effective scheduling avoids long wait times for patients and maintains a consistent flow of appointments for physicians. In this section, you will learn about scheduling and cancelling appointments.

Scheduling an Appointment

The process of scheduling begins with blocking off times when providers are not seeing patients in the clinic. Examples of blocked times include lunchtime, attendance at a conference, or time spent seeing patients in the hospital (**Figure 4.11**).

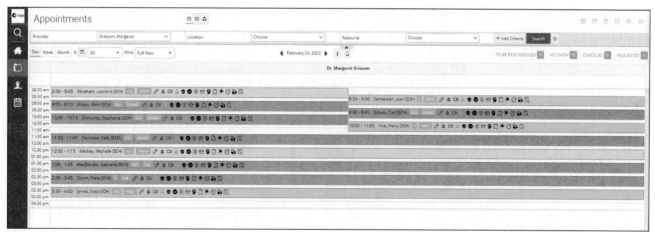

Courtesy of OmniMD

Figure 4.11 This schedule shows Dr. Grissom's appointments for the day. *Is there time for the doctor to have a lunch break? Are there open times in the morning and afternoon for emergencies? How many types of appointments can you identify in this list?*

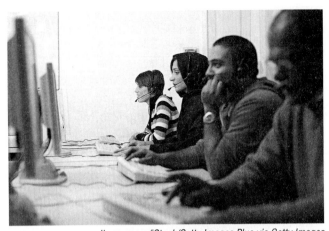

Figure 4.12 When scheduling appointments, you must verify several items of information about the patient. *How many of these items can you list?*

The length of an appointment is the next consideration. Healthcare facilities determine the standard time allowed for each type of appointment. Many appointments are 15 minutes in length, but a physical exam may last one hour. Your scheduling system will block the correct amount of time when you enter the type of appointment. If not, you will need to reserve the correct amount of time for each appointment. Leave a few open appointment times in the morning and in the afternoon. This allows for emergencies and catch-up time if the scheduled appointments run late.

When scheduling a patient's appointment over the phone, request the reason for the appointment and the patient's full name (**Figure 4.12**). Ask for the spelling if you are unsure. Search for the patient record and confirm the date of birth. When you have the correct patient record, check for the current address and phone number. Then ask the patient for the preferred provider and appointment time.

A scheduling program will search for the next available appointment times or show you the schedule for a date you have entered. It may take a few attempts to find an available appointment at a time that is convenient for the patient. Once you have set an appointment, repeat the day, date, and time for the patient before ending your call. If the patient makes the appointment at the clinic, provide a reminder card with these details and the name of the physician.

Online Scheduling

Some offices use online scheduling systems in addition to phone scheduling. These allow patients to view available times and book their appointments online (**Figure 4.13**). Doctors can access their schedules from any digital device at any time.

To make an appointment, a patient must set up an account with a secure username and password. The patient selects the clinic location, a specific doctor, and the type of appointment. The software program calculates the amount of time required for the appointment and displays available dates and times. Once the patient selects a time, the appointment is added to the doctor's schedule, and the screen shows the patient pre-visit instructions, if applicable.

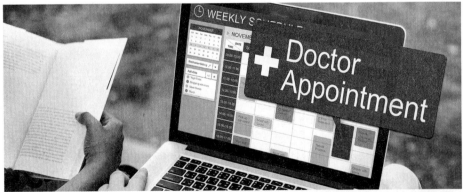

Figure 4.13 Online scheduling systems allow patients to schedule their own appointments, but types of appointments may be limited.

Many patients appreciate the opportunity to schedule an appointment even when the clinic is closed. However, some patients report frustration with online systems. They might spend time using the website only to learn the type of appointment they need must be scheduled by phone.

Handling Cancellations

If a patient calls to cancel an appointment, remain polite and positive and ask why the appointment needs to be cancelled. Record the cancellation in the schedule and list the cancellation and reason in the patient's chart. Offer to reschedule the appointment. If the patient needs continuing care, you may need to call back to remind the patient to reschedule.

If your office needs to cancel appointments because of an emergency or because a doctor is ill, you do not need to give the specific reason. Contact the patient as soon as you know about the schedule change and try to reschedule while you have the patient on the phone.

4.2-4 HOSA Connections

HOSA—Future Health Professionals provides professional development opportunities designed for health science students. Being a member of HOSA will benefit your career development. Participating in HOSA's competitive events can strengthen both your general career skills and your health informatics skills. Review the *Competitive Events* section of the HOSA website for descriptions of events related to health informatics services, such as Medical Spelling or Medical Math.

Begin recording your HOSA activities. Note the years you participate and what activities you complete for your local chapter and state organization. Make this part of your career portfolio. You will use this information to complete job and scholarship applications.

Lesson 4.2 Review

 Complete the *Map Your Reading* graphic organizer for the section you just read.

1. When receiving a new patient, you will enter information into the patient's (4.2-1)
   A. appointment reminder
   B. patient registration form
   C. patient privacy notice
   D. insurance claim form

2. Why do workers need to speak privately with patients and keep others from viewing patient information? (4.2-1)
   A. Patient information must remain confidential.
   B. Patients do not want others to know their diagnoses.
   C. Individuals might gossip.
   D. They want the record to remain accurate.

3. Alphabetic filing begins by using the patient's (4.2-2)
   A. medical record number
   B. first name
   C. last name
   D. most recent appointment

4. When scheduling appointments, you should *not* (4.2-3)
   A. ask patients to spell their names
   B. confirm the day, date, and time
   C. confirm date of birth
   D. fill every single appointment time

5. What are the benefits of HOSA? Choose all that apply. (4.2-4)
   A. Participation in competitive events
   B. Stronger career skills
   C. Professional development opportunities
   D. Participation in local and statewide activities

Chapter 4 Review and Assessment

Chapter Summary

4.1-1 Personal traits are an individual's unique combination of qualities and characteristics. Health informatics workers must be accurate, organized, trustworthy, and self-controlled. They exhibit competence when they keep patient records confidential and strive for accuracy.

4.1-2 Health informatics workers focus on information rather than hands-on patient care. Health informatics services careers are organized into five career families: Operations and Medical Records Administration, Coding and Revenue Cycle, Informatics and Data Analytics, Compliance and Risk Assessment, and Information Technology Infrastructure.

4.1-3 Those working in health informatics services frequently use computers and must have a willingness to learn new skills and adapt to ongoing changes in technology. For example, the number of medical transcriptionists and coders is declining as technology automates these job tasks.

4.1-4 Education and training vary depending on the type of health informatics services job. In general, advancing in health informatics services involves getting more education, training, and experience.

4.1-5 Medical assistants, medical scribes, and health educators have more interaction with people compared to other health informatics workers.

4.2-1 Setting up a new patient record includes completing a registration form and a medical history form, providing a privacy statement, and getting the patient's signature for permission to bill the insurance provider. Health informatics workers take several steps to keep patient information private.

4.2-2 Healthcare facilities may use several different filing systems. The alphabetic filing system organizes patient records by the first letter of the last name. Other filing systems are numeric, geographic, chronologic, and by subject.

4.2-3 When scheduling an appointment by phone, you will need to verify the patient's name and correct spelling, date of birth, home address, and the reason for the appointment. Confirm the correct provider and available appointment times, then schedule the appointment.

4.2-4 HOSA—Future Health Professionals offers competitive events that can help prepare students for health informatics services careers.

Maximize Your Professional Vocabulary

1. **Dice Roll Review.** Number each term from this chapter from one to six. Continue numbering until all terms have been assigned a number. Form groups of four to six students. One student starts as the "caller." Each player takes a turn to roll the die. The caller asks for the definition of any term matching the number rolled. A point is awarded for each correct response. At the end of the first round, a new student has the caller job, and play continues.

2. **Terms Tabloid.** Write a fictional story about healthcare using at least 10 terms from this chapter. Replace the terms with blank spaces. Trade papers with another student and try to fill in the blanks in each other's stories. Have you used the vocabulary terms correctly?

Reflect on Your Reading

1. Review the bubble diagram you created in the *Connect with Your Reading* activity at the beginning of this chapter. Pick one health informatics worker from the bubble diagram you created. Revise your diagram, if needed, to include a health informatics worker. Was this person a competent health informatics worker, or not? Use evidence from your reading to support your conclusion.

Review and Recall

1. Which is the least important personal trait for working in health informatics services? (4.1-1)
   A. Enthusiasm
   B. Competence
   C. Willingness to learn new skills
   D. Organized

2. Which statement best describes why health informatics workers must make accurate entries in patient medical records? (4.1-1)
   A. Misspelled words are confusing.
   B. Misfiled records can be lost.
   C. A patient's health depends on it.
   D. Accurate records reflect high-quality work.

Match each health informatics services job family with one of its occupations (3–6). (4.1-2)

A. Informatics security manager	3. Operations and Medical Record Administration
B. Benefits coordinator	4. Coding and Revenue Cycle
C. Patient registrar	5. Informatics and Data Analytics
D. Clinical informatics coordinator	6. Compliance and Risk Management

7. Which of the following represents the most dramatic technological change in health informatics services? (4.1-3)
   A. Health insurance requirements
   B. The electronic health record
   C. Increased computer security
   D. Protected health information

8. What is the lowest educational requirement for entry-level health informatics services jobs? (4.1-4)
   A. Bachelor's degree
   B. Associate's degree
   C. Master's degree
   D. High school diploma

9. Which occupation offers the smallest amount of interaction with people? (4.1-5)
   A. Medical scribe
   B. Health educator
   C. Data analyst
   D. Medical assistant

10. Which of these would *not* be found in a patient medical record? (4.2-1)
    A. Home address
    B. Current medications
    C. Health history of aunts and uncles
    D. Insurance information

11. Which filing system assigns a unique number to each patient? (4.2-2)
    A. Numeric
    B. Alphabetic
    C. Geographic
    D. By subject

12. Robert Williams received a call to confirm his medical appointment, but it turned out to be an appointment for a different Robert Williams at the same clinic. What steps did the health informatics worker fail to take? Choose all that apply. (4.2-3)
    A. Check the patient's last name.
    B. Check the patient's date of birth.
    C. Check the patient's first name.
    D. Check the patient's home address.

13. Carter is scheduling patients for Dr. Solara. He is proud of filling each 30-minute spot throughout the day, so that Dr. Solara will not be sitting around waiting for patients. What advice applies to this situation? Choose all that apply. (4.2-3)
    A. Always block meetings and meal breaks before scheduling patients.
    B. Record the reason for a cancellation.
    C. Leave some appointments open to accommodate emergencies.
    D. Check to confirm there is enough time for each type of appointment.

14. Which HOSA competitive event best relates to health informatics services? (4.2-4)
    A. Medical Spelling
    B. CERT Skills
    C. CPR and First Aid
    D. Prepared Speaking

Build Core Skills

1. **Writing.** Suppose you are the administrator of a hospital, clinic, or other healthcare facility. Write a paragraph describing your ideal health informatics worker. What are the personal traits, characteristics, and interests that would lead someone to succeed in a health informatics services career?

2. **Problem Solving.** Suppose you have a summer internship organizing the filing system for your professor's research project. Describe the type of filing system you will use and explain the reasons for your choice.

3. **Speaking and Listening.** Suppose you are a college student studying health information management. You are speaking at your former high school and want to encourage the high school students to join HOSA—Future Health Professionals. What will you say to explain the benefits of membership in HOSA?

4. **Reading.** Suppose you have recently graduated from a medical coding training program. You know employers like to hire credentialed workers, so you decide to seek certification as a certified coding associate (CCA). Your program instructor mentioned the American Health Information Management Association (AHIMA) offers certification testing and credentials. Visit the AHIMA website to find answers to the following questions about the certification process:
   - Besides completion of a training program, what else is necessary to be eligible for certification?
   - How much does the exam cost, and how long is the exam?
   - The exam will cover coding and reimbursement procedures. What are the other four topics included in the exam?
   - Once certified, how will you keep your certification current?

Activate Your Learning

1. Your cousin, Nolan, recently moved to Star Prairie. He will see a new doctor to get a sports physical for school. You have agreed to help him complete the new patient registration and medical history forms he needs to bring to his appointment. Review the information about patient records in this chapter.

Then find sample patient registration and medical history forms and use the information provided to complete the forms. Submit each completed form for your instructor's review.
- Your aunt, Rita, works as a preschool teacher at Playtime Child Care Center at 14 Ruby Lane in Star Prairie, TX 74260. Rita has diabetes, but otherwise her health is good. Her birthdate is April 3, 1981, and her Social Security number is 111-11-1111. Rita is Nolan's only living parent.
- Nolan's birthdate is March 20, 2006. His Social Security number is 000-00-0000. Sadly, he does not have a cell phone. Your mom, Eve Sherman, is the emergency contact. Her number is 123-701-3500.
- Rita has rented a condo at 400 S. Main Street. The phone number is (123) 701-0197. Rita provided the insurance card shown.

DC Health Plan

Group number 06172   Member number 03654

Member name: Rita James 01

Nolan James 02

1600 Allen Blvd   Washington, DC 65432

Claims questions: 1-800-789-6756

Goodheart-Willcox Publisher

- Nolan experienced congestion during the months of March and April. He wishes his acne would clear up, and Rita is worried about hockey season because Nolan had a concussion during a game last year. Nolan has a bee-sting allergy and carries an EpiPen®. He has no other identified health concerns. He is physically active and exercises daily.

Think and Act Like a Healthcare Worker

1. Madison is calling Dr. Solara's patient to schedule a biopsy, so she already knows what the appointment is for and how much time is needed. Write the questions Madison must ask this patient to complete the scheduling process.

2. Imagine you are training a new clinic scheduler. Review the information about scheduling in this chapter. Then analyze Dr. Solara's schedule. List three scheduling errors and explain what should be done to correct each error.

8 am	Hospital Rounds
15	
30	
45	
9 am	Jane Brooks, sports physical
15	
30	Lamar Smith, back pain
45	Jim Sykes, skin rash
10 am	Al Sims, complete physical exam
15	
30	
45	
11 am	Barb Engles, insect bite
15	Martel Brown, fever and flu
30	Gina Downs, pelvic pain
45	Robert Alquist, new patient
12 pm	Lunch
15	
30	
45	
1 pm	
15	
30	Josh Oines, remove stitches
45	Noah Collins, sports physical
2 pm	Betty Franks, knee pain
15	Hannah Jacobs, sore throat
30	Kerry Long, blood pressure check
45	
3 pm	
15	
30	
45	
4 pm	Marquis Linton, complete physical exam
15	
30	
45	
5 pm	Quinton Zelman, new patient
15	
30	Angie Olson, back pain
45	

Goodheart-Willcox Publisher

3. Imagine that you are working in a healthcare office and see a coworker's computer screen. On the computer screen is a sticky note with your coworker's computer password. What is wrong with this situation? What are the risks?

Go to the Source

1. Use online resources to learn more about careers in health informatics services. Select two careers that interest you and complete a career profile page for each career. Use at least one website that ends in .gov and one that ends in .org. Record the following information for each career:
   - name of career
   - tasks involved in this career
   - personal traits and abilities needed
   - educational requirements
   - type of credential needed and how it is obtained
   - work conditions
   - wages and benefits
   - job outlook for the future
   - the websites you accessed

   How do the two careers compare? Why might you prefer one to the other?

2. Reference Appendix A: Career Personality Types. Which two personality types are most like you? Search the O*NET website for the two health informatics services careers you researched in the previous activity. Do the interest types listed for these careers match your personality types? What conclusions can you draw based on your findings?

3. Research HOSA—Future Health Professionals competitive events. Use the HOSA website for this activity. Which events develop health informatics skills? Select and note your top choice event. List the reasons for your choice.

4. **Portfolio Builder.** Create an activity record for logging your HOSA participation. Record dates of membership and activities in which you participate. In addition, track other school activities such as music or athletic participation. Note take-aways, such as new skills or something you gained from the experience. Place this record in your career portfolio.

HOSA Event Prep: Health Informatics

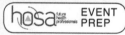

Gina has a nursing background, but really has a passion for research. While at a conference, she discovers nursing informatics. At the conference, one of the university hospitals presented about how they used their nurse informatics department and pediatric team to research asthma triggers and how to prevent asthma attacks in children. Gina discovered how she could use her nursing degree, passion for research, and associate's degree in informational technology all together. She decided to go to graduate school and pursue a master's degree in nursing informatics.

Think About It

1. Explain how nursing informatics would allow Gina to use her nursing degree, passion for research, and associate's degree in information technology.

2. Using reliable and valid online resources, research nursing informatics. What are typical job titles in this field?

3. What qualities do you think are most important in a health informatics worker? Why?

4. Is health informatics a career pathway that interests you? Why or why not?

Career Skills in Therapeutic Services

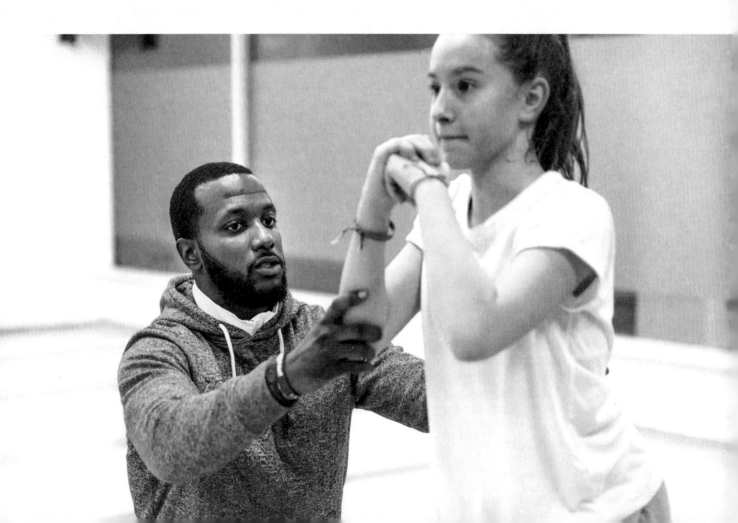

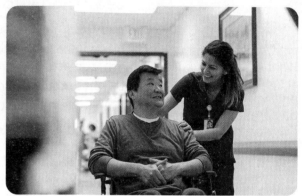

If you ask health science students what their career plans are, many will say they want to be a nurse. But did you know there are many areas of nursing? Nursing positions range from labor and delivery, neonatal nursing, pediatrics, surgical, emergency nursing, to geriatrics. Nurses can also work at schools as school nurses and even teach health science. There are many educational levels of nursing, including an LPN/LVN, associate's degree, bachelor's degree, master's degree, or even doctorate in nursing. One can soar as high as desired in nursing education. Nurses have their own licensing requirements and board and can even be practitioners. In HOSA—Future Health Professionals competitive events, competitors can actually practice nursing skills as they compete. This can expose students to skills nurses may use and give them a head start.

Go to the HOSA website to learn more about the HOSA *Clinical Nursing* event. Find out the purpose of the event, what is involved in the event, and what knowledge is demonstrated in the event.

As you prepare for HOSA competitive events, be sure to check the website and talk with your HOSA advisor for the most up-to-date guidelines and procedures. Once you have learned about the *Clinical Nursing* event, answer the following questions:

1. How might participating in this event benefit you personally and your future career? Explain.
2. Are you interested in participating in this event? Why or why not?

SDI Productions/E+ via Getty Images

Connect with Your Reading

Make a list of the first 10 healthcare occupations that come to mind. As you read this chapter, take note of how many jobs on your list are therapeutic services careers. The therapeutic services pathway includes the largest number of healthcare careers. Since these workers focus on treating patients, they are the people you most often meet when you receive care.

Map Your Reading

For this diagram, you will need to fill in the main headings as they appear in the text. As you read each section, answer the accompanying questions. Then answer the questions that follow.

1. Consider your own personal traits. Which of the traits described in this chapter do you possess?
2. Select any career discussed in this chapter. Describe how it suits your aptitudes and interests.

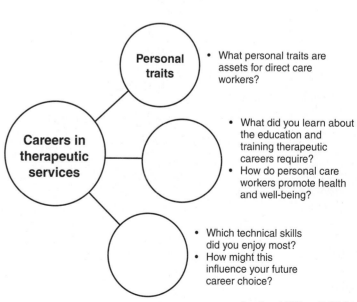

- **Personal traits** — What personal traits are assets for direct care workers?

- **Careers in therapeutic services**

- What did you learn about the education and training therapeutic careers require?
- How do personal care workers promote health and well-being?

- Which technical skills did you enjoy most?
- How might this influence your future career choice?

Chapter opener image: ti-ja/E+ via Getty Images

Goodheart-Willcox Publisher

Personal Traits and Career Choices in Therapeutic Services

ESSENTIAL QUESTION

What jobs are found in the therapeutic pathway, and how do personal traits benefit this work?

Learning Outcomes

After studying this lesson, you will be able to

5.1-1 identify personal traits of healthcare workers and explain how therapeutic workers apply them.

5.1-2 describe education, training, and career outlook for therapy careers.

5.1-3 examine the different types of dental careers.

5.1-4 identify the education, training, and career outlook for medical careers.

5.1-5 compare and contrast job opportunities in the field of nursing.

5.1-6 describe the roles that personal services workers fulfill in providing therapeutic services.

Professional Vocabulary

Essential Terms

clinical training   hands-on work with patients that students do under the supervision of a licensed healthcare provider

empathy   the ability to recognize and identify with another person's feelings and thoughts

postgraduate   education and training completed after receiving a bachelor's degree

residents   (1) individuals living in long-term care facilities; (2) medical school graduates who are completing the last portion of their medical training before becoming licensed physicians

tact   the ability to communicate difficult or embarrassing information without giving offense

technical training   education lasting two years or less and leading to an industry certificate, a technical diploma, or an associate's degree

therapeutic   treatment given to maintain or restore health

Important Terms

clients

certified nursing assistant (CNA)

dementia

fellowship

intern

licensed practical nurse (LPN)

morticians

outsource

patients

physician assistant (PA)

registered nurse (RN)

tier

Introduction

Are you a "people person"? Are you the one who listens to your friends' problems? Do you enjoy showing another person how to do a task? Do you get satisfaction from helping someone who is sick? Careers in the **therapeutic** services pathway focus on interacting with patients to provide care and treatment. Because these careers require close contact with patients, you need a strong interest in people to find job satisfaction in therapeutic careers. Many therapeutic workers have social or "helper" personalities according to their John Holland career personality assessments.

Healthcare Professions: The Therapeutic Career Path

Tina always loved children, so she took a child development class in high school and became an assistant teacher at a local childcare center. During her senior year, she also took a nursing assistant class to gain more skills and experience. She would have to live on her own and support herself after graduation, so she needed a full-time job. She knew that the more job skills she had, the better her chances for getting that full-time job.

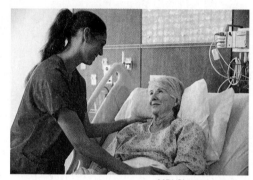

MBI/Shutterstock.com

After graduation, Tina worked at an assisted living facility for one year and then moved on to work at a university hospital. Several years later, she is still in that hospital position. She is the person with the most experience on her floor. In addition to her nursing assistant duties, she teaches the orientation class for all newly hired nurses and university student nurses who complete clinical training on her floor. Notice that all of Tina's jobs—teaching children, caring for residents and patients, and teaching her fellow employees—involve working with people.

5.1-1 Personal Traits

Can you remain calm and patient under stress? Therapeutic workers must handle patient emergencies, sometimes daily. Even when you are helping a person who could bleed to death in a few minutes, you must respond calmly.

When you work with people who are sick, you cannot expect them to be polite and concerned about your feelings. You must be patient when a difficult client keeps complaining about his food. You must be patient when a resident with **dementia** (dih-MEHN-chuh), a condition that causes memory loss, repeatedly asks you what day it is. You must be patient when a coworker takes frustration out on you. Caring for people who are sick is stressful work.

Empathy

Therapeutic workers must have **empathy** for their patients. Understanding the emotions of your patient will help you deliver compassionate care. Successful therapeutic workers know that patients' mental, social, and spiritual needs are just as important to wellness as the physical needs for which they are receiving medical treatment.

Healthcare workers communicate with a diverse group of patients and must show social and cultural competence in their interactions with others. Empathy and a willingness to listen to others improves communication and patient care.

 ## Healthcare Professions: Serving People

Selena is a therapeutic worker. One Friday evening, Selena is preparing to leave work when she is called on to help a patient. The patient, an older woman, requires surgery to amputate (AM-pyoo-tayt), or surgically remove, her leg due to spreading cancer. The patient asks Selena if she can talk to

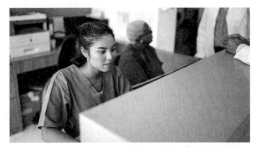

FG Trade/E+ via Getty Images

the pastor at her church. Even though Selena's shift has ended, she looks in the patient's medical record and calls the religious contact listed there. Selena arranges for a visit and lets the patient know when she will see her pastor. After she has helped the patient, Selena heads home.

Tact

Successful healthcare workers use **tact** when communicating with patients. Could you respond without embarrassment to a patient who asks if he will be able to have sex after his surgery? Could you politely ask a patient with digestive issues to describe her bowel movements? Could you find the right words to convince a visitor not to feed special homemade brownies to her grandmother with diabetes? All these situations require healthcare workers to communicate clearly yet without offending others.

Accepting Criticism

Accepting criticism can be a difficult experience for anyone. It is human nature to feel hurt and angry when criticized and to want to "defend" your position. Even when people know they have made a mistake, they have a strong urge to fight back by blaming something or someone else. Too often, people retaliate with their own criticism and create a hostile work environment.

Criticism, however, is part of working in healthcare. For therapeutic workers, a client who is in pain or frustrated by physical limitations caused by illness may give undeserved criticism. These situations require patience. It helps to remember that criticism is not really about you, but about the emotions of your patient. Sometimes you are just the convenient target of those emotions. Learning how to accept criticism is a valuable skill that will improve your work performance.

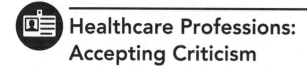

Healthcare Professions: Accepting Criticism

Dalmar and Lynn both work as personal care attendants. Dalmar notices that Lynn always wears gloves. She even wears them from one resident's room to the next. Dalmar mentions that Lynn needs to change her gloves when she moves to a new resident, even if she did not provide direct care. Dalmar is surprised by Lynn's angry reaction: "You're not my boss! I don't have to listen to what you say!"

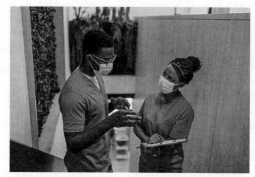

mixetto/E+ via Getty Images

Actually, Lynn was embarrassed and felt stupid for not knowing the standard precautions guidelines. Instead of becoming defensive, she should have taken a deep breath and waited until she calmed down. Then she could really think about Dalmar's advice. When she realized Dalmar was helping her protect residents from the risk of infection, she apologized for her outburst and thanked Dalmar for his help. The next day she registered to retake the infection control training class so she could feel confident about following the guidelines correctly.

During a performance evaluation, a boss is looking not only at what workers do well, but also at how they can improve. Successful workers think about possible areas for improvement in their job performance before an evaluation. They ask their boss questions during the evaluation to clarify suggestions that do not seem accurate or are confusing. Finally, they create a plan to improve their job performance and stick to that plan.

At the next evaluation, these workers can show their boss exactly what they have done to improve job performance. Would you value a worker who takes your suggestions and applies them without arguing, complaining, or becoming defensive? You can be sure that healthcare managers do. Showing improvement on the job is an important skill for receiving promotions and pay raises at work.

Dependability

Dependability seems like an obvious trait of a successful healthcare worker, but for therapeutic workers, it is essential. Since patients rely on you, regular work attendance and prompt responses to patient needs are crucial to providing quality patient care. Suppose a healthcare worker named Matt heard the call buzzer for one of his patients but was in the middle of charting. He finished the charting but forgot about the buzzer. When he remembered and checked on his patient, he found the man unconscious on the floor of his hospital room. The patient had to use the bathroom and was embarrassed that he might wet the bed. Even though he was at risk of falling, he tried to get to the bathroom on his own. Matt's failure to respond promptly to a patient's call led to that patient being injured.

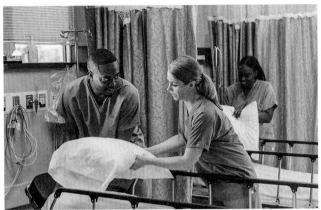

kali9/E+ via Getty Images

Figure 5.1 Healthcare workers are dependable and function as team players. *What does it mean to be a dependable therapeutic worker?*

Your fellow workers depend on you to be a team player (**Figure 5.1**). When you are absent from work, another trained employee must take your place. Paperwork can sometimes wait, but patient care never can. Frequent absences place a burden on fellow workers and create resentment.

For therapeutic workers, being dependable also requires a commitment to maintaining personal health. Because you are working with people who may have weakened immune systems, you must be healthy when you are providing care. Without good health, you cannot be a dependable worker. Are you willing to eat a healthy diet, get regular physical activity, and get adequate sleep so your team and patients can rely on you?

5.1-2 Therapy Careers

Therapeutic workers strive to change the health status of a patient over time. Therapy means treatment, and workers in therapeutic services use a variety of treatments to improve patient health. These treatments may improve physical, mental, or emotional health.

The therapeutic services pathway includes the largest number of healthcare careers. Since therapeutic services require the most worker-to-patient interaction, facilities cannot easily **outsource** these jobs to a different country. However, many hospitals, behavioral health facilities, and long-term care organizations do outsource some services. To save money, they use local agencies to provide medical, nursing, therapy, support, and other services. In this type of outsourcing, outside staff members provide care or treatment within the healthcare organization or under its name.

The job outlook for therapeutic workers is changing because of the rising costs of healthcare. Therapeutic work is increasingly being assigned to lower-paid workers to cut costs. For example, physician assistants, medical assistants, dental hygienists (hI-JEHN-ists), and physical therapy aides complete tasks that were previously performed by doctors, nurses, dentists, or physical therapists. This trend has created a new **tier**, or level of careers, for workers with **technical training** lasting two years or less. Professionals with more training still complete the patient evaluation and create treatment plans. Technical workers, however, often deliver part of the treatment. As a result, technical workers may actually have more contact with patients.

Therapists

All therapists use a special set of knowledge and skills to assist people with impaired functions. Physical illness or injury, emotional disorders, or the aging process can limit a person's abilities. *Congenital* disorders that are present at birth or disabilities that develop over time can also cause impairments. Therapists help patients become as self-sufficient and productive as possible.

They evaluate the needs of each patient and develop a treatment plan to improve the person's health status. They specialize in specific types of treatments, which results in a large number of specialties (**Figure 5.2**).

Therapists work in many different settings, including hospitals, clinics, schools, private offices, clients' homes, gyms, outdoors, and at private swimming pools. Therapy work can be both physically demanding and emotionally challenging. A therapist must remain patient when clients make slow progress. A lack of progress can be frustrating for the therapist and the client, but seeing improvement is very satisfying.

The field of therapy is expanding. For example, massage therapy is growing as more people learn about its health benefits. Trained and licensed therapists have the best opportunity for employment. However, many massage therapists work part-time until they build a client base large enough to support full-time employment.

Types of Therapists	
Specialist	**Services Provided**
Athletic trainer	Prevents and treats muscle and bone injuries
Audiologist	Assesses and treats hearing, balance, and related ear conditions
Exercise physiologist/ kinesiotherapist	Plans and implements fitness programs
Massage therapist	Performs therapeutic massage of soft tissues and joints
Mental health therapist	Counsels individuals and groups to promote mental and emotional health
Occupational therapist	Plans rehabilitative programs to restore vocational and daily living skills
Physical therapist	Plans rehabilitative programs to relieve pain, improve mobility, and increase strength
Radiation therapist	Administers radiation to treat cancer
Recreational therapist (art/music/dance therapist)	Provides treatment services and recreational activities for people with disabilities or illnesses
Rehabilitation counselor	Designs rehabilitation programs that include personal and vocational counseling, training, and job placement
Respiratory therapist	Treats and cares for patients with breathing disorders
Speech-language pathologist	Assesses and treats people with speech, language, voice, and fluency disorders
Vision rehabilitation therapist	Provides instruction for adaptive living skills to adults who have blindness or visual impairments

Figure 5.2 Each type of therapist has unique responsibilities and may work in a variety of healthcare settings.

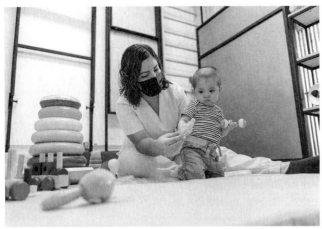

aldomurillo/E+ via Getty Images

Figure 5.3 Recreational therapists provide treatment services and recreational activities for people of all ages.

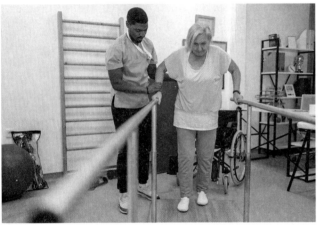

Phynart Studio/E+ via Getty Images

Figure 5.4 Residents in rehabilitation care facilities might receive physical therapy as part of their treatment.

Recreational therapy includes many types of treatment. These therapists use sports, games, arts, crafts, and music to help patients build confidence and restore physical and social function (**Figure 5.3**). Recreational therapists are not the same as the recreational workers, who conduct games for fun at parks and other locations. Therapists use patient medical records and interviews with the healthcare team to design specific treatment activities. For example, a treatment plan might include helping a right-handed girl who cannot use her right arm anymore learn to throw a ball with her left arm.

Currently, most therapists work in hospitals and nursing homes, but alternative settings are becoming more common. Adult day care programs, assisted living facilities, and physical rehabilitation sites also provide many job opportunities. Some recreational therapy programs may employ activity aides, rather than certified therapists, as a cost-control measure.

Therapeutic workers use different terms to identify the people they treat based on the care setting. **Patients** receive treatment in hospitals and clinics. **Clients** receive treatment in privately owned offices, treatment facilities, or their own homes. **Residents** live in long-term care facilities such as group homes, assisted living facilities, and nursing homes (**Figure 5.4**).

Patients sometimes use alternative therapies such as Reiki (RAY-kee), acupuncture, and traditional Chinese medicine to complement Western treatments. Patients feel their clinical treatment plans benefit from complementary therapies, and demand for such therapies is growing. If you want to provide alternative therapies, look for an accredited training program that leads to certification. The National Certification Commission for Acupuncture and Oriental Medicine (NCCAOM) is a national organization with a certification process to show employers you are competent. In most states, NCCAOM certification is a requirement for licensure.

The need for therapists is increasing due to the aging population of the United States. Older adults have an increased incidence of heart attack and stroke, both of which require therapy in the recovery process. Those who are 75 years of age and older have more disabling conditions. As a result, they require more therapeutic services. In addition, more patients with critical conditions or severe injuries are surviving because of medical advancements. These patients may need extensive therapy. However, federal legislation that limits reimbursement for therapy services may slow growth in therapy careers.

Education and Training for Therapy Careers

Most therapists need a bachelor's or graduate degree to practice. Therapy assistants often need an associate's degree. Therapy aides may require a specialized training course of one year or less.

Regardless of the type of degree, therapeutic workers develop their skills during **clinical training**. This volunteer work is part of their educational program. Although clinical training is required for all therapeutic workers, each type of therapy requires a unique education and training program supervised by a licensed healthcare provider. Note the differences in training and work responsibilities for the physical therapy and occupational therapy career ladders shown in **Figure 5.5**.

Workers can specialize within their chosen field of therapy as they learn new treatments or work with a specific patient population. For example, occupational therapists can train to become lymphedema (limf-uh-DEE-muh) therapists, who treat patients who have swollen limbs due to excess fluid in the tissues.

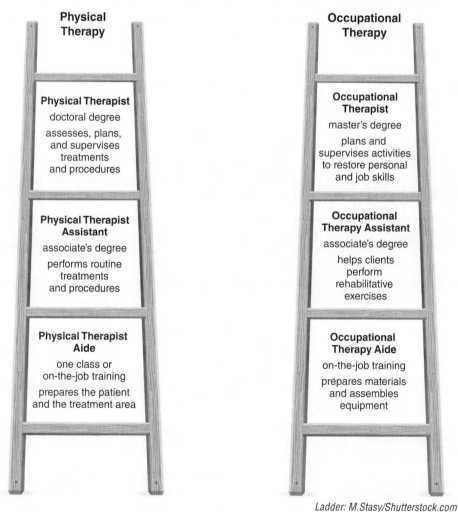

Physical Therapy

Physical Therapist
doctoral degree
assesses, plans, and supervises treatments and procedures

Physical Therapist Assistant
associate's degree
performs routine treatments and procedures

Physical Therapist Aide
one class or on-the-job training
prepares the patient and the treatment area

Occupational Therapy

Occupational Therapist
master's degree
plans and supervises activities to restore personal and job skills

Occupational Therapy Assistant
associate's degree
helps clients perform rehabilitative exercises

Occupational Therapy Aide
on-the-job training
prepares materials and assembles equipment

Ladder: M.Stasy/Shutterstock.com

Figure 5.5 Jobs at the top of the career ladder require more training and education, which generally means more responsibilities at work. In addition to their patient responsibilities, physical and occupational therapists supervise the work of their assistants and aides.

Physical therapists may specialize in working with patients who have spinal cord injuries or infants who have birth disorders, birth injuries, or delays in motor development.

5.1-3 Dental Careers

Job opportunities in dental careers are increasing rapidly. Why do you think this is? Did you think about our aging population? Older adults are keeping their natural teeth rather than getting dentures these days. This is a major reason for growth in the dental field.

Dentists

General dentists complete a bachelor's degree with an emphasis on science. They take the highly competitive dental admissions test before entering dental school. During their four years of dental school, students continue to study science and learn lab techniques for patient treatment. During the final two years of dental school, students treat patients in special clinics. They work under the supervision of a licensed dentist. Graduates must pass a licensing exam to practice dentistry.

Dentists can specialize in treating specific dental conditions by completing two to four years of additional **postgraduate** education after finishing dental school. For some specialties, a two-year postgraduate residency is required. During this time, the dentist practices the specialty under the supervision of an experienced specialist (**Figure 5.6**).

Dental Specialties

Public health dentist
- Provides dental health education and disease prevention

Prosthodontist
- Replaces missing teeth

Endodontist
- Treats the tooth root/root canal

Oral and maxillofacial pathologist/radiologist/surgeon
- Treats diseases and injuries to the mouth and jaw

Periodontist
- Treats diseases of the gums

Pediatric dentist
- Treats children

Orthodontist
- Straightens teeth

Goodheart-Willcox Publisher

Figure 5.6 Within the field of dentistry, there are specialties that you can pursue. *Can you identify some advantages and disadvantages of career specialization?*

Dentistry requires skill both in diagnosing dental conditions and working with your hands. Many dentists work in private practice. This means they also need good business sense, self-discipline, and communication skills to run their own businesses.

Hygienists, Therapists, and Assistants

While dentist jobs will be available as older dentists retire, much growth in dental careers is currently focused on dental hygienists and dental assistants. Hygienists complete an associate's degree. They work directly with patients to clean teeth, take oral X-rays, assess patient gum health, and teach patients good oral care practices. While there will be job openings for dental hygienists, about one-half of all hygienists work part-time. Dental hygiene is ideal for someone interested in a flexible work schedule.

A growing number of states are licensing dental therapists. These mid-level workers hold a master's degree and often work in areas where there is a shortage of dentists. They work under the supervision of a dentist. They can examine patients and provide routine dental treatments, such as fillings, sealants, and extracting first teeth.

Dental assisting is another fast-growing occupation. On-the-job training is still common in most states, but more dentists are looking for employees who have completed a six-month or one-year dental assisting training program. Requirements for licensure vary widely from state to state, so research your specific state regulations when preparing for this career.

Like medical assistants, dental assistants can perform a wide range of duties:

- Chairside assistants work directly with the dentist in the treatment area. They set up instrument trays, prepare the patient, and hand materials and instruments to the dentist.
- Laboratory assistants make casts of the teeth and mouth from impressions, clean and polish removable appliances, and make temporary crowns (**Figure 5.7**).
- Office assistants schedule and confirm appointments, receive patients, keep treatment records, send bills, receive payments, and order dental supplies and materials.

With additional education and work experience, dental assistants may work as claims approvers for insurance companies, dental office managers, or dental sales representatives.

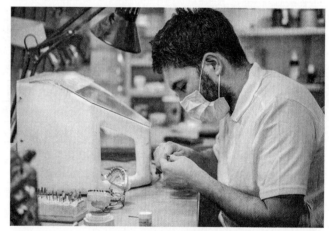

South_agency/E+ via Getty Images

Figure 5.7 Dental assistants can work in dental labs where they create crowns, mouthguards, retainers, and other dental appliances for patients.

5.1-4 Medical Careers

So, you want to become a doctor. To many students, the life of a physician seems glamorous. Physicians work in a highly respected profession and earn a high rate of pay. While this is true, you should consider every aspect of the profession before pursuing medicine.

Physicians

There are two types of physicians: the medical doctor (MD) and the doctor of osteopathic (ahs-tee-oh-PA-thihk) medicine (DO). Both MDs and DOs may use all accepted methods of treatment, including drugs and surgery. However, DOs place emphasis on the body's musculoskeletal system, preventive medicine, and holistic patient care. They are most likely to be primary care physicians. Medical doctors can work in one or more specialties (**Figure 5.8**). The *American Board of Medical Specialties* certifies physicians in 40 different specialties and 87 subspecialties.

Education and Training

The education and training requirements for physicians are among the most demanding of any occupation. Preparation begins with a bachelor's degree in a field of the student's choice. Science coursework is important, but a well-rounded education is an asset for anyone entering the field of medicine. Some students volunteer at local hospitals or clinics to gain practical experience in the health professions.

Application to medical school is highly competitive. Students must score well on the Medical College Admissions Test (MCAT). College transcripts and letters of recommendation are important. Schools also consider an applicant's character, personality, and leadership qualities. These can be demonstrated through extracurricular activities, including healthcare experiences. Most schools require an interview with members of the admissions committee.

Examples of Medical Specialties	
Specialty	**Treatment Areas**
Allergy and immunology	Immune system disorders such as asthma and AIDS
Anesthesiology	Pain relief for surgery
Dermatology	Disorders of the skin, hair, and nails
Diagnostic radiology	Use of radiation, ultrasound, and other methods to diagnose disease
Emergency medicine	Quick evaluation and action to prevent death
Family medicine	Comprehensive healthcare for the individual and family
General surgery	Disorders of the abdomen, digestive tract, and other systems
Internal medicine	Comprehensive care for adults and older adults
Medical genetics and genomics	Treatment for genetically linked diseases
Neurology	Diagnosis of brain and nervous system disorders
Nuclear medicine	Anatomic and molecular imaging for diagnosis
Obstetrics and gynecology	Care of pregnant people; evaluation and treatment of female reproductive health
Ophthalmology	Disorders of the eye
Pathology	Examination of tissue to diagnose disease
Pediatrics	Diseases and disorders in children
Physical medicine and rehabilitation	Treatment of patients with physical disabilities
Preventive medicine	Health promotion and disease prevention
Psychiatry	Diseases and disorders of the mind
Radiation oncology	Diagnosis of and treatment for cancerous tumors
Urology	Diseases of the kidney or bladder

Goodheart-Willcox Publisher

Figure 5.8 The Association of American Medical Colleges has identified more than 160 medical specialties and subspecialties.

The first two years of medical school are mostly classroom work, but the last two years include clinical or hands-on patient work under the supervision of a physician (**Figure 5.9**). During this time, students rotate through different specialties such as surgery, pediatrics, and neurology. They learn about each field so they can decide which interests them most. You may see these medical students in hospitals, but they have not finished their training and are not yet licensed doctors. Upon graduating from medical school, students add the MD or DO to their names and become residents.

After School

As they are finishing medical school, students apply for a residency program and hope they will be matched with the program of their choice. The term *resident* comes from the time when most residents lived on the hospital grounds to be on call at all times.

The term **intern** describes a student doctor completing rotations through various specialties in the first year of residency. To become licensed as specialists, these new doctors still have many more years of study, depending on their chosen field. For example, an internal medicine doctor will study for three more years, and a neurologist will study for six or seven more years. Some highly specialized programs and subspecialties, such as endocrinology or pediatric cardiology, can require even more training. These types of programs are known as **fellowships**.

Have you added up the years of education and training? A physician completes 11 to 14 years of training after high school before being licensed to practice medicine. This is a huge investment of time and money. Doctors do receive a small salary during residency, but most physicians have large school loans to repay when they begin to earn an income.

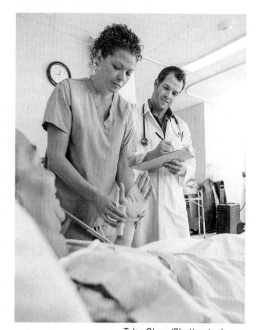

Tyler Olson/Shutterstock.com

Figure 5.9 Medical students receive hands-on training with physician supervision. *How does experience working in several different specialty areas benefit medical students?*

Finding a Job

Job prospects are best for primary care physicians and those willing to practice in rural and low-income areas. These medically underserved areas typically have difficulty attracting medical professionals. Physicians in specialties that treat the rapidly growing older population will also have better opportunities for employment. Emerging specialists such as hospitalists, cancer immunologists, and medical virtualists will create new opportunities.

Physician Assistants

Physician assistants (PAs) practice medicine under the supervision of a physician (**Figure 5.10**). They can diagnose, treat, and prescribe medication for patients. Each state determines the duties a PA may perform. Many PAs work in primary care areas such as internal medicine, pediatrics, or family medicine. They may also train to work in medical specialties. PAs work an average of 40 hours a week. They may work nights and weekends in a hospital setting. Physicians, by comparison, work long and irregular hours averaging more than 50 hours a week.

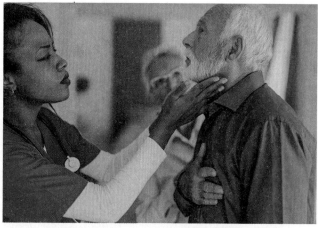

milan2099/E+ via Getty Images

Figure 5.10 A physician assistant works under the supervision of a physician. *What duties can a physician assistant perform?*

Whether you choose a physician or a physician assistant career, you must have a strong desire to serve patients, good bedside manner, emotional stability, and the ability to make decisions in an emergency. Do you enjoy learning? As a physician or PA, you will need to study medical advancements constantly to provide quality care for your patients.

While the job prospects for physicians are good, the job prospects for physician assistants are even better. Physician assistants begin their training with a bachelor's degree. Many PAs have prior experience as registered nurses, emergency medical technicians, and paramedics. Physician assistant schooling includes two years of classroom and lab training, along with clinical rotations in several areas. Graduates earn a master's degree and pass a national examination to become certified.

Other Doctors in Therapeutic Services

When you hear the word *doctor*, you probably think of an MD. However, many other therapeutic healthcare professionals also hold doctoral degrees. *Optometrists*, *chiropractors*, *veterinarians*, and *pharmacists* also have doctoral degrees. The Doctor of Optometry (OD), Doctor of Chiropractic (DC), and Doctor of Veterinary Medicine (DVM) use the word *doctor* in their title, but the Doctor of Pharmacy (PharmD) does not.

Advanced practice nurses and physical therapists may also obtain doctoral degrees. They may complete several years of education and training beyond a bachelor's degree to prepare for a chosen healthcare profession or to advance their professional skills.

5.1-5 **Nursing Careers**

You may plan to become a pediatric nurse, but why limit yourself? The nursing field has an incredible variety of job opportunities. Nursing has the largest number of job openings and employs more workers than any other healthcare occupation (**Figure 5.11**).

Nursing also has a well-developed career ladder. At the entry level, home health aides work to assist their clients with daily activities. After completing a nursing assisting class and passing a certification test, a person becomes a **certified nursing assistant (CNA)**. CNAs work in assisted living facilities, nursing homes, and hospitals providing basic nursing care to patients and residents.

At the next level, a **licensed practical nurse (LPN)** or *licensed vocational nurse (LVN)* completes a one-year technical training program and can perform additional nursing tasks such as giving injections, monitoring catheters, and dressing wounds. Each state determines the specific care skills an LPN may perform. There are still many job openings for LPNs. LPNs may also continue nurses' training for a second year and complete an associate's degree in nursing.

A **registered nurse (RN)** has either an associate's degree in nursing (ADN) or a bachelor's of science in nursing (BSN). Regardless of their degree,

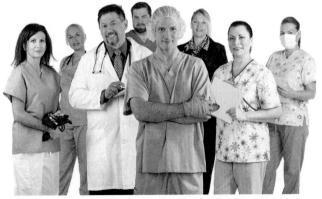

Alina555/E+ via Getty Images

Figure 5.11 The field of nursing offers many healthcare job opportunities. *What are some job titles that appear on nursing's career ladder?*

these nurses take the same examination and have the same license to practice. Individuals who complete a BSN receive more training in areas such as communication, leadership, and critical thinking. These skills are becoming more important as nursing practice becomes more complex. A bachelor's degree or higher is often necessary for administrative, research, consulting, and teaching positions.

Advanced practice nurses need at least a master's degree. These positions include clinical nurse specialists (CNSs), nurse practitioners (NPs), registered nurse anesthetists (a-NEHS-theh-tists) (RNAs), and certified nurse midwives (CNMs). Many programs now offer a doctor of nursing practice (DNP) degree as well. Nurses who are already working can often take advantage of tuition reimbursement from their employers to advance their education and earn a bachelor's, master's, or doctoral degree.

Using orders from the physician and input from other team members, nurses establish a care plan for the patient and make sure the plan is carried out. They perform a variety of tasks, including but certainly not limited to the following:

- administering medications, carefully checking dosages, and avoiding interactions between certain types of medication
- starting, maintaining, and discontinuing intravenous (IV) lines
- administering therapies and treatments
- observing the patient and recording those observations
- consulting with physicians and other healthcare clinicians

Registered nurses also delegate or assign nursing tasks appropriate to the training of their team members and supervise the work of the LPNs and CNAs on their care team.

Today's nurses are assuming more technically challenging roles. As a result, nurses are becoming more specialized in the work they perform (**Figure 5.12**).

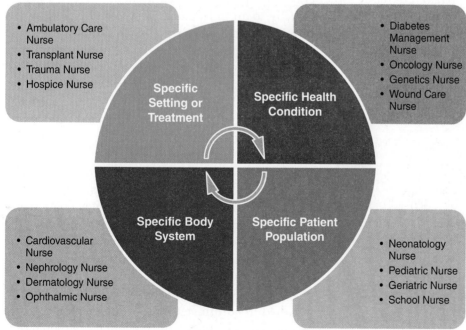

Goodheart-Willcox Publisher

Figure 5.12 Nurses are becoming increasingly specialized, so their duties can vary widely. This diagram shows examples of nursing careers arranged by four categories of specialization.

The duties of RNs vary widely and are often determined by their work setting or the patient population they serve. Registered nurses can specialize by

- working in a particular setting or with a particular type of treatment;
- specializing in a specific health condition;
- working with a specific body system; and
- working with a specific patient population.

Some nurses have jobs that require an RN license but include little or no direct patient care. A forensic (fuh-REHN-zihk) nurse does provide care to people who have been subjected to crimes, collects evidence after crimes occur, and provides care to patients within the prison system. However, infection control nurses track and work to reduce infectious outbreaks in healthcare facilities. Nurse informaticists manage and communicate nursing data to improve healthcare decisions. These nurses do not provide direct care to patients.

If you have an interest in caring for people, take the time to research a career in nursing. Because there are so many opportunities in this field, you are almost certain to find one that fits your skills and interests.

5.1-6 Personal Services Careers

As people age, they often require more assistance with personal care. Because most individuals want to stay in their homes as they age, there is a growing need for personal care services delivered in client's homes or smaller residential facilities within communities. The following service workers play a therapeutic role in the health and well-being of clients, residents, and their families.

Personal Care Attendants/Home Health Aides

There are many job openings for personal care attendants. These workers provide personal service directly to an individual. They usually work in clients' homes, where they provide basic healthcare and household assistance for older patients and those with disabilities (**Figure 5.13**). Providing companionship and noticing changes in the client's condition are key components of the job. Some workers live in the client's home, while others travel to the homes of several clients at scheduled times.

Although no formal education is needed to become a personal care attendant, many agencies and some states require candidates to have licensure or certification. Agencies employ some workers, but many are self-employed. The client or the client's family hires the specific care worker. Home health aides typically have some medical training and are certified. While they provide the same services as a personal care attendant, they may also be trained to administer medication or monitor vital signs. The job outlook is excellent for personal care workers, but pay remains low for these positions.

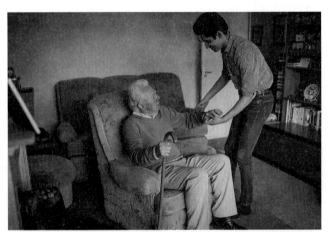

DGLimages/iStock/Getty Images Plus via Getty Images

Figure 5.13 Personal care attendants provide a variety of care services, often inside a client's home.

Cosmetologists

Cosmetologists are also personal care workers. Cosmetology enhances a client's appearance through treating the hair, skin, and nails. You may picture these workers at businesses in our communities, but they may also have connections to a healthcare residential facility. Many cosmetologists spend part of their workday at a residential care facility providing the same services they offer in a salon. Some travel to clients' homes to provide haircare or other services. A few work in funeral homes providing hair and makeup care for memorial services. Cosmetologists complete an approved training program that includes supervised clinical experience before they obtain state licensure to work in the field. Licensing requirements vary by state. Job openings are growing in this occupation as current workers transition to other careers or retire.

While training programs for home health aides and cosmetologists focus on the skills required to provide care services, personal care workers will also benefit from small business training. If self-employed, they must negotiate fees, collect payments, secure liability insurance, prepare marketing materials, and keep careful and confidential records of client information and business transactions.

Mortuary Science Workers

You might not associate death with healthcare services, but funeral home directors provide an important service for grieving families. Funeral directors, also called **morticians** (mor-TIH-shuhns) and *undertakers*, manage funeral homes and arrange the details of a funeral. They provide transportation of the deceased and submit paperwork and legal documents. They assist the family in planning wakes, memorial services, and burials. Because funeral practices vary among cultures and religions, morticians must be sensitive to family needs when determining whether a body will be entombed, cremated, or buried.

Funeral directors complete an associate's or bachelor's degree in mortuary science. Following an apprenticeship of one to three years, they must pass a qualifying exam to become licensed. Because the mood is consistently somber, the work of a mortician can be stressful. Funeral directors must arrange the details of a funeral within 24 to 72 hours of death and may be responsible for multiple funerals on the same day. Employment opportunities in this field are more favorable for those willing to relocate for available job openings.

Technical Workers in Therapeutic Services

The number of therapeutic technical workers is increasing. According to the Bureau of Labor Statistics, the following therapeutic healthcare careers require an associate's degree or less training:

- dental hygienist and dental assistant
- home health aide
- occupational therapy aide and assistant
- pharmacy technician (**Figure 5.14**)
- physical therapy aide and assistant
- veterinary technician

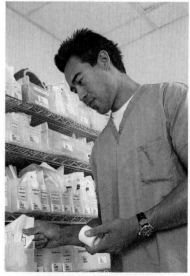

bikeriderlondon/Shutterstock.com

Figure 5.14 Pharmacy technician is one example of a technical position in the therapeutic pathway.

These careers offer opportunities for students who do not wish to pursue a professional degree. Typically, the job prospects for these careers will be good.

Therapeutic services offers a multitude of job choices. Whether you want on-the-job training or are ready to study for several years, you can find a career in therapeutic services.

Lesson 5.1 Review

 Complete the *Map Your Reading* graphic organizer for the section you just read.

1. Therapeutic workers can recognize and identify with another person's feelings and thoughts. This trait is called (5.1-1)
   A. tact
   B. calmness
   C. stamina
   D. empathy

2. When discussing a sensitive subject, workers use (5.1-1)
   A. tact
   B. calmness
   C. stamina
   D. empathy

3. Making a plan to improve work performance following an evaluation shows the ability to (5.1-1)
   A. become a team player
   B. overcome disappointment
   C. find fault with a supervisor
   D. accept criticism

4. Therapeutic healthcare services focus on changing which of the following? Choose the best answer. (5.1-2)
   A. Emotional well-being
   B. Social interaction
   C. Physical stamina
   D. Health status

5. To reduce costs, healthcare facilities are using more _____ workers. (5.1-2)
   A. certified
   B. professional
   C. licensed
   D. technical

6. Which of the following is a technical therapeutic occupation? (5.1-3)
   A. Physician
   B. Nurse practitioner
   C. Dental hygienist
   D. Pharmacist

7. Which of these professionals completes the longest education and training program? (5.1-4)
   A. Ophthalmologists
   B. Registered nurses
   C. Pharmacists
   D. Dentists

8. Which type of nurse delegates tasks to the LPNs and CNAs on a nursing team? (5.1-5)
   A. Certified nursing assistant
   B. Registered nurse
   C. Licensed practical nurse
   D. All of these.

9. _____ is not a job task of a personal care attendant. (5.1-6)
   A. Providing companionship
   B. Giving pain injections
   C. Preparing meals
   D. Assisting with dressing

Technical Skills in Therapeutic Services

Learning Outcomes

After studying this lesson, you will be able to

5.2-1 demonstrate dressing and undressing a patient with a weak arm and verbalize your reaction to providing close personal care.

5.2-2 list preprocedure and postprocedure care actions and explain their purposes.

5.2-3 practice performing passive range of motion for the hand.

5.2-4 explain the steps for filling a prescription.

5.2-5 relate the purpose for and demonstrate proper technique for putting on and removing sterile gloves.

5.2-6 explain how HOSA participation can build your professional skills and which competitive events can improve your therapeutic skills.

Professional Vocabulary

Essential Terms

contamination   the unwanted presence of harmful substances or microorganisms

range of motion (ROM)   the full extent of movement for a joint

Important Terms

contraindicated

sterile technique

> **? ESSENTIAL QUESTION**
>
> *How well do the technical skills in this lesson match your work interests and preferences?*

Introduction

In difficult situations, do you find yourself taking care of others? If a family member gets sick, are you the one who cares for them? A desire to help and take care of people is important for those in the therapeutic services career pathway. You have likely encountered therapeutic workers at the dentist's office, in hospitals, and at doctors' offices. Therapeutic services workers are dedicated to helping others through direct contact with patients.

If you want to help patients by providing care and treatment to improve their health, consider a therapeutic services career. In this lesson, you will learn the patient interaction guidelines that promote patient safety and comfort while protecting patient rights. You will also practice a common therapeutic task from the fields of nursing, therapy, and pharmacy. As you practice these new skills, think about your preferences. Do any of these career fields appeal to you?

When asked about his job as a nursing assistant, Darius smiled his slow grin and said, "I like it." Darius' journey to a therapeutic career began back in high school. His girlfriend's mom was a nurse, and she talked to him about healthcare job opportunities. He decided to take the *Introduction to Healthcare Careers* class

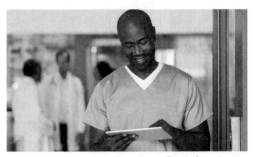

shapecharge/E+ via Getty Images

offered at his high school. He liked the idea of a diagnostics job and thought he might like to become an X-ray technician.

Around that same time, Darius' friend from the football team, who was interested in nursing, convinced him to sign up for the nursing assistant class. There were some things Darius was unsure of as he studied the duties of a nursing assistant. He was not sure of his ability to give a bed bath, but training at a nursing home helped him master these tasks. His clinical instructor at the nursing home gave him some good insights into caring for another person.

After passing his state certification test, Darius got a part-time job at the nursing home where he completed his training. Within a few months, he realized he really enjoyed caring for people, and his employer had already noticed his skills. His calm demeanor; patience with people; and slow, easy grin made him a favorite with the residents. As a result of his education, training, and experience in the field, Darius chose the therapeutic pathway and a career as a registered nurse.

5.2-1 Dressing and Undressing

Many therapeutic workers provide close personal care for their patients. As a nurse or therapist, you need to feel comfortable with providing a caring touch to another person. Practicing basic steps for dressing and undressing will help you develop this skill. In this activity, you will help a patient with a weak arm put on and take off a button-front shirt. Notice how it feels to invade a patient's personal space.

The first step is getting authorization from your supervisor. Sometimes, normal care tasks are **contraindicated** (kahn-truh-IHN-duh-kay-ted). This means the patient has a particular condition that makes normal care tasks uncomfortable or dangerous. For example, a patient with an open foot sore could not soak his foot in water during bathing. Bacteria in the water could enter his body through the open sore. So, taking a bath is contraindicated for this patient. In the skill that follows, your patient has a weak arm. This means you will take special steps to protect the arm when dressing or undressing the patient.

Once you have authorization, you can prepare for dressing your patient. Begin by performing hand hygiene before entering the patient's room. Either wash your hands or use hand gel. Assemble your supplies and knock on the patient's door before entering the room. Always introduce yourself and make sure you have the correct patient by saying the patient's name and checking the ID band. Explain your care task and provide privacy by closing the door and lowering window blinds Now you can begin providing care. For this activity, practice both putting on and removing a shirt as one task.

Dressing

1. Put on gloves if required for infection control. Do either you or your patient have non-intact skin? Is there a possibility of exposure to blood or other body fluids?
2. Your patient is mobile (able to sit, stand, and walk independently) and sitting on the edge of the bed or in a chair. Assist her to sit up and forward in the chair.
3. Your patient has a weak right arm. Insert your hand through the right sleeve of the shirt and grasp the patient's hand. Then slide the shirt onto the weak arm and shoulder (**Figure 5.15**).
4. Bring the shirt around the patient's back. Then ask the patient to slide the stronger arm into the other sleeve (**Figure 5.16**).
5. Adjust the shirt and close the buttons.

Pretend that your patient changes her mind and wants to wear a different shirt, so you will remove the shirt you just put on. Reverse the steps to remove the shirt.

Undressing

1. Continue to wear gloves if required.
2. Assist your patient to sit up and forward if seated in a chair.
3. Unfasten buttons and remove the shirt from the stronger arm first.
4. Bring the shirt around the patient's back and slide the sleeve off the weaker arm last. Do not force any arm movements or pull on your patient's arm.

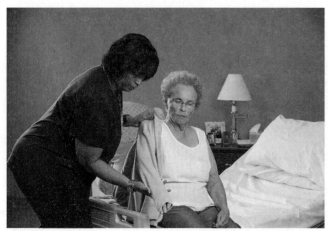

© Tori Soper Photography

Figure 5.15

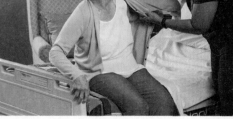

© Tori Soper Photography

Figure 5.16

When you have finished the procedure, make sure your patient is in a safe and comfortable position. Place the call signal within reach. Clean and store your equipment. For safety reasons, check to see that the room is free of clutter or spills. Open the window blinds and the door. Next, wash your hands. Finally, report and record the completion of your care task.

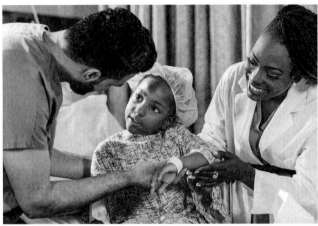

kali9/E+ via Getty Images

Figure 5.17 Preprocedure and postprocedure actions are intended to improve a patient's care. *What pre- or postprocedure actions are shown in this image?*

5.2-2 Patient Interaction Guidelines

As you followed the steps for dressing and undressing, did you notice you were learning additional requirements associated with patient care, such as identifying your patient and providing privacy? You should follow specific steps before and after any care procedure. Preprocedure actions promote safety and courtesy while protecting the patient's or resident's rights. Postprocedure actions provide for patient comfort, safety, and communication among healthcare team members. Caregivers learn the following steps to perform before and after every care procedure (**Figure 5.17**).

Preprocedure Actions

Memorize these steps and complete them before providing care.

1. Seek authorization and special care instructions from your supervisor.
2. Perform hand hygiene.
3. Gather your supplies.
4. Knock and identify yourself by name and title.
5. Identify and greet the patient.
6. Explain the procedure. Answer questions and ask for permission to provide care.
7. Provide privacy.
8. Perform hand hygiene and use standard precautions.
9. Follow safety precautions for the use of equipment.

Postprocedure Actions

Memorize these steps and complete them after providing care.

1. Make sure the bed wheels are locked. Provide for the patient's comfort and good body alignment.
2. Leave the call button within the patient's reach.
3. Lower the bed and position the side rails as required.
4. Open the curtain or door according to the patient's preference.
5. Wash your hands.
6. Report and record your care actions.

5.2-3 Range-of-Motion (ROM) Exercises

Range-of-motion (ROM) exercises preserve joint and muscle function for a patient whose movement is limited (**Figure 5.18**). These exercises put each joint through its full range of motion and repeat each movement three to five times. When they are not used, muscles become weak, and joints become stiff.

General Guidelines for ROM Exercises

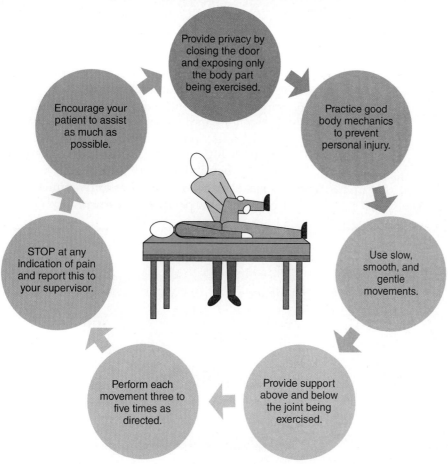

Goodheart-Willcox Publisher

Figure 5.18 Follow these general guidelines for performing all range-of-motion exercises. *When might range-of-motion exercises be used?*

Eventually, a contracture may occur (**Figure 5.19**). In this condition, the muscle is permanently shortened, and the affected joint cannot move.

In some cases, patients do their own exercises. This is called *active ROM*. Sometimes patients can do the exercises but need assistance to achieve full range. This is called *active assistive ROM*. *Passive ROM* means the patient needs another person to move each joint.

Before working with a patient, healthcare workers must check with their supervisor to find out which range-of-motion exercises will be performed and if there are any limitations to the exercises. For example, after a hip or knee replacement, certain exercises are restricted.

Healthcare workers must also be aware of their scope of practice regarding ROM exercises. For example, in some states or certain facilities, nursing assistants are not allowed to perform ROM exercises for the neck.

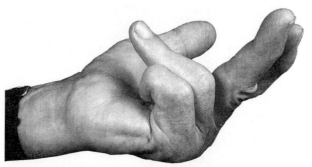

Biophoto Associates/Science Source

Figure 5.19 In the condition known as a *contracture*, an unused muscle is permanently shortened, and use of the joint is lost. The type of contracture pictured here, in which the bent fingers cannot be straightened, usually affects the pinkie and ring fingers and occurs most frequently among older males.

Practice performing passive ROM for the hand by following these steps:

1. Complete the preprocedure actions you learned in the previous section.
2. Position the patient comfortably.
3. Hold the patient's hand with one of your own. Use your other hand to hold the patient's thumb. Move the thumb gently away from the index finger and back again. Then touch the thumb to the tip of each finger (**Figure 5.20A**). Never force the joint beyond its limit. ROM exercises should not produce pain.
4. Hold the patient's fingers together with one hand. With your other hand, move each finger apart and back again (**Figure 5.20B**).
5. Support the patient's wrist with one hand. Use your other hand to bend the patient's fingers, making a fist. Tuck the thumb under the fingers (**Figure 5.20C**). Then straighten each finger and the thumb individually (**Figure 5.20D**).
6. Repeat each movement three to five times.
7. Complete your postprocedure actions.

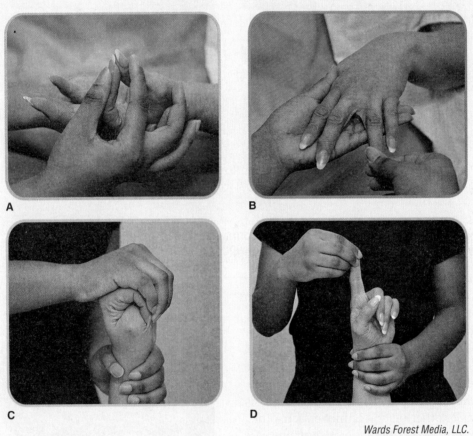

A

B

C

D

Wards Forest Media, LLC.

Figure 5.20

5.2-4 **Preparing a Medication**

The pharmacy technician is also a therapeutic healthcare worker. Filling a prescription is one of the most important and common duties a pharmacy technician performs. With the increased use of electronic medical records, many prescriptions are automatically sent to the pharmacy. Patients bring other prescriptions to the pharmacy. There are specific steps involved with filling a prescription. Note that each step that begins with a plus sign (+) is a point at which the technician rechecks the prescription to avoid medication errors. Attention to detail is very important in the work of a pharmacy technician.

+ The technician's first task is to make sure the prescription lists the correct information. It must list the patient's full name, the medication name and dosage, directions for taking the medication, the physician's signature, and refill information. Since more than one customer may have the same name, the technician checks additional information to make sure it is the correct patient. The prescription must also be current, not outdated.

Next, the technician translates the physician's written prescription. During this step, the technician consults with the pharmacist to interpret any prescriptions that are difficult to read. Computerized systems have greatly reduced the problem of reading a physician's poor handwriting. Finally, the technician enters a nonelectronic prescription into the computer program.

The computer prints a prescription label, which the pharmacist checks for accuracy. The pharmacist also checks other medications the patient is taking. If drug interactions are possible, the pharmacist contacts the physician.

PROCEDURE   Filling a Prescription

A technician should follow these steps to fill the prescription:

1. Select the correct medication from the stock shelf area. + Check the bottle label and national drug code number in the computer to make sure it matches the prescription.
2. Count out the necessary amount of the medication and fill the vial, taking care not to touch the medication. Select and attach the correct lid based on size and the patient's preference for a childproof or easy-open lid.
3. + Attach the label to the vial and initial the bottom right-hand side of the printed label.
4. Attach auxiliary labels. These give additional information, such as whether the medication needs to be taken with water or on an empty stomach.
5. + Set the medication on top of the original prescription.
6. Present the medication to the pharmacist for final approval (**Figure 5.21**).

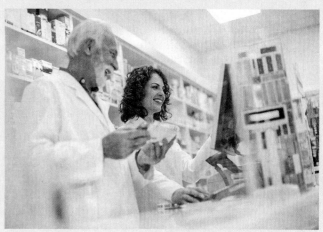

GoodLifeStudios/E+ via Getty Images

Figure 5.21   A pharmacy technician must get final approval on prescriptions from his or her supervising pharmacist.

When the patient picks up the prescription, the pharmacist checks it one more time. The pharmacist consults with each patient to answer questions and explain information about the medication. When the pharmacist has finished, the technician can ring up the sale. In some cases, the technician also gets the signature of the person picking up the prescription as part of required recordkeeping.

5.2-5 **Sterile Gloving**

DeShawn is a medical assistant at a healthcare clinic. Today he is assisting the physician with open wound care for a patient. Unlike gloving for standard precautions, this procedure requires **sterile techniques**. This means sterile instruments will be used, and a sterile field will be created. DeShawn will perform very thorough handwashing and put on sterile gloves. He will take extra steps to prevent **contamination** of gloves and equipment as he assists the physician. Open wounds and surgical procedures provide an easy route for microorganisms that cause infection to enter the body. Sterile techniques seek to eliminate all potential microorganisms in a sterile field and keep objects as free from microorganisms as possible.

PROCEDURE | **Putting On and Removing Sterile Gloves**

Follow these steps for putting on and removing sterile gloves:

Putting On Sterile Gloves

1. Remove all rings and watches and perform hand hygiene.
2. Select a package of sterile gloves. Check for correct size and expiration date. Make sure the package is dry and has no holes or tears.
3. Place the glove package on a dry, flat, clean work surface at waist level.
4. Peel the outer package apart and place the inner package on your work surface.
5. Open the top flap away from your body and the bottom flap toward your body. Touch only the outside edges of the packaging.
6. Open the side flaps without touching the inside of the wrapper. Fingers of gloves should face away from you. Cuffs will face toward you (**Figure 5.22**).

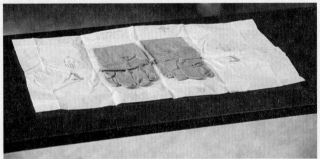

© Tori Soper Photography

Figure 5.22

7. Use the thumb and index finger on your nondominant hand to grasp the wrong side of the glove at the cuff on the glove for your dominant hand. Lift and carefully pull the glove over your hand (**Figure 5.23**). Do not touch any surfaces. Do not touch the outside of the glove.

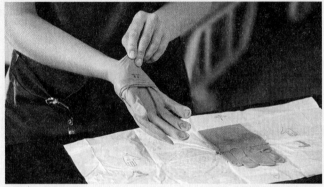

© Tori Soper Photography

Figure 5.23

8. Carefully slide the fingers on your gloved hand under the cuff on the right side of the remaining glove. Do not let your thumb touch the glove (**Figure 5.24**).

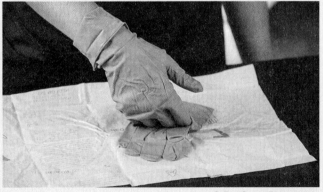

© Tori Soper Photography

Figure 5.24

(continued)

9. Carefully insert your bare hand into the glove without touching the outside surface and use your gloved fingers to pull the second glove over your hand. Examine gloves to make sure there are no tears or holes.
10. Interlock gloved fingers to prevent touching nonsterile items. Take care to keep your hands above your waist.

Removing Sterile Gloves

1. Grasp the outside of one cuff with the other gloved hand. Avoid touching your skin.

2. Pull the glove off, turning it inside out, and hold it in the palm of the gloved hand. Do not touch the contaminated side of the glove with your bare hand.
3. Slide the index finger of your bare hand inside the other glove cuff and peel the glove off, turning it inside out over the glove removed first. Again, be careful not to touch the contaminated side of the glove with your bare hand.
4. Dispose of contaminated gloves into the appropriate waste container.
5. Perform hand hygiene.

5.2-6 HOSA Connections

HOSA provides many opportunities to build your professional skills, as well as your therapeutic skills. When you attend HOSA state and international conferences you will wear professional clothing and interact with other members in a professional development setting. General sessions, speaker sessions, and voting sessions introduce you to the work of a professional organization. Several HOSA competitive events such as nursing assisting or sports medicine can strengthen your therapeutic skills. Read about all of these in the *competitive events* section of the HOSA website.

Lesson 5.2 Review

 Complete the *Map Your Reading* graphic organizer for the section you just read.

1. Because many therapeutic workers provide close personal care for their patients, they must become _____ with giving a caring touch to another person. (5.2-1)
   A. efficient C. comfortable
   B. resigned D. concerned
2. When dressing and undressing a patient with a weak arm, the _____ arm goes into the sleeve first when dressing and comes out of the sleeve last when undressing. (5.2-1)
   A. weak C. right
   B. strong D. left
3. Which of the following do preprocedure and postprocedure care steps preserve? Choose all that apply. (5.2-2)
   A. Patient safety C. Patient privileges
   B. Patient comfort D. Patient rights
4. The purpose of performing range-of-motion exercises is to preserve _____ function. (5.2-3)
   A. joint and muscle
   B. tendon and ligament
   C. blood flow and heartrate
   D. bone and cartilage

5. The pharmacy technician may prepare a medication, but a _____ answers patient questions. (5.2-4)
   A. physician
   B. triage nurse
   C. pharmacist
   D. pharmacy consultant
6. When are sterile gloves used? Choose the most correct answer. (5.2-5)
   A. Preventing infection
   B. Protecting the worker
   C. Infection can enter the body easily
   D. Microorganisms are present in the environment
7. Which of the following describes a professional skill rather than a technical skill? Choose all that apply. (5.2-6)
   A. Appropriate clothing
   B. Attending a conference voting session
   C. Performing first aid
   D. Appropriate behavior

Chapter 5 Review and Assessment

Chapter Summary

5.1-1 Therapeutic services workers enjoy working with people. They interact with patients to provide care and treatments.

5.1-1 Therapeutic workers must be skilled at showing empathy and using tact when communicating with patients.

5.1-1 Healthcare workers are dependable and willing to accept criticism.

5.1-2 As a cost-saving measure, therapeutic tasks are increasingly being delegated to workers with technical training such as therapy assistants and pharmacy technicians.

5.1-3 Job opportunities in dental careers are rapidly increasing as the use of dentures in older adults is declining.

5.1-4 The education and training requirements for physicians are among the most demanding of any occupation.

5.1-5 Nursing has the largest number of job openings and employs more workers than any other healthcare occupation. Nurses can receive technical training or professional levels of education and training.

5.1-6 Personal care workers assist with personal care and household tasks to preserve client health and well-being.

5.2-1 Since many therapeutic workers provide close personal care for their patients, they must become comfortable with giving caring touch to another person.

5.2-2 Preprocedure and postprocedure actions provide for patient safety and comfort while protecting patient rights.

5.2-3 Range-of-motion exercises preserve joint and muscle function for a patient with limited movement. Support the resident's hand as you gently move each joint through its full range of motion.

5.2-4 The pharmacy technician completes several checks to maintain accuracy when filling a prescription.

5.2-5 Sterile gloves are used when caring for open wounds, during surgical procedures, and any time there is an easy route for infection to enter the patient's body.

5.2-6 Attending HOSA conferences provides opportunities for building professional skills, and competitive events such as nursing assisting and sports medicine can improve therapeutic skills.

Maximize Your Professional Vocabulary

1. **Your Own Words.** Read the text passages that contain each of the terms in the chapter. Then write the definitions of each term in your own words. Double-check your definitions by re-reading the text and using the text glossary.

2. **Hollywood Squares Terms Review.** The teacher will select nine students to be the "celebrities" and then divide the remaining students into two teams. Each celebrity holds a large card marked with an O on one side and an X on the other. Three students sit on chairs placed at the front of the classroom, three sit on the floor in front of the chairs, and three stand behind to simulate the tic-tac-toe board. Contestants from each team take turns selecting a celebrity to answer a question for them. The contestants must then agree or disagree with their celebrity's answer. Each team tries to create a row of Xs or Os to win. Rotate contestants after each vocabulary question and rotate celebrities after each game to allow all students to participate.

Reflect on Your Reading

1. Review the list of 10 occupations you created for the *Connect with Your Reading* activity. How many of those occupations are in the therapeutic pathway? Use the career chart available on the National Consortium for Health Science Education (NCHSE) website to check your list.

2. For each therapeutic occupation on your list, indicate whether it requires technical training (two years or less) or professional training (four years or more). Mark the occupations on your list you believe will provide good job opportunities in the future. Be prepared to discuss your list with your classmates.

Review and Recall

1. Ruby's patient is experiencing significant pain and complains loudly about Ruby's care. Ruby thinks about what the patient is experiencing and reacts calmly to the patient's complaints. Which two personal traits is Ruby exhibiting? (5.1-1)
   - A. Tact
   - B. Patience
   - C. Empathy
   - D. Stamina

2. Mital must convince the mother of her patient with diabetes not to bring unhealthy treats to the hospital. This task requires (5.1-1)
   - A. tact
   - B. patience
   - C. empathy
   - D. stamina

3. Select all the traits exhibited by dependable healthcare workers. (5.1-1)
   - A. Responds promptly to patient needs
   - B. Maintains personal health
   - C. Uses all sick leave
   - D. Is a team player

4. It is important for therapeutic workers to be able to _____ so they can improve their job performance and have a successful career. (5.1-1)
   - A. delegate
   - B. accept criticism
   - C. attend training
   - D. outsource

5. Therapeutic workers develop their skills during _____ as part of their educational program. (5.1-2)
   - A. clinical training
   - B. postgraduate studies
   - C. volunteer work
   - D. classroom work

6. _____ make casts of the teeth and mouth from impressions, clean and polish removable appliances, and make temporary crowns. (5.1-3)
   - A. Chairside assistants
   - B. Laboratory assistants
   - C. Office assistants
   - D. Dentists

7. The term _____ describes a student doctor completing rotations through various specialties in their first year of residency. (5.1-4)
   - A. resident
   - B. fellow
   - C. intern
   - D. trainee

8. Which of the following is considered an advanced practice nurse? (5.1-5)
   - A. Registered nurse
   - B. Certified nursing assistant
   - C. Nurse practitioner
   - D. Licensed practical nurse

9. What is the lowest educational requirement for personal care attendants? (5.1-6)
   - A. Master's degree
   - B. Bachelor's degree
   - C. Associate's degree
   - D. High school diploma

10. Sometimes normal care tasks are _____ for patients, meaning the task could be uncomfortable or dangerous for them. (5.2-1)
    - A. contaminated
    - B. unauthorized
    - C. contraindicated

11. Which actions promote safety and courtesy while protecting the patient's or resident's rights? (5.2-2)
    - A. Preprocedure
    - B. Postprocedure

12. Which actions provide for patient comfort, safety, and communication among healthcare team members? (5.2-2)
    - A. Preprocedure
    - B. Postprocedure

13. _____ exercises preserve joint and muscle function for a patient who is unable to move independently. (5.2-3)
    - A. Active ROM
    - B. Active assistive ROM
    - C. Passive ROM
    - D. None of these.

14. What information should be listed on a prescription? (5.2-4)
    - A. Patient's height, weight, and ethnicity
    - B. Patient's full name, medication name, dosage, directions, and refill information
    - C. Patient's address and pharmacy address
    - D. All of these.
15. In sterile gloving, you should *not* (5.2-5)
    - A. put on both gloves
    - B. remove all rings
    - C. wash your hands first
    - D. touch the outside of the glove
16. Which of these HOSA competitive events will strengthen therapeutic skills? (5.2-6)
    - A. Prepared speaking
    - B. Job-seeking skills
    - C. Nursing assisting
    - D. Parliamentary procedure

Build Core Skills

1. **Writing.** Review the section in this chapter that discusses personal traits for therapeutic workers. Think about your own life and write a paragraph about a personal experience in which you were empathetic, dependable, or showed the ability to accept criticism.
2. **Problem Solving.** Which type of medical specialist would each of these people see?
    - A. Jim, a three-year-old, has a high fever.
    - B. Mr. Jones is experiencing symptoms of depression following his divorce.
    - C. Mr. Rogers needs to learn what a particular shadow on his X-ray means.
    - D. Kim's eyes are not focusing and they are red and itchy.
    - E. Regina has developed Parkinson's disease.
3. **Critical Thinking.** Create a five-point chart to compare two occupations: physician and physician assistant. As you prepare your chart, consider the following topics: education and training, work environment, job outlook, job tasks and responsibilities, and earnings. Based on your comparison, which occupation would you like to·pursue? Why?
4. **Critical Thinking.** Review the section in this chapter on nursing careers to identify the job tasks for a certified nursing assistant, licensed practical nurse/licensed vocational nurse, registered nurse, and nurse practitioner. Review the career ladder for nursing.

Then list all nurses qualified to complete each of the following tasks:
- A. making a hospital bed
- B. diagnosing a patient condition
- C. giving a vaccination
- D. writing a prescription
- E. providing wound care
- F. assisting with ambulation
- G. feeding a patient
- H. training nursing students

5. **Speaking and Listening.** Review the preprocedure actions found in the text. Then read the statements made by the healthcare worker. Identify two verbal items that are missing.

   Hi, Mrs. Bridges. My name is Dan. I am going to help you with your exercises this morning. Do you have any questions?
6. **Critical Thinking.** Review the information about ROM exercises. Then state the purpose for ROM and explain the three basic types of ROM exercises.

Activate Your Learning

1. Review the steps for dressing and undressing a patient. Then practice putting on and removing a shirt for a patient with a weak left arm.
2. Review the steps for filling a prescription. Then copy the sample label shown here and practice filling the following prescription for Jane Doe.

Star Prairie Clinic
Dr. John Smith
333 Clinic Street
Star Prairie, TX 74260
123-701-3000
Medication: 500mg M&M tablets
Three times each day for three days
to treat fungal infection
NO REFILLS
Signature: *Dr. John Smith*

Prescription

Star Prairie Pharmacy   Date _____
123 Clinic St.
Star Prairie, TX 74260
123-701-5000
Patient's Name _____
Medication _____
Direction _____
_____
# of tablets _____
NO REFILLS   Rx# 345678

Label
Goodheart-Willcox Publisher

3. Explain when sterile gloves are used. Then, practice the steps for putting on sterile gloves without contaminating them. Next, remove the gloves without further contaminating your hands or clothing.

Think and Act Like a Healthcare Worker

1. Sasha was excited to get a part-time job in a dental office. She always wanted to become a dental hygienist and knew this would be the perfect opportunity to expand her knowledge and skills while still in high school. Two months later, she was having doubts about her career choice. She did not think she could perform the same tasks every day as part of her job. Reference Appendix A: Career Personality Types. Which John Holland personality type finds satisfaction in dental careers? What are the primary work tasks of the dental hygienist? What would you suggest Sasha do next to prepare for a satisfying healthcare career?

Go to the Source

1. Use the internet to learn more about careers in therapeutic services. Select two careers of interest to you and complete a career profile page for each career. Use at least one website that ends in .gov and one that ends in .org. Record the following information for each career:
   • name of the career
   • tasks involved in this career
   • personal traits and abilities needed
   • educational requirements
   • type of credential needed and how it is obtained
   • work conditions
   • wages and benefits
   • job outlook for the future
   • the websites you accessed

   How do the two careers compare? Why might you prefer one to the other?
2. Research HOSA competitive events. Use the HOSA website for this activity. Which events develop therapeutic skills? Select and note your top choice event. List the reasons for your choice.

HOSA Event Prep: Clinical Nursing

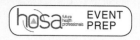

Norma, a nurse practitioner at the children's hospital, is seeing Charli, a five-year-old patient with fever, cough, congestion, and irritability. This patient weighs 25 kg. Vital signs are temperature—102.2 degrees, pulse—112 bpm, respirations—40 breaths per minute, blood pressure—100/50 mmHg, oxygen saturation—90% on room air (RA). Lungs sound coarse with stridor (high-pitched sound), and the patient has a harsh, barky cough. Norma orders a
   • chest X-ray;
   • complete blood count (CBC);
   • cool, humidified oxygen to keep saturation above 95%;
   • albuterol treatments every four hours;
   • amoxicillin 10 mg/kg by mouth (PO) three times a day (TID); and
   • acetaminophen 10 mg/kg every four hours as needed (PRN) for a fever over 101 degrees.

The patient has an allergy to Zithromax®. Amoxicillin comes in 125 mg/5 mL. If there is no improvement in 12 hours, Norma will admit Charli to the medical floor.

Think About It

1. There is a record of vital signs for the patient, Charli. These were likely taken before Norma saw Charli. Which types of nurses or other healthcare workers might measure and record vital signs before a patient sees a doctor, physician's assistant, or nurse practitioner?
2. Some nurses are practitioners and perform tasks previously limited to medical doctors. Which actions in Charli's care would be performed by Norma because she is a nurse practitioner?
3. What qualities do you think are most important in a nurse? Why?
4. Is nursing a career that interests you? Why or why not?

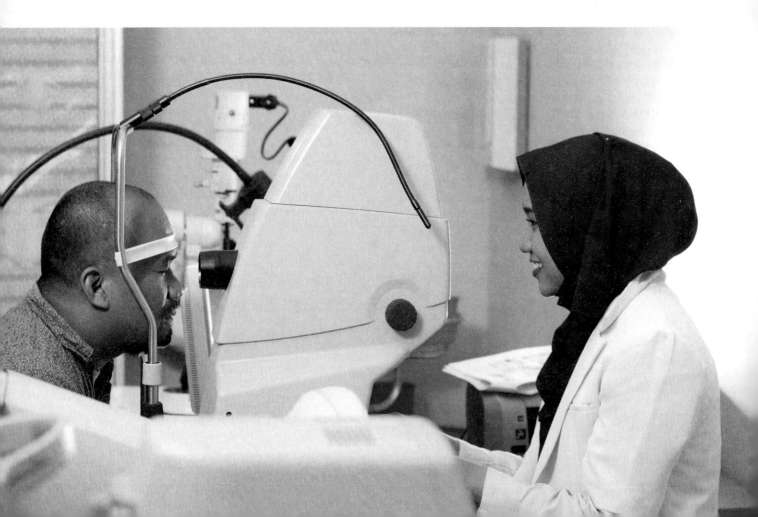

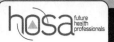

Many medical procedures and visits occur in a clinic or medical practice. A day in a medical office can be routine but also unpredictable. There will be appointments left open for emergencies or illnesses that cannot wait. A patient could come in for a checkup but have high blood pressure or chest pain. Staff in a medical practice must be adaptable and stay calm when the situation is critical. Medical assistants begin exams by measuring vital signs, height, and weight and interviewing the patient. Medical assistants work in a variety of practices and assist physicians in procedures and exams. They can also be office managers. If this sounds interesting, you can learn more and compete in the HOSA—Future Health Professionals *Medical Assisting* event.

Go to the HOSA website to learn more about the HOSA *Medical Assisting* event. Find out the purpose of the event, what is involved in the event, and what knowledge is demonstrated in the event.

As you prepare for HOSA competitive events, be sure to check the website and talk with your HOSA advisor for the most up-to-date guidelines and procedures. Once you have learned about the *Medical Assisting* event, answer the following questions:

1. How might participating in this event benefit you personally and your future career? Explain.
2. Are you interested in participating in this event? Why or why not?

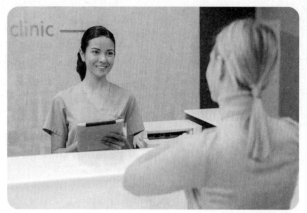

Pressmaster/Shutterstock.com

 ## Connect with Your Reading

Think of a time you or someone you know was injured, such as a car accident or athletic injury. Which healthcare professionals helped figure out or diagnose the damage? Patients meet some diagnostic healthcare workers, but never see everyone who plays a part in their diagnosis. Can you identify diagnostic workers who are unseen, as well as those who are seen by patients?

 ## Map Your Reading

Draw the radial diagram and fill in the main headings as they appear in the text. As you read each section, answer the accompanying questions. Then answer the questions that follow.

1. Consider your own personal traits. Which of the traits described in this chapter do you possess?
2. Select any career discussed in this chapter. Describe how it suits your aptitudes and interests.

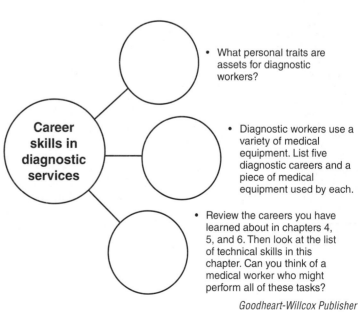

- What personal traits are assets for diagnostic workers?

- Diagnostic workers use a variety of medical equipment. List five diagnostic careers and a piece of medical equipment used by each.

- Review the careers you have learned about in chapters 4, 5, and 6. Then look at the list of technical skills in this chapter. Can you think of a medical worker who might perform all of these tasks?

Goodheart-Willcox Publisher

Chapter opener image: SVRSLYIMAGE/Shutterstock.com

Personal Traits and Career Choices in Diagnostic Services

ESSENTIAL QUESTION

What jobs are found in the diagnostic pathway, and how do personal traits benefit this work?

Learning Outcomes

After studying this lesson, you will be able to

6.1-1 identify personal traits of healthcare workers and explain how diagnostic workers apply them.

6.1-2 describe careers, changing technology, and the importance of tests completed in the clinical laboratory.

6.1-3 explain the variety of medical imaging professions.

6.1-4 identify careers related to vision and hearing health.

Professional Vocabulary

Essential Terms

diagnostic   pertaining to the identification of a disease or syndrome

discretion   the ability to know when to keep sensitive information private

integrity   adherence to ethical principles and professional standards

invasive procedure   a test or treatment that requires incisions to the skin or the insertion of instruments or other materials into the body

noninvasive procedure   a test or treatment that does not require incisions to the skin or the insertion of instruments or other materials into the body

radiographers   healthcare professionals who create medical images or treat diseases by passing radiation, such as X-rays or gamma rays, through an object

sonographers   healthcare professionals who create medical images or treat diseases using high-frequency sound waves

Important Terms

audiologist

cardiovascular
  technologists

nuclear medicine
  technologists

ophthalmologist

optometrist

otolaryngologist

phlebotomist

public health laboratory
  professionals

radiation therapist

stamina

Introduction

Unlike doctors, nurses, or other therapeutic workers, those who work in the diagnostic services career pathway are often unseen. These behind-the-scenes workers help determine diagnoses through clinical tests and medical imaging.

Diagnostic workers often interact with machines more than with patients. If you are interested in healthcare technology and equipment, the diagnostic services pathway may be for you.

This lesson illustrates the important role diagnostic healthcare workers perform in clinical laboratory and imaging careers. You will learn about opportunities in vision- and hearing-related careers and understand how some healthcare workers complete both diagnostic and therapeutic tasks.

Healthcare Professions: The Diagnostic Worker

Briana always knew she wanted to work in healthcare, specifically as a nurse. She signed up for challenging science and math classes. She enjoyed all the health science courses available to her until it was time to register for a nursing assistant class. Briana wanted to help people, and her aunt always talked positively about her own nursing career.

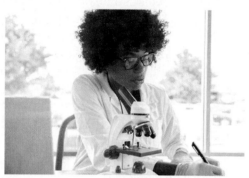

Courtney Hale/E+ via Getty Images

However, the more Briana thought about the nursing assistant class, the more uncertain she became.

Briana shared her concerns with her family and health science teacher. They had observed her preference for working in an organized environment with a predictable schedule. Since Briana enjoyed her science lab classes, Briana's health science teacher suggested medical laboratory careers. Briana did some research and met with her school counselor to learn more about college programs in her state. She decided not to take the nursing assistant course and went on to major in clinical laboratory science.

The more courses Briana completed in college, the more convinced she became that medical technology was the career for her. She even noticed that other students in her courses had similar interests and aptitudes. When asked how she found such a good career match, Briana says she just "fell into it." The reality is Briana took important steps to find a good career fit. Instead of sticking to her first career choice, she paid attention to her own uncertain feelings about nursing. She talked to people who knew her well to get their advice. She took the time to research careers with an open mind, and it paid off.

Today Briana is a medical technologist at a major research hospital. She has met her goal of helping people, but she does this by analyzing laboratory findings that lead to detecting and diagnosing disease, not by interacting directly with patients. Briana is a diagnostic healthcare worker.

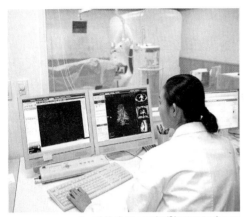
A and N photography/Shutterstock.com

Figure 6.1 Diagnostic workers use equipment such as this MRI machine to provide images that will lead to a diagnosis.

6.1-1 Personal Traits

Do you enjoy working with equipment? Are you interested in operating machines? **Diagnostic** workers are experts in using machines to create the best possible images for identifying a disease or syndrome correctly (**Figure 6.1**). Mechanical aptitude is important for this career pathway. Diagnostic workers follow detailed instructions to complete laboratory tests and record and organize data in precise ways. They must be accurate and reliable, and must remain calm and focused in stressful situations.

Being willing to admit your mistakes and correct your errors demonstrates honesty and **integrity**. Workers with integrity do what is right even when they think no one will notice. Honest healthcare workers earn the trust and respect of their patients and fellow workers.

 Healthcare Professions: Personal Traits

It was a busy day in the lab. Jack was labeling blood specimens in preparation for testing when a fellow worker interrupted him with a question. When he turned back to the labels, Jack could not remember which specimen belonged to which patient. Now he had to contact both patients and have them return

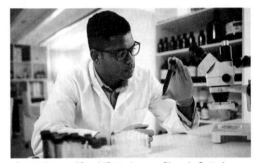
PeopleImages/iStock/Getty Images Plus via Getty Images

to the clinic to leave a second specimen. As you can imagine, they were not pleased. However, a correct diagnosis relies on the accuracy of the diagnostic test, and on the integrity of the healthcare worker.

Workers with a realistic, "doer" personality can perform repeat procedures with a high degree of accuracy. This can be an asset in the diagnostic field. However, as diagnostic tests become more computerized, the role of the diagnostic worker is becoming more analytical. This means the work involves more thinking and reasoning. Workers with an investigative, "thinker" personality will enjoy the problem-solving parts of diagnostic work. This might involve asking questions, such as: *How can I position this patient to get the clearest image without causing further injury? If I arrange images in a specific order, will the physician be able to examine the characteristics of the entire tumor? How can I organize the data to make the results easier to read and interpret?*

When diagnostic workers interact with patients, they should demonstrate a pleasant and relaxed manner. Patients may be in pain or worried about the results of their test. Workers need to be *articulate* (ar-TIHK-yuh-leht), or able to communicate clearly and effectively, so they can explain the test and answer the patient's questions about it. These workers must also show **discretion** by not revealing information outside their scope of practice.

For example, Mital performed an ultrasound for a patient with a suspected miscarriage. She used discretion by turning the screen away from her patient. She spoke calmly to the patient but did not reveal what the screen showed. An ultrasound technician does not diagnose; that is the job of the physician. Mital provided information about when the results would be sent to the patient's physician and encouraged the patient to contact her doctor.

Many diagnostic careers require physical **stamina**, or *endurance*. Diagnostic workers may be on their feet operating equipment the entire workday. They may also need to lift and position patients for imaging tests or transport heavy equipment to a patient to complete an imaging test.

The diagnostic worker must be committed to lifelong learning because technology is always advancing. Diagnostic workers learn to use automated equipment and computerized instruments capable of performing many tests simultaneously. They may specialize in the fast-growing fields of microbiology, immunology, and molecular biology. In addition to traditional X-ray radiography, diagnostic workers who specialize in medical imaging may learn ultrasonography (uhl-trah-sah-NAHG-rah-fee), magnetic resonance imaging (MRI), computed tomography (toh-MAHG-ruh-fee), or other specialized imaging techniques (**Figure 6.2**).

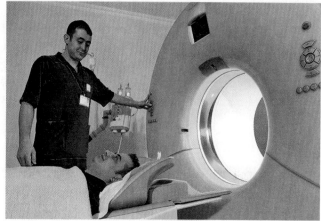

Medioimages/Photodisc/Thinkstock

Figure 6.2 Computed tomography (CT) is just one type of imaging technology with which diagnostic workers may be familiar. *What are some other types of imaging technology?*

6.1-2 Clinical Laboratory Careers

Clinical laboratory workers perform diagnostic laboratory testing. These tests play an important role in medical care. They are often the least expensive healthcare procedures, but they influence more than 70 percent of healthcare decisions. They provide objective information that is used for many purposes. Test results can assess a patient's risk of developing a disease, monitor the course of a disease, or measure a patient's response to medical treatment.

Lab technicians and technologists examine and analyze body fluids and cells to

- look for bacteria, parasites, and other microorganisms;
- analyze the chemical content of fluids;
- match blood for transfusions; and
- test for levels of medication in the bloodstream to measure a patient's response to treatment.

Depending on the test and methods used, diagnostic tests can be performed at a centralized laboratory, hospital bedside, physician's office, medical clinic, workplace, and even at home. Clinical lab workers are no longer confined to a hospital lab and can work in a variety of settings such as blood banks, dialysis centers, and medical laboratories.

Technology in Clinical Laboratory Careers

Technological advances have made tests easier to use and more accurate. Point-of-care tests speed up the process of diagnosis and treatment. For example, a rapid strep test can confirm a positive streptococcal (strehp-tuh-KAHK-uhl) infection in the physician's office. People can purchase pregnancy tests at a pharmacy and use them at home. During the COVID-19 pandemic, local pharmacies became test sites for both rapid tests and molecular lab tests. These new types of tests provide flexibility and convenience for patients.

Progress in technology is changing the practice of medicine. Lab technologists can perform gene-based and other molecular diagnostic tests that predict the likelihood a patient will develop a specific disease even before symptoms appear. For example, genetic testing for specific gene mutations can indicate an individual's risk for developing breast or ovarian cancer. This allows physicians to focus on prevention or early treatment and reduces the negative effects of a disease.

Diagnostic tests that involve the molecular analysis of genes, proteins, and metabolites (substances made or used in metabolism) will lead to more personalized medical care. Doctors will use test results to select the best medication in the right amount for a particular patient and avoid adverse reactions to treatment.

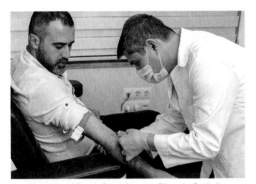

ozgurdonmaz/iStock/Getty Images Plus via Getty Images

Figure 6.3 A phlebotomist is one kind of diagnostic worker who may work in a clinical laboratory. Phlebotomists draw blood for testing.

Clinical Laboratory Job Titles

In a healthcare laboratory, you may meet a **phlebotomist** (fleh-BAHT-uh-mihst) or a medical assistant. Both can draw your blood and receive specimens for testing (**Figure 6.3**). You may not meet the clinical laboratory technician. You are also unlikely to meet the medical laboratory scientist. In this section, you will learn about several clinical laboratory careers.

- **Medical laboratory scientists.** Medical laboratory scientists are often called *clinical laboratory scientists, medical technologists,* or *medical laboratory technologists.* Lab technologists use microscopes, cell counters, and other specialized laboratory equipment. Manual dexterity and normal color vision are assets for these workers. Computer skills are essential as the use of automated equipment and computerized instruments capable of performing several tests simultaneously become more common. Technologists working in large laboratories often become specialists in specific testing procedures (**Figure 6.4**).

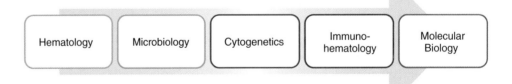

Hematology | Microbiology | Cytogenetics | Immuno-hematology | Molecular Biology

Goodheart-Willcox Publisher

Figure 6.4 There are many specialty areas within the field of clinical laboratory science. *Can you use your knowledge of medical terms to determine which of these specialties works with cells? blood? molecules? bacteria and viruses? blood transfusion?*

- **Public health laboratory professionals.** Public health laboratory professionals are highly educated specialists with knowledge of one or more scientific disciplines. They have advanced skills in laboratory practice and use their skills to solve complex problems that affect human health. When health risks emerge, public health laboratories analyze the threat, provide prevention and treatment information, and act to protect the public. These labs are found in every state and can focus on environmental health concerns and disease detection. **Figure 6.5** shows the variety of services provided by a public health laboratory scientist.

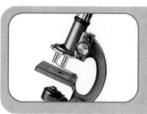
Environmental Health
Testing drinking water and air quality to screen for harmful substances.

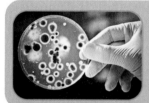
Food Safety
Detecting and preventing the spread of foodborne illness

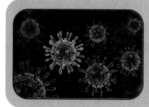
Infectious Diseases
Identifying outbreaks of infectious disease and detect new diseases

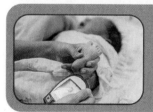
Newborn Screening
Screening babies for potentially life-threatening metabolic and genetic disorders

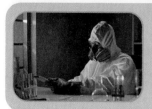
Preparedness and Response
Identifying suspect agents such as anthrax

Top to bottom: Nenad Zivkovic/Shutterstock.com, Alexander Raths/Shutterstock.com, Christina Krivonos/Shutterstock.com, Atiwat Witthayanurut/Shutterstock.com, nimito/Shutterstock.com

Figure 6.5 Public health laboratories provide a wide range of services to benefit the residents of each state.

- **Clinical laboratory technicians.** Clinical laboratory technicians may be called *medical technicians* or *medical laboratory technicians.* Lab technicians perform tests and laboratory procedures that are less complex. Technicians may prepare specimens, operate automated analyzers, or perform manual tests under the supervision of a technologist. Because clinical laboratory workers handle infectious specimens, they must be skilled in infection control and sterilization techniques. Personal protective equipment is required for laboratory work.

Job opportunities for laboratory technicians and technologists are expected to be excellent. Technologists need a bachelor's degree in medical technology or a life science for entry-level positions. A graduate degree promotes advancement to the positions of lab supervisor, manager, or director. Technicians generally need an associate's degree from a technical or community college or a certificate from a hospital training program. Phlebotomists and medical assistants are also in high demand. These workers complete technical training to receive a program certificate or diploma. Some states may require licensure for these positions, and employers prefer to hire certified workers.

6.1-3 Medical Imaging Careers

Medical imaging has come a long way since 1895, when Wilhelm Roentgen accidentally discovered an image cast from his cathode ray generator (**Figure 6.6**).

Imaging Techniques

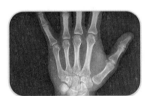

X-Ray: produces images of the structures inside your body, particularly your bones

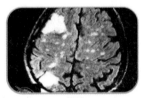

Magnetic Resonance Imaging (MRI): produces clear images of soft tissues in the body

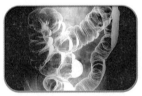

Fluoroscopy: shows a continuous X-ray image of moving body structures on a monitor, much like an X-ray movie

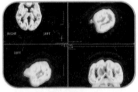

Positron Emission Tomography (PET): shows functional processes in the body and can show the development of a condition

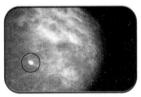

Mammography: uses a low-dose X-ray system to examine the breasts

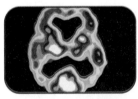

Single Photon Emission Computed Tomography (SPECT): shows how blood flows to tissues and organs

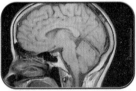

Computed Tomography (CT): uses a narrow beam of X-rays and high-powered computers to generate images of bones and soft tissues in the body

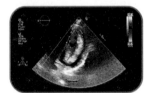

Sonography: uses sound waves to create a computerized picture

Left to right, top to bottom: tsmejust/Shutterstock.com, muratart/Shutterstock.com, Living Art Enterprises, LLC/Science Source, Donna Beeler/Shutterstock.com, xpixel/Shutterstock.com, PROF J. LEVEILLE/Science Source, wenht/iStock/Thinkstock, Radiological Imaging/Shutterstock.com

Figure 6.6 Radiographers use a wide variety of imaging techniques for diagnosing medical conditions.

Medical imaging professionals make a significant contribution to the healthcare industry. Doctors use the images they obtain to diagnose health issues quickly and treat patients sooner than ever before. Imaging professionals work with a rapidly expanding number of imaging procedures and technologies. In addition to knowledge of medical equipment and technology, these jobs may require direct contact with patients. Therefore, medical imaging professionals must be caring and empathetic to patients' needs. **Figure 6.7** shows how clinical laboratory and medical imaging professionals can advance in their careers and the level of education needed for each step.

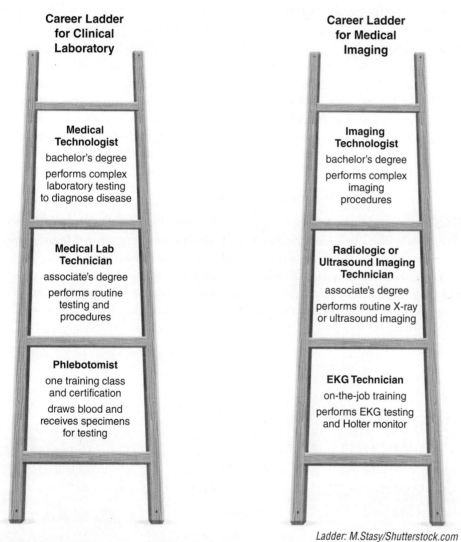

Career Ladder for Clinical Laboratory

Medical Technologist

bachelor's degree

performs complex laboratory testing to diagnose disease

Medical Lab Technician

associate's degree

performs routine testing and procedures

Phlebotomist

one training class and certification

draws blood and receives specimens for testing

Career Ladder for Medical Imaging

Imaging Technologist

bachelor's degree

performs complex imaging procedures

Radiologic or Ultrasound Imaging Technician

associate's degree

performs routine X-ray or ultrasound imaging

EKG Technician

on-the-job training

performs EKG testing and Holter monitor

Ladder: M.Stasy/Shutterstock.com

Figure 6.7 Tests performed by diagnostic healthcare workers influence more than 70 percent of healthcare decisions. Review the tasks for each of the jobs in these career ladders. *Which diagnostic career interests you the most? What education and training are required for that job?*

Radiology

Today, **radiographers** perform a wide variety of imaging exams. Radiologic technicians, previously called *X-ray technicians*, perform X-ray imaging examinations (**Figure 6.8**). Radiologic technologists use other methods of examination, such as mammography, computed tomography (CT), and magnetic resonance imaging (MRI). Radiographers produce X-ray images, or *radiographs*, of the human body for use in diagnosing medical conditions. Their duties include

- positioning a patient to obtain the proper projection for the body part being imaged;
- aligning the X-ray beam to limit radiation exposure and using shielding techniques to prevent exposure;
- selecting the correct control settings to get clear, detailed images;
- working with physicians to decide if additional images need to be taken; and
- storing and retrieving images.

Today X-ray images are captured digitally, which results in sharper images. These images can be enhanced on a computer and sent or stored electronically. This means images may be readily available to several caregivers.

Radiologic technologists perform more complex imaging procedures than radiologic technicians. A fluoroscopy, for example, requires the patient to drink a special solution that will result in an image clearly showing soft tissues in the body. Technologists who specialize in mammography use low-dose X-rays to produce images of the breast to screen for abnormalities.

Specialization in computed tomography or magnetic resonance imaging is becoming more common. Computed tomography takes multiple cross-sectional X-rays. The computer processes these to produce virtual images showing what a surgeon would see during an operation. Computed tomography allows doctors to examine the inside of a patient's body without operating. Magnetic resonance imaging uses radio frequency to produce an image contrast.

The job of the **radiation therapist** has evolved with advancements in radiography. Radiation therapy is a treatment that projects high-energy X-rays at targeted cells to shrink and eliminate cancerous tumors.

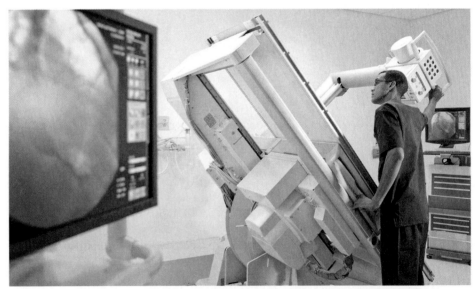

Juice Flair/Shutterstock.com

Figure 6.8 Radiographers perform a wide variety of imaging exams. *Can you identify three imaging techniques used by radiographers?*

As part of a medical radiation oncology team, a radiation therapist uses CT or other imaging techniques to pinpoint a tumor's location. Using this information, the oncology physician develops a treatment plan for the patient. Then the radiation therapist uses the treatment plan to position the patient and deliver the radiation treatment. The radiation therapist monitors the physical and emotional reactions of the patient. Because patients with cancer experience high levels of stress, radiation therapists must maintain a positive attitude and provide emotional support.

Nuclear Medicine

Nuclear medicine technologists administer radioactive substances as part of the imaging process. Nuclear medicine scans can detect disease based on metabolic changes and focus on physiology, or how the body is functioning. These scans can detect tumors, abnormal bulges in blood vessels called aneurysms (AN-yuh-rihz-uhms), poor blood flow to tissues, and other conditions.

Two types of nuclear medicine scans are positron emission tomography (PET) and single-photon emission computed tomography (SPECT). PET scans create a 3D image of the body and can show the process of glucose metabolism in the brain. PET scans can detect cancer, heart conditions, and brain disorders. SPECT scans create a similar image but use different radioactive chemicals. These scans can show blood flow through the brain and help doctors diagnose brain injury.

Sonography

Diagnostic medical **sonographers** use sound waves to generate an image (**Figure 6.9**). Sonography or ultrasonography is often associated with imaging during pregnancy, but there are many other uses for this method of medical imaging. Areas of specialty for sonographers include the following:

- abdomen—evaluation of all the soft tissues, blood vessels, and organs of the abdominal cavities such as the liver, spleen, urinary tract, and pancreas
- breast—frequently used to evaluate breast abnormalities found with mammography
- obstetrics/gynecology—evaluation of the female reproductive system
- echocardiography (ehk-oh-kard-ee-AHG-ruh-fee)—evaluation of the anatomy and blood flow of the heart
- vascular technology—evaluation of the blood flow in peripheral and abdominal blood vessels
- neurosonography—evaluation of the brain and spinal cord
- ophthalmology—evaluation of the eye

Because sonography does not involve the risk of radiation exposure, it is considered safer than imaging methods that use X-rays. However, its use is limited because it cannot image through air. As a result, sonography is not used for lung or bowel imaging.

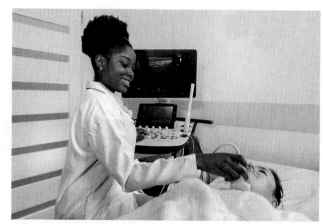

Andrey_Popov/Shutterstock.com

Figure 6.9 Sonographers can specialize in certain areas of the body. *Why is sonography safer than radiography?*

Heart and Brain Imaging

Cardiovascular technologists and technicians assist physicians in diagnosing heart and blood vessel disorders. Cardiac diagnostics may require **invasive** or **noninvasive procedures**. For example, cardiovascular technologists assist physicians with cardiac catheterization procedures, which are invasive (**Figure 6.10A**). During this procedure, a small tube or *catheter* is threaded through an artery from the groin to the heart. The catheter can locate blocked blood vessels and may open them using a balloon angioplasty process. Catheterization procedures can also help locate areas of heart tissue that are causing abnormal rhythms. Cardiovascular technologists may also assist physicians during open-heart surgery or during the insertion of pacemakers or stents.

Cardiographic technicians perform electrocardiogram (EKG) tests and Holter monitor procedures using electrode patches attached to the skin. These tests measure the electrical impulses of the heart and help detect abnormal rhythms of the heartbeat. They are noninvasive procedures (**Figure 6.10B**). These technicians may also perform stress tests to measure the effect of physical exertion on the function of the heart.

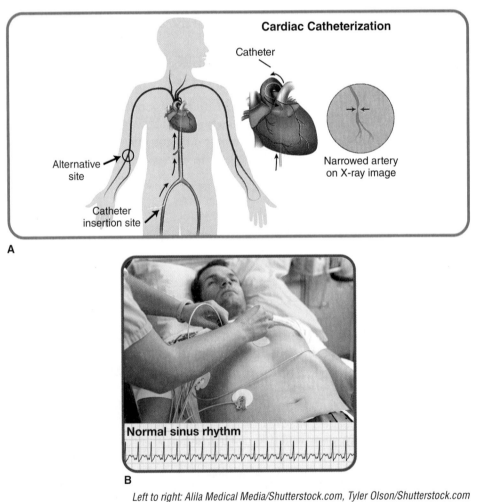

Left to right: Alila Medical Media/Shutterstock.com, Tyler Olson/Shutterstock.com

Figure 6.10 Cardiac catheterization (A) and electrocardiograms (B) provide valuable information about the functioning of the heart. Catheterization is an invasive procedure. EKG is a noninvasive procedure. *What makes a procedure invasive?*

Electroencephalographic (ee-lehk-troh-ehn-sehf-uh-luh-GRAF-ihk) (EEG) technologists, electroneurodiagnostic (ee-lehk-troh-noo-roh-dI-ag-NAHS-tihk) (END) technologists, and polysomnographic (pahl-ee-sahm-nuh-GRAF-ihk) technologists all perform tests that measure brain activity and responses. Results of these tests can help doctors diagnose brain-related disorders such as tumors, strokes, epilepsy, and sleep disorders. All these tests are noninvasive procedures.

Most imaging workers are employed in hospitals, but a growing number work in medical clinics and in medical and diagnostic laboratories. While a 40-hour workweek is common, hospital employees often work overtime, evening, and weekend hours, and maintain on-call schedules. Medical imaging professionals who are trained in more than one kind of imaging will have more job opportunities.

Medical imaging technicians typically complete a technical training program through a community college or hospital-sponsored program. Unlike other healthcare technicians, most EKG technicians are trained on the job. Employers prefer to train workers who are already in the healthcare field, such as nursing assistants. The majority of imaging technologists complete an associate's degree, but four-year bachelor's degree programs are becoming more common.

6.1-4 Vision- and Hearing-Related Careers

The fields of audiology and ophthalmology use many diagnostic tests to assess changes in hearing and vision. You may have observed that several medical careers have overlapping diagnostic and therapeutic roles. For example, physicians both diagnose and treat diseases. Some technicians in the ophthalmologist's (ahf-thal-MAHL-uh-jihst) office perform tests to diagnose vision changes, while others fit eyeglasses or contact lenses to treat vision changes.

Ophthalmology

An **ophthalmologist** is an eye specialist, and an **otolaryngologist** (oh-toh-lair-uhn-GAHL-uh-jihst) is an ear, nose, and throat specialist. Many patients never see these doctors when they have their hearing or vision checked. Routine vision testing and correction are performed in the office of an **optometrist**.

An optometrist holds a doctor of optometry (O.D.) degree that requires a minimum of seven years of postsecondary study. Optometrists pass state and national examinations to maintain licensure. In addition to vision care, they can test for glaucoma and diagnose eye conditions caused by diabetes and high blood pressure. Each state determines their scope of practice. As a result, optometrists in certain states may perform limited surgical procedures. They refer patients with eye diseases and those who need surgery to an ophthalmologist.

Optometrists, who often operate independent businesses, need business-management skills and the ability to deal tactfully with patients. Job opportunities for optometrists are expected to grow rapidly, but there is tough competition for admission to the limited number of required training programs.

Optometrists often employ optometric technicians so they can serve a larger number of patients. These technical jobs have a variety of titles and may have separate duties, depending on the organization of the office (**Figure 6.11**).

Audiology

An **audiologist** works with people who have hearing and balance conditions. Audiologists can identify the symptoms of hearing loss as well as related sensory and neural conditions. They use audiometers (awd-ee-AHM-eh-ters) and other equipment to assess patients' hearing disorders and develop treatment plans. Treatments may include cleaning the ear canal, fitting hearing aids, and programming cochlear implants. Audiologists also work to develop and present programs about hearing-loss prevention for factory workers and students.

Audiologists complete eight years of postsecondary training and receive the doctor of audiology degree (Au.D.). Like optometrists, they are licensed and complete continuing education to learn new diagnostic and treatment technologies. While employment is expected to grow in this field, there are relatively few job openings due to the small size of this field. For instance, there are more than twice as many optometrists compared to audiologists in the United States.

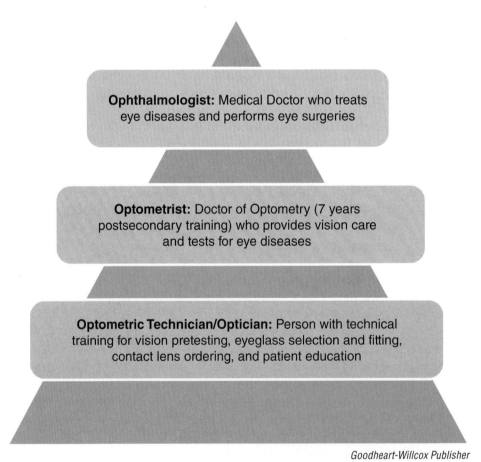

Goodheart-Willcox Publisher

Figure 6.11   The diagnostic pathway includes vision-related careers such as the ones shown here. *What is the difference between an ophthalmologist and an optometrist?*

Audiologists may employ assistants who work with patients to fit hearing aids. These technicians may be called *hearing aid specialists* or *audioprosthologists* (aw-dee-oh-prahs-THAHL-oh-jihsts). They generally have six months to two years of supervised training or a two-year college degree. These technicians must pass licensing tests in most states and can seek national certification.

Diagnostic services careers are worth a closer look if you enjoy working with equipment and are interested in learning about advances in technology. Whether you want to work directly with patients or prefer a laboratory setting, there are many interesting job opportunities in the diagnostic career pathway.

Lesson 6.1 Review

 Complete the *Map Your Reading* graphic organizer for the section you just read.

1. Which of these personal traits are important for diagnostic workers? Choose all that apply. (6.1-1)
   A. Mechanical aptitude
   B. Charisma
   C. Stamina
   D. Discretion

2. Which clinical laboratory worker prepares specimens, operates automated analyzers, and performs manual tests under supervision? (6.1-2)
   A. Medical laboratory scientists
   B. Clinical laboratory technician
   C. Public health laboratory professional
   D. Radiographer

3. Which level of education do most medical imaging professionals complete? (6.1-3)
   A. Associate's degree
   B. Bachelor's degree
   C. Master's degree
   D. High school diploma

4. Which nuclear medicine scan can show blood flow through the brain? (6.1-3)
   A. CT scan
   B. X-ray
   C. PET scan
   D. SPECT scan

5. Which diagnostic worker performs routine vision testing and correction? (6.1-4)
   A. Optometrist
   B. Ophthalmologist
   C. Audiologist
   D. Otolaryngologist

Technical Skills in Diagnostic Services

ESSENTIAL QUESTION

How well do the technical skills in this lesson match your personal work interests and preferences?

Learning Outcomes

After studying this lesson, you will be able to

6.2-1 state the purposes for different patient positions and practice positioning patients.

6.2-2 explain the reasons for and demonstrate the steps for completing a vision screening.

6.2-3 identify equipment used and demonstrate the steps in preparing and assisting with a routine physical examination.

6.2-4 explain how HOSA participation can build your healthcare network and which competitive events can improve your diagnostic skills.

Professional Vocabulary

Essential Terms

body alignment   a position of the body in which the spine is not crooked or twisted

networking   interacting with others to exchange information and develop professional contacts.

occluder   an implement used to block light to the eye

Important Terms

audiometer
ophthalmoscope

otoscope
percussion hammer

Introduction

Clinical technologists can perform literally thousands of different laboratory tests. Imaging specialists operate extremely advanced technological equipment as they assist in diagnosing or monitoring a patient's illness or injury. The basics of health assessment begin with measuring vital signs and checking for vision or hearing concerns. In this lesson, you will learn how to complete a vision screening. You will also learn the body positions used for examination and diagnostic imaging and the steps for assisting with a routine physical examination. As you practice these skills, consider whether you would enjoy a career in diagnostic services.

6.2-1 Positioning a Patient

Medical examinations and imaging procedures require specific patient positions. In simple terms, a person needing examination on the front part of the body will lie on their back. Each position has a specific name, and position descriptions become more detailed as imaging requirements become more specialized.

For example, suppose a physician orders an upright chest X-ray with two views of an ambulatory (able to walk independently) patient. *Upright* means that the patient will stand during the X-ray. The standard positions are *posterior/anterior* (P/A), which means back to front, and *lateral*, which means from the side. The radiographer positions the patient standing and facing the X-ray image receptor for a posterior/anterior projection (the X-rays pass through the patient's body from back to front) and a left lateral projection (the patient stands with the left side closest to the image receptor, and the X-rays pass through the body from right to left). Body positioning may also involve steps like moving the patient's arms out of the imaging area.

Positions also describe patients resting in bed. Those who cannot move independently need to be repositioned frequently to prevent skin breakdown. As you position patients, pay close attention to **body alignment**. Position your patient so the spine is not twisted or crooked. Imagine a line going down the middle of the patient's body. The line should be straight in any position (**Figure 6.12**). Proper body alignment makes the patient more comfortable by relieving strain on muscles and joints.

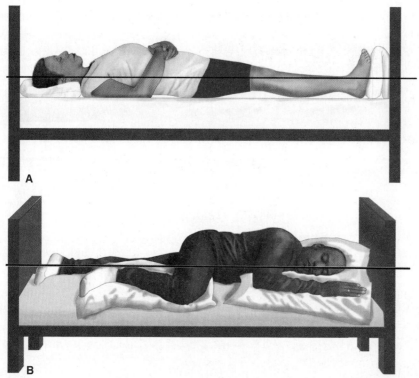

© Body Scientific International

Figure 6.12 When a patient is in proper body alignment, the spine is not twisted or crooked, regardless of the position. In the supine position (A), the patient's hip, shoulder, and ear will form a straight line. In Sims' position (B), you can draw an imaginary line connecting the patient's nose, sternum, and pubic bone. Note that pillows provide comfort and help the patient to maintain correct alignment.

You may position patients on a wide variety of tables for surgery, examinations, or imaging procedures. You must learn how to operate each kind of table to provide for patient safety. Tables are cleaned or disinfected and often covered with table paper before the patient enters the examination room.

As you position a patient, ensure privacy by closing the door or pulling the curtain. Drape or cover the patient to avoid unnecessary exposure. Watch the patient closely and observe safety precautions to prevent falls and injuries. Always provide for your own safety by using proper body mechanics.

Figure 6.13 provides the descriptions and uses for a few basic patient positions. Remember to use your beginning and end-of-procedure steps as you practice positioning a patient.

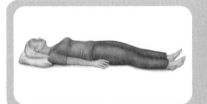

Supine/Dorsal Recumbent Position
- Lying on the back with the bed flat
- Used for physical examinations and surgeries of the chest, heart, and abdomen

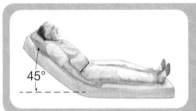

Fowler's Position
- A sitting position with the head of the bed elevated
- High Fowler's is 60–90 degrees, Fowler's is 45–60 degrees, low or semi-Fowler's is 30–45 degrees
- Used for eating in bed and reading or watching TV
- Used to make breathing easier and for examining legs or feet

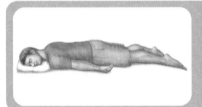

Prone Position
- Lying face down
- Used when examining the spine or back

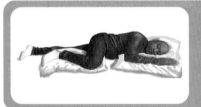

Sims' Position
- Halfway between lateral position and prone position, with upper knee bent
- Used for rectal examinations and enemas

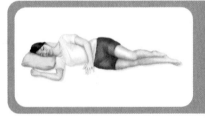

Lateral/Lateral Recumbent Position
- Lying on the side
- Used to relieve pressure on the spine, tailbone, and hips and to reduce back pain

© Body Scientific International

Figure 6.13 These patient positions are each used in specific situations, such as surgery, exams, or imaging procedures.

6.2-2 Screening Vision and Hearing

Vision and hearing screenings help identify children who need further evaluation, diagnosis, and treatment for vision and hearing conditions. Many state departments of public health set guidelines for the routine screening of school-age children. Because vision and hearing are important to learning, screenings help identify barriers to a child's ability to learn. Identifying children with hearing or vision conditions when they are just entering school can prevent or reduce many learning issues. Screening all children is the most practical approach to identifying those who need professional services.

Adults receive vision exams at the office of an optometrist or ophthalmologist. The purpose is to prescribe appropriate corrective lenses. In addition, providers will complete screening tests for other eye disorders such as color blindness, glaucoma, and macular degeneration. A routine physical exam may also include vision screening. The physician will refer the patient to an eye doctor for additional testing if needed.

Visual acuity tests in the school setting screen for distance vision, or *near-sightedness* (myopia). The child reads letters and pictures on a Snellen chart mounted on a wall 20 feet away. Depending on age, a child is expected to read either the 20/40 or 20/30 line accurately. Normal vision for adults is 20/20. Several different types of charts are used for this screening (**Figure 6.14**). For small exam rooms, the chart is projected on the wall at the correct size.

Adult vision screening also tests near vision, or *farsightedness* (hyperopia). Adults read paragraphs from a chart held 14-16 inches from the eyes. The paragraphs move from smaller to larger font on the Jaeger eye chart. The smallest print patients can read determines their near visual acuity.

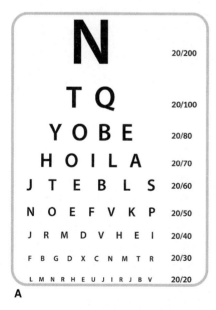
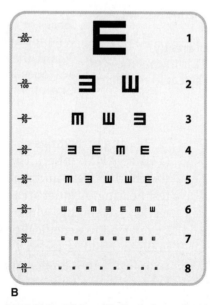
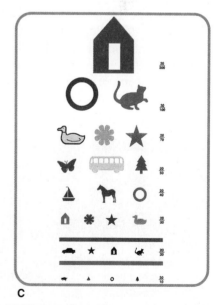

Left to right: Paul Stringer/Shutterstock.com, Roman Sotola/Shutterstock.com, Courtesy of Ennovation CO

Figure 6.14 Distance vision can be tested using several different Snellen charts. These include a simple letter chart (A), the tumbling E chart (B), and a simple shapes chart for younger children (C).

Follow these steps to conduct a vision screening for a child or adult using an alphabet eye chart:

1. Complete your beginning procedure steps, including washing your hands. Use the correct chart for the child's age and development. A good way to determine this is to ask the child if they recognize the alphabet letters on the chart. If the child does recognize the letters, proceed with the alphabet eye chart. If not, you will have to use a different eye chart.

2. Greet the child/adult and explain the testing procedure. Use age-appropriate language and review the steps to be sure the person understands. Check to make sure the person is the correct distance from the chart. Note if the person is wearing glasses and ask teens and adults if they are wearing contact lenses.

3. Have the child keep both eyes open while you occlude or cover the left eye using a tool called an **occluder**. Adults will occlude their left eye and read the chart using corrective lenses as needed.

4. Ask the person to identify the letters or pictures in order starting with the first line. Move across the line from left to right. To pass a line, the child must read more than half the letters correctly. An adult must have one or fewer mistakes.

5. Move to the next line and have the person read right to left to avoid memorization.

6. Continue to the 20 line as long as the individual reads letters at a passing rate.

7. If the individual reads the 20 line correctly, record the visual acuity as 20/20. This means the person can see from a distance of 20 feet to read the letters on the 20 line.

8. If the person failed a line, have them repeat it in the opposite order from the first reading. If they fail twice, record the visual acuity as the next highest line.

9. Repeat steps three through eight with the other eye.

10. Record the individual's visual acuity for the left eye (OS) and right eye (OD). If required, repeat the exam using both eyes and record the visual acuity for both eyes (OU). Record whether they wore corrective lenses (glasses or contact lenses) during the screening. You may be asked to screen children or adults with and without corrective lenses. Record any difficulties you observe, such as the person leaning forward or squinting to see more clearly. Complete step 11 if you are screening a child but continue to step 12 for an adult.

11. Compliment the child on participation, but do not comment on the test results. Clean or discard the occluder. Complete your end-of-procedure steps.

12. Direct the person to sit in a chair located in a well-lighted area. Give them the Jaeger chart and ask them to hold the chart 14 to 16 inches from their eyes.

13. Ask the person to read the paragraphs aloud with both eyes open. Record the smallest print the individual can read correctly. You may also be directed to screen with and without corrective lenses or to test each eye separately as you did with the Snellen wall chart.

14. Thank the individual and ask if they have any questions. Clean or discard the occluder. Complete your end-of-procedure steps.

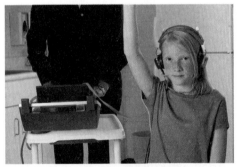

Brian Eichhorn/Shutterstock.com

Figure 6.15 Hearing screenings can detect hearing problems, but a professional hearing exam is needed to identify the cause of hearing loss and to determine appropriate treatment.

Hearing screenings conducted in schools use an **audiometer** (awd-ee-AHM-eht-er). This machine has a set of headphones for the child to wear and makes sounds at different frequencies to test hearing. A quiet area is necessary for accurate results. This test is a screening, which means students who fail the test will be referred to a medical professional for follow-up testing. Generally, a child is tested twice with at least one week between each test before a referral is made. An upper respiratory infection can cause temporary hearing loss. An exam by a medical professional is necessary to determine the cause of hearing loss (**Figure 6.15**).

6.2-3 Preparing and Assisting with a Routine Physical Examination

Physicians perform a variety of physical examinations to determine a patient's health status or investigate and diagnose a health condition. Today, a medical assistant named Andre will assist Dr. Khan with a routine physical examination for Mr. Garcia. Andre's duties include preparing the exam room, greeting the patient, completing prescreening, and preparing the patient for the doctor's examination. He will assist as needed during the examination and complete follow-up steps with the patient. Finally, he will clean and restore the room in preparation for its next use.

Andre considers the type of examination and what equipment the physician will need. You already know about the equipment used for vision screening. The physician may also need equipment for measuring vital signs, a **percussion hammer** to check reflexes, an **otoscope** to examine ears, a laryngeal mirror and tongue depressor to examine the mouth and throat, and an **ophthalmoscope** and penlight to examine the eyes (**Figure 6.16**). The patient will wear a gown. Disposable covers, drapes, gloves, specimen containers, and tissues will also be used. Finally, Andre will need containers for disposing of soiled equipment, used linens, and contaminated waste materials.

Andre is the first and last person the patient sees. He must make the patient feel at ease, assist the patient as needed, and clearly explain procedures to the patient so the examination goes smoothly. Patient education is important since Andre provides directions for the vision screening, describes the steps for giving a urine specimen, and explains how to undress and robe for the exam.

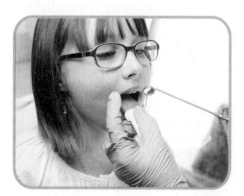
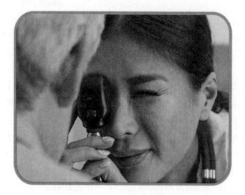
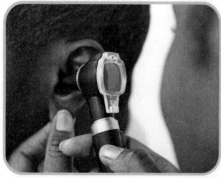
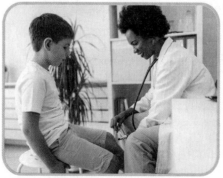

Left to right, top to bottom: Doro Guzenda/Shutterstock.com, Rocketclips, Inc./Shutterstock.com, Andrey_Popov/Shutterstock.com, Lordn/Shutterstock.com

Figure 6.16 Healthcare workers use several kinds of equipment for assessing patient health. *Can you identify the equipment for examining the ears, eyes, and mouth and for testing reflexes?*

During the exam, Andre remains quiet so the physician can hear as she examines the patient. Andre will position the patient for the exam and assist as needed to maintain safety. He follows the direction of the doctor and may assist by handing equipment at the doctor's request.

When the examination is complete, Andre assists the patient as needed to leave the exam table and redress. He will provide follow-up treatments ordered by the physician, such as a vaccination. He escorts the patient to the front desk to schedule future appointments. Then he returns to clean the exam room by discarding disposable materials into the appropriate waste containers and cleaning and storing equipment.

PROCEDURE

Preparing and Assisting with a Routine Physical Examination

Andre completes the following steps for preparing and assisting with a routine physical examination:

1. Perform hand hygiene before entering the exam room. Put fresh paper on the exam table and set out a fresh gown and the disposable drapes needed for the exam. Assemble equipment and place on a tray, providing easy access for the physician. Cover equipment with a towel.

2. Access the patient's medical record and locate the health history and physical examination form. Check for any special instructions or precautions, such as a disability that limits patient positioning.

3. Andre greets Mr. Garcia in the waiting room and brings him to the exam room. He introduces himself using appropriate preprocedure actions. He provides instructions for Mr. Garcia as he completes prescreening tasks, such as measuring height, weight, and vital signs. Andre verbalizes and records these measurements, then asks Mr. Garcia questions to update his health history such as noting any changes in medications or new signs or symptoms.

4. Next Andre explains the steps for cleaning the genital area and giving a urine specimen. He gives Mr. Garcia a specimen container and directs him to the bathroom. He shows him where to place the covered container when finished.

5. When the patient returns, Andre explains what clothing to remove and shows him where it can be placed. He tells Mr. Garcia to wear the gown open in back, sit on the exam table, and use the drape to cover his legs. Then

he pulls out the step on the exam table and asks Mr. Garcia if he will need any help. He leaves the room and closes the door to provide privacy.

6. Andre knocks on the door when he returns and checks to see that Mr. Garcia is ready for the exam. Then he notifies Dr. Khan.

7. Andre positions Mr. Garcia in the horizontal recumbent position, also called the dorsal or supine position. He assists Dr. Khan as requested during the exam and follows standard precautions as needed. He helps Mr. Garcia sit up when the exam is finished and makes sure he is not dizzy before he climbs down from the exam table. Then he tells Mr. Garcia he can get dressed again and provides privacy or assists him if needed.

8. Andre gives Mr. Garcia instructions about his care as directed by Dr. Khan. He checks for questions and verifies that Mr. Garcia understands the doctor's instructions before guiding Mr. Garcia back to the waiting room exit and saying goodbye.

9. Andre returns to the exam room and wears gloves to dispose of the table cover and other disposable drapes and supplies in the appropriate waste containers. He follows the correct cleaning and sterilizing procedures for reusable equipment and disinfects the counters and exam table surfaces. Now he can remove and discard his gloves and wash his hands.

10. Finally, Andre replaces the used supplies and covers the exam table and pillow with clean paper. Andre performs hand hygiene before moving on to his next task.

6.2-4 HOSA Connections

HOSA conferences provide a great opportunity for **networking**. At these conferences, you will meet healthcare professionals and fellow HOSA members from around your state or the entire nation. Get to know these people because they may be your future employers or coworkers. As your career advances, you will use this network of healthcare workers to seek out information and advice about career opportunities. Create a list of your healthcare network. Record the names, work roles, and contact information for people in your healthcare network. Keep your list with your career portfolio materials. Try the *Clinical Laboratory Science* or *Pathophysiology* competitive events to strengthen your diagnostic skills. You can read about these events in the competitive events section of the HOSA website.

Lesson 6.2 Review

 Complete the *Map Your Reading* graphic organizer for the section you just read.

1. For correct body alignment, you should imagine a straight line going down the _____ of a patient's body. (6.2-1)
   A. side
   B. front
   C. back
   D. middle

2. Which machine makes sounds at different frequencies to test hearing? (6.2-2)
   A. Stethoscope
   B. Audiometer
   C. Otoscope
   D. Laryngeal mirror

3. During a physical examination, a medical assistant should do all of the following *except* (6.2-3)
   A. talk to the physician
   B. hand the physician instruments on request
   C. position the patient for the exam
   D. escort the patient to the front desk

4. Which of the following are advantages of the networking HOSA provides? Choose all that apply. (6.2-4)
   A. Meeting future employers
   B. Getting advice about career opportunities
   C. Accessing information about different careers
   D. Connecting with future coworkers

Chapter 6 Review and Assessment

Chapter Summary

6.1-1 Diagnostic healthcare workers exhibit honesty and integrity when they are willing to admit mistakes, correct errors, and strive to do what is right even when no one sees their efforts. Diagnostic workers show discretion by not sharing test results and by encouraging patients to contact their physician for a diagnosis. Mechanical aptitude, physical stamina, and the ability to learn new technologies and follow detailed instructions with precision and accuracy lead to success in diagnostic careers.

6.1-2 Diagnostic workers include clinical lab technologists who perform the lab tests that influence more than 70 percent of healthcare decisions.

6.1-3 Imaging specialists such as radiographers and sonographers use a wide variety of imaging techniques that help providers diagnose disorders in both the structure and function of the human body.

6.1-4 Audiologists and ophthalmologists both diagnose and treat hearing and vision disorders.

6.2-1 Healthcare workers always check for correct body alignment when positioning patients. Workers use a variety of patient positions to accommodate patient examination and improve patient comfort.

6.2-2 Vision and hearing screenings reduce learning issues by identifying children who need further evaluation, diagnosis, and treatment.

6.2-3 Medical assistants assemble a variety of equipment and supplies such as an otoscope, percussion hammer, laryngeal mirror, penlight, ophthalmoscope, tongue depressor, and disposable covers and drapes in preparation for assisting with a routine physical examination.

6.2-4 HOSA provides valuable opportunities for networking. Several competitive events can help strengthen a person's diagnostic skills.

Maximize Your Professional Vocabulary

1. **Diagnostic Dialogue.** Work in pairs to create a vocabulary chart that lists each vocabulary term under one of these categories: *Careers*, *Personal Traits*, *Knowledge (Things to Know)*, and *Skills (Things to Do)*. As your instructor reads a term definition, you and your partner will compete against each other to cross off the correct term first. Whoever crosses off the most terms is the winner.

2. **Walk the Plank.** Write each of the vocabulary terms for this chapter on a card. Line up the cards in a row on the floor. "Walk the plank" by stepping on each card as you define its term. How many terms caused you to "fall off the plank" because you could not define them? Take these terms and review their meanings. Then create a new plank and try "walking the plank" again until you can define all the terms.

Reflect on Your Reading

1. Review the diagnostic careers discussed in this chapter. Check the Bureau of Labor Statistics website data on healthcare careers to see which diagnostic career area has the best opportunities for employment. Would you consider a career in this area? Be prepared to explain the reasons for your choice.

Review and Recall

1. Which personal trait helps diagnostic workers keep up to date with advancing technology? (6.1-1)
   A. Calm
   B. Endurance
   C. Integrity
   D. Lifelong learning

2. Lab technicians and technologists examine and analyze specimens to (6.1-2)
   A. look for microorganisms
   B. test for blood levels of medications
   C. match for blood transfusions
   D. All of these.
3. Which type of medical imaging uses sound waves to generate an image? (6.1-3)
   A. Nuclear medicine
   B. Sonography
   C. X-rays
   D. EKG
4. Which conditions do audiologists diagnose and treat? Choose all that apply. (6.1-4)
   A. Hearing conditions
   B. Balance conditions
   C. Vision conditions
   D. Skeletal conditions
5. Which body position is used for rectal examinations and enemas? (6.2-1)
   A. Sims' position
   B. Lateral position
   C. Fowler's position
   D. Prone position
6. To pass a line on a vision screening, a child must read _____ of the letters correctly. (6.2-2)
   A. all
   B. one-fourth
   C. more than one-half
   D. one-half
7. When assisting with a physical examination, what should a medical assistant do first? (6.2-3)
   A. Dispose of soiled linens
   B. Check the patient's medical record
   C. Perform hand hygiene
   D. Verbalize and record measurements
8. Which HOSA competitive events are most likely to strengthen diagnostic skills? Choose all that apply. (6.2-4)
   A. Clinical Laboratory Science
   B. Pathophysiology
   C. CERT Skills
   D. CPR and First Aid

Build Core Skills

1. **Critical Thinking.** Some healthcare jobs involve both diagnostic and therapeutic tasks. Identify the following workers as *D* for diagnostic, *T* for therapeutic, or *D/T* for both diagnostic and therapeutic. List a job task to illustrate your choice for each worker.
   A. audiologist
   B. dentist
   C. physician
   D. nursing assistant
   E. dental hygienist
   F. optometrist
   G. radiation therapist
   H. emergency medical technician
2. **Critical Thinking.** Review the chapter section about personal traits. Identify which trait each diagnostic worker is showing.
   A. A radiologic technician moves and adjusts equipment to get a clear image.
   B. An ultrasound technician encourages the patient to ask the physician what the echocardiogram reveals.
   C. A medical lab technician recognizes an error in a lab procedure and repeats the procedure.
   D. An X-ray technician operates mobile radiography equipment and moves it throughout the hospital to quickly set up and create patient images at the point of care.
3. **Critical Thinking.** Use this list of clinical laboratory workers to identify which lab worker typically performs each task.
   List of clinical laboratory workers
   - Clinical laboratory technician
   - Medical laboratory scientist
   - Phlebotomist
   - Public health laboratory professional
   Tasks
   A. Draw blood
   B. Identify diseases outbreaks
   C. Receive specimens for testing
   D. Operate automated analyzers
   E. Perform genetic testing
   F. Perform molecular diagnostic tests
   G. Perform newborn screening tests
   H. Prepare specimens
   I. Provide disease prevention and treatment information
   J. Test drinking water

4. **Writing.** Write a paragraph explaining the concept of personalized medical care. How is it different from the current medical care model? Include technological advances in your explanation.

5. **Speaking and Listening.** Review the chart of services provided by public health laboratories in Figure 6.5. Describe three instances in which you have personally benefited from the work of a public health laboratory employee.

6. **Critical Thinking.** Identify an imaging technique that could be used in each of the following patient situations:
   A. Jane, age 40, is being seen for a regular physical examination.
   B. John is complaining of heart palpitations.
   C. Lea is a patient with a history of heart disease. She is complaining of pain in her calf muscle but has no apparent injury.
   D. Dylan is receiving treatment to shrink a brain tumor.
   E. Lily has passed out a few times in the past couple of months, and the doctor wants to rule out a seizure disorder.

7. **Reading.** List the healthcare workers you meet when receiving a routine eye exam. Reread the section on vision-related careers. If necessary, search online for additional information. Identify the required level of training for each worker.

8. **Critical Thinking.** Diagnostic careers involve working with laboratory equipment and imaging machines. Do you like to repair cars or machinery, build items from wood or other materials, or operate a cash register or video equipment? What is the connection between these activities and diagnostic careers? How can you use the answers to these questions to guide your health career selection process?

9. **Reading.** Suppose you have recently graduated from a medical laboratory technician training program. You know employers like to hire credentialed workers, so you decide to seek certification as a medical laboratory technician (MLT). Your program instructor mentioned that the American Medical Technologists (AMT) offers certification testing and credentials.

Visit the AMT website to answer the following questions about the certification process:
   A. What level of education is required to be eligible for certification?
   B. How much does the exam cost, and how long is the exam?
   C. There are several topics addressed in the exam. Which topic includes blood typing?
   D. Once certified, how will you keep your certification current?

10. **Critical Thinking.** Cardiovascular technologists and brain-imaging specialists perform many procedures to diagnose and treat a variety of conditions. Indicate whether each of these procedures is *I* for invasive or *N* for noninvasive.
   A. Polysomnogram
   B. Electrocardiogram
   C. Cardiac catheterization
   D. Electroencephalogram
   E. Coronary stent placement
   F. Holter monitoring

Activate Your Learning

1. Set up a vision screening area by carefully measuring the correct distance for the chart you are using. Select an occluder and practice instructing and screening "patients" for visual acuity. Record results for each individual. What steps are taken when a child "fails" a vision screening?

2. Assemble the equipment and supplies used in a routine physical exam. Identify each item and explain how it is used. Then practice the steps for preparing and assisting with a routine physical examination.

3. Review the guidelines for positioning patients. Then assemble supplies and follow the procedure steps in this chapter to practice patient positioning.

4. Use the HOSA website to research the HOSA competitive events listed in this chapter. Select and note which event would be your first choice. Explain why you chose this event.

5. **Portfolio Builder.** Begin to build your career network. List all the people you know who could help you with educational information, volunteer opportunities, job shadowing, or employment in the field of healthcare. Save this list in your career portfolio.

Think and Act Like a Healthcare Worker

1. Yolanda is assisting the school nurse with vision screening for first-grade students. As each class enters the screening room, students wait in line for their turn to be screened. Halfway through one of the classes, Dillen steps up and recites each alphabet line before Yolanda can even point to the letters. What has happened? How can Yolanda respond in a way that encourages Dillen's continued participation and provides an accurate screening of his vision?

Go to the Source

1. Use online resources to learn more about diagnostic services careers. Select two careers of interest to you and complete a career profile for each one. Use at least one website that ends in .gov and one website that ends in .org. Record the following information for each career:
   - name of career
   - tasks involved in this career
   - personal traits and abilities needed
   - educational requirements
   - type of credential needed and how it is obtained
   - work conditions
   - wages and benefits
   - job outlook for the future
   - the websites you accessed

   How do the two careers compare? Why might you prefer one to the other?

HOSA Event Prep: Medical Assisting

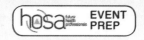

When Georgia completed her medical assisting program, she decided she wanted to work in a practice where she would get to know her patients. She also wanted to work with children. She discovered a new practice starting up with pediatrician Sara Sims, MD. Dr. Sims hired Georgia as her medical assistant. Each day Georgia helps care for children ages newborn to 18. Her daily schedule usually includes around five well-child exams, five to six asthma appointments, a few injuries, a couple of foreign objects in ears and noses, and other kids with illnesses. Dr. Sims also reserves the first hour after lunch and at the end of the day to meet with expectant parents. The hardest part of Georgia's job is vaccinations. She hates seeing the kids cry getting their shots. Before lunch and going home, Georgia also reviews all voicemails and emails to make sure Dr. Sims can intervene when needed quickly.

Think About It

1. Which values and interests led Georgia to become a medical assistant in a pediatrician's office? Is this job a good fit for her? Why or why not?

2. Using reliable and valid online resources, research the responsibilities of a medical assistant. What personal traits are important for medical assistants? What skills do medical assistants need to know?

3. Is medical assisting a career that interests you? Why or why not?

Chapter 7 Career Skills in Support Services

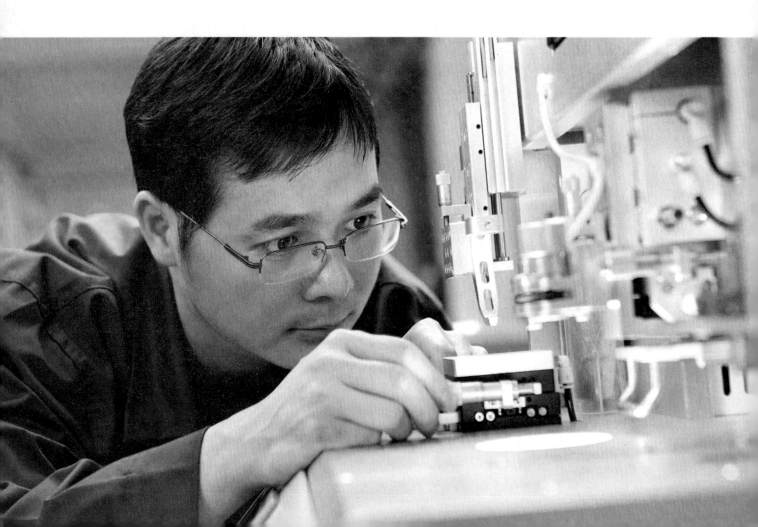

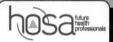

HOSA Event Prep: Creative Problem Solving

In medicine, answers are not always easy to find. Sometimes a healthcare team must work together to find solutions. Problem solving may involve managing limited resources or deciding when a patient should receive a resource. Thinking outside the box and brainstorming ideas help solve problems when answers are not clear. HOSA—Future Health Professionals has a team event called *Creative Problem Solving*. In this event, teams receive a problem to solve. Teams are given time to review challenges, brainstorm solutions, and present their ideas to a panel of judges. Problem solving is a great skill to learn early in life.

Go to the HOSA website to learn more about the HOSA *Creative Problem Solving* event. Find out the purpose of the event, what is involved in the event, and what knowledge is demonstrated in the event.

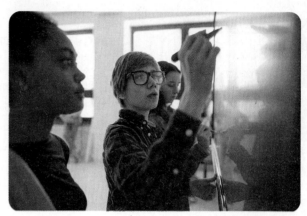

As you prepare for HOSA competitive events, be sure to check the website and talk with your HOSA advisor for the most up-to-date guidelines and procedures. Once you have learned about the *Creative Problem Solving* event, answer the following questions:

1. How might participating in this event benefit you personally and your future career? Explain.
2. Are you interested in participating in this event? Why or why not?

Halfpoint/Shutterstock.com

Connect with Your Reading

While a wide variety of occupations focus on support services, these occupations are often invisible to patients. Connect the following items to a healthcare facility department or to a healthcare employee to help you envision healthcare support services occupations: a hospital bill, dinner, sterilized surgical equipment, a television ad for a hospital, an interview, a newsletter, a time study, a health club, and a group home. Share your responses with a classmate and discuss your results.

Map Your Reading

Draw the radial diagram and fill in the main headings as they appear in the text. Create a question or two for each heading to help you identify the main point of each section. As you read each section, answer the questions you have written. Then answer the questions that follow.

1. Consider your own personal traits. Which of the traits described in this chapter do you possess?
2. Select any career discussed in this chapter. Describe how it suits your aptitudes and interests.

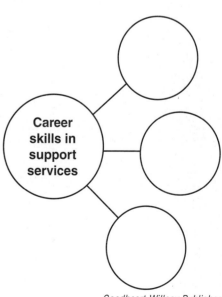

Career skills in support services

Chapter opener image: 7postman/iStock/Getty Images Plus via Getty Images

Goodheart-Willcox Publisher

Personal Traits and Career Choices in Support Services

ESSENTIAL QUESTION

What jobs are found in the support services pathway, and how do personal traits benefit this work?

Learning Outcomes

After studying this lesson, you will be able to

7.1-1 relate the common goal of support services workers.

7.1-2 illustrate traits of successful support services workers.

7.1-3 describe support service careers in business operations.

7.1-4 examine careers in maintaining a safe and healthy facility environment.

7.1-5 explain types of careers in nutrition and wellness.

7.1-6 identify careers in community and social services.

Professional Vocabulary

Essential Terms

central services hospital department responsible for receiving, storing, cleaning, disinfecting, sterilizing, and distributing medical and surgical supplies and equipment

compassion sympathy for the distress of others accompanied by a desire to help

environmental services hospital department responsible for housekeeping, laundry, and facility maintenance

initiative ability to decide independently what to do and when to do it

support services career pathway that focuses on creating a therapeutic environment for providing patient care

sanitation procedures and practices that maintain cleanliness and preserve public health

Important Terms

case managers
clinical engineers
dietetic technician
dietitians
environmental engineers

fitness trainers
health and wellness
    managers
human resources
industrial engineers

marketing
paramedics
public relations
transport technicians

Introduction

You may not always see them, but support services workers are important members of a healthcare facility's staff. Their work contributes to the successful operation of a healthcare facility. You will find support services workers in administration, food preparation, and facility maintenance. These departments support high-quality patient care. In addition, you will learn about supportive healthcare careers available in your community.

7.1-1 Support Services Professionals

The **support services** career pathway includes many different healthcare occupations. Yet, all support services workers help create a therapeutic environment for providing patient care. From administrators to counselors, and fitness experts to maintenance engineers, these professionals are all part of the support services pathway.

The support services pathway also offers a variety of entry-level positions. These include dietary aide, housekeeper, transport technician, and central services technician. Entry-level positions offer valuable work experience in the healthcare setting. Students can use part-time jobs in these occupations to supplement their income while they train for their chosen healthcare career.

Healthcare Professions: The Support Services Worker

When Gloria headed off to college, she decided to study dietetics (dI-uh-TEH-tihks). She loved to cook, so she thought a career working with menus and food would be a good fit. Her own family members followed a healthy diet to manage their health conditions, and she wanted to help other people do the same thing. After a couple years of college, however,

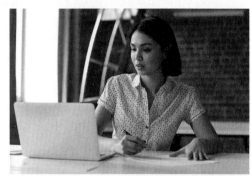

fizkes/iStock via Getty Images Plus via Getty Images

Gloria was bored and discouraged. She was a good student but did not enjoy all the chemistry-based science courses. She began to wonder if she would really like analyzing diets and planning menus. She was looking for something more creative.

Gloria always gave the best parties. She was good at organizing groups of people and could always talk her friends into following her plans. She thought business and marketing might be more exciting than dietetics, so she changed her major and finished her degree.

Two years later, Gloria had a job in business, but it was just a job. She was a good worker, but she did not find organizing the sale and shipment of products satisfying. Around this time, Gloria volunteered to help a colleague organize a fundraiser to benefit patients with AIDS. She planned an Oscar party event, which was a huge success. This was a project she really enjoyed, it was for a worthwhile cause, and it got her thinking.

Today, Gloria has a satisfying job in marketing at a nonprofit children's hospital. She is passionate about the care her organization provides for its patients. She loves planning children's fairs, annual proms for the teen patients, and other special events to enhance the experiences of children who spend so much of their young lives as hospital patients. Gloria is a healthcare worker. Her career is just one example of the wide variety of careers that make up the healthcare support services pathway.

7.1-2 Personal Traits

Do you like organizing people and events? Are you a natural leader? Then you might enjoy a career in healthcare administration, marketing, or public relations. People in these careers make sure that the business side of a healthcare facility is successful. They manage finances, plan for future growth, and make sure potential patients know about their facility and its services. To succeed in these careers, you need a strong sense of **initiative** and self-motivation. You must be able to see the "big picture" for the future of your organization and be willing to set personal goals to achieve success.

Are you enthusiastic about improving the lives of others? Do you enjoy analyzing the challenges in their lives? Do you feel empathy and **compassion** for others? Then you might enjoy a career in social work or counseling. Healthcare professionals in these areas have strong communication skills. They use their problem-solving abilities to help people figure out insurance coverage or locate community resources to meet individual needs. The work they perform allows patients to improve their personal relationships and live healthier lives.

Is food your passion? Do you like to help people maintain and improve their health and fitness? Then you might enjoy a career in nutrition or fitness training. These workers are enthusiastic and have a positive attitude about helping their clients and patients improve health and wellness.

Do you get satisfaction from doing a job the right way every time? Are you a responsible and reliable worker? Then you might find satisfaction in maintaining a healthcare facility (**Figure 7.1**). Building maintenance workers make sure heat, water, and electricity are available even during a power outage. When you consider healthcare careers, a maintenance engineer may not be the first one that comes to mind. However, patients who rely on ventilators to breathe know that this work is important.

Do you like solving problems and working with your hands? If you are fascinated with understanding how things work, you might enjoy a career in maintaining and repairing medical equipment. From the simple tasks of calibrating scales and sphygmomanometers (blood pressure cuffs) to maintaining the most complex imaging equipment, these workers ensure the accuracy of diagnostic tests and the success of treatments that require sensitive equipment. Workers' attention to detail in this area supports a positive outcome for patients.

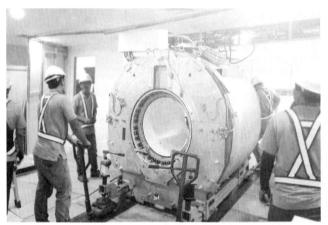

Radiological Imaging/Shutterstock.com

Figure 7.1 Medical equipment engineers provide vital services to healthcare facilities. *What personal traits are useful for this career?*

7.1-3 Sustaining Successful Business Operations

Successful businesses need capable leaders. Healthcare businesses are no different. Healthcare administrators like clinical managers and financial officers provide leadership for facilities by overseeing daily operations and financial planning. Marketing specialists and public relations workers promote the services provided by the facility. Professionals in human resources make sure the facility hires qualified workers.

Administration

Healthcare administrators, or managers, oversee the daily operation of a healthcare facility. In a small facility such as a nursing home, one administrator may manage everything. In a large hospital facility, however, several assistant administrators oversee daily operations in each clinical area, such as nursing, surgery, therapy, and medical records. Other assistant administrators oversee human resources, finances, and facility operations. Each of these assistants reports to the top administrator in the facility.

Healthcare administrators may work in large hospitals, outpatient care centers, physicians' offices, nursing facilities, or home health agencies. Since healthcare facilities often operate around the clock, facilities may call on administrators at all hours to address problems. Administrators work long hours and may travel to attend meetings or oversee satellite facilities (**Figure 7.2**).

Successful healthcare managers and administrators have strong leadership skills. They like to sell ideas and tend to be energetic and sociable. Managers strive to maintain positive communication between governing boards, medical staff, and department heads. They analyze and evaluate information to solve problems. They monitor equipment and oversee spending. They make sure the facility complies with federal, state, and local regulations. Managers in charge of a specific department or function have unique job tasks (**Figure 7.3**).

sturti/E+ via Getty Images

Figure 7.2 Both large and small facilities require the skills of a healthcare administrator. Some administrators oversee several facilities within the same healthcare system.

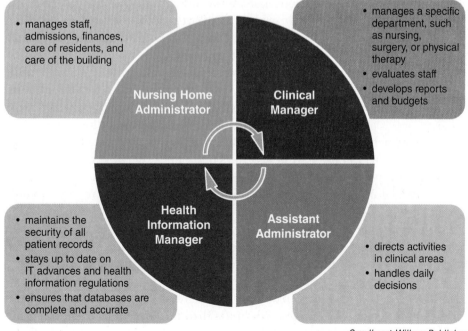

- **Nursing Home Administrator**
  - manages staff, admissions, finances, care of residents, and care of the building

- **Clinical Manager**
  - manages a specific department, such as nursing, surgery, or physical therapy
  - evaluates staff
  - develops reports and budgets

- **Health Information Manager**
  - maintains the security of all patient records
  - stays up to date on IT advances and health information regulations
  - ensures that databases are complete and accurate

- **Assistant Administrator**
  - directs activities in clinical areas
  - handles daily decisions

Goodheart-Willcox Publisher

Figure 7.3 Specific types of healthcare managers have unique job tasks.

Entry-level healthcare managers and administrators need a bachelor's degree in healthcare administration, public health, or business administration. Larger healthcare facilities commonly require a master's degree. Becoming a clinical department head requires a degree in the department's field, a few years of work experience, and an advanced administration degree. For example, a hospital nursing supervisor is usually an experienced RN with a bachelor's degree in nursing. To become eligible for a nursing administrator position, the RN obtains a master's degree in administration. Nursing home administrators are licensed by each state. They complete a training program, examination, and continuing education. Some states also require licensure for administrators of assisted living facilities. However, there is no license requirement for administrators in other areas of medical and health services management.

While the largest numbers of managers work in a hospital setting, the largest job growth will occur in the offices of health practitioners. Demand for managers in medical group practices is increasing. Job opportunities will be especially good for applicants with work experience in healthcare.

Marketing and Public Relations

Medical **marketing** professionals develop specific marketing plans to encourage future patients to use their organization's services. These marketing professionals create the healthcare ads you see. They work for regional medical centers, physicians' groups, private and public hospitals, and other healthcare organizations.

Marketing positions usually require a bachelor's or master's degree. Courses in business law, management, economics, accounting, finance, mathematics, and statistics provide important background knowledge for this career. The completion of an internship is also an advantage in the job market. Employers look for workers who are creative and can use new technologies to promote healthcare (**Figure 7.4**).

Individuals who specialize in healthcare **public relations** oversee the internal and external communications for a healthcare facility. They must have excellent communication skills. They interact with physicians, nurses, managers, administrators, and patients. Their job tasks include writing for staff newsletters and handling calls from the media. Their most important function is handling all communication with the public. Public relations specialists must be highly organized and prepared to deal with a variety of situations.

Public relations professionals work in a variety of healthcare settings. In larger facilities, they may supervise several public relations assistants who help with daily operations. Most healthcare public relations positions require a bachelor's degree combined with a public relations internship. Employers usually prefer a degree in journalism, public relations, or advertising. Individuals may seek professional credentials through the Public Relations Society of America or the International Association of Business Communications.

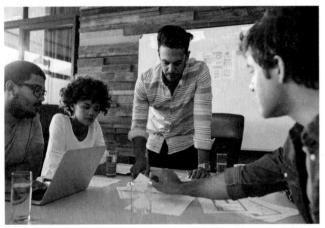

Jacob Lund/Shutterstock.com

Figure 7.4 Marketing professionals use their creative and technical skills to promote healthcare. *What information might be included in a marketing presentation for a healthcare facility?*

While the demand for marketing and public relations specialists is increasing, the job market is competitive. The number of qualified applicants is expected to exceed the number of job openings.

Human Resources

Human resources professionals find the most qualified employees. They match them to the jobs for which they are best suited and try to keep them at the company. In addition, these professionals oversee employee benefits such as health insurance, vacation, sick leave, and retirement benefits. Human resources workers also organize training programs to improve worker skills. There are many types of human resources managers and specialists. Small facilities will employ a generalist who is responsible for all the human resources functions. However, a large facility will employ several specialists to oversee specific tasks in human resources (**Figure 7.5**).

A bachelor's degree is the entry-level requirement for human resources professionals. Courses in behavioral science, business management, and finance provide a foundation of general knowledge. Because this field includes a wide variety of tasks, specialists will need additional training. For example, many labor relations jobs require graduate study in labor relations, labor law, and contract negotiations.

Human resource assistants are entry-level workers who keep records of a healthcare facility's employees. They update information in the records, complete reports for managers, and assist in the hiring of new employees. These assistants are usually high school graduates who receive training on the job.

Regardless of job title and training, all workers in human resources must interact well with people and keep employee information private (**Figure 7.6**). A wide variety of software keeps track of worker records and benefits, so computer skills are essential. Since human resources managers and specialists work with and supervise people of various ages and cultural backgrounds, the ability to speak multiple languages is also an asset.

Human resources workers can improve their knowledge and job opportunities by seeking training and certification from professional organizations. For example, the Society for Human Resource Management offers two levels of certification: Professional in Human Resources (PHR) and Senior Professional in Human Resources (SPHR). Certification usually requires completing coursework and passing certification exams along with demonstrated work experience. The field of human resources is growing. College graduates and those who have earned certification should have the best job opportunities.

Tasks of Human Resources Specialists	
Specialists	**Duties**
Placement Specialists	• Help set up interviews • Match employers with qualified job seekers
Labor Relations Specialists	• Interpret and administer labor contracts • Handle grievance procedures
Employment Interviewers	• Refer suitable candidates to employers • Interview potential applicants for job openings
Recruitment Specialists	• Find, screen, and interview applicants for job openings • Test applicants, contact references, and extend job offers

Goodheart-Willcox Publisher

Figure 7.5 Human resources specialists perform a variety of different tasks depending on their position.

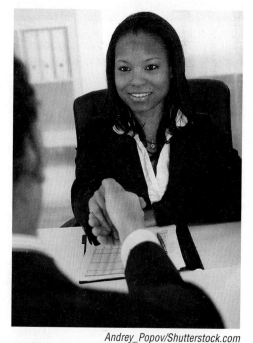

Andrey_Popov/Shutterstock.com

Figure 7.6 Interviewing potential job candidates is a major function of the human resources specialist. *What skills are needed for this particular job task?*

Maintaining a Safe and Healthy Facility Environment

Facility maintenance is a large task that requires many types of workers. Engineers maintain heating, air, and ventilation systems. Equipment repair technicians keep diagnostic and therapeutic equipment functioning accurately. Housekeepers and central services workers clean and sanitize the facility and its equipment to prevent the spread of infection. Transport technicians move patients to different areas of the facility and move specimens to the laboratory.

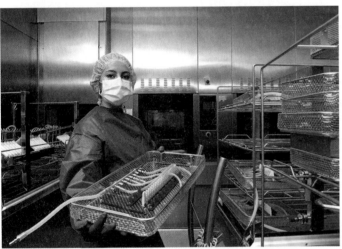

Photo-Art-Lortie/Shutterstock.com

Figure 7.7 Central services technicians work to prevent the spread of infection. *Can you describe some of their job tasks?*

Central Services

The **central services**, or *central supply*, department in a hospital receives, stores, and distributes medical and surgical supplies and equipment. Central services technicians play an important role in preventing the spread of infection (**Figure 7.7**). These technicians must know all the tools used in an operating room and be proficient in sterilizing and packaging surgical instruments.

Technicians may be trained on the job, but many complete a technical training program. Employers prefer workers certified by the Certification Board for Sterile Processing and Distribution or by the International Association of Healthcare Central Service Materials Management. Through these agencies, technicians receive continuing education and can complete coursework for job specialties such as instrumentation specialist, central supply manager, or ambulatory surgery technician.

Engineering and Maintenance

A variety of engineering professionals support the work of a healthcare facility. Most positions require a bachelor's degree in a specific type of engineering. Healthcare engineering and maintenance managers maintain the entire physical plant, including repairs to the facility and its equipment. The plant includes the building and all its heating, ventilation, electrical, and air conditioning systems. In addition, the engineering manager makes sure the facility complies with all regulatory agency rules. Managers typically have several years of work experience in a healthcare facility in addition to their bachelor's degree. Specialized engineers who work in healthcare include:

- **Environmental engineers.** Environmental engineers are concerned with safe drinking water, air quality, and other issues affecting public health. They work for universities, public health agencies, research agencies, and various commercial industries as compliance officers. Other positions include county public health directors, hazardous waste specialists, and water quality scientists.

- **Clinical engineers**. Clinical engineers have a college degree in biomedical engineering. Their primary job is to use medical technology to improve healthcare delivery. They consult with physicians and medical equipment companies and provide advice about design improvements for specialized medical equipment. They also train and supervise biomedical equipment technicians. These technicians usually have an associate's degree. They are responsible for equipment installation, routine inspections, and calibration of diagnostic instruments. They may earn a national certification and go through specialized training to understand laboratory and radiology equipment.
- **Industrial engineers**. Industrial engineers work primarily with people and processes rather than machines and products. They identify the most efficient ways to use space, time, workers, and other resources. For example, they may forecast the number of hospital patients to be treated in future years so that human resources can plan for adequate staff hiring. The results of industrial engineers' work improve patient care and reduce the costs of providing care.

Maintenance technicians and housekeepers also work in this department. Technicians are responsible for routine plumbing and electrical repairs and may need technical training in these areas. Housekeepers clean and sanitize areas such as patient or resident rooms, bathrooms, offices, lounges, and hallways using proper cleaning techniques. They usually receive on-the-job training and must be familiar with healthcare **sanitation** standards. Some facilities refer to this department as **environmental services**, which includes the combined functions of housekeeping and laundry.

Patient Transport

Transport technicians take patients to and from diagnostic imaging appointments (**Figure 7.8**). They may also transport specimens for laboratory analysis. These technicians maintain transportation devices such as wheelchairs and gurneys and perform general cleaning and storage of patient-related equipment. Technicians are trained on the job. They need strong customer service and interpersonal skills for communicating with a variety of patients. They must also work efficiently under stress, such as when they are transporting trauma patients.

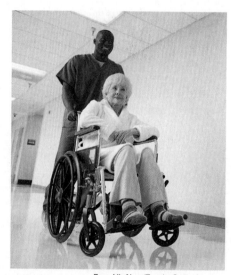

FangXiaNuo/E+ via Getty Images

Figure 7.8 Transport technicians may use a wheelchair to take hospital patients to and from imaging and surgery appointments.

7.1-5 Promoting Nutrition and Wellness

While your first thought may be that healthcare treats injury and illness, it also works to improve patient health and well-being through diet and physical activity. As the focus on promoting healthy lifestyles increases, a variety of career opportunities is emerging.

Food Services

If you have recently been a hospital patient, you know that hospital food service has changed dramatically from what you may have expected. Instead of standardized menus delivered at scheduled times, patients now order room-service meals from a restaurant-style menu at whatever times they choose to eat.

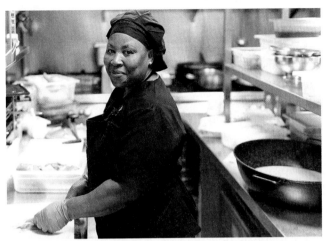

Figure 7.9 Hospital food service workers use their talents to prepare appealing, healthy meals for patients and staff. *What are some dietary specifications they must consider when preparing meals for patients?*

Customized menus meet special dietary needs, such as those for patients with heart conditions. In addition to a traditional cafeteria, visitors and employees may eat at the hospital bistro or even a commercial restaurant located within the medical center. Large facilities may employ an executive chef, as well as more traditional cooks and kitchen aides (**Figure 7.9**).

Dietitians (dI-uh-TIH-shuhns) are food and nutrition experts. They are therapeutic workers who advise patients about what foods to eat to improve a specific health condition. They are also support workers who develop meal plans for patients and residents in healthcare facilities. Many dietitians educate the public on food and nutrition topics (**Figure 7.10**).

Dietitians earn a bachelor's or master's degree in dietetics, food service management, or food and nutrition. Students must complete a supervised internship and pass an exam to become licensed as registered dietitians (RDs). The job market for dietitians is expected to grow as their work helps prevent illnesses such as diabetes and heart disease. An aging population and an increase in diabetes diagnoses at all ages will fuel the need for more dietitians.

A **dietetic technician** holds an associate's degree and works under the supervision of a dietitian or food services manager. Technicians plan and produce meals based on established guidelines, teach principles of food and nutrition, or help clients make healthy food choices. These employees work in hospitals, nursing homes, and long-term care facilities. Schools, day care centers, and government agencies such as prisons also hire them.

A sense of creativity combined with a strong knowledge of food and nutrition help dietetic technicians prepare food patients will enjoy. Employment for dietetic technicians is expected to grow, with the largest number of positions located in nursing homes, residential care facilities, and hospitals. Dietary services departments also employ cooks, dishwashers, cafeteria attendants, and dietary aides. Regardless of job title, all dietary workers must meet high standards for cleanliness and safety to avoid food contamination and injury.

Health and Wellness

A national trend toward adopting healthy lifestyles is driving an increase in the need for **fitness trainers** and instructors. Health clubs, community recreation departments, and large businesses that want to maintain a healthy workforce employ these healthcare workers.

Specializations Within the Field of Dietetics		
Clinical Dietitian	**Management Dietitian**	**Community Dietitian**
• Provides medical nutrition therapy • Creates nutritional programs for patients or residents	• Plans meal programs • Oversees kitchen staff or other dietitians	• Educates the public about food and nutritional issues • Works in public health or nonprofit agencies

Goodheart-Willcox Publisher

Figure 7.10 Different specialists in the field of dietetics perform specific tasks.

Fitness instructors receive training in specific exercise methods such as Pilates or yoga. They complete certification programs to teach a specific type of class. CPR certification is also a requirement. An increasing number of employers require fitness workers to have an associate's or bachelor's degree related to a health or fitness field, such as exercise science, kinesiology, or physical education. Programs often include courses in nutrition, exercise techniques, and stress reduction.

Employment for fitness instructors is expected to grow in the coming years. Aging baby boomers will be encouraged to remain active to help prevent injuries and illnesses associated with aging, so retirement communities and residential care facilities will need instructors (**Figure 7.11**). Businesses and insurance organizations continue to recognize the benefits of health and fitness programs for employees. Incentives to join gyms or other types of health clubs are expected to increase the need for fitness trainers and instructors. Other careers in health and wellness include the following:

- **Health and wellness managers.** Health and wellness managers work for small businesses and corporations. They develop and coordinate programs to improve employee wellness. Companies began to establish wellness programs to reduce healthcare costs. These managers oversee employee nutrition, exercise, stress management, and other health-related workshops and programs. They have at least a bachelor's degree and may have advanced degrees. They need business-management skills in addition to knowledge about principles of health and wellness. Their job tasks and routines are changing to support a larger remote workforce.
- **Health and wellness coaches.** Health and wellness coaches focus on the progress of an individual client toward reaching personal health and wellness goals. In addition to a knowledge of healthy lifestyles, these individuals are skilled at teaching, encouraging, and motivating their clients to work toward improved health. They complete coursework to develop coaching skills and can be certified through the National Board for Health and Wellness Coaching.

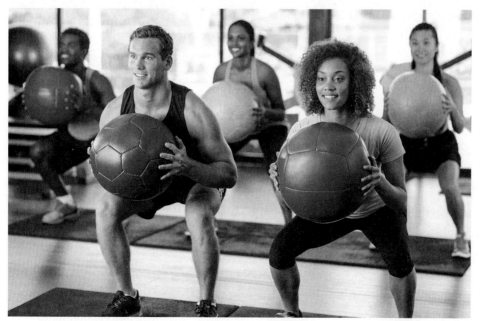

Lee Torrens/Shutterstock.com

Figure 7.11 Fitness instructors work at health clubs, but also at residential healthcare facilities. They lead programs and classes for all ages.

7.1-6 Providing Community and Social Services

Community settings provide many supportive healthcare services. Counselors and social workers, healthcare emergency responders, and human services workers provide healthcare support services where you live.

Counseling and Social Work

Counselors and social workers help community members who face challenges in their everyday lives. These careers require an advanced degree such as a master's or PhD. Direct-service social workers help people solve and cope with problems, while clinical social workers diagnose and treat patients with mental, behavioral, or emotional issues. Mental health clinics, schools, hospitals, and private practices employ social workers. Social workers generally work full time and may need to work evenings and weekends.

Counselors specialize in the specific needs of a patient population such as marriage and family therapy, substance abuse counseling, or career counseling. Counselors have at least a master's degree and usually must be certified or licensed to work (**Figure 7.12**). They work in private practice, mental health centers, hospitals, and colleges. They generally work full time and may work evenings and weekends, since counseling sessions are scheduled to accommodate clients who may have job or family responsibilities.

Rehabilitation Counselor	• Helps people with emotional and physical disabilities live independently • Helps clients overcome the effects of disabilities as they relate to employment
Marriage and Family Therapist	• Helps people manage or overcome issues with their family and relationships • Helps clients develop strategies to improve their lives
Mental Health Counselor	• Helps people manage or overcome mental and emotional disorders • Helps clients develop strategies to improve their lives
Substance Abuse and Behavioral Disorders Counselor	• Advises people who have alcohol use disorder or other types of addiction • Provides treatment and support to help clients recover from addiction
Guidance and Career Counselor	• Helps students develop social skills and succeed in school • Helps people choose a career or educational program

Goodheart-Willcox Publisher

Figure 7.12 Different types of counselors provide services for people who need help with a variety of issues.

Employment is expected to grow in all areas of counseling because this form of treatment is becoming an accepted part of healthcare. Increasingly, insurance companies provide reimbursement for mental health counselors and marriage and family therapists as a less costly alternative to psychiatrists and psychologists.

Case managers oversee the care of a client. They will assess the client's needs, develop a plan for meeting health needs, and connect the client with the resources required to improve and maintain health. While case managers do not provide direct treatment to a resident or client, they are critical to coordinating the resources a client needs. They follow up on care plans and evaluate a client's progress over time.

Case managers often work for government agencies and hospitals. They have at least a bachelor's degree and usually have a background in healthcare, counseling, or social work. Many employers require the Commission for Case Manager certification, and internships are part of the training program. Job growth is expected as an aging population will require more health services.

Social and human services assistants support the work of counselors, social workers, and case managers. They might work directly with clients to help them find benefits and access community resources such as food stamps or Medicaid health coverage (**Figure 7.13**). They may supervise homes for clients recovering from alcohol or drug abuse or they may support individuals with developmental disabilities living in a group home setting. They monitor and keep case records on clients and report progress to supervisors and case managers.

These assistants often have technical college training. They work for nonprofit organizations, private for-profit social services agencies, and state and local governments. Employment is expected to grow for social and human services assistants. This is due to an increase in the older adult population and an increase in the number of people sent to drug treatment programs rather than prison.

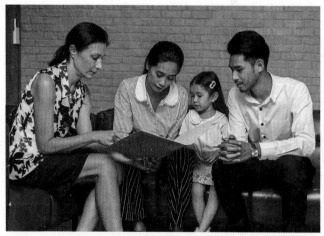

JOKE_PHATRAPONG/Shutterstock.com

Figure 7.13 Social service workers help clients locate and access community resources. *What are some examples of these resources?*

Emergency and Disaster Response

Firefighters, police officers, and **paramedics** respond to emergencies to restore a safe environment and treat illness and injury before patients reach a healthcare facility. These workers routinely face personal risk in responding to emergency situations and receive specialized training for their roles. All these individuals also receive training to respond to medical emergencies. Emergency medical technicians and paramedics staff the ambulance. They have training beyond the level of first responders. First responders complete a training program to become certified, while EMTs and paramedics complete a postsecondary education program and must be licensed according to the guidelines in each state.

Disaster relief workers respond to natural disasters like fires and hurricanes. Their actions save lives, preserve property, and provide humanitarian care. These workers lead evacuations, establish temporary shelters, and work to restore power to affected areas. They also bring food, medicine, and other supplies to support displaced residents. Government agencies and nonprofit organizations such as the American Red Cross employ relief workers. Some relief workers are full-time employees, while others are on call to respond when a disaster occurs. Still, many others volunteer in response to an emergency. Full-time workers have at least a bachelor's degree. Part-time workers have specialized emergency medical skills or technical skills, such as an electrician who can help restore power. Like emergency workers, they are willing to work in stressful conditions and find satisfaction in helping people in difficult or even desperate situations.

Lesson 7.1 Review

 Complete the *Map Your Reading* graphic organizer for the section you just read.

1. The goal of healthcare support services is to (7.1-1)
   A. treat illness and injury
   B. diagnose illness and injury
   C. create a therapeutic environment for providing patient care
   D. document patient care

2. Self-motivation and _____ lead to success in healthcare marketing, public relations, and administration careers. (7.1-2)
   A. compassion
   B. initiative
   C. support
   D. engineering

3. Medical _____ professionals create plans that encourage future patients to use their organizations and the services they provide. (7.1-3)
   A. administrative
   B. finance
   C. marketing
   D. human resources

4. _____ professionals manage training opportunities, oversee employee benefits, and hire new employees. (7.1-3)
   A. Public relations
   B. Housekeeping
   C. Marketing
   D. Human resources

5. Healthcare facilities depend on _____ professionals to keep a healthcare building and equipment safe and working properly. (7.1-4)
   A. engineering
   B. central services
   C. housekeeping
   D. administrative

6. Food service professionals include dietitians, who counsel patients and develop meal plans for patients, and _____, who plan and prepare meals for residents. (7.1-5)
   A. transport technicians
   B. dietetic technicians
   C. maintenance technicians
   D. equipment technicians

7. Which support services workers provide health services in a community setting? Choose all that apply. (7.1-6)
   A. Human resources workers
   B. Social and human services workers
   C. Emergency and disaster response workers
   D. Counseling and social workers

Technical Skills in Support Services

Learning Outcomes

After studying this lesson, you will be able to

7.2-1 practice bedmaking techniques that prevent contamination and protect the patient's skin.

7.2-2 identify standard and therapeutic diets and explain the function of a therapeutic diet.

7.2-3 describe actions and behaviors that create safe and pleasant environments for feeding meals to residents.

7.2-4 practice the steps for safely transporting patients in a wheelchair.

7.2-5 explain how HOSA participation can provide service-learning opportunities and which competitive events can improve your support services skills.

ESSENTIAL QUESTION

How well do the technical skills in this lesson match your personal work interests and preferences?

Professional Vocabulary

Essential Terms

service-learning an educational experience that integrates academic achievement with community service

therapeutic diet a special food plan ordered by a physician to help treat a disease

Important Terms

aspiration
consistency
dehydration

edema
mitered corners

United States Department of Agriculture (USDA)

Introduction

The job skills of support services workers vary greatly. This lesson focuses on tasks performed by environmental workers who maintain a clean and safe facility. You will practice making a hospital bed. You will learn how dietary aides follow safe food-handling techniques and see how therapeutic diets improve patient health. Finally, you will practice safe wheelchair transport techniques. As you practice these skills, consider the valuable tasks that support services workers perform.

7.2-1 Bedmaking

Brett works as a housekeeper at a major university hospital. In addition to cleaning and disinfecting patient rooms, he will make the hospital bed in preparation for a new patient. He has already removed used linens and disposable items and has completed terminal cleaning to sanitize and disinfect the patient room.

He will make a closed bed to keep the bed clean until a new patient is admitted. He brings only the linens he needs into the room. Extra linens are considered contaminated and must be laundered again. He is careful not to let the bed linens touch his uniform. He does not shake them out but unfolds them gently. In addition to hand hygiene, these steps help avoid contamination.

Brett makes a bed with smooth **mitered corners** (tight-fitting triangular folds) and no wrinkles in the sheets. Wrinkled sheets are uncomfortable and can lead to skin breakdown and open sores.

Brett works efficiently to save time and uses good body mechanics to avoid personal injury. He raises the bed to a working height, organizes bed linens in the order used, and limits the number of times he moves to the opposite side of the bed during the bedmaking process. He follows these steps to make a closed bed.

PROCEDURE | **Making a Hospital Bed**

Begin with hand hygiene and wear gloves if required by your facility.

1. Select clean linens, including a bottom sheet, top sheet, pillow, pillowcase, and bedspread. Place them on the clean overbed table.
2. Raise the bed to a comfortable working height and lower the side rails.
3. Place the bottom sheet on the bed and pull the corners of the nearest side over the corners of the mattress. Smooth down the sides.
4. Move to the other side of the bed and repeat the previous step to secure the bottom sheet if you are using a fitted bottom sheet. When using a flat bottom sheet, you will save time and energy by finishing all steps on one side of the bed before moving to the other side.
5. Place the top sheet with the centerfold at the middle of the bed and the wide hem at the top of the mattress. Open the sheet, keeping it centered, and place the bottom edge over the foot of the bed (**Figure 7.14A**).
6. Repeat the previous step with the bedspread. Usually, the top sheet is placed right side down, and the bedspread is right side up.

7. Tuck the bedspread and top sheet together under the foot of the mattress. Make a mitered corner on both sides (**Figure 7.14B through F**).
8. Fold the top of the bedspread and sheet back to make a cuff at the head of the bed. Check to make sure the linens are smooth, with no visible wrinkles, and that seams will face away from the patient's skin.
9. Place the pillow on the bed and grasp the closed end of the pillowcase. Turn the case inside out over your hand and grasp the pillow with the same hand. Pull the case down over the pillow. Avoid shaking the pillow or sheets when making a bed to reduce surface contamination from dust particles (**Figure 7.14G and H**).
10. Place the pillow on the bed with the open end of the case facing away from the door (**Figure 7.14I**).
11. Return the bed to its lowest position. Move the call light and bedside table back into place. Remove gloves, if worn. Wash your hands.

(continued)

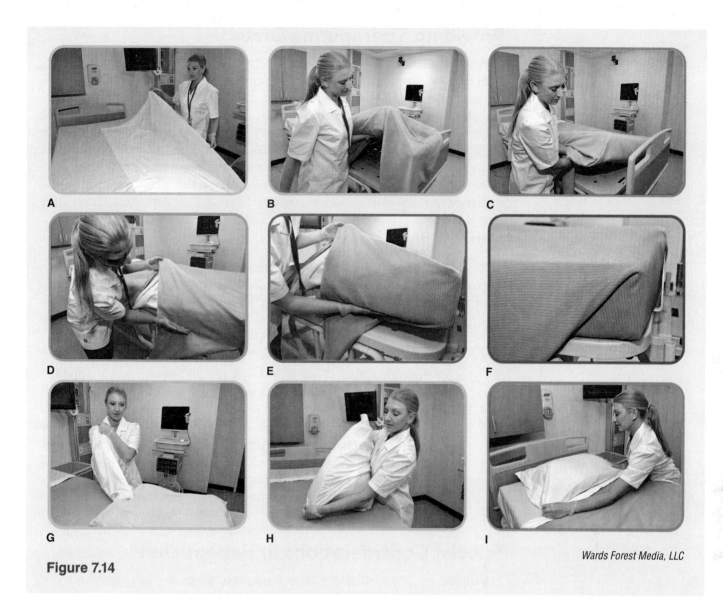

A

B

C

D

E

F

G

H

I

Figure 7.14

7.2-2 Patient Diets

Your diet includes the food and fluids you regularly consume as a part of daily living. Healthy diets follow guidelines recommended by the **United States Department of Agriculture (USDA)**, the federal agency regulating food quality and nutrition. They provide the nutrients needed to maintain or improve your general health. Most residents in healthcare facilities follow the general diet, or *house diet*. There are no food restrictions in this diet, but the facility may follow NAS (no added salt) or NCS (no concentrated sweets) guidelines in meal planning and preparation. In addition to the house diet, there are three standard diets: clear liquid, full liquid, and texture modified (**Figure 7.15**).

Standard Diets

Clear liquid diet	• tea, broth, gelatin, soda, and some fruit juices • for residents experiencing stomach or intestinal distress
Full liquid diet	• clear liquids plus milk, ice cream, sherbet, custards, and other foods that are liquid at room temperature • for residents with digestive disorders or difficulty chewing, and for recovery from illness
Texture modified diet	• same as a regular diet, but food has been chopped fine, ground, or puréed • for residents having difficulty chewing or swallowing

Goodheart-Willcox Publisher

Figure 7.15 These diets, along with the house diet, are considered standard diets. *What is the house diet?*

Providing Therapeutic Diets

Physicians order a **therapeutic diet** to help treat a disease or medical condition. A therapeutic diet may increase some food amounts, omit some foods as in the case of a food allergy, and restrict some foods to carefully measured amounts. A dietitian plans and manages all therapeutic diets. However, following therapeutic diet guidelines is the responsibility of all dietary workers. When a dietary aide serves a resident a meal, the tray must contain the right meal for the right resident. For example, the aide must know whether to meet a resident's request for sugar in coffee or use a sugar substitute. Correct diets are essential to maintaining good health, so dietary workers take care to serve only the foods that are permitted (**Figure 7.16**).

Swallowing Issues

Residents who have difficulty swallowing may drink thickened liquids. This helps prevent aspiration, or the inhalation of a liquid into the lungs. A special thickening product is added to bring liquids to the required consistency, which is the way the liquid flows. Dietary workers must recognize the following consistencies and may be asked to prepare thickened liquids according to a resident's care plan:

- **Nectar-like or nectar-thick liquids.** These fluids can be sipped from a cup or through a straw. They will slowly fall off a spoon that is tipped. Examples include buttermilk, cold tomato juice, and eggnog.
- **Honey-like or honey-thick liquids.** These fluids can be eaten with a spoon but do not hold their shape on a spoon. They can be sipped from a cup but are too thick for a straw. Examples include thick yogurt, tomato sauce, and honey.
- **Spoon-thick, pudding-thick, or pudding-like liquids.** These very thick fluids must be eaten with a spoon. They hold their own shape on a spoon and cannot be sipped from a cup. Examples include thickened applesauce and thick milk pudding.

Special Considerations in Patient Diets

Culture, religious beliefs, or other food preferences may also influence residents' dietary guidelines. For example, vegetarians do not eat meat, fish, or poultry, and some do not eat eggs or dairy products. Muslims do not eat pork, Mormons do not drink beverages that contain caffeine, and Roman Catholics have meat restrictions on Fridays during Lent and on some religious holidays.

Therapeutic Diets		
Type of Diet	**Description**	**Function**
High calorie, high protein	Encourages small but frequent intake of high-protein and high-calorie foods; may include nutritional supplements	Provides extra energy; promotes weight gain; helps wounds heal
Reduced sodium	Restricts the use of table salt and omits processed foods that are high in sodium	Reduces excess fluid retention in body tissues
Low fat, low cholesterol	Restricts the type of fats or the total amount of fats per day	Helps patients with liver, gallbladder, or heart disease; promotes weight loss
Carbohydrate controlled	Limits total intake of carbohydrates and/or calories, limits intake of refined carbohydrates, or balances carbohydrate intake throughout the day	Promotes weight loss; helps patients manage diabetes

Goodheart-Willcox Publisher

Figure 7.16 Therapeutic diets serve specific functions for promoting resident wellness.

According to the Omnibus Budget Reconciliation Act (OBRA), these preferences must be accommodated.

The passage of OBRA shifted the focus of long-term care from "rules and routines" to resident-centered care. The dining experience offers a significant opportunity to focus on residents' preferences. Making healthy food choices, socializing with friends, interacting with attentive staff, and enjoying a tasty meal are important. They are powerful elements in maintaining the quality of a patient's or resident's everyday life. OBRA includes these dining requirements:

- Meals must meet the individual nutritional requirements of each resident.
- Dining with other residents is recommended.
- Residents who are relearning independent eating skills must have a private eating area available.
- Food must be served at the proper temperature.
- Food must be appealing to look at and seasoned according to the resident's preference.

Serving a Meal

Allie works as a dietary aide in an assisted living healthcare facility. She is careful to follow sanitary food handling practices so that she does not contaminate the residents' meals. Clean hands and clean surfaces begin every task that Allie undertakes. It is Allie's job to follow meal guidelines for each resident carefully, and to make the dining experience pleasant and enjoyable. She follows these steps to serve a meal to 20 residents:

- Make coffee and set out meal tickets for each resident. The tickets display the menu choices prepared by the dietitian to meet the dietary requirements of each individual resident.
- Restock the kitchen with additional beverages, snacks, equipment, and supplies as needed. Record items on the inventory sheet so they will be reordered when supplies run low.
- Assist residents to complete their menu selections on the meal tickets. According to Allie, learning the unique needs of each resident is important. Low vision, hearing loss, and arthritis can make this task challenging for some people. Your assistance reduces frustration and keeps mealtime pleasant.
- Plate food according to each resident's ticket selections. To prevent food contamination, Allie always wears gloves when handling food. She is careful to ladle the correct amounts as well as the correct foods for each resident's tray.
- Serve each resident. Assist with slicing meats as requested by the resident. Alert residents if the food is hot. Observe residents and be alert for any eating issues, such as choking on meat.
- Clear tables when residents have finished eating. Scrape all dishes and discard leftover food.
- Run the dishes through the sanitation machine, making sure the machine is set for the temperatures and time that will sanitize correctly.
- Clean and sanitize tables, then set the tables in preparation for the next meal (**Figure 7.17**).

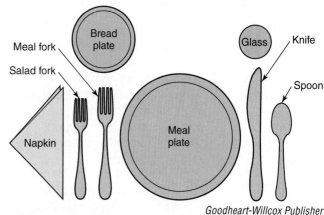

Goodheart-Willcox Publisher

Figure 7.17 This is the correct layout for a basic table setting.

7.2-3 Feeding Residents

Independent eating is always encouraged. When residents cannot maintain good nutrition through self-feeding, feeding assistants or nursing assistants provide support (**Figure 7.18**). Both types of assistants receive training in the complete dining experience. They know the elements of good nutrition and learn to recognize signs of malnutrition and fluid imbalance. They use adaptive equipment and techniques to encourage healthy eating. These workers understand that positive social interaction enhances the dining experience and improves dietary outcomes.

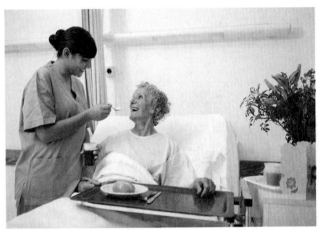

Wavebreakmedia Ltd/Wavebreak Media/
Getty Images Plus via Getty Images

Figure 7.18 When independent eating is not possible, a feeding assistant will help a patient with the meal.

Signs of Fluid Imbalance	
Edema (Too Much Fluid)	**Dehydration (Too Little Fluid)**
• Swelling or puffiness in feet, ankles, and hands • Congestion or wheezing • Weight increase • Decrease in urine output because the body is retaining fluid	• Dry mouth and lips, trouble swallowing, and appetite loss • Tongue that is thick and coated • Skin that is dry and itchy • Decrease in urine output because there is not enough fluid (urine is concentrated, darker in color, and has a strong odor) • Unusual fatigue and weakness • Onset of confusion • Weak or rapid pulse

Goodheart-Willcox Publisher

Figure 7.19 Healthcare professionals need to watch for these signs of fluid imbalance.

Creating a Positive Dining Environment

Making the dining experience pleasant and relaxed is an important goal when assisting with feeding. Provide for the resident's comfort by asking the nurse's aide to toilet and transfer the person before mealtime. Check to see that the resident is neatly dressed and has eyeglasses, dentures, and hearing aids if necessary. Wash the resident's hands and position the eating utensils within easy reach. Make sure the resident's head is upright to make swallowing easier. If permitted, raise the head of the bed to high Fowler's position for residents eating in bed. Use clothing protectors to keep clothing clean but ask for the resident's preference before using one. Remember that a clothing protector is not a bib. Since infants wear bibs, the term is considered demeaning for an adult.

Provide companionship as well as assistance during feeding. Checking your cell phone, talking with other aides about your weekend plans, or complaining about personal problems during a resident's meal is poor etiquette at the very least. It is also not consistent with high-quality care and may lead to neglect of the resident. Focus on talking to your resident even if the resident does not answer you. The sound of your caring voice will increase the resident's appetite and improve digestion.

Fluid Imbalance

Watch for signs of fluid imbalance as you assist residents. The amount of fluid consumed should be equal to the amount eliminated through urine output, stool, perspiration, and respiration. Too much fluid in body tissues results in **edema** (eh-DEE-muh), and too little fluid causes **dehydration**. Since fluid balance regulates functions such as body temperature and digestion, you must be alert to signs of dehydration or edema (**Figure 7.19**).

Preventing dehydration is challenging for older residents because a person's sense of thirst declines with age. First, check the resident's care plan for information on fluids to be encouraged and fluids to be restricted.

Then offer fluids frequently, especially when the weather is hot, or the resident has a fever. Keep fresh water within reach to encourage drinking water throughout the day. Pay attention to the resident's preferences and offer the beverages that appeal to the resident.

7.2-4 Providing Wheelchair Transport

Many different healthcare workers transport patients. Clinic nurses, radiology technicians, therapy aides, nursing assistants, and even hospital volunteers may transport a patient in a wheelchair. In large facilities, the transport technician takes patients in wheelchairs and on gurneys from one part of the hospital to another for diagnostic tests, medical appointments, and surgeries. In any situation that involves wheelchair transport, safety is the number-one priority.

Become familiar with the parts and operation of the wheelchair before you try to transport a person (**Figure 7.20**). Practice opening and folding the chair, adjusting and removing the footrests, and setting the brake. Drive cautiously through doorways and down hallways, being especially careful at intersections. Bend your knees and keep your back straight as you begin to push the chair. These good body mechanics help prevent back injury. Allow plenty of turning room to avoid smashing a footrest against the wall.

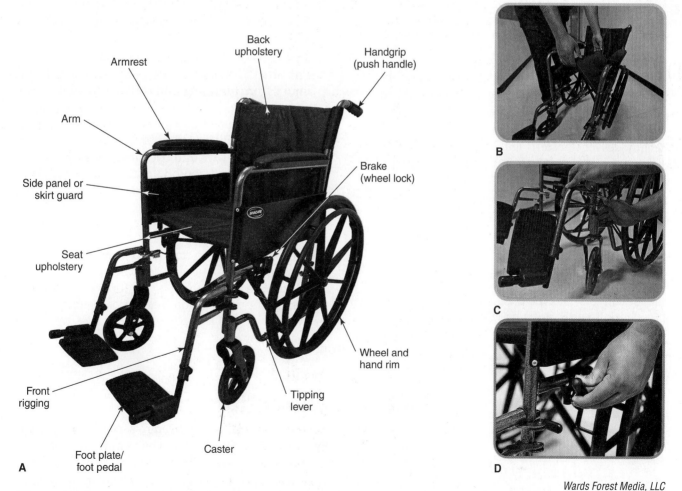

Wards Forest Media, LLC

Figure 7.20　Becoming familiar with a wheelchair means learning its parts (A) as well as practicing opening and folding it (B), adjusting the footrests (C), and setting the brake (D).

Learn how to turn and reverse the wheelchair smoothly (**Figure 7.21**). You should move wheelchairs in reverse when entering elevators, traveling down steep ramps, and rolling over bumps to avoid throwing the patient out of the chair. If you need to move up onto a curb, use the wheelchair's tipping lever. Step on the lever to raise the front casters onto the curb. Then roll the wheels up and over the curb.

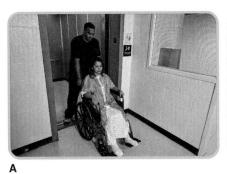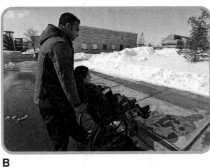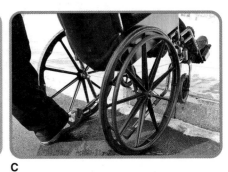

A **B** **C**

Wards Forest Media, LLC

Figure 7.21 Wheelchairs must be backed into elevators (A) and in several other situations. You should practice moving a wheelchair up onto a curb using the tipping lever (B and C).

PROCEDURE **Providing Wheelchair Transport**

The following steps for transporting a patient in a wheelchair assume that the patient can transfer independently. Patients who need help to stand and move to the wheelchair will need the assistance of one or two aides who are trained in the use of transfer belts and techniques for transferring to and from a wheelchair.

1. Follow standard precautions by washing your hands.
2. Rotate the footrests to the side of the chair.
3. Position the chair close to the patient.
4. Set the brakes. For safety reasons, this is the single most important step in using a wheelchair. Set the brakes during any transfer.
5. Make sure the patient is wearing nonskid shoes or slippers. Ask the patient to sit in the chair and check to see that the patient is seated comfortably. Tuck loose clothing away from the wheels.
6. Adjust the footrests and ask the patient to keep arms tucked in close to the body. This will avoid injury from bumping into walls or furniture in narrow spaces.
7. Release the brakes and push forward, keeping your knees bent and your back straight.
8. Remember to turn and back into elevators, over bumps, and down ramps. For the comfort of your passenger, the chair should never tilt forward.
9. When you reach your destination, set the brakes again. Move the footrests out of the way and allow the patient to stand and move away from the chair.
10. Make sure your patient is comfortable and notify the appropriate person that the patient has arrived.
11. Wash your hands.

7.2-5 HOSA Connections

HOSA is a great place to experience healthcare through service to your community. Look for **service-learning** opportunities as you acquire new healthcare skills. When you learn how to test vision and hearing and then use your skills to assist your school nurse in completing vision and hearing screening, you have a great service-learning experience. Remember that your community can include your school, city, state, country, or the world.

Is there a healthcare concern of special importance to you—providing healthy drinking water, ensuring vaccinations for children, or increasing physical activity levels? Take your health science knowledge and create a service-learning activity to address your concern. This will give you the satisfaction of improving your community while strengthening your own healthcare work skills.

Keep a log of your service activities in your career portfolio (**Figure 7.22**). This list will help you identify the healthcare skills you have learned and serve as a record of service hours completed. You may refer to this list as you write college entrance essays or complete scholarship applications.

Healthy Lifestyles, Community Awareness, and other HOSA competitive events will strengthen your support services skills. Read about them in the competitive events section of the HOSA website.

Sample Volunteering and Community Service Log					
Date	Hrs.	Type of Service	Place	Supervisor's Signature & Phone #	Skills Acquired
List the date.	List the number of hours.	Describe the type of service.	Describe the place.	Have supervisor sign.	Describe skills acquired.
List the date.	List the number of hours.	Describe the type of service.	Describe the place.	Have supervisor sign.	Describe skills acquired.
List the date.	List the number of hours.	Describe the type of service.	Describe the place.	Have supervisor sign.	Describe skills acquired.

Goodheart-Willcox Publisher

Figure 7.22 Keep a log of community service activities in your career portfolio to track service hours and identify healthcare skills.

Lesson 7.2 Review

 Complete the *Map Your Reading* graphic organizer for the section you just read.

1. What is the first and last step to making a hospital bed? (7.2-1)
   A. Folding the sheets
   B. Washing your hands
   C. Raising the bed to waist-level
   D. Shaking the pillows to remove and replace the pillowcase

2. In addition to the house diet, which of the following are the three standard diets? Choose all that apply. (7.2-2)
   A. Clear liquid
   B. Full liquid
   C. Non liquid
   D. Texture modified

3. Physicians order a _____ to help treat a disease or medical condition. (7.2-2)
   A. specialty diet
   B. therapeutic diet
   C. house diet
   D. general diet

4. Providing _____ during feeding is just as important as providing assistance. (7.2-3)
   A. independence
   B. a positive environment
   C. background music
   D. a bib

5. Which steps of wheelchair operation should you practice before transporting a patient? Choose all that apply. (7.2-4)
   A. Opening and folding the chair
   B. Setting the brake
   C. Adjusting and removing the footrests
   D. Spinning the wheels

6. Which HOSA competitive event will strengthen your support services skills? (7.2-5)
   A. Employability Skills
   B. Healthy Lifestyles
   C. Pharmacology
   D. Growth and Development

Chapter 7 Review and Assessment

Summary

7.1-1 Support services careers encompass a wide variety of healthcare occupations, but all support service workers help create a therapeutic environment for providing patient care. Support services offer entry-level job opportunities in patient transport, food services, and central services.

7.1-2 Self-motivation and a sense of initiative will lead to success in marketing, public relations, and healthcare administrative careers. Counseling and social work careers need workers who are empathetic and compassionate. Responsible and reliable workers support patient well-being in central services, engineering and maintenance, nutrition and wellness careers, and environmental health careers.

7.1-3 Administrators as well as workers in human resources, marketing, and public relations sustain the business operations of a healthcare organization.

7.1-4 A variety of engineering professionals, including maintenance, environmental, clinical, and industrial engineers, support the work of a healthcare facility. Environmental services and central supply workers contribute to a safe and healthy facility.

7.1-5 Dietitians, food services workers, and health and wellness workers promote nutrition and wellness in healthcare facilities and in local communities.

7.1-6 Case managers, social workers, and emergency workers provide emergency and social services within communities.

7.2-1 When making a bed, prevent contamination by not "shaking out" the bed linens. Prevent skin irritation by eliminating wrinkles in the bed linens.

7.2-2 The house diet has no dietary restrictions. In addition to the house diet, there are three additional standard diets: clear liquid, full liquid, and texture modified used in healthcare facilities. Physicians might order a therapeutic diet, such as a reduced-sodium or high-protein diet, to help treat a disease or medical condition.

7.2-3 Making the dining experience pleasant and relaxed is an important goal when assisting with feeding.

7.2-4 Setting the brake is the single most important step when using a wheelchair to transport patients. In addition, keep footrests out of the way when patients move to and from the chair, always reverse to avoid having the chair tip forward, and remember to use good body mechanics to avoid personal injury.

7.2-5 HOSA competitive events, like Healthy Lifestyles and Community Awareness, will strengthen your support services skills. HOSA offers many opportunities to build healthcare skills through service-learning.

Maximize Your Professional Vocabulary

1. **Vocabulary Sorting.** Sort each of the professional vocabulary terms under one of these headings: *skills and techniques*, *careers*, *conditions/diagnoses*, *departments*, and *regulatory agencies*. Be ready to explain your choices. Use any remaining words in a sentence to see if they might fit under or connect with any of the headings.

2. **Terms Presentation.** Prepare a presentation about two of the terms from the list. In your presentation, explain each term as it might apply to your own life. Then, provide a more scientific explanation of the term. Answer any question your classmates may have after your presentation.

Reflect on Your Reading

1. Consider the occupations you came up with in the *Connect with Your Reading* activity at the beginning of this chapter. Many of these occupations were located in a healthcare facility. However, many support services occupations exist in businesses other than hospitals and clinics. List five of these occupations. What do you think motivates these support services employees to work in the field of healthcare?

Review and Recall

1. Which of the following are entry-level positions in support services? Choose all that apply. (7.1-1)
   A. Dietary aide
   B. Transport technician
   C. Healthcare administrator
   D. Housekeeper

2. Social workers and counselors need (7.1-2)
   A. empathy
   B. compassion
   C. communication skills
   D. All of these.

3. Entry-level positions in human resources require at least a(n) (7.1-3)
   A. associate's degree
   B. high school diploma
   C. bachelor's degree
   D. master's degree

4. Which support services professional identifies the most efficient ways to use space and resources? (7.1-4)
   A. Industrial engineer
   B. Clinical engineer
   C. Environmental engineer
   D. Maintenance technician

5. Which support services professional focuses on helping individual clients reach personal health and wellness goals? (7.1-5)
   A. Fitness instructor
   B. Health and wellness coach
   C. Health and wellness manager
   D. Dietitian

6. Postsecondary education is required for which professionals? Choose all that apply. (7.1-6)
   A. First responders
   B. Paramedics
   C. Emergency medical technicians
   D. All of these.

7. When making a bed, you should avoid (7.2-1)
   A. making a mitered corner
   B. washing your hands
   C. shaking pillows or sheets
   D. smoothing the bed linens

8. Drinking thickened liquids helps prevent (7.2-2)
   A. aspiration
   B. heart disease
   C. foodborne illness
   D. frustration during eating

9. Which of the following is *not* part of serving a meal to residents? (7.2-3)
   A. Alerting residents food is hot
   B. Clearing tables
   C. Leaving while residents are eating
   D. Assisting with slicing meat

10. When pushing a wheelchair, you should (7.2-4)
    A. keep your knees straight
    B. bend your back
    C. move as fast as possible
    D. allow plenty of turning room

11. Which of the following are advantages of keeping a service log? (7.2-5)
    A. A log lists healthcare skills you have learned.
    B. A log serves as a record of service hours.
    C. You can list service hours and experiences on scholarship applications.
    D. All of these.

Build Core Skills

1. **Writing.** Create a newsletter, marketing ad, or brochure promoting a healthcare facility, such as a nursing home, hospital, clinic, or assisted-living facility. Make your writing clear, but brief, and include graphics to appeal to the public.

2. **Reading.** Use online resources to research NAS (no added salt) and NCS (no concentrated sweets) diets. Determine the specific guidelines for each of these commonly used diets. Compare and contrast the guidelines for and health benefits of these diets across the life span. Discuss your findings with a classmate.

3. **Critical Thinking.** Imagine you observe the following conditions in residents or patients. Use an "E" for *edema* to mark the signs typical of fluid retention. Use a "D" for *dehydration* to mark the signs of too little fluid.
   A. unusual fatigue or weakness
   B. wheezing or congestion
   C. coated, thick tongue
   D. rapid pulse
   E. puffy feet, ankles, and hands
   F. dry, itchy skin
   G. onset of confusion
   H. trouble swallowing and loss of appetite

4. **Problem Solving.** Whom would you go to for help in a healthcare facility to solve the following problems? For each situation, identify the support services worker who can address it.
   A. A patient needs help paying for healthcare.
   B. A patient wants to participate in a program to prevent falls.
   C. A resident's call light is not working.
   D. A patient needs a ride to the imaging department.
   E. The medical clinic needs to expand.
   F. A patient with diabetes needs nutritious snacks.
   G. You need an ad campaign to promote your healthcare facility.
   H. There are no paper towels in a patient's room.
   I. You need suggestions for streamlining average time for each patient encounter in a new ER addition.
   J. Surgical tools needed for an appendectomy must be sterilized.
   K. You want the public to know your hospital received the highest rating for patient safety.
   L. A potential employee needs to be interviewed.
   M. The bone-density machine needs recalibration.

5. **Speaking and Listening.** Work in a group to create a video that illustrates a poor atmosphere in a healthcare facility's resident dining area. Each person in the group should have a role, such as playing a resident or healthcare worker, writing the video, or working behind-the-scenes with the camera. Be sure to show examples of healthcare workers who act or speak inappropriately. Show your video to the class and explain how the examples you chose could influence the resident's quality of care.

6. **Critical Thinking.** Which therapeutic diet would help address each patient health concern?
   A. Slow wound healing
   B. Manage diabetes
   C. Manage heart disease
   D. Low energy
   E. Reduce excess fluid in tissues
   F. Promote weight loss

Activate Your Learning

1. Plan a meal that follows a specific therapeutic diet. Using a paper plate, create a visual that shows the meal's components. Identify the specific diet you followed and include a description of health conditions this diet improves. Analyze the meal's visual appeal based on variety of color, texture, temperature, shape, and flavor.

2. Review the steps for making a bed. Assemble the necessary supplies and practice bedmaking.

3. Review the steps for wheelchair transport. Then take turns practicing this skill with a classmate.

Think and Act Like a Healthcare Worker

1. You are preparing to assist Mrs. Allen with eating her breakfast. For each of the categories that follow, list the steps you should take to provide a meal that is as pleasant and relaxed as possible.
   - Provide for the comfort of the resident
   - Provide for safety and sanitation
   - Provide companionship

Go to the Source

1. Use online resources to learn more about support services careers. Select two careers of interest to you and complete a career profile for each one. Use at least one website that ends in .gov and one website that ends in .org. Record the following information for each career:
   - name of the career
   - tasks involved in this career
   - personal traits and abilities
   - educational requirements
   - type of credential needed and how it is obtained
   - work conditions
   - wages and benefits
   - job outlook for the future
   - the websites you accessed

   How do the two careers compare? Why might you prefer one to the other?

2. **Portfolio Builder.** Create a community service log using the example shown in Figure 7.22. Chart your service during a time period designated by your instructor. Add the log to your career portfolio.

3. Use the HOSA website to research the competitive events listed in this chapter. Select and note which event is your top choice and list reasons for your choice.

HOSA Event Prep: Creative Problem Solving

hosa future health professionals · EVENT PREP

Jefferson County is a small community hospital with limited resources. They have four family practice physicians and three pediatricians. Their surgeon retired and has not been replaced. They do not deliver babies and only have a three-bed intensive care unit (ICU) and a 30-bed medical/surgical unit. The nearest large hospital that has a trauma center, surgeons, a large labor and delivery unit, and a neonatal ICU is 40 miles away. In June 2020, the county had a large outbreak of COVID-19. They were seeing 20–50 patients a day with COVID-19 symptoms. All their beds were full, and the ICU was using the only two ventilators they had. One day, two people presented with severe respiratory distress and would soon need respiratory support. What would you do in this situation?

Think About It

1. Use valid online resources to research how hospitals coped with a ventilator shortage during the COVID-19 outbreak.

2. List one creative solution you identified through your research.

3. Do you think you would enjoy working in a team to research and find creative solutions to healthcare issues? Name a healthcare professional who would use creative problem solving at work.

Chapter 8

Career Skills in Biotechnology Research and Development

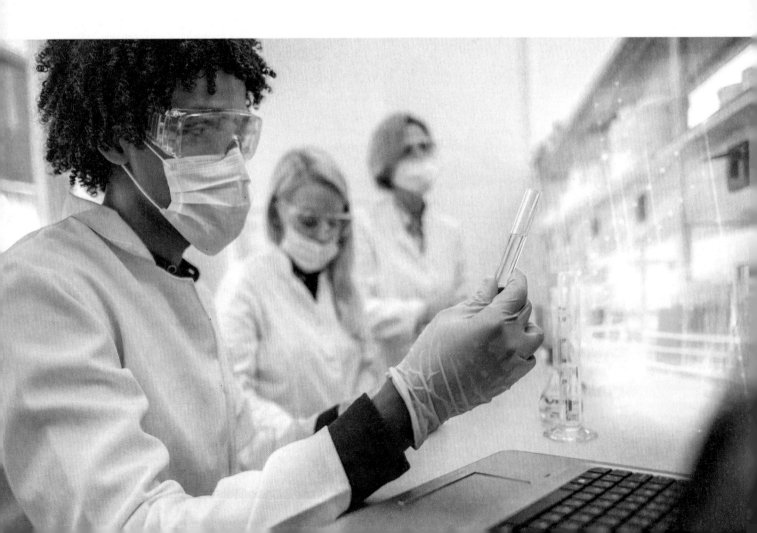

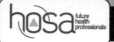

Medicine is always changing and getting better. Research is vital to making progress. All fields of medicine rely on research to improve their practice. When you do research, there are many ways it can be presented. One way is through a poster presentation. Poster presentations allow the presenter to use visuals and words to communicate their message. The *Research Poster* competitive event allows the student to pick a topic and then research and present findings.

Go to the HOSA website to learn more about the HOSA *Research Poster* event. Find out the purpose of the event, what is involved in the event, and what knowledge is demonstrated in the event.

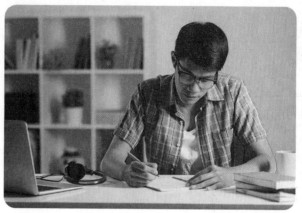

As you prepare for HOSA competitive events, be sure to check the website and talk with your HOSA advisor for the most up-to-date guidelines and procedures. Once you have learned about the *Research Poster* event, answer the following questions:

1. How might participating in this event benefit you personally and your future career? Explain.
2. Are you interested in participating in this event? Why or why not?

Dragon Images/Shutterstock.com

 ## Connect with Your Reading

Make a list of five improvements made to medical care during your lifetime. These may be procedures, equipment, or treatments. Compare and discuss your list with a classmate. Did you list the same improvements or different ones?

Next, identify the types of workers involved in creating each new procedure, piece of equipment, or treatment on your list. Once again, compare your list with a classmate. Consider these workers as you read about biotechnology, research, and development careers in this chapter.

 ## Map Your Reading

Draw a radial diagram as shown with one circle for each main heading in the chapter. Write the chapter title in the large circle and fill in the main headings as they appear in the text. Create a question or two for each heading to help you identify the main point of each section. As you read each section, answer the questions you have written. Then answer the questions that follow.

1. Consider your own personal traits. Which of the traits described in this chapter do you possess?
2. Select any career discussed in this chapter. Describe how it suits your aptitudes and interests.

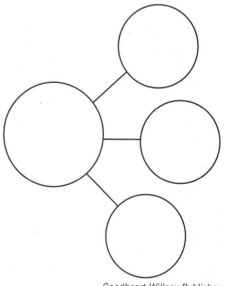

Chapter opener image: bluecinema/E+ via Getty Images

Goodheart-Willcox Publisher

Personal Traits and Career Choices in Biotechnology Research and Development

ESSENTIAL QUESTION

What jobs are found in the biotechnology research and development pathway, and how do personal traits benefit this work?

Learning Outcomes

After studying this lesson, you will be able to

8.1-1 identify traits of successful biotechnology research and development workers.

8.1-2 describe the field of biotechnology and scientific advances that have shaped it.

8.1-3 explain the basic differences between clinical and research laboratories.

8.1-4 categorize the wide variety of biotechnology research and development employment opportunities.

Professional Vocabulary

Essential Terms

assay   analysis done to determine the presence and amount of a substance or the potency of a drug

biotechnology   the manipulation of living organisms to produce useful products

biotechnology research laboratories   research facilities that develop new products or treatments and are located on college campuses, in hospitals, and in private biotechnology companies

clinical laboratories   facilities that examine materials taken from the human body to discover information related to diagnosis, prognosis, prevention, or treatment of disease

clinical trial   research conducted with patients to evaluate a new medical treatment, drug, or device

Important Terms

algorithms
aptitude
bioassays
bioinformatics scientists
biomedical engineers
bioreactors
centrifuges
consultants
epidemiologists
fermentors
forensic DNA analysts
genetic counselors

geneticists
good laboratory practices (GLPs)
good manufacturing processes (GMPs)
health and safety specialists
hypothesis
manufacturing process engineers
placebo
point-of-care testing

quality assurance specialists
quality control technicians
sales representatives
standard operating procedures (SOPs)
technical service representatives
waived tests

Introduction

Whether they develop a new drug, build a surgical robot, market artificial heart valves, or maintain sterile conditions where medicines are produced, biotechnology research and development workers fill a wide variety of work roles. In this lesson, you will learn about job opportunities in the biotechnology research and development pathway.

Healthcare Professions: The Biotechnology Research and Development Worker

Annika was excited about finally finishing her PhD program. After completing her undergraduate degree and six years of postgraduate research, she was ready for the next step in her career. However, that step was causing a problem.

Annika had enjoyed science in high school and had chosen that field for her college coursework. Part-time

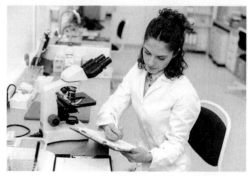

GoodLifeStudio/E+ via Getty Images

work in a research lab during her undergraduate years convinced her that research was the direction her career should take. Her postgraduate work in stem cell research was energizing, and she spent many hours perfecting her laboratory research and scientific writing skills to prepare for a career in biotechnology research.

When asked why she chose research instead of medicine, Annika always explained that physicians help one person at a time. Researchers, on the other hand, can help many people and change the delivery of healthcare with their discoveries. Her program supervisor and lab director encouraged her to pursue an academic research career. That had always been her goal, but lately she was not quite sure.

Annika observed the high level of commitment shown by academic research lab directors and saw how the work consumed them. She had also experienced that singular focus when her postgraduate research consumed her life. Did she really want her career to be the main focus of her life? Maybe she should consider a career working for a pharmaceutical or other biotechnology company. She could still use her research skills, but would have more time to pursue personal goals. Either way, Annika knew she would find her career niche in the expanding field of biotechnology research and development.

8.1-1 Personal Traits

Do you enjoy science classes? Do you find lab experiments interesting? If so, you might find a satisfying career in **biotechnology** research and development. If you pay attention to details and take pride in performing work precisely and accurately, then you have qualities required for successful work in a research laboratory.

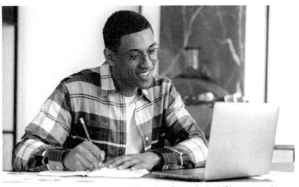

Kateryna Onyschchuk/Shutterstock.com

Figure 8.1 If you have organized class notes like Davante, you may have a natural aptitude for skills needed by lab workers.

For example, Davante's friends teased him about his class binder. He had the best notes in the class and routinely made lists of tasks to complete every assignment (**Figure 8.1**). His teacher commented he had the most organized binder she had ever seen. Though Davante did not know it, he had an **aptitude**, or natural inclination, for documenting experimental data. Habits that came naturally to him are strengths of skilled lab workers.

Do you like to figure out why things happen or come up with your own ideas to solve problems? Then you may enjoy the challenge of working as a lab scientist developing and testing new biotechnology products. Are you persistent but also patient? Since it takes many years to develop and test new products, these qualities will keep you from becoming discouraged during the research process.

Do you enjoy working with computers? As a result of DNA sequencing, large databases of biological information are becoming common in research settings. Biotechnology research and development scientists will need computation skills for working with large data sets.

Can you be discrete about sharing information? In a competitive research environment, teamwork moves a project forward and can help increase the documentation of results. However, sharing research ideas and information inappropriately can cost a researcher years of work. If that information is leaked, someone else might publish similar research findings first.

Nora, a lab technician for a biotechnology research company, says that honesty is important for all research workers. Inaccurate test results caused by poor lab practices or falsified research data can cause real harm to patients. Physicians rely on research results that are valid, legitimate, and accurate when they develop treatment regimens for their patients. Validity is important in scientific research because patients expect new treatments to be beneficial. In Nora's lab, a broken beaker in step seven means starting over from step one to prepare the designated formulation. That means Nora might have to stay late to finish so that the steps in the research study are not interrupted and the results are reliable.

Are you a likeable person with great listening skills? Do you like a team-oriented environment and enjoy working with people who have different personalities? Then you might find your career in biotechnology sales and support. While sales representatives focus on building relationships with potential customers, they must also become **consultants** for any healthcare worker who uses the products they sell. This means they give professional advice or provide training seminars for those healthcare workers. Sales reps need self-motivation, enthusiasm, and resilience to be successful in selling products. They also need good time-management and organizational skills to educate and support the people who use their products.

8.1-2 **Advances in Biotechnology**

You might choose a career in biotechnology so you can cure diseases, feed the hungry, or improve the environment. People who work in this field discover new drugs and manufacture medical devices. They also improve food crops and preserve the environment. Biotechnology is a growing industry that provides job opportunities for people who have studied biological sciences and have good laboratory and computer science skills.

What exactly is biotechnology? This field uses advances in life sciences to create products that come from the living things we call organisms. The science of biotechnology uses the DNA molecules found in the cells of all living organisms (**Figure 8.2**). People have used the concept of biotechnology—modifying living organisms for human purposes—for many years. Historically, people have domesticated animals or cultivated plants using artificial selection or hybrid development during breeding. Modern biotechnology, however, began in the 1970s. Scientists modified a DNA molecule by "recombining" DNA from two different organisms. They combined an insulin gene with a bacterium cell. Then they multiplied it millions of times to harvest the insulin. Insulin treats diabetes. This manufactured insulin is more plentiful and less expensive than insulin extracted from animals. Biotechnology was also used to sequence the human genome and clone mammals.

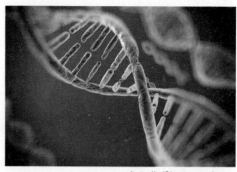

vitstudio/Shutterstock.com

Figure 8.2 In the field of biotechnology, DNA molecules become the building blocks for research tools and diagnostic tests.

Today, people use biotechnology to formulate drugs and create **assays** and other biological research tools. Using biotechnology, scientists develop the diagnostic tests that are used in medical research, diagnosis, and treatment (**Figure 8.3**). Currently, researchers are working to develop gene therapies with the goal of curing genetic diseases. They are using stem cells to develop treatments for spinal cord injuries and chronic diseases like sickle-cell disease. As medicine becomes more personalized, providers will use a patient's own genomic sequence to tailor medical treatment.

Biotechnology research and development also includes the development of new medical products and devices. MRI machines, DNA sequencers, surgical robots, and automated specimen analyzers are all examples of advancements made through biotechnology research and development.

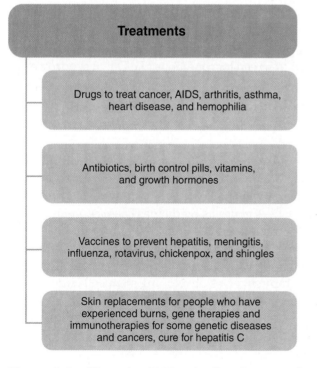

Treatments

- Drugs to treat cancer, AIDS, arthritis, asthma, heart disease, and hemophilia
- Antibiotics, birth control pills, vitamins, and growth hormones
- Vaccines to prevent hepatitis, meningitis, influenza, rotavirus, chickenpox, and shingles
- Skin replacements for people who have experienced burns, gene therapies and immunotherapies for some genetic diseases and cancers, cure for hepatitis C

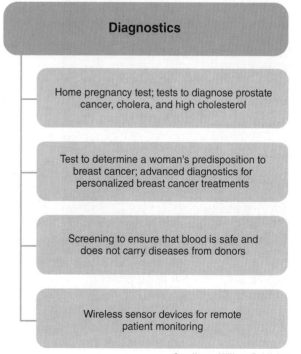

Diagnostics

- Home pregnancy test; tests to diagnose prostate cancer, cholera, and high cholesterol
- Test to determine a woman's predisposition to breast cancer; advanced diagnostics for personalized breast cancer treatments
- Screening to ensure that blood is safe and does not carry diseases from donors
- Wireless sensor devices for remote patient monitoring

Goodheart-Willcox Publisher

Figure 8.3 Since the 1970s, the list of accomplishments achieved through biotechnology research and development in the area of human health has continued to grow. *Can you name additional advances in diagnosis and treatment?*

8.1-3 Types of Biotechnology Laboratories

Clinical laboratories test patients. They are located in medical facilities, at the Department of Public Health in each state, and at the federal Centers for Disease Control and Prevention (CDC). Each lab is certified by the Centers for Medicare and Medicaid Services (CMS). The five levels of certification explain what types of tests a laboratory can perform. These range from simple tests with little risk to complex tests requiring highly trained workers.

Small clinics and physician offices perform **waived tests**. These are tests the CDC or FDA has determined are so simple there is little risk of error. Waived tests include blood glucose metering, urinalysis using reagent strips, rapid strep test, and urine specimen pregnancy tests, to name a few.

The development of small, simple-to-use analyzers has increased **point-of-care testing**. This allows tests to be performed where care is delivered, including nursing homes, emergency rooms, intensive care units, and surgery suites. Portable analyzers can measure hemoglobin, glucose, and cholesterol. Most point-of-care tests are also waived tests.

Biotechnology research laboratories develop products and treatments. They are located on college campuses, in hospitals, and in private biotechnology companies. The FDA oversees biomedical research and regulates the development of human drugs and medical devices.

Medical biotechnology labs use monoclonal (mah-noh-KLOH-nuhl) antibody technology, bioprocess technologies, and genetic engineering technologies. Biotechnology research develops tests that diagnose patients. Examples include

- tests to confirm a diagnosis, such as the rapid test to detect strep throat;
- tests for carrier status of inherited disorders, such as cystic fibrosis or sickle-cell anemia; and
- methods for prenatal testing, such as chorionic villus sampling or blood tests to screen for conditions like Down syndrome.

Biotechnology research also develops patient treatments. Examples include the following:

- Enzyme replacement therapy produces enzymes that are given like medicine. For example, pancreatic enzymes are given to people with cystic fibrosis to help them absorb fat and proteins. They replace missing enzymes caused by blocked pancreatic ducts.
- Gene therapy uses genes as medicine. The new gene takes over for a faulty gene. For example, a treatment called *Glybera* compensates for lipoprotein lipase (LI-pays) deficiency (LPLD), which can cause severe pancreatitis.
- Stem cell therapy involves developing stem cells into specific tissue to replace or supplement tissue in a patient. For example, bone marrow transplants replace faulty cells with healthy donor cells.

Biotechnology research developed DNA fingerprinting (**Figure 8.4**). Also known as *DNA typing* or *DNA profiling*, this test uses DNA to show whether two subjects are related or to identify humans, other animals, or plants. In forensic science,

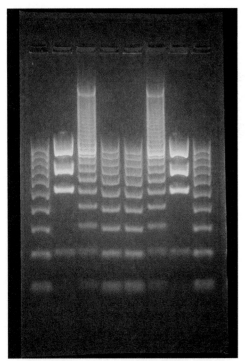

Jarrod Erbe/Shutterstock.com

Figure 8.4 In DNA fingerprinting, probes with radioactive labeling attach to complementary DNA segments of the same length and "mark" the segments to make them visible. An X-ray image of the membrane shows where the probes attached to the DNA fragments. The barcode-like result shown here is the DNA fingerprint.

the DNA fingerprint can eliminate a suspect, prove someone is innocent of a crime, or show that someone was present at a crime scene. In addition to forensic applications, DNA fingerprinting can also identify human remains and organisms that cause disease.

8.1-4 Biotechnology Research and Development Career Choices

Biotechnology research and development includes many different career opportunities. These careers might focus on research and development, manufacturing and services, sales and technical support, or quality and regulation.

Careers That Focus on Research and Development

Laboratory assistants, technicians, and scientists work in academic research labs. These biotechnology workers develop and test new products and medications.

Laboratory Support Workers

Laboratory support positions employ entry-level workers. These jobs require a high school diploma. These workers maintain the basic equipment used in a lab. They clean and store glassware, maintain inventory and reorder supplies, and test glassware to verify it is sterile.

Other entry-level positions focus on the plants or animals used in research. For example, animal caretakers provide daily care for laboratory or farm animals used in biotechnology research. In addition to feeding, cleaning, and grooming the animals, caretakers maintain records to comply with research regulations. They may administer medication to the animals in their care. This entry-level job requires a high school diploma and documented experience in caring for animals. Students can gain experience by volunteering at an animal shelter, zoo, or veterinary clinic (**Figure 8.5**).

Animal caretakers do lots of walking, lifting, and carrying. While they love animals and like working with them, seeing the effects of illness can be stressful. Forty-hour workweeks are typical for laboratory support workers. Working nights, weekends, and holidays is common in a research setting. Jobs related to caring for animals are expected to increase quickly and provide very good job opportunities.

Lab Technicians

Lab assistants and technicians usually have an associate's degree in biological science. Many technicians work to complete a bachelor's degree as well.

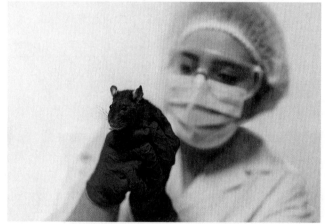

anstudiophoto/Shutterstock.com

Figure 8.5 Animal caretakers provide for the daily care of laboratory animals used in biotechnology research.

These employees work with scientists on biotechnology experiments. They follow directions using a high degree of accuracy according to **standard operating procedures (SOPs)**. These procedures spell out the exact steps used when completing any laboratory task. Workers know and follow **good laboratory practices (GLPs)**, which are regulations that describe how laboratories must operate.

Lab technicians prepare biological samples such as blood or bacteria. They complete experiments under the supervision of medical scientists and analyze and graph data from the experiments. They may assist in medical research by giving new medications to lab animals.

Successful lab technicians have excellent math skills and can work carefully at repetitive tasks to maintain accuracy. Greater demand for biotechnology research is expected to increase the need for lab technicians. Applicants with lab experience will have the best job opportunities.

Research Associates

Laboratory technicians with a bachelor's or master's degree and at least a few years of lab experience may become research associates. In addition to supervising the work of technicians and assistants, they may be responsible for developing the SOPs for the lab. Associates often have experience in specific biotechnology laboratory techniques or specialized areas of research. They are responsible for writing reports or making presentations about their research. They may also develop new protocols for research projects. Research associates work in many areas of biotechnology, including developing new products, testing new medications, and developing processes for manufacturing new products.

Medical Scientists

Medical scientists have a PhD and sometimes an MD. They plan and direct studies that investigate human diseases and methods for preventing or treating those diseases. Medical scientists can form a **hypothesis** and develop the experiments needed to test that hypothesis, or *theory*. They lead the teams of research associates and lab technicians who will carry out their experiments.

When their research leads to a new treatment or medication, scientists conduct a **clinical trial** using patient volunteers in cooperation with the volunteers' physicians (**Figure 8.6**). Patients in a drug-related clinical trial receive either the trial drug or a **placebo** (pluh-SEE-boh), which is a harmless substance that contains no medication. Patients do not know if they are taking the drug or the placebo. Scientists analyze data from all the patients in the trial to see if the trial drug worked better than the placebo. They also determine which patients had the most or least desirable outcomes. Finally, scientists write about their findings and publish them in a formal lab report, case study, or research article.

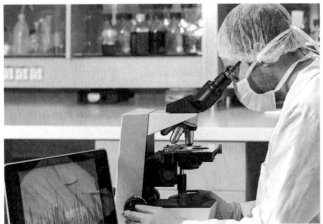

Belushi/Shutterstock.com

Figure 8.6 Medical scientists analyze research data and publish research study results that lead to new or improved treatments.

Medical scientists who work at universities also write and submit grant proposals to organizations such as the National Institutes of Health or the National Science Foundation to secure funding for their research. Scientists employed in the private sector develop new medications or medical instruments and typically have less freedom to select their areas of research. While they do not have to write grant proposals, they do have to justify their research plans to company managers. Scientists employed by government agencies also conduct research on human diseases and health. They may focus on exploratory research using nonhuman subjects or on overseeing clinical trials (**Figure 8.7**).

Careers That Focus on Manufacturing and Services

Once a product has been developed and tested, the manufacturer prepares for full-scale production. Once again, the government regulates the manufacturing process to ensure the manufacture of safe and reliable medical products. Medical manufacturers must follow GLPs as well as **good manufacturing processes (GMPs)** in the production process.

Medical manufacturing companies produce a wide variety of products. Pharmaceuticals and vaccines make up a large segment of the industry. Companies also produce **bioassays** that measure the effect of a substance on living cells for use in conducting medical research. Tests for screening or detecting genetic illnesses or chronic diseases are continually being developed and improved. For example, a colonoscopy is effective in detecting colon cancer. However, many people avoid the test because of the unappealing test preparation process. Scientists have developed an alternate screening process that is less invasive and eliminates the colon-cleansing preparation.

Medical devices and equipment represent another area of medical manufacturing. Picture all the equipment you encounter as a patient in a hospital or clinic. In addition, consider all the equipment used in medical laboratories. This includes digital microscopes, **centrifuges** (SEHN-truh-fyooj-ehs) for separating fluids, and analyzers for DNA or blood to name just a few.

Material Handlers

Material handlers are entry-level workers in biotechnology manufacturing. They work in warehouses, unpacking and checking incoming supplies and packing products for shipment. They may work with biological products that have a limited life span and with products that require a temperature-controlled environment. For example, some products may be packed in dry ice to maintain proper temperature during the shipping process. Material handlers feel comfortable lifting heavy materials and can operate conveyors, forklifts, and other equipment.

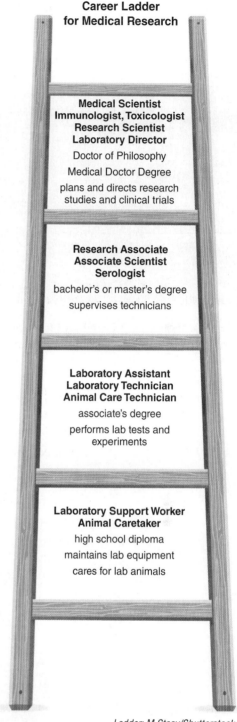

Career Ladder for Medical Research

Medical Scientist Immunologist, Toxicologist Research Scientist Laboratory Director
Doctor of Philosophy
Medical Doctor Degree
plans and directs research studies and clinical trials

Research Associate Associate Scientist Serologist
bachelor's or master's degree
supervises technicians

Laboratory Assistant Laboratory Technician Animal Care Technician
associate's degree
performs lab tests and experiments

Laboratory Support Worker Animal Caretaker
high school diploma
maintains lab equipment
cares for lab animals

Ladder: M.Stasy/Shutterstock.com

Figure 8.7 The career ladder for medical research workers.

Requiring only a high school diploma, this job provides an opportunity to learn about a company and its products. Employees may take advantage of company educational benefits to continue their studies and advance to other jobs within the company.

Manufacturing Assistants, Technicians, and Engineers

Manufacturing assistants have a high school diploma or an associate's degree. They work with **fermentors** and **bioreactors** to produce drugs or enzymes for use in the biotechnology industry (**Figure 8.8**). They may work in a "clean room" and wear special clothing to maintain a sterile environment. They operate equipment to fill, label, and package products. They may be exposed to disease-causing bacteria or viruses or poisonous chemicals, so their ability to follow safety procedures is critical.

Manufacturing technicians oversee the assistants' production work (**Figure 8.9**). Technicians typically have an associate's or bachelor's degree along with work experience in biotechnology manufacturing. They frequently use automated and robotic equipment and are responsible for sterilizing equipment, setting up the machines used to fill sterile containers, and completing routine equipment maintenance. They monitor equipment to ensure that SOPs and GMPs are followed. Since medications must be produced using the exact procedures approved by the FDA, mistakes during the process cost companies time and money. Medications cannot be sold if correct procedures have not been followed and documented.

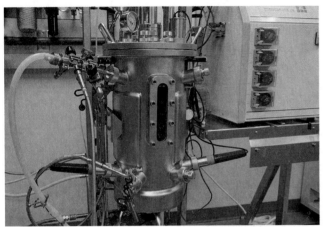

PT Hamilton/Shutterstock.com

Figure 8.8 Bioreactors are used for making pharmaceutical products such as antibiotics and insulin.

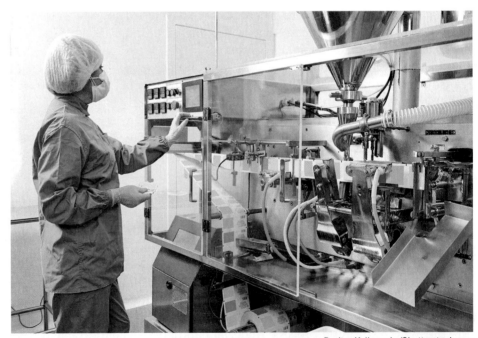

Dmitry Kalinovsky/Shutterstock.com

Figure 8.9 This manufacturing assistant is producing pharmaceuticals. *Why is she wearing PPE (personal protective equipment)?*

Engineers have at least a bachelor's or master's degree, and some have a PhD. **Manufacturing process engineers** design the methods and equipment used to manufacture a product. They apply scientific principles to the production of goods to make better products at the lowest possible cost.

Biomedical engineers combine their knowledge of biology and engineering to design and develop products such as artificial organs, prostheses, and machines for diagnosing medical conditions. These engineers can analyze the needs of patients and enjoy problem solving to design medical products. They frequently work directly with patients, therapists, physicians, and medical scientists. Because of this, they must be skilled communicators who incorporate the ideas of other professionals during the design process. Rapid advances in technology are expected to create new job opportunities for biomedical engineers.

Biotechnology workers can also provide services in crime laboratories. For example, **forensic DNA analysts** work in crime labs to extract and match DNA from samples that are used as evidence to solve crimes (**Figure 8.10**). DNA samples from crime scenes can help identify and convict people who have committed crimes. Analysts use samples of human tissue from blood, urine, or saliva to create a DNA profile unique to each individual.

Since forensic analysts work in law enforcement, they must pass drug tests and background checks. In addition to a bachelor's or master's degree in biological sciences, analysts need to complete coursework in crime detection and investigation. Forensic analysts also need strong speaking and writing skills. Their laboratory notes are submitted as court documents, and they may be called to testify in court cases.

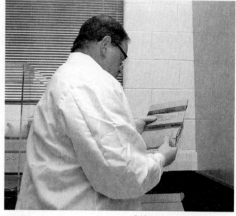

©iStock.com/Supersport

Figure 8.10 Forensic DNA analysts find information that may be used as evidence.

Careers in Sales and Technical Support

Sales representatives contact and meet potential customers to sell their company's products. They need a bachelor's degree in marketing or science combined with additional training in medical sales. Medical sales reps study medical terminology, anatomy, disease states, and specific product knowledge. They complete exams to prove their knowledge of company policies and government regulations.

Sales reps are excellent communicators. They listen to the needs of their clients and can demonstrate a product, answer technical questions about its use, and check to make sure it is working correctly. In some cases, they train the healthcare workers who will use their products. They also use writing skills as they analyze sales data, write sales reports, and keep careful records of sales contacts. The field of sales is appealing to individuals who enjoy traveling and working with people.

Technical service representatives have strong technical and science skills, but they are also good at working with customers. They usually have a bachelor's degree in biological sciences and have often worked as lab technicians. They solve technical problems that customers encounter. Reps usually communicate by phone or email, but they may go to the customer's business to install products. These reps know about product updates and receive training for all the company's new products. They track customer complaints to identify problems with a product and report those problems to supervisory staff. They may also complete research and lab work to find solutions to technical problems.

Careers That Focus on Quality and Regulation

Health and safety specialists focus on making the workplace safe for all employees by ensuring that safety regulations are followed. As part of the emergency response team, the health and safety specialist responds to hazardous spills, fires, and accidents that occur in the workplace.

A bachelor's degree in environmental science, safety, or hazardous materials technology prepares you for this career. Health and safety specialists write safety procedures for their companies and train employees regarding safety regulations and emergency procedures. They are also responsible for the safe storage, use, and disposal of any hazardous materials used at their company. A health and safety specialist needs strong communication skills and the ability to work with all company employees, especially during an emergency. While certification through the Institute of Hazardous Materials Management is not required, employers prefer certified job applicants.

Quality assurance specialists make sure that the manufacturing process follows required guidelines and procedures. They analyze data, write reports, and document every step in the manufacturing process. Their work shows the FDA that regulations have been followed so that a product will be approved for sale. Entry-level qualifications include a bachelor's degree in biology, engineering, or computer science and work experience in a manufacturing environment. These workers need good lab skills, attention to detail, and excellent organizational skills.

Quality control technicians perform inspections at every step in the manufacturing process. They examine raw materials used in manufacturing to make sure they meet quality requirements. Technicians also monitor the work environment to make sure that clean or sterile conditions are maintained (**Figure 8.11**). They test the finished product and check its packaging and labeling.

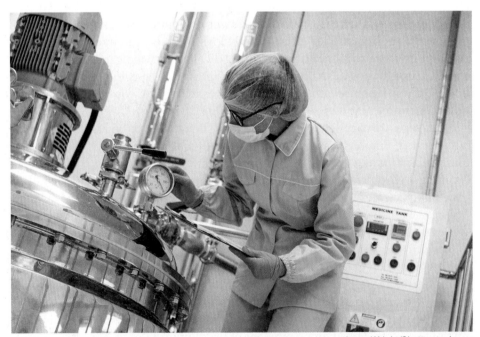

Jasen Wright/Shutterstock.com

Figure 8.11 Biotechnology manufacturing follows strict regulations to produce products that are safe for human use. *What is the role of a quality control technician in following these regulations?*

Technicians need a bachelor's degree in the biological sciences and some work experience in biotechnology lab work or manufacturing. They may specialize in biotechnology, microbiology, or chemical analysis. However, all technicians need good lab and problem-solving skills. They must continue to learn the changing regulations affecting the biotechnology industry. A working knowledge of SOPs, GLPs, and GMPs is expected. With experience, technicians can advance to analyst positions, which also require technical writing skills. Certification is voluntary and is available through the American Society for Quality.

Additional Career Opportunities

Bioinformatics scientists use their computer skills to organize the expanding overload of data created by improved DNA sequencing technologies. These workers combine biology and computer science to develop organized databases of biological information and to write **algorithms** or sets of rules that computers follow to process and analyze the information. For example, they may write a program to track and analyze influenza outbreaks across the country or one that evaluates the genetic codes of thousands of individuals to develop personalized medicine. These scientists have at least a master's degree with an extensive background in life science and computer science.

Epidemiologists (ehp-ih-dee-mee-AHL-uh-jihsts) study the spread of diseases. You will find them working in public health, research, and hospital settings. Epidemiologists solve medical mysteries by answering the question "What caused it?" Research epidemiologists figure out how to eliminate or control a disease, while clinical epidemiologists investigate outbreaks of infection. Epidemiologists have a master's degree in public health with an emphasis in epidemiology. Advanced epidemiologists have a PhD. Epidemiologists are meticulous, analytical, and logical. They possess a strong desire to help people. Indeed, their work has the potential to save many lives.

Geneticists (juh-NEHT-ih-sihsts) are laboratory scientists who study genes, heredity, and the variation of organisms. **Genetic counselors**, however, use genetic science to advise families affected by inherited diseases. They need a master's degree and must complete extensive coursework in biology, genetics, and counseling. These professionals meet with clients to gather medical information (**Figure 8.12**). They construct a detailed health history to inform clients about possible genetic disorders and help them understand and manage existing disorders. They connect families with resources that can assist them, such as support organizations or healthcare specialists. Counselors can work in a variety of specialty areas, such as cancer counseling, prenatal counseling, or pediatrics. Most employers require certification by the American Board of Genetic Counseling, and some states require licensure.

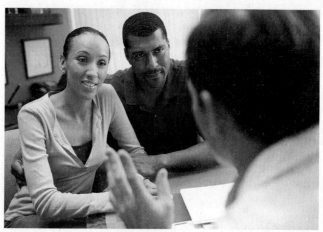

MBI/Shutterstock.com

Figure 8.12 Genetic counselors may work in specialty areas such as cancer counseling, prenatal counseling, or pediatrics. *How might counselors help a couple wanting to start a family?*

Healthcare Professions: Computer Graphic Design

Jesse never expected to work in the field of health science. He is a creative individual who enjoys working with computers. During high school, he did some photo retouching. Then a class speaker from a career college got him interested in computer graphics, animation, and game design. While attending college, he learned about an internship

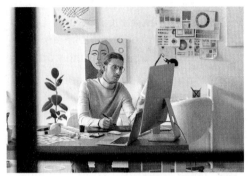

hobo_018/E+ via Getty Images

opportunity from a friend. That internship led to a full-time job working for a foundation that conducts biomedical research.

Today Jesse is a graphic web user interface designer. He works to promote the foundation's goal to make science accessible, exciting, and relevant for students of all ages. He does this by designing computer games that teach scientific concepts. He develops educational games so that students learn by playing, making complex medical concepts user-friendly. The results are interactive and intuitive games that do not overwhelm people with instructions. Jesse loves the flexible and collaborative work environment that gives him access to experienced medical scientists as consultants during game development. He loves his job and says, "I still pinch myself because I can't believe work is this fun!"

Lesson 8.1 Review

 Complete the *Map Your Reading* graphic organizer for the section you just read.

1. Which of the following are essential personal traits for biotechnology workers? Choose all that apply. (8.1-1)
   A. Honesty
   B. Computer skills
   C. Physical stamina
   D. Discretion

2. Which of the following best describes the concept of biotechnology? (8.1-2)
   A. Modifying living organisms for human purposes
   B. Conducting research
   C. Sharing research data
   D. Using science to solve crimes

3. Using a portable analyzer to measure glucose in an emergency room is an example of (8.1-3)
   A. point-of-care testing
   B. monoclonal antibody technology
   C. stem cell research
   D. DNA typing

4. Which of these careers requires more than a high school diploma? Choose all that apply. (8.1-4)
   A. Animal caretaker
   B. Laboratory support worker
   C. Geneticist
   D. Health and safety specialist

Technical Skills in Biotechnology Research and Development

Learning Outcomes

After studying this lesson, you will be able to

8.2-1 provide an overview of biosafety guidelines.

8.2-2 analyze laboratory safety measures observed in clinical and biotechnology labs.

8.2-3 demonstrate basic biotechnology skills, such as measuring mass and volume, testing urine, and using high-quality laboratory documentation.

8.2-4 summarize key skills for medical sales representatives.

8.2-5 explain how HOSA participation can build your leadership skills and which competitive events can improve your biotechnology research and development skills.

ESSENTIAL QUESTION

How well do the technical skills in this lesson match your personal work interests and preferences?

Professional Vocabulary

Essential Terms

biohazard a biological agent, infectious organism, or insecure laboratory procedure that constitutes a danger to humans or the environment

business-to-business selling exchanging goods between businesses rather than between businesses and individuals

electronic balances measuring instruments that display the weight of a substance digitally and are used to weigh chemicals in labs

laboratory documentation written records of observable, measurable, and reproducible findings obtained through examination, testing, research studies, and experiments

micropipette an instrument designed for the measurement of very small volumes

sales presentation a prearranged meeting in which a salesperson presents detailed information and often a demonstration of a product

Important Terms

customer objections
exposure control plan
meniscus
urinalysis

Introduction

Many employees in the biotechnology research and development pathway work in laboratory or manufacturing environments where safety and accuracy are critical. Research and development workers follow specific guidelines and protocols to ensure safety and validity. However, everyone involved in this pathway—from research planning to sales—needs to be concerned with the safety and effectiveness of the products they offer. For that reason, healthcare marketing professionals provide advanced training and technical support to their customers to ensure highly specialized products are used correctly.

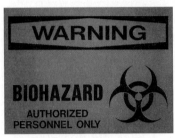

David W. Leindecker/Shutterstock.com

Figure 8.13 Entrances to areas containing biohazardous materials display the universal biohazard symbol. This means biological material that could pose a risk to human health may be present.

8.2-1 Biosafety Guidelines

All laboratory workers focus on safety measures that protect them from physical and chemical hazards created by fires, faulty electrical equipment, and toxic chemicals. Medical laboratory workers in both clinical and research settings must also focus on safety measures that protect against infectious agents. The term **biohazard** and the presence of the biohazard symbol warn workers of a risk to health or the environment from biological agents (**Figure 8.13**). Workers must know and use the appropriate measures to prevent exposure.

Biological agents are classified according to their level of risk. Biosafety Level One (BSL-1) agents represent the lowest level of risk, while Biosafety Level Four (BSL-4) agents pose the highest level of risk. There are four corresponding levels of biological containment to protect against biohazards. Each level of containment has guidelines for laboratory facilities. These include safety equipment requirements as well as laboratory practices and techniques.

For example, a BSL-1 lab is common in high schools and colleges that teach introductory microbiology courses. Students wear lab coats and gloves, and chemical disinfectants and steam autoclaving are used to decontaminate surfaces and equipment. Autoclaving uses pressurized steam to sterilize instruments, glassware, and other materials (**Figure 8.14**).

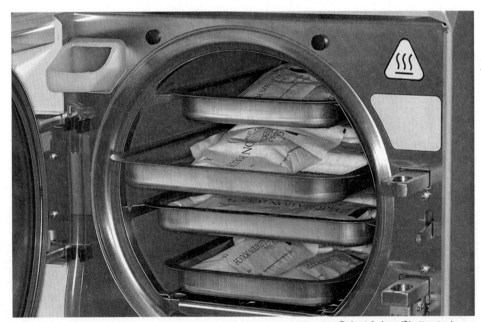

Robert A. Levy/Shutterstock.com

Figure 8.14 Autoclaves use pressurized steam to sterilize lab equipment. *Why are autoclaves important equipment for a lab?*

A BSL-2 lab has restricted access. Workers wear gloves, lab coats, and face protection. Autoclaves decontaminate waste materials, and a biological safety cabinet is available (**Figure 8.15**). Positive air pressure keeps infectious materials inside the cabinet, and air is drawn away from the worker into a vent or filter. BSL-3 and BSL-4 labs use separate buildings with double-door entry and directional inward airflow, as well as many special procedures and protective devices.

8.2-2 Laboratory Safety Protocols

Before beginning any lab procedure, healthcare workers must be trained in standard precautions and the use of personal protective equipment (PPE). They learn how to use a safety shower or eyewash station that limits exposure to biohazards. Laboratory workers also learn work practice controls. These controls are safe work habits that limit the possibility of exposure, such as handwashing after removing gloves. Every laboratory develops an **exposure control plan** that explains how to handle specimens, contaminated equipment, work surfaces, and waste materials safely. The following safety protocols apply to all lab settings:

- Wear pants or a skirt that fully covers your legs and shoes with closed toes. Tie your hair back and away from your face. Do not wear loose clothing, dangling chains or earrings, or large rings.
- Wash your hands before and after all lab procedures, after removing gloves, and before leaving the lab.
- Wear a lab coat or gown and gloves. Wear appropriate face protection, such as goggles, a face shield, or a mask, when working with strong chemicals or when splashing is possible.
- Know the locations of exit doors, a fire extinguisher and fire blanket, the safety shower, and the eyewash station so you can respond to an emergency or accident.
- If a reagent (chemical substance used in experiments) splashes your face or eyes, wash for several minutes at the eyewash station (**Figure 8.16**). Use the safety shower if a reagent splashes on any exposed skin or soaks through your clothing.
- Follow exposure control plan guidelines to treat contaminated work surfaces and clean up spills immediately.
- Report all accidents and exposure incidents to the lab supervisor *immediately* after using the eyewash or shower.

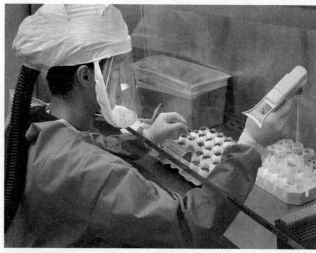

CDC/Douglas E. Jordan/Science Source

Figure 8.15 A biological safety cabinet protects lab workers by preventing infectious materials from escaping into the lab.

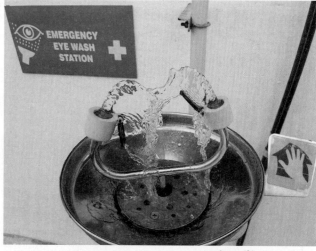

mark_vyz/Shutterstock.com

Figure 8.16 Wash for several minutes at the eyewash station if a reagent splashes your face or eyes.

Lab workers also follow rules of laboratory etiquette that promote a safe and pleasant work environment. These rules include the following:

- No eating, gum chewing, or drinking is permitted in a lab setting. Do not bring food, beverages, tobacco products, or cosmetics into the lab.
- Clean your work area before and after lab procedures and whenever needed. Put away all supplies and equipment before leaving the lab.
- Leave your lab coat, equipment, samples, and reagents in the lab.
- Do not allow visitors into the lab work area unless they are properly dressed and have been instructed in patient confidentiality and safety precautions. Follow facility guidelines for visitors.

8.2-3 Tasks Performed by Laboratory Workers

Valid results rely on accurate measurements. Especially in biotechnology lab settings, technicians frequently measure miniscule (very small) amounts, and small mistakes can cause major errors. Labs use metric units of measurement (**Figure 8.17**). In addition to taking correct measurements, lab workers must complete tests correctly and keep accurate records.

Measuring Mass

Biotechnologists measure reagents, which are chemical substances used in preparing a product or detecting a component in another substance. A common example is a reagent strip used by a lab worker to test a urine specimen. The chemical reagents in this case are attached to a plastic strip and react to a specific substance. The strip is inserted in the sample, and when the specific substance is present, it reacts with the chemical reagent and produces a color change. The color change indicates the amount of the substance present in the sample.

Metric Units Used in the Lab			
Size	**Prefix**	**Symbol**	**Meaning**
Larger	kilo	k	1,000
Base unit	meter	m	1
	gram	g	1
	liter	L	1
Smaller	centi	c	.01
	milli	m	.001
	micro	μ	.000001
	nano	n	.000000001

Goodheart-Willcox Publisher

Figure 8.17 Lab workers use metric units of measurement.

Because biotechnology reagents are often measured in small amounts or masses, lab workers use precision instruments such as **electronic balances** for lab measurements. There are several different types of balances (**Figure 8.18**). Tabletop balances measure amounts weighing between 1 gram (g) and 1,000 grams. Analytical balances are more precise and can measure amounts between 10 milligrams (mg) and 1,000 milligrams. A microbalance will measure even smaller amounts. Follow these steps for measuring mass using an electronic balance:

1. Turn the balance on and press the control bar. Wait for zeros to appear, showing that the scale is ready for use.
2. Use a weighing container for all substances. Place the empty weighing container on the balance pan and close the doors.
3. Tare the container by briefly pressing the control bar. The display will show zero with the container sitting on the pan. This allows the mass of your sample to be read directly. You will not need to subtract the empty weight from the filled container weight.
4. Remove the weighing container and add the substance to be weighed. Be careful not to spill chemicals on the balance.
5. Return the filled weighing container to the balance pan and close the chamber doors. Read the display to find the mass of your sample.

Measuring Volume

Volumes are measured using graduated cylinders, pipettes (for smaller amounts), and **micropipettes** (for very small amounts). Flasks and beakers hold substances, but are not used for measuring volume because they are not very accurate.

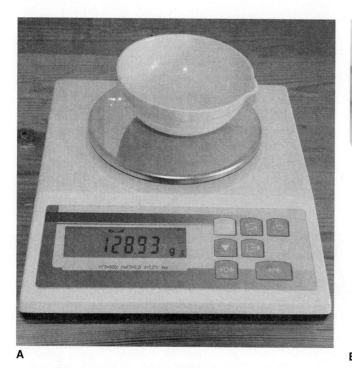

A

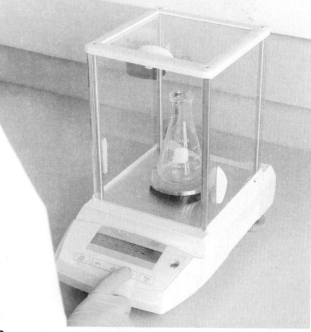

B

Figure 8.18 A tabletop balance (A) measures amounts weighing between 1 gram and 1,000 grams, while an analytical balance (B) measures amounts between 10 milligrams and 1,000 milligrams.

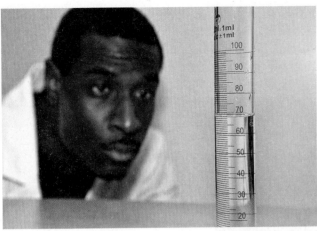

Figure 8.19 Graduated cylinders measure volumes between 10 mL and 5 L. For accuracy, always read the volume at eye level from the lowest point of the meniscus. *What measurement is shown here?*

Always use the smallest cylinder or pipette possible for your specific measurement because the markings on a smaller instrument are more precise. This will ensure accuracy and minimize error. For example, when measuring 9 milliliters (mL), a 10-mL pipette is more accurate than a 25-mL pipette. Use a graduated cylinder for measuring volumes between 10 mL and 5 liters (L) (**Figure 8.19**). Follow these protocols for measuring volume in a cylinder:

1. Check the total volume of the cylinder and the value of each marking on the cylinder.
2. Place the cylinder on a level surface and add the substance to be measured.
3. Locate the **meniscus** (meh-NIHS-kuhs). This is a curve at the surface caused when liquid sticks to the walls of the cylinder. It is lower in the middle of the cylinder.
4. Read the volume measurement at eye level from the lowest point of the meniscus.

Pipettes measure volumes from 1 mL to 50 mL. Micropipettes measure very small volumes in microliter (μL) amounts (**Figure 8.20**). Micropipettes measure volumes from 0.1 μL to 1 mL and are available in different sizes. For example, a P-1000 measures from 100 μL to 1,000 μL (1 mL), while a P-10 measures from 0.5 μL to 10 μL.

Follow these steps for measuring volume in a pipette or micropipette:

1. Select the correct pipette/micropipette size for your measuring task and set the dial to your desired volume.
2. Push the micropipette directly into the correct size tip. Do not touch the tip to avoid contamination.

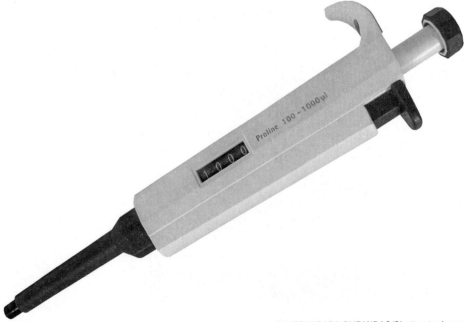

Figure 8.20 Micropipettes measure very small volumes. *What volumes can be measured with this pipette?*

3. Open the cap or lid of the tube from which you are taking liquid.
4. Depress the plunger of the micropipette to the first stop and hold it in position.
5. Place the tip in the solution to be measured. Draw fluid into the tip by *slowly* releasing the plunger. Close and return the tube to the storage rack.
6. Using your free hand, open the cap of the tube you are filling. Gently touch the micropipette tip to the inside wall of the tube to create surface tension that helps draw the fluid out of the tip.
7. Carefully press the plunger of the micropipette to the first stop and then to the second stop to expel all the fluid. Hold the plunger in this position (**Figure 8.21**).
8. Remove the micropipette from the tube, keeping the plunger depressed to avoid drawing liquid back into the tip.
9. Release the plunger and press the ejector button to discard the micropipette tip into the appropriate waste container. Use a new tip for each reagent.

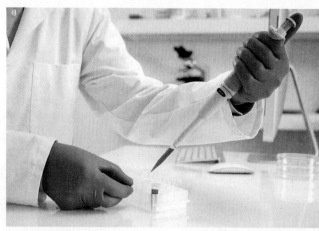

8percentgrey/Shutterstock.com

Figure 8.21 A pipette measures volumes between 1 mL and 50 mL. *Why is the pipette tip touching the inside of the receiving tube?*

Testing Urine

Urinalysis (yer-ih-NAL-uh-sihs) is the examination of urine to observe its physical, chemical, and microscopic properties. Because abnormal urine tests are often the first indication of disease, urine tests are common in clinical labs. Physical testing includes observing and recording color, odor, transparency, and specific gravity. Next, a chemical reagent strip checks pH, protein, glucose, ketones, bilirubin, and blood. Reagent strips can test as few as two or as many as 10 different parameters (**Figure 8.22**).

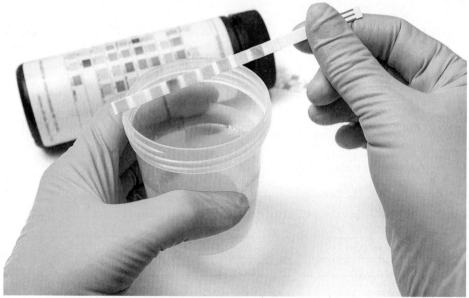

Alexander Raths/Shutterstock.com

Figure 8.22 The color change in a reagent strip indicates the amount of a substance that is present in the sample, such as the amount of glucose present in a urine sample.

Finally, microscopic testing examines the formed elements in urine. A centrifuge spins out the solid particles. These are examined under a microscope to check for the presence of blood cells, bacteria, and other elements.

Testing urine with a reagent strip is a waived clinical test often performed in a medical clinic by the medical assistant. It is a rapid test that can be read and recorded in a few minutes.

PROCEDURE — Testing Urine Using a Reagent Strip

Follow these steps to test urine using a reagent strip.

1. Assemble all supplies and begin with hand hygiene. Then put on gloves and other PPE as required by the healthcare facility.
2. Test only fresh urine specimens for accurate results. Verify that the name on the specimen container matches the name on the lab report.
3. Gently rotate the specimen container between your gloved hands to mix the urine.
4. Hold the reagent strip at the clear end, away from the test areas. Dip the strip into the specimen so all the test areas are immersed. Remove the strip quickly and run the edge against the rim of the specimen container to remove excess urine.
5. Hold the strip in a horizontal position to avoid mixing the reagent chemicals.
6. Begin timing and compare the test squares to the color chart in chronological order and at the times specified on the color chart.
7. Record the results of each test on the lab report (**Figure 8.23**).
8. Discard the test strip and contaminated disposable supplies.
9. Discard the specimen according to facility protocols and disinfect the work area.
10. Remove and dispose of gloves and other PPE. Wash hands.
11. Enter results into the patient medical chart.

Laboratory Report

Patient Name:

Date:

Substance Tested	Normal Value	Observed Value
glucose	negative	
billirubin	negative	
ketones	negative	
blood	negative	
pH	4.5 to 8.0	
protein	negative to trace	
urobilinogen	0.1 to 1.0 mg/dL	
bacteria (nitrite)	negative	
leukocyte esterase	negative	
specific gravity	1.005 to 1.030	

Goodheart-Willcox Publisher

Figure 8.23

Completing Laboratory Documentation

The FDA's handbook says that if something is not written down, it was not done. That is the guideline for all **laboratory documentation**. In a clinical laboratory, lab information systems (LIS) use specialized software to track the testing of samples and record test results. More complex systems also track patient check-in, order entry, specimen processing, result entry, and patient demographics. The LIS stores this information in its database for future reference. Once a provider has reviewed lab results, patients receive a letter and can often access the results more quickly using a secure online portal and a personal password. When patients review a lab report, they see reference values to compare with their own test results. Results that are outside the normal or reference range signal that further investigation is needed (**Figure 8.24**).

In a biotechnology lab, the information management system processes reports and records data for large batches of samples. The information system must follow good manufacturing procedures and meet FDA reporting requirements.

Researchers also record each step taken in their research. Documentation is an essential skill for all biotechnology workers because excellent lab work is worthless without proper documentation. Lab notes record not only procedures and observations, but also the equipment and materials used.

Lipid Panel Results

Component	Your Value	Standard/Reference Range
Hours Fasting	**8–12 hours**	
Cholesterol	**175** mg/dL	*<=199 mg/dL<=199 mg/dL*
	<200 Desirable	
	200–239 Borderline High	
	>239 High	
Triglycerides	**68** mg/dL	*<=149 mg/dL<=149 mg/dL*
	<150 Normal	
	150–199 Borderline High	
	200–499 High	
	>499 Very High	
HDL	**57** mg/dL	*>=40 mg/dL>=40 mg/dL*
LDL Calculated	**108** mg/dL	*<=99 mg/dL<=99 mg/dL*
	<100 Optimal	
	100–129 Near Optimal	
	130–159 Borderline High	
	160–189 High	
	>189 Very High	

Goodheart-Willcox Publisher

Figure 8.24 Patients can access test results through the online portal of their healthcare system. They compare their results with the standard or reference results on the lab report. *Which item is outside of the reference range in this lab report?*

In addition, high-quality notes will indicate that these items were used in the correct manner. All recorded information must be legible and complete. Much like the documentation in patient medical records, lab documentation is permanent rather than erasable. Information may be corrected but not removed from the record (**Figure 8.25**).

8.2-4 Sales and Technical Support Skills

Healthcare marketing includes researching, planning, promoting, selling, and distributing goods and services to meet the needs of healthcare facilities and individual consumers. Because healthcare requires many specialized products that use advanced technologies, training and technical support are often part of a company's marketing plan.

Sales representatives for medical companies focus on **business-to-business selling**. This means the customer may be a large organization with multiple facilities. However, the process of selling still includes gathering information about the customer and advising the customer about which products would best suit the organization's needs.

After contacting a potential customer, you need to prepare your **sales presentation** using the following steps.

Determine Needs

For a presentation to be effective, you must first identify the customer's needs. Does the facility need to save time, provide better results for its patients, or simplify a procedure? Listening is your most important communication skill during this part of the sales process. It is a good idea to spend time "selling" the appointment for a sales presentation by learning the customer's needs and then telling customers what they will receive from your presentation. For your customers, knowing that you intend to meet their needs is more important than knowing what product you intend to show.

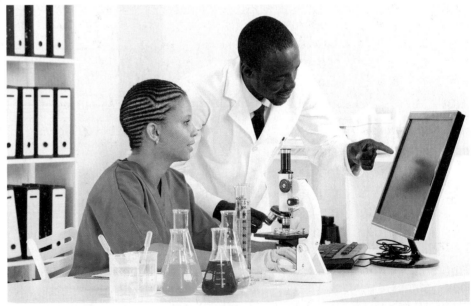

michaeljung/Shutterstock.com

Figure 8.25 Excellent lab work is worthless without proper documentation. *What items will lab notes include?*

Present the Product

In this step, you educate the customer about the product's features and benefits. Solid planning and preparation are essential. A physician who sees that a sales rep does not know a product very well will not want to consult with that rep in the operating room. The sales presentation must also be well organized. Healthcare workers are busy people who cannot afford to waste time.

Tailor your presentation to a specific customer. In today's market, the physician may be your first customer, but the purchasing agent or a product approval committee may also need to agree to a purchase. While product quality and performance might be the doctor's priority, equipment cost and maintenance will be the purchasing agent's focus. Develop your presentation to meet the needs of both customers.

Be prepared to provide a sales quote. This is a written document specifying the exact product and its cost. Sales quotes are valid for a limited time, so the customer must order within that time for the price to be honored.

Finally, know your presentation backward and forward so you can concentrate on the customer. Observe the customer during your presentation to pick up subtle clues. Does the customer look confused? Then take a moment to clarify. Does the customer have a question? Stop your presentation and take time to answer it. This keeps the customer's attention on the presentation. If you lose the customer's attention, you will not make a sale.

Overcome Objections

Be prepared for **customer objections**. These are concerns, doubts, or other reasons the customer gives for not making a purchase. When a potential customer voices an objection, listen carefully. Maintain eye contact and let the customer talk. Acknowledge the customer's objection by responding with, "I understand your point," or "Yes, other customers had similar questions." These comments do not mean that you agree with the customer, but they show that you care about the customer's concerns. When you disagree with customers or tell them they are wrong, they become defensive. That rarely leads to a sale.

Frequently, customers' objections are actually questions. Once you figure out the basic cause of the objection, you can respond to the concerns and questions. For example, a customer objecting to the design of a product may really want to know how difficult it will be to adapt to a new product design. Respond to this concern by explaining the experiences of other customers. You might say, "Yes. Other customers had that same concern about the new design, but they found they adapted quickly and easily to the change" (**Figure 8.26**).

How to Handle Customer Objections	
Objection	**Response**
Price: "I can get the product cheaper from someone else."	Break your prices into smaller parts to show the unique services you will provide that others may not provide.
Fear of change: "It's easier to keep doing things the way we always have."	Explain what competitors are doing and show how change can make a positive improvement.
Authority: "My partner/boss/spouse needs to approve this."	Become a part of the decision by meeting with those who have decision-making authority. Assist your customer in answering questions about the product.
Timing: "I'm too busy right now. Call back in a few months."	Show the customer how easy it will be to work with you and how much your products will benefit them.

Goodheart-Willcox Publisher

Figure 8.26 Anticipate objections and role-play your responses as you prepare your sales presentation.

Close the Sale

This means getting the customer's positive agreement to buy. This could be a purchase contract for services or an approved purchase order for products. Suggest other options your customer might appreciate, such as a discount for purchasing multiple items (**Figure 8.27**).

Maintain Your Customer Relationship

Successful sales reps use many techniques for communicating with customers and presenting products, but their most important skill is following through on commitments made to customers. Something as simple as making a phone call when you promised to or remembering to check a price and call the customer back builds a trusting relationship. Although this requires a high level of personal organization and commitment, it results in long-term success in sales.

8.2-5 HOSA Connections

You can continue to receive the benefits of HOSA membership beyond high school by joining the postsecondary/collegiate division. You will be able to continue participating in competitive, service, and leadership events throughout your college years. When you finish your healthcare training, consider supporting and mentoring future healthcare workers as an alumni or professional member (**Figure 8.28**). HOSA allows you to continue your personal and professional development as you enhance the delivery of healthcare by assisting in the preparation of qualified healthcare workers.

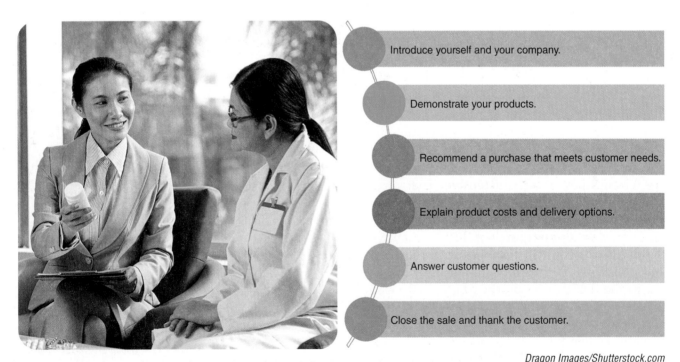

Introduce yourself and your company.

Demonstrate your products.

Recommend a purchase that meets customer needs.

Explain product costs and delivery options.

Answer customer questions.

Close the sale and thank the customer.

Dragon Images/Shutterstock.com

Figure 8.27 Healthcare sales representatives follow these steps when they present a product.

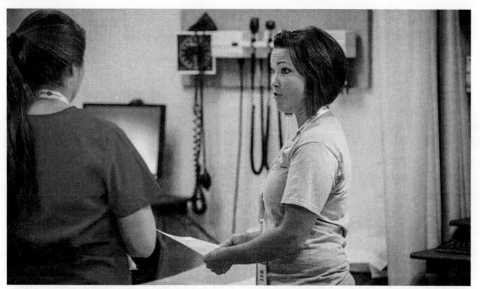

Courtesy of HOSA-Future Health Professionals

Figure 8.28 Mentor future healthcare workers as an alumni or professional member of HOSA.

In the meantime, consider serving on a committee, leading a service project, or becoming a HOSA officer. Just like other professional organizations, HOSA offers excellent opportunities for developing your leadership skills. In addition, competitive events such as Biomedical Debate, Biotechnology, or Medical Innovation will strengthen your biotechnology, research, and development skills. You can read about these events in the competitive events section of the HOSA website.

Lesson 8.2 Review

 Complete the *Map Your Reading* graphic organizer for the section you just read.

1. Which biosafety level represents the lowest level of risk? (8.2-1)
   A. BSL-4
   B. BSL-2
   C. BSL-3
   D. BSL-1

2. Which of the following is *not* a laboratory safety protocol? (8.2-2)
   A. Wear closed-toe shoes.
   B. Wash your hands after removing gloves.
   C. Wait an hour before reporting accidents.
   D. Know the locations of exit doors.

3. Which step for measuring mass should you complete first? (8.2-3)
   A. Tare the scale.
   B. Read the display.
   C. Place the empty container on the balance pan.
   D. Fill the container with the substance to be weighed.

4. What is the first step in selling a medical product to a customer? (8.2-4)
   A. Tailor your presentation to the customer.
   B. Overcome objections.
   C. Provide a purchase contract.
   D. Determine the customer's needs.

5. Which HOSA competitive event would best strengthen biotechnology skills? (8.2-5)
   A. Medical Innovation
   B. Clinical Specialty
   C. CPR and First Aid
   D. Medical Spelling

Chapter 8 Review and Assessment

Chapter Summary

8.1-1 Employees in biotechnology research and development possess a variety of personal traits from precision and accuracy to self-motivation and resilience. Workers in the research, development, and manufacturing of medical products are problem-solvers whose use of honesty and discretion produce valid results. Employees in medical sales and support are team players who enjoy working with people. They must be self-motivated, well-organized, and resilient workers.

8.1-2 Biotechnology uses advances in the life sciences to create products that come from living things. Biotechnology is an evolving field that is constantly shaped by medical advances.

8.1-3 Different types of biotechnology laboratories focus on different tasks. Clinical laboratories test patients, while biotechnology research laboratories develop products and treatments.

8.1-4 The biotechnology industry employs a variety of people and contains many different career paths. Careers in biotechnology research and development may focus on research and development, manufacturing and services, sales and technical support, or quality and regulation.

8.2-1 Biotechnology laboratories are classified according to their level of risk from exposure to biological agents.

8.2-2 All lab workers must follow laboratory safety protocols. Workers use standard precautions and PPE to prevent exposure and can operate a safety shower or eyewash station to limit exposure. They follow the lab's exposure control plan to handle specimens and waste materials safely.

8.2-3 Lab workers need to know how to perform certain technical skills. Lab workers measure mass using electronic balances and volume using graduated cylinders, pipettes, or micropipettes. Medical assistants can perform a rapid urine test using a reagent strip. Documentation is an essential skill for all biotechnology workers because excellent lab work is worthless without proper documentation.

8.2-4 Sales representatives for medical companies focus on business-to-business selling. They meet with prospective buyers and deliver a sales presentation to sell medical products.

8.2-5 Participation in HOSA can help students develop biotechnology research and development skills. Members can develop leadership skills and contribute to HOSA even after high school.

Maximize Your Professional Vocabulary

1. **Write It, Define It.** Select one or more of the professional vocabulary terms from the chapter. Write the terms you chose on slips of paper. Put the slips of paper in a basket or bowl with all your classmates' terms. Pass the bowl or basket around the class, each student selecting a term at random. When you select a term, define it and explain how it connects it to biotechnology research and development in the field of healthcare. Keep passing the bowl or basket of words around until they have all been taken.

2. **Career Story.** Write a short story describing the development of a new and beneficial healthcare product or medication, from the research stage to the use of the new product. In your description, highlight the biotechnology research and development workers who play a role in the story and include professional vocabulary terms where appropriate.

Reflect on Your Reading

1. Look at the biotechnology workers you listed in the *Connect with Your Reading* activity. Organize them under these headings: *Research and Development Careers*, *Manufacturing and Services Careers*, *Sales and Technical Support Careers*, *Quality and Regulation Careers*, and *Additional Career Opportunities*. Were any of your headings empty? Complete your chart by adding at least two career opportunities for each section of the chart.

Review and Recall

1. Which of the following is true of biotechnology sales representatives? (8.1-1)
   A. They rarely use organization skills.
   B. They need to know a little bit about the products they sell.
   C. They need enthusiasm and resilience.
   D. They do not work in teams.

2. Which biotechnology advancement aims to cure genetic diseases? (8.1-2)
   A. Gene therapy
   B. Recombinant DNA
   C. Domestication
   D. Assays

3. Which of the following are waived tests? Choose all that apply. (8.1-3)
   A. Blood glucose metering
   B. Urinalysis
   C. Culture and identification
   D. Rapid strep test

4. Which biotechnology worker develops products such as artificial organs, prostheses, and machines for diagnosing medical conditions? (8.1-4)
   A. Quality assurance specialist
   B. Sales representative
   C. Biomedical engineer
   D. Medical scientist

5. Which of the following labs would have restricted access? Choose all that apply. (8.2-1)
   A. BSL-1
   B. BSL-2
   C. BSL-3
   D. BSL-4

6. Which of the following are examples of good laboratory etiquette? Choose all that apply. (8.2-2)
   A. Chewing gum while working
   B. Taking reagents home
   C. Cleaning your work area
   D. Leaving your lab coat in the lab

7. Which instrument would be most appropriate for measuring 8 mL of a substance? (8.2-3)
   A. 9-mL pipette
   B. Graduated cylinder
   C. 25-mL pipette
   D. Micropipette

8. When a customer raises an objection, you should (8.2-4)
   A. argue about it
   B. ignore it
   C. agree with it
   D. acknowledge it

9. How can you keep receiving the benefits of HOSA membership even after high school? (8.2-5)
   A. Participation through college
   B. Mentorship as an alumni
   C. Helping to prepare healthcare workers
   D. All of these.

Build Core Skills

1. **Critical Thinking.** Review the personal traits section in this chapter, as well as personal traits for other healthcare pathways. Analyze your own personal traits and describe which healthcare career pathways most closely match your own personal traits.

2. **Reading.** Research a healthcare-related biotechnology company located in your community or state. What product or products does the company produce? Are the products still in the development and testing stage or are they available for purchase? How have the company's products improved healthcare?

3. **Critical Thinking.** Research one of these topics: SOPs, GLPs, or GMPs. Use online resources to learn the definition, purposes, settings, and examples that describe your topic. Form a group of three students whose combined research includes all the topics. Prepare a three-section T-chart using *SOP*, *GLP*, and *GMP* as your horizontal headings and *definition*, *purposes*, *settings*, and *examples* as your vertical headings. Record your information. Analyze your information to identify similarities and differences. Post your T-chart and compare the results of all the research groups.

4. **Writing.** Write a two-paragraph explanation that compares and contrasts clinical and research labs.

5. **Problem Solving.** For each of the following urine descriptions, identify the part of a urinalysis (physical, chemical, or microscopic testing) that would identify the abnormal sign.
   - high bacteria count
   - strong smell
   - high pH level
   - presence of ketones
   - presence of red blood cells
   - cloudy liquid
   - high protein level
   - presence of bilirubin and blood
   - medium to dark color
   - high glucose level

6. **Problem Solving.** Review DNA fingerprinting as explained in the chapter and use online resources to create a list of situations in which DNA fingerprinting techniques would be useful. Explain how DNA fingerprinting would be helpful in those situations.

7. **Speaking and Listening.** Develop a sales presentation for the fictional product you previously created for your career story. Include responses to at least three common objections you might face.

8. **Critical thinking.** Use the Important Terms list at the beginning of Lesson 8.1 as a guide and write the biotechnology worker who performs each task.
   A. Design equipment used to manufacture a product
   B. Monitor work environment to maintain sterile conditions
   C. Design prostheses and machines for diagnosing medical conditions
   D. Extract and match DNA to solve crimes
   E. Investigate outbreaks of infection
   F. Sell medical products
   G. Advise families affected by inherited diseases
   H. Provide customer service to resolve equipment problems
   I. Respond to hazards in the workplace
   J. Document required procedures in the manufacturing process

9. **Critical Thinking.** For each of the following word pairs, write a statement that illustrates the relationship between the words.
   Example: centrifuge and urinalysis—During a microscopic urinalysis, a centrifuge is used to separate the liquid in the urine from solid components such as blood cells or mineral crystals.
   A. Algorithms and computers
   B. Bioassays and medical research
   C. Biohazard and biological containment
   D. Bioreactors and pharmaceuticals
   E. Hypothesis and medical scientists
   F. Meniscus and lowest point
   G. Placebo and clinical trial
   H. Validity and scientific research

Activate Your Learning

1. Review lab protocols and the steps for measuring mass and volume as described in the chapter. Assemble the necessary supplies and practice measuring the mass and volume of substances provided by your instructor.

2. Select a medical product of your choice. Research your product. Then prepare a sales presentation for your product and present it to your classmates.

3. Search for biohazard symbols in the school setting. What biohazards exist? Where are they located? What precautions are used to prevent exposure?

Go to the Source

1. Use online resources to search for information about prosthetics. In addition to limbs and braces, what other products have been developed to replace or support body parts?

2. Use online resources to learn more about careers in biotechnology research and development. Select two careers of interest to you and complete a career profile page for each one. Use at least one website that ends in .gov and one website that ends in .org. Record the following information for each career:
   - name of career
   - tasks involved in this career
   - personal traits and abilities needed
   - educational requirements
   - type of credential needed and how it is obtained
   - work conditions
   - wages and benefits
   - job outlook for the future
   - the websites you accessed

   How do the two careers compare? Why might you prefer one to the other?

3. Review all the HOSA competitive events listed on the HOSA website and select two. Explain how your participation in these events will help you achieve your personal and professional development goals.

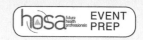

HOSA Event Prep: Research Poster

Mary, a nurse educator in pediatrics, wanted to improve pain management in younger surgical patients. She did a two-week study about how nurses used the pain scale and managed pain in their patients. She noticed that some of the nurses automatically gave pain medicine when a patient's pain reached a five, while others waited until the pain was a nine or the patient asked for medicine. The patients who received pain medicine automatically when their pain was a five were more active and ambulated (walked) in the hospital more. They were also discharged from the hospital an average of 1.5 days earlier than the other groups. The patients who were medicated when their pain was a nine had more complications and less ambulation and were discharged an average of two days later. They also had more problems with nausea. The group who received medicine only when they asked did better than the group that received medicine at a 9, but they did not ambulate as well. Mary wanted to showcase the importance of proactive pain management, so she decided to create a poster and do a five-minute presentation on the importance of managing pain in the young postoperative patient.

Think About It

1. Analyze the steps Mary used to conduct a study that would accurately measure patient responses to different methods of pain management. Why do you think Mary took each of these steps?

2. Imagine you were creating the poster to present Mary's research. What information would you include on the poster? Why?

3. What do you think are the major components of an effective research poster?

Chapter 9

Health Maintenance for Health Professionals and Patients

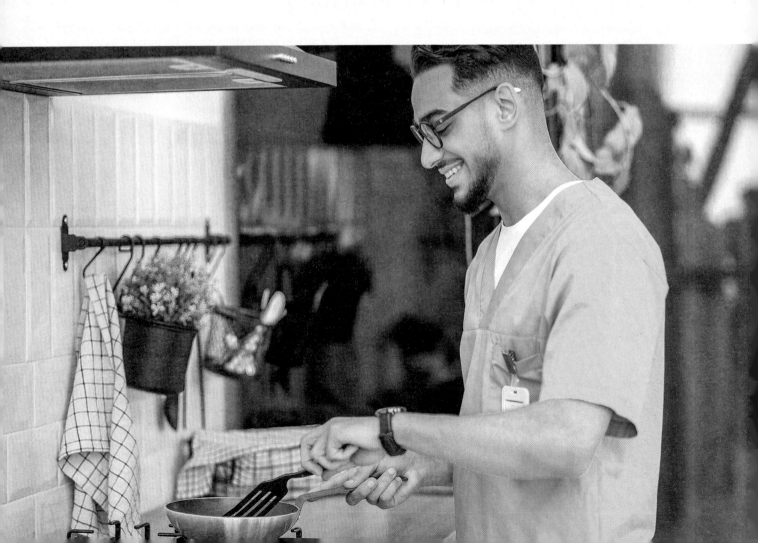

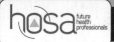

HOSA Event Prep: Healthy Lifestyle

Involvement in HOSA supports healthy living by providing opportunities to develop future career skills, encouraging health maintenance practices, creating opportunities for positive social interactions, and teaching students to persevere. In the competitive event *Healthy Lifestyle*, future health professionals can learn more about healthy living across the life span. They set a SMART goal related to personal health in any dimension of wellness, then document their progress toward a healthier lifestyle through a portfolio. As a future healthcare worker, you will benefit personally from practices that maintain your own wellness. In addition, your knowledge of wellness will benefit your patients as you work with them to improve their habits and lifestyle choices.

Go to the HOSA website to learn more about the HOSA *Healthy Lifestyle* event. Find out the purpose of the event, what is involved in the event, and what knowledge is demonstrated in the event.

As you prepare for HOSA competitive events, be sure to check the website and talk with your HOSA advisor for the most up-to-date guidelines and procedures. Once you have learned about the *Healthy Lifestyle* event, answer the following questions:

1. How might participating in this event benefit you personally and your future career? Explain.
2. Are you interested in participating in this event? Why or why not?

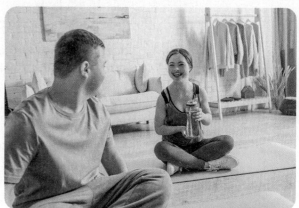

LightField Studios/Shutterstock.com

Connect with Your Reading

What do you think of as "wellness" and "illness"? In two columns, list the ways people keep themselves well and things that make people ill. Share your ideas with a partner. Do your thoughts match your partner's? Did you gain any new ways of thinking about wellness and illness? How might these two concepts relate to health maintenance?

Map Your Reading

Fold a sheet of paper in half vertically and horizontally to make four sections. Label the sections *physical*, *intellectual*, *social*, and *emotional*. As you read, take notes about how each aspect of development changes from birth to old age and ways to support wellness or avoid illness in each area. These ideas will apply to both you and your future patients in a healthcare career.

Physical	Intellectual
Social	Emotional

Goodheart-Willcox Publisher

Chapter opener image: Dmytro Zinkevych/Shutterstock.com

Physical Health, Wellness, and Self-Care Practices

ESSENTIAL QUESTION

In what ways can your behaviors impact your overall health?

Learning Outcomes

After studying this lesson, you will be able to

9.1-1 describe physical development, wellness, and their impact on healthcare.

9.1-2 explain the importance of choosing nutritious foods.

9.1-3 identify the impact physical activity has on health and wellness.

9.1-4 explain how maintaining a healthy weight benefits your overall health.

9.1-5 describe the importance of healthy sleep habits.

9.1-6 identify self-care methods to manage stress in a healthy manner.

9.1-7 describe the impact healthy relationships have on overall health.

Professional Vocabulary

Essential Terms

nutrients   molecules such as carbohydrates, proteins, fats, vitamins, and minerals used by the body to grow and maintain body processes

physical wellness   involves balancing diet, physical activity, sleep, and other activities to keep your body healthy

stress   physical, mental, or emotional pressure caused by change

Important Terms

calories	nutrient-dense	sleep deficit
carbohydrates	obesity	
fats	protein	

Introduction

Many healthcare workers are helpers by nature. Perhaps your desire to help others drew you to this field. This focus on helping others can keep people from maintaining their own health. Do you skip meals or eat fast food simply because it is convenient? Are you just too busy to get regular physical activity? Do you get by on a few hours of sleep each night because 24 hours is just not enough time in one day? Are you so busy focusing on problems in your friends' lives that you avoid your own until they reach a crisis point? If you answered *yes* to any of these questions, you should consider taking a closer look at your personal health maintenance practices. The first step to good health is putting yourself first. Are you actively working to stay healthy?

In this lesson, you will learn about ways both healthcare workers and consumers maintain good health through self-care. Personal health may not be your main focus as you prepare for your future career, but it is important for healthcare workers. Healthcare workers have a responsibility to practice healthy behaviors as a positive role model for clients. Healthcare workers also have an obligation to wellness. Those who work directly with patients cannot risk transmitting illnesses. If healthcare workers are not healthy enough to perform their tasks safely, they cannot work (**Figure 9.1**).

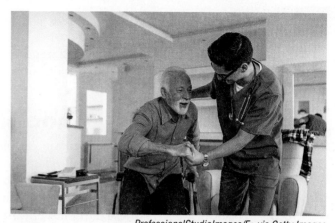

ProfessionalStudioImages/E+ via Getty Images

Figure 9.1 Healthcare workers need physical wellness to care for patients safely. *What might happen if this worker was lacking strength or physical fitness to assist this patient with mobility?*

9.1-1 Physical Development and Wellness

Physical wellness means listening to your body's need for proper nutrition, daily physical activity, sleep, and safety. Physical health and wellness include the development and functioning of your body. When your body is healthy, it can better resist illness and injury. Physical wellness and self-care activities keep your body ready to participate in daily activities.

Understanding normal stages of development helps parents and healthcare workers recognize issues and anticipate a person's needs and challenges. Physical development is monitored even before birth. Physical growth of the body follows two general patterns. Development starts at the head and works its way down. Infants learn to lift their head, then push themselves up, then sit up, and finally walk. Development also radiates from the midline of the body outward. Infants learn to use the large-motor muscles of their torso and arms before they can control the fine-motor skills of their fingers. Children develop more independence as they gain control of their body. They will experience several growth spurts, particularly at puberty. The development of secondary sexual characteristics will also begin at this time. Physical growth in terms of height and body mass is not complete until young adulthood. The metabolism will begin to slow at this point, so it is important to maintain healthy diet and physical activity habits. This will also help slow the gradual loss of bone and muscle mass that generally occurs in old age.

Children use play and daily activity to support healthy growth and physical development (**Figure 9.2**). Delays in physical development should be shared with the pediatrician. They can indicate a serious health condition, such as muscular dystrophy or Down syndrome. Physical health and wellness behaviors are strongly tied to the development or avoidance of many preventable diseases. For example, lack of physical activity increases the risk for cardiovascular disease, diabetes, osteoporosis, and cancer.

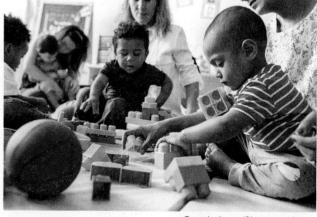

Rawpixel.com/Shutterstock.com

Figure 9.2 Children learn many physical skills through play. Play is an essential part of children's development.

Maintaining your physical health includes several basic components. These include choosing nutritious foods, getting physical activity, maintaining a healthy weight, getting adequate sleep, managing stress, and maintaining healthy relationships. Staying healthy will allow you to work at your best.

9.1-2 Choosing Nutritious Foods

The food you eat provides your body with important nutrients for health and body development. Self-care includes choosing a variety of foods to get all the nutrients your body needs. Scientists have identified six main nutrients essential for maintaining good health (**Figure 9.3**). When your diet lacks any of these nutrients, optimal body function is interrupted, and signs of poor nutrition, or *malnutrition*, may appear over time. Malnutrition leads to the development of conditions such as goiter, caused by a lack of iodine; rickets, caused by a vitamin D deficiency; and anemia, due to a lack of folate, vitamin B_{12}, or iron. Some nutrients that are lost in food manufacturing or that people do not eat enough of are supplemented in certain foods. These *fortified* foods help prevent deficiency diseases. For this reason, table salt is fortified with iodine, cow's milk is fortified with vitamin D, and processed grain foods are fortified with B vitamins and iron.

Carbohydrates
- major source of human energy
- easily digested

- dietary sources: bread, pasta, crackers, cereals, potatoes, corn, peas, fruits, sugar, and syrups

Fats (Lipids)
- concentrated form of energy
- aid in the absorption of fat-soluble vitamins
- give food flavor

- dietary sources: butter, margarine, oils, cream, fatty meats, cheeses, and egg yolks

Protein
- builds and repairs body tissue
- provides heat and energy

- dietary sources: complete proteins — meats, fish, milk, cheese, and eggs incomplete proteins— cereal, nuts, and dried beans

Vitamins
- important for metabolism, tissue building, and regulating body processes

- dietary sources: fruits, vegetables, some grains, meat, and dairy

Minerals
- regulate body fluids
- contribute to growth
- aid in building tissues

- dietary sources: meat, fish, poultry, dairy, whole grains, and some fruits and vegetables

Water
- essential for the digestion of food
- makes up the majority of blood plasma
- helps body tissues absorb nutrients
- helps move waste material through the body
- dietary sources: 6 to 8 cups of water each day and water present in foods

Goodheart-Willcox Publisher

Figure 9.3 These six essential nutrients are necessary to maintain health and proper body function.

Sometimes foods provide energy, but without much nutritional value. The phrase *empty calories* describes these foods. Alcohol, soft drinks, and candy have empty calories. Highly processed snack foods are usually high in solid fats and added sugar, and the empty calories add up quickly. At seven calories per gram, alcohol adds up faster than carbohydrates or proteins (**Figure 9.4**). An average adult female who is not pregnant or lactating needs approximately 2,000 calories per day. An average adult male has more muscle mass to support and requires approximately 2,500 calories per day. These calories and nutrients should come from a variety of **nutrient-dense** foods. These are foods high in vitamins, minerals, complex carbohydrates, lean proteins, and healthy fats, but low in calories. About 3,500 excess calories adds 1 pound of body fat.

Food Energy Values by Macronutrients	
Macronutrients	**Energy Content**
Protein	4.0 calories/g
Carbohydrates	4.0 calories/g
Fat	9.0 calories/g

Goodheart-Willcox Publisher

Figure 9.4 Different macronutrients provide different amounts of energy to the body. *Which nutrient provides the greatest number of calories per gram?*

Nutrients

Nutrients are substances used for energy, structure building, and chemical reactions taking place in the body. Your digestive system gathers them from the foods you eat. Without a variety of foods, you will not have all the vitamins and minerals required for good health.

Nutrients categorized as macronutrients provide energy for the human body. **Calories** are the units used to measure energy gained from your food. You need the *macronutrients* of carbohydrates, proteins, and fats in larger quantities to provide energy and nutrition. The *micronutrients* of vitamins and minerals are needed in smaller amounts for chemical reactions within the body. Micronutrients do not provide energy for the body. A healthy diet provides both energy and nutrition daily. Choosing healthy foods reduces the risk of many diseases such as diabetes, heart disease, cancer, and osteoporosis. If calories are restricted too much, a person will not receive the nutrients that they need. Excess calories beyond what the body needs will be stored as body fat for padding, warmth, and a future source of energy.

Carbohydrates

Different foods provide your body with different nutrients. **Carbohydrates** are mostly plant-based compounds of carbon, hydrogen, and oxygen. Your body breaks down foods with carbohydrates into glucose, a form of sugar that is your body's first source of energy. Many people in the US consume more added sugar than what they need. Whole grains are good sources of carbohydrates. These complex carbohydrates, or *starches*, must be broken down to make sugar for energy. Whole grains also supply dietary fiber. Fiber does not provide energy, but helps move food through your bowels, lowers blood cholesterol, and may prevent some cancers.

Fats

Fats are compounds from plant and animal sources that provide triglycerides for metabolism. They are necessary in your diet to build insulation, pad vital organs, transport fat-soluble vitamins, make hormones, and store energy.

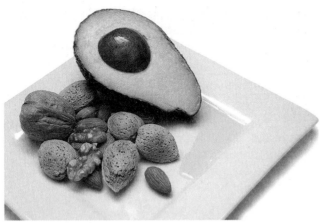

Sandra Caldwell/Shutterstock.com

Figure 9.5 Unsaturated fats can be found in avocados and nuts like almonds and walnuts.

Approximately 30 percent of total calories should come from fat, and less than 10 percent should come from saturated fats. *Saturated fats* are typically solid at room temperature and are found in meats, full-fat dairy products, and baked goods. *Unsaturated fats* and omega-3 fatty acids protect your heart and support good health. They are usually liquid at room temperature and are often found in nuts and fish (**Figure 9.5**). Trans-unsaturated fatty acids, or *trans fats*, are often chemically produced and should be limited as much as possible. Many companies have removed *trans* fats from their food products. Saturated and *trans* fats can raise blood cholesterol levels and increase your risk for developing heart disease and cancer.

Dietary *cholesterol* is a fatty substance that comes from animal food sources, such as red meat, eggs, and milk. It is necessary for some body processes, but you do not want too much. There are three kinds of blood cholesterol. Low-density lipoprotein (LDL) is a type of cholesterol that impacts risk for cardiovascular disease. High-density lipoprotein (HDL) helps prevent heart disease. Triglycerides are the fat in blood plasma that can impact health when elevated. A lipid profile test is used as a tool to decide whether someone needs medical nutrition therapy or medication to lower their risk for heart disease or stroke.

Protein

Meat, fish, poultry, nuts, dry beans, and dairy foods are major sources of **protein**. The amino acids in protein provide the building blocks for your body to repair and make new cells. Your body requires about 20 different amino acids. Different sources of protein provide different combinations of these amino acids. Nine of them are considered *essential amino acids* because your body does not make them, and they must come from your diet. Protein deficiency can be an issue for people who do not eat enough food, follow restrictive diets, or are recovering from illness.

Vitamins and Minerals

Vitamins and minerals are micronutrients that have no energy value, but they are important to your body processes. For example, calcium works with vitamin D to build strong bones and is important for your nerve and cell functions. Iron helps your body's red blood cells carry oxygen. Potassium regulates your fluid balance, making it important for reducing blood pressure. Magnesium regulates biochemical reactions in your body, making it important to many functions such as nerve-impulse conduction and muscle contractions. Both vitamin A and vitamin C are important for your immune system. Vitamin A is also important for good eyesight and healthy skin, while vitamin C helps you repair wounds and build healthy connective tissues. These are the micronutrients most often lacking in US diets and should be included when making food choices.

Guidelines for Healthy Eating

The US Department of Agriculture (USDA), in combination with the Department of Health and Human Services (HHS), sets guidelines for healthy eating and develops consumer materials about a healthy diet. The *Dietary Guidelines for Americans* reflect the public's current dietary needs to promote health, prevent chronic disease, and maintain a healthy weight (**Figure 9.6**). The guidelines apply to people of all ages and are not considered therapeutic. In other words, they are not intended for the treatment of a medical condition.

Research shows that 42 percent of adults in the US have **obesity**, which is an excessive accumulation of body fat. Most people also have one or more chronic diet-related health conditions, such as heart disease, stroke, type 2 diabetes, hypertension, liver disease, cancer, dental caries, and metabolic syndrome. The standard American diet contains too much fat, sodium, and added sugars and not enough fruits, vegetables, and whole grains.

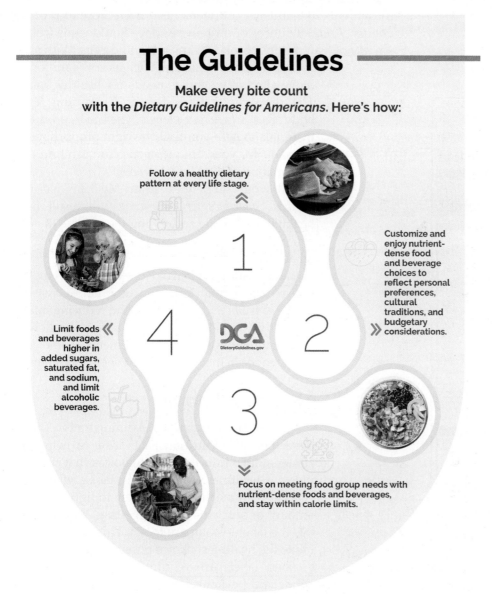

The Guidelines

Make every bite count
with the *Dietary Guidelines for Americans*. Here's how:

Follow a healthy dietary
pattern at every life stage.

1

Customize and
enjoy nutrient-
dense food
and beverage
choices to
reflect personal
preferences,
cultural
traditions, and
budgetary
considerations.

Limit foods
and beverages
higher in
added sugars,
saturated fat,
and sodium,
and limit
alcoholic
beverages.

4

DGA
DietaryGuidelines.gov

2

3

Focus on meeting food group needs with
nutrient-dense foods and beverages,
and stay within calorie limits.

Courtesy of the US Department of Agriculture

Figure 9.6 These are some key goals of the *Dietary Guidelines for Americans*. *How can you "make every bite count"?*

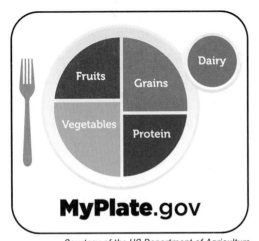

Courtesy of the US Department of Agriculture

Figure 9.7 The MyPlate diagram shows what proportions of the food groups people should eat. *Why do you think the USDA chose to display this information on a plate?*

Nutrition Facts

1 serving per container

Serving size   **1 cup (245g)** ——— Serving size

Amount per serving	
Calories	**208**

——— Calories per serving

	% Daily Value*
Total Fat 3g	4%
Saturated Fat 2g	10%
Trans Fat 0g	
Cholesterol 12mg	4%
Sodium 162mg	7%
Total Carbohydrate 34g	12%
Dietary Fiber 0g	0%
Total Sugars 34g	
Includes 17g Added Sugars	34%
Protein 12g	
Vitamin D 0mcg	0%
Calcium 419mg	32%
Iron 0.2mg	1%
Potassium 537mg	11%

——— Limit these nutrients

——— Get enough of these nutrients

——— Percent (%) Daily Value (DV)

* The % Daily Value (DV) tells you how much a nutrient in a serving of food contributes to a daily diet. 2,000 calories a day is used for general nutrition advice.

Courtesy of the US Food and Drug Administration

Figure 9.8 Nutrition Facts labels are required on most packaged foods. They allow you to compare foods and work toward a healthier diet.

Health effects from a lack of nutrients include osteoporosis from a lack of vitamin D and calcium, as well as hypertension from a lack of potassium. Vitamin D and calcium can be found in fortified milk. Fruits, such as oranges and bananas, and vegetables, such as spinach and potatoes, are high in potassium. People should eat more nutrient-dense foods and avoid added sugars, saturated fat, and sodium.

The MyPlate graphic, developed by the USDA, is a visual guide for a healthy eating pattern that provides the correct balance of nutrients (**Figure 9.7**). It shows the proportions of foods to eat from the five food groups. Vegetables should be the focus of the meal, with 2 to 3 cups taken in per day. Fruits are a good source of carbohydrates, vitamins, and minerals. Including 2 to 4 cups of fruit per day can provide vitamin C, folate, and potassium. A quarter of each plate can come from grains. An average adult male needs 6 to 8 ounces of grains per day. Active individuals like athletes and teens need even more to provide energy. About 6 ounces of protein per day should come from a variety of lean meats, seafood, beans, nuts, and eggs. With each meal, a source of calcium, such as cow's milk or a dairy alternative, meets needs for healthy bones. The proportions are different for various ages, body sizes, and activity levels. The USDA produces materials to help you find the right proportions of nutrients for your unique needs. You can find this information at the MyPlate website.

Following guidelines from MyPlate and the *Dietary Guidelines for Americans* will result in a healthier diet while addressing the public's dietary concerns. The dietary guidelines give advice on what to eat and drink to meet nutritional needs, promote health, and avoid disease. They emphasize reducing total food consumption, increasing intake of fruits and vegetables, and reducing intake of sodium and added sugars. If everyone followed these guidelines, what improvements would you expect to see in the health of the general population?

Nutrition Labels

The US Food and Drug Administration (FDA) developed the Nutrition Facts label to help consumers make informed food choices that contribute to a healthier diet. Reading labels when you shop or plan meals makes it easy to figure out the amount of nutrients you are getting. You can also use the label to compare foods. This allows you to make the healthiest choice possible.

Food labels are required on most packaged foods and beverages (**Figure 9.8**). They show the average serving size people typically eat and highlight calories and serving sizes with larger print.

Because of their link to obesity and heart disease, added sugars and types of fat are shown. In the percent Daily Value, 5 percent is considered low, and 20 percent or more is high. This is because the label represents the amount in just one serving. Look for foods that are higher in dietary fiber, vitamin D, calcium, iron, and potassium. Choose a variety of foods to get all the nutrients you need.

Pay attention to your total daily intake of saturated fats, added sugars, and sodium. Excess intake of these can contribute to heart disease, diabetes, and other chronic diseases. There is not a Daily Value for *trans* fats, protein, or sugar, but you can use information on the ingredients list to help identify healthier choices. A product's ingredient list shows ingredients that weigh the most first and those that weigh the least last (**Figure 9.9**).

Beware of foods where the ingredients lists begin with sugars (sugar, corn syrups, or sucrose), fats and oils (vegetable oil, soybean oil, or partially hydrogenated oils), or salt (sodium, disodium, monosodium glutamate (MSG), or Himalayan pink salt). If these ingredients appear early in the ingredient list, the food is probably a less healthy choice.

A long ingredient list may also signal a less healthy food choice. In many cases, a long list indicates fewer natural ingredients and a highly processed food. Look for foods with a short ingredient list and ingredient names you recognize.

Ingredients: Roasted Peanuts, High Maltose Corn Syrup, Sugar, Whole Grain Oats, Tapioca Syrup, Palm Kernel Oil, Rice Flour, Cashews Roasted in Safflower Oil, Almonds, Fructose, Whole Grain Wheat, Canola Oil, Maltodextrin, Salt, Soy Lecithin, Reduced Minerals Whey, Nonfat Milk, Partially Defatted Peanut Flour, Honey Roasted Almond Butter (almonds, honey, maltodextrin, palm oil, mixed tocopherols), Barley Malt Extract, Cashew Butter (cashew nuts, safflower oil), Baking Soda, Natural Flavor. Mixed Tocopherols Added to Retain Freshness.
CONTAINS PEANUT, CASHEW, ALMOND, WHEAT, MILK, SOY; MAY CONTAIN PECAN AND MACADAMIA INGREDIENTS.

A

INGREDIENTS: SUGAR, CORN SYRUP, NONFAT **MILK**, HIGH FRUCTOSE CORN SYRUP, SOYBEAN OIL, CONTAINS 2% OR LESS OF: FULLY HYDROGENATED COTTONSEED OIL, MOLASSES, CORN STARCH-MODIFIED, NATURAL FLAVOR (WITH **MILK** AND **SOYBEAN**), CARAMEL COLOR, MONOGLYCERIDES, SODIUM PHOSPHATE, SODIUM CITRATE, SALT, XANTHAN GUM, VANILLIN (ARTIFICIAL FLAVOR), YELLOW 6, TBHQ (ANTIOXIDANT), RED 40.

B

INGREDIENTS: UNBLEACHED ENRICHED FLOUR (WHEAT FLOUR, NIACIN, REDUCED IRON, THIAMINE MONONITRATE (VITAMIN B1), RIBOFLAVIN (VITAMIN B2), FOLIC ACID), SOYBEAN OIL*, SALT, PARTIALLY HYDROGENATED COTTONSEED OIL*, YEAST, BAKING SODA.
CONTAINS: WHEAT.
*ADDS A TRIVIAL AMOUNT OF SATURATED FAT

C

INGREDIENTS: TOMATO PUREE (WATER, TOMATO PASTE), WATER, LESS THAN 2% OF: DEXTROSE, TOMATO FIBER, CITRIC ACID, SPICE, NATURAL FLAVORS.

D

Goodheart-Willcox Publisher

Figure 9.9 Review these ingredient lists. *Which shows the most highly processed food? Which shows the least processed food? Which shows the food with the highest level of sugar? Why are ingredient lists important to people with food allergies?*

9.1-3 Physical Activity

Physical activity is an important component of self-care to improve and maintain your overall health. It reduces your risk of heart disease, stroke, cancer, diabetes, and other chronic diseases. Regular physical activity also helps you feel, function, and sleep better; reduces anxiety; helps with managing weight; and decreases depression.

Many people today are inactive, or *sedentary*. People sit too long at desks in school, in office chairs at work, and in front of screens at home. The use of technology contributes to a sedentary lifestyle. How much time do you spend sitting in front of your "screens," including your computer, smartphone, tablet, television, or game console? Because many individuals no longer have a job that provides regular physical activity, people need to choose physical activities that keep their bodies healthy. While the number of adults engaging in 30 minutes of aerobic physical activity per day is slowly increasing, the number of adolescents meeting physical activity guidelines has decreased.

The best physical activity is the one you will actually do. Make plans to be physically active daily. Work toward 30 to 60 minutes of moderate or vigorous physical activity each day. You can break this into shorter intervals or do it all at once. You do not need to run a marathon to have a healthy level of physical activity. The following are all examples of healthy options for moderate physical activity:

- walking 2 miles in 30 minutes
- bicycling 5 miles in 30 minutes
- dancing quickly for 30 minutes
- playing basketball for 15 to 20 minutes

If necessary, you can increase your physical activity using the suggestions in **Figure 9.10**.

Calories Burned per Hour of Physical Activity	
Physical Activity	**Calories Burned per Hour**
Playing volleyball	250
Walking	300
Dancing fast	380
Bicycling	550
Running	650
Jumping rope	680
Playing basketball	700

Goodheart-Willcox Publisher

Figure 9.10 This table shows different types of physical activity and the calories burned per hour. *How many calories are burned in 30 minutes of walking?*

9.1-4 Managing Your Weight

Even if everyone ate the same foods, people would all still be different shapes and sizes. Many factors, including genetics, access to healthy foods, age, and habits, impact how much people weigh. No matter body size, it is important to have self-care habits that promote overall well-being and health.

Maintaining a healthy weight makes you feel better. Excess weight can put extra strain on your joints and can increase the risk of joint pain and arthritis as you grow older. Excess weight gain can also increase people's risk of developing many diseases, including type 2 diabetes, heart disease, and some types of cancer. Dropping below a healthy weight range has negative health effects as well. It weakens your immune system and increases your risk of infection. Dangerously low weight reduces your body's ability to absorb nutrients, leading to a variety of harmful conditions such as osteoporosis, anemia, fatigue, and exhaustion.

Weight management begins with healthy food choices based on your body's individual needs. It is about learning how much food and which foods your body needs, then making healthy changes to your diet and sticking with them over time. The best strategy is to watch your serving sizes and choose a diet low in added sugars and solid fats. Eating a variety of food types and colors helps provide your body with all the nutrients it needs. If you find you use food as a distraction when bored or sad, you can seek the help of a counselor to substitute alternate activities.

Physical activity is another important tool for managing weight. You can manage weight by balancing the amount of food energy taken in and the amount of body energy used. Moderate activities such as jogging or riding a bike burn about 550 calories per hour (**Figure 9.11**).

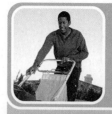

Tips for Staying Active

- Choose activities that fit your schedule and your personality.
- Team up with a friend and motivate each other.
- Get active during the time of day when you have the most energy.
- Use routine chores such as walking the dog or mowing the lawn to increase your exercise levels.
- Walk up the stairs instead of taking the elevator.
- When you care for young children, join them in playing tag or kickball.
- Just get yourself moving every day!

bikeriderlondon/Shutterstock.com

Figure 9.11 The best physical activity for you is one that you will actually do. Consider these tips for increasing your physical activity.

9.1-5 Sleep Habits

Many people do not recognize that sleep is a part of healthy weight management and physical wellness. Self-care habits should include getting enough sleep.

Healthy Sleep

Because so many things seem more interesting or important, people often give up on getting more sleep. However, sleep is just as essential as nutrition and physical activity for health and happiness. Sleep is a restorative activity that allows your body to reset. The quality and amount of sleep you get directly affects your mental alertness and productivity, emotional stability and creativity, physical energy, and even weight. The amount of sleep you need depends primarily on your age. For example, infants and children require 10 to 18 hours of sleep per day, while teens need 8½ to 9¼ hours. The average adult sleeps fewer than 7 hours each night, although most adults need 7½ to 9 hours for optimal functioning.

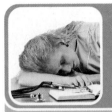

**Tips for
Better Sleep**

- exercise each day
- set a regular bedtime
- no caffeine after 4:00 p.m.
- turn off all technology one hour before bedtime
- avoid all-nighters
- wake up with a bright light in the morning

DenisNata/Shutterstock.com

Figure 9.12 Try these techniques for improving your sleep if you feel tired during the day.

Sleep Deficit

Many teens know they need even more sleep than adults do, but typical school schedules present a challenge. Teens' internal biological clocks, or *circadian rhythms*, tell them to fall asleep and wake up later. They may naturally fall asleep after midnight but still need to wake up early for school. This limits their sleep to 6 or 7 hours per night on a regular basis and creates a **sleep deficit**. This accumulation of missed sleep affects everything from paying attention in class to everyday mood. Teens with sleep deficits experience lower grades, reduced athletic performance, increased sadness and depression, and a higher risk of car crashes caused by driving when drowsy.

Even if you think you are getting enough sleep, the following signs will tell you otherwise:

- difficulty waking up in the morning
- an inability to concentrate
- a tendency to fall asleep during class
- feelings of moodiness and even depression

Your commitment to good health includes paying attention to sleep deficits. Try some of the tips listed in **Figure 9.12** to improve the quantity and quality of your sleep.

Healthcare Professions: Students and Sleep

Jake claimed he had a serious case of "senioritis." With one month of school left, he lacked the ambition to do homework and even get out of bed on time each morning. He was ready to give up on his plan for graduation and college. Maybe he would take the GED and enter the military instead. That was not really what he wanted, but it seemed easier somehow.

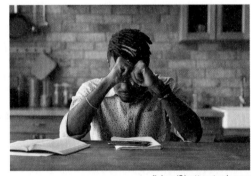

fizkes/Shutterstock.com

Jake was working about 30 hours a week at a local restaurant, and his shift ended at midnight. He got home by 1:00 a.m. and crashed on the couch. When the alarm went off in the morning, he was too tired to get up and head to school. He claimed he needed his job to pay for everyday expenses and future college costs.

Jake's part-time job was taking priority over his high school graduation and future college education. Why do you think he was so set on keeping a late work schedule? Could he have compromised and worked fewer hours during school and more hours during the summer? This would have been a logical choice, but Jake had a serious sleep deficit. Do you recognize the signs of sleep deprivation in his mood and mental focus?

9.1-6 Managing Stress Through Self-Care

Stress is your body's response to change, such as a new challenge or situation. It creates hormonal, respiratory, cardiovascular, and nervous system responses. The physical and emotional signs, such as sweaty palms, a red face, tense muscles, a burst of energy, fear, or nervousness, can be uncomfortable. Everyone faces stressful situations, such as dealing with illness, taking an important test, or even getting married. Stress can be positive or negative. While everyone feels some form of pressure in their life, healthcare workers face a unique set of stressors:

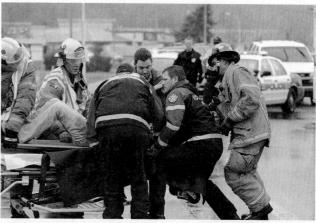

TFoxFoto/Shutterstock.com

Figure 9.13 Emergency workers must remain calm even in life-threatening situations. *What are some other stressful healthcare occupations?*

- working with people who are ill or injured
- staying calm in life-threatening situations (**Figure 9.13**)
- performing tasks that require a high degree of accuracy
- remaining alert at all times

Physical health and emotional health are interdependent—each one affects the other. Staying physically healthy will help reduce emotional stressors, and emotional stress must be recognized and managed appropriately so it does not affect your physical health. Cortisol is the body's primary stress hormone. It plays a role in the body's sleep-wake cycles, blood-sugar levels, inflammation, and blood pressures. Chronic stress can cause trouble sleeping, headaches, digestive issues, and hypertension.

 ## Healthcare Professions: Effects of Stress

Jean was sailing through her workday. Her schedule was light, and she was catching up on tasks that needed to be finished. Then came the news: her hospital was experiencing low occupancy due to the poor economy and was planning to cut back on staff hours. Suddenly, Jean's mood changed dramatically. A knot formed in her stomach, her heart began to pound, and her back started to hurt—all common signs and symptoms of stress. Jean was paying off school loans, and her budget was tight. She could not afford to lose any income. Will Jean choose positive or negative methods for coping with her stress?

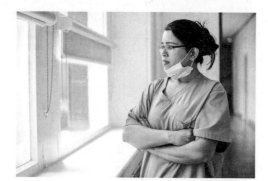

Rawpixel.com/Shutterstock.com

Too many people choose overeating, smoking, or using drugs or alcohol in response to stress. The problem is that all these behaviors mask the problem.

Over time, they also increase risk for serious health conditions. The following self-care methods for coping with stress will benefit your health:

- Physical activity increases endorphin production and improves mood and sleep.
- Both laughter and prayer can inhibit the release of cortisol, reducing the negative impact of stress on the immune system.
- Meditation provides a sense of calm that enhances emotional and physical well-being.
- Spending time on a hobby may reduce blood pressure and relieve symptoms of depression.
- Spending time with your family pet or people who care about you can help.

9.1-7 Healthy Relationships

Research shows that positive relationships with family and friends can help you recover more quickly from illness and may help you live longer. It is important that the relationship is positive and brings more happiness than stress to your life. Having healthy relationships is a self-care behavior that allows both people to feel supported and connected but not totally dependent on the other person. Signs of a healthy relationship include feeling safe, valued, and respected (**Figure 9.14**).

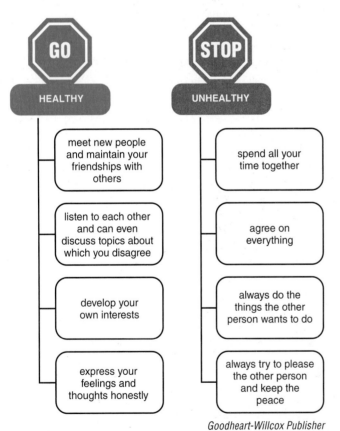

Goodheart-Willcox Publisher

Figure 9.14 As you develop new social relationships, be alert for these signs.

Communication and Boundaries

Communication and boundaries are important to maintaining healthy relationships. You should be able to speak openly and be respected for expressing your feelings. You should be able to express what you are or are not comfortable with and not feel pressured to do something you do not want to do. This includes physical, social, and sexual boundaries. When conflicts arise, both people should listen to each other and look for ways to compromise. You should also trust each other and not limit the ability to spend time with other people. You should maintain your own interests and feel comfortable spending time apart.

For teens who are in romantic relationships, sexual abstinence is the healthiest choice. Sexual abstinence is the only 100 percent effective method of preventing sexually transmitted infections (STIs) and pregnancy. STIs can be spread through any kind of sexual activity. Youth ages 15–24 make up one-half of the 20 million new STI cases each year. People in a sexual relationship should discuss their sexual histories and whether they have STIs. Some STIs can still be spread when there are no symptoms.

Condoms can reduce the risk of spreading STIs. Not being able to discuss this topic with a partner means the relationship is probably not ready for this level of intimacy.

Healthy Emotional Relationships

You should not neglect your own health or feel pressured to change who you are to please someone else. A healthy relationship should not make you worry about how the other person will react when you disagree with them. You should not feel controlled or limited by the other person. They should never call you names, put you down, or make you feel bad about yourself.

If you are unhappy with your relationship, you can try to improve it through open communication or counseling. Do not remain in a negative relationship out of guilt or fear of being alone. If you are in an unsafe relationship or are unable to leave, talk to an adult you trust about a safe way to leave.

Lesson 9.1 Review

 Complete the *Map Your Reading* graphic organizer for the section you just read.

1. When should a person's physical development begin to be monitored? (9.1-1)
   A. Before birth
   B. After birth
   C. Around 1 year of age
   D. Around 5 years of age
2. What should a healthy diet contain? Choose all that apply. (9.1-2)
   A. Fats
   B. Carbohydrates
   C. Protein
   D. Empty calories
3. The MyPlate graphic, developed by the USDA, helps balance (9.1-2)
   A. calories
   B. food groups
   C. protein intake
   D. carbohydrates
4. A _____ lifestyle does not provide enough physical activity to stay healthy. (9.1-3)
   A. highly active
   B. sedentary
   C. regularly active
   D. moderately active

5. Weight should be managed by balancing _____ and physical activity. (9.1-4)
   A. stress
   B. sleep
   C. calories
   D. protein
6. Staying up late and waking early causes _____ that can make it difficult to concentrate. (9.1-5)
   A. circadian rhythms
   B. weight gain
   C. stress
   D. sleep deficits
7. _____ is a physical and emotional response to change that can have negative health effects. (9.1-6)
   A. Stress
   B. Circadian rhythm
   C. Obesity
   D. Endorphin production
8. Healthy relationships allow both people to feel supported and connected, but not overly (9.1-7)
   A. active
   B. dependent
   C. sedentary
   D. independent

Public Health and Preventive Care Strategies

ESSENTIAL QUESTION

How does public health support health maintenance and preventive care?

Learning Outcomes

After studying this lesson, you will be able to

9.2-1   describe public health strategies for preventing disease.

9.2-2   explain how public health has responded to health disparities.

Professional Vocabulary

Essential Terms

preventive care   practices that help detect or prevent the start of serious diseases

public health   a branch of medicine focused on protecting and improving health of people and their communities

social determinants of health (SDOH)   nonmedical factors related to where a person is born and lives that influence their health status

Important Terms

community health
  education outreach
  programs
food insecurity

health disparities
oral health
personal hygiene

population health
screening tools
socioeconomics

Introduction

Along with understanding the fundamentals of wellness and disease prevention, healthcare workers must practice and promote healthy behaviors with their clients. Lifestyle choices play a role in the development of many diseases affecting patients today.

Public health is a branch of medicine focused on protecting and promoting the health of all people through organized community efforts. They use a variety of assessment, education, prevention, and policy-making strategies. Public health interventions save lives and money. In addition to promoting healthy behaviors through social media and public policies, public health offers health clinics and relevant educational programs in a variety of community settings. Their goal is to control epidemics and target treatments toward chronic health issues. Their work on immunization clinics, motor vehicle safety, workplace safety, nutrition, tobacco use, child health, and family planning has had a significant impact on health in the US.

9.2-1 Public Health and Preventive Care Strategies

Preventive care focuses on ways to avoid the start of a condition, so that fewer treatments and cures are needed. These routine habits are part of a healthy lifestyle. Preventive care includes personal hygiene, regular checkups at the doctor and dentist, and recommended immunizations. Preventive care is important for healthcare workers so they will be healthy and can work with people who are ill. Preventive care is an important part of public health efforts.

Personal Hygiene

Since the 1800s, public health has been promoting good hygiene as a way to reduce your risk of infection. Personal hygiene also benefits general health and is part of the professional appearance standards expected of healthcare workers. **Personal hygiene** includes bathing, brushing your teeth, washing your hands, and other grooming habits (**Figure 9.15**). Personal hygiene affects the first impression you create. You need to demonstrate to patients that you know how to care for yourself so they will trust you to care for them. You want to avoid body odor, bad breath, and skin conditions that feel awkward when in close contact.

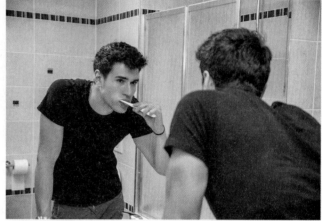

ArtOfPhotos/Shutterstock.com

Figure 9.15 Daily grooming promotes health and helps make a good first impression.

Begin with personal cleanliness, including your hair, hands, and fingernails. How often a person needs to bathe will depend on physical activity and the endocrine system. Some people need to bathe and wash their hair daily, while others find this too drying. How often you need to comb your hair depends on your hair and how you style it but check that it looks neat each morning. Keep your nails short and avoid wearing artificial nails. This reduces the risk of carrying infections in cracks and under edges where it is difficult to clean. Use deodorant but avoid strong perfumes or cologne that might trigger a patient's nausea, allergies, or asthma.

Wash clothing and bed linens on a regular basis. This reduces body odor and skin conditions. If you live with someone who smokes or a furry pet, washing will also help remove these allergens. Air out clothing that will not be washed. Shoes can be washed, wiped clean, or brushed to remove dirt. Shoelaces can also be removed and washed as needed.

Maintaining your personal hygiene is a matter of finding a routine that fits into your lifestyle. You will need to set aside time for doing laundry. You may need to create a schedule if you share a bathroom. You cannot skip hygiene if you want to work in healthcare.

Routine Health Screenings and Examinations

Public health organizes and conducts medical, dental, and mental health screenings and routine physical exams for people who need them most. Regular doctor visits and diagnostic tests are an essential part of preventive care.

Your age, risks factors, and current health affect how often you should see a doctor. Doctors recommend that most people have a wellness visit annually, and adults should have a complete physical every three years up to age 50. After that, an annual physical is recommended. Children, older adults, and people with chronic diseases or other risk factors should see their doctor annually or more often, as recommended.

Regular checkups help your doctor identify health conditions early before they become more serious. They are also important for maintaining a good relationship with your primary care physician, so you are comfortable sharing information. Doctors may not notice subtle changes, but patients should bring things they notice to their doctor's attention.

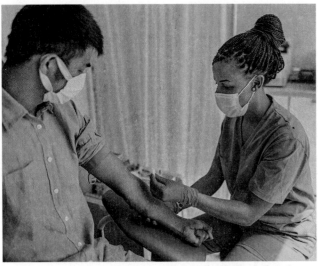

Figure 9.16 Blood tests, which are performed by diagnostic workers such as phlebotomists and medical assistants, can provide important health information.

Recommended for Everyone

The US Preventive Services Task Force (USPSTF) recommends preventive services that will be most useful. **Screening tools** assess the risk for many conditions. Screening usually begins with measuring height, weight, and vital signs. Sets of questions assess for depression, drug and alcohol use, safety in the home, and abuse. All adults should receive tobacco-use screening and guidance for quitting annually. High blood pressure screenings should begin at age 18 and be repeated every three years until age 40, when it should become an annual screening.

Blood tests are often part of these checkups. They can reveal health issues, such as high cholesterol or diabetes, that require treatment (**Figure 9.16**). Screenings for hepatitis B, human immunodeficiency virus (HIV), chlamydia, and gonorrhea are recommended beginning at age 15.

Recommended for Some Groups

Specific tests and preventive care are recommended for certain groups of people. Children are screened for vision and hearing. Behavioral counseling on safer sex is recommended for those who are sexually active. Pre-exposure prophylaxis (PrEP) is recommended for those at risk for HIV. People with female anatomy should receive cervical cytology and human papillomavirus (HPV) screenings for cervical cancer every three to five years after 21 years of age. People should have a colonoscopy every five to 10 years after age 45 to check for colorectal cancer and remove small growths. The task force suggests a moderate benefit of mammograms to screen for breast cancer every other year for people with female anatomy beginning at 50 years of age. There are also moderate benefits for females 65 years of age and older being screened for osteoporosis, a disease that causes bones to break easily.

Infants, children, and those who are pregnant or have other health risks will have additional recommendations. Your doctor will look at family history, health history, ethnic group, work or environmental risk factors, and any DNA test results in determining the best schedule for preventive screening tools.

Vaccinations

As a healthcare worker, you will be required to have certain vaccinations. School-entry vaccinations were first required in 1850 to prevent smallpox, and vaccinations have been a part of public health's efforts to prevent the spread of infections among children since 1955. The CDC recommends immunization against 15 different diseases between birth and age 18. It is important to follow the recommended vaccination schedule. This will allow immunity to develop during childhood before you are exposed to potentially life-threatening diseases. Vaccines have been shown to be safe and effective.

Not following the vaccine schedule causes risks to both the person who is unvaccinated and the community. People who are unvaccinated can carry and spread contagious illnesses even without symptoms. They also provide an opportunity for illnesses to grow and mutate. You should not rely on "herd immunity" to protect against infection. Approximately 90–95 percent of the population would need to be immunized for those without immunization to be somewhat protected, and you cannot know everyone's immunization status. During a disease outbreak, people who are unvaccinated should stay away from others until the end of the disease incubation period. Those who develop early signs or symptoms of a contagious disease should self-isolate until they have been tested or see their doctor.

The need for vaccinations continues throughout your life. Adults should keep their vaccinations up to date because immunity from childhood vaccines can wear off over time. You are also at risk for different diseases as an adult. Annual flu vaccination and a tetanus booster shot every 10 years should continue through old age. Additional vaccines may be needed based on your job, travel, lifestyle, health, or age.

Oral Health

Oral health includes the health of the teeth, gums, tongue, and mouth. Oral health is a predictor of overall health because it is directly connected to other chronic health conditions such as heart disease. Public health has been educating people about oral health since about 1950.

Oral health affects people in many ways. Healthy teeth help people eat, speak, smile, and show emotions. Oral disease can cause pain, disability, illness, and low self-esteem. The good news is that many oral diseases, such as cavities, are preventable. Fluoride in water and fluoride varnish applied to baby teeth can reduce cavities in children. Dental sealants and fluoride toothpaste can prevent cavities on permanent teeth. Because of fluoride, tooth loss is declining. Baby boomers will be the first generation to keep their natural teeth through old age.

You should brush and floss your teeth at least twice a day. This reduces plaque, bacteria, and breath odor. Do not forget to brush your tongue and rinse with mouthwash. Regular dental cleaning and X-rays can also protect oral health. Dental hygienists remove plaque that can cause gum disease. X-rays provide early warning of decay and bone loss (**Figure 9.17**). During a dental exam, you are also screened for oral cancer, mouth ulcers, impaired taste, and dry mouth. Preventive oral care can reduce the impact of conditions such as emphysema, reflux, osteoporosis, and HIV on oral health.

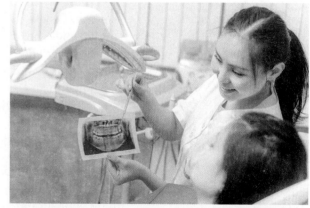

Mark Agnor/Shutterstock.com

Figure 9.17 Dental cleanings prevent gum disease and X-rays can detect tooth decay and bone loss before they cause symptoms.

- Availability of resources to meet daily needs for housing, food, and safety
- Social norms and attitudes around discrimination and racism
- Exposure to crime, violence, and chaos
- Quality of education and job training
- Access to insurance and healthcare services
- Access to transportation options
- Literacy and exposure to languages
- Access to opportunities for financial growth
- Access to social media and technology
- Availability of community-based recreational activities

Goodheart-Willcox Publisher

Figure 9.18 Many aspects of socioeconomics have an impact on health. *Which one has the largest impact on your life, either positive or negative?*

9.2-2 Supporting Public Health

Chronic diseases began replacing infectious diseases as major health issues in the US in the mid-1900s. Public health responded by shifting their focus from prevention to proactively improving population health. **Population health** refers to the physical, mental, and social well-being of groups of people and the differences in health between these groups. Chronic diseases, such as heart disease, cancer, diabetes, and tooth decay, affect a higher percentage of people with lower social status and income. Studies also show different outcomes for preventive and proactive care depending on a person's position in society. **Socioeconomics**, or the combined force of social class and income, is influenced by unequal access to resources and unfair privileges for some groups in society.

Social determinants of health (SDOH) are the conditions in which people grow, live, and work that affect their health, well-being, and quality of life (**Figure 9.18**). These personal, social, economic, and environmental factors affect their interactions, feelings of safety, and access to opportunities. They create **health disparities**, which are unexpected differences, or *inequalities*, in health outcomes for a group of people due to their unequal position in society. Some marginalized populations have higher rates of preventable disease, death, and disability. You will see these differences between people who have different racial or ethnic backgrounds, genders and sexes, sexual orientations, ages, disabilities, social classes and incomes, and geographic locations.

Health disparities have a negative effect on a whole population's health. This results in added healthcare expenses, reduced quality of life, and premature death. Examples of health disparities are:

- People with an African-American background have a much greater risk for preterm births, infant mortality, asthma, hypertension, heart disease, diabetes, and early death.
- People with a Native American background have higher rates of obesity, mental health conditions, and chronic liver disease.
- People with a Hispanic background have higher rates of liver cancer and may be less likely to seek and receive healthcare due to language barriers.
- People who are lesbian, gay, bisexual, or transgender are more likely to experience physical violence, sexual assault, substance use, HIV infection, and suicide.
- Veterans have higher rates of PTSD, depression, and suicide.
- Those living with disabilities have higher rates of obesity.

Community Health Education Outreach

Although more people have health insurance today, many people still do not make or keep appointments for preventive healthcare. Public health has many educational and community-based programs and strategies designed to reach people outside of traditional healthcare settings. **Community health education outreach programs** serve populations that are less likely to use preventive health services and tend to have more healthcare needs.

The programs use existing social structures in schools, community centers, and worksites to encourage informal social interaction for sharing information in a nonthreatening way. They also encourage discussions that can improve health programs and policies in the community. They recognize that a well-functioning healthcare system requires a strong connection to the community it serves.

These programs provide health screenings, case management, and better access to health services. They also offer educational programs that can be tailored to a population. They might educate the community about unintended pregnancy, substance use, or physical activity at schools and community centers. Discussions about chronic diseases, obesity prevention, mental health, and tobacco use might be offered at community centers and religious organizations. Work centers may offer weight-management clinics, injury and violence prevention, mental health or substance use support groups, and chronic disease checkups. They are not worried about overlap between settings. Instead, they hope they will reach their intended population through at least one of these community-based programs. Their activities can improve health outcomes for individuals and communities.

Addressing Food Insecurity

Food insecurity is the lack of consistent access to enough healthy food to support physical health. This issue is widespread but more often affects marginalized groups such as people of color, people with low incomes, households with children, and people who live in rural areas. Food insecurity is increased by insufficient resources, such as income and transportation. Areas without access to healthy and affordable food, or *food deserts*, exist in both rural and urban areas. Zoning policies, segregation, and profit margins all play a role in creating food deserts. More than 30 million people live in areas classified as a food desert.

Food access programs, such as government-funded food assistance and food pantries, serve as a safety net. They are short-term solutions that do not address barriers to food security. Public health is working with communities to build alternative food systems that support marginalized groups. Food insecurity is being addressed by building community gardens, starting food co-ops, and organizing regional programs that increase access and local control over food resources.

Lesson 9.2 Review

 Complete the *Map Your Reading* graphic organizer for the section you just read.

1. Good personal _____ benefit(s) your health and gives others the impression you can take care of their health needs. (9.2-1)
   A. screenings
   B. hygiene
   C. examinations
   D. habits

2. What is the purpose of screening tools in a checkup? (9.2-1)
   A. They avoid the need for annual checkups.
   B. They reduce the amount of work the doctor must do during a checkup.
   C. They help the patient to feel the checkup was thorough.
   D. They check for health issues the doctor may need to address.

3. Which of these statements about herd immunity is true? (9.2-1)
   A. A very high percentage of vaccination is required to protect those who are unvaccinated.
   B. Herd immunity demonstrates vaccine safety.
   C. It provides maximum protection against communicable diseases.
   D. Only natural immunity leads to herd immunity, not vaccination.

4. Community health education centers provide health education and services at which of the following? Choose all that apply. (9.2-2)
   A. Schools
   B. Community centers
   C. Your home
   D. Worksites

Mental and Behavioral Health

ESSENTIAL QUESTION

How do mental and behavioral health influence wellness?

Learning Outcomes

After studying this lesson, you will be able to:

9.3-1 describe mental development and its impact on behavioral health.

9.3-2 discuss common issues that affect mental and behavioral health.

9.3-3 identify maladaptive and risky behaviors that can negatively affect health.

9.3-4 recognize the signs for risk of suicide.

9.3-5 identify how to seek support for mental health conditions.

9.3-6 describe how healthcare workers can aid in managing grief.

Professional Vocabulary

Essential Terms

behavioral health   involves the daily habits, choices, and actions that affect mental and physical wellness.

mental health   involves how people think, feel, behave, and cope when faced with life challenges

Important Terms

adverse childhood events (ACEs)

anxiety

depression

maladaptive behaviors

opioids

trauma-informed

Introduction

In this lesson, you will learn about mental and behavioral development. You will also learn about ways to recognize mental health conditions and improve mental health and wellness.

9.3-1 Mental and Behavioral Development

Mental and behavioral health are related, but not the same. **Mental health** is your psychological and emotional well-being that affects how you think and feel. **Behavioral health** describes how your responses to different situations impact the health of your mind, body, and spirit. All people have the same basic needs that drive behavior. Abraham Maslow identified five levels of needs (**Figure 9.19**). He recognized that needs exist in a *hierarchy*, meaning some are typically met before others. For example, after meeting basic physical needs, attention can shift to safety and security needs.

If you feel protected from harm, you can focus on developing relationships for love and belonging. Once you feel accepted, you can work toward self-actualization. Different ages and cultures may meet these needs in different ways.

Influences on Behavior

Needs influence your behavior. Erik Erikson was a psychoanalyst who identified basic conflicts that must be resolved in psychosocial development (**Figure 9.20**). Infants must rely on others to meet their basic physical needs. They test different behaviors, such as crying and cooing, to see what works. Children want to explore and push for more independence. Family rules keep them safe and help them fulfill their needs.

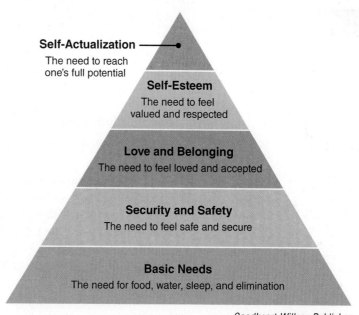

Goodheart-Willcox Publisher

Figure 9.19 The five levels of need, as determined by Abraham Maslow. *Why are these arranged in a hierarchy?*

Erikson's Stages of Psychosocial Development		
Age	**Stage Description**	**Main Challenge**
Infancy birth to 18 months	Infants experience rapid growth but are not yet able to control their bodies or fend for themselves. They need to be fed, bathed, clothed, and kept safe and warm by caregivers. They have difficulty expressing their needs.	Learning to trust others to meet needs for food, care, and affection
Early childhood 18 months–3 years of age	Toddlers begin to control their bodies and assert independence, but need others to keep them safe by providing limits.	Developing self-control and autonomy without a loss of self-esteem to build will power
Preschool 3–5 years of age	Preschoolers use growing independence to explore the world and exert control over their environment.	Developing initiative and a sense of purpose without guilt
School age 6–11 years of age	Children begin school and experience extended separation from parents. They form new friendships and learn to cope with demands to perform well in school.	Needing praise and reassurance in accomplishments so they do not feel inferior to others
Adolescence 12–18 years of age	Adolescents go through a period of self-discovery, with increasing responsibilities and independence in relationships, money control, and decision-making. Peers have more influence than parents. Experimenting may lead to risky behaviors.	Needing loyalty, acceptance, and self-identity to avoid role confusion
Early adulthood 20–40 years of age	Young adults feel the stress of building a new career and a family apart from their parents.	Needing intimacy and love versus isolation
Middle adulthood 40–65 years of age	Middle adults may face the pressures of parenthood, aging parents, and work responsibilities.	Being productive and caring for others so they do not become self-absorbed
Late adulthood 65 years of age and older	Older adults look back on life as friends and family are aging. Health may begin to decline, and they experience loss. Older adults may face shrinking financial resources and social opportunities with retirement.	Accepting accomplishments and loss without despair

Goodheart-Willcox Publisher

Figure 9.20 Erik Erikson identified eight stages of psychosocial development.

Children must learn to create their own structure and form their own supportive relationships as they gain independence from their family.

Many factors can affect the relationships children form. For example, autism spectrum disorder (ASD) is a developmental disability that impacts a child's ability to form relationships with others. Approximately one in 54 children born today will develop ASD. Other factors that affect behavior and development include illness, adolescence, and adverse childhood experiences (ACEs).

Illness

Healthcare workers must remember that illness affects patients' basic needs, behaviors, and reactions to others. Sudden illness or surgery can create feelings of insecurity, pain, and stress. Medications and illness can alter patients' mental states or affect their ability to interact with others or the environment. Try to anticipate the needs of your patients and their families. Be sensitive to their need for privacy or self-expression. Reactions will vary and may be influenced by age and culture. It is important to be patient and encourage patients to talk about their feelings.

Adolescence

Adolescence and young adulthood are a critical period of transition. Physical, social, and emotional behavior patterns established during this period determine health and risks for chronic diseases later in life. Issues that can appear during this time include substance use, nutrition and weight concerns, sexually transmitted infections, unintended pregnancy, academic struggles, depression, and many other challenges. The influence of society, media messages, peer groups, family, and environment can either support or threaten health and wellness.

Adverse Childhood Experiences (ACEs)

Social, economic, and physical environments influence lifestyle choices and the likelihood of **adverse childhood experiences (ACEs)**. ACEs are challenges such as violence, abuse, neglect, and household dysfunction that can create toxic stress and lead to poor physical health. The first signs are mental and behavioral health issues. Those with four or more ACEs have a higher risk for the leading causes of death in adulthood: heart disease, stroke, cancer, chronic obstructive pulmonary disease (COPD), diabetes, Alzheimer's disease, and suicide.

It is important to provide services to those affected by ACEs. Being **trauma-informed** helps people who work with youth recognize its symptoms. Behaviors such as acting out at school, risk-taking, recurring stomachaches, overly emotional reactions to a negative event, hurting people, self-isolation, obsessive diet or physical activity, and binge eating can be calls for help. Providing appropriate support and counseling as soon as possible can help reduce the effects on health.

Identifying Concerns

Some physicians assess stressors and check in with youth using the BATHE technique, shown in **Figure 9.21**. When issues are identified, they can refer them to support services such as counseling and community resources. They can also talk about the importance of the mind-body connection in holistic care and the benefits of meditation for coping with stress.

The BATHE Technique		
Aspect	**Action**	**Example**
Background	Establish background, ask about things in their life.	"What is going on in your life right now?"
Affect	Ask how this issue affects them.	"How do you feel about that?"
Troubles	Ask what troubles them most.	"Which of these creates the most problems for you?"
Handling	Find out how they are handling the situation.	"How have you been managing this situation?"
Empathy	Express empathy.	"That seems very difficult."

Goodheart-Willcox Publisher

Figure 9.21 The BATHE technique helps physicians assess stressors their patients are experiencing.

9.3-2 Issues Affecting Mental and Behavioral Health

Emotional, psychological, and social well-being interact to form mental health. Mental health is more than the absence of a mental health condition. Mental health or wellness is the ability to function well and respond with resilience to life's challenges. Biological, environmental, and socioeconomic factors all influence mental health. Poor mental health is associated with stressful home and work conditions, discrimination, instability, and physical illness.

Mental Health Conditions

Mental health conditions interfere with everyday living and are the leading cause of disability in the US. According to the National Institute of Mental Health, one in five US adults is affected by a mental health disorder each year. Nearly one-half of those are cases of depression.

Mental health conditions affect how a person feels, thinks, and acts and interfere with regular activities and daily functioning. Some mental health conditions relate to organs of the nervous system and brain, but others do not. People with mental health conditions are more likely to experience chronic conditions that also affect physical health. Prevention and early treatment of mental health conditions can improve physical and emotional wellness. They can also reduce substance use disorders, homelessness, and community violence. To develop mental well-being, a person needs to feel like a productive, contributing member of their community and feel able to cope with normal life stresses. This develops over time in a stable, safe, and supportive environment. Two of the most common mental health conditions are anxiety and depression.

Anxiety

Anxiety is a feeling of nervousness, uneasiness, or dread. Some anxiety is a natural response to stress about the unknown. An anxiety disorder is a persistent and exaggerated feeling of uneasiness, worry, and fear that lasts for many months and interferes with your life. There are many types of anxiety disorders, such as post-traumatic stress disorder (PTSD), obsessive-compulsive disorder (OCD), phobias, and social anxiety disorder.

Symptoms of anxiety include an increased heart rate, rapid breathing, sweating, trouble concentrating, apprehension, tingling sensations, restlessness, and difficulty sleeping. The symptoms usually come on slowly and build as the stressful situation gets nearer. An anxiety attack can be severe and is sometimes mistaken for a heart attack.

To manage anxiety, try taking slow, deep breaths, then counting down as you exhale. Practice *mindfulness* by being aware of your thoughts and sensations without reacting to them. Use positive self-talk about your ability to manage stress. Remind yourself that the symptoms will pass, and you will be okay. Do things that you find relaxing, such as a hot bath or walking outside. Avoid alcohol, smoking, and caffeine. Consider lifestyle changes to reduce sources of stress in your life. Psychotherapy treatments and medications are also available.

Depression

Depression is the most common mental health condition among teens. **Depression** is a long-lasting and overwhelming feeling of sadness. It is more than the normal sadness that follows an adverse event. Major depressive disorder, or *clinical depression*, is characterized by persistent symptoms of depression that occur nearly every day and last for a period of two weeks or more. Depression affects your thoughts, feelings, and daily activities, including eating, sleeping, and going to school or work. Many factors, including changes in hormones or chemicals in the brain, can cause depression. **Figure 9.22** provides a helpful mnemonic for identifying depression symptoms.

You can help people experiencing depression just by letting them know you are there for them. They need to feel valued, supported, and listened to. You can say, "It seems like you've been going through a lot lately. Is there anything I can do to help?" Remind them that asking for help is a normal part of life.

Symptoms of Depression	
Symptom	**Description**
Sleep changes	May sleep a lot more or experience insomnia
Overwhelming feelings	Sadness, guilt, or hopelessness that lasts for several weeks
Memory problems	Difficulty remembering details, concentrating, or making decisions
Behavioral changes	May stop doing activities that used to be enjoyable
Eating changes	May eat excessively or lose appetite and stop eating
Restlessness	Inability to stick with one task for a long period of time; irritable

Goodheart-Willcox Publisher

Figure 9.22 The acronym *SOMBER* can help you identify symptoms of depression.

9.3-3 Maladaptive and Risky Behaviors

Maladaptive behaviors are some of the nonproductive ways people deal with emotional challenges. These patterns of thinking and behavior may help reduce anxiety in the short term, but they do not help in the long term. Examples include the rituals of a person with OCD, the self-injury of a person with depression, or the social and emotional withdrawal by a person with an anxiety disorder. Maladaptive behaviors can be harmful to the people who do them and to others. They do not help people solve problems or adapt to life's demands.

Risky behaviors can cause physical and mental harm. Some people turn to risky behaviors to escape stress or depression. For example, people with mental health conditions are twice as likely to use substances, including alcohol, prescription drugs, over-the-counter medications, cough medicine, marijuana, and household products such as inhalants. The risk of harm is increased for teens and young adults because their brain and body are still developing. Schools and health-care providers use a questionnaire to screen for risk-taking behaviors (**Figure 9.23**).

Excessive Alcohol Use

Excessive alcohol use includes binge drinking and heavy drinking. Alcohol misuse also includes any alcohol use by people who are underage, pregnant, planning to drive, or taking medications that interact with alcohol. When people drink alcohol, it is quickly absorbed in the stomach and small intestines, then slowly removed from the blood by the liver. Intoxication happens when the liver does not keep up with the rate of absorption. This results in impaired brain function, reduced reaction time and judgment, and loss of balance and motor skills. Alcohol is a depressant, so a rapid rise in blood alcohol levels can result in a coma or death.

Most people know using alcohol or drugs affects the ability to drive, but they do not consider the other impacts of impaired judgment and loss of inhibition. For example, studies have established a link between alcohol and sexual assault. Nearly one in four female college students and one in 16 males reported experiencing unwanted sexual contact while under the influence of alcohol or drugs. They also report an increased likelihood of taking risks they would not normally have taken if they were not under the influence.

Not drinking alcohol or taking drugs is the best way to protect yourself from these risks. In a national survey, one in 13 students reported being drugged at a party. Do not accept drinks from others and be wary of food or drinks that may contain drugs. Do not mix drugs and alcohol, as this can intensify the effects. Avoid risky situations and surround yourself with people who respect your decisions.

Many people who drink excessively do not meet the definition for an *alcohol use disorder*, or alcoholism, but misusing alcohol still has negative effects. If alcohol use causes trouble in a person's relationships, education, or social activities, or if someone cannot limit their alcohol use, help is needed. Binge drinking, which is the rapid consumption of several drinks within two hours or less, can cause alcohol poisoning, or *acute intoxication*. This is a medical emergency and can result in coma or death. If someone has too much to drink, do not put the person in the shower or bed and assume the person will be okay. When someone who was drinking or taking drugs cannot stay awake, has irregular breathing, looks sweaty, is incoherent and vomiting, or is unconscious, call 911. Acute intoxication causes more than 80,000 deaths per year.

Smoking and Vaping

Tobacco use remains the number-one cause of preventable deaths in the US. Smoking and secondhand smoke cause emphysema, chronic bronchitis, and other lung diseases, as well as high blood pressure and a variety of cancers. Nicotine is addictive, and smoking damages nearly every organ of the body, not just the lungs. Although some progress has been made in reducing

Example Risk Assessment	
Risk Assessment Questions	**Response**
I would enjoy skydiving.	Yes/No
I enjoy wild and crazy parties.	Yes/No
I hide my activities from adults.	Yes/No
I take more risks when I am in a hurry.	Yes/No
I sometimes do frightening things just for fun.	Yes/No
I prefer friends who are exciting and unpredictable.	Yes/No
I do things on an impulse without thinking them through.	Yes/No
When I start doing something foolish, I just can't stop myself.	Yes/No
I often create problems by acting or speaking without thinking.	Yes/No
I like doing things where you can't predict how they will turn out.	Yes/No

Goodheart-Willcox Publisher

Figure 9.23 Risk assessments are used as a screening tool.

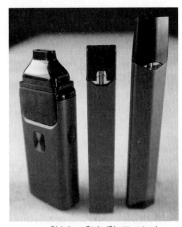

Chicken Strip/Shutterstock.com

Figure 9.24 Vaping is a risky behavior that has the potential for many unknown side effects.

cigarette smoking, there has been less progress reducing cigarette smoking among people with lower income. On average, people who smoke die at least 10 years earlier than people who do not. The US Preventive Services Task Force recommends that pediatricians educate school-age patients and parents about the risks of tobacco and secondhand smoke. Raising prices and restricting access for minors has also helped reduce tobacco use.

As the use of cigarettes has decreased, the use of electronic cigarettes and vaping have increased. The aerosol inhaled during vaping contains nicotine, flavorings, and other chemicals (**Figure 9.24**). Although these products are known to be harmful, their health impacts are not fully understood. In the lungs, aerosol is absorbed more readily than tobacco smoke. Flavorings in aerosol, which were approved for consumption in food products, were never tested on the lungs. Known short-term effects include headaches, respiratory tract irritation, and changes in appetite. Vaping products have not been studied enough to know the long-term impacts.

The FDA began regulating the sale of electronic cigarettes and vaping devices in 2016, but the number of teens who use them has continued to rise. Teens who vape are often younger than teens who smoke cigarettes. Vaping can also be a gateway to the use of other tobacco products, such as cigarettes, and marijuana. THC, the active ingredient in marijuana, is much more potent when vaped than when smoked. Vaping THC oil was related to a sudden increase in lung injuries and deaths in 2019. In 2020, the FDA restricted the use of flavorings for electronic cigarettes due to their appeal to kids and began enforcing new age restrictions on the sale of tobacco. It is now illegal to sell any tobacco product, including cigarettes, cigars, electronic cigarettes, and vaping devices, to anyone under 21.

Opioid Crisis

In 2017, the Department of Health and Human Services (HHS) declared the widespread misuse of opioids a public health emergency. In 2018, 10.3 million people misused prescription opioids. Approximately 136 people die every day from an opioid-related drug overdose. Forty percent of these involve prescription opioids. An increasing number of newborns experience withdrawal syndrome due to opioid use and misuse during pregnancy.

Opioids are a class of drugs often used to manage pain. Examples are the prescription drugs oxycodone, codeine, and morphine. There is a misconception that prescription drugs are safer than street drugs. Even when taken as prescribed by a doctor, opioids can have many side effects. It is important not to take (or allow someone else to take) another person's prescription drug. You do not know how the drug will react in your body.

There is a serious risk of addiction, tolerance, abuse, and overdose for people taking opioids. The risk is higher if people illegally purchase drugs online or from street dealers, who may cut the drugs with other harmful substances. Synthetic opioids, such as fentanyl and carfentanil, can be 50 to 100 times more powerful than morphine. Opioid or other drug use can lead to a *substance use disorder*. The lives of people with a substance use disorder are significantly affected by their use, and people feel a strong urge to take more of the drug each time it wears off. These cravings can happen long after quitting. Withdrawal symptoms can include restlessness, nervousness, muscle and bone pain, diarrhea, vomiting, and chills. A person who takes opioids regularly may require higher doses to achieve the same results. High doses of opioids can stop breathing and cause death. Injecting the drug also increases risk for infectious diseases, such as HIV and hepatitis.

Misusing prescription opioids is the strongest risk factor for future use of the illegal drug heroin. Heroin-related deaths have increased dramatically in the past 10 years. A person may need to receive treatment several times to stop using heroin.

The US Department of Health and Human Services (HHS) has a five-point strategy to combat this opioid crisis (**Figure 9.25**). Through research and education, they hope to improve opioid-prescribing practices and identify high-risk individuals early. They also hope to increase access to substance use treatment.

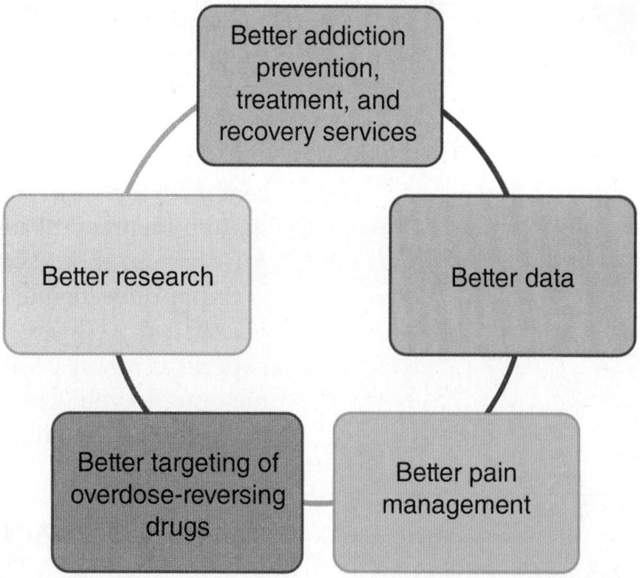

9.3-4 Suicide

If left untreated, mental health conditions, such as depression and substance use disorders, can increase risk for suicide. Suicide rates have increased by 30 percent in the last 20 years and are the second leading cause of death for teens and young adults. Those with a family history of suicide, substance use, chronic illness, or stress have an increased risk for suicide.

Behaviors that signal someone may be about to attempt suicide are giving away possessions, acquiring a means for attempting suicide, and saying goodbye to friends and family. These behaviors are an emergency. You should call 911, call the 988 Suicide & Crisis Lifeline, or see a healthcare provider immediately. Let friends know you are there for them and there are people they can talk to. Listen and encourage them to talk about their feelings. Suicidal thoughts are a symptom, and therapy and coping skills can improve them over time. Suicide is a permanent solution to what is often a temporary problem.

9.3-5 Seeking Support

Keep in mind that mental health conditions are real illnesses. People cannot be talked out of having poor mental health, but emotional support can help with managing symptoms. If you or a friend are feeling depressed or having unhealthy thoughts, seek help. Do not wait. Ask your doctor or a mental health professional for an evaluation or treatment. When treating mental health conditions, remember to set realistic goals and be patient.

Different mental health conditions respond to different types of treatment. Some people benefit from talk therapy, or *psychotherapy* (**Figure 9.26**). Others may respond better to medication. Electroconvulsive therapy (ECT) can help interrupt signals in an overactive brain. Being physically active can trigger the brain's natural secretion of neurotransmitters and endorphins, which are helpful for some people.

Better addiction prevention, treatment, and recovery services

Better research

Better data

Better targeting of overdose-reversing drugs

Better pain management

Goodheart-Willcox Publisher

Figure 9.25 The HHS strategy for combatting the opioid crisis includes five key areas of focus.

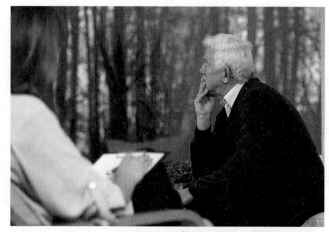

Photographee.eu/Shutterstock.com

Figure 9.26 Talk therapy is often used to treat mental health conditions such as depression.

Research shows that mood-regulating drugs, such as antidepressants, can reduce symptoms for many people by balancing neurotransmitters in the brain. These drugs work differently for different people because of the complex causes of mood disorders. They are most effective over a long period of time because they help stimulate neuron growth that connects the emotion centers of the brain. There is a risk, especially with children and young adults, that antidepressant medications can increase thoughts of suicide, so antidepressant use should be monitored closely.

Support for mental health conditions is available. You can encourage mental health and wellness through support, community connections, and positive experiences. Stay positive, avoid risky behaviors, and focus on things that have meaning to you. Use physical activity, meditation, relaxation techniques, and coping skills to manage stress and recognize when you need help.

9.3-6 Managing Grief

All people experience a major loss or stress at some point in life, but healthcare workers may be exposed to more loss than people in other careers. The stages of deep sorrow, or *grief*, identified by Dr. Elisabeth Kübler-Ross, apply to times of major loss or crisis (**Figure 9.27**). These include death, breakups, and diagnosis of a major illness. Not all people experience these stages in the same way or have the same timing, but the stages provide some understanding of what to expect. It can help to know your experience is normal, although you may still need support from others to get through it. Some people may not progress through all the stages. As a healthcare worker or friend, recognizing the stages will help you understand people's needs and not take it personally if they lash out.

The Stages of Grief	
Stage	**What It May Be Like**
Denial People refuse to believe the truth.	Ignoring the facts or sad news "There must be a mix-up." "I feel fine. I'm sure their estimates are off."
Anger People become angry when they can no longer deny the truth.	Feeling upset with doctors and others "Why me?" "This is your fault." "That doctor's a quack. He didn't keep me well."
Bargaining People accept death but want more time.	Trying to make deals with the doctor, family members, or a higher power "If I stop smoking, can you just keep me alive until my grandchild is born?" "I will take my medicine and exercise if you can give me a few more years."
Depression People realize that death will come soon.	Extreme sadness that interferes with life activities Crying easily Poor memory and concentration Sleeping a lot; restless when awake
Acceptance People understand and accept that they are going to die.	Acceptance of the loss as real and beginning to move on Making a will and getting affairs in order Ability to talk about life after the person is gone Shifting concern to those who will be left behind

Goodheart-Willcox Publisher

Figure 9.27 The stages of grief can help someone understand what to expect after a major loss.

Hospice care is available for people with six months or less to live. Hospice is a philosophy of care that supports dignity and comfort in death. Palliative care is provided to relieve pain, but the focus is no longer on finding a cure. Some facilities are dedicated specifically to providing hospice care, but a care team may provide this type of care in any setting. Working with patients at the end of life can be very rewarding but also stressful for caregivers. Supportive care and self-awareness are important to the well-being of families and healthcare workers. Hospice social workers, chaplains, support groups, and other grief services are available to anyone who is experiencing loss due to death, even if the loved one was not a hospice patient. Nonprofit hospices have a charitable mission of serving those in need.

Lesson 9.3 Review

 Complete the *Map Your Reading* graphic organizer for the section you just read.

1. ACEs such as violence and abuse can create _____ that leads to poor health. (9.3-1)
   A. toxic stress
   B. mindfulness
   C. risky behavior
   D. impaired judgment

2. Some anxiety is a normal response to stress, but _____ continue(s) for a long time and interfere(s) with your life. (9.3-2)
   A. stress management
   B. ACEs
   C. maladaptive behaviors
   D. an anxiety disorder

3. _____ is the most common mental health condition among teens. The symptoms are persistent, lasting for two weeks or more. They are often caused by changes in hormones. (9.3-2)
   A. Anxiety
   B. Depression
   C. Risky behavior
   D. Maladaptive behavior

4. Which of these behaviors can cause physical harm? Choose all that apply. (9.3-3)
   A. Smoking
   B. Vaping
   C. Binge drinking
   D. Opioids

5. Which statement about opioid use is false? (9.3-3)
   A. Drug cravings stop shortly after quitting.
   B. Forty percent of opioid deaths involve prescription opioids.
   C. High doses of opioids can stop breathing and cause death.
   D. There is a serious risk of addiction, tolerance, abuse, and overdose for people taking opioids.

6. Which of the following behaviors signal that someone may attempt suicide? Choose all that apply. (9.3-4)
   A. Giving away possessions
   B. Impulsively adopting a pet
   C. Saying goodbye to family and friends
   D. Having a history of substance use

7. Which of the following are treatment options for managing the symptoms of mental health conditions? Choose all that apply. (9.3-5)
   A. Psychotherapy
   B. Electroconvulsive therapy
   C. Antidepressants
   D. Meditation

8. Which of these is a philosophy of care that supports dignity and comfort in death? (9.3-6)
   A. Grief counseling
   B. Palliative care
   C. Hospice
   D. Psychotherapy

Holistic Health and Wellness Practices

?

ESSENTIAL QUESTION

How do holistic approaches support health and wellness?

Learning Outcomes

After studying this lesson, you will be able to

9.4-1 describe the holistic approach to health and wellness.

9.4-2 apply techniques for intellectual wellness.

9.4-3 describe social wellness techniques and their impact on healthcare.

9.4-4 compare types of complementary and alternative medicine for supporting wellness.

Professional Vocabulary

Essential Terms

complementary and alternative medicine (CAM)   healthcare practices, products, and supplements that are not a part of Western medicine

holistic health   provides care for the whole person with a balance between the body, mind, spirit, and emotions; acknowledging that a change in one aspect affects the others

intellectual wellness   involves keeping your brain active through stimulating and creative activities that expand your knowledge and skills

social wellness   involves building positive relationships and interacting in a meaningful way with those around you

Important Terms

alternative medicine

cognitive development

complementary medicine

professional distance

Introduction

In this lesson, you will learn about health maintenance and wellness through holistic health. You will learn to distinguish between physical, intellectual, emotional, and spiritual health. You will explore health issues and tools for achieving wellness. This includes the use of complementary and alternative medicine practices for wellness, disease prevention, and stress reduction.

9.4-1 Holistic Health

Health and wellness are more than just not being sick. While preventing illness is important, **holistic health** focuses on wellness as a balance between the body, mind, spirit, and emotions (**Figure 9.28**). The human body works as a system, trying to maintain this balance. Signs and symptoms of illness are the body's way of showing something is out of balance that needs to be adjusted.

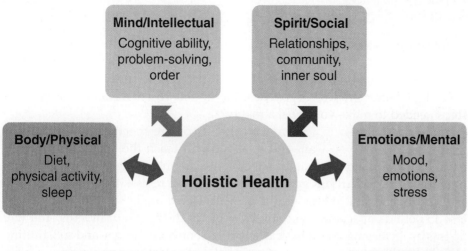

Goodheart-Willcox Publisher

Figure 9.28 Holistic health promotes a balanced relationship between the mind, body, spirit, and emotions.

When you have a headache, you look for the source of the problem. Is it hunger, tiredness, or stress? Treating the problem, by eating, sleeping, or relaxing, is better for wellness than taking a pain reliever to make the symptoms go away. You need to bring the body back in balance to maintain wellness. When there is too much emphasis on one area of wellness, the other areas become unbalanced, and good health suffers. Have you ever stayed up late to study for a test? You focused on learning, which is part of intellectual wellness, but neglected sleep, which is part of physical wellness. All aspects of wellness are important to your overall health.

9.4-2 Intellectual Wellness

Intellectual wellness refers to cognitive or mental abilities that affect how the brain functions. This includes critical thinking, problem solving, curiosity, creativity, and the desire to learn new things. Intellectual wellness does not necessarily mean earning good grades in school. It involves applying learning for the health and welfare of yourself and others. **Cognitive development** is the process of gaining thinking, reasoning, and learning abilities. This begins in infancy, using the senses and motor abilities to understand the world. Toddlers begin to understand symbols, use language, and develop memory and imagination. Elementary-age children use logic and problem-solving skills. Adolescents can understand abstract concepts and think about their process of thought. Formal thought operations are not fully developed until early adulthood.

Intellectual ability and memory are a combination of heredity and environment. Common issues that affect cognitive development include learning disorders, developmental delays, or a lack of exposure to new experiences. It is possible to make up for early delays by providing a supportive and stimulating environment.

You can support your intellectual wellness by keeping your mind active and seeking out learning opportunities. Explore subjects that interest you. Stimulate your brain with games, puzzles, and interaction with people different from yourself. Expose yourself to new ways of thinking and question the world around you. Create an organized environment for your mind that supports its functions. Clear your mind with meditation. Avoid distractions that pull you away from your goals. Engage in solving problems that challenge your brain. What do you do to keep your mind active?

Setting Goals

Setting goals and working toward them provides a sense of satisfaction that helps you maintain your motivation. It is not enough to just set a goal; you must also take action to achieve it. Have you heard yourself say, "I just know I could get better grades" or "eat healthier"? Did you make a plan or take the steps needed to make your goal a reality?

You are most likely to achieve your goal if you are specific about it. *SMART goals* explain what you want and how you will reach the goal. This acronym reminds you to set goals that are specific, measurable, achievable, relevant, and time bound. A SMARTER goal also evaluates and revises the plan as the goal evolves. If you want to lose weight, a SMART goal might say that you want to lose 15 pounds by losing 1 pound per week for the next four months. You will do this by increasing your physical activity to one hour per day and substituting more vegetables and water for your current diet of fast food and soda.

You can break big goals down into smaller, more manageable pieces (**Figure 9.29**). It is easy to say you want to be a doctor, but a long list of goals and accomplishments actually makes you an MD. First, list steps for reaching the long-term goal. These will be completed over the next few months or years.

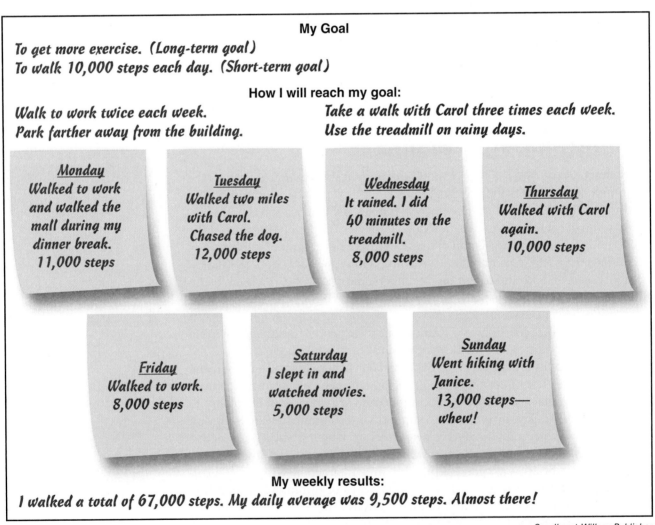

My Goal

To get more exercise. (Long-term goal)
To walk 10,000 steps each day. (Short-term goal)

How I will reach my goal:

Walk to work twice each week.
Park farther away from the building.

Take a walk with Carol three times each week.
Use the treadmill on rainy days.

Monday
Walked to work and walked the mall during my dinner break.
11,000 steps

Tuesday
Walked two miles with Carol.
Chased the dog.
12,000 steps

Wednesday
It rained. I did 40 minutes on the treadmill.
8,000 steps

Thursday
Walked with Carol again.
10,000 steps

Friday
Walked to work.
8,000 steps

Saturday
I slept in and watched movies.
5,000 steps

Sunday
Went hiking with Janice.
13,000 steps— whew!

My weekly results:
I walked a total of 67,000 steps. My daily average was 9,500 steps. Almost there!

Goodheart-Willcox Publisher

Figure 9.29 Sue is working on health maintenance. Notice that her goal is specific, measurable, achievable, relevant, and time bound. She is tracking her progress each day as she works to achieve this goal.

Then break the first long-term step into short-term steps to complete in the next few days or weeks. Continue in this pattern until you accomplish your goal.

As you work toward achieving a goal, keep track of your progress in a visible way. Cross steps off a list or post signs where you can see them to keep your goal in mind. Celebrate each milestone on the way to reaching your goal.

Be realistic about your goals. Is the goal of interest to you, or are you setting it based on someone else's expectations? Are you willing to spend your time, energy, and money to achieve your goal? Does your goal match your personal priorities? You cannot reach a goal if you are not motivated enough to stick with it.

Managing Your Time

Effective time management contributes to mental wellness by helping people reach their goals and reduce stress. No one gets more than 24 hours in a day, but an organized person can accomplish more in four hours than a disorganized person completes in a whole day.

Effective time management begins with priorities. Make a list of tasks and obligations. List your most important items first. Can you remove any items that are not important enough to demand your time? Effective time managers know how to say *no* when a request does not match their personal priorities.

Organize Your Tasks

Organize your work into long-term and short-term tasks in much the same way you set your personal goals. You should break a long-term task, such as writing a term paper, down into smaller steps so you can complete sections of the project over several days. Start with your due date and work backward to schedule the smaller steps. Make your to-do list for the day, and you are ready to begin working.

Schedule Your Time

Schedule a time to work each day. Pick the time when you are most alert and energetic and begin with your most difficult tasks first. Avoid interruptions at all costs. Checking messages, replying to texts, and posting or checking status updates all interfere with your focus and delay your work. Once you have completed the difficult tasks, cross them off your list. You will feel a big sense of accomplishment, and finishing the remaining tasks will seem easier.

Consider this daily schedule developed by a first-year medical student:

- 6:00 to 6:30 a.m.: breakfast/shower
- 6:30 to 8:30 a.m.: study
- 8:30 to 10:30 a.m.: class
- 10:30 to 11:30 a.m.: study
- 11:30 a.m.to 12:30 p.m.: lunch
- 12:30 to 1:30 p.m.: class
- 1:30 to 2:30 p.m.: class
- 2:30 to 6:00 p.m.: study
- 6:00 to 11:00 p.m.: relax

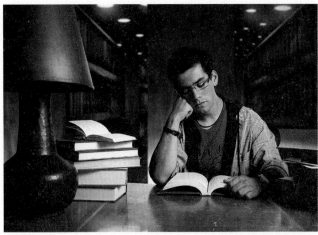

Fer Gregory/Shutterstock.com

Figure 9.30 A disciplined study schedule is important if you want to succeed in school. *What environment works best for you to focus on studying?*

Notice that this student finishes studying by 6:00 p.m. each evening and has several hours of free time. He is earning excellent grades. He is successful because he commits to getting up early every day and makes it a priority to dedicate time to studying (**Figure 9.30**). He goes to a remote corner of the library where he will not see anyone he knows. He studies for 50 minutes, takes a short walk to refresh his focus, then gets right back to work. While his schedule is not magical, this student's time-management skills are excellent. He has taken control of his time and is focused on his primary goal of graduating from medical school.

A practical system for organizing the tasks in your life will go a long way toward preventing procrastination. You may be putting off work because it seems overwhelming, but procrastination increases your stress.

Time-Management Tools

It takes trial and error to develop a time-management system, but it will greatly improve school and work performance. First, you will need a place to store the dates, tasks, appointments, and details of the projects that make up your life. This is a good opportunity to use technology. Capture this information in a device you carry with you each day, such as a smartphone or tablet. You will have all the information in one place, so you do not have to remember it. Have the calendar send you reminders to keep you on track.

While technology is helpful, some people prefer a low-tech option that focuses on the plan itself. A paper calendar or piece of notebook paper avoids the need to enter reminders into a device and is easy to modify. Post the schedule on your bulletin board or take a picture of it so it can travel with you.

Whichever system you choose, list your priorities for each day and note specific appointment times. Break larger projects into smaller steps, then work backward from the due date, as shown for the case study assignment in **Figure 9.31**. You will get satisfaction from crossing off completed items.

Weekly Plan						
Sun	**Mon**	**Tues**	**Wed**	**Thurs**	**Fri**	**Sat**
1—lunch at Scott's; bring salad 6—Study group for micro test	Work on med terms 8–1—field trip; meet in 2705 5–9—work	Ask teacher about case study questions Finish med terms homework	Med terms homework is due Ch. 14–16 3:15—haircut 5–9—work	Practice case study reading Study for micro test 6—HOSA fundraiser at Bariosos	Present case study Microbiology test Ch. 12	Get cash for the week Do laundry 12–6—work

Goodheart-Willcox Publisher

Figure 9.31 A weekly plan helps you balance the schedule of daily activities. *What days of the week are the busiest for you?*

Solving Problems

Organized workers take the routine problems and conflicts of life in stride. They use their prioritizing and time-management skills to handle decisions and problems automatically. Sometimes, however, you will encounter a problem that gets in the way of reaching your goals. When the right choice is not obvious, problem-solving skills can help you overcome this challenge (**Figure 9.32**). These skills help you make the best decision available for a given situation. You can use problem-solving skills throughout life to improve both personal and career decisions.

Individuals who maintain intellectual wellness use problem-solving skills to limit the impact of stressful situations. They are good planners and managers of their own lives. They begin by identifying personal priorities, then rank their responsibilities in order of importance. When there is conflict between responsibilities, they look at the long-term impact of each choice to make the best decision.

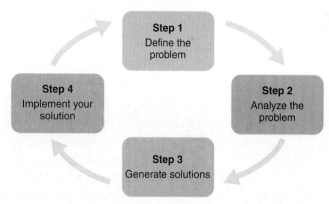

Goodheart-Willcox Publisher

Figure 9.32 Continue to cycle through the problem-solving steps until you find a workable solution.

9.4-3 Social Wellness

Social wellness is the ability to interact and form meaningful relationships with a support system of family and friends. Social skills develop over time and with practice. Young children spend most of their time with family. They learn to trust others and pick up social cues from those experiences. When they enter school, their social circle expands. They learn to cooperate and communicate with a wider variety of personalities and cultures. They develop empathy and appreciation of differences. As they join team sports, clubs, and jobs, they take on more complex social roles and leadership positions. They get better at interpreting nonverbal cues and expressing their emotions in appropriate ways. The process of social and emotional development benefits from good role models and open, honest communication.

Internal Skills for Managing Social Wellness

For social wellness, it is important to focus on things that are within your control. Internal skills for social wellness require self-awareness and self-control. You can control your inner motivations and emotions.

Inner Motivations

Your inner spirit is the part of social wellness that involves identifying and following your inner motivations. Sometimes called the *soul*, the inner spirit is the place your strongest beliefs live. This is where you look for answers to life's mysterious questions, such as *Why am I here?* or *What will happen to me when I die?* From these strong beliefs, you develop your values. Values tell you what is important and what is right in terms of moral and ethical behavior. You use values to prioritize, make important life decisions, and guide interactions with other people. When your decisions and behaviors are consistent with your values, you feel a sense of inner peace and spiritual wellness. Having strong inner motivations helps keep you on track.

Focusing on your inner spirit does not need to involve religion, but it is your connection to something greater than yourself. People use prayer, reflection, meditation, or specific spiritual practices to foster spiritual balance and maintain their connection to a higher power or belief system. Your religious faith, values, beliefs, ethical principles, and morals all define your spirituality.

Managing Emotions

Emotions affect your relationships with others. Identifying and naming your feelings and emotions can improve your social wellness. Naming your emotions allows you to talk about and decide what to do with them. Feelings come and go. It is in their nature to change, and they often do so quickly. When you pay attention to your body's signals, you can better identify your feelings and manage them. For example, a tight jaw, clenched teeth, and pounding heart may signal anger. Emotions can last longer than feelings. Think about the love of a parent for a child. A parent may feel frustrated by a child's actions but will continue to love and support the child's needs.

Emotions can also affect your physical wellness. Identify negative thinking and shift to a positive mind-set of what you can improve (**Figure 9.33**). Practice positive self-talk with a daily pep talk and do not say anything to yourself that you would not say to someone else you care about.

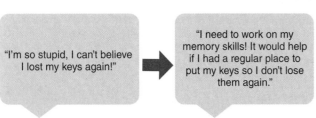

Goodheart-Willcox Publisher

Figure 9.33 Convert negative thinking into positive thinking and self-talk. *How can you change one of your negative thinking patterns?*

External Skills for Managing Social Health

Skills for managing social relationships include social awareness and interpersonal skills. Your connections with others can have a positive effect on your physical health. For example, social wellness appears to strengthen the immune system. People with strong social connections get fewer colds and fewer cavities. Strong social ties also reduce stress, help you cope with difficult life events, and are linked to longer life.

Build a Network

Building a network of social supports is especially protective during challenging times, such as illness or a death in the family. Use caution, however, with social media networks. They help connect people who are far away, but they are not a replacement for face-to-face relationships. On social media, people choose what pictures they post. It may appear that everyone else's life is picture-perfect and amazing, while your own falls short. Most people do not post their failures, but this does not mean they do not happen. People may also express themselves without thinking of others. Limit how long and often you are tuned in to social media. When it stresses you out, put it away and talk to someone face-to face or on the phone.

Connect with Community

Social wellness usually includes care and concern for one's community. It is healthy to belong to different groups and be involved in a diverse community. Both community service and service learning provide excellent opportunities to improve your community and develop new connections with others.

As a future healthcare worker, you can try out different types of work and different healthcare settings through volunteer opportunities.

Maintain Professional Distance

To maintain social wellness, healthcare workers must also develop the skill of maintaining **professional distance**. This means healthcare workers are caring toward their patients but do not try to become their friends. Ideally, healthcare workers get satisfaction from helping others become healthy, but they do not need the approval or friendship of the people they serve. You demonstrate an appropriate worker-patient relationship when you focus on the patient's health-related goals and not on how much the patient likes you.

 Healthcare Professions: Understanding Holistic Health

Marco was a social worker who could not figure out what was wrong. He had no energy and no ambition, but he did not know why he felt this way. His social life was fine. He had a solid group of friends in his biking club and often went home to spend time with his family. He was not experiencing problems at work and usually enjoyed his counseling groups

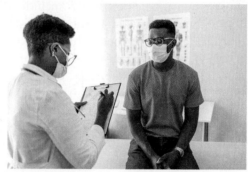

Ijubaphoto/E+ via Getty Images

and working with the students and families at his school. He was not feeling angry, frustrated, or sad, and was not facing any unusually stressful situations. What could be wrong?

Marco finally decided to see his doctor and learned he had a double ear infection. After a course of antibiotics, Marco was back to normal and enjoying life again.

Marco knew that his body, mind, spirit, and emotions all affect wellness. When he did not feel well, he checked his social and mental health for signs of imbalance. Unlike most people, he was so attuned to these areas that he missed his body's signs of physical illness.

Keeping your physical, intellectual, social, and mental health in balance maintains your energy and enthusiasm for life. It pays off as you work toward accomplishing your goals, and it provides a sense of satisfaction when you achieve them.

9.4-4 Complementary and Alternative Medicine (CAM)

The use of **complementary and alternative medicine (CAM)** has been increasing in the United States. This includes a diverse group of practices and products that are not yet considered part of conventional Western medicine.

Complementary medicine practices are used along with mainstream medicine to promote wellness, prevent disease, manage disease symptoms, and reduce stress. Patients using CAM report an increased sense of control over their health and improved emotional well-being. Taking an active role in your own healthcare can have other positive effects. Patients involved in their care are more likely to ask questions that keep them healthy. All CAM practices should be openly discussed in a healthy doctor-patient relationship.

There are many ways of grouping CAM practices. The National Center for Complementary and Integrative Health (NCCIH) groups these practices into five categories: alternative medical systems, mind-body interventions, biologically based treatments, manipulative and body-based methods, and energy therapies.

Alternative Medical Systems

Alternative medicine refers to entire systems of theory and healthcare practices that have developed independent of Western medicine. These include manipulative medicine, acupuncture, Ayurveda, traditional Eastern or Chinese medicine, holistic medicine, homeopathic medicine, and naturopathy. Although these are called "alternative," some are accepted practices with proven benefits. Osteopathic doctors use a holistic approach in their medical care, balancing treatment of the body, mind, spirit, and emotions instead of just treating a disease. Acupuncture can relieve nausea and pain from cancer treatments that are difficult to control with Western medications (**Figure 9.34**). Others, such as homeopathy, are not supported by scientific research. Always discuss new healthcare practices with your doctor before starting treatment.

Juri Pozzi/Shutterstock.com

Figure 9.34 Acupuncture is a type of alternative medicine that involves inserting needles into the skin or body tissues.

Mind-Body Interventions

Mind-body interventions, such as meditation, prayer, and yoga, are based on the mind and do not require other products or devices. Medical imaging has studied prayer and meditation techniques and showed they do stimulate parts of the brain responsible for mental focus, higher thinking, and reasoning. These techniques can relieve stress, increase body awareness, and slow breathing and heart rate.

Biologically Based Treatments

Biologically based treatments include natural products, such as herbs, oils, dietary supplements, and biologics, as well as specialized diets. There are a wide variety of alternative diets. Many, such as the Mediterranean and Ornish diets, promote low-fat, high-fiber, plant-based diets proven to be generally healthy. Others, such as the Atkins diet, follow different theories for weight management that have not yet been proven through long-term, large-scale studies.

Some herbs, vitamins, and mineral supplements are scientifically proven to be effective, but others are not. Be wary of any claims that sound too good to be true. Herbal supplements and other alternative treatments are less regulated than medications and are not held to the rigorous FDA testing and quality-control standards (**Figure 9.35**).

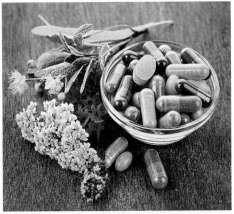

Elena Elisseeva/Shutterstock.com

Figure 9.35 A lack of regulation for herbal supplements and alternative treatments means patients need to communicate with healthcare providers about their use and what is safe or effective.

Keep in mind that the label "natural" does not automatically mean a product or treatment is safe. Diets and herbal supplements can affect a person's body and other medications. It is important that patients discuss all alternative treatments and practices with their care provider.

Manipulative and Body-Based Methods

Manipulative and body-based methods involve movement of the body. Massage therapy and chiropractic adjustments of the spine are common and accepted methods for managing muscle aches and pinched nerves. Many insurance companies provide coverage for massage therapy and chiropractic manipulations to treat certain conditions. Wellness rebates may cover the cost of tai chi, Pilates, or yoga. Many patients report a sense of wellness and a better mind-body connection using these alternative therapies.

Energy Therapies

Energy healing involves the manipulation of invisible energy fields of the body. Reiki, qi gong, and therapeutic touch are the most well-known. The focus is opening blocked channels of energy and returning balance to bioelectrical fields within the body. These treatments are intended to prevent disease from taking hold in the physical body. The existence of energy fields and their manipulation need more scientific study, but these treatments do not cause harm as long as they do not delay other needed treatment.

CAM Regulation

Many CAM practices fall outside the system for medical regulation. The National Certification Commission for Acupuncture and Oriental Medicine provides credentialing and licensing standards for some CAM professions in some, but not all, states. Some states regulate chiropractors, osteopaths, and massage therapists. Without a licensing or credentialing system, patients often find it difficult to judge which providers are qualified. Patients also need information to judge which practices are safe or effective. Research funded by the National Center for Complementary and Integrative Health (NCCIH) aims to increase the amount of reliable information in this area.

Lesson 9.4 Review

 Complete the *Map Your Reading* graphic organizer for the section you just read.

1. Holistic health is a balance between wellness of the body, mind, spirit, and which other aspect? (9.4-1)
   A. Emotions
   B. Intellect
   C. Morals
   D. None of these

2. SMART goals should have which of these characteristics? Choose all that apply. (9.4-2)
   A. Specific
   B. Measurable
   C. Accurate
   D. Relevant
   E. Team-oriented

3. Social wellness is the ability to interact and form meaningful (9.4-3)
   A. boundaries
   B. communication
   C. networks
   D. relationships

4. Although they can reduce stress and support health, it is important to discuss _____ practices such as herbal medicine and homeopathy with your doctor. (9.4-4)
   A. complementary and alternative medicine (CAM)
   B. holistic
   C. biologically based treatment
   D. mind-body intervention

Chapter 9 Review and Assessment

Chapter Summary

9.1-1 Physical health and wellness include the development and functioning of your body. Understanding normal stages of growth and development helps you know what to expect and anticipate needs. An infant's physical development progresses from the head down and from the midline outward. Large-motor skills develop before fine-motor skills. Physical wellness means listening to your body's need for proper nutrition, daily physical activity, and sleep, as well as keeping yourself safe.

9.1-2 The body needs macronutrients (carbohydrates, proteins, and fats) in larger quantities and micronutrients (vitamins and minerals) in smaller amounts. Healthy choices include complex carbohydrates, unsaturated fats, and essential amino acids.

9.1-3 Physical activity has many benefits, including managing weight, reducing anxiety, and decreasing depression.

9.1-4 Maintaining a healthy weight reduces your risk for some chronic diseases. Managing weight involves balancing energy taken in through food with energy exerted during physical activity.

9.1-5 Sleep is an essential activity that allows the body to reset. A sleep deficit has negative effects on health.

9.1-6 Stress management is important for all people, but especially healthcare workers. Positive ways to manage stress include physical activity and meditation.

9.1-7 Healthy relationships improve a person's health. Skills for healthy relationships include good communication and clear boundaries.

9.2-1 Public health uses health assessment, education, and policy-making strategies to protect health and prevent disease. They promote good hygiene, oral health, and preventive care. Preventive care is expected of healthcare workers so they will be healthy and able to work with people who are ill.

9.2-1 It is a patient's responsibility to see their doctor and dentist regularly and keep their vaccinations up to date to maintain good health. Recommended annual diagnostic tests, which may include blood tests and cancer screenings, depend on your age group and health status.

9.2-2 Public health works proactively to improve population health by reducing health disparities. Community health education outreach programs bring health education and services into the community for those who do not regularly visit a healthcare provider. Food insecurity is being addressed by building alternative food systems.

9.3-1 Needs influence behavior. Mental health and behavior patterns established during adolescence and adverse childhood experiences influence the risk for behavioral health issues. Being trauma-informed helps care providers recognize symptoms and provide support.

9.3-2 Mental health is marked by resilience and the ability to function well. Poor mental health is associated with stressful conditions, instability, and the inability to function in daily life.

9.3-3 People may use risky behaviors, such as binge drinking, vaping, and misusing opioids, to escape from stress or depression. These risks are increased for teens.

9.3-4 Suicide is the second leading cause of death for teens and young adults. Recognizing warning signs can help prevent suicide.

9.3-5 Seeking treatment and support can help people with mental health conditions. Mental health conditions are real illnesses and need treatment like any other health condition.

9.3-6 Understanding the stages of grief can help people process grief and help others who have experienced a loss.

9.4-1 Holistic health focuses on wellness as a balance between the body, mind, spirit, and emotions.

9.4-2 You can support intellectual wellness and cognitive function by creating an organized environment, setting and working toward goals, managing your time, and engaging in problem solving.

9.4-3 Self-awareness, self-control, social awareness, and interpersonal skills support social wellness. People use values to help prioritize, make important life decisions, and guide interactions with others. Strong social connections lead to longer, happier, and healthier lives. Healthcare workers must learn to establish professional distance in their work relationships.

9.4-4 Complementary and alternative medicine (CAM) can reduce stress, increase wellness, and support Western medicine practices. It is important to discuss CAM practices with your healthcare provider.

Maximize Your Professional Vocabulary

1. **Poster.** Choose a term from this chapter to study. Create a poster for the term that includes its definition, a synonym, an antonym, another term with the same root, a sentence using the term, and a picture that helps you understand the term. If there is not a true antonym for the term, substitute a term that might be confused with the term you chose.

Reflect on Your Reading

1. Revisit the answers you gave for the *Connect with Your Reading* activity. What new ideas have you gained about wellness and illness? How would you define the concept of *health maintenance*?

Review and Recall

1. In what order does physical development progress? Choose all that apply. (9.1-1)
   A. From head to toe
   B. From front to back
   C. From fine-motor to large-motor skills
   D. From the center of the body outward

2. Which substances are used for energy, structure building, and chemical reactions taking place in the body? (9.1-2)
   A. Nutrients
   B. Calories
   C. Malnutrition
   D. Processed foods

3. Regular _____ helps you manage weight, reduce anxiety, and decrease depression. (9.1-3)
   A. meditation
   B. physical activity
   C. sleep deficit
   D. circadian rhythm

4. Excess _____ can put extra strain on your joints and increase the risk of joint pain and arthritis as you grow older. (9.1-4)
   A. sleep
   B. stress
   C. weight
   D. physical activity

5. A person who gets six to seven hours of sleep on average has (9.1-5)
   A. healthy sleep habits
   B. less stress
   C. increased energy
   D. a sleep deficit

6. Physical activity, laughter, meditation, spending time on a hobby, and spending time with family and friends are all good methods for managing (9.1-6)
   A. weight
   B. relationships
   C. stress
   D. sleep

7. Communication and _____ are important to maintaining healthy relationships because they allow you to speak openly and be respected. (9.1-7)
   A. laughter
   B. cortisol
   C. emotions
   D. boundaries

8. Public health encourages people to go to the doctor and dentist for regular exams and follow the _____ schedule as part of preventive care. (9.2-1)
   A. X-ray
   B. dental
   C. immunization
   D. health

9. _____ serve(s) populations that are less likely to use preventive health services. (9.2-2)
   A. Doctor's offices
   B. Community health education outreach programs
   C. Complementary and alternative medicine
   D. Western medicine

10. Which aspect of health describes how your behaviors and responses to different situations impact the health of your mind, body, and spirit? (9.3-1)
    A. Behavioral
    B. Physical
    C. Emotional
    D. Spiritual

11. Which of these is the ability to function well and respond with resilience to life's challenges? (9.3-2)
    A. Healthy behaviors
    B. Mental health
    C. Mental health conditions
    D. Mindfulness

12. Patterns of thinking and behaviors that reduce anxiety in the short term, but do not help in the long term, are called _____ behaviors. (9.3-3)
    A. mindfulness
    B. unhealthy
    C. disordered
    D. maladaptive

13. If left untreated, mental health conditions, such as depression, and substance use disorders can increase risk for (9.3-4)
    A. anxiety
    B. positive behaviors
    C. suicide
    D. mental health

14. Which of these is a type of talk therapy? (9.3-5)
    A. Electroconvulsive therapy
    B. Psychotherapy
    C. Meditation
    D. Relaxation techniques

15. As a healthcare worker or friend, recognizing the stages of _____ will help you understand people's needs. (9.3-6)
    A. anger
    B. mental health conditions
    C. anxiety
    D. grief

16. Which of these focuses on wellness as a balance between the body, mind, spirit, and emotions? (9.4-1)
    A. Holistic health
    B. Spiritual wellness
    C. Emotional wellness
    D. Social wellness

17. _____ goals are specific, measurable, achievable, relevant, and time bound. (9.4-2)
    A. REAL
    B. ACCURATE
    C. SMART
    D. ALL

18. Which of the following are skills for managing social wellness? Choose all that apply. (9.4-3)
    A. Time management
    B. Building a network
    C. Professional distance
    D. Connecting with the community

19. _____ practices are used along with mainstream medicine to promote wellness, prevent disease, manage disease symptoms, and reduce stress. (9.4-4)
    A. Holistic medicine
    B. Alternative medicine
    C. Western medicine
    D. Complementary medicine

Build Core Skills

1. **Reading.** Research and review reading strategies for learning content. Then select an article related to one of the topics in the *Physical Health and Wellness* section. Use the strategies you learned to read and comprehend the article you found. Evaluate the source of the reading and the purpose for writing it. Skim through the headings to understand the topic and its organization. Turn the headings into questions, then take notes that include your questions and their answers. Write the notes in your own words, including any new terms you circled or underlined. Review the notes you have made and underline the key points to separate them from details.

2. **Problem Solving.** Investigate what options are available in your area for supporting preventive healthcare. What programs are available through healthcare facilities? your school? community health education outreach programs? others?

3. **Math.** Find the Nutrition Facts label for your favorite snack. How many servings would it take to get 100 percent of your Daily Value for calcium? iron? vitamin A? vitamin C? For each of these calculations, how many calories would you be taking in?

4. **Writing.** Write a three- to five-paragraph essay about the benefits of holistic health. Include a SMART goal for physical, intellectual, emotional, or spiritual wellness.

5. **Speaking and Listening.** Practice using the BATHE technique with a classmate. Use the questions in Figure 9.21 to ask about their level of stress at school. Actively listen to their responses. You and your classmate can make up answers if you do not want to share.

6. **Critical Thinking.** Name your favorite cartoon character and analyze which stage of psychosocial development the character is in. Use one of their conflicts to support your answer. What behavioral health issues might this character be at risk of developing and why?

7. **Reading.** Visit the National Institutes of Health (NIH) website's physical wellness toolkit. Read their strategies for improving physical health. What is one new technique that might work for you?

8. **Problem Solving.** Jean was easily stressed by bad news at work. What physical, social, and spiritual wellness techniques could make her more resilient to stress? What negative outcomes might this avoid?

9. **Writing.** Keep a food diary for one week. Compare your intake to the *Dietary Guidelines for Americans*. What is one guideline you need to work on? Write a paragraph summarizing your findings and plan for improvement.

10. **Math.** Choose a physical activity in Figure 9.10. How many hours would you need to do this activity to burn off 1 pound of body fat?

11. **Speaking and Listening.** Think about negative self-talk you have had recently. Change this to a positive affirmation that focuses on your strengths. Repeat this to yourself aloud 10 times in the morning, 10 times in the evening, and any time you are in a stressful situation. After one week, do you notice any change in your mental or spiritual wellness?

12. **Critical Thinking.** What are three complementary and alternative medicine practices that could help with back pain? Which of these would you be most likely to try, and why?

Activate Your Learning

1. Examine the weekly plan in Figure 9.31. Imagine your English teacher just assigned a one-page paper on Monday, and it is due Friday. How will you break this into smaller tasks? Where in this schedule will you fit the required tasks to complete it?

2. Participate in HOSA's *Healthy Lifestyle* leadership event. Download the event guidelines from the HOSA website. You will set a specific goal and document your efforts to practice a healthier lifestyle through physical activity, nutrition, or avoiding risky behaviors.

Think and Act Like a Healthcare Worker

1. Imagine you are a pediatrician. Your teenage patient has lost some weight and complains of difficulty sleeping. Lab tests are negative for physical illnesses. What questions would you ask regarding healthy behaviors?

Go to the Source

1. Go to the MyPlate website to generate a daily meal plan. Insert your personal data (age, sex, weight, height, and physical activity level) to find your recommended caloric intake, then read the suggestions for your daily meal plan. Consider the value of this website for a preschooler, parent, or teenager. If you were a dietitian or nutrition counselor, how could you use this website to help your clients? Report back to the class with your observations and insights.

2. Review Figure 9.22. Then visit the National Institute of Mental Health website and the Mayo Clinic website. Use the information there to answer the following questions.

   A. What are additional facts about depression not covered in the text?

   B. Select one form of depression. What are signs and symptoms of this form? What are some potential causes? Who is most at risk? How is it diagnosed? What treatments are recommended?

   C. How could you best support someone experiencing depression?

HOSA Event Prep: Healthy Lifestyle

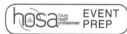

Jessica, a nurse who works in a busy cardiologist office, wants to improve her heart health. Jessica knows she is most likely to follow through on her lifestyle changes if she has someone else joining in with her. Since February is *Go Red for Women*, a campaign for women's heart health, her office has activities planned all month. On the first Friday, she is asking the whole office to wear red. She has also set up blood pressure checks every Friday. For Valentine's Day, she has planned exercise classes for couples and heart-healthy date night ideas. She plans on attending a seminar at the end of the month on healthy heart habits that last a lifetime. She documents her progress as she participates in these heart healthy activities and evaluates which activities she will continue and any additional changes she can make.

Think About It

1. Explain how Jessica's plans support heart health.

2. What is the value of documenting your progress toward a health goal?

3. What is another health goal you could advocate for yourself or your patients, and how would you go about it?

Chapter 10 Preparing for Healthcare Employment

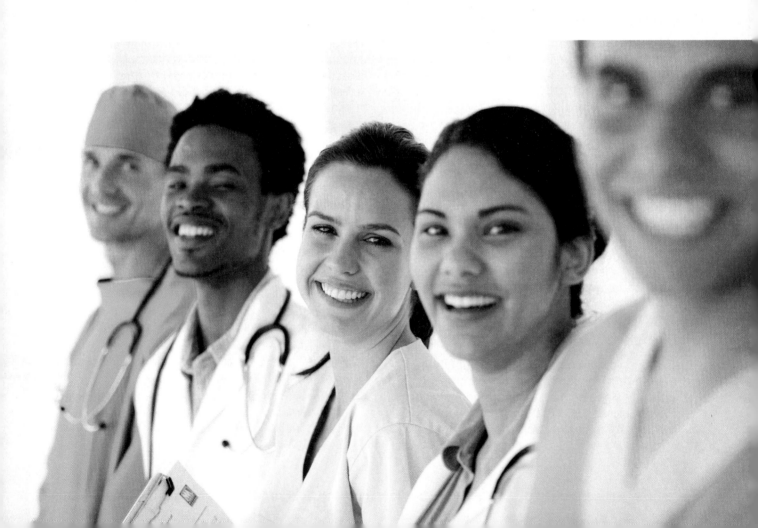

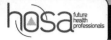

Being confident and successfully expressing why your skills make you the best candidate is often what lands the job. For many, the hardest part is expressing pride in oneself or one's accomplishments and skills, especially during the first time interviewing for a job in healthcare. You may not feel like you have the skills needed to make you the best candidate right out of training. However, knowing how to showcase the knowledge you have and your potential could spark the interest of the one who may be hiring you. HOSA's event *Job Seeking Skills* helps provide early practice on résumé building, personal statements, making a digital portfolio, and interviewing in the healthcare field.

Go to the HOSA website to learn more about the HOSA *Job Seeking Skills* event. Find out the purpose of the event, what is involved in the event, and what knowledge is demonstrated in the event.

As you prepare for HOSA competitive events, be sure to check the website and talk with your HOSA advisor for the most up-to-date guidelines and procedures. Once you have learned about the *Job Seeking Skills* event, answer the following questions:

1. How might participating in this event benefit you personally and your future career? Explain.
2. Are you interested in participating in this event? Why or why not?

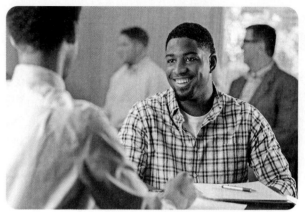

SDI Productions/E+ via Getty Images

 Connect with Your Reading

Knowledge. Skills. Attitude. All three are important to job success. Which one do you think most often causes young workers to lose their jobs? Pick one and create a scenario to support your choice.

 Map Your Reading

Create a mind map for the content in this chapter. Write the name of the chapter in the middle circle and connect a circle for each of the three lessons. Create additional spokes to add main ideas and important details as you read each lesson.

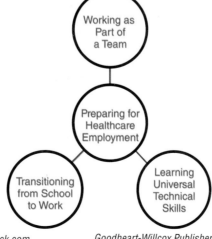

Goodheart-Willcox Publisher

Chapter opener image: ESB Professional/Shutterstock.com

Working as Part of a Team

Learning Outcomes

After studying this lesson, you will be able to

10.1-1 enumerate characteristics of effective teams.

10.1-2 describe types of teams used in healthcare facilities.

10.1-3 illustrate the guidelines team members follow for delegating tasks, sharing information, and building positive relationships.

10.1-4 summarize sources of team conflict and steps for resolving conflict.

10.1-5 identify qualities of an effective leader.

Professional Vocabulary

Essential Terms

collaborate   to work together; to consult with each other

delegate   to direct another healthcare worker to perform a care task that is within that worker's training and experience and within the scope of practice of the licensed provider giving the direction

interdisciplinary healthcare team   a group of professionals from different health science training backgrounds working in coordination toward a common goal for the patient

multidisciplinary healthcare team   a group of healthcare workers from different healthcare specialties, each providing specific services to the patient

personal leadership style   an individual approach to giving directions, implementing plans, and motivating people

Important Terms

case manager	primary care teams	team nursing
delegation	primary nursing	teleconferencing
functional nursing	secondary care teams	work styles

Introduction

Healthcare workers know that they must have top-notch job skills and perform their duties accurately. They may not realize that they also need to be highly skilled at working in a team. The healthcare industry is increasingly using teams of workers to improve healthcare delivery.

Teams deliver patient care in all kinds of healthcare settings. Healthcare professionals can improve patient safety and quality of care for a larger number of patients when they work in teams. Teams also reduce the cost of patient care by employing workers with different levels of training. For example, a nursing team that includes a registered nurse, licensed practical nurse, and certified nursing assistant can care for more patients than a single registered nurse. Using the combined skills of many health professionals reduces medical costs for patients and helps bring healthcare to underserved areas.

As a healthcare worker, you need to know your roles and responsibilities within a team and understand how to be an effective team member. In this lesson, you will learn about types of teams used in healthcare, how to resolve team conflict, and team leadership styles.

10.1-1 Effective Teams

Myesha, a medical coder, is part of an **interdisciplinary** (ihn-ter-DIH-suh-plih-nair-ee) **healthcare team** in her medical clinic. The team members include doctors, nurses, therapists, medical assistants, insurance representatives, and even the housekeepers she works with in the office. Each member of the team has different skills and knowledge and contributes to the patient's care in a different way (**Figure 10.1**). Myesha knows she must code patient procedures in a reasonable amount of time so the clinic will receive payment for its services. She knows who is responsible for each part of patient care and whom to ask if the medical records lack the information needed.

As part of a diverse interdisciplinary team, Kia—the medical assistant—organizes appointments so patients do not wait for long periods of time and the doctor does not have to wait for the next patient to arrive. When there is an emergency or delay, Kia adjusts the schedule and continues to meet the needs of patients. Calming a frustrated patient can be a challenge. As the first person who answers the phone, Kia must quickly assess the level of each caller's need. If every call went directly to the doctor, the doctor would spend the day talking on the phone instead of assessing and treating patients. Sometimes Kia calls 911 if there is an emergency, but often she can have a nurse return the patient's call. Despite many interruptions to her work, Kia is careful to keep accurate and complete patient records so the billing process goes smoothly.

Adam also works at the medical clinic as an education specialist. All the people on Adam's team are from the same discipline. They are all educators. The team members have similar responsibilities that include developing educational workshops. They schedule students and teachers to attend the workshops and organize equipment and supplies for teaching. When the team members meet, they coordinate teaching schedules and evaluate the outcomes of their teaching methods to make improvements. They all benefit from working together.

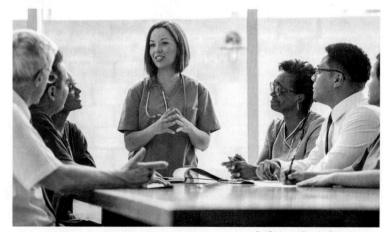

FatCamera/E+ via Getty Images

Figure 10.1   Each member of an interdisciplinary healthcare team has specific roles and responsibilities. *How does teamwork improve patient care?*

Knowing your own roles and responsibilities is the first step in becoming an effective team member. You must also know the roles and responsibilities of the other members of your team. The responsibilities of each team member are part of scope of practice, which includes certain tasks the team member is qualified to perform. For example, when Kia directs a phone call to the nurse, she communicates a patient's need that she is not qualified to meet. By knowing each team member's scope of practice, she can choose the correct person to help the patient.

Directing information to the correct person is a teamwork-related skill. Skilled team members monitor the activities of other members. They know their strengths and weaknesses and organize tasks with each person's strengths in mind. For example, Kia knows the doctor on her team is excellent at assessing and diagnosing a patient but has a hard time remembering names. She always prompts the doctor's memory by introducing a patient at the beginning of an exam.

Members of effective teams remain positive despite personal differences. A positive attitude is critical to the success of a team. In addition to knowing the strengths and weaknesses of other members, everyone on the team must know how to fit their different personalities together to create a comfortable work environment. Understanding and respecting the feelings and beliefs of each team member is just as important as performing the duties of your job correctly.

 ## Healthcare Professions: Working in a Team

When Adam designs a workshop for students, he naturally thinks of creative activities students will enjoy. Another team member considers the information that must be presented for students to learn a scientific concept. A third team member creates a schedule and determines what lab supplies to order. By using the personal strengths of each team member, the team can work efficiently. Team members rely on each other to complete different tasks when preparing for the workshop. They are happy to focus on the tasks they enjoy most. A positive attitude toward teamwork and mutual trust among team members make this team successful.

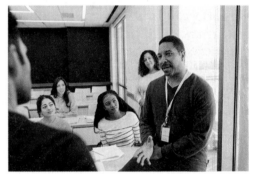

SDI Productions/E+ via Getty Images

10.1-2 Types of Healthcare Teams

Many physician specialties have developed during the past 50 years. As a result, many different doctors can work with a single patient. A patient might see a podiatrist, dermatologist, cardiologist, obstetrician, and so on. Each specialist could have a different office. In the past, each office maintained its own set of records and did not share patient records with other offices. Unless the patient talked about other doctors, many physicians were unaware a patient was receiving any other treatment. The patient was being treated by a **multidisciplinary healthcare team**, but care was not coordinated, especially because patient records were not shared.

If a general practice physician referred a patient to a specialist, the physician would receive a consult report but could not access complete patient records.

In healthcare today, the interdisciplinary healthcare team approach is becoming more common. Interdisciplinary teams coordinate patient care. They improve patient outcomes by preventing conflicting treatments and avoiding duplication of services. This saves money. Communication between interdisciplinary team members improves when all providers can access patient records.

Interdisciplinary Teams

Interdisciplinary teams consist of different types of healthcare professionals just like multidisciplinary teams. However, interdisciplinary team members **collaborate** as they work together to provide a coordinated plan of treatment for the patient. Interdisciplinary teams are either *primary* or *secondary*. Primary care teams function in clinical and community settings, while secondary care teams provide hospital services.

Primary care teams include the primary care physician, physician assistants, and nurse practitioners who see the patient in the clinic setting. Depending on patient needs, the team may also include nutritionists, pharmacists, social workers, or others. The team decides which additional healthcare practitioners are needed to promote patient health and wellness. For example, a community-based health team may add dentists, health educators, or mental health professionals. A rehabilitation team would include physical, occupational, and speech therapists.

Secondary care teams deliver services to hospital patients. For example, surgical teams include surgeons, surgical technicians (**Figure 10.2**), nurse anesthetists, and operating room nurses. Cardiologists, dietitians, and exercise therapists make up cardiovascular teams. An infection control team might consist of infectious disease specialists, a pharmacologist, a social worker, and so on.

Collaboration is key in the interdisciplinary team model (**Figure 10.3**). Regardless of the healthcare team or setting involved, team members communicate regularly. Hospital-based teams go on rounds together or hold conferences to communicate about patients in their care. A team working in an outpatient office or clinic communicates frequently to keep team members up to date about which patients have been seen and which treatments they have received. Team members work together to plan and carry out patient treatments. The physician diagnoses and prescribes medications, the nurse practitioner educates the patient about the illness and treatment, and the social worker counsels the patient on community resources available.

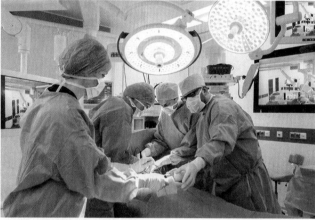

Gorodenkoff/Shutterstock.com

Figure 10.2 The surgical team is a secondary care team. *In addition to the surgeon, can you identify other members of this team?*

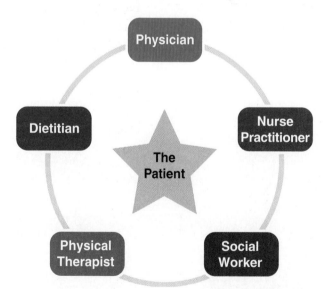

Goodheart-Willcox Publisher

Figure 10.3 Healthcare team members collaborate by communicating with each other and with the patient as they coordinate the plan of treatment for the patient. *Who is the most important member of this team?*

Teleconferencing allows healthcare professionals to interact and collaborate over long distances. As a result, healthcare team members can be spread over a wide geographic area. This is important when providing care to patients in rural areas. Telemedicine allows a primary physician to seek a specialist's opinion without sending the patient hundreds of miles to see that specialist. Similarly, an anesthesiologist (an-ehs-thee-zee-AH-luh-jihst) working at a major medical center in another city can use telemedicine to supervise a nurse anesthetist in a small community hospital.

Nursing Teams

Nurses function as members of the healthcare team. They also have their own teams to provide the round-the-clock care required in hospitals and long-term care facilities. The most basic nursing team includes the nurse (RN, LPN, or LVN) and the nursing assistant (CNA). The nurse carries out the doctor's orders, and the nursing assistant completes care tasks assigned by the nurse. The nurse has the authority to delegate tasks that are within the nursing assistant's scope of practice.

Nursing teams also include supervisors. The charge nurse supervises all the nurses for a specific shift. The head nurse oversees a department, and the director of nursing (DON) supervises all the nursing care within a facility.

Nurses provide care using a variety of nursing care models. Each healthcare facility determines which model its nurses will use. Home healthcare often uses a **case manager** model. The RN serving as the case manager develops a care plan along with the client and the client's family. The nursing assistant follows this plan when visiting the client, and the case manager supervises the care provided.

In a **primary nursing** model, one RN, LPN, or LVN cares for several patients or residents. This nurse is responsible for planning and carrying out all aspects of care while patients are in the care unit. Other nurses will follow this care plan when the primary nurse is not working, but the primary nurse has 24-hour responsibility for planning patient care. Patients report higher levels of satisfaction with this model.

A **functional nursing** model assigns tasks. Each nurse is responsible for completing a set of assigned tasks for every patient or resident. So, one nurse may administer medications, while another nurse delivers special treatments. The nursing assistant takes all vital signs and assists with meals. Patient care becomes fragmented with this system, and patients do not like this model as much.

An RN functions as the team leader in the **team nursing** model (**Figure 10.4**). Nursing staff members report to the team leader, and together the group divides nursing care tasks. Team members complete tasks based on their training and expertise, but the team leader is still accountable for all the care provided. Planning for patient care uses the input and expertise of all team members (RN, LPN, and CNA). In this model, the team leader needs clinical nursing skills and must also be an effective group leader. When a nursing team communicates effectively, patient needs are met quickly. Patients are very satisfied with this model, especially when nursing team members stay the same for each patient.

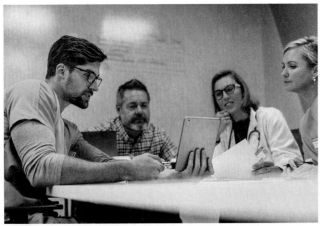

Jacob Lund/Shutterstock.com

Figure 10.4 In the team nursing model, tasks are divided up according to each member's training and expertise.

10.1-3 Healthcare Team Interaction

As healthcare team members work with each other, they follow a set of important guidelines for assigning tasks to each team member. This process is called **delegation**. Even the sharing of patient information follows a set of established guidelines or protocols. Following these guidelines ensures that patient care is safe and effective. It protects each patient's right to confidentiality.

Productive relationships among team members promote high-quality patient care. In addition, having a positive attitude at work makes your workday more pleasant and calm. Since people spend about one-third of their lives at work, learning how to build and maintain positive team relationships is worth the time and effort.

Delegating Tasks

Healthcare workers who supervise other workers may have the right to delegate some work tasks. To **delegate** means to make another person responsible for completing a specific task for you. For example, licensed nurses (RNs or LPNs) may delegate tasks to nursing assistants or medical assistants. Physicians may delegate tasks to physician assistants or nurse practitioners. State laws and facility policies guide the practice of delegation. Physicians and nurses have the authority to delegate tasks, but they are still responsible for the quality of patient care.

A worker's scope of practice always determines which tasks are delegated (**Figure 10.5**). If a nurse delegates a task a nursing assistant is not qualified to perform and fails to supervise the assistant, the nurse is liable if the patient is harmed. However, if a nurse delegates a task within the assistant's scope of practice, but the assistant does not complete the task correctly, then the assistant is liable for patient injury.

Delegation	
CAN Delegate	**CANNOT Delegate**
Tasks That Physicians CAN Delegate to Physician Assistants and Nurse Practitioners	**Tasks That Physicians CANNOT delegate to Physician Assistants or Nurse Practitioners**
Examining patients	Assuming responsibility for total care of the patient
Interpreting diagnostic test results	Supervising other physician assistants and nurse practitioners
Obtaining and recording patient medical data	Prescribing medication
Performing therapeutic procedures, such as injections and wound sutures	Performing tasks outside the physician's scope of practice
Instructing and counseling patients	
Tasks That Registered Nurses or Practical Nurses CAN Delegate to Nursing Assistants	**Tasks That Registered Nurses or Practical Nurses CANNOT Delegate to Nursing Assistants**
Assisting with activities of daily living	Administering medications
Measuring vital signs	Receiving verbal orders from doctors
Ambulating patients	Supervising other nursing assistants
Changing bed linens	Inserting or removing catheters
Repositioning patients	

Goodheart-Willcox Publisher

Figure 10.5 This table shows the types of tasks that physicians and registered nurses and practical nurses can and cannot delegate to others on their team. *Why do you think some of these tasks can be delegated while others cannot?*

Workers protect patients and themselves when they carefully consider work assignments. Healthcare workers never refuse a task because they do not want to do it. However, they may refuse a task for valid reasons, including the following:

- The task is illegal or unethical.
- The task is outside their scope of practice.
- They cannot perform the task safely because they lack clear directions, proper equipment, or adequate supervision.
- They have not been trained for the task.
- The task is not part of their job description at the facility where they are working.

Healthcare team members follow the organizational chain of command when reporting problems. They also follow a chain of command for accepting work assignments. They know when they can take directions from another worker and when they cannot. For example, a nursing assistant may not supervise or delegate tasks to another nursing assistant.

Sharing Information

A healthcare worker's scope of practice also guides the process of sharing information. For instance, a dental assistant does not diagnose patient conditions. When a patient asks if a tooth can be repaired, the dental assistant refers the question to the dentist (**Figure 10.6**). If a physician calls to give orders regarding patient care, an RN or LPN must take the phone call.

Healthcare workers are cautious about what patient information they share and with whom. They must protect the privacy of each patient's medical information according to the guidelines of the HIPAA Privacy Rule. As a general guideline, physicians will disclose an individual's information for three purposes: treatment, payment, and healthcare operations such as quality assessment or medical reviews.

Healthcare workers only share medical information that is important to a patient's care with other members of the healthcare team. For example, a physician will give orders for patient care following surgery but will not discuss any previous medical procedures unless they affect current care. A nurse caring for a patient who has had an appendectomy (removal of the appendix) does not need to know about the patient's history of depression unless the patient shows signs of depression that require nursing observation and care.

Healthcare workers must also follow guidelines for sharing medical information with a patient's friends and family members. If the patient does not object, a healthcare provider may share information with family, friends, or others involved in providing or paying for that person's care. However, they may only discuss the information the third party needs to know about the care. Healthcare providers have policies regarding this type of information sharing. These policies may require a patient's verbal or written permission to share information. If a patient objects to the sharing of his or her information, providers are not allowed to share it.

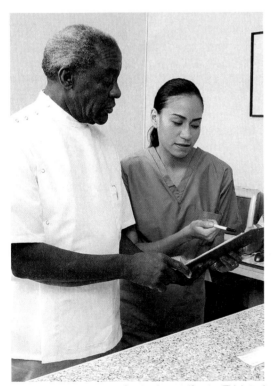

Creatas Images/Creatas/Thinkstock

Figure 10.6 Because of her scope of practice, this dental assistant must ask the dentist to answer diagnostic questions from patients.

Building Positive Team Relationships

Team members rely on each other as they work together to provide quality care. When team members do not work well together, workers' stress levels increase. This causes the quality of care to decrease. Successful healthcare teams make a constant effort to maintain positive working relationships.

Team members understand that each member is unique. Members will have different ages, sexes, socioeconomic statuses, lifestyle preferences, beliefs, education, and cultural backgrounds. These differences affect each person's attitudes and work preferences. Team members must be sensitive to and respectful of these differences to build positive relationships.

Productive and positive relationships result when team members are friendly and willing to assist each other (**Figure 10.7**). They keep their communication positive and encourage rather than criticize fellow team members. Finally, they work hard and perform job tasks to the best of their ability. Their actions show that they are reliable and can be trusted.

10.1-4 Team Conflict and Conflict Resolution

When a group of people works closely together, there will always be differences of opinion. This can create conflict within a team. Unresolved conflicts can cause problems for both employees and patients. Ineffective teamwork reduces the quality of healthcare.

Effective team members know the factors that lead to conflict and can handle disagreements without damaging their working relationships. They are committed to resolving conflict quickly so that quality of care is not compromised. Some people are naturally good at this type of cooperation and collaboration. Many people, however, learn conflict-resolution skills in the same way they learn medical skills—through training and experience.

Identifying Factors That Lead to Team Conflict

Team members are unique individuals with differing viewpoints and work habits (**Figure 10.8**). This is generally a good thing. Teams can accomplish more work with a variety of talents. A team needs practical workers and creative thinkers, detailed people and "big picture" people, reserved workers and outgoing workers. However, these differences can also lead to conflict.

Dos and Don'ts for Building Positive Relationships	
Do	**Don't**
Be sensitive to the feelings of all team members	Expect everyone to participate equally
Be willing to compromise	Demand that others compromise before you will
Be honest	Give up at the first sign of disagreement
Listen to all members	Assume that everyone thinks the way you do
Be patient	Assume that all of your expectations will be met

Goodheart-Willcox Publisher

Figure 10.7 Building positive relationships is important for everyone on the healthcare team. *Which of these practices do you already follow when building your own relationships?*

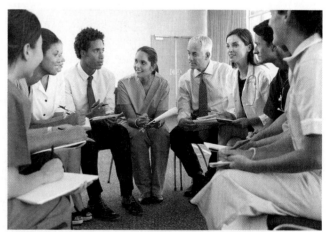

Monkey Business Images/Shutterstock.com

Figure 10.8 Team members are individuals, so they will bring unique opinions and work styles to a project. *Explain how this is a benefit to the team and why it might also cause problems.*

Team conflict is a disagreement or difficulty that occurs between two or more members of a team. As a result, the whole team works less effectively.

Many conflicts arise from differences in individual viewpoints and the ways people like to work. It is easy to think that other team members should "see things your way." However, there is more than one right way to accomplish most tasks, and you can learn a lot by observing other team members. They may get great results using a different method than what you use. The "my way is right" mind-set only causes more conflict.

Team members often try to analyze each other's behavior using their own personal viewpoint. For example, if you are naturally talkative, do you assume a quiet person is angry or upset? Another person's behavior does not necessarily mean what you think it does. Using your own viewpoint to interpret the behavior of others is often the root of misunderstandings between team members. Misunderstandings can lead to conflict.

When a team member wants to do something in a new or different way, try not to be judgmental. It is easy to label this person a troublemaker and begin to gossip or complain about the person's ideas. However, these "troublemakers" are actually good for the team. When they challenge the team, team members can reevaluate, consider, and maybe even learn a new and better way to accomplish a task.

Just as individuals have different learning styles, team members have different **work styles** (**Figure 10.9**). Once you identify the work preferences of fellow team members, you can take advantage of style differences when dividing work tasks. This allows all members to contribute and avoids misunderstandings. Ignoring work styles leads to ineffective teamwork and frustrated team members. Do you see your own preferences in the list of contrasting work styles in Figure 10.9?

Avoiding potential conflicts begins with each team member. Analyze your own behavior and avoid the patterns that lead to serious conflict with other members. Learn to recognize the work-style preferences of each team member and use them to provide positive results.

Resolving Team Conflict

People are imperfect communicators, so conflicts among team members do happen. Your first goal when managing conflict is to recognize and correct simple misunderstandings. Begin by checking your own motivation and attitude. Are you trying to prove you are right or make things right? Successful team members focus on fixing problems and achieving the common goals of the team.

Work Preferences

A team member may		A team member may
• complete one task before starting a new one	OR	• work on several projects at once
• work alone	OR	• work with others
• work with details	OR	• create ideas
• know exactly what to do	OR	• figure it out along the way
• receive lots of direction	OR	• work with little supervision
• prefer quiet and order	OR	• thrive on noise and activity

Goodheart-Willcox Publisher

Figure 10.9 People have different work preferences. *Which work preferences do you identify with?*

Look at how your team is functioning. When you see these behaviors, your team needs to focus on conflict resolution:

- gossip, blaming, and complaining
- hoarding of information that should be shared
- late work, poor quality work, and absenteeism

Resolving conflict begins with setting clear goals for the team. What is the team supposed to accomplish? What are each member's individual roles and responsibilities? How will the team share information, and how can members get help when needed? As you work to resolve a conflict, remember to listen to other points of view (**Figure 10.10**). You can certainly speak up and share your ideas and opinions, but always state your view positively. Blaming or ridiculing another team member only increases conflict.

If necessary, ask your team leader to help you focus on the facts of your situation. Your leader can mediate your dispute and work with you to negotiate a resolution.

Finally, be willing to accept the team's decision even if it is not your first choice. As you move forward, do not allow disagreements to become personal. Instead, focus on doing your part as a team member. Complete your work to the best of your ability. Ask for help when you need it and volunteer to help others as well. Practice using the key skills shown in **Figure 10.11** for managing and resolving conflict.

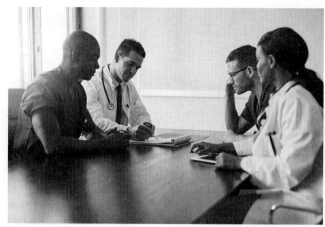

Ground Picture/Shutterstock.com

Figure 10.10 Successful teams resolve conflicts and move onto more important tasks. *What are some signs that your team needs to focus on conflict resolution?*

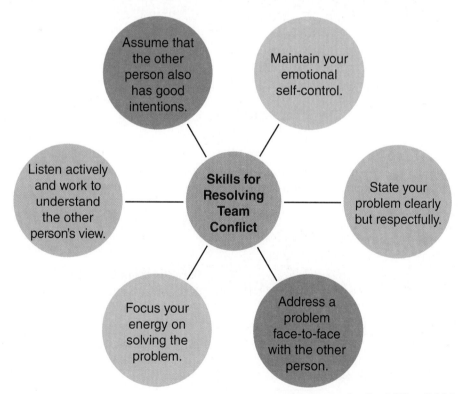

Goodheart-Willcox Publisher

Figure 10.11 The behaviors described here will help team members resolve conflicts and keep a positive working relationship in the process.

10.1-5 Team Leadership

All people assume leadership roles at various times in their personal and work lives. When you choose to lead, you usually will find a leadership task that fits your personality. These leadership opportunities feel comfortable, and you will feel confident about your skills.

For example, Sally works as a medical secretary at a local healthcare clinic. When she joins the local chamber of commerce as a representative of her company, she acts as the organization's secretary. She is comfortable taking notes and feels confident producing accurate minutes of each meeting.

Emily, on the other hand, dreaded being assigned the team leader role for a group project. Although Emily was a good leader in her classroom every day as she helped other students struggling with the course content, she believed she could never be a successful leader. Because of Emily's quiet nature, managing a team and organizing the work of her classmates felt uncomfortable. How could she be effective doing something she did not like?

Leadership Styles

Each individual has a **personal leadership style** that relies on unique preferences and attributes. Like the connection between personality and career choices, there is a connection between personality and leadership styles. Do any of the descriptions in **Figure 10.12** match your leadership preferences?

Characteristics of Leadership Styles		
John Holland Type	**Leadership Style**	**When to Use**
Realistic Doer Likes mechanical, hands-on activities	Role Model • Takes action • Sets an example by doing what is asked of others	When team members lack motivation and are not focused on accomplishing tasks
Investigative Thinker Is an analytical problem solver	Pioneer • Analyzes and compares other situations • Develops a long-term view of the future	When long-term change is needed
Social Helper Is cooperative and people-oriented	Facilitator • Encourages and mentors people • Builds personal relationships and cares for others	When there are sensitive situations or when support from others is necessary
Enterprising Persuader Is a competitive leader	Innovator • Tries new things and likes change • Creates new work-related opportunities	When the group is stuck in the same routines
Conventional Organizer Pays attention to detail	Monitor • Observes and organizes the work of different people • Sets clear goals and manages resources	When there is a lack of organization and expectations are unclear
Artistic Creator Exhibits creativity and originality	Motivator • Shows passion for key issues • Supports the current cause	When the group has lost its sense of identity

Goodheart-Willcox Publisher

Figure 10.12 There are six John Holland types of leaders, each with their own characteristics and leadership styles. *Which type of leader are you?*

Knowing your personal leadership style helps you assess how effective you will be at accomplishing a leadership task. Because different tasks require different styles, you may need to expand your leadership skills to accomplish your goals. In the same way you learn the technical skills and knowledge required for your job, you can also learn the skills required for various leadership roles.

Leadership Skills

Effective leadership uses many familiar skills (**Figure 10.13**). Developing leadership skills begins with developing all the skills that make you a good worker. When you take on or are assigned a leadership role, remember that a true leader unites people and works to achieve a positive result. Effective leaders do not focus on themselves. They do not try to prove they are better than others or make a show of being in charge. Instead, they model the behavior they want to see in team members. They encourage and help team members perform work tasks effectively.

From informal team working sessions to formal business gatherings, effective leaders frequently conduct meetings. These leaders usually set the agenda that lists the topics to be discussed and acted upon. In formal meetings, they may guide the meeting's progress using parliamentary procedure.

Based on Robert's Rules of Order, parliamentary procedure is a set of rules that maintains order and allows all members to participate in the meeting. Leaders know how to call a meeting to order, handle a variety of motions, and address a motion to adjourn or end the meeting. In a well-run meeting, people take turns speaking and discuss only one idea at a time.

Members present their ideas by making a motion. Everyone has an opportunity to discuss or debate each motion before voting to accept or reject it. Ideally both the leader and members of the group are familiar with several different kinds of motions. If everyone speaks clearly and uses parliamentary procedure correctly, the group is more likely to accomplish business in a productive, timely manner.

Effective leaders also accept the challenge of learning new leadership skills. They develop self-confidence and learn to make decisions in the face of disagreement. Team leaders make the best choice after considering all the information, but they understand some team members may not like the decision. Effective leaders know their personal leadership preferences, but they are willing to learn different styles of leadership that fit their current leadership task.

Leadership Skills	
Familiar Skills for Leaders	**How Leaders Put Those Skills to Use**
Effective leaders practice personal health maintenance.	They set realistic goals and manage their time to effectively achieve their goals.
Effective leaders are effective workers.	They have developed excellent technical skills for the job tasks they perform.
Effective leaders use an organized system for managing the tasks of everyday work and life.	They use problem-solving techniques to make decisions when conflicts and problems arise.
Effective leaders are team players.	They use a positive attitude and assertive communication skills to improve relationships with coworkers.

Goodheart-Willcox Publisher

Figure 10.13 Effective leaders practice and adapt their skills.

Healthcare Professions: Leadership Styles

Margo spent multiple hours planning her hospital department's budget. She analyzed previous purchases, reviewed equipment usage trends, and tried to anticipate future needs. Before committing to major purchases based on her plan, she sought the advice of her supervisor, Janelle. Janelle told her to move forward with major purchases without even looking at Margo's plan. Janelle wanted to discuss a change in the color of scrubs worn on each hospital unit. Margo was dumbfounded. She could not believe her boss was more interested in uniforms than a major spending initiative.

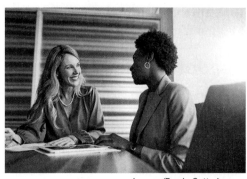

gradyreese/E+ via Getty Images

A few weeks later, Margo attended a leadership training workshop and learned about leadership styles. Now her supervisor's actions and her own reactions made more sense. Margo learned she has a pioneer style, which causes her to focus on future plans. Janelle has a role-model style of leadership. She prefers to focus on smaller activities that can be decided and completed now. Neither leadership style is right or wrong. However, effective leaders learn to change their preferred style to fit the current task.

Great leaders are developed rather than born. They build excellent work skills and are willing to step beyond their comfort zone to learn new skills for leading others' work. They know effective leaders promote positive changes by inspiring others. They work to become innovators, motivators, and facilitators rather than pessimists, opponents, or referees.

Lesson 10.1 Review

 Complete the *Map Your Reading* graphic organizer for the section you just read.

1. Knowing your _____ is the first step in being an effective team member. (10.1-1)
   A. education and training
   B. experience and work history
   C. roles and responsibilities
   D. cultural background

2. The two main types of interdisciplinary healthcare teams are (10.1-2)
   A. case manager and functional nursing
   B. multidisciplinary and monodisciplinary
   C. team nursing and primary nursing
   D. primary and secondary

3. Which term refers to the assignment of tasks to each team member? (10.1-3)
   A. Delegation   C. Supervision
   B. Election   D. Resolution

4. To avoid conflict, team members should consider each other's different (10.1-4)
   A. personal styles
   B. work styles
   C. personal opinions
   D. group opinions

5. Effective leaders _____ the work behaviors they want to see in team members. (10.1-5)
   A. model   C. dictate
   B. change   D. invent

Learning Universal Technical Skills

Learning Outcomes

After studying this lesson, you will be able to

10.2-1 explain why temperature, pulse, respiration, and blood pressure are called vital signs and demonstrate steps for measuring vital signs, including height, weight, oral temperature, radial pulse, respiration, and blood pressure.

10.2-2 describe the steps for graphing vital signs.

10.2-3 articulate how to obtain the appropriate first aid training and certification for your healthcare career.

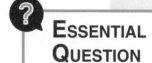

ESSENTIAL QUESTION

What universal technical skills do healthcare workers need to master?

Professional Vocabulary

Essential Terms

first aid emergency treatment given before regular medical services can be obtained

vital signs the key measurements that provide information about a person's health; they include temperature, pulse, respiration, and blood pressure

Important Terms

apical pulse
automated external defibrillator (AED)
blood pressure
cardiopulmonary resuscitation

continuous compression resuscitation (CCR)
hypertension
hypotension
radial pulse

rectal temperature
respiration
sphygmomanometer
stethoscope
temporal artery thermometers

Introduction

Many healthcare workers measure and record vital signs for patients. Obtaining certification in first aid may also be a requirement for employment. Learning these technical skills builds a good foundation for entry-level healthcare employment.

10.2-1 Measuring Vital Signs

The term *vital* means "needed for life." **Vital signs** measure height, weight, temperature, pulse (heartbeat), respiration (breathing), and blood pressure. Healthcare workers must know the normal ranges for each vital sign and techniques for accurately measuring them. Healthcare workers must also know how to record vital sign measurements in the medical record and when to report changes that may indicate a need for prompt medical care.

Height and Weight

Height and weight are measured periodically. The relationship between a person's weight and height provides information about that person's overall health. Physicians can compare a baseline height and weight to future changes.

Height is typically measured on admission to a healthcare facility or at a yearly exam. Individuals with osteoporosis, a degeneration of the spinal column, will have more frequent height measurements.

Weight, however, is measured at most physician visits and on admission, transfer, and discharge at a healthcare facility for a variety of reasons:

- Weight indicates nutritional status.
- When a patient retains fluid, weight will increase. This is an indication of heart and kidney function.
- Unexplained weight loss can signal a disease such as cancer or diabetes.
- Since many medications are prescribed based on body weight, a change in weight may require a change in medication dosage.

Healthcare facilities use several types of scales (**Figure 10.14**). Both the mechanical scale and digital scale are commonly used for patients who can stand independently. To use a mechanical scale, you slide metal weights along a bar until the bar is balanced. Once turned on, a digital scale automatically measures a patient's weight and displays it on a screen. Height measurements are recorded in feet (') and inches ("), or meters (m) and centimeters (cm). Weight is recorded in pounds (lb) or kilograms (kg).

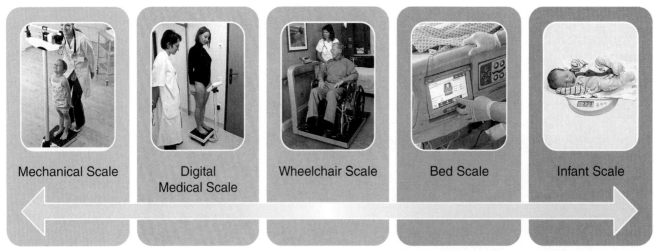

Mechanical Scale   Digital Medical Scale   Wheelchair Scale   Bed Scale   Infant Scale

Left to right: bikeriderlondon/Shutterstock.com, Frédéric Astier/Science Source, Courtesy of Doran Scales, Inc.,Voisin/Phanie/Science Source, Sokolova Maryna/Shutterstock.com

Figure 10.14 Different patients require different types of scales. *When might it be necessary to use the bed scale?*

Measuring Height and Weight Using a Mechanical, Upright Scale

Follow these steps to measure height and weight using a mechanical, upright scale:

1. Complete your beginning procedure steps, including washing your hands.
2. Place paper toweling on the stand area of the scale. Move both weights to the zero position.
3. Ask the patient to remove their shoes and coat and put aside anything they are carrying. Help the patient onto the scale platform, facing the balance bar. Check to see that the patient is not holding on to you or the scale.
4. Move the large weight to the right until the balance bar drops down on the lower guide. Slide the weight back one notch (**Figure 10.15**). Move the small weight on the upper scale bar to the right until the balance pointer is centered between the two scale bars.

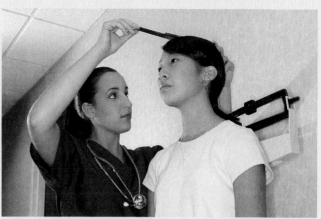

Thinkstock Images/Stockbyte/Thinkstock

Figure 10.16

Read the number at the place where the movable ruler bar meets the stationary ruler bar. This is the patient's height (**Figure 10.17**).

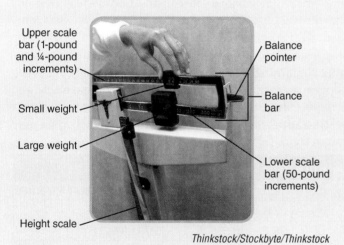

Upper scale bar (1-pound and ¼-pound increments)

Balance pointer

Small weight

Balance bar

Large weight

Lower scale bar (50-pound increments)

Height scale

Thinkstock/Stockbyte/Thinkstock

Figure 10.15

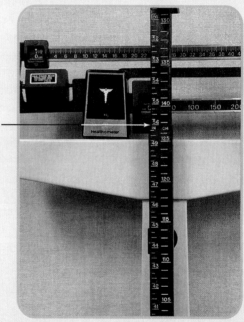

moodboard/moodboard/Thinkstock

Figure 10.17

5. Read the numbers on the upper and lower scale bars where each weight is positioned. Add these two numbers together. This is the patient's weight.
6. Help the patient turn and face away from the scale bar. Keep safety in mind by observing the patient and assisting as necessary to prevent falls. Slide the height rod up until you can open the measuring bar without hitting the patient. Seek assistance if you cannot safely operate the height bar when a patient is taller than you.
7. Slide the height rod down until it touches the top of the patient's head (**Figure 10.16**).

8. Help the patient step off the scale.
9. Record the patient's name, the time you took measurements, and the height and weight measurements.
10. Discard the paper toweling, lower the height rod, and slide the weights to zero.
11. Complete your end-of-procedure steps.

When patients cannot stand independently, you can use a wheelchair scale to measure weight. Wheelchair scales allow you to roll the chair onto a platform, which weighs the patient and the chair. Next, you weigh the empty chair. Subtracting the weight of the chair from the first measurement gives you the patient's weight. Patients who must stay in bed can be measured and weighed using a bed scale. You can weigh infants using a special scale that features a tray to support the infant.

Temperature

The human body balances the heat it loses and the heat it produces to maintain a temperature that varies only slightly. When you are hot, you sweat to cool the body, and when you are cold, you shiver to warm the body. Physical activity, sleeping, and anything that creates excitement cause temperatures to change slightly. These are normal variations. However, an abnormally increased temperature signals a fever. Fever is a sign the body is fighting infection. **Figure 10.18** shows the normal ranges for temperatures taken in different body locations for children and adults. Note that normal temperature readings vary depending on the body location. Healthcare workers report temperatures outside these normal ranges. They also report changes outside the typical range of temperatures for a particular patient. Even though a temperature may be within average normal ranges, it can still signal illness when it is not normal for a specific patient.

You can measure temperature at various sites in the body. Measurement in the mouth, called *oral temperature*, is common. For accuracy, an oral temperature cannot be measured if a person has recently had something to eat or drink. In this case, wait at least 15 minutes before taking the oral temperature.

Glass thermometers (not containing mercury), such as the one in **Figure 10.19**, and digital electronic thermometers measure oral temperature. Digital electronic thermometers measure temperature in just a few seconds. They are easier to read because the temperature appears in large numbers on the viewing screen.

Normal Temperature Ranges for Adults and Children (° Fahrenheit)				
Method	**0 to 2 Years**	**3 to 10 Years**	**11 to 65 Years**	**Greater Than 65 Years**
Oral	N/A	95.9–99.5°F	97.6–99.6°F	96.5–98.5°F
Rectal	97.9–100.4°F	97.9–100.4°F	98.6–100.6°F	97.1–99.2°F
Axillary	94.5–99.1°F	96.6–98.0°F	95.3–98.4°F	96.0–97.4°F
Tympanic	97.5–100.4°F	97.0–100.0°F	96.6–99.7°F	96.4–99.5°F
Temporal Artery	97.9–100.0°F	97.5–100.0°F	98.2–100.2°F	96.6–98.8°F

Note: Tympanic thermometers are used with infants 6 mo. and older. Temporal artery thermometers are used with infants 3 mo. and older.

Goodheart-Willcox Publisher

Figure 10.18 Normal temperature ranges vary based on age and body site where the temperature is taken.

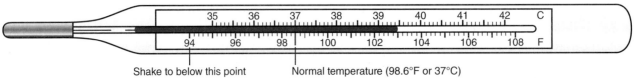

Goodheart-Willcox Publisher

Figure 10.19 To read temperature on a glass thermometer, hold the thermometer at eye level and rotate until you see the indicator line. Add 0.2 degrees for each mark on the thermometer. *What temperature is shown on this thermometer?*

Follow these steps to take an oral temperature using a digital thermometer:

1. Complete your beginning procedure steps, including washing your hands. Wear gloves for this procedure.
2. Make sure the person has not had anything to eat or drink within the last 15 minutes.
3. Cover the thermometer's probe with a sheath/probe cover (**Figure 10.20**). Turn the thermometer on and wait until it beeps or the "ready" sign appears on the viewing screen.

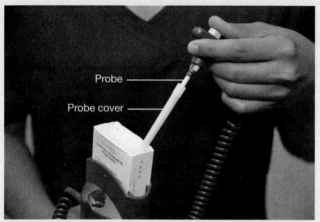

Probe

Probe cover

Wards Forest Media, LLC

Figure 10.20 *What is missing from this image?*

4. Ask the patient to open their mouth and carefully place the thermometer under the tongue and to one side. Have the patient gently close their mouth to hold the thermometer in place and breathe through the nose.
5. Hold the thermometer in place until it blinks or beeps.
6. Ask the patient to open their mouth and carefully remove the thermometer while holding it at the stem end.
7. Remove the sheath or eject the probe cover and discard it in an approved waste container.
8. Read the temperature on the display screen.
9. Turn off the thermometer. Clean as required by facility policy and push the probe back into the thermometer case. Remove gloves and wash hands.
10. Record the patient's name, time you took the temperature, temperature, and method used (in this case, *O* for *oral*). Report an abnormal temperature immediately.
11. Complete your end-of-procedure steps.

Some situations require a different method of temperature measurement, such as axillary (armpit), tympanic (eardrum), or temporal artery (forehead). For example, young children may bite an oral thermometer, and an unconscious person cannot hold an oral thermometer in the mouth. **Figure 10.21** shows a variety of thermometers.

A **rectal temperature** is taken by placing the thermometer in the rectum. Rectal and temporal artery temperatures are the most accurate temperature readings. For this reason, a physician may indicate a patient's temperature should be measured rectally in critical situations.

Hospitals and clinics frequently use **temporal artery thermometers**. They are safe to use with infants through adults, read temperature quickly, and are easy to use and store. While more expensive than a digital thermometer, they are becoming a popular choice for home use as well.

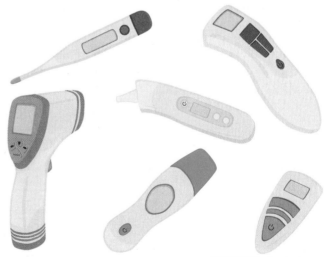

OLEG525/Shutterstock.com

Figure 10.21 Today you see many types of thermometers. *Can you tell which one takes a tympanic temperature? temporal artery temperature? Which one is a noncontact thermometer?*

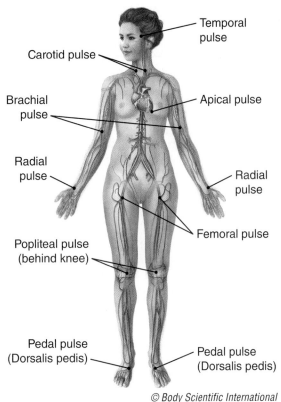

Temporal pulse
Carotid pulse
Brachial pulse
Radial pulse
Apical pulse
Radial pulse
Femoral pulse
Popliteal pulse (behind knee)
Pedal pulse (Dorsalis pedis)
Pedal pulse (Dorsalis pedis)

© Body Scientific International

Figure 10.22 This figure shows pulse points on the body. *Which pulse requires a stethoscope for its measurement?*

Noncontact forehead thermometers are popular for quickly screening large numbers of people, such as at the entrance to a hospital.

To take a temperature using a temporal artery thermometer, simply place the probe on the center of the forehead and slide the thermometer sideways to the hairline. You will read the temperature on the screen within a few seconds. If the patient is sweating, take the temperature on the neck just behind the ear lobe. When using a noncontact thermometer, make sure the person's forehead is clear and dry. Follow the manufacturer's directions for distance and position of the thermometer.

Pulse

Pulse measures heartbeats. With each beat, blood moves through the arteries in a wave or pulse. When you touch or *palpate* an artery near the surface of the skin, you will feel these waves. All your arteries have a pulse, but you can feel the pulse in only a few of the arteries (**Figure 10.22**).

You measure pulse rate by counting the number of beats or pulses in one minute. This tells you the heart rate, which is how fast the heart is beating. In addition to measuring pulse rate, you will assess pulse rhythm and pulse volume, or *amplitude*. Pay attention to the pattern of pulsations and the pauses between them. Normally, pulse rhythm is smooth and regular, with the same amount of time between each pulsation. Pulse amplitude measures the force or quality of the pulse; it describes how the pulse feels. A normal pulse is easy to feel, and each pulsation is strong. You can describe pulse using terms such as *weak, thready, normal, full,* or *bounding*. Report and record any pulse rate that is higher or lower than normal, is irregular, or feels weak or faint.

Pulse rate varies with age (**Figure 10.23**). An infant's heart beats much faster than an adult's does. Physical activity affects pulse rates because the heart speeds up to supply more oxygen to body tissues. Heart rates also increase due to anger, excitement, illness, pain, or fever. Medications may increase or decrease heart rate. Low body temperature, lowered oxygen levels, physical conditioning, and sleep will decrease heart rate.

Average Resting Pulse Rate Per Minute	
Group	**Average Resting Pulse Rate**
Adults	60–100 bpm
Teenagers	60–100 bpm
Children	70–120 bpm
Infants	120–160 bpm
Well-conditioned athletes	40–60 bpm

Goodheart-Willcox Publisher

Figure 10.23 Pulse rate measures heartbeats. *How do age and physical conditioning influence resting pulse rates?*

Two common sites for pulse measurement are the radial artery and the apex of the heart. These are known as *radial pulse* and *apical pulse*. You can measure **radial pulse** by placing two or three fingers over the radial artery on the inside of the wrist.

Follow these steps to measure radial pulse:

1. Complete your beginning procedure steps, including washing your hands.
2. Rest the patient's arm on a table or the bed. Locate the radial pulse on the thumb side of the wrist using two or three fingers. Do *not* use your thumb because you may feel your own pulse.
3. Count the number of pulses for one full minute to assess rhythm and amplitude. For pulse rate only, you may count pulses for 30 seconds and multiply by two.
4. Record the patient's name; time you took the pulse; and pulse rate, rhythm, and amplitude. Report an abnormal pulse rate, rhythm, or amplitude immediately.
5. Complete your end-of-procedure steps.

You can measure **apical pulse** by listening over the apex (lower tip) of the heart using a stethoscope. A **stethoscope** makes sound louder (**Figure 10.24**). You will hear, rather than feel, each beat of the patient's heart. The apex is located in the left fifth intercostal space on the midclavicular line, or approximately 2 inches below the left nipple. An apical pulse is taken when a patient has a weak or irregular pulse that may be difficult to feel. An apical pulse is also used to measure heart rate in infants.

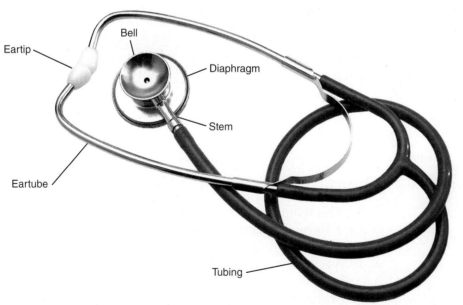

Eartip

Bell

Diaphragm

Stem

Eartube

Tubing

Alex Hinds/Hemera/Thinkstock

Figure 10.24   Before using a stethoscope, clean the earpieces, bell, and diaphragm with alcohol wipes. Rotate the diaphragm until you can hear sound through the earpieces.

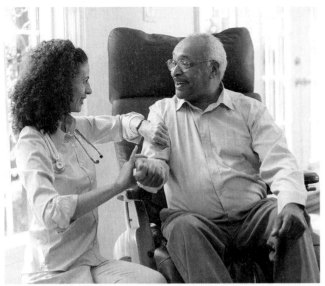

Fuse/Thinkstock

Figure 10.25 To check a patient's respiration, pretend to continue taking a pulse reading as you observe and count the patient's breaths.

Respiration

Counting breaths for one minute is the simplest way to assess a person's respiratory function. As you watch a patient's chest move, count one breath in (inhalation) and one breath out (exhalation) as a single **respiration** or breath. If it is difficult to see chest or abdominal movement, place your hand near the collarbone to feel the patient's breathing. Try to measure respiration right after measuring pulse. Keep your fingers on the patient's wrist as though you are still counting the pulse (**Figure 10.25**). You do not want the patient to know you are measuring respirations because a person can consciously change breathing rates, which will result in an inaccurate measurement. Your measurements will be more accurate when patients do not know that their breaths are being counted.

A healthy resting adult will breathe about 12 to 20 times per minute. During normal breathing, the chest rises and falls evenly in a regular rhythm and breathing is quiet and easy.

PROCEDURE | **Measuring Respirations**

Measure respirations using the following steps:

1. Complete your beginning procedure steps, including washing your hands.
2. Measure respiration right after measuring pulse. Without telling the patient, begin counting each rise and fall of the chest as one breath. For regular respirations, you may count for 30 seconds and multiply by two. If breathing is irregular, you should count respirations for a full minute.
3. Record the patient's name, time you measured the respiration, and respiratory rate. Report a respiratory rate that is greater than 24 or less than 10 breaths per minute. Report any breathing that is irregular, very deep or very shallow, difficult, or painful.
4. Complete your end-of-procedure steps.

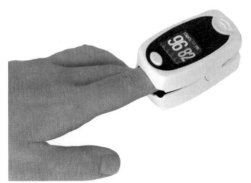

James Kappernaros/Shutterstock.com

Figure 10.26 Pulse oximeters measure oxygen saturation and heart rate. *Are this adult patient's readings within normal ranges?*

Oxygen Saturation

A pulse oximeter measures the amount of oxygen in blood (**Figure 10.26**). Oxygen saturation indicates how much oxygen the blood is carrying as a percentage of the maximum it could carry. A normal reading is 95–100 percent. A pulse oximeter will also show pulse rate.

You may take an oximeter reading as part of vital signs measurement. This is especially important for patients with blood disorders, circulatory diseases, and lung issues. These health conditions negatively affect blood oxygen saturation levels. You will also use oximeters when patients are receiving oxygen.

Remove nail polish before using a pulse oximeter. The oximeter uses infrared light, and nail polish will absorb light and interfere with the oxygen measurement. Clip the oximeter to the tip of the finger. Hold the hand still and wait for the reading to appear. Within seconds, the pulse rate and oxygen saturation level will appear on the screen. Record this measurement in the patient's chart. Report any readings outside the normal range.

Blood Pressure

Blood pressure is the force of blood pushing against the inside of the blood vessel (artery) walls. When you take someone's blood pressure, you record two measurements: systolic and diastolic. Systolic (sihs-TAHL-ihk) pressure is the force caused by the contracting heart muscle pushing blood through the arteries. Diastolic (dI-uh-STAHL-ihk) pressure is the lesser force of the blood when the heart muscle relaxes. Blood pressure is measured in millimeters of mercury (mmHg) and is recorded as a fraction. Write the higher (systolic) number first and the lower (diastolic) number second. A systolic pressure of 115 mmHg and a diastolic pressure of 70 mmHg are written as 115/70.

Blood pressure readings provide vital information about a person's current health and future risk for disease. Normal blood pressure varies throughout the day, with readings being lower in the morning and when lying down. Readings are typically higher when sitting or standing, after eating a meal, and when exercising. Stress, anxiety, and pain all increase blood pressure. **Figure 10.27** shows several factors that influence blood pressure, including some related to lifestyle choices.

When blood pressure is too low (**hypotension**), the body tissues do not get enough nutrients and oxygen. When blood pressure is too high (**hypertension**), the heart works harder to push blood through the arteries.

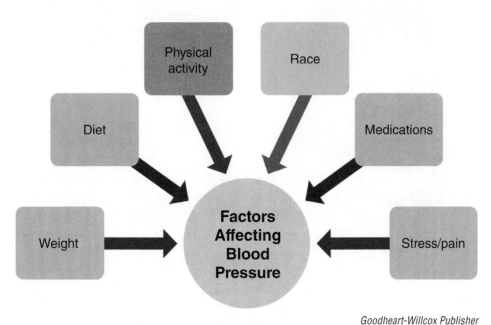

Figure 10.27 Many factors influence blood pressure readings. *How many of these factors are related to lifestyle choices?*

Blood Pressure Classifications for Adults	
Classification	**Range**
Hypotension	<90/60 mmHg
Normal	90–120/60–80 mmHg
Elevated	120–129/<80 mmHG
Hypertension	Stage 1: 130–139/80–90 mmHG
	Stage 2: >140/90 mmHg

Goodheart-Willcox Publisher

Figure 10.28 Blood pressure readings provide important information about a person's current health and future disease risk. *What risks are associated with hypotension and hypertension?*

Eventually, this causes damage to the heart muscle. High blood pressure also stresses the kidneys and blood vessels, which can lead to kidney failure and stroke. **Figure 10.28** lists the readings that indicate normal blood pressure, hypertension, and hypotension.

A **sphygmomanometer** (sfihg-moh-muh-NAHM-eht-er) measures blood pressure and comes in two types: aneroid and digital (**Figure 10.29**). Aneroid sphygmomanometers are very common. They use a small mechanical device with a convenient dial to measure pressure. Aneroid sphygmomanometers do require recalibration, which means the equipment must be checked regularly to ensure its measurements remain accurate. The manometer, or *gauge*, should point to zero when the cuff is deflated. When using an aneroid sphygmomanometer, you are trying to "hear" the blood pressure.

Digital sphygmomanometers are more convenient, especially in noisy places. Instead of sound, digital instruments use vibration to determine diastolic and systolic pressures. When blood pressure is high, arterial walls vibrate as blood flows through them. Digital sphygmomanometers detect the changes in these vibrations as the pressure in the cuff is released.

You will hear sounds through the stethoscope as you auscultate (AW-skuhl-tayt), or listen to, a blood pressure on an aneroid sphygmomanometer. These sounds are named for Nikolai Korotkoff (koh-RAHT-kohf), the Russian surgeon who first identified them. As you slowly release the valve, you will hear tapping sounds that gradually become louder.

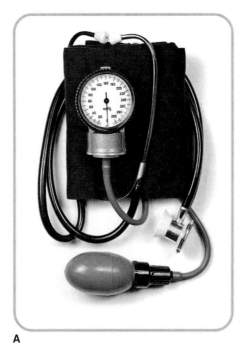
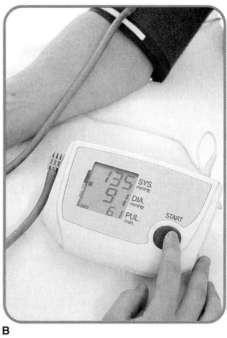

A   B

Dmitry Naumov/Shutterstock.com, Khamidulin Sergey/Shutterstock.com

Figure 10.29 Shown here are (A) aneroid and (B) digital sphygmomanometers. *Which piece of equipment works better in a noisy setting?*

The first tapping sound indicates the systolic pressure. Next, you will hear a sequence of swishing and tapping sounds. Finally, the sound will become muffled and very soft. The last sound indicates the diastolic pressure.

Sphygmomanometers consist of a bulb that is squeezed to fill the cuff with air, a manometer that measures pressure in the cuff, the cuff itself, and flexible tubing to connect all the parts. Cuffs come in different sizes, designed to fit children, adults, large adults, and the thigh. The cuff must fit correctly, or the blood pressure reading will not be accurate. The manometer measures the pressure of the air in the cuff (**Figure 10.30**). The longer dark lines mark increments of 10 mmHg, and the short lines in between mark increments of 2 mmHg.

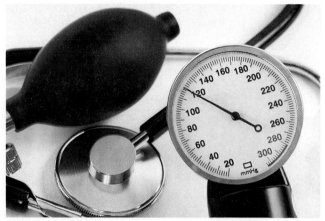

Tatiana Popova//Shutterstock.com

Figure 10.30 Each long line on the manometer gauge represents 10 mmHg. *What pressure measurement is shown on this gauge?*

PROCEDURE | **Measuring Blood Pressure**

The most common place to measure a person's blood pressure is the brachial artery of the upper arm. Measuring blood pressure requires practice until you can operate the equipment smoothly and assess the sounds accurately. Use the following steps to measure a patient's blood pressure:

1. Complete your beginning procedure steps, including washing your hands.
2. Help the patient into a sitting or lying-down position so the forearm is level with the heart and the palm is facing upward. Expose the upper arm by rolling up the sleeve or removing the shirt if the sleeve is tight. For accuracy, the patient should be resting quietly for five minutes before blood pressure is measured.
3. Use alcohol wipes to clean the stethoscope. Rotate the diaphragm until you can hear through it.
4. Locate the patient's brachial artery pulse by straightening the arm. Place your fingers across the inside of the antecubital space located at the inner bend of the elbow.
5. Place the arrow mark on the blood pressure cuff over the brachial artery. Wrap the cuff around the patient's upper arm so the bottom of the cuff is at least 1 inch above the elbow. The cuff must be even and snug. Place the stethoscope earpieces in your ears.

6. Pump the bulb until the pressure is 30 mmHg higher than the systolic pressure. You can achieve this by using one of the following methods:
   A. Place the stethoscope over the brachial artery. Inflate the cuff until you hear the pulse stop. Inflate 30 mmHg more.
   B. Hold the bulb in one hand and palpate the radial artery with the other hand. Inflate the cuff until you no longer feel the radial pulse. Inflate 30 mmHg more.
7. With the stethoscope positioned over the brachial artery, release the valve slightly by turning it counterclockwise. This will allow air to escape from the cuff slowly.
8. Note the reading on the manometer when you hear the first Korotkoff sound. This is the systolic pressure.
9. Continue to deflate the cuff and note the reading when you hear the last Korotkoff sound. This is the diastolic pressure.
10. Deflate the cuff completely and remove it from the patient's arm.
11. Record the patient's name, time you measured the blood pressure, and blood pressure reading. Report an abnormal blood pressure immediately.
12. Store the sphygmomanometer. Clean and store the stethoscope.
13. Complete your end-of-procedure steps.

Does it make a difference which arm you use to take a blood pressure reading? A good guide is to determine whether a person's pulse feels stronger in one arm compared to the other. You will have an easier time measuring blood pressure in the arm with the stronger pulse. Do not use an arm that is injured, in a cast, or has an IV. If a patient has had a mastectomy with lymph node removal, use the arm on the other side of the body. In the case of a double mastectomy, seek a doctor's advice about the best option for measuring blood pressure.

Do not partially deflate the cuff and then reinflate it while taking a blood pressure measurement. This will result in an inaccurate reading. If the cuff is partially deflated, release all the air in the cuff and wait 30 seconds before trying again. Remember that the cuff pressure is uncomfortable for the patient. Be accurate, but also efficient with your blood pressure measurement.

If, while practicing, you take a blood pressure measurement that is very high or extremely low, check again. Remember, you are just learning this skill. Remain calm, but ask the person to have a healthcare professional check their blood pressure if the measurement varies from the normal range.

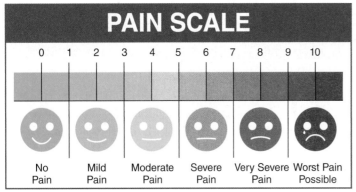

EgudinKa/Shutterstock.com

Figure 10.31 A pain scale can help patients communicate their level of discomfort to their healthcare provider.

Pain Assessment

Unlike vital signs, pain cannot be measured. It is a symptom, rather than a sign. Still, pain level is an important factor in assessing your patient's well-being. Begin by observing your patient. Are the patient's teeth clenched and eyes closed? Is the patient clutching her ankle, holding her arms over her stomach, or rubbing her forehead? Facial expressions and gestures can provide clues to pain. Is your patient crying or moaning? Document these observations and all complaints of pain. Ask your patient to assess pain level using a pain scale (**Figure 10.31**). When a patient cannot communicate verbally, compare the patient's facial expressions to the pain scale to make the most objective assessment of pain. Finally, remember that some individuals are stoic about pain. Because of personality or culture, they are unwilling to express pain. Do not assume a patient has no pain because the patient does not talk about it.

10.2-2 Graphing Vital Signs

Vital signs are routinely recorded in a patient's medical record. Today, most facilities use electronic health records, which automatically graph vital signs. Healthcare workers enter the measurements in a table in the electronic record. Selecting the chart view displays the measurements in a graph. Graphic charts provide a visual diagram of a patient's progress and can be easier to read than a list of numbers containing the same information. Newer technologies connect vital signs equipment with the patient's medical record. When the equipment measures the patient's vital signs, the readings are transmitted directly to the patient's electronic health record. This avoids possible recording errors.

Figure 10.32 shows two formats of the vital signs taken for a patient who has just returned from surgery.

Before the development of electronic records, all vital signs were graphed on paper charts and written by hand. This process took time and great attention to detail when locating the correct spot on a grid. When recording temperatures, healthcare workers would also flag any temperature not taken orally. For example, an oral temperature is recorded as 98.6°F, but a rectal temperature is recorded as 99.6°F followed by the letter *R* in a circle. A temporal artery temperature may read like an oral temperature or a rectal temperature depending upon the individual thermometer. Record the temperature reading followed by the letters *TA* in a circle.

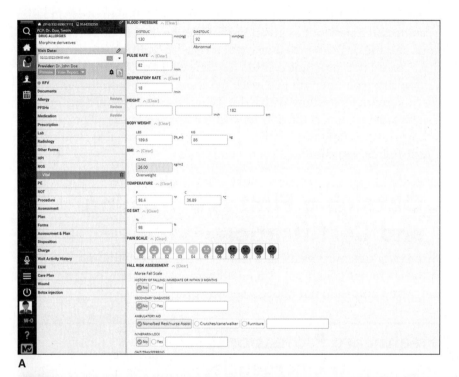

A

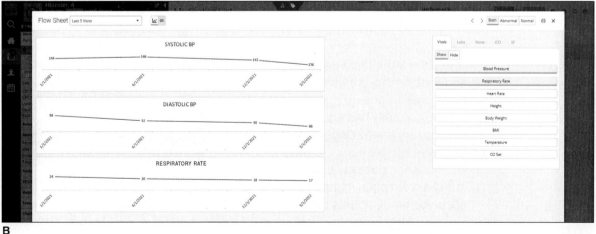

B

Figure 10.32 Vital signs are entered into a table like this one. In an electronic health record, the chart view displays vital signs in a graph form. This makes it easier to see a patient's progress over time. *What does the red text indicate in the table?*

Remember that temperature readings vary based on the site. For example, a rectal temperature will be higher than an oral temperature because it measures temperature closer to the core of the body. For this reason, healthcare workers also note additional vital signs information that may affect readings. These include items such as the site for measuring temperature, or which arm was used for taking a blood pressure measurement. Facilities that still use handwritten charts often require workers to note medications that affect vital signs or hospital events such as admission, delivery, surgery, and discharge on the graphic chart (**Figure 10.33**). Specific graphic forms vary by facility, but the basic steps for graphing vital signs remain the same:

1. Fill in patient identification information and dates.
2. Note the admitting date (ADM) and number the days after admission. Day 1 is the first day after admission.
3. Note the date of surgery (OR) and number the days after surgery (PO for *postoperative*). If a patient has given birth, note the date of delivery (DEL) and number the days after delivery (PP for *postpartum*).
4. Find the correct date and time column for your vital sign reading (x-axis). Move down the column until you reach the correct number on the left side (y-axis) and mark the reading with a dot. When you have made dots for each vital sign reading, connect the dots for each vital sign to make a line graph.
5. Flag temperatures not taken orally by writing the correct abbreviation on the graph. Circle the abbreviation for emphasis.

10.2-3 Obtaining First Aid Training and Certification

Healthcare workers must be alert to changes in patient status and prepared to report those changes. Sometimes a healthcare worker will detect a patient emergency when others do not notice a serious problem.

Healthcare Professions: Identifying Emergencies

Erin works in a long-term care facility. She knows the normal signs of health for the residents in her care and realizes that a change in status can signal an emergency. For example, Mr. Lyon usually has above-normal blood pressure readings, Mrs. Siemens is always hungry at mealtime, and Mr. Frederick complains about his arthritis most often in the evening. Erin observes her residents closely to notice when something is different.

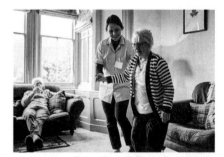

Dean Mitchell/E+ via Getty Images

Could Mrs. Siemens' tiredness and indigestion be signs of a heart attack? Does Mr. Frederick's slurred speech indicate a stroke? Does Mr. Lyon's drop in blood pressure mean something is wrong? Erin reports signs and symptoms that are unusual or alarming, so her residents receive needed emergency care at the earliest opportunity.

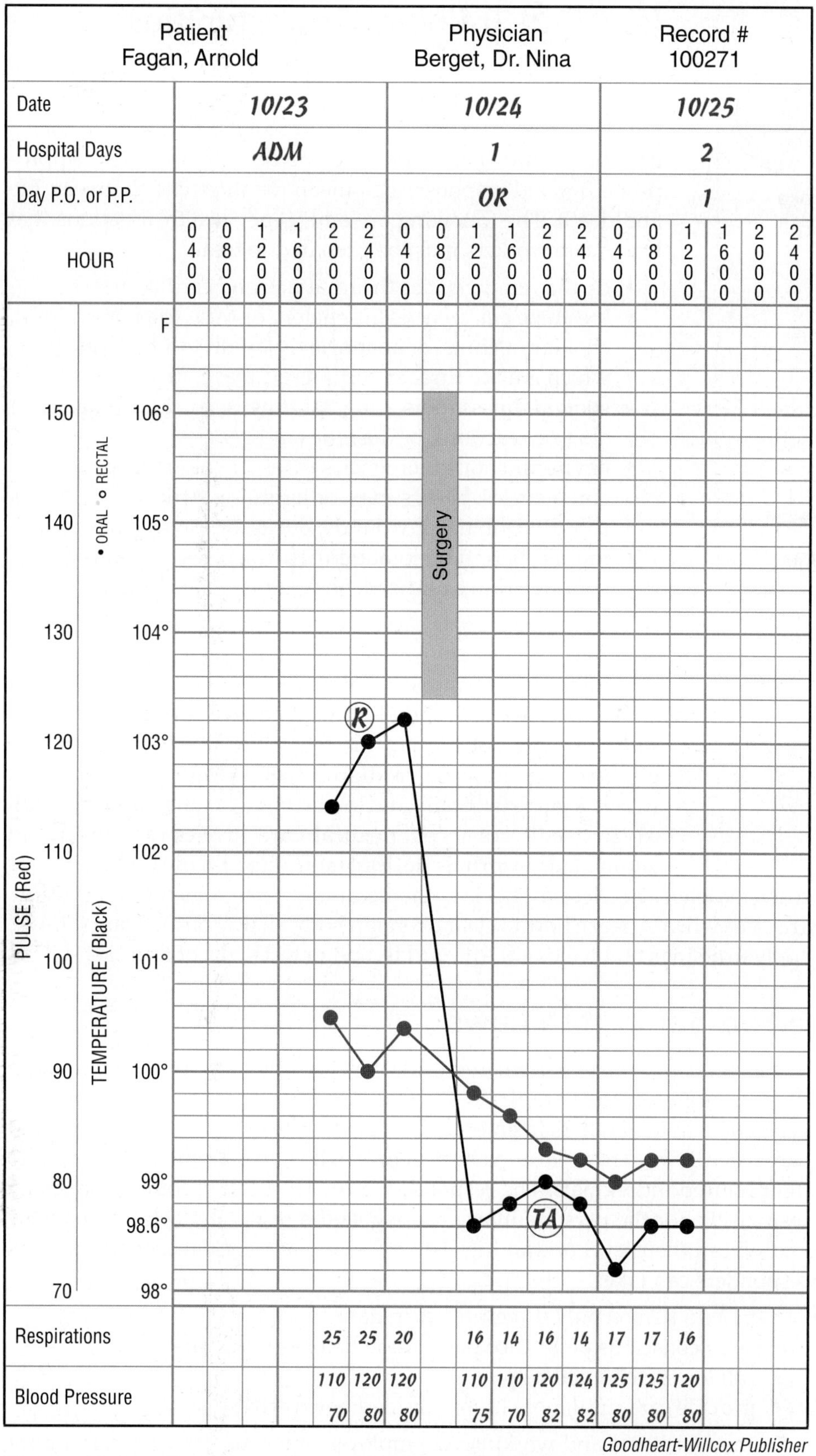
Patient
Fagan, Arnold
Physician
Berget, Dr. Nina
Record #
100271
Date
10/23
10/24
10/25
Hospital Days
ADM
1
2
Day P.O. or P.P.
OR
1
HOUR
0400 0800 1200 1600 2000 2400 0400 0800 1200 1600 2000 2400 0400 0800 1200 1600 2000 2400
PULSE (Red)
150
140
130
120
110
100
90
80
70
TEMPERATURE (Black)
• ORAL ∘ RECTAL
F
106°
105°
104°
103°
102°
101°
100°
99°
98.6°
98°
Surgery
R
TA
Respirations
25 25 20 16 14 16 14 17 17 16
Blood Pressure
110/70 120/80 120/80 110/75 110/70 120/82 124/82 125/80 125/80 120/80
Goodheart-Willcox Publisher

Figure 10.33 The red line traces pulse; the black line traces temperature. Respirations and blood pressure have been listed below. Hand-charting of vital signs requires close attention to detail to produce an accurate record.

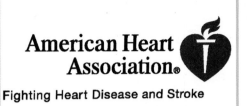

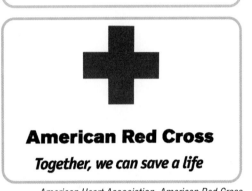

American Red Cross

Together, we can save a life

American Heart Association, American Red Cross

Figure 10.34 The American Red Cross and the American Heart Association offer many training courses and certification for CPR and first aid. *How will you determine which course to take?*

First Aid Training Opportunities

Healthcare workers must also be prepared to act in the case of a sudden illness or injury. All workers can seek **first aid** training. The goal of first aid is to minimize the effects of an injury or illness until more advanced medical help arrives. Appropriate first aid responses can mean the difference between life and death. The following are emergency health situations that healthcare workers must be prepared to treat:

- cardiac emergencies (heart attack and cardiac arrest)
- breathing emergencies (respiratory distress, respiratory arrest, choking, asthma, or anaphylaxis [an-uh-fuh-LAK-sihs]), which is a life-threatening allergic reaction)
- sudden illness (poisoning, fainting, seizures, stroke, allergic reactions, or diabetic emergencies)
- environmental emergencies (heat- or cold-related emergencies, bites, stings, or lightning strikes)
- soft tissue injuries (wounds, burns, or external bleeding)
- muscle, bone, and joint injuries (fractures; dislocations; sprains; strains; or head, neck, and spinal injuries)

The American Heart Association and the American Red Cross offer several levels of first aid training courses (**Figure 10.34**). At a minimum, health science students should learn basic first aid procedures for responding to a medical emergency. Course skills include, but are not limited to, checking an injured or ill person; performing **cardiopulmonary resuscitation** (CPR), which keeps the brain and other vital organs supplied with oxygen until advanced medical care arrives; and using an **automated external defibrillator** (dee-FIHB-ruh-layt-er), or AED, to deliver an electric shock to the heart and restore its normal rhythm. Trainees will also learn how to clear a foreign body airway obstruction (FBAO), apply dressings and bandages to wounds, and detect signs of a stroke.

Good Samaritan Laws

When people encounter emergencies, they are often afraid to help because they feel unprepared or are afraid of being sued. Good Samaritan laws encourage people to help others in emergencies. Each state establishes its own Good Samaritan laws. These laws protect people who provide emergency care to ill or injured individuals. The responder cannot be sued or found financially responsible for the person's injury as long as the responder acted reasonably and within their level of training. The following are some reasonable actions responders can take:

- move a person only if their life is in danger
- ask a conscious person for permission before giving care
- call for professional help
- provide care until more highly trained help arrives

In many schools and workplaces, employers sponsor first aid training for employees. They may establish an emergency response team of volunteers who can assist when an emergency occurs. The Good Samaritan law continues to protect these workplace volunteers.

Training for Healthcare Workers

Many healthcare workers complete a more extensive training program designed for professional rescuers, and certain healthcare workers have a duty to respond to an emergency. Individuals who perform rescues as a part of their jobs have a legal duty to respond and rescue in an emergency. In addition, when emergency medical technicians (EMTs) are on duty, they are legally responsible for the care they provide to people who have experienced an accident or sudden illness. The training for EMTs includes each of the following:

- making primary assessments
- giving ventilations
- performing advanced CPR and AED
- using epinephrine autoinjectors and asthma inhalers
- using emergency oxygen and breathing devices
- responding to opioid overdoses

Certification

Whether you are learning basic first aid or professional rescue techniques, you can earn certification to show you have passed a test demonstrating your new skills. The American Red Cross and the American Heart Association are the two agencies that certify first aid skills. To become certified, your first aid course must be taught by an approved trainer. You must complete the entire course curriculum and pass a written test as well as a skills demonstration.

Scope of Practice

In all situations, healthcare workers should provide emergency care within their scope of practice based on their training and certification (**Figure 10.35**).

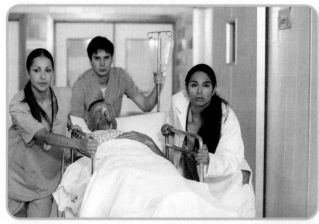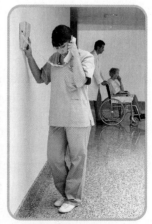

Wavebreakmedia Ltd/Wavebreak Media/Thinkstock, wavebreakmedia/Shutterstock.com

Figure 10.35 Healthcare workers in a hospital must alert personnel in the hospital when an emergency occurs. In contrast, healthcare workers at an assisted living facility should call 911 if an emergency occurs. *What concept does this illustrate?*

They also follow their facilities' policies for responding to emergencies. For example, Cindy works as a CNA in a hospital. When she identifies a patient emergency, a special code alerts hospital personnel to respond with medical assistance. Janice, on the other hand, works at an assisted living facility. She is required to maintain first aid certification. In an emergency, she calls 911 and provides appropriate first aid until emergency medical personnel arrive. Both workers must know a patient's wishes for resuscitation before providing life support. For example, patients who have a no code, or *do not resuscitate (DNR)*, order have chosen not to receive resuscitation in the event of respiratory or cardiac arrest.

Job Requirements

You will want to seek the appropriate training and certification required for your current or future career. For example, emergency medical responder programs require professional level coursework and training. Some college nursing programs include a professional level course in their entrance requirements. Nursing assistants may or may not be required to complete first aid training based on individual state certification requirements, but employers appreciate CNAs who take the initiative to seek this training on their own. Employers often require home care and assisted living aides to maintain first aid certification since they may be the only ones available to act when a medical emergency occurs. Individuals who work as lifeguards are required to take a specialized water safety training course.

Current Resources

The most important step you can take to prepare for an emergency is completing a CPR and first aid training course. Continue to take refresher courses to maintain your certification. Care procedures change as newer and more effective treatments for illness and injury are developed. The AED is an example of an improvement in emergency care. **Continuous compression resuscitation (CCR)** is a technique developed to encourage more people to act immediately when they witness cardiac arrest in an adult.

The American Heart Association has developed a first aid and CPR mobile app that provides text and video care instructions. Since it can be downloaded and stored on a mobile device, you can access the app even without internet. Recently, a person who was injured in an earthquake used basic first aid knowledge and the information in his phone to care for his wounds and respond to signals of shock while he waited for rescue personnel to arrive.

The American Red Cross also has a free first aid mobile app with advice for everyday emergencies. It offers videos and interactive quizzes for reviewing first aid information. In addition, you can access the complete American Red Cross first aid training manual through the agency's website for further reading and study.

1. Vital signs measure _____ functions of the body. (10.2-1)
   A. unique
   B. essential
   C. important
   D. routine

2. In what units should a patient's weight be recorded? Choose all that apply. (10.2-1)
   A. Pounds
   B. Milligrams
   C. Ounces
   D. Kilograms

3. When measuring weight, which of these should a healthcare worker do first? (10.2-1)
   A. Move the large weight to the right until the balance bar drops.
   B. Move the small weight to the right until the balance pointer is centered.
   C. Read the numbers on the upper and lower scale.
   D. Move both weights to the zero position.

4. Martin is measuring the oral temperature of his teenage patient. Which of these temperatures will need to be reported as well as recorded? (10.2-1)
   A. 96.8 degrees
   B. 98.6 degrees
   C. 99.0 degrees
   D. 98.0 degrees

5. Patients should not have anything to eat or drink for at least 15 minutes before taking a(n) _____ temperature. (10.2-1)
   A. rectal
   B. tympanic
   C. temporal artery
   D. oral

6. A radial pulse is measured inside the wrist, while an apical pulse is measured at the apex of the (10.2-1)
   A. heart
   B. lung
   C. carotid artery
   D. femur

7. Which of these pulse points is *not* palpated? (10.2-1)
   A. Radial
   B. Brachial
   C. Apical
   D. Carotid

8. Which of the following patient health concerns require oxygen saturation monitoring? Choose all that apply. (10.2-1)
   A. Blood disorders
   B. Poor circulation
   C. Lung issues
   D. Patients who are not receiving oxygen

9. Respiration measures (10.2-1)
   A. heartbeats per minute
   B. amount of oxygen in the blood
   C. breaths per minute
   D. pressure of blood against artery walls

10. In a blood pressure reading of 120/80, the number 120 represents _____ pressure. (10.2-1)
    A. diastolic
    B. more important
    C. less important
    D. systolic

11. Which condition indicates blood pressure is too low, meaning the body tissues do not get enough nutrients and oxygen? (10.2-1)
    A. Hydrotension
    B. Hydratension
    C. Hypotension
    D. Hypertension

12. You should record the _____ when taking a temperature. (10.2-2)
    A. age of the patient
    B. suspected cause for symptoms
    C. site of the measurement
    D. type of thermometer

13. Which of the following healthcare workers could take a basic first aid course as preparation for a job? (10.2-3)
    A. Home health aide
    B. Physician
    C. Emergency medical technician
    D. Registered nurse

Transitioning from School to Work

ESSENTIAL QUESTION

What employability skills do healthcare workers need for transitioning to work?

Learning Outcomes

After studying this lesson, you will be able to

10.3-1 define employability skills and name several examples.

10.3-2 describe each step in the process of acquiring a job.

10.3-3 relate the work behaviors that lead to job and career success.

10.3-4 explain how to leave a job responsibly and list the components of a letter of resignation.

Professional Vocabulary

Essential Terms

cover message   a short letter sent with a résumé to introduce the job applicant and give the reasons for applying to a particular job

employability skills   tasks related to choosing a career, acquiring and keeping a job, changing jobs, and advancing in a career

incompetence   a lack of qualifications or ability to perform job tasks

interview etiquette   accepted appearance and behavior for the interview process

letter of resignation   a written document that formally states an employee's decision to leave a job

personal and professional development   steps taken to improve personal, educational, and career-related performance

professional organization   an association formed to unite and inform people who work in the same occupation

Important Terms

advocate

Background Information Disclosure (BID) form

barred

Federal Insurance Contributions Act (FICA)

federal withholding tax

gross pay

net pay

network

personal data page

references

Social Security

Introduction

Preparing for a job includes more than completing an education and training program. Workers need employability skills to locate a job, get hired, succeed in their jobs, and advance in their careers.

10.3-1 Employability Skills

While education and training prepare you for a job, **employability skills** help you find and keep a job. Of course, employability skills include completing job applications and interviews. However, soft skills like professionalism, trustworthiness, and a positive attitude, are equally important for getting and keeping a job. Healthcare workers need customer service skills to communicate respectfully with patients. They use emotional intelligence to express their own feelings appropriately and show empathy toward patients and coworkers. Personal skills like time management and a good work ethic also contribute to job success. As you study communication skills and learn about the chain of command in healthcare systems, you will continue to build your employability skills.

Perhaps you have completed a couple of health science classes or have passed your nursing assistant test and are ready to find a job. You will need to think creatively to locate an entry-level opportunity in the healthcare field because most healthcare jobs require a degree and license or certification. However difficult finding that first job might be, work experience in healthcare is an asset when you apply for future professional positions. Entry-level work experience also helps you decide about your future career goals.

 ## Healthcare Professions: Work Experience

Brittany completed a nursing assistant class during high school and worked at a nearby nursing home all through college. In her sophomore year, she changed her mind about majoring in nursing and pursued a business degree instead. After graduation, she looked for a sales job in the medical field. The employer who hired her said that her previous CNA job set her apart from all the other applicants. That job gave her work experience in the field and proved that she could be a successful healthcare employee.

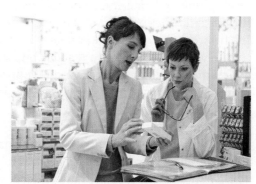

Image Point Fr/Shutterstock.com

10.3-2 Getting a Job

Getting hired for a job that builds your healthcare work history might take some time and effort. Yet, work experience in a healthcare setting teaches valuable skills for your future healthcare career.

The Job Search

Your first job does not have to directly relate to your future career. It should, however, provide opportunities to learn skills you can use in your professional life. For example, becoming a dietary aide may not teach you physical therapy skills, but it will teach you how to interact with residents. You will observe how physical limitations affect their lives. Likewise, a dental receptionist learns the scheduling process and skills for communicating with patients, and a pharmacy assistant learns a great deal about pharmacology and medical record keeping. The skills learned in these entry-level positions are important skills for higher-level careers such as professional therapist, dentist, and pharmacist.

Begin your job search by listing all the settings where healthcare is delivered. Then make a list of the businesses in your area. Search their websites to find available jobs for which you are qualified. Job-search websites can help you identify healthcare businesses in your area and alert you to those currently hiring. However, be aware that creating an account with a site could bring unwanted spam mail, and it may take a lot of searching on a national site to locate healthcare jobs in your specific area.

You can also post your résumé to large job websites or social media platforms, including those specifically for healthcare. Employers and recruiters search these websites for potential employees. You will get better responses if you already have a healthcare certification and some job experience. Before posting your résumé information to a social media website, make sure your social media does not contain personal information that would hurt an employer's first impression of you.

Ask your health science teacher and school counselor for names of businesses that hire entry-level workers. Enrolling in a youth apprenticeship program or other work-based learning experiences can offer job opportunities not typically open to high school students. Check the job postings at your school. Local papers still advertise a few jobs, so you should look there as well. Stop by the chiropractor's, dentist's, or veterinarian's office. Ask if they are hiring and if you can fill out an application. Most important, use your personal network. Many times, jobs are filled based on "who you know" before they are ever posted.

A **network** is the group of people you know who work in healthcare. Is your friend's mom a dentist? Ask her about a job. Have you asked your own optometrist about job openings? The best job opportunities develop when people you know tell you their company is hiring and offer to recommend you. Make a list of all the people you know who already work in healthcare. Take the time to connect with them. These contacts can lead to a job.

The Application Process

Applying for a job includes different steps for each employer. Searching job listings on a company website and applying online is common today. You may be asked to attach your résumé at the end of the application, so refer to your career portfolio and update your résumé so you have a current copy ready. Many companies hire a firm to operate their online job application process. Be cautious about the personal information you supply. Check for a secure website before providing any identifying information.

Smaller companies may require a paper application form. Some job advertisements will ask you to send your résumé along with a letter expressing your interest in a particular job (**Figure 10.36**). This letter is called a **cover message**, or *letter of application*.

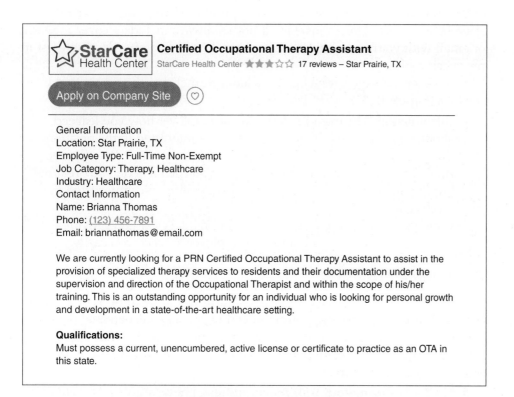

General Information
Location: Star Prairie, TX
Employee Type: Full-Time Non-Exempt
Job Category: Therapy, Healthcare
Industry: Healthcare
Contact Information
Name: Brianna Thomas
Phone: (123) 456-7891
Email: briannathomas@email.com

We are currently looking for a PRN Certified Occupational Therapy Assistant to assist in the provision of specialized therapy services to residents and their documentation under the supervision and direction of the Occupational Therapist and within the scope of his/her training. This is an outstanding opportunity for an individual who is looking for personal growth and development in a state-of-the-art healthcare setting.

Qualifications:
Must possess a current, unencumbered, active license or certificate to practice as an OTA in this state.

Goodheart-Willcox Publisher

Figure 10.36 Online applications are common. Be ready to attach your résumé and always include a cover message.

Cover Message

When you mail a résumé or post it online, you should include a cover message to introduce yourself and explain why you are applying for the job. This message summarizes your main qualifications and expresses positive interest in the job. Just like your résumé and application form, your cover message must be error-free. Unless instructed not to, always include a cover message or email with your online application. This shows extra effort and interest in the specific job.

Your cover message uses a business letter format and should contain three sections (**Figure 10.37**):

- **Introduction.** The introduction tells the employer how you learned about the job or company and why you are interested in the position.
- **Body.** The body of the message explains how your skills will meet the organization's needs. Do not repeat all the facts on your résumé but include enough information to get the employer interested in reading it.
- **Conclusion.** In your conclusion, ask for an interview and provide the contact information needed for the employer to reach you easily.

Personal Data Page

Whether you complete an application form at the beginning of your job search or after an interview, you will need to access your personal data. The easiest way to do this is to prepare a **personal data page** for your career portfolio and use it for completing job applications. Include the following information in your personal data page:

- **Contact information.** Your name, address, phone number, and email; you will also need to know your Social Security number but should submit that after you are hired.
- **Education.** List the names and locations of all the schools you have attended and the years you attended. List any diplomas or degrees you were awarded and your grade-point average. Many applications do not request all this information, but this will prepare you for the ones that do.
- **Work experience.** List all your work experience, including volunteer work. Write the name, address, and phone number of each employer and include the years you worked there. Record your job title, duties, the name of your supervisor, and beginning and ending wage.
- **Skills.** List whatever skills you have that apply to the jobs you are seeking. For example, fast and accurate keyboard skills are important in a medical office.
- **References.** Create a list of three or four **references**. These are people who know you well and are willing to discuss your skills and job qualifications with potential employers. Former employers, teachers, club advisors, or coaches make good references. Your relatives and friends do not make good references because they are considered biased. Do not list them as references. Write the name, title, address, and phone number for each reference. You must ask permission from all these individuals before listing them as references.

Sam Sanchez
4035 Starlight Ct.
Star Prairie, TX 74260

November 3, 2023

Human Resources
PO Box 123
Star Prairie, TX 74260

Greeting — Dear Hiring Manager:

Introduction — I am writing in response to your posting for a certified pharmacy technician. After reading your job description, I am confident that my skills and aptitudes are a perfect match for this position.

Body — I began working in a pharmacy during my senior year of high school through the health youth apprenticeship program. During my senior year, I completed a full year of pharmacy technician coursework. Upon graduation, I took the state certification exam and became a certified pharmacy technician last June.

My youth apprenticeship mentor ranked my attention to detail and responsible work attitude as outstanding on my work program evaluations. In addition to my pharmacy coursework, I have completed courses in medical terminology, body structure and function, and computer concepts. I was an active member of HOSA, attending state conferences and competing in pharmacology and prepared speaking.

Conclusion — I would welcome the opportunity to discuss this position with you. If you have questions or would like to schedule an interview, please contact me by phone at 123-217-2130 or by e-mail at SSanchez@gmail.com. I have enclosed my résumé for your review, and I look forward to hearing from you.

Sincerely,

Sam Sanchez

Sam Sanchez

Enclosure

Figure 10.37 This cover message is in letter format because it will be mailed. If applying by email, begin with the greeting and list your contact information at the end of the message. When responding to an online job ad, always attach your résumé along with your cover message.

Application Form

Whether you complete your application online or on paper, you will follow the same guidelines. Neatness, accuracy, and correct spelling are all very important. Sloppy applications are discarded. Even if you are well qualified for the job, you will not be considered if your application is sloppy. Employers think sloppy applications indicate that people will be sloppy in their work. Complete paper applications by printing in ink but use cursive handwriting for your signature. Have your personal data page nearby to use as a reference.

Complete every question on the job application form. If some questions do not apply to you, write *does not apply* or *N/A* in the space so the employer knows you did not skip the question. For questions related to salary, write *negotiable.* If you write a higher wage than what the job pays, you may be eliminated from consideration. Remain positive when stating your reasons for leaving previous jobs. Examples might include *reduction of workforce* or *return to school.* Negative comments about former employers will not help your employment prospects.

For privacy reasons, you should not list your Social Security number on a job application form. In this case, you can write *available upon job offer.* If you are hired, the business will need your Social Security number before you can be paid. Use these same guidelines when applying online.

In the field of healthcare, you may need to complete a **Background Information Disclosure (BID) form** or caregiver background form. This process eliminates workers who have a history of harming others. The background check protects clients, patients, and residents. A Social Security number is required for completing a background check.

Make positive choices about your current behavior. Students who have had fights can be **barred**. This means they cannot work in healthcare if the charges result in a criminal record. Many companies also do an internet search. Be very careful about posting personal information on social media (**Figure 10.38**). People have been eliminated from hiring processes and lost current jobs because of information or photos they posted online.

Drug prescreening is common in healthcare. A pre-employment drug test determines if a future employee uses illegal substances or abuses prescription medication. Getting the job will depend on passing the test. Some facilities have a random test policy, and any employee can be tested at any time without prior notice. Other facilities test when a problem is suspected.

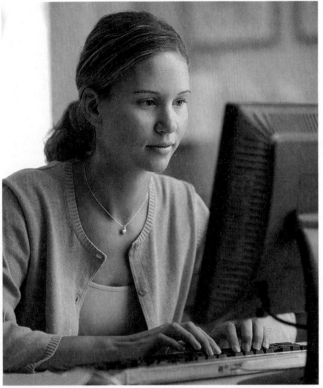

Blend Images/Shutterstock.com

Figure 10.38 Other people can see what you post online—even potential employers. Use good judgment about what you post to social media and elsewhere.

The Job Interview

The job interview is a conversation between you and a possible future employer. The employer wants to know if you will be a good fit for the healthcare facility, and you want to know if you will enjoy working at this facility. You should prepare for your interview by learning as much as you can about the business. Search online and talk with someone who works there. Read the job description carefully.

Consider your knowledge and experience. Then prepare examples you can talk about to illustrate your job qualifications. The employer will want to know you have the technical skill for the job but will also be looking for examples of your communication, teamwork, and problem-solving skills. Do not be afraid to talk about school classes, clubs, or athletic team experiences that demonstrate these skills.

Next, prepare a few questions to ask about the healthcare facility and the position. Avoid asking questions about pay and benefits before you have been offered the job. Be prepared to answer typical interview questions by practicing your answers at home. Know that some personal questions are considered illegal in the interview process (**Figure 10.39**).

Questions you might ask

What are the specific duties of this position?
What skills are most important in this position?
What are the working hours?
What do you consider your facility's most important assets?
How is your facility organized, and how does your department fit into the organization?
What types of services are provided at your facility?
What is the next step in your hiring process?

Questions to avoid asking until you have a job offer

How much does this job pay?
How much vacation time do I get each year?
Will I have to work overtime?
Do you pay bonuses?

NEVER ask:
Can I use your phone to call my ride?
I hated my last boss. How does management work here?
This job sounds pretty neat. How come the last person left?

Questions they might ask

What are your strengths/weaknesses?
What makes you a good employee?
Describe your work experiences.
Why do you want to work for this organization?
Tell me something about yourself.
What subjects did you enjoy in school and why?
How do you manage your time?
What does success mean to you?

Questions they cannot legally ask

Do you have children?
Are you single or married?
How old are you?
How tall are you? or How much do you weigh?
Do you have any disabilities?
How's your family's health?
Have you ever been arrested?
Do you go to church?
ANY question about nationality/color/religion

Goodheart-Willcox Publisher

Figure 10.39 Reviewing these four categories of questions will help you prepare for the question-and-answer format used in job interviews.

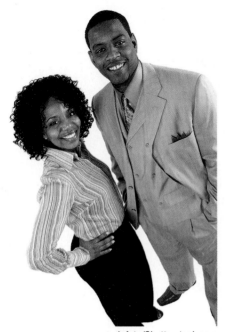

zulufoto/Shutterstock.com

Figure 10.40 Professional, business-like attire is required for a job interview.

Practicing proper **interview etiquette** includes choosing business-like attire (**Figure 10.40**). You are not dressing for a party or school. Avoid jeans, T-shirts, tank tops, tennis shoes, hats, and sunglasses. Limit jewelry, wear only light makeup, and avoid fake nails and colored nail polish. Since you will not know facility policy, limit visible piercings and tattoos.

People expect healthcare facilities to be clean, so make sure you are as well. Your hair, clothing, nails, hands, and shoes should all look clean and neat. Strong fragrances can be irritating and unpleasant when you are ill or have allergies. Demonstrate that knowledge by limiting your use of scented products.

Bring your career portfolio with you. Have extra copies of your résumé to leave with the employer. Arrive a few minutes early and alone. Do not bring a friend or family member with you because that person may make a bad impression. Turn off your phone or just do not bring it if you are tempted to check messages. Greet the interviewer with a smile and offer a firm, but not gripping, handshake. Do not feel offended if the person does not want to shake hands. Since the COVID-19 pandemic, people may be less comfortable with a handshake.

Your goal is to convince the employer you are the right person to hire. Let your appearance say you take work seriously and think this interview is important. Let your behavior say you will be easy to talk with, easy to work with, and a positive addition to the staff. Thank the interviewer for taking the time to speak with you.

Send a thank-you email the next day (**Figure 10.41**). If you want the job, express your interest again in the thank-you email. Add any information you forgot to provide during the interview.

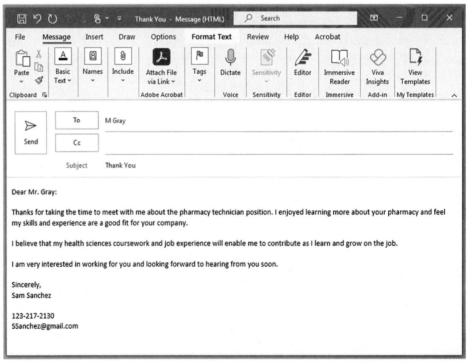

Goodheart-Willcox Publisher

Figure 10.41 Send a thank-you note within a day of your interview. An email is generally acceptable now, but you can also send a written note if you think that would be appreciated.

10.3-3 Succeeding on the Job

Congratulations, you got the job. You filled out several applications and had a few interviews. Finally, your work paid off, and you have a job. Breathe a sigh of relief and pat yourself on the back. Then take a deep breath and get ready to succeed on the job.

Steps to Success

You are probably thinking about all the benefits a job will bring you, such as your first paycheck, work experience for your résumé, and the chance to learn new skills. However, to succeed on the job, you will need to focus on meeting your employer's expectations. Your employer will evaluate your work and decide your future job responsibilities. This work experience will influence your future career opportunities.

Feeling nervous about your first day at work is normal. Get plenty of rest and allow extra time to get to work. On your first day, you may attend an orientation and complete employment forms. Your supervisor or a coworker may train you. During your first week, try to focus on these guidelines:

- Be on time. Show up to work on time and take only the time allowed for breaks and lunches.
- Dress appropriately and be well groomed every day. Learn the facility's dress code policies and follow them exactly.
- Learn as many names as possible. Focus on the names of your supervisor and coworkers in your immediate area.
- Listen closely and follow instructions. Show enthusiasm for and interest in learning your job duties. Ask questions if you do not completely understand a task.
- Work hard and be productive. Make a positive first impression by focusing on accuracy. Do your best work.

As you gain experience, learn any facility policies that affect your work. Demonstrate an increase in the work you complete and a decrease in the supervision you need. Show initiative and become self-directed in your work. Employers will expect you to complete your own job and then seek out other tasks you are qualified to complete while waiting for your next instruction. Workers who stand around waiting become a burden to their supervisors. Finally, be positive and enthusiastic. No one enjoys working with a complainer.

Learning your duties leads to job success, but working well with other people is just as important. You can expect to be assigned tasks you do not want to do. Since the work needs to be done, accept this and do a good job without complaining. Supervisors have different personalities and leadership styles. Make the effort to cooperate with your supervisor. Listen respectfully and follow through on your supervisor's suggestions (**Figure 10.42**).

Keep your eyes and ears open to observe how your facility operates. Observe the social interactions of your coworkers. Always be friendly and cooperative, but resist the temptation to gossip, repeat rumors, or take rumors seriously. In other words, avoid workplace drama.

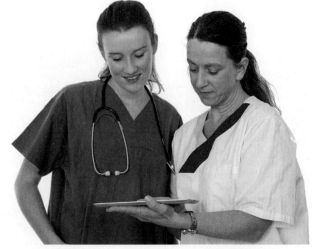

Firma V/Shutterstock.com

Figure 10.42 Listen respectfully and follow through on your supervisor's suggestions.

These job-success skills are just as important as knowing how to perform the tasks you are assigned. Ninety percent of job firings are due to personal reasons such as poor conduct and problems working with others. The following are the most common reasons employers give for firing employees:

- not showing up for work on a regular basis (especially problematic in the healthcare setting where patients require around-the-clock care)
- laziness on the job (taking long breaks, leaving the work area without reason, texting friends while working, or avoiding less pleasant job tasks)
- personality conflicts (not getting along or collaborating effectively with the supervisor or coworkers)
- violating facility rules (smoking, using alcohol, and ignoring safety regulations)
- **incompetence** (the inability to perform job tasks)

Professional Standards for Healthcare Workers

When you follow steps for success, you are practicing professional behaviors that apply to all workers. However, healthcare workers have an additional set of behaviors that support patient rights and advance directives. Following these professional standards protects you, your employer, and your patients.

As you study these standards, you will recognize some of the beginning and end-of-procedure steps you generally perform. Notice how these standards fulfill the ethical guidelines and legal obligations required in the delivery of healthcare.

- **Work within your scope of practice.** This means you will perform only the procedures for which you have been trained and are legally permitted to perform. You must refuse to perform any procedure for which you are not qualified. This is a legal obligation.
- **Use correct, approved methods for all procedures.** Follow the approved procedure manual for your place of employment. Complete procedures according to the methods learned in your training program.
- **Seek proper authorization for all procedures.** Your supervisor may authorize a procedure by assigning a patient care task to you. Some healthcare professionals, such as nurses, will receive verbal authorization from a physician or therapist. For other workers, such as those in a pharmacy, a written order provides authorization for a procedure.
- **Treat the correct patient.** Check the name or scan the barcode on the patient's wristband in the hospital setting. Verify the patient's birthdate and scan a photo ID at the clinic reception area. Address patients by name in all healthcare settings.
- **Obtain the patient's consent.** Patients have the right to refuse treatment. Adults ages 18 and older give their own consent, while parents or guardians give consent for minors. You must explain each procedure and get the patient's permission before proceeding. For some procedures, like surgery, written consent is required (**Figure 10.43**).

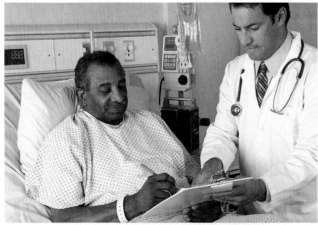

MBI/Shutterstock.com

Figure 10.43 Some healthcare procedures require written consent from the patient.

- **Maintain confidentiality.** Choose a private area when reporting patient information to your supervisor. Keep written records where unauthorized individuals cannot view them. Do not discuss patient information with other patients, your friends and family, or even other healthcare workers who are not part of the care team. Do not discuss medical information with parents of patients ages 18 and older unless the patient has signed a HIPAA release form.
- **Provide high-quality care at all times to all people.** Healthcare workers do not accept tips because the quality of healthcare is not based on payment. Patients receive high-quality care regardless of their social or economic status, race, age, religion, sex, nationality, or other protected category.
- **Report errors to your supervisor immediately.** Take responsibility for your actions by reporting errors and correcting your errors whenever possible. This is important because mistakes made by healthcare workers can affect a patient's health status.
- **Stay calm.** Even during an emergency, healthcare workers must remain calm to reassure patients and think clearly. When you are frustrated by the actions of a coworker, calm yourself before trying to resolve the problem. Follow the chain of command by reporting a problem to your supervisor rather than complaining to your coworkers.
- **Act with integrity.** Healthcare workers with integrity fulfill their legal and ethical obligations. They are loyal and dedicated employees. They provide empathetic care and maintain a positive attitude.

Understanding Your Paycheck

When you enter the world of work, you begin to earn an income. Knowing how your income is calculated is important. You will want to understand why money is taken out of your paycheck in the form of deductions.

 ## Healthcare Professions: Understanding Paychecks

Stacy could not wait to check her bank account on the first payday at her new job. After two weeks of work, she had carefully calculated her wages. She was excited to celebrate her hard work by splurging on a few special purchases. However, she received a shock when she looked at her deposit. It was less than half of the wages she had earned. She needed some information to help her understand her paycheck.

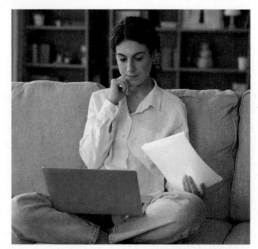

fizkes/Shutterstock.com

Every business has an established pay-period schedule. You may be paid each week, every other week, twice each month, or once each month. Pay will lag behind actual hours worked. This allows the business time to calculate the hours you have worked, determine the appropriate deductions, and prepare paychecks or transfer automatic deposits to employee accounts. In Stacy's situation, she was paid for the first week she worked. On her next check, she will receive pay for her second and third weeks of work. She will then have been working a total of four weeks.

Gross pay is the amount you will earn if you calculate the number of hours you have worked multiplied by your hourly wage. Your **net pay** (take-home pay) is that amount with deductions subtracted (**Figure 10.44**). At least two deductions will appear on your pay statement: Federal Insurance Contributions Act (FICA) and federal withholding tax.

The **Federal Insurance Contributions Act (FICA)** is a tax to fund **Social Security**. Social Security provides retirement income, disability, and survivors' benefits. It also supports Medicare, which is a health insurance plan for older adults and citizens with disabilities.

Federal withholding tax is a tax on your personal income. Taxes are payments citizens are required to make so governments can provide a wide range of public services. Some of these services include police and fire protection, libraries, parks and recreation, hospitals, schools, road maintenance, garbage collection, and unemployment insurance. Additional deductions may be made for state income tax, retirement savings plans, union dues, or insurance premiums.

Plan your spending based on net income rather than gross income. When you file your tax return, you may receive a refund if more money was withheld than required for the tax you owe. When you change jobs, you will usually receive one final paycheck from the facility at which you no longer work. That is pay that lagged behind the hours you actually worked, which appeared to be missing from your first paycheck.

My Statement

Employee Irma M. Payne	Employee Identification 123-45-6789	Check # 164	Net Pay $1,102.98
Employee Address 012 Canal Street Star Prairie, TX 74260			

	Pay Type– Gross Pay	Deductions	Current	Year-to-date
	$1,353.33	Federal Withholding	$106.00	$2,120.00
		State Withholding	$40.82	$816.40
		Fed OASDI/EE or Social Security	$83.91	$1,678.20
		Fed MED/EE or Medicare	$19.62	$392.40
		Medical	$0.00	$0.00
		401k	$0.00	$0.00
		Totals	$250.35	$5,007.00

Pay Period 10/12/2023 – 10/26/2023

Goodheart-Willcox Publisher

Figure 10.44 Deductions are listed on your pay statement so you can understand how your net pay amount was determined.

Continuing Personal and Professional Development

Healthcare is always changing. Successful healthcare workers adapt to workplace changes by pursuing personal and professional development activities. For example, Darius is studying the hospital's new protocols for environmental safety. Briana is taking a training class to operate the lab's new analyzer. Nan is completing training in the protection of human subjects during clinical research. Addison hired a personal trainer to improve her fitness level so she can handle the long hours of standing for her surgical technologist position.

These are all healthcare workers. While their jobs may be very different, they have one thing in common. They are lifelong learners. All of them have already completed the education and training needed for their healthcare position. Yet they continue to learn new skills to enhance their personal and professional development.

Personal and professional development includes all activities that increase your knowledge and skills. They can improve your employment opportunities and help you accomplish your goals. You could seek an advanced degree or attend a conference. You could participate in training sessions to learn new job skills or complete independent study. All these are part of personal and professional development. You might also request additional responsibilities at your current job. Addison became a preceptor who guides future surgical technologists during their clinical training at her hospital. If you choose to further your education, see if your employer will reimburse your tuition costs. For example, Janice is taking a medication training so she can deliver medications to residents (**Figure 10.45**).

Many healthcare workers must obtain additional training to maintain licensure or certification for the jobs they perform. For example, Janice just renewed her CPR certification. This is a requirement of her nursing assistant position at an assisted living facility. Professional development may lead to new job opportunities or job advancement. For example, Logan works as a medical assistant, but continues to attend college to achieve his long-term career goal of becoming a physician assistant.

Rapid advances in medical care and continuing changes in technology make professional development necessary for long-term success in healthcare careers. It keeps your knowledge current and helps you perform your job effectively. Learn to view your professional development as an opportunity to expand your knowledge and skills rather than a burden.

Membership in a **professional organization** supports your career development in several ways. First, professional organizations may offer certification and provide continuing education related to your specific career field. For example, the American Health Information Management Association (AHIMA) issues credentials such as the Registered Health Information Technician (RHIT) certification. Employers look for this certification when hiring health informatics workers. The association also promotes lifelong learning for health informatics professionals. They offer online training, specialty advancement institutes, workshops, and seminars.

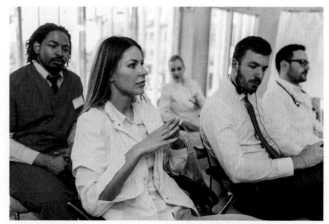

adriaticfoto/Shutterstock.com

Figure 10.45 Your employer may offer workshops and presentations that provide valuable professional development opportunities.

Continuing education credits offered by professional organizations allow you to renew your certification. A continuing education unit (CEU) typically represents one hour of instruction or other learning activity. CEUs can be granted for completing assignments or passing tests, as well as class or workshop attendance. Your certifying agency decides which CEUs count toward your license or certificate, so always check their requirements before taking a class or attending a workshop.

Second, membership in a professional organization provides a networking opportunity for learning about job openings and staying updated on changes in your work environment. These organizations provide information and encouragement to newer members of the profession. For example, AHIMA maintains an online networking tool its members can use to share, problem-solve, and stay informed on the latest trends in all HIM-related topics.

Third, organizations **advocate** for, or *promote*, your profession. They may publish journals and write public relations materials to inform consumers and government officials about the profession. Their members may serve on committees to establish best practices for your profession. Currently, AHIMA is working to improve the benefits of information technology in healthcare by focusing on the appropriate use of health data, privacy and security, and system interoperability.

Finally, professional organizations offer you an opportunity to develop your leadership skills (**Figure 10.46**). Volunteer to serve on a committee or become an officer of your organization. Your participation will broaden your knowledge and understanding of issues affecting your profession beyond your everyday work environment. At the same time, you will improve your teamwork capabilities and strengthen your management skills. This may lead to future job advancement.

Healthcare professionals can choose from a wide variety of professional organizations. Some are large and well known, such as the American Medical Association or the American Nurses Association. Many others are smaller and more specific, such as the Opticians Association of America or the Association of Surgical Technologists. Some organizations focus on serving special populations, such as Doctors without Borders or Healing the Children. The National Library of Medicine offers an extensive directory of organizations on its website. Search this list to locate health organizations and information about career fields that interest you.

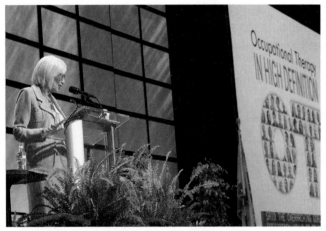

AOTA President Florence Clark, PhD, OTR, FAOTA, presiding over a meeting of the American Occupational Therapy Association in 2013. Copyright American Occupational Therapy Association. Used with permission.

Figure 10.46 Rising to a leadership position in a national organization can be a very rewarding experience. Here, the president of the American Occupational Therapy Association (AOTA) presides over an AOTA meeting.

Maintaining Your Career Portfolio

Your career portfolio should include the following items:

- a personal statement
- your résumé
- a personal data page
- a list of career contacts
- a sample application form and cover message
- copies of your current licenses and certificates

- a sample letter of resignation
- documentation of continuing education, awards, achievements, and service-learning activities
- letters of recommendation
- memberships in professional organizations (list and describe leadership roles)
- copies of career assessments

As you work in healthcare, keep your portfolio current. Add contact information for your employers and supervisors. Update your address and enter all your continuing education information. Keeping all your work records in one location simplifies the process of applying for a new job or renewing your license or certification. When you apply for a scholarship or a reimbursement of course costs, you will have all the information in one place.

10.3-4 Changing Jobs

Changing jobs is common, but always leave your job in a responsible manner. People change jobs for a variety of reasons, including improving pay or working conditions, moving to a new city, or dealing with company layoffs.

Leaving Your Job

When you are considering a job change, think carefully about your options and weigh the pros and cons of leaving your current job for another position. Resist the urge to leave your current place of employment immediately. Complete the search for a new job before leaving your current one. Save enough money to cover your expenses until you receive a paycheck from a new job.

 ## Healthcare Professions: Making a Job Change

Sophia worked at her first job during her junior and senior years of high school. Working part-time in a pharmacy was an excellent learning experience that fit right in with her plan to become a pharmaceutical sales representative. Now she was heading off to college in another city and needed to make a job change. She left her current job with the understanding that she could work during school breaks when she returned home. The pharmacy would be looking for workers to fill in for regular employees who were taking vacation breaks. In addition, her current supervisor recommended her to the supervisor at a pharmacy located in her college town. Eventually, she was able to work at that location as well. It was a win-win situation for Sophia.

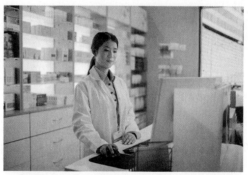

gorodenkoff/iStock/Getty Images Plus via Getty Images

Sometimes changes at work are out of your control. When problems arise, try to see the situation from the employer's view and avoid making decisions when you are upset.

For example, Jac was a hard-working employee at a medical equipment manufacturing company. Earning a regular paycheck was important because he had a large payment due each month for his new truck. When the number of orders for products decreased, his hours were cut. Jac was angry. "How can they do this to me?" he thought. "I need the money!" He stormed into his supervisor's office to complain. After learning that she could not give him more hours, he was still so angry that he quit his job. As a result, Jac has no income and no employer reference for seeking a new position.

Always leave a job under the best possible circumstances. Be sure to tell your employer before you tell your coworkers. Give at least two weeks' notice before leaving so your employer can find your replacement. If it is helpful and appropriate, offer to train your replacement. Give notice to your employer in person but also provide a **letter of resignation**. Your letter can be brief, but it should always be positive (**Figure 10.47**). Include the following elements in the letter:

- the date of your last day of work
- the reason you are leaving, stated positively
- a thank you for the opportunity to work at the facility
- a description of how the job has been a benefit to you

Sam Sanchez
4035 Starlight Ct.
Star Prairie, TX 74260

August 5, 2023

Shondra Lorenz
Pharmacy Manager
Star Prairie Pharmacy

Dear Shondra:

While I am happy to be heading to college, I am sorry that I will need to leave my job as a technician here at Star Prairie Pharmacy. My last day of work will be August 20.

This job has taught me so much about daily pharmacy operations. I feel well prepared for my college-level pharmacy courses because I was able to learn so much about the classifications of medications as well as their functions.

Thank you so much for being a caring boss and a great mentor. Completing an apprenticeship at Star Prairie was a fantastic learning experience.

Sincerely,

Sam Sanchez

Sam Sanchez

Goodheart-Willcox Publisher

Figure 10.47 Provide a letter of resignation in addition to talking with your employer in person. *What elements should a letter of resignation include?*

Keep a sample letter of resignation in your career portfolio to remind you of these elements when you prepare to leave a job.

Work just as hard in your last two weeks as you always have. Let your employer remember you as a good worker. Remain positive with your coworkers. You may work with these people again in a different job. Resist any temptation to complain about your current job or brag about your new one. Instead, thank your coworkers for their help and support before you leave.

Lesson 10.3 Review

 Complete the *Map Your Reading* graphic organizer for the section you just read.

1. Which of the following is *not* considered an employability skill? (10.3-1)
   A. Completing job interviews
   B. Following professional standards
   C. Completing a course of study
   D. Maintaining a positive attitude

2. Working with your healthcare _____ can contribute to success in locating job openings. (10.3-2)
   A. resumé
   B. technical skills
   C. network
   D. cover message

3. Healthcare workers protect patient rights when they follow _____ for the delivery of healthcare. (10.3-3)
   A. personal knowledge
   B. professional standards
   C. professional skills
   D. personal standards

4. As a new employee, your job success is determined by how well you meet the expectations of your (10.3-3)
   A. own self
   B. coworkers
   C. employer
   D. facility

5. When leaving a job, always give _____ notice and provide a letter of resignation. (10.3-4)
   A. one week's
   B. two weeks'
   C. one month's
   D. two months'

Chapter 10 Review and Assessment

Chapter Summary

10.1-1 Effective team members know the roles, responsibilities, and scope of practice for each team member. They maintain positive working relationships and respect the feelings and beliefs of each team member.

10.1-2 Interdisciplinary teams use collaboration to coordinate patient care. Primary care teams are found in clinic and community settings, while secondary care teams provide hospital services. Nursing teams use case manager, primary, functional, and team nursing models.

10.1-3 Healthcare supervisors may delegate tasks that are within a worker's scope of practice. Only the medical information important to a patient's care will be shared with team members. Patient information is not shared with friends or family members without the consent of the patient.

10.1-4 Team conflict is a disagreement or difficulty that occurs between two or more members of a team. Resolving team conflict requires positive communication and commitment to accomplishing the goals of the team.

10.1-5 All people assume leadership roles at various times in their work lives. While each person has a preferred leadership style, effective leaders model good work habits and learn new leadership skills to motivate and inspire others.

10.2-1 Vital signs measure essential body functions and include height, weight, body temperature, pulse rate, respiration rate, and blood pressure. Measurements of height and weight indicate normal/abnormal development. The mouth is a common site for taking a temperature. Wear gloves and use a sheath to cover the thermometer when taking an oral temperature. Pulse rate measures heartbeats. Respiration measures the number of breaths in one minute. Pulse oximeters measure the amount of oxygen in the blood. Blood pressure measures the force of blood pushing against the inside of the artery walls. Taking accurate vital sign measurements requires following procedure steps carefully. Report all abnormal vital signs measurements.

10.2-2 Vital signs measurements are documented in the patient's medical record. Electronic health record software will graph the measurements entered in the record. Hand charting and graphing requires more time and attention to detail.

10.2-3 The American Red Cross and the American Heart Association offer first aid training and certification. Basic first aid training and certification provides valuable skills for health science students.

10.3-1 Employability skills help workers acquire a satisfying job, succeed at that job, and advance in their chosen career path.

10.3-2 Use healthcare websites, job websites, and your healthcare network to locate an entry-level job. Write a cover message and a complete application form. Make all three neat and error-free. Learn as much as you can about the business and follow proper etiquette during a job interview.

10.3-3 Performing your job duties competently and working well with other people are important to job success. Healthcare workers also follow a special set of professional standards that support patient rights and protect both patients and workers.

10.3-4 Find your new job before leaving your current job. Give at least two weeks' notice. Provide a letter of resignation listing your last day of work and a positive reason for leaving.

Maximize Your Professional Vocabulary

1. **Taking on Terms.** Review the professional vocabulary list and select the five most difficult terms and the five most familiar terms. Use each of these terms correctly in a sentence. Then share your sentences with your classmates.

Reflect on Your Reading

1. Which job attribute most often causes young people to lose their jobs? If you chose attitude, you are correct. Discuss your job experiences with classmates. What job experiences support this data?

Review and Recall

1. Which of the following is the primary consideration for effective teamwork? (10.1-1)
   A. Coordination of tasks
   B. Scope of practice for each team member
   C. Personal strengths
   D. Positive attitude

2. The RN needs group leadership skills in (10.1-2)
   A. case manager nursing
   B. functional nursing
   C. primary nursing
   D. team nursing

3. Gene's doctor arrives at his hospital room to discuss his test results and treatment options. Which of these actions comply with HIPAA Privacy Rule guidelines? Choose all that apply. (10.1-3)
   A. Assume his wife will want to know the results and include her in the conversation.
   B. Ask visitors to wait in another area until the conversation is finished.
   C. Ask Gene who should be included in the conversation.
   D. Mention to a nurse assisting with Gene's appendectomy that Gene has a history of depression.

4. Alonzo and Quinn work on the same nursing team. Alonzo accuses Quinn of doing his care tasks and making him look bad to the rest of the team. Quinn claims he is just helping the team so they complete care tasks more quickly. What are the best steps to take to resolve this conflict? Choose all that apply. (10.1-4)
   A. Assign Quinn more care tasks than Alonzo
   B. Create guidelines for getting help with care tasks when needed
   C. Accuse Alonzo of intentionally working slowly to reduce his workload
   D. Ask the team leader for guidance

5. Alannah will lead a meeting for department heads to agree on budget requests for the coming year. Which leadership style is a good fit for this task? (10.1-5)
   A. Monitor
   B. Innovator
   C. Role model
   D. Facilitator

6. Along with temperature, pulse, respiration, and blood pressure, which of the following is frequently monitored with vital signs? (10.2-1)
   A. Oxygen saturation
   B. Electrocardiogram
   C. Complete blood count
   D. Lipid panel

7. When graphing temperature readings, which of these measurement locations is *not* flagged or noted? (10.2-2)
   A. Rectal
   B. Oral
   C. Temporal
   D. Tympanic

8. Which two agencies develop first aid training courses? (10.2-3)
   A. American Red Cross
   B. Local EMS departments
   C. Local healthcare facilities
   D. American Heart Association

9. Eric works as a nursing assistant and is frustrated because the facility keeps running out of gloves. He would like to barge into the manager's office and complain loudly but reports the shortage to his immediate supervisor instead. Which employability skill is he demonstrating? (10.3-1)
   A. Job competence
   B. Time management
   C. Chain of command
   D. Good attitude

10. You bring your career portfolio to a job interview. Which item is *not* in your portfolio? (10.3-2)
    A. Letters of recommendation
    B. Samples of projects that demonstrate skills
    C. Awards received
    D. HIPAA regulations

11. Anaya does not understand why she needs to wear gloves when taking an oral temperature. She can take a temperature without exposing her skin to the patient's saliva. Which professional standard should she follow in this situation? (10.3-3)
    A. Use correct, approved methods for all procedures.
    B. Work within your scope of practice.
    C. Seek proper authorization for all procedures.
    D. Provide high-quality care at all times and to all people.

12. Which of the following is *not* part of a letter of resignation? (10.3-4)
    A. Date of your last day of work
    B. A thank-you for the opportunity to work at the facility
    C. Your reason for leaving stated positively
    D. Your concerns about the facility's management policies

Build Core Skills

1. **Critical Thinking.** Describe a disagreement or conflict you have experienced recently. Using each guideline in Figure 10.11, rate your conflict-resolution behaviors on a scale of one to five. Five indicates that you followed the guideline, and one indicates that you did not. Draw conclusions about your conflict-resolution skills.

2. **Problem Solving.** Review the following situations. Make changes as needed so that they reflect an appropriate delegation of tasks.
    A. A nursing assistant tells a coworker to complete vital signs for his patients.
    B. A pharmacy technician answers a patient's question about the side effects of her medication.
    C. The supervising RN asks the nursing assistant to finish delivering medications to patients.
    D. A nursing assistant answers the phone and writes down the patient orders for a physician in a hurry to get to a surgical appointment.
    E. A physician assistant writes a prescription.
    F. An RN asks a fellow RN to administer medication to her patients while she responds to a patient emergency.

3. **Math.** Review the figure showing normal temperature ranges, found in the vital signs section of this chapter. Compare the oral, temporal, and axillary temperatures. Write a sentence that summarizes your findings.

4. **Critical Thinking.** Pretend you are interviewing for a job as a phlebotomist at your local medical clinic. Show your knowledge of etiquette as you answer the following questions:
    • What will you wear to the interview?
    • What will you take with you to the interview? What will you not take with you?
    • How do you greet the interviewer?
    • How do you end the interview, and what do you do after the interview?

5. **Reading.** Read the following statements taken from a job application form.

> **Please Read Before Signing:**
> The information that you provide on this application is subject to verification. Falsifications or misrepresentations may disqualify you from consideration for employment or, if you are hired, may be grounds for termination later.
> With my signature below, I certify that all information on this application is true, correct, and complete to the best of my knowledge and contains no willful falsifications or misrepresentations. I authorize all former employers to release job-related information they may have about me, and I release all persons or companies from any liability or responsibility for providing such information.
> Signature
> Date

You may be required to sign a job application form that looks like this. Will you know what are you signing? Define the following terms: *verification, falsification, misrepresentation, grounds for termination, certify, willful, authorize,* and *liability*. With these definitions in mind, rewrite the passage in your own words. Do you understand what you are signing?

6. **Speaking and Listening.** Refer to Figure 10.39 in your text. Select any three questions an interviewer might ask, prepare your responses, and practice answering the questions aloud. Be prepared to give your answers during a classroom interview simulation.

7. **Math.** Sue works as a pharmacy technician earning $15.00 per hour. She worked 40 hours during her two-week pay period. What is her gross pay? Calculate these deductions: federal withholding tax = 10%; FICA = 6.2%; Medicare = 1.45%. Subtract those deductions from her gross pay. What is her net pay?

8. **Critical Thinking.** List the professional standard that applies to each of these situations.
    A. A friend of your grandmother is a resident at the nursing home where you work. Your grandmother asks you what is wrong with her friend.
    B. As your patient is discharged from the hospital, he offers you a tip for the good care you provided.
    C. At lunch in the hospital cafeteria, your friend begins to tell you about the diagnosis and treatment for a specific patient who is not in your care.

Activate Your Learning

1. Review the guidelines for observing standard precautions and measuring vital signs. Then assemble supplies and follow the procedure steps in this chapter to practice measuring temperature, radial pulse, respiration, and blood pressure. Practice locating and measuring your own apical pulse.

2. **Portfolio Builder.** Create your personal data page. Include all the information listed in the text. Place your completed page in your career portfolio.

3. **Portfolio Builder.** Locate an advertisement for a health science job that interests you. Create a cover message using the sample in the text as a guideline. Place the completed letter in your career portfolio.

4. **Portfolio Builder.** Complete a sample job application form for practice. Follow the guidelines in the text. Place the completed form in your career portfolio.

5. **Portfolio Builder.** Write a sample letter of resignation using Figure 10.47 as a guide.

6. **Portfolio Builder.** Organize your career portfolio. Include all the items listed in the text.

Think and Act Like a Healthcare Worker

1. Read the following situations. Determine which leadership style would be most helpful to accomplish each task or activity. Justify your answer, especially if more than one style could apply to the situation. Refer to Figure 10.12 if needed.

   - The clinic needs more space, and a new addition is being proposed. The board of directors has asked Martina to spearhead the project and share potential plans.
   - Ashley works in a local nursing home. One of her coworkers is having difficulty relating to fellow employees and several residents. Ashley has offered to work with this person to make the work environment more positive for everyone.

2. Shannon has been working at an assisted living center for a month. She likes working with the residents, but getting along with the rest of the staff has been difficult. Shannon is the youngest worker at the assisted living center. Every time she asks a question, Shannon feels like the other employees are annoyed, and she thinks they are talking about her. Sometimes she just feels like giving up and quitting. Create a dos and don'ts chart with specific steps Shannon can take to improve relationships with her coworkers.

3. Liam graduated from college with a degree in biology and will start medical school in the fall.

He has been working as a personal care assistant at a medical clinic during the summer. One of his patients requires an ear cleaning. Liam has never done this procedure. He asks Jesse, a fellow personal care assistant, to do the ear cleaning procedure. Jesse, who has been trained and has performed many ear cleanings, completes the procedure while Liam observes. Review the professional vocabulary list for this chapter. Select two terms that relate to this scenario and explain how they apply.

Go to the Source

1. Locate three professional organizations related to a healthcare career of your choice. Research their websites to identify two professional development opportunities offered by each organization.

2. Review the leadership styles described in Figure 10.12. Identify your preferred leadership style. Select a HOSA leadership opportunity of interest to you. How will this experience demonstrate the skills, characteristics, and responsibilities of a leader?

HOSA Event Prep: Job Seeking Skills

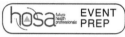

When Deandre was in high school, he participated in his school's health science program and found a passion for treating injuries. He was a part of the student sports medicine program. After high school, he worked to get his bachelor's degree and was accepted into a physical therapy program. During PT training, he worked with a group of physical therapists who specialize in sports medicine. When he graduated, he decided to apply to be a physical therapist for a group of sports medicine specialists. Even though this would be his first job, he used his experiences to highlight what he could offer to the group. His eagerness to learn and seek experiences impressed the group, so they hired him to work at their clinic.

Think About It

1. Explain how Deandre successfully interviewed for a physical therapy position and got hired for the job, even though he had recently graduated and had little job experience.

2. Imagine you are interviewing for a job at a company you really want to work for. What skills would you highlight, or what training do you think would benefit you for the position?

3. What skills do you think are most important for finding a job in healthcare? Why?

4. Do you think these job seeking skills can help you in the future with your career path? Why or why not?

Foundational Knowledge and Skills for Health Science

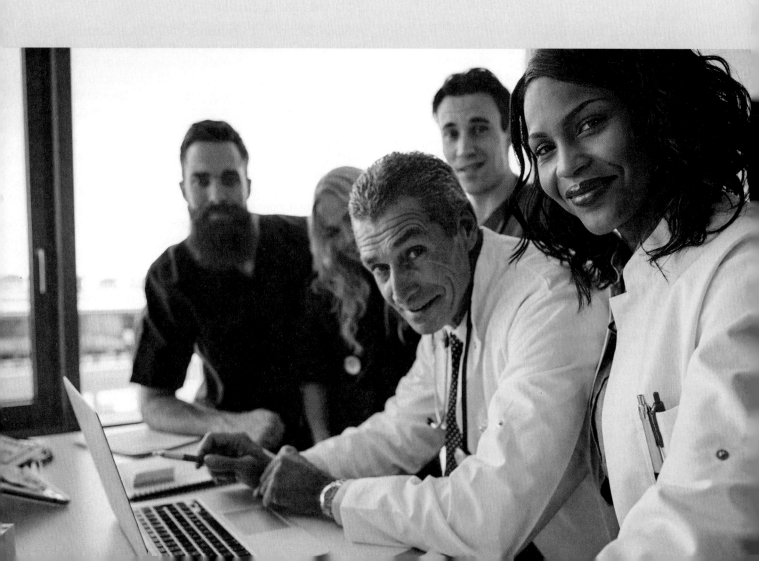

Healthcare Insider

P.M. Xiong, Bachelor of Science, Healthcare Management—Patient Care Coordinator

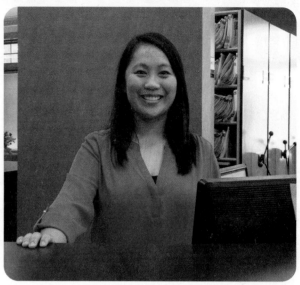

Photograph taken by Susan Blahnik

I find my job to be very rewarding! The opportunity to meet new people and get to know them is the best part of my job. Making patients feel comfortable while they are visiting the dental office is essential. Many people are afraid of the dentist due to bad experiences. While working at the dental office, I realized that I wanted to manage my own office one day. I made the decision to go back to school to continue my education while working full time. It was very difficult to work full time, go to school full time, and be a mom to two young kids. But it was all worth it in the end.

Discussion Activity

P.M. Xiong is a health informatics worker. She works with data and information every day. She finds her job rewarding because she can make patients feel comfortable at the dental office.

1. What will make a job rewarding for you?
2. How do you know that P.M. Xiong is committed to her career?
3. How much time and effort do you want to spend in preparing for your career?

Communication

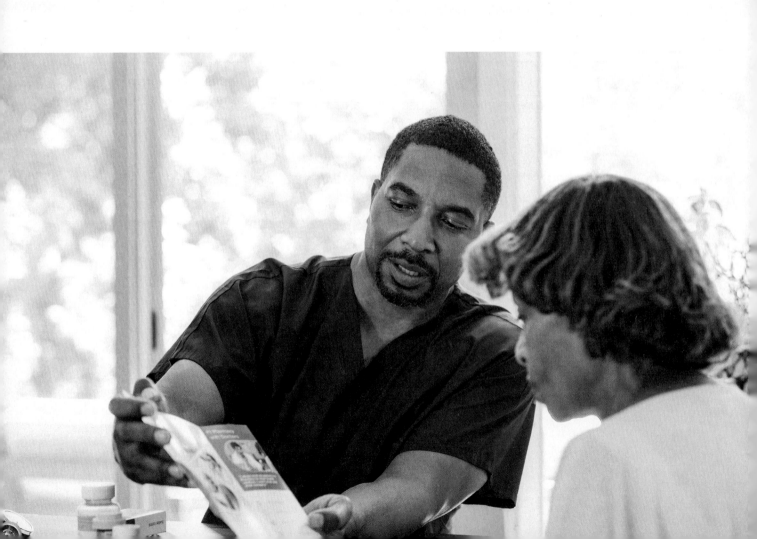

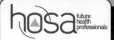

HOSA Event Prep: Prepared Speaking

Healthcare workers must have good communication skills. They must speak confidently to assure their patients and gain their trust. Speaking skills are a talent and a professional skill. Knowing what to say and when is important when providing care for patients. Healthcare workers may also deliver speeches or talks about health. HOSA—Future Health Professionals has an event that will help you practice your speaking skills. In the *Prepared Speaking* event, competitors give a speech on a HOSA theme.

Go to the HOSA website to learn more about the HOSA *Prepared Speaking* event. Find out the purpose of the event, what is involved in the event, and what knowledge is demonstrated in the event.

As you prepare for HOSA competitive events, be sure to check the website and talk with your HOSA advisor for the most up-to-date guidelines and procedures. Once you have learned about the *Prepared Speaking* event, answer the following questions:

1. How might participating in this event benefit you personally and your future career? Explain.
2. Are you interested in participating in this event? Why or why not?

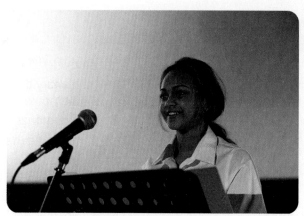

DGLImages/iStock/Getty Images Plus via Getty Images

Connect with Your Reading

Communication is a vital skill for all healthcare workers. Even simple errors can result in life- and health-threatening situations. Consider the occupations within each health science pathway. For each pathway, name an occupation and predict a problem that might occur due to an error in communication. For example, in the therapeutic pathway, a nursing assistant might record but fail to report a patient's elevated blood pressure.

Map Your Reading

Write the essential question for each lesson in this chapter. After reading each lesson, answer the essential question using main points from the sections under each subheading. Then list any unfamiliar terms and write definitions using your own words.

Speaking and Listening Skills

Learning Outcomes

After studying this lesson, you will be able to

11.1-1 identify the goal of the communication cycle and explain its elements.

11.1-2 summarize four common communication styles.

11.1-3 describe the four parts of the SBAR communication format.

11.1-4 articulate guidelines for conducting patient interviews that relate to professional protocols, the patient's age and stage of development, and your questioning techniques.

11.1-5 provide examples of telephone etiquette.

Professional Vocabulary

Essential Terms

assertive communication   a communication style characterized by confidence and consideration for others

communication   the act of sharing a message, thought, or idea so it is accurately received and understood

open-ended question   a question that requires more than a one- or two-word response

telephone triage   a system for assessing patient needs to determine if patients require emergency treatment, an appointment with a doctor, or self-care at home

Important Terms

active listening	feedback	SBAR system
communication style	patient interview	
etiquette	protocol	

Introduction

Often, communication mistakes are minor. Other times, however, they can lead to serious errors in patient care with devastating results for patients and their families. Patient information is shared with multiple healthcare workers during the process of diagnosis, treatment, and payment. Communicating with care and accuracy is critical to patient outcomes. Healthcare workers need effective communication skills for interacting with patients, patients' family members, and fellow healthcare workers (**Figure 11.1**).

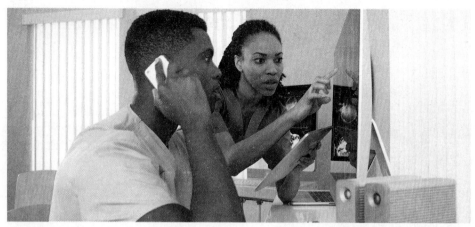

Rocketclips, Inc./Shutterstock.com

Figure 11.1 Healthcare workers must have excellent communication skills. *Why is it important to communicate patient information accurately?*

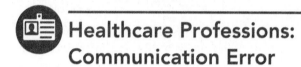

Healthcare Professions: Communication Error

Abby left work in a rush to make a late-afternoon appointment at the medical clinic. With a full-time job and three grandchildren to care for, she was always on the run. This is why she did not think much about the clicking noise and fluttery feeling in her ear when she first noticed it. Now, however, it was happening almost every day, and she wanted to make sure it was not a serious condition.

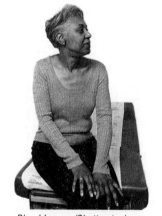

Blend Images/Shutterstock.com

After a short wait at the clinic, the medical assistant took Abby back to the exam room. Following some initial questions, she waited about 15 minutes for the doctor. When he arrived, the doctor looked in her ears and told her the audiologist (aw-dee-AH-luh-jihst) would give her a hearing test. Following the test, the audiologist took her back to the exam room to wait.

Abby assumed the doctor would return to discuss the hearing test with her. She waited about 30 minutes, but it was getting later and quieter in the clinic. When she noticed the lights turning off in the hallway, Abby left the room to find the assistants closing the office for the day. They were embarrassed about forgetting her and blamed the audiologist for not telling them she was waiting in the exam room. She headed home without any idea whether her symptoms were serious or not.

This was just a minor misunderstanding, a simple mistake in communication. Although this situation was frustrating for Abby, it was not a critical problem. She learned the next day that her hearing was fine, and stress caused her symptoms.

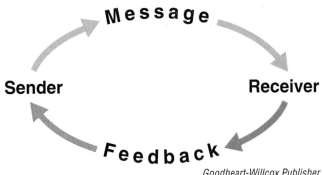

Message

Sender

Receiver

Feedback

Figure 11.2 The communication cycle is shown here. The sender begins the communication process, and the receiver provides feedback to show understanding of the message. *Why is feedback so important for communication?*

Communication Cycle

Communication is the process of sharing a message, thought, or idea. The key element in communication is understanding. Effective communication shares understanding between the person sending the message and the person receiving it. Communication flows in a cycle that eventually returns to the sender (**Figure 11.2**).

The sender begins the communication cycle by creating the message. Effective communicators consider their audience, or those receiving the message. The information being communicated must be organized, relevant to the receiver, and delivered in a format and language the receiver understands.

The sender determines the best format for a message. This can be a written form, such as a letter, memo, or report. Alternatively, the sender may choose spoken communication, as in a presentation, performance, conversation, or verbal instructions. The sender may choose to communicate in the form of pictures, charts, or video.

The sender also decides the best method for delivering the message. Messages can be delivered verbally in face-to-face conversation or by telephone. Written communications can be mailed, emailed, faxed, texted, or posted in a place where receivers can access the information. Websites, books, magazines, and brochures are only a few ways of distributing written material to a large group of people. The sender considers several questions when deciding the best method for delivering a message:

- How many people will receive the message?
- How close (in distance) is the sender to the receiver?
- Is it important to have a written record of the information?
- How quickly does the receiver need to have the information?
- How much formality is required for the message to follow the guidelines of protocol?

Protocol (PROH-tuh-kawl) refers to the appropriate conduct, etiquette, or procedures for communication. Healthcare communication follows many protocols for delivering accurate patient information to providers and insurers while preserving the privacy of health information.

The receiver hears or reads the message in whatever format and method the sender has chosen. However, communication does not end at this point.

The receiver also participates in the communication process. Paying attention to the message and the sender is not only courteous (KER-tee-uhs), or polite, but also necessary to the communication process. Unless the receiver understands the message and responds in some way, there is no communication.

The receiver responds to the message by providing **feedback** that closes the communication loop. Through feedback, the sender learns the receiver has understood the message as it was intended. If there is no feedback, the sender does not know if the message was even received, much less understood. When the receiver responds with questions, the communication continues in its cycle of sender-message-receiver-feedback until there is a clear understanding.

11.1-2 Communication Skills and Styles

Effective communication requires speaking and listening, reading and writing, and observation skills. It also requires familiarity with communication styles.

Listening Skills

Listening is the most neglected of all communication skills, yet it is the most vital skill for understanding a message. Because you can hear or process words at a much faster rate than they are spoken, your mind can easily wander while listening to someone. Good listeners practice **active listening**. They pay attention to and concentrate on understanding what a speaker is saying. When they notice a distraction, they purposefully refocus their attention on the speaker.

 ## Healthcare Professions: Poor Listening Skills

Jeff approached his boss, Kara, for some advice on how to complete his written report. Kara assured him she was happy to answer his questions. However, she was trying to complete her own reports before the final deadline. Since she was proud of her multitasking skills, she continued to type while attempting to answer Jeff's questions. After a couple of minutes, Jeff excused himself and went back to his office. It seemed clear to him that Kara was busy with her own work and did not have time to answer his questions. He did the best he could on his report, but he made a couple of mistakes that cost the company extra time and money to correct.

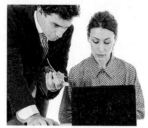

Feel Photo Art/Shutterstock.com

Obvious factors such as a noisy environment, phone call, or interruption from another person can interfere with good listening. An effective listener must also be alert for personal reactions that disrupt attention. For example, do you avoid listening carefully because you think you already know what the speaker is going to say? Do you focus on what you will say in response rather than paying attention to the speaker's message, especially if you disagree? Good listeners practice the following steps to improve not only listening, but also understanding a message:

- **Face the sender.** Maintain eye contact if this is comfortable for the speaker.
- **Eliminate, or at least limit, outside distractions.** Keep your attention on the speaker and not on your reaction to the speaker's words.
- **Wait for the speaker to finish before responding.** Do not interrupt or finish the speaker's sentence.
- **Be comfortable with a brief silence.** This allows the speaker to think for a moment and encourages the speaker to provide further information.
- **Keep track of information that needs clarification.** You can provide feedback by repeating the speaker's words. This is called reflecting. Alternatively, summarize what the speaker has said or ask further questions to improve your understanding.

Speaking Skills

Effective speaking requires more than a large vocabulary. The way you speak counts just as much as the words you use. Consider the following techniques used by effective speakers and practice them to improve your healthcare communication skills:

- **Always speak clearly and distinctly.** You may not realize you speak more softly at the beginning or end of your sentences or run words together. Maybe you talk very quickly, making it difficult to understand everything you are saying. Try recording your voice in conversation. How clear and distinct is your speech?
- **Speak to the listener.** Look at your audience, whether that is one person or a crowd of many people. Making eye contact will help you hold the attention of your audience and show your interest in them.
- **Carefully choose words your audience will understand.** Use correct grammar and pronunciation in the work setting. Formal language is appropriate in healthcare facilities and indicates worker competence (**Figure 11.3**).
- **Talk "with" your listener rather than "at" your listener.** Speak in a friendly and courteous tone of voice. Use positive language and keep your messages short and clear. Introduce a constructive idea rather than focusing on criticism. Then check for understanding by asking for opinions so the listener can provide feedback.

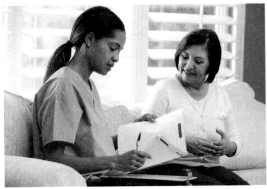

MBI/Shutterstock.com

Figure 11.3 Using correct grammar and pronunciation is especially important when giving information to patients who speak a language other than your own. *How can you effectively communicate with these patients?*

The Four Communication Styles

Tone of voice and nonverbal signals are just as important as the words people use. **Communication style** is a combination of all three of these aspects (**Figure 11.4**).

Communication Style Self-Assessment				
Style	**Passive**	**Aggressive**	**Passive/Aggressive**	**Assertive**
How it sounds	Apologetic; soft/tentative tone of voice	Loud, demanding tone of voice; uses "you" statements to accuse or humiliate others	Sarcastic tone of voice; says *yes* but means *no*	Firm tone of voice; uses "I" statements to express feelings and opinions clearly
How it looks	No eye contact; stooped posture	Tense and rigid posture; points fingers at others	Appears satisfied with decision, but will complain about it later	Direct eye contact; relaxed posture
How it feels	I'm shy; I'll go with the flow; my feelings aren't important.	My feelings are most important; I think I'm superior.	I'm uncomfortable saying what I think.	I think we are equal; we are both important.
How it turns out	I feel angry and resentful.	No one trusts me; they just avoid me.	I don't have real friends anymore.	I expressed my opinion even if it didn't go my way this time.

Goodheart-Willcox Publisher

Figure 11.4 This table shows communication styles and their characteristics.

Every person has a preferred communication style based on personality and environment, including individual experiences. Do you recognize your style in any of the following descriptions?

- **Passive.** You may be shy or very easygoing. You usually say, "I'll just go with whatever the group decides." You want to avoid conflict. This attitude creates problems because you are sending the message that your thoughts and feelings are not as important as those of other people. When you are too passive, you allow other people to disregard your wants and needs. That can make you feel angry and resentful, increasing your stress level.
- **Aggressive.** You may ignore the feelings and opinions of others. You may even humiliate and intimidate others. While you appear to get what you want, your aggression can destroy trust. Others may avoid you or oppose your ideas because they do not trust you.
- **Passive-Aggressive.** You may say *yes* when you want to say *no*. You may be sarcastic or complain about others behind their backs. Feeling uncomfortable about stating your needs and feelings can lead to passive-aggressive behavior. This communication style damages relationships and makes it harder to meet goals.
- **Assertive.** You state your opinions and feelings clearly. You stick up for your rights and needs but respect the rights of others in the process. This style tells people your needs and opinions are important. Assertiveness is a healthy communication style because it is effective and diplomatic, or tactful. It can help you manage stress levels.

How can you recognize **assertive communication**? People who use assertive communication make eye contact. They stand up straight and look like they are ready to talk and listen. They give their opinions, but they do not try to argue and do not become mean or sarcastic. They listen to criticism and consider it carefully, but they do not let it make them feel inferior or inadequate. They understand that being assertive includes respecting the opinions of others and not always getting what you want.

Healthcare Professions: Passive Communication

Nadia, a registered nurse at the hospital, was worried about her patient, Mr. Benning. Instead of feeling better after his surgery, his pain was increasing. He did not look quite right either. Nadia believed something was seriously wrong with her patient. She decided to call the doctor.

"Hello, Doctor Black," she said. "This is Nadia, one of the nurses. Mr. Benning is in pain that he says is at 10. I just don't feel right about him."

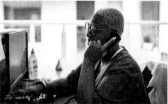

FG Trade/E+ via Getty Images

The doctor replied that Nadia should increase the dose of Tylenol® for Mr. Benning.

Now Nadia was frustrated. She really wanted the doctor to examine her patient, but what could she do?

Do you recognize Nadia's style? Because she used a passive style, Nadia did not communicate her concerns and opinions about her patient's needs. She did not even tell the doctor that she wanted her patient to be evaluated for a serious complication.

Communicating assertively in a healthcare environment increases the level of patient care. Several healthcare facilities have developed training programs to teach assertive communication skills to employees.

11.1-3 SBAR Communication System

The **SBAR system** is a method that helps healthcare workers communicate with each other more clearly. The system creates a standardized communication format that is very useful for reporting changes in a patient's status. SBAR is an acronym that stands for *Situation*, *Background*, *Assessment*, and *Recommendation*. Each term means something specific in a healthcare setting:

- **Situation.** What is currently happening? Begin by identifying yourself, your occupation, and your location. Then identify your patient by name and date of birth. Describe the patient's current status and your reason for communicating.
- **Background.** What are the circumstances leading to this situation? Give a brief summary of relevant past medical history. Provide details of the patient's status, including vital signs, pain scale, and level of consciousness.
- **Assessment.** What is the problem? Note any signs that are outside the normal ranges, your impressions, and any additional concerns.
- **Recommendation.** What should be done to correct the problem? Explain what you want to happen and how soon you think it should happen. Suggest possible actions and then clarify your expectations.

 Healthcare Professions: SBAR System

The SBAR system helps healthcare workers communicate with each other. Using SBAR to communicate with the physician, Nadia might communicate her concerns more clearly:

Situation. Dr. Black, my name is Nadia. I'm the RN on 6 west caring for your patient, Mr. Benning, DOB 12/06/51. He is here for a GI bleed. He is currently complaining of chest pain, looks pale, and is sweating profusely.

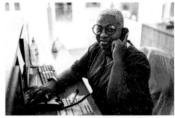
FG Trade/E+ via Getty Images

Background. Mr. Benning received two units of red blood cells this morning. At 3:00 p.m., he had blood drawn, and his hematocrit (hih-MA-tuh-krit) is 31. His vital signs are BP, 88/52; pulse, 120; respiration, 24. His pain is a 10 on a scale of 10. I just administered 2 L/min oxygen by nasal cannula (KAN-yoo-luh).

Assessment. It looks like he may have internal bleeding or an MI (myocardial infarction), but I think additional tests are needed to know for sure.

Recommendation. I would like an order for an EKG, a blood test to check hemoglobin and hematocrit, medication for increased pain, and I need you to evaluate him without delay. What questions do you have for me?

Learning to communicate assertively has many benefits. It reduces anxiety and increases self-esteem. It helps you achieve your goals and make decisions more easily. Most importantly, communicating assertively in a healthcare setting by using a system such as SBAR can improve patient outcomes.

11.1-4 Interviewing a Patient

A **patient interview** is useful when taking a patient's medical history. During interviews, you want patients to feel comfortable about explaining their symptoms. When healthcare workers conduct a patient interview, they follow a specific set of protocols.

Following Professional Protocols

Successful interviews begin with courtesy. Knock before entering the exam room. Remember that patient interviews are conducted in private. Greet your patient using a formal title, such as *Mr. Soto,* and introduce yourself by giving your name and job title. Use first names only when requested. Limit interruptions and be prepared with your forms and questions. Avoid going straight to the computer and barely looking at the patient.

The next steps in the interview process help build trust. Use your positive nonverbal communication skills. Sit so you face the patient at eye level and make eye contact as the patient speaks. Patients need to feel that you understand their symptoms. If you are not looking at them as they are talking, you will be perceived as not listening, even if you have heard every word. Keep a distance of 2 to 4 feet to avoid invading the patient's personal space.

Show respect by keeping an open mind about what the patient tells you. Differences in culture or experience can impair effective communication with your patient. Examine your own values and beliefs to minimize any personal biases that could interfere with the interview. Healthcare workers apply a "therapeutic use of self." This means they remain nonjudgmental as they use their interpersonal skills to help their patients (**Figure 11.5**). Avoid talking about your own problems. Professional healthcare workers set aside their own difficulties when they care for others.

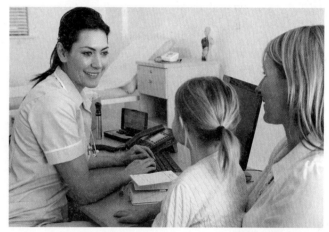

MBI/Shutterstock.com

Figure 11.5 Use positive body language and remain nonjudgmental during a patient interview.

Considering the Patient's Age and Stage of Development

Healthcare workers use their knowledge of lifespan development to interact effectively with patients of all ages. They might provide toys for a preschooler who wants to touch everything in the exam room. Offering to let a child help by holding bandages and speaking to the child at eye level allows the child to feel more in control while you treat an injury. Adolescents may want to speak privately with their healthcare provider and will appreciate the opportunity to make choices about their own care as ethical and legal guidelines allow. Adults need clear explanations that do not make them feel childish. Because they are busy, a printout of the treatment plan is helpful. Older adults may gradually be losing their independence and will want to continue making their own healthcare decisions as long as possible. Reviewing the stages of human development will help you learn more about the needs of patients throughout their lives.

Asking Open-Ended Questions

Communicating with patients involves using techniques that encourage a patient to share information. Always begin by asking **open-ended questions**. Of course, if a patient has trouble breathing or speaking, you will want to receive a short response, but more information is beneficial in most patient interactions. For example, if you ask, "Would you say you are in good health?" the patient will reply *yes* or *no*, and the conversation will be over. If you say, "Tell me about your health," the patient is more likely to name a problem or give a description.

Avoid asking questions that begin with the word *why*. Perhaps you are caring for a patient who finds it difficult to communicate. While discussing how he feels about his illness, he stops talking mid-sentence. If you ask, "Why did you stop?" he is likely to reply, "I don't know," and your conversation will be over. If instead you acknowledge his feelings by saying, "You seem uncomfortable," he will see that you are empathetic and may talk further about his feelings.

Rephrasing what the patient has said is another method for encouraging conversation. If a patient says, "I don't know how I'll be able to pay for this hospitalization," try rephrasing this in the form of a question, such as, "You're worried about finances?" This shows you are listening and encourages further communication.

Address sensitive topics at the end of the patient interview, after you have built a connection with the patient. Practice asking sensitive questions before the interview so you can ask them calmly with a patient. You will become more comfortable with practice, and this will make patients more willing to voice problems and concerns (**Figure 11.6**).

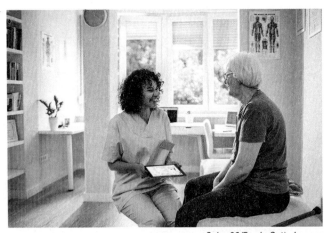

Geber86/E+ via Getty Images

Figure 11.6 You can learn more about a patient's health concerns by asking open-ended questions and showing sensitivity.

The Patient Interview Process

Follow these steps as you complete a patient interview:

1. Gather your tools. These may include forms, a computer tablet, a pen, and equipment for measuring vital signs.
2. Introduce yourself and state your role at the healthcare facility. For example: "Hi, Mr. Soto. I'm Alexa, Dr. Black's medical assistant. I would like to ask you a few questions to update your medical history, and I want to take your vital signs before the doctor sees you."
3. Verify the patient's name and birth date. Then update the patient's medical history. Note any surgeries or family medical history that might mean a patient has more risk for a particular medical condition.
4. Record a list of medications the patient is currently taking, including vitamins and herbal supplements. This allows the physician to check for drug-related symptoms or drug interactions. For each medication, list the amount, dosage, frequency, and time of day the medication is taken. Spell out each medication to make sure you have the correct one. A patient may give you a list of medications, but you should verify each item on the list to make sure it is current.

5. Measure and record vital signs.
6. Ask the reason for the patient's visit. This is the time to use your open-ended questions. Do not rush. If you give your patient time to think, you will receive answers that are more reliable. Record the patient's responses in detail. If your computerized record uses a drop-down menu, make sure the correct symptoms have been checked. Then add details in the comment section.
7. Review the patient's information and reason for seeing the doctor. This will verify your data and act as a polite ending to the interview. Let the patient know how soon to expect the doctor and excuse yourself, closing the door as you exit.

11.1-5 Communicating by Telephone

Patients often use the telephone to contact their healthcare facility. Healthcare workers strive to create a positive experience for callers. This earns goodwill for your facility. More importantly, however, your telephone communication skills will affect health outcomes for patients as you quickly connect them to the correct healthcare resource, provide clear directions, or even respond to a medical emergency.

Telephone skills begin with polite behavior called **etiquette** (EH-tih-keht). In healthcare facilities, telephone skills also include screening, prioritizing, and documenting calls, tasks that all become part of healthcare delivery.

Courteous Conversation

The increasing use of social media means individuals do not practice the art of conversation very often. A positive telephone conversation is more challenging than a face-to-face encounter. This is because you cannot observe nonverbal cues such as facial expressions or body language. As a result, your verbal skills become even more important.

Answer the phone with a smile (**Figure 11.7**). Smiling makes your tone of voice more cheerful and positive. Remember that your tone of voice sends a strong signal in a phone conversation. You may be very busy when the telephone interrupts your work, but you should not let your irritation come through in your voice. Instead, use a pleasant tone that is low in pitch. Speak at a moderate speed and more slowly when giving directions. Practice pronouncing words clearly and distinctly since people cannot read your lips. Eating, drinking, and chewing gum will ruin your conversation. Avoid them when you communicate by phone.

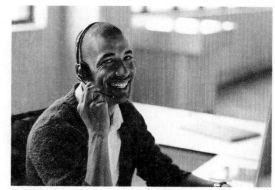
kuplcoo/E+ via Getty Images
Figure 11.7 When talking on the phone, try smiling to convey a cheerful and positive attitude.

Basic telephone etiquette requires you to answer the phone as soon as possible. You should answer no later than the third ring. Remember, you are working in a healthcare facility, and this may be an emergency call. Use your facility's standard greeting to identify your facility and yourself. This lets callers know they have dialed correctly. A typical greeting might be, "Hello, Sun View Medical. This is April, the medical assistant. How may I help you?" In larger facilities, automated messages will guide the direction of a call and provide a direct-dial number for emergency calls.

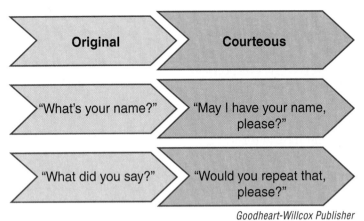

Original	Courteous
"What's your name?"	"May I have your name, please?"
"What did you say?"	"Would you repeat that, please?"

Goodheart-Willcox Publisher

Figure 11.8 These are some examples of using courteous language.

Use courteous phrasing when asking questions. "How may I help you?" is better than "What do you want?" Compare the questions in **Figure 11.8** to note the difference courteous phrasing can make.

As a routine courtesy, you should thank callers before you hang up. Allow them to hang up first to be certain they have finished speaking.

Courtesy also counts when using the "hold a call" feature on a telephone. First, make sure the call is not an emergency or another physician calling to speak to one of your physicians. Then ask for permission before placing a caller on hold. Take a callback number and a message if the person cannot remain on hold.

While this sounds simple, in a healthcare setting, you will often handle many phone calls and patients at once. Remember to check back every minute or two with the caller who is on hold. If you cannot connect the call, continue to ask if the caller wants to remain on hold or leave a callback number.

Above all, you should understand how to use the telephone equipment in your office properly. There is nothing more frustrating than waiting on hold, being disconnected, and having to start the call process all over again. If you mistakenly disconnect a patient who is on hold, call the person back and apologize before completing the call.

Call Screening and Telephone Triage

Every call received at a healthcare facility must be screened to determine who will respond to the caller. Most calls involve scheduling an appointment, which a medical assistant or personnel working at a centralized appointment desk will handle. Calls from other physicians or from the physician's family are handled according to the physician's preferences. You will need to learn these preferences to manage calls appropriately. Follow your facility's policy for responding to calls from salespeople or insurance companies. In a smaller office, the medical assistant may respond to these calls. In a larger facility, they may be transferred to a specific department such as *Business Services*.

Approved personnel, such as medical assistants or nursing staff members, can manage routine patient requests for prescription refills ordered by the physician, test results, and progress reports from other healthcare personnel. Typically, a physician will review the updated information in a patient's chart and speak with patients who do not report satisfactory progress. However, you should always tell the physician about calls in which the patient reports new symptoms or a seriously worsening condition. Do not wait for the doctor to discover this information in the patient's chart.

When a patient calls to report symptoms of illness, you must be able to tell the difference between a panicked caller and a medical emergency. To evaluate the different calls coming into a healthcare facility, you will need to use **telephone triage** (TREE-ahj). In a clinic setting, a specific triage nurse may handle triage, or it may be part of the medical assistant's duties (**Figure 11.9**).

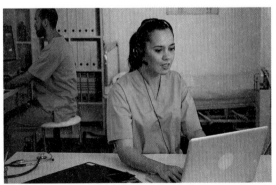

DC Studio/Shutterstock.com

Figure 11.9 A triage nurse questions callers to determine whether a medical emergency exists. *Why might clinics employ a triage nurse as well as a medical receptionist?*

The process of triage includes asking a series of questions to determine whether emergency medical personnel should be called or if the patient can wait to see the physician at the next available appointment time. You will be most effective in triaging calls if you remain calm as you learn what happened and what symptoms the patient is experiencing. The following conditions represent true emergencies and require immediate care:

- chest pain or any other severe pain
- difficulty breathing
- loss of consciousness
- a fever above 102°F
- heavy bleeding
- severe vomiting or diarrhea

Privacy rules guide the phone conversations of healthcare workers. Use care when discussing patient information so others cannot overhear it. Know when and with whom patient information may be shared. For example, the patient must provide permission for information to be shared with family members. In some facilities, it is a breach of privacy to acknowledge that a specific person is even a patient. Be cautious about sharing test results over the phone. Is this within your scope of practice? Some facilities designate specific staff members to communicate test results. In some cases, the physician will make these calls.

Documenting Phone Conversations

Since all phone communication with patients must be documented in their medical records, you will need an efficient system for recording messages and conversations. A phone message should include at least the following information:

- caller's name
- date and time of call
- phone contact number for the caller
- a short description of the caller's question or concern
- person to whom the message is directed
- your name or initials so the message recipient can check with you for questions (**Figure 11.10**)

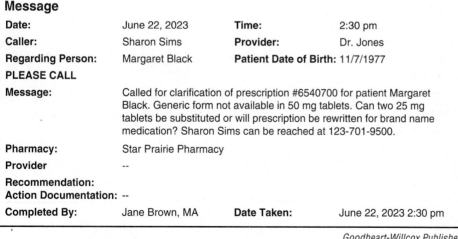

Message			
Date:	June 22, 2023	**Time:**	2:30 pm
Caller:	Sharon Sims	**Provider:**	Dr. Jones
Regarding Person:	Margaret Black	**Patient Date of Birth:**	11/7/1977
PLEASE CALL			
Message:	Called for clarification of prescription #6540700 for patient Margaret Black. Generic form not available in 50 mg tablets. Can two 25 mg tablets be substituted or will prescription be rewritten for brand name medication? Sharon Sims can be reached at 123-701-9500.		
Pharmacy:	Star Prairie Pharmacy		
Provider	--		
Recommendation:			
Action Documentation: --			
Completed By:	Jane Brown, MA	**Date Taken:**	June 22, 2023 2:30 pm

Figure 11.10 One efficient method for recording phone messages is shown here.

When a patient calls the healthcare facility, you will enter the message you took into the patient's chart. When you contact a patient, write a summary of your conversation to document the call in the patient's chart. Remember that the medical record is a legal document of the care provided. As a result, you should be concise, accurate, and complete when documenting your phone calls with patients (**Figure 11.11**).

Message

Date:	June 22, 2023	**Time:**	2:30 pm
Caller:	Judy Bleeker	**Provider:**	Dr. Jones
Regarding Person:	Judy Bleeker	**Patient Date of Birth:** 2/3/1990	

PLEASE CALL

Message: Pt called to cancel appt for ear recheck. Says she is feeling better. Advised to continue medication and keep appt to make sure eardrum is normal. Patient says, "That seems like a wasted trip. I'm not coming." Advised Dr. Brenner. Judy Bleeker can be reached at 456-812-0611.

Pharmacy:	--		
Provider	--		
Recommendation:			
Action Documentation:	--		
Completed By:	Jane Brown, MA	**Date Taken:**	June 22, 2023 2:30 pm

Message

Date:	June 22, 2023	**Time:**	2:30 pm
Caller:	Judy Bleeker	**Provider:**	Dr. Jones
Regarding Person:	Judy Bleeker	**Patient Date of Birth:** 2/3/1990	

PLEASE CALL

Message: Pt called to cancel appt. Judy Bleeker can be reached at 456-812-0611.

Pharmacy:	--		
Provider	--		
Recommendation:			
Action Documentation:	--		
Completed By:	Jane Brown, MA	**Date Taken:**	June 22, 2023 2:30 pm

Goodheart-Willcox Publisher

Figure 11.11 *Which of these entries was probably made shortly after the phone call? Which entry provides a better defense in a court case?*

Lesson 11.1 Review

 Complete the *Map Your Reading* graphic organizer for the section you just read.

1. The communication loop closes when the receiver provides _____ to the sender. (11.1-1)
   A. messages
   B. responses
   C. information
   D. feedback

2. Because it is direct, but still tactful, _____ is considered the healthiest style of communication. (11.1-2)
   A. passive
   B. aggressive
   C. passive-aggressive
   D. assertive

3. Which of the following is *not* a part of the SBAR communication format? (11.1-3)
   A. Situation
   B. Background
   C. Assessment
   D. Referral

4. Use _____ questions when interviewing patients to encourage them to share more information about their symptoms. (11.1-4)
   A. open-ended
   B. direct
   C. meaningful
   D. specific

5. A pleasant tone, courteous phrasing, and clear pronunciation are all parts of telephone (11.1-5)
   A. skills
   B. etiquette
   C. performance
   D. screening

6. Healthcare workers _____ phone calls to identify medical emergencies. (11.1-5)
   A. address
   B. answer
   C. triage
   D. redirect

Reading and Writing Skills

Learning Outcomes

After studying this lesson, you will be able to

11.2-1 state the purpose of technical communication and relate the steps in reading and writing a technical document.

11.2-2 practice appropriate format and etiquette for business letters, memos, and emails.

11.2-3 identify examples of scientific communication and list three guidelines for scientific writing.

Professional Vocabulary

Essential Terms

scientific communication a type of technical communication used by scientists and nonscientists to provide information and promote understanding

technical reading a skill used to comprehend science, business, or technology publications

technical writing a type of writing used in the workplace to inform or persuade a specific audience

Important Terms

business letters	memorandums	proposals
clear writing	objective writing	recommendation reports
correspondence	precise writing	target audience

> **? ESSENTIAL QUESTION**
>
> *What reading and writing skills do healthcare workers need for effective communication?*

Introduction

Can you think of a healthcare job that does not require reading? Reading and comprehension skills are vital to workplace success. Effective employees not only read, but also understand the memos, reports, directions, and records associated with healthcare documentation and procedures.

Effective writing is clear, concise, and accurate. When writing, you must organize your thoughts and present your ideas in a logical manner. In a healthcare setting, the accuracy and clarity of a written document can affect the life and well-being of patients.

11.2-1 Technical Communication

The world of work requires the ability to read technical materials. Workplace reading includes various technical documents, including correspondence, instruction manuals, government regulations, and professional journals. Product labels, records, reports, and proposals also require technical reading skills (**Figure 11.12**). In addition to these, workplace writing can involve marketing materials, patient education brochures, and the guidelines for many different procedures. Technical communication helps workers accomplish tasks by providing the necessary information.

In addition, technical communication focuses on new technologies. Healthcare workers study the documents that explain technological advances so they can use new equipment and procedures to improve healthcare. Technical communication also informs providers about new developments in the field of healthcare and the progress of experiments related to the diagnosis and treatment of disease.

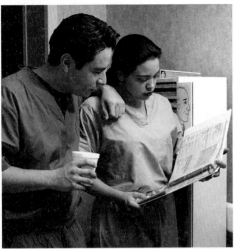

Creatas/Creatas/Thinkstock

Figure 11.12 Healthcare workers use technical reading skills to understand and interpret manuals, procedures, and other materials.

 ## Healthcare Professions: Reading and Writing

Salina was feeling desperate. As the dietary manager at a long-term care facility, her job duties included reading the newly published nutrition guidelines. Once she read the guidelines, Salina would have to write a set of instructions for her staff to follow as they prepared healthy snacks, or nourishments, for the residents. There was so much information to read! How could she put all that information into a single set of instructions? She realized that she needed some help to complete this task. Salina needed to learn the skills for technical reading and technical writing.

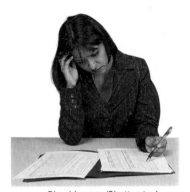

Blend Images/Shutterstock.com

Reading Technical Documents

When you read technical documents, you must focus on understanding the facts and logic presented. Technical documents require a special reading strategy because they are filled with detailed information and use technical terms specific to their topic. Taking the time to learn **technical reading** skills allows you to keep up with the latest advances in healthcare. These skills also improve patient and worker safety as you handle hazardous chemicals, administer patient medications, and operate new equipment.

Technical reading requires attention and concentration. To read successfully, select the time of day when you are most alert. Pick a location with few distractions, such as a quiet conference room at work or a quiet corner of the library. Silence your cell phone to avoid interruptions. Your own bedroom may offer peace and quiet, but do not get too comfortable. Relaxing on your bed to read technical material usually leads to falling asleep. Know your preferences regarding background music: does it distract you or help you focus?

Read technical documents slowly. They are packed with information, and you will miss the details if you read quickly. When you lose concentration, you may continue to read, but you will not remember the content. You may need to pace yourself and take short breaks from your reading about every 15 minutes. Summarize what you have just read before continuing.

As you read technical documents, do not skip the graphics. Tables, charts, graphs, and even photographs provide detailed information you will need to accomplish your task or solve your problem. Once you have finished reading a document, consider doing some additional reading from other sources to clarify your understanding.

Look more closely at Salina's task of providing instructions for making healthy snacks. Salina needs to read the revised *Dietary Guidelines for Americans*. She locates the guidelines on the United States Department of Agriculture (USDA) website. The full document is available online, but it is 149 pages long. Salina follows these steps for reading a technical document:

1. **Read with a purpose.** Salina's purpose is to develop a set of instructions for her staff to follow when preparing healthy snacks for residents. She needs to know what foods and beverages will promote good health and what foods and beverages need to be restricted or omitted from the residents' diets.

2. **Scan the entire document.** Salina begins the scanning process by reviewing the table of contents and reading the executive summary. The executive summary is helpful because it makes key recommendations about foods to reduce in the diet and foods and nutrients to increase in the diet. She takes notes on the key recommendations that affect her residents.

3. **Use the table of contents, headings, and index to locate specific information.** Returning to the table of contents, Salina selects two chapters for focused reading (**Figure 11.13**).

4. **Take notes about important ideas.** Salina carefully reads each chapter. She takes frequent breaks and summarizes important information in her own words as she takes notes.

5. **Learn the meanings of unfamiliar words.** Salina studies the "Terms to Know" sections in the document. She makes a list and looks up the meanings of unfamiliar terms.

6. **Paraphrase by writing important information in your own words.** Finally, Salina reviews her notes and selects the main information her staff needs to know (**Figure 11.14**).

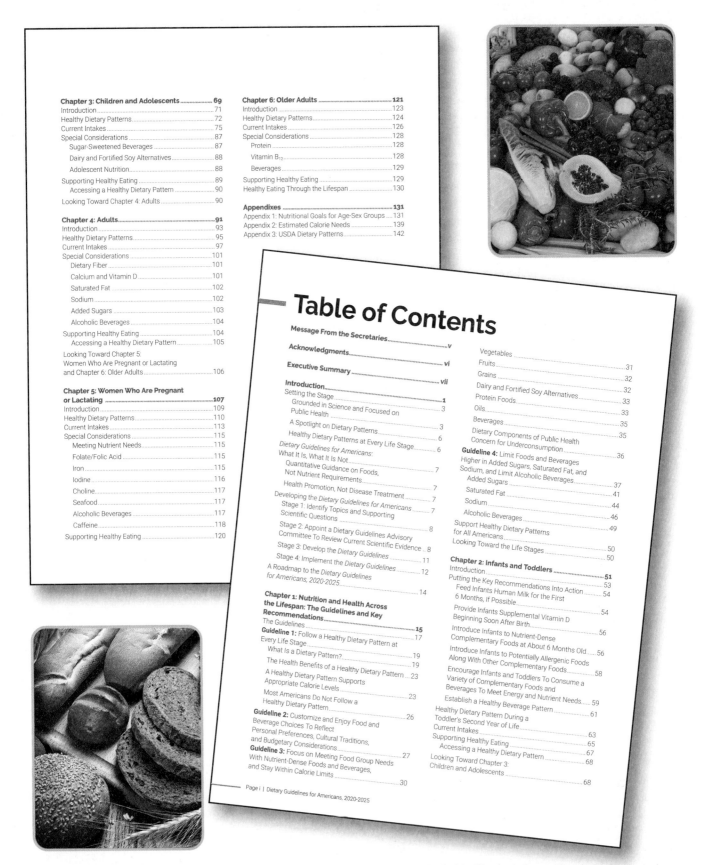

Table of Contents

Page i | Dietary Guidelines for Americans, 2020-2025

Courtesy of the USDA; Food images: Tischenko Irina/Shutterstock.com, Brian Chase/Shutterstock.com

Figure 11.13 The table of contents from the USDA guidelines that Salina reviewed. *If you were Salina, which two chapters would you choose for focused reading?*

Copyright Goodheart-Willcox Co., Inc.

Dietary Guidelines

Chapters 1 and 6	Terms to clarify
Snacks should contribute to a healthy dietary pattern.	Dietary pattern
Limit foods and beverages that are higher in added sugars, saturated fat, and sodium.	Nutrient dense
	Added sugars
Reduce added sugars in beverages, snacks, and desserts.	Saturated fats
Limit refined-grain desserts and sweet snacks.	Hydration status
Limit saturated fats and trans fats because they increase the risk of cardiovascular disease.	
Choose low-fat dairy products and lean meats.	
Limit sodium because it raises blood pressure.	
Avoid salted snack foods.	
Stay below 2300 mg/day of sodium.	
Increase vegetable intake, whole fruit intake, and low-fat dairy in snacks.	
Encourage fluids to prevent dehydration.	
Offer foods to support recommended intake of calcium, vitamin D, potassium, fiber, protein, and vitamin B_{12}.	

Figure 11.14 Salina chose to read chapters 1 and 6 of the *Dietary Guidelines*. For each chapter, she took notes, listed, and clarified the meanings of unfamiliar terms, highlighted the most important information, and underlined the main points.

Salina follows several links on the USDA website to find additional resources. Since most of her residents are senior citizens, she reads a report about fruit and vegetable consumption among older adults and another about the quality of older adults' diets. In the material Salina reads, charts provide information about specific foods to include and avoid in her residents' diets (**Figure 11.15**).

Technical documents will rarely entertain you. However, when you use technical reading skills and have a desire to learn, these documents will inform you. In this way, technical reading skills lead to improved care for patients and improved job performance for you.

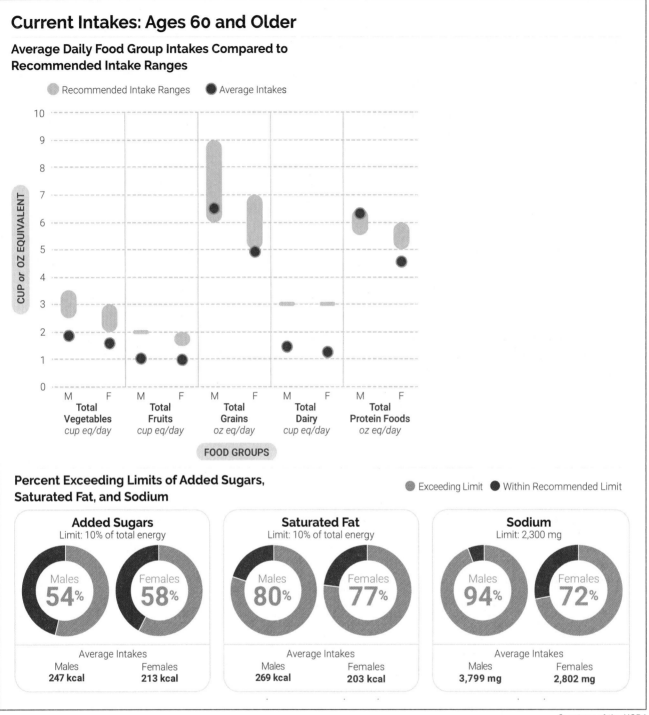

Current Intakes: Ages 60 and Older

Average Daily Food Group Intakes Compared to Recommended Intake Ranges

● Recommended Intake Ranges   ● Average Intakes

CUP or OZ EQUIVALENT

| | M | F | M | F | M | F | M | F | M | F |
| Total Vegetables cup eq/day | Total Fruits cup eq/day | Total Grains oz eq/day | Total Dairy cup eq/day | Total Protein Foods oz eq/day |

FOOD GROUPS

Percent Exceeding Limits of Added Sugars, Saturated Fat, and Sodium

● Exceeding Limit   ● Within Recommended Limit

Added Sugars
Limit: 10% of total energy

Males **54%**   Females **58%**

Average Intakes

| Males | Females |
| 247 kcal | 213 kcal |

Saturated Fat
Limit: 10% of total energy

Males **80%**   Females **77%**

Average Intakes

| Males | Females |
| 269 kcal | 203 kcal |

Sodium
Limit: 2,300 mg

Males **94%**   Females **72%**

Average Intakes

| Males | Females |
| 3,799 mg | 2,802 mg |

Courtesy of the USDA

Figure 11.15 Salina reviewed the data in each of the charts found in the USDA guidelines. They provided important details about food choices for her residents. *What do these graphics tell you about the dietary patterns of older adults?*

Writing Technical Documents

Technical writing meets a specific need. Rather than expressing the writer's thoughts or experiences, a technical document informs or persuades a specific audience. Salina's technical writing informed her staff about dietary guidelines so they could prepare nourishments for residents of their healthcare facility.

When a medical equipment manufacturer prepares a brochure explaining the benefits of a new imaging machine, the technical writer hopes to persuade healthcare facilities to purchase that machine (**Figure 11.16**).

Technical writing targets a specific group. Frequently, the writer must collect expert-level information and then translate and summarize it into language easily understood by the intended audience. For example, when writing patient-education materials about hyperlipidemia (hI-per-lih-puh-DEE-mee-uh), you could say that it involves abnormally elevated levels of lipids, such as cholesterol or triglycerides. However, most patients would better understand that hyperlipidemia is too much fat in your blood.

Technical writing is clear and concise. A physician writes a prescription for "125 mg amoxicillin (uh-mahk-suh-SIH-lihn) po q 8h," not "The patient needs some of that pink liquid that treats bacterial infections." Technical documents use headings, lists, and graphics to direct the reader to specific information. When replacing a filter in the heating system, a technician can quickly locate the directions by finding the maintenance section in the table of contents. She can simply scan the headings, looking for "Replacing a Filter." She does not need to read the entire manual to complete her task.

Technical writers follow these basic steps:

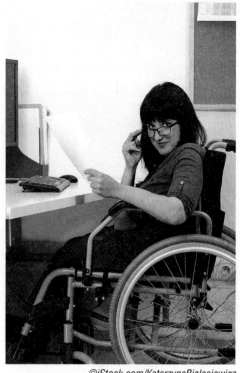

©iStock.com/KatarzynaBialasiewicz

Figure 11.16 Technical writers create materials meant to inform or persuade an audience.

1. **Plan.** During the planning stage, clearly define the document's purpose and identify the characteristics of the specific group known as your **target audience**. Then gather the information needed to write the document. Gathering information may involve reading, doing research and surveys, and even conducting interviews.
2. **Draft and revise.** First, select a format that fits the purpose of the document. For example, instructions will use numbered lists. Reports may need a summary or abstract, and a proposal will include a request for a plan of action or the purchase of goods or services. Keep the purpose and audience in mind while writing your first draft. During the revision process, verify the information is accurate, well organized, and written clearly. Finally, focus on the document design. Are the headings easy to spot? Do bulleted or numbered lists highlight important information? Do the graphics make the data easy to understand?
3. **Edit and publish.** Editing removes errors in spelling and grammar. It produces a professional document that represents your company. Having another person edit your work will catch errors your brain automatically corrects. Reading aloud may help you hear awkward phrases or incomplete sentences. Remember to cite your sources. Submit your document before the deadline so there is adequate time for publishing.

Salina already knew the purpose for her writing. Before writing, she considered her audience, the dietary aides who worked in her facility. They would need some background information about why there were new guidelines. They would also need instructions for selecting appropriate snacks for residents. Finally, they would need to know foods to avoid to promote residents' health. Using the information in her notes, Salina prepared a first draft.

During the revision process, Salina followed a checklist of tips for technical writing and made changes to her document (**Figure 11.17**). She then asked one of her dietitians to proofread it for readability and errors.

Draft and Revise

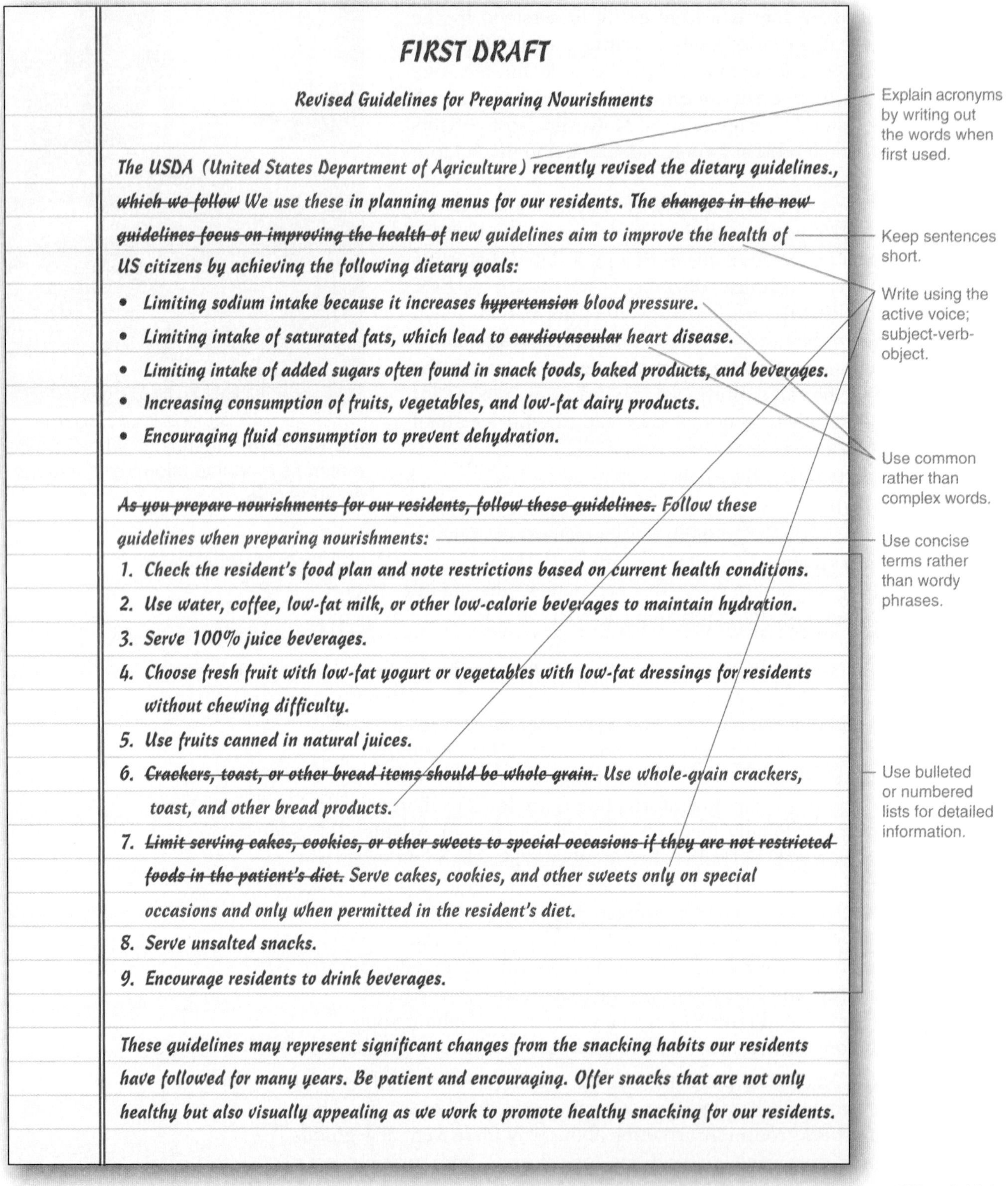

FIRST DRAFT

Revised Guidelines for Preparing Nourishments

The USDA (United States Department of Agriculture) ~~recently revised the dietary guidelines., which we follow~~ We use these in planning menus for our residents. The ~~changes in the new guidelines focus on improving the health of~~ new guidelines aim to improve the health of US citizens by achieving the following dietary goals:

- Limiting sodium intake because it increases ~~hypertension~~ blood pressure.
- Limiting intake of saturated fats, which lead to ~~cardiovascular~~ heart disease.
- Limiting intake of added sugars often found in snack foods, baked products, and beverages.
- Increasing consumption of fruits, vegetables, and low-fat dairy products.
- Encouraging fluid consumption to prevent dehydration.

~~As you prepare nourishments for our residents, follow these guidelines.~~ Follow these guidelines when preparing nourishments:

1. Check the resident's food plan and note restrictions based on current health conditions.
2. Use water, coffee, low-fat milk, or other low-calorie beverages to maintain hydration.
3. Serve 100% juice beverages.
4. Choose fresh fruit with low-fat yogurt or vegetables with low-fat dressings for residents without chewing difficulty.
5. Use fruits canned in natural juices.
6. ~~Crackers, toast, or other bread items should be whole grain.~~ Use whole-grain crackers, toast, and other bread products.
7. ~~Limit serving cakes, cookies, or other sweets to special occasions if they are not restricted foods in the patient's diet.~~ Serve cakes, cookies, and other sweets only on special occasions and only when permitted in the resident's diet.
8. Serve unsalted snacks.
9. Encourage residents to drink beverages.

These guidelines may represent significant changes from the snacking habits our residents have followed for many years. Be patient and encouraging. Offer snacks that are not only healthy but also visually appealing as we work to promote healthy snacking for our residents.

Margin tips:
- Explain acronyms by writing out the words when first used.
- Keep sentences short.
- Write using the active voice; subject-verb-object.
- Use common rather than complex words.
- Use concise terms rather than wordy phrases.
- Use bulleted or numbered lists for detailed information.

Figure 11.17 After her focused reading, Salina created the first draft of the document for her staff. Note the changes she made (in red text) and the corresponding technical writing tips she used to revise her document.

She made a few corrections and improvements based on her colleague's suggestions. After completing the final draft, Salina considered other changes to make the document easier to read. She increased the size of the headings to show the different sections of the document. She also added color blocks to make the numbered steps stand out from the rest of the document. Then she determined how many posters and what sizes would work best before ordering copies of her document.

When you are familiar with a subject, you may use technical terms in your document. That is fine if you are writing for colleagues with similar knowledge and career experience. However, technical writing is most successful when it puts complex information into simple language adapted for a specific audience. Your purpose and your audience should always remain the focus of your technical writing.

11.2-2 Writing Letters, Memos, and Emails

Effective written communication is an essential skill for all healthcare workers. There are many times you will need to communicate with patients, coworkers, insurance companies, pharmacies, and other organizations through written communication, such as letters, memos, and emails. It is important to convey your message clearly and professionally.

Letters

As a healthcare worker, you will write **business letters** for a variety of purposes. For example, business letters may tell a patient the results of a test or provide consultation reports to other healthcare professionals. Business letters may also explain patient treatments to insurance companies or announce changes in schedules and services for your healthcare facility. Regardless of their audience or content, effective business letters follow the same basic guidelines (**Figure 11.18**).

Your letters will go to people outside your organization. For this reason, you should choose your words carefully, keep a formal tone, and focus on the purpose of your **correspondence**, or written communication. Provide enough background information to keep your reader informed. Maintain goodwill with your reader by being honest, polite, and prompt in your correspondence.

Memos

Memos, short for **memorandums** (meh-muh-RAN-duhms), are less formal than letters (**Figure 11.19**). You send memos to people within your organization, so you can use a more personal tone in your writing. Your memos serve as a written record of an event or problem. They may also be used to evaluate your performance. Managers look for correspondence that shows you are solving problems, building relationships, and getting the job done.

Smile a Mile Dental
123 Crown Lane
Amalgam, ID 53216 — heading: complete address of the sender

June 23, 2023 — dateline (at approximately 15th line)

Mr. John Weiser
623 Willow Lane
Amalgam, ID 53216 — inside address (at approximately 20th line)

double space

Dear Mr. Weiser: — salutation: greeting and name that matches the name in the inside address

double space

We are very happy to welcome you to the eastside location of our dental practice. We appreciate the opportunity to care for you and your family in our new facility. Our team will work to provide you with high-quality, gentle dental care.

double space

During your first visit, Doctor Smile will examine your teeth, review necessary X-rays, and assess your oral health. You will meet other members of our team as they assist with your examination. Doctor Frown has forwarded your past records. — body: content of your message

double space

If you need further care, a treatment plan will be prepared for you. You will be able to review this plan and associated cost estimates. You will also have an opportunity to ask questions about the recommended treatment.

double space

Thank you for choosing Smile a Mile Dental. We look forward to meeting you at your appointment on July 7, 2023, at 2:00 p.m.

double space

Sincerely, — closing (leave 4–5 lines after for signature)

Serena Smile — handwritten signature

Serena Smile, DDS — typed signature

double space

SS/dw — reference initials

double space

Enc. (2) — enclosure notation

double space

c: Dr. Frown — copy notation: indicates a copy has been sent to other people

Goodheart-Willcox Publisher

Figure 11.18 A business letter includes specific components, some of which are explained here. The inside address of a letter should consist of the title, name, and complete address of the person to whom you are writing. The closing should always be friendly, but business-like. Never use "thank you" as your closing. Reference initials consist of the uppercase initials of the letter's sender and lowercase initials of the letter's typist.

MEMORANDUM

To: Jean Lee, Office Manager
From: Jeff Brown
Date: 06/03/23
Re: Vacation leave

I would like to use vacation time on September 1, 2, and 5 to attend my sister's wedding. Please let me know at your earliest convenience if you can meet this request. I will need to make airline reservations for the trip. Thank you for your help.

Goodheart-Willcox Publisher

Figure 11.19 Memos are usually short and focus on a particular topic. *In what situations might you use a memo instead of a business letter?*

Memos start with the word *memo* or *memorandum* at the top of the page. The headings *To, From, Date,* and *Subject* are followed by the message of the memo. Follow your employer's preferred format for these communications. Readers expect memos to be brief and cover only one topic. Always explain your topic carefully and include all the necessary details. This is especially important when you are using a memo to document the decisions made by a group. Use the guidelines for effective correspondence in all your written communication (**Figure 11.20**).

Electronic communication has dramatically increased the speed of personal and business correspondence. Sometimes, however, speed can result in carelessness and loss of privacy for patients. Health informatics workers must always protect the privacy of patient information when using electronic systems for communication and other tasks. Workers must also use appropriate etiquette and follow facility procedures when using technology to communicate with patients, doctors, and fellow healthcare workers.

Effective Correspondence	
Characteristics	**Purpose**
No unnecessary words	Avoids wasting the reader's time
Accurate and complete information	Avoids mistakes and misunderstandings
Professional appearance (uses Block Style Format and Standard English)	Makes you and your employer appear competent
Logical organization of information	Avoids frustrating or confusing the reader

Goodheart-Willcox Publisher

Figure 11.20 Each characteristic of effective correspondence has a clear purpose.

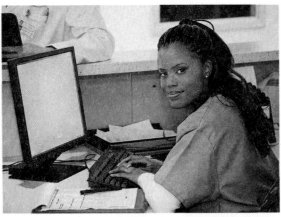

Sean Locke Photography/Shutterstock.com

Figure 11.21 Health informatics workers use electronic communication. They may receive dozens of messages each day. *How quickly should you respond to an email?*

Emails

Electronic mail (email) communication has become vital to daily business operations in healthcare facilities (**Figure 11.21**). Email has replaced traditional paper options for sending memos, announcements, and reports. It sends secure, digital lab results and discharge summaries to the physician's office. Health informatics workers use electronic communication systems to code services and submit claims for payment to health insurance providers and the Centers for Medicare and Medicaid Services.

Email is sent by means of a secure transmission process such as encryption to protect patient privacy. A secure web portal can also be used. In this case, physicians and patients both sign into a secure website to send messages back and forth within that site. Typically, the healthcare facility sends a generic "do not reply" email message to the patient. The patient uses a password to access the healthcare system web portal to view messages and test results.

Workers protect the privacy and security of patient information by keeping their passwords private. They do not reply to phishing requests for information. Emails and websites with grammatical errors, typos, poor graphics, or unknown logos may not be legitimate. Do not click on untrusted attachments or links, since they could contain a virus, malware, or ransomware. These cyberattacks can alter files, change device settings, steal stored information, and block future access. Report anything suspicious to your IT department immediately.

Each healthcare organization stores, monitors, and manages its email communications. Employers have the right to read any message sent through their computer system by an employee. Since emails belong to the organization, employees must use them for business purposes only. Many businesses also monitor internet use by employees. Online shopping and writing negative posts about your employer while at work could cost you your job.

Managing email communications has become challenging because employees may receive dozens of messages each day. Therefore, your emails must be clear and accurate, but also brief and to the point. Address only one concern in each email so recipients can organize their messages more easily. Because your recipient cannot read your nonverbal signals, you should choose your words carefully to send the correct message in a professional tone. Avoid sending a message when you are angry or frustrated. Since your email may be forwarded to others, review your words before you hit the send button.

When you send an email to a friend, your message's format may be unstructured and casual. As you reply to each other, you do not need to repeat your name as you would if writing a business letter. However, email communication in a healthcare setting is more formal and follows the rules of business communication because it may become part of the legal record of patient care.

The format of an email is similar to a printed memo. Follow these guidelines as you write an email message:

- **To.** In this line, key in the names of your main recipients. These are the people who will be replying to your email or those with a primary interest in your message.
- **Copy (CC).** Use this line to add people who will want to read the information but are not expected to reply.

- **Blind Copy (Bcc).** Generally, it is courteous to let the recipient know all the people who are receiving your message. However, you can use the Blind Copy, or *Bcc*, feature when emailing a large number of people outside your organization. This courtesy protects the privacy of everyone's contact information and reduces clutter at the beginning of the message.
- **Subject.** Provide a clear and concise statement for your subject line. Avoid general statements such as *Hello* or *For Your Information*. Include a subject that reflects the topic or content of your email so readers can keep track of their replies.
- **Salutation.** Keep your salutations formal by using the word *Dear* in front of the recipient's name for all communication sent outside your facility. If you are on a first-name basis with the intended recipient, you may use the first name in email communication. However, in all communication, you should follow the guidelines set by your healthcare facility.
- **Message.** Format your message the same way you would a letter or memo. Use correct spelling, punctuation, and grammar. Keep your message short and simple. Avoid using all capital letters, as this can be interpreted as shouting your message. Use an attachment to provide details, if necessary.
- **Closing.** Use a friendly but business-like closing such as *Sincerely* or *Cordially*. Less formal emails to coworkers may end with *Thanks* or *Thank you*.
- **Signature.** Include your full name and contact information, including your job title and department, at the bottom of your email. Since many programs display only the sender's name, include your email address in your signature. You can set up your program to insert this information automatically. Include a confidentiality footer with every email. This statement is required for sensitive, confidential, or protected health information. It also adds privacy protection to emails sent to an incorrect address (**Figure 11.22**).

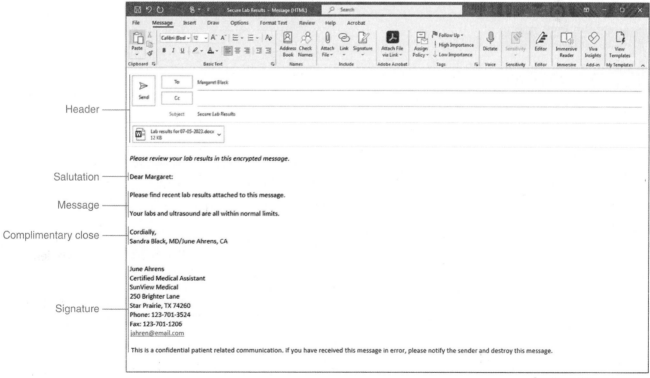

Goodheart-Willcox Publisher

Figure 11.22 Emails sent in a healthcare facility must follow specific guidelines.

Before sending any patient information to another provider or insurance company, be certain you have a written release from the patient. When sending personal information to a patient, direct it to the correct email address. Double-check the address before you send the message. If a mistake is made, unauthorized individuals may gain access to protected health information.

Also follow professional etiquette guidelines for handling the emails you receive. Respond to incoming emails as quickly as possible, but at least within 24 hours. If you need more time to write your response, send a short message indicating you will respond as soon as possible. Use the *out-of-office* feature when you are not at work. This feature will generate an automatic reply that lets people know when you will return.

When you respond to a message, stick to the original topic in your reply. To switch to a new topic, create a new email and mention the new topic in the subject line. This allows both the sender and the recipient to organize and file the messages by topic.

Some healthcare facilities use a messaging system so employees can communicate with each other quickly via computer. These in-office messages tend to be far less formal than emails, but always follow your facility's guidelines (**Figure 11.23**).

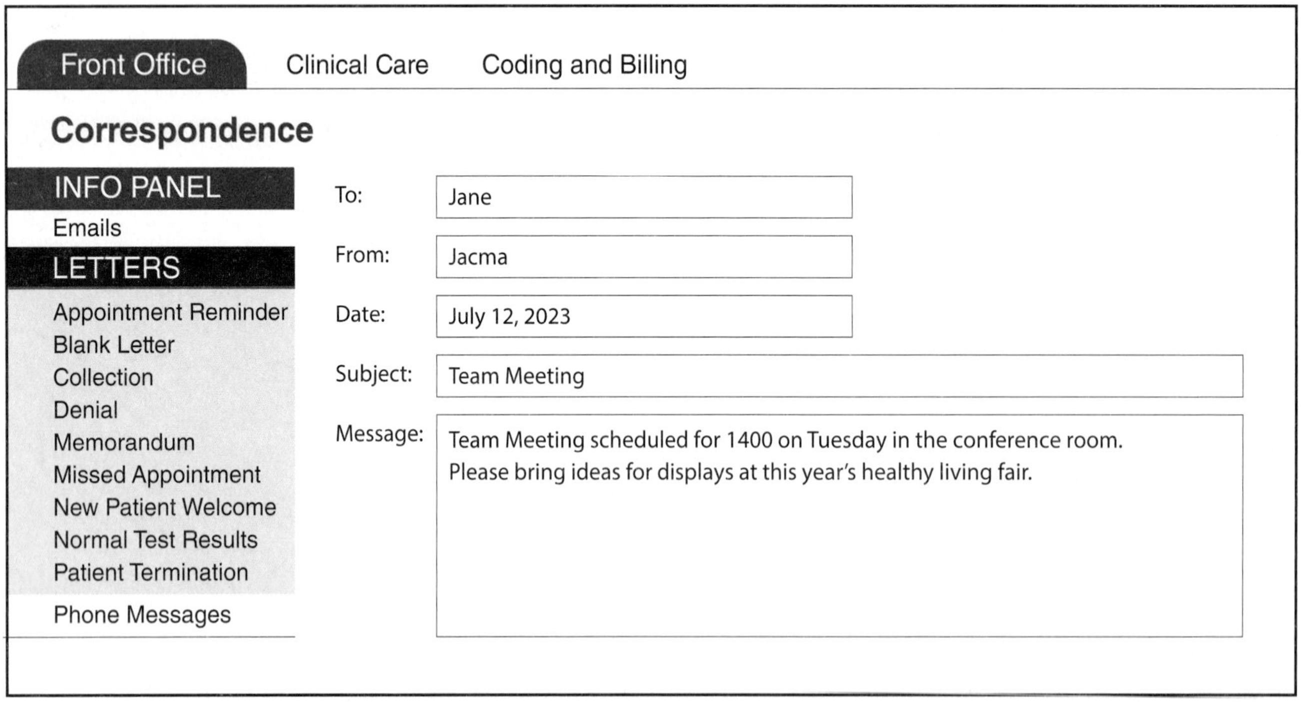

Goodheart-Willcox Publisher

Figure 11.23 Email memos sent to coworkers can be written more casually than business emails.

Scientific Communication

Scientific communication is a specific subset of technical communication. Scientific communication can be a simple explanation of a medical condition in language a child can understand, or it can be a complex report detailing innovative research for sharing with fellow researchers involved in similar studies.

Healthcare Professions: Scientific Communication

Dr. Workman was putting in some long hours in front of his computer. The deadline for a major grant proposal was approaching quickly, and he needed to finalize all sections of the document before submitting his team's proposal. The research team members had been meeting frequently to outline the content for each section and collect the data to support their research request. They spent many hours discussing and developing measurable goals hoping the foundation would grant the funds needed to continue their research project.

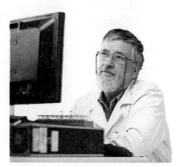

l i g h t p o e t/Shutterstock.com

Now it was up to Dr. Workman to make sense of all that information and present it in a logical and convincing way. How could he make the review team at the foundation see the value of his team's research and the urgency for focusing on this new study? Dr. Workman is a scientist by training, but he is also a writer. He uses scientific communication skills both to fund his research and to document the results of that research.

Understanding is a primary goal of scientific communication. When the public—people who are not scientists—are your audience, you must communicate information in ways that help readers understand scientific concepts. Medical writers usually have strong backgrounds in science. They can read and interpret scientific research documents. They can also focus on their purpose and tailor material to their audience to produce documents readers can understand.

While most of a scientist's time might be spent in a laboratory with other scientists, a research scientist also writes reports for administrators and explains ideas to supervisors. Writing skills help scientists share their knowledge, secure research funding, and improve their employment options. In addition to research papers, scientific writing can include **proposals** and **recommendation reports**.

Proposals and Recommendation Reports

Proposals, as their name indicates, propose or suggest something. Sales proposals attempt to sell a product or service. Research proposals seek approval for a research study. Grant proposals ask for funding for a project, and planning proposals try to persuade the audience to take a certain action.

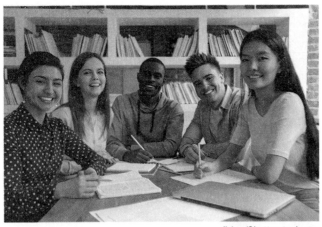
fizkes/Shutterstock.com

Figure 11.24 Successful proposals, such as grant requests, persuade your target audience to invest in your solution. *What two elements do all proposals have in common?*

When HOSA members wanted to conduct a service project promoting healthy physical activity for elementary school students, they needed money. This money would go toward renting buses to get to the elementary school, buying pedometers and other supplies to complete the activities with the students, and hiring the bus chaperone required by their school district. Their advisor suggested they write a service-learning grant. They spent the next four weeks refining their ideas and completing the grant proposal (**Figure 11.24**). Two months after submitting their proposal, they received an award letter and $2,000 to fund their project.

Proposals can be brief and informal. A request to order thermometers from a different supplier, written to the head of your department, may be just one or two pages. On the other hand, a research grant proposal to conduct a specific project for several years may be hundreds of pages. The requirements of your audience determine the detail and formality of your writing, yet all proposals have two things in common. They describe a problem and suggest a solution. Successful proposals persuade the audience to invest in their solutions.

Recommendation reports also consider problems and solutions. They provide a written answer that shows how to meet a need in the workplace. Because there can be more than one solution to a problem, a recommendation report identifies the best solution. These reports can recommend which equipment to purchase or the best location for a new hospital.

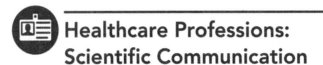

Healthcare Professions: Scientific Communication

Addison is a surgical technologist. She also serves on a healthcare team researching the installation of an MRI scanner in the surgical suite of the hospital where she works.

First, the team met to discuss and list the difficulties of doing surgical procedures without the guidance of ready images. Next, they visited other surgical suites with imaging equipment and interviewed healthcare workers at each site to learn the benefits and possible drawbacks of surgical suite imaging. Finally, they obtained cost

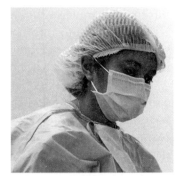
PIJITRA PHOMKHAM/Shutterstock.com

estimates for the purchase and installation of new imaging equipment. Now they are ready to write a recommendation report that does the following:

- defines the problem
- explains and compares the possible solutions along with the criteria used to evaluate the solutions
- makes a recommendation by choosing the best solution after considering all factors, including costs, patient outcomes, and effects on healthcare workers

Scientific Writing Guidelines

Scientific writing follows specific guidelines. Scientific writing presents data or ideas with enough detail to let the reader judge the validity of the conclusions by using the facts in the document. To achieve this goal, scientific writing must be objective, precise, and clear.

Objective writing draws a conclusion from the facts. It makes no assumptions. It does not use intuition or emotions to form conclusions.

Correct: "The data shows that . . . "

Incorrect: "We believe that . . . "

Objective writing can use the active voice, but it avoids beginning a sentence with *I* or *we*. This keeps the focus on the data and procedures instead of the researcher.

Correct: "Blood pressure measurements indicate . . . "

Incorrect: "We think the blood pressure measurements mean that . . . "

Precise writing uses concrete rather than figurative language. Be as specific as possible to avoid confusion.

Correct: "Inflate the cuff to 140 mmHg."

Incorrect: "Inflate the cuff until it feels tight like a tourniquet."

Precise writing requires quantitative descriptions that can be measured rather than qualitative descriptions that list characteristics.

Correct: "Blood pressure measurements increased by 20 mmHg at each reading."

Incorrect: "Blood pressure measurements showed a steady increase."

Clear writing uses simple language to explain ideas that may be complex.

Correct: "The text uses effective strategies to explain hypertension."

Incorrect: "Utilization of efficacious strategies to elucidate hypertensive symptoms is a hallmark of the text."

Clear writing also avoids wordiness.

Correct: "Discomfort with the procedure may elevate blood pressure readings."

Incorrect: "It is interesting to note the fact that discomfort with the procedure may elevate blood pressure readings."

Always follow these guidelines when writing scientific reports.

For example, Chaunté is reviewing data from patient records to select patients who could benefit from wellness programs. She looks for changes in average blood pressure readings over a period of several years. She selects 10 patients and records average blood pressure readings for each patient at 20, 40, and 60 years of age. She assembles her data and writes a report (**Figure 11.25**).

Patient #	Avg. BP at age 20	Avg. BP at age 40	Avg. BP at age 60
1	110/75	120/80	135/85
2	118/72	128/78	148/92
3	98/68	108/72	115/72
4	140/88	145/95	155/98
5	115/70	120/74	145/95
6	135/85	150/105	120/80
7	130/80	125/75	130/80
8	110/72	130/78	120/75
9	128/78	135/84	148/95
10	113/67	125/75	150/100

Title: Hypertension Data Review

Introduction: Our goal is to help patients make lifestyle changes that reduce hypertension. The purpose of this study is to review patient data so we can select patients who will benefit from learning how to reduce hypertension.

Method: I selected 10 patients and reviewed their average blood pressure readings at ages 20, 40, and 60. I entered the data into a table (see table above).

Results: The blood pressure readings of most patients increased with age. One patient had hypertension and three patients had prehypertensive readings at age 20. Two patients had hypertension and four patients were prehypertensive by age 40. At age 60, five patients had hypertension and two patients had readings indicating prehypertension.

Conclusions: It looks like age really increases your blood pressure. We could really help the patients!

Goodheart-Willcox Publisher

Figure 11.25 Chaunté's first draft report.

After reviewing the guidelines for scientific writing, Chaunté makes several changes to her report to make her writing more objective, precise, and clear (**Figure 11.26**).

Explaining complex scientific results in objective language takes time, thought, and practice. Remember that you are not trying to impress your audience with your own intelligence. You are trying to expand their scientific knowledge by drawing valid conclusions supported by facts learned through research.

Title: Hypertension Data Review

Introduction: SunView Medical wants to help patients make lifestyle changes that reduce hypertension. The purpose of this study is to review patient data to select patients who will benefit from learning how to reduce hypertension.

Chaunté removed the words our, we, and I from her report because scientific writing focuses on data rather than the researcher.

Method: Ten patient records were selected. Average blood pressure readings at ages 20, 40, and 60 were entered into the following table.

Patient #	Avg. BP at age 20	Avg. BP at age 40	Avg. BP at age 60
1	110/75	120/80	135/85
2	118/72	128/78	148/92
3	98/68	108/72	115/72
4	140/88	145/95	155/98
5	115/70	120/74	145/95
6	135/85	150/105	120/80
7	130/80	125/75	130/80
8	110/72	130/78	120/75
9	128/78	135/84	148/95
10	113/67	125/75	150/100

Chaunté moved this table to the "method" section of her report to show the quantitative data she collected.

Results: Between ages 20 and 60, eight patients had increased blood pressure readings, one remained the same, and one had decreased readings. One patient had hypertension and three patients had prehypertensive readings at age 20. Two patients had hypertension and four patients were prehypertensive by age 40. At age 60, five patients had hypertension and two patients had readings indicating prehypertension.

Hypertension Data Review

Chaunté replaced the word most with an exact number because scientific writing uses concrete language and quantitative descriptions. She drew a bar graph to make the results easier to visualize.

Conclusion: Data shows that 40 percent of 20-year-old patients could benefit from learning about lifestyle changes to reduce blood pressure. It is anticipated that improving lifestyle choices of the youngest patients will provide long-term health benefits by eventually reducing the incidence of prehypertension and hypertension at all ages.

Chaunté rewrote her conclusion to include specific data because scientific writing draws conclusions from data rather than intuition or emotion.

Goodheart-Willcox Publisher

Figure 11.26 After reading the guidelines for scientific writing, Chaunté makes some changes to her report. *Can you suggest ways to make Chaunté's conclusion even clearer?*

Lesson 11.2 Review

 Complete the *Map Your Reading* graphic organizer for the section you just read.

1. The purpose of technical writing is to _____ the reader. (11.2-1)
   A. inform
   B. entertain
   C. impress
   D. alert

2. Writing information using your own words is called (11.2-1)
   A. promoting
   B. paraphrasing
   C. restating
   D. reviewing

3. Which of the following is *not* an element of technical writing? (11.2-1)
   A. Inspires emotion
   B. Meets a specific need
   C. Is clear and concise
   D. Targets a specific group

4. Which of the following does *not* describe technical communication? (11.2-1)
   A. Provides entertainment
   B. Explains new technologies
   C. Provides information
   D. Describes research results

5. Which is the first step in technical reading? (11.2-1)
   A. Read slowly.
   B. Take notes in your own words.
   C. Look up unfamiliar terms in the glossary.
   D. Read the executive summary.

6. Follow the rules for business communication when sending emails because (11.2-2)
   A. emails may become part of the legal record of patient care
   B. it shows professionalism
   C. it provides more consistent communication
   D. All of these.

7. Which phrase illustrates a guideline for scientific writing? (11.2-3)
   A. We believe that . . . .
   B. The data shows that . . . .
   C. It is interesting to note the fact that . . . .
   D. The measurements increased . . . .

Observation Skills

Learning Outcomes

After studying this lesson, you will be able to

11.3-1 provide examples of body language.

11.3-2 differentiate between signs and symptoms when communicating patient observations.

11.3-3 explain four techniques used during a physical examination.

11.3-4 produce orderly and concise observations.

> **? ESSENTIAL QUESTION**
>
> *What observation skills do healthcare workers need to know and practice?*

Professional Vocabulary

Essential Terms

body language   nonverbal communication that occurs through conscious or unconscious gestures and movements

sign   evidence of a health condition that can be seen or measured

symptom   an indication of a disease or disorder experienced by the patient, such as pain

Important Terms

assess	minimum data set (MDS)	percussion
auscultation	nursing diagnosis	shift report
differential diagnosis	objective observations	subjective observations
inspection	pain scale	
medical diagnosis	palpation	

Introduction

Observation is a skill that involves looking for messages that are not spoken but can be found in nonverbal signals. Healthcare workers use observation when assessing their patients. They look for obvious signs of illness or distress but are also alert to situations where a patient's verbal and nonverbal messages do not match.

11.3-1 Observing Body Language

Effective communicators pay attention to **body language** as well as the words a person says. A smile or sneer, a raised eyebrow or frown, a shrug or clenched fist—all of these facial expressions and gestures communicate a message as clearly as words. Be aware of the nonverbal signals you send and receive, or you may communicate the wrong message.

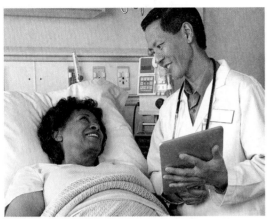

MBI/Shutterstock.com

Figure 11.27 Healthcare workers should maintain eye contact and be as friendly as possible as they talk with patients.

Body language is usually the expression of what the sender truly feels because it happens as a result of subconscious thought. A patient may say she is fine, but her clenched teeth and shallow breathing send a different message. Try reflecting the feelings you observe back to the patient to allow the patient to express them. For example, ask the patient with clenched teeth where her pain is located.

In addition to observing the unconscious body language of patients, healthcare workers also consciously use their own body language to improve patient care. Effective healthcare workers look at the patient, but also turn and lean slightly toward the patient to show interest and caring. They nod or say *yes* to acknowledge what the patient is saying. They use a warm and open facial expression to encourage the patient to speak freely (**Figure 11.27**).

In certain situations, healthcare workers might even use gestures and facial expressions to show they are currently busy but are aware of the patient's needs. For example, if Kia is talking on the phone when a patient arrives for an appointment, she will greet the patient with a smile. She will nod her head and make a quick hand gesture to indicate she will speak with the patient as soon as she can. This type of body language reassures the patient, who might otherwise feel ignored.

11.3-2 Communicating Observations

In the process of diagnosis, physicians use reading skills as they review entries in the patient record. They use speaking and listening skills as they interview patients using open-ended questions. Perhaps most importantly, they use the powerful skill of observation as they examine patients.

 Healthcare Professions: First Day Nerves

Trinity was surprised she was feeling nervous. After 12 years of preparation, she was starting her first full-time job as a medical doctor. Of course, she had already worked with many patients during her internship and residency, but this felt different. Today she would see patients as a newly licensed, board-certified physician working independently instead of under the supervision of another doctor.

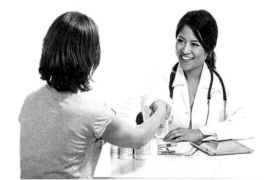

kurhan/Shutterstock.com

Starting today, patients would rely on her examination, diagnosis, and treatment to restore their good health. It was a sobering realization, but it was exciting at the same time. Helping people and curing disease had been Trinity's dream job for as long as she could remember.

Checking her schedule, she reviewed the first patient's record and headed to the exam room. She knocked, entered, smiled, and said, "Hello, I'm Dr. O'Dell. What seems to be the problem?"

Healthcare workers use nearly all their senses when they observe a patient:

- **Sight.** Healthcare workers look for the **signs** of injury or illness using **inspection**. Also called **objective observations**, signs can be seen (as with bruises, swelling, rashes, or cuts) or measured (as with vital signs, such as temperature and blood pressure).

- **Hearing.** Listening to a patient's statements or complaints reveals **symptoms**. Also called **subjective observations**, symptoms cannot be seen or measured by a healthcare worker. For example, only the patient can detect stomachache, back pain, and fatigue. Healthcare workers will not learn about symptoms unless the patient tells them.

  In the process of examination, healthcare providers also use hearing as they listen to respirations and abnormal body sounds. Through **auscultation** (aw-skuhl-TAY-shuhn), healthcare workers hear the sounds of the heart and lungs, listen to bowel sounds, and hear the flow of blood through arteries.

- **Touch.** Healthcare providers use **palpation**, or touching and applying pressure, to measure pulse rates and assess blood flow to many areas of the body. They also use palpation to identify abnormal conditions such as swelling, unusual hardness, body parts that are out of place, and the location of pain. They can feel dryness, perspiration, heat, and unusual skin texture through touch.

  Percussion is a method of tapping body parts with fingers, hands, or small instruments while listening for sounds coming from body organs. Through percussion, healthcare workers learn the size, density, and position of internal organs. They can also detect the presence or absence of fluid in specific body areas.

  Using percussion on a body part is like playing a drum. A healthcare provider can interpret differences in sound to determine the kind of tissue within the body. For example, healthy lungs sound hollow because they are filled with air. Bones and joints sound solid, but the abdomen sounds like a hollow organ filled with air, fluid, or solids.

- **Smell.** Healthcare workers pay attention to body odors, as well as unusual breath, wound, urine, or *stool* (waste material released during a bowel movement) odors. While the concept of using odors in patient assessment may not be appealing, odors provide important signals about a patient's health. For example, breath that smells fruity may mean the patient is experiencing *ketoacidosis*, a serious condition that can lead to diabetic coma and needs further medical care.

Performing a Physical Examination and Assessment

During a physical examination, the medical provider follows four basic steps: inspection, palpation, percussion, and auscultation (**Figure 11.28**). Moving from head to foot, the provider checks each area of the body and documents findings in the patient's medical record.

Examinations may be preventive, as in the case of a yearly physical, or may be done to determine the cause of problematic symptoms a patient is experiencing.

When a patient *presents* (comes to the provider) with signs of illness, the provider begins the process of forming a **differential diagnosis**. The physician completes a physical examination and takes a medical history. The results of the examination along with the patient's medical history are used to formulate a list of all the possible causes of the patient's symptoms. The differential diagnosis narrows the list of possible disorders.

Next, the physician works to develop a **medical diagnosis**. The physician orders specific diagnostic tests to confirm the cause or identify other previously overlooked causes before beginning treatment. The physician interprets the results of these tests to determine the medical diagnosis.

Physical examinations vary according to the needs of each patient. Specialists focus on a particular body system or organ. For example, a cardiologist will focus an examination on the patient's heart-related symptoms. The patient's chief complaint, or most important health concern, also guides the examination. For example, a patient who has trouble hearing may be given Weber and Rinne tests to screen for conductive hearing loss.

Nursing staff members also **assess**, or evaluate, patients to determine a **nursing diagnosis** and develop a patient care plan. This diagnosis may be made using patient and family interviews, medical records, and a physical examination to identify a patient's condition. The nursing diagnosis states the patient's condition and the cause of the condition. For example, a nursing diagnosis could be "impaired mobility caused by stroke." The nursing staff members use the diagnosis to develop a care plan that identifies solutions for this condition and techniques that team members will use to help the patient improve.

As the care plan is implemented, staff members use observation skills to evaluate the patient's progress. A nursing assistant, for example, looks for changes in the patient's skin to prevent the development of skin ulcers and reports any observations of skin redness and warmth at pressure points. The nursing process—which consists of assessment, problem identification, planning, implementation, and evaluation—relies on careful observation to promote patient recovery (**Figure 11.29**).

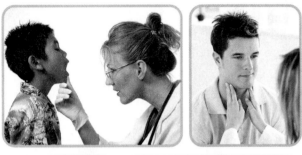
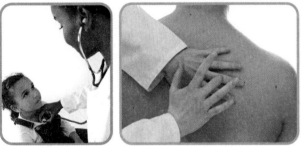

Geo Martinez/Shutterstock.com, wavebreakmedia/Shutterstock.com, Darren Baker/Shutterstock.com, Bencemor/Shutterstock.com

Figure 11.28 The four basic steps in a physical examination are shown here. *Which of these steps uses a stethoscope?*

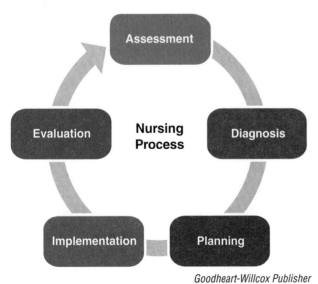

Goodheart-Willcox Publisher

Figure 11.29 Nurses use the steps in the nursing process to develop and evaluate patient care plans.

When a resident enters a long-term care facility, a special **minimum data set (MDS)** assessment is completed. This minimum data set is part of a government requirement for the clinical assessment of all residents in a long-term care facility (**Figure 11.30**). The MDS provides a comprehensive evaluation of each resident's functional capabilities. This helps long-term care staff identify health conditions. MDS assessments are required for residents on admission to the facility and at the end of their stay.

Licensed healthcare professionals, usually registered nurses employed by the long-term care facility, complete the MDS. These professionals transmit MDS information electronically to the state MDS database and, from there, it becomes part of the national MDS database at the Centers for Medicare and Medicaid Services (CMS). CMS uses the data to generate reports concerning resident status and indicators of quality care.

Sample Categories of the Minimum Data Set

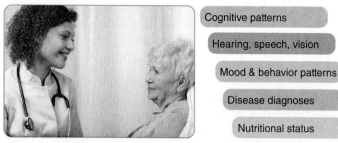

Cognitive patterns

Hearing, speech, vision

Mood & behavior patterns

Disease diagnoses

Nutritional status

Photographee.eu/Shutterstock.com

Figure 11.30 The minimum data set assessment provides a comprehensive evaluation for each long-term care resident. Selected examples of assessment categories are listed. *How is the assessment data used?*

11.3-4 Reporting and Recording Observations

All healthcare workers are responsible for reporting unusual events or changes in a patient's behavior or physical condition. For example, an observant receptionist may notice a person in the waiting room who is having trouble breathing and needs immediate help. Take your reporting obligation seriously and do not wait for someone else to report an unusual situation. You may prevent a more serious problem by quickly calling attention to unusual behavior.

In a care facility, health team members report changes in a patient's or resident's status throughout the shift by giving a verbal report to a supervising team member. In general, the following patient or resident observations are reported:

- changes in the person's condition (vital signs, skin color, breathing, or behavior—confusion, agitation, restlessness, or lethargy)
- reactions to a new treatment or therapy
- complaints of pain or discomfort such as weakness, dizziness, or nausea
- refusal of treatment
- request for a clergy visit

You should report specific indications and symptoms of pain, as well as specific signs and symptoms of infection (**Figure 11.31**). Always ask the patient about pain. Do not assume the patient will tell you. Use a **pain scale** to help you assess a patient's level of pain.

Observations to Be Reported

Report These Signs and Symptons of Infection

- Elevated temperature
- Sweating/chills
- Skin is hot, cold, red, or swollen
- Drainage from wounds or body cavities
- Discharge of mucus or pus

Report These Indications and Symptoms of Pain

- Chest pain
- Radiating pain
- Pain when moving
- Pain during urination or bowel movement
- Any pain is not normal; report all complaints of pain

Goodheart-Willcox Publisher

Figure 11.31 Shown here are observations to be reported, including observations related to infections and pain.

When you make a report, state the patient's name and room number. Make your report orderly and concise by giving actual vital sign measurements and reporting only what you observe. Because others cannot observe or measure symptoms, you should always report exactly what a resident tells you when complaining of symptoms.

Correct: Jane Smith in Room 602 has a right arm that is red, swollen, and warm to the touch.

Correct: Jane Smith in Room 602 says her left ear aches.

Incorrect: Mrs. Smith has an ear infection.

Incorrect: Mrs. Smith's vital signs don't look good.

At the end of each shift, workers present a **shift report** that tells the oncoming staff the information necessary for a smooth continuation of patient care. During the shift report, the oncoming staff members learn about new patients or residents and their care plans. Outgoing staff highlight changes in the care plans for current patients, such as new medication orders or treatments, and share changes in patient status, such as a change in appetite or level of alertness.

Record all observations in the patient record and, just as importantly, record the fact that you reported an observation. For example: *Right arm is red, swollen, and warm to touch. Reported to charge nurse.*

Abbreviations are less common when charting in an EHR, but remember to use only the abbreviations approved by your facility whether you are documenting by hand or electronically. If you do not know the meaning of an abbreviation that appears in a resident's care plan, look it up or ask your supervisor for clarification. Never guess or assume you know the meaning.

Lesson 11.3 Review

 Complete the *Map Your Reading* graphic organizer for the section you just read.

1. Which of the following is *not* an example of body language? (11.3-1)
   A. Grimace
   B. Groan
   C. Clenched teeth
   D. Frown

2. Which of the following is a sign rather than a symptom? (11.3-2)
   A. Abdominal pain
   B. Sore left arm
   C. Fractured bone
   D. Headache

3. Which examination technique uses tapping and listening for sounds? (11.3-3)
   A. Palpation
   B. Percussion
   C. Auscultation
   D. Inspection

4. Which examination technique uses the sense of sight? (11.3-3)
   A. Palpation
   B. Percussion
   C. Auscultation
   D. Inspection

5. Which of the following observations is orderly and concise? (11.3-4)
   A. Temperature is high.
   B. Patient's ear hurts.
   C. Patient has an ear infection.
   D. Temperature is 101°F.

Barriers to Communication

Learning Outcomes

After studying this lesson, you will be able to

11.4-1 provide examples of environmental barriers, sensory impairments, and cognitive impairments that can create barriers to effective communication.

11.4-2 explain how responding to unmet needs may improve communication.

11.4-3 describe the indicators of low health literacy and appropriate responses from healthcare workers.

11.4-4 illustrate ways that cultural differences between patients and healthcare workers may create a communication barrier.

Professional Vocabulary

Essential Terms

communication barrier   anything that blocks or interferes with the exchange of information

health literacy   a person's ability to obtain and understand health-related information and make informed decisions using that information

Important Terms

aphasia	environmental barriers	sensory impairments
cognitive impairments	medical interpreter	
cultural differences	prostatectomy	

> **?**
> **ESSENTIAL QUESTION**
> *What barriers do healthcare workers face in communication?*

11.4-1 Barriers to Effective Communication

In spite of people's best efforts to communicate clearly, a multitude of barriers can interrupt communication. Recognizing possible **communication barriers** and using techniques to overcome these barriers goes a long way toward making communication truly effective.

Environmental Barriers

Environmental barriers are distractions in the surrounding area that cause people's attention to wander. Healthcare workers learn to ignore many of these barriers, but they can distract patients. People talking in the hallway, an overhead speaker announcement, or the radio or TV playing in a patient's room can create barriers. Checking your messages or answering a phone call when caring for a patient also creates a barrier. Check your environment and eliminate or reduce as many distractions as possible before you begin to communicate with your patient.

Sensory Impairments

Sensory impairments such as hearing loss, vision loss, or speech difficulties also create communication barriers. Learn to recognize these barriers and adjust your communication style accordingly. An older hospital patient who directs the TV remote at you and presses the volume button while you are talking is sending a clear message that you need to talk louder. Does your patient turn one ear toward you, ask you to repeat things, or just smile and nod? Do you check for understanding or just assume that the patient has heard you? **Figure 11.32** shows a variety of techniques to improve communication when sensory impairments create barriers.

Cognitive Impairments

Cognitive impairments occur when a patient's ability to think is affected by pain or medication or when the patient is confused or disoriented. They also occur when a patient has dementia or **aphasia**, the loss of ability to understand or express speech. All these conditions create barriers to effective communication. Sometimes common sense will guide your methods.

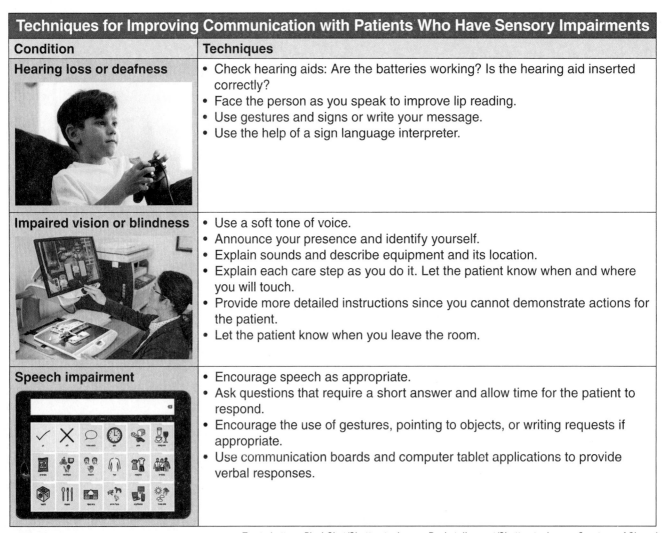

Techniques for Improving Communication with Patients Who Have Sensory Impairments	
Condition	**Techniques**
Hearing loss or deafness	• Check hearing aids: Are the batteries working? Is the hearing aid inserted correctly? • Face the person as you speak to improve lip reading. • Use gestures and signs or write your message. • Use the help of a sign language interpreter.
Impaired vision or blindness	• Use a soft tone of voice. • Announce your presence and identify yourself. • Explain sounds and describe equipment and its location. • Explain each care step as you do it. Let the patient know when and where you will touch. • Provide more detailed instructions since you cannot demonstrate actions for the patient. • Let the patient know when you leave the room.
Speech impairment	• Encourage speech as appropriate. • Ask questions that require a short answer and allow time for the patient to respond. • Encourage the use of gestures, pointing to objects, or writing requests if appropriate. • Use communication boards and computer tablet applications to provide verbal responses.

Top to bottom: Pixel-Shot/Shutterstock.com, Reshetnikov_art/Shutterstock.com, Courtesy of Cboard

Figure 11.32 Shown here are some examples of ways to improve communication when sensory impairments create a barrier.

Consider a physician who catches himself asking his patient to consider the pros and cons of a caesarean delivery in the middle of a strong labor contraction. Of course, the physician waited and resumed the conversation when the patient was not in as much pain.

The following techniques will improve communication with patients who have cognitive impairments:

- Identify yourself and greet your patient by name.
- Use simple language and short sentences.
- Speak slowly and clearly but not loudly. Hearing is not the issue.
- Provide plenty of time for the patient to respond.
- If you repeat the message, use the same words both times.
- Check for understanding and provide additional written information if appropriate.
- Use pictures and objects or demonstrate actions when patients do not understand verbal instructions.

11.4-2 Unmet Needs

Considering the stress, worry, and pain that illness brings to patients and the stressful environments that healthcare workers can experience, you will encounter some difficult interactions. While you cannot directly change the behavior of another person, the way you interpret and react to a situation can lead to solving the problem.

The first step in dealing with difficult people is to not label them as difficult. Using that label creates a barrier that keeps you from looking more closely at the reason for the behavior you want to change. People usually have a reason for acting the way they do. However, they might not be able to explain their reason logically or even know the reason.

People who are being "difficult" typically need something. Look at the situation from the patient's point of view and ask yourself what has changed in the patient's environment. Try to diagnose the individual's unmet need. Is it physical, social, emotional, or intellectual? Once you figure out what that need is and satisfy it to the best of your ability, the behavior may change.

For example, Mrs. Li usually enjoys a relaxing bath, but she has recently refused her bath, saying she is too tired or in too much pain. Yet, she is not too tired or in too much pain to participate in other activities at the care center. This has gone on too long, and now she really needs that bath.

Taking a careful look at the bath schedule, you see that Jake, a new employee, was assigned to give Mrs. Li her baths around the same time she began to refuse them. You review her chart and notice that all her physicians are female. You speak with Mrs. Li privately to ask if she would like a female bath aide. She looks relieved and immediately says yes. She did not want to make Jake feel bad, but she was embarrassed to have a male aide help her bathe.

Suppose you have just worked 11 hours of a 12-hour nursing shift and are feeling exhausted. Mr. Amin, who is recovering from a partial **prostatectomy** (surgical removal of the prostate gland), presses his call light every couple of minutes. He complains about everything: your care, the food, and even the other patients in his room. You would like to tell him to grow up and act his age. Instead, you take a deep breath and put yourself in his place. He is the head of a large company and is used to giving orders to other people. How do you think he feels lying in bed and waiting for someone else to take care of him? Consider his surgery. What other feelings might he be experiencing?

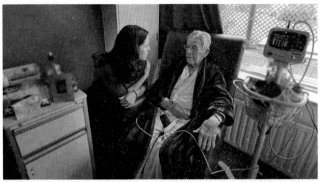

ChameleonsEye/Shutterstock.com

Figure 11.33 Listening to your patients' needs and concerns will help you understand why they may be acting uncooperatively.

Feelings of helplessness, frustration, and fear may be expressed with loud and angry complaints. Try not to take it personally. These complaints certainly are not about you. They are caused by the emotional stress the patient is experiencing. Remain calm and listen to your patient's requests. Offer as many choices as possible to help your patient regain a sense of control. Instead of avoiding a demanding patient, use your observation and listening skills to learn more about the patient (**Figure 11.33**). You may be surprised by the power of careful listening. It allows your patient to express worries, which may begin to calm the patient's fears.

11.4-3 Low Health Literacy

Health literacy is how well people can find, understand, and use basic health information and services to make good decisions about their care. A person's education, age, background knowledge, culture, and access to resources affect health literacy. Older adults, marginalized individuals, people with limited English skills, and people with less than a college education are most likely to have low health literacy skills.

 Healthcare Professions: Avoiding Errors

Nguyen Xuan is an older Vietnamese man. He is preparing to get dentures so he can eat better. He sits patiently, waiting for his name to be called, but never hears it. After a long wait, he checks with the receptionist. Apparently, his name was so poorly pronounced he missed his appointment. After another wait, he finally sees the dentist.

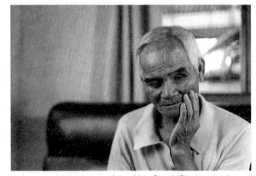

Love You Stock/Shutterstock.com

After the exam is complete, the dentist says two teeth will need to be pulled before the dentures can be fitted. Nguyen receives a prescription for pain medication and is told to bite down on the gauze pads until the bleeding stops.

Nguyen fills the prescription, which says to take two pills by mouth every four to six hours as needed for pain. He returns to the dentist the next day complaining that the pain medication is not working. The dentist finds one capsule inserted in each of the open wounds where the teeth were pulled. What went wrong, and how could it have been avoided?

In a therapeutic health career, part of your role will be educating your patients about their treatment. Keep in mind that a person who speaks a different language may not understand your directions for their care or taking medication.

Poor eyesight or arthritis may keep someone from reading information about an upcoming surgery. Patients may have different ideas about wellness and dismiss symptoms as normal. Education will play a big role in your patient's well-being.

It is your job to provide health information in a way your patient can read and understand. Healthcare workers do this by assessing a patient's level of literacy and adapting their communication accordingly. They may need to use simpler language or hand gestures to explain care procedures or medication administration. Showing the patient how much medicine to take is more helpful than assuming that the patient knows how to calculate and measure doses in the metric system. Use an interpreter when needed. Suggest that the patient bring another person to listen and take notes. Use handouts at an appropriate reading level and highlight important information. Demonstrate procedures and ask the patient to show them back to you. Ask patients to repeat back what they understand in their own words and clarify as needed. Provide a direct phone number for future questions. Check in with a phone call after a day or two to see if new questions arise. These actions can help prevent complications for your patient (**Figure 11.34**).

Health literacy influences all aspects of healthcare. It affects a person's ability to determine how much medicine to give a child, how to choose a health insurance plan, how to prepare for a surgical procedure, and even how to navigate a healthcare facility. For example, how many people going to the hospital for an X-ray will know the department they are looking for is called *radiology* or *imaging*?

Medical care is complicated, but understanding how to care for yourself is more important than ever before. Today, patients are released from the hospital as soon as possible, and more procedures are performed on an outpatient basis to keep costs down. As a result, the ability to understand any healthcare information given to you is essential for when you return home. Healthcare workers have an obligation to provide high-quality care. Communicating effectively with patients is an important part of that care.

11.4-4 Cultural Differences

Cultural differences can create communication barriers. Language barriers are obvious. When you and your patient speak different languages, you might ask for the help of a family member or friend of the patient. With the patient's permission, that person can interpret, but be aware that culture may limit what a family member is willing to communicate. Cultural differences are less obvious.

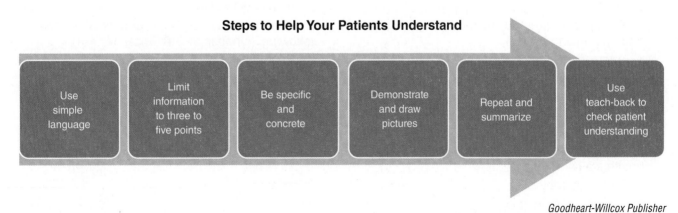

Steps to Help Your Patients Understand

Use simple language · Limit information to three to five points · Be specific and concrete · Demonstrate and draw pictures · Repeat and summarize · Use teach-back to check patient understanding

Goodheart-Willcox Publisher

Figure 11.34 Healthcare workers improve health literacy by helping patients understand the information and instructions they give.

For example, one nurse assumed her patient's daughter would communicate care instructions to her father because the daughter spoke fluent English as well as Korean. When her father continued to risk a fall by getting out of bed, the nurse found a Korean nurse to speak with him. He was unaware of his diagnosis or the risk of falling. The daughter explained that her brother would arrive the next day and talk to her father. Culture dictated that it was not her place to tell her father what he should do.

Developing an attitude of humility and a willingness to listen to your patients is a first step to developing competence in communicating with others. As you gain experience, consider these differences and communication suggestions.

When there is no one to interpret, greet your patient with a smile. Use gestures and pictures, or demonstrate your message, but do not speak loudly. Increasing your volume does nothing to improve a patient's understanding if you do not speak the same language. If necessary, request help from a **medical interpreter** who can translate complex terminology to ensure your patient's needs are met.

In addition to language, cultural differences in communication affect the use of gestures, touch, and sense of time. To you, a thumbs-up may signal that everything is OK, but it is a rude sexual gesture in Islamic culture. You may hug a coworker as a sign of encouragement and empathy, but hugging could make a coworker from an Asian background very uncomfortable. Some patients stop taking their medication after a few days because they feel better. You may need to explain the long-term outcomes by using the patient's interpretation of time. For example, you can tell a grandmother that taking the medicine every day will keep her feeling strong enough to hold her new grandchild.

Lesson 11.4 Review

 Complete the *Map Your Reading* graphic organizer for the section you just read.

1. Noise in the environment, vision or hearing conditions, and cognitive impairments create _____ to effective communication. (11.4-1)
   A. enhancements
   B. difficulties
   C. improvements
   D. barriers

2. When dealing with challenging patients, you might improve communication by searching for and responding to (11.4-2)
   A. additional symptoms
   B. irrational behavior
   C. unmet needs
   D. your own personal reactions

3. _____ skills involve understanding health information and are the strongest predictor of health status. (11.4-3)
   A. Health literacy
   B. Cultural competence
   C. Social media
   D. Technical reading

4. Which is *not* a step taken by healthcare workers to improve patient understanding? (11.4-3)
   A. Use gestures to indicate how to take the medicine.
   B. Show the amount of medicine to take.
   C. Provide an extra copy of the medication label.
   D. Ask the patient to show you how much medicine to take.

5. Cultural differences may include which of the following? Choose all that apply. (11.4-4)
   A. Speaking a different language
   B. Use of gestures
   C. Sense of personal space
   D. Sense of time

Developing Cultural Competence

Learning Outcomes

After studying this lesson, you will be able to

11.5-1 enumerate general guidelines for working with diverse populations.

11.5-2 describe the process of developing individual rapport with patients.

11.5-3 illustrate how age might influence coworker communication preferences.

11.5-4 explain how personal bias, prejudice, and stereotypes affect patient interaction.

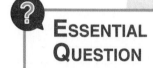

ESSENTIAL QUESTION

How can healthcare workers show cultural competence to improve patient care?

Professional Vocabulary

Essential Terms

cultural competence the ability to interact effectively with people of different cultures

personal bias an unfair preference for, or dislike of, something or someone

prejudice a strong feeling or belief about a person or subject that is not based on reason or actual experience

stereotype the assumption that everyone in a particular group is the same

Important Terms

conscious

rapport

unconscious

Introduction

Cultural competence is the ability to interact effectively with people of different cultures. It begins with understanding that patients and coworkers may think differently than you think. One employer refused to hire any nursing assistants who would not look her in the eye during the interview. She believed these applicants could not be trusted. Two excellent caregivers failed the test because they looked down as a sign of respect. An attitude of cultural humility allows healthcare workers to listen and learn from patients and coworkers. Cultural humility requires respecting patient views that differ from your own.

You begin to develop your knowledge and skills for working with diverse populations by following basic guidelines for showing sensitivity to cultural differences. Continue to expand your knowledge by learning about the cultural backgrounds and individual customs of your coworkers and patients.

Direct eye contact
shows interest,
honesty, and attention
to the speaker in
some cultures.

In other cultures,
avoiding eye contact
shows respect.

In some cultures,
direct eye contact
between a man and a
woman may be seen
as sexual.

Goodheart-Willcox Publisher

Figure 11.35 Customs
involving eye contact vary in
different cultures.

Finally, as you get to know the individual personalities and beliefs of patients and coworkers, adjust your own communication style to accommodate their individual preferences.

11.5-1 Learning General Guidelines

You will never know the cultures and customs of all your future patients and coworkers. In this way, you will never be truly culturally competent. Since cultural beliefs and values change over time, you can provide more effective care by showing cultural humility. This means you choose to learn from your patients. You can develop patient-provider relationships that benefit patient care when you listen to and respect patients' views. As you work in healthcare, following these general guidelines will help you avoid unintentionally insulting patients and colleagues.

Eye Contact

Sit next to—instead of facing—a patient or coworker who appears uncomfortable with direct eye contact. **Figure 11.35** shows several different cultures' beliefs about eye contact.

Body Language

With physical distance and touching, you should always follow the lead of the person with whom you are speaking (**Figure 11.36**). Be sensitive to those who are uncomfortable with close contact and ask permission before touching a patient during an examination.

Closer Contact Areas of the World	**Distant Contact Areas of the World**
• Africa	• North America
• Indonesia	• Northern Europe
• Latin America	• Great Britain
• Mediterranean	• Middle East
• Southern Europe	• Asia

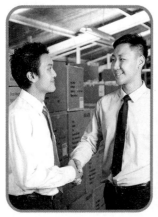 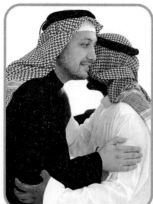 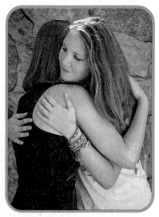

Kzenon/Shutterstock.com, Zurijeta/Shutterstock.com, Olga Rosi/Shutterstock.com

Figure 11.36 In closer cultures, friends of the same sex may hold hands, and kissing is a common greeting. In more distant cultures, the handshake is a common greeting, with hugs reserved for close friends and family members.

Use gestures cautiously because they can have very different meanings in different cultures. Ask patients about their reactions to a gesture if you are uncertain.

Do not interpret pain or fear based solely on facial expressions. A person's cultural and personal background influences appropriate expressions of physical or emotional feelings (**Figure 11.37**). Remember that pain is an individual experience. Do not assume a patient is exaggerating pain. Always check for all possible causes for pain.

Sense of Time

Understand that healthcare facilities operate on "clock" time, but many people operate on "activity" time. For example, arriving at 3:30 p.m. for a 2:45 p.m. appointment is late to a clinic, but it is still midafternoon to a person with "activity" time orientation. These patients will not see themselves as late. Someone with "activity" time orientation might simply come to the appointment when the morning work is finished rather than when the clock says it is time.

In this situation, avoid showing frustration. Respectfully explain why clock time is important to your clinic. For example, you could say, "Our clinic policy is to reschedule appointments when patients are more than 15 minutes late. This prevents long waits for patients."

Speech and Communication

Address patients and coworkers formally, using a title such as Mr. or Mrs. and their last name. Then follow their lead if they ask you to use their first name. Ask patients how they would like to be addressed if you feel uncertain.

Match the volume and speed of your speech to those of the patient. This will make the patient feel more comfortable. Avoid interrupting and showing impatience, which is disrespectful in nearly every culture.

Use an interpreter when language differences interfere with the patient's ability to understand healthcare information or your ability to understand the patient's description of signs and symptoms. Provide written information and directions in the patient's own language whenever possible.

While many people in the United States prefer independent decision-making, many cultures defer to a head of the household to make decisions for family members. For example, a woman may look to her husband for permission to speak.

Pain Responses

People of Northern European, Asian, and American Indian backgrounds tend to have more stoic responses to pain.

People of Hispanic, Middle Eastern, and Mediterranean backgrounds tend to have more expressive responses to pain.

Goodheart-Willcox Publisher

Figure 11.37 Expressions of pain may vary by a patient's cultural background.

Modesty

Provide complete privacy for all patients when they are changing clothing. Knock before entering the exam room to avoid interrupting a patient who is changing. Keep the patient covered as much as possible during the examination, diagnosis, and treatment process. Use a provider of the same sex when culture forbids a person of the opposite sex from touching a patient. For example, in some cultures, males may not touch females who are not immediate family members.

Your challenge, as you improve your cultural competence, is to develop a balance between understanding specific cultural groups and using skills and attitudes that are not specific to any cultural group.

Learning your patients' religious customs, views on death and dying, and ways of explaining illness and its causes is valuable to the delivery of healthcare. For example, in the United States, many people value telling patients the truth, whether the news is good or bad. However, this is not the case for all cultures. Did you know that some cultures believe talking about death actually leads to death? You will need to do more research as you work with individual patients.

11.5-2 Developing Individualized Approaches to Care

Even though you are a product of your culture, you are also a unique individual with your own set of preferences. Never presume to know a patient's preferences based on your personal understanding of the patient's culture.

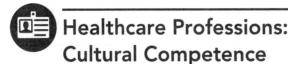

Healthcare Professions: Cultural Competence

Celia works as a nutritionist in a senior apartment complex. Two of the residents who have an Asian background have terminal illnesses. Celia is familiar with the customs of families who have Asian heritage in her community and assumes the families of these two residents will not share the diagnosis with their loved ones. One family did not tell the resident about the terminal diagnosis. They were happy she lived out her last days without the burden of knowing she was dying. However, the other family shared the terminal diagnosis. Celia was surprised when the resident said goodbye and thanked her for her careful work and helpful manner. The resident's family was happy the resident was able to make final arrangements and say goodbye to everyone.

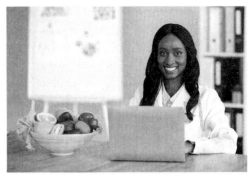

Prostock-studio/Shutterstock.com

Spend time learning about the specific cultural beliefs of groups in your community but also try to develop individual **rapport** (ra-POR) or empathetic understanding with the patients you serve. A positive relationship enhances the delivery of healthcare. When you make patients feel comfortable and show respect and caring, they will begin to trust you. When patients trust you, they will share their healthcare concerns, and your diagnosis, treatment, and care will be far more effective.

Developing rapport begins with making patients feel comfortable. Do you focus your attention on patients when talking to them, or are you looking at the computer screen to enter their information? Could you learn a couple of simple phrases to greet patients in their own language? Do you assume patients know whom they will see and what these individuals will do as part of patient care, or do you take the time to explain? Do all patients know how to learn the results of their lab tests and when those results will be available? Do you make sure patients clearly understand follow-up procedures before they leave the facility? Taking the time to show these courtesies to all patients illustrates cultural competence. Notice that culturally competent medical receptionists are just as important as culturally competent care providers.

As you develop rapport with the patients you serve, try to know them as individuals. Take the time to ask about their views and preferences. Record these for future reference and use them in your interactions with your patients. This shows respect, care, and concern. This kind of individualized approach to care leads to a higher quality of care. Healthcare professionals sometimes use mnemonic tools to remember detailed guidelines. As you record health history, you can use the UNIQUE mnemonic shown in **Figure 11.38** to learn your patients' individual preferences.

		UNIQUE Mnemonic for Charting Patient Preferences
Letter	**Assessment Categories**	**Sample Questions**
U	Uncover cultural background	1. Where were you born? 2. How long have you lived in the United States? 3. What is your age? (also note gender)
N	Note religious and spiritual traditions	1. How might religious observances affect your treatment? 2. Do you avoid any particular foods or change your diet during religious observances?
I	Identify healthcare beliefs and treatment preferences	1. What do you believe causes illness/preserves good health? 2. What traditional/home health remedies do you use? 3. Are there any healthcare procedures that are unacceptable to you? 4. What alternative healing methods do you use?
Q	Questions and concerns for care	1. Do you find it easier to talk with a man or a woman? someone older or younger? 2. What do you want to accomplish from today's visit/treatment?
U	Unmet language needs	1. What language do you prefer to speak/read? 2. Do you need an interpreter? 3. Do you prefer printed or spoken instructions?
E	Environment	1. With whom do you live? 2. Who helps you when you are ill? 3. When do you usually eat? 4. Can you shop and cook for yourself?

Goodheart-Willcox Publisher

Figure 11.38 You can use the mnemonic *UNIQUE* to help with charting patient preferences.

11.5-3 Exhibiting Cultural Competence with Coworkers

As the workforce becomes more diverse, people must expand their viewpoints regarding the delivery of care. Expecting others to think exactly as you do invites misunderstanding and damages working relationships. You need to extend the same respect, care, and concern to coworkers that you show to patients. Your differences could be as simple as age. Older workers and patients may prefer to communicate with a letter or face to face. Middle-age workers may be comfortable with phone or email, while younger workers prefer to use text messaging and social media. Older workers may not realize younger workers need to learn how to mail a letter. Younger workers may not understand why their older patients and fellow workers want to "waste time" talking when it is so much faster to text. Take the time to know your colleagues' beliefs and preferences so you can work as a team, taking advantage of each member's unique skills (**Figure 11.39**). Of course, this teamwork leads to a higher quality of care for your patients. Remember that providing the best care for your patients is the primary goal of all coworker communication.

11.5-4 Barriers That Affect Patient Interaction

Healthcare workers have their own cultural beliefs, attitudes, and viewpoints that can influence their feelings about and their diagnosis and treatment of patients. These personal preferences can be **conscious**, meaning you are aware of them, or **unconscious** preferences you do not know you have. Though most healthcare workers do not purposely ignore the beliefs and preferences of their patients, all workers can benefit from examining their own personal biases and prejudices to learn how these affect their interactions with patients.

Personal Bias

Your **personal biases** may interfere with patient care if you are unaware of them. For example, consider pain treatment. If you expect patients to be stoic and put up with pain, do you ignore those who express pain because they are just being "difficult"? On the other hand, if you expect patients to express pain, do you ignore stoic patients because you assume their silence means they have no pain?

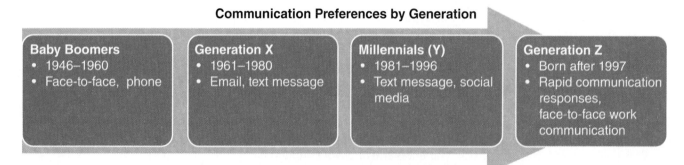

Communication Preferences by Generation

Baby Boomers
- 1946–1960
- Face-to-face, phone

Generation X
- 1961–1980
- Email, text message

Millennials (Y)
- 1981–1996
- Text message, social media

Generation Z
- Born after 1997
- Rapid communication responses, face-to-face work communication

Goodheart-Willcox Publisher

Figure 11.39 Each generation has preferred methods for communicating healthcare information. As individuals learn new technologies, their preferences may change.

Prejudice

Prejudice is a pre-established opinion based on a lack of individual knowledge or irrational feelings. Prejudice can lead to an unfounded dislike, fear, or mistrust of a person or cultural group.

Suppose a female patient of Hispanic background came to the surgical recovery room. As her sedation wore off, she began to scream and complain of terrible pain. The nurse, Alphonso, administered the prescribed pain medication, but the patient's screaming continued. He checked her vital signs and examined the surgical site but did not find any unusual signs. He was frustrated with the patient's loud cries. He thought to himself, "Looks like another loud complainer. I wish she would quit exaggerating her pain."

After another hour of her cries, Alphonso finally decided to call the surgeon. An examination showed pressure on nerves near the patient's surgical site, which was causing excruciating pain. Further surgery was completed to fix this problem. This time, the patient was calm and cooperative in the recovery room. Alphonso's prejudice caused him to mistrust the patient's expression of pain. Fortunately, he eventually reported her pain, and the patient received the necessary treatment.

Stereotypes

When you believe **stereotypes**, you view everyone in a cultural group as identical to each other. Some stereotypes may seem harmless, but stereotypes can influence patient care and have serious consequences.

For example, Mrs. Carter is an African-American mother with young children. Like many families, her family has health insurance through her husband's employer. Yet when she approaches the clinic reception desk, she is asked for her Medicaid card. She is irritated that the reception staff automatically assumes she is poor. You should avoid making assumptions and using harmful stereotypes such as this one.

Lesson 11.5 Review

 Complete the *Map Your Reading* graphic organizer for the section you just read.

1. When working with diverse populations, watch for clues about (11.5-1)
   A. eye contact
   B. body language
   C. modesty
   D. All of these.

2. Developing rapport with patients involves learning their _____ preferences. (11.5-2)
   A. individual
   B. cultural
   C. patient
   D. medical

3. Which of the following illustrates a communication challenge that may be generational? (11.5-3)
   A. Using inappropriate language
   B. Ignoring body language
   C. Using complex language
   D. Having to learn how to mail a letter

4. Automatically asking a patient for a Medicaid card illustrates (11.5-4)
   A. prejudice
   B. assimilation
   C. acculturation
   D. stereotyping

Chapter 11 Review and Assessment

Chapter Summary

11.1-1 The communication cycle begins with a sender delivering a message. The receiver responds with feedback. This continues until the receiver understands the intended message.

11.1-2 Four common communication styles include passive, aggressive, passive-aggressive, and assertive.

11.1-3 Using the SBAR system, you will tell what is currently happening with the patient (Situation) and give a brief summary of recent medical history (Background). Next, state the problem (Assessment), and finally, say what you believe needs to happen (Recommendation).

11.1-4 During a patient interview, show courtesy and a respectful manner. Consider the patient's age and stage of development. Use open-ended questions to encourage conversation.

11.1-5 Telephone skills include phone etiquette, call screening, triage, and documentation.

11.2-1 Technical communication meets a specific need and targets a specific audience to inform or persuade them. Technical writing is clear and concise.

11.2-2 Digital communication in healthcare settings follows the same guidelines for effective correspondence and professional etiquette found in traditional letters and memos.

11.2-3 Scientists may write research or grant proposals and recommendation reports as part of their work. Scientific writing is objective, precise, and clear.

11.3-1 Body language uses nonverbal signals such as gestures and facial expressions.

11.3-2 Signs are indicators of disease or injury that can be seen or measured. Symptoms, such as pain, are not visible but are experienced by the patient.

11.3-3 During a physical examination, physicians use inspection, auscultation, palpation, and percussion.

11.3-4 Orderly and concise observations give actual vital sign measurements and report only what is observed, not what you think the observation means.

11.4-1 Environmental barriers to patient communication include distractions, sensory impairments, and cognitive impairments.

11.4-2 Angry or uncooperative patients often have an unmet need that is causing their behavior. Identify the unmet need to provide a possible solution.

11.4-3 Therapeutic workers need to consider health literacy when educating patients about their treatment plan.

11.4-4 Using a different language creates the most common cultural barrier to communication, but differences in the meaning of gestures or touch and differences in beliefs about healthcare can also become barriers.

11.5-1 When working with diverse populations focus on preferences related to eye contact, body language, sense of time, modesty, speech, and communication.

11.5-2 Developing rapport with patients begins with courteous and attentive behavior that makes patients feel comfortable. It continues with learning more about the patient's individual beliefs and preferences.

11.5-3 Age of coworkers can affect communication preferences. However, learning coworkers' individual preferences leads to better working relationships.

11.5-4 Healthcare workers need to learn their personal biases, prejudices, and stereotypes so that inaccurate beliefs do not negatively affect patient care.

Maximize Your Professional Vocabulary

1. **That's My Term.** The instructor will distribute one professional vocabulary term card or definition card to each student. Students will take turns reading a definition card. The student with the term card that matches the definition being read will stand up and say, "That's My Term."

Reflect on Your Reading

1. Share your predictions about communication errors made by healthcare workers with your classmates. How many different healthcare occupations were included in all the scenarios? How many of the scenarios resulted in life-threatening situations? Write three guidelines for avoiding these errors.

Review and Recall

1. Which of the following best describes the goal of communication? (11.1-1)
   A. Communication flows in a cycle.
   B. Effective communication considers the audience.
   C. Effective communication shares understanding.
   D. The sender decides the best method for delivering a message.

2. Lucia usually agrees with whatever her friends decide but complains to others after the decision is made. Which style does this illustrate? (11.1-2)
   A. Passive   C. Assertive
   B. Aggressive   D. Passive-aggressive

3. *My patient is experiencing abdominal pain near the umbilicus and moving to the lower right pelvic area. She will need additional tests.* This statement represents (11.1-3)
   A. Situation   C. Assessment
   B. Background   D. Recommendation

4. Sheena walked into the exam room to meet her new patient saying, "Hi, Bob. I'm Sheena." Patting him on the back, she offered him a chair and began wrapping the blood pressure cuff around his arm. Identify patient interview protocols that were not followed. Choose all that apply. (11.1-4)
   A. Use a formal title when greeting a new patient.
   B. Identify yourself by name.
   C. State your job title.
   D. Avoid invading the patient's personal space.

5. Choose the best response for Juan when answering the phone. (11.1-5)
   A. "Hi, this is Sunview Medical. I am Juan, the medical assistant. Can I have your name? How can I help you?"
   B. "Hi, this is Juan. How can I help you? What is your name?"
   C. "Juan here. What do you need? Your name?"
   D. "Sunview Medical. Who do you need? OK, I'll put you right through."

6. Which statements indicate phone call screening? Choose all that apply. (11.1-5)
   A. "Let me connect you with the appointment desk."
   B. "Are you having any breathing problems?"
   C. "I will send that refill request to your pharmacy."
   D. "Hi, Dr Jones. Yes, Dr. Smith is in her office. I can connect you now."

7. *Apnea index was 0.4 per hour and apnea-hypopnea index was 7.3 per hour. Arousal index was 0.7 per hour. There were no REM events. Mr. Ramos read this information in his sleep study report in his online medical chart.* Which element of technical writing is a mismatch in this reading experience? (11.2-1)
   A. Technical writing informs the audience.
   B. Technical writing targets a specific group.
   C. Technical writing is clear.
   D. Technical writing is concise.

8. Which of the following is *not* an element of a business email? (11.2-2)
   A. To   C. Salutation
   B. Subject   D. Enclosure notation

9. Scientific writing must be all of the following *except* (11.2-3)
   A. objective   C. acute
   B. precise   D. clear

10. Which of the following show unprofessional body language? Choose all that apply. (11.3-1)
    A. Focus only on the computer screen.
    B. Roll your eyes at the patient's complaints.
    C. Lean toward patients while they are speaking.
    D. Nod to acknowledge what the patient says.

11. Which of these are objective observations? Choose all that apply. (11.3-2)
    A. Bruise   C. Stomachache
    B. Swelling   D. Rash

12. Healthcare workers can detect emphysema in the lungs using this exam technique. (11.3-3)
    A. Inspection   C. Auscultation
    B. Palpation   D. Percussion

13. Choose the best record of an observation. (11.3-4)
    A. Forehead feels hot.
    B. Temperature is 101°F. Reported to head nurse.
    C. Temperature feels high.
    D. Temperature is 101°F.

14. Your patient is leaning toward you and turning his head as you speak. Eventually, he just smiles and nods before leaving. What type of communication barrier might you suspect? (11.4-1)
    A. Cognitive impairment
    B. Sensory impairment
    C. Environmental
    D. Low health literacy

15. Mrs. Neubauer refuses to eat her lunch. She glares stubbornly at any care provider who tries to convince her. Which action might be useful in this situation? (11.4-2)
    A. Ask yourself what has changed in the patient's environment.
    B. Threaten to call the doctor if she does not eat.
    C. Assess the patient's level of pain and discomfort.
    D. Offer other acceptable food choices.

16. You are filling a prescription for an older patient. The patient squints at the label on the medication vial. Which actions will improve health literacy for this patient? (11.4-3)
    A. Provide printed information in larger font.
    B. Use an easy-open lid on the medication vial.
    C. Speak with the patient in a quiet area.
    D. Tell the patient how to take the medication.

17. Which action improves communication when cultural differences create a barrier? (11.4-4)
    A. Talk loudly and slowly.
    B. Use pictures.
    C. Maintain personal space.
    D. Assume your patient agrees with you.

18. Which of these guidelines does *not* illustrate cultural competence? (11.5-1)
    A. Provide complete privacy for a patient to change clothing.
    B. Use an interpreter.
    C. Interrupt the patient to clarify the message.
    D. Address patients and coworkers formally.

19. Select the actions that will help develop rapport with patients. Choose all that apply. (11.5-2)
    A. Learn a few phrases to greet patients in their own language.
    B. Focus your attention on the computer screen.
    C. Record patients' preferences and use them.
    D. Provide written instructions so you do not have to explain them.

20. Which is a common communication preference of older workers and patients? (11.5-3)
    A. Face-to-face conversation
    B. Email
    C. Text
    D. Instant messaging

21. Ignoring patients who express pain because they are just being "difficult" is a sign of (11.5-4)
    A. personal bias
    B. prejudice
    C. stereotyping
    D. cultural competence

Build Core Skills

1. **Critical Thinking.** List three of the skills for effective listening described in the text. Rate yourself on each skill and provide an example to explain your rating.

2. **Speaking and Listening.** Review the following phone conversation and identify errors made by the speaker.
   "Hi! Who do you want to talk to? What's your problem? Say that again. Like, Dr. Jeffers won't be in till, like, tomorrow. What's your name? You'll have to come in then. Bye."

3. **Problem Solving.** Screen and triage the following list of phone calls in order of importance. Use numbers to indicate the level of importance of each phone call. Number one is most urgent, and number four is least urgent.
   A. A mother calls to say her four-year-old has a stomachache, but no fever.
   B. A man calls to say he has tightness in his chest and pain down his arm.
   C. A father calls to say his daughter was stung by a bee, and her hand is beginning to swell.
   D. An older, crying woman calls saying her husband fell in the bathroom and is slurring his words.

4. **Writing.** Work with a partner to compile and organize information and then write a technical report that would be used in a healthcare setting. This might be a hospital menu or patient brochure. Exchange your completed documents with another group. Edit and evaluate the other team's document. What criteria did you use? Share your findings with the class.

5. **Critical Thinking.** Which of the following statements represent the objective, clear, and precise style of writing required for scientific communication? Be prepared to explain your responses.
   A. It is believed that chronic dry eye disease causes dryness and itchy eyes.
   B. According to data results from the National Institutes of Health, losing 5% of one's body weight can cut one's risk of heart problems and related health problems, such as diabetes, 25% or more.
   C. Adults with low levels of vitamin D are two times more likely to suffer from heart disease.
   D. Lower bone density can occur in people who don't like milk.
   E. Pneumonia occurs more often in people with COPD.

F. After the first year of quitting smoking, the risk of heart disease drops by 50%.

6. **Critical Thinking.** Use the internet to find photos of people expressing various emotions. Can you correctly identify the emotion shown in each photo by evaluating the person's nonverbal communication? Print three of the photos you selected and bring them to class. Ask your classmates to identify the emotion in each photo. Then discuss your responses.

7. **Critical Thinking.** Which of the following questions are open-ended? Rewrite any of the questions that can be answered with a one- or two-word response so they are open-ended.
   A. What symptoms bring you to the emergency room today, Mr. Wright?
   B. Do you have pain?
   C. Are you taking any medications, Pablo?
   D. When are you most likely to feel faint?

8. **Critical Thinking.** Review each patient description. Mark signs with an "x" and symptoms with a "v." For each sign, determine which diagnostic technique (inspection, auscultation, palpation, percussion) would identify the medical issue.
   A. patient complains of wrist pain
   B. patient has a wet cough
   C. patient has a sore on his tongue
   D. patient has a lump under the skin near the wrist
   E. patient complains of severe pain on the right side of the abdomen

9. **Writing.** Clarence is an older man who is uncooperative when the nurse wants to take his blood pressure. Since his wife died, Clarence has gained a considerable amount of weight. He has had to rely on restaurant food because his late wife did all the cooking. Identify Clarence's potential unmet needs and propose ways to meet those needs.

10. **Reading.** Use the internet to research a cultural group represented in your community. What are the cultural beliefs of this group? Be sure to research specific healthcare-related beliefs in this group.

Activate Your Learning

1. Prepare a sample business letter using the topic described here. Follow the guidelines shown in Figure 11.18.
   Letter topic: Introduce patients to Dr. James Brace, who will be joining the Smile a Mile dental practice. Dr. Brace's specialty is orthodontics. Include the date on which he will begin seeing patients, and explain how patients can schedule an appointment. This letter is written by you on behalf of Dr. Serena Smile.

2. Prepare a sample memorandum using the topic described here. Follow the guidelines shown in Figure 11.19.
   Memorandum topic: Announce to the staff that Smile a Mile employees will have holidays on both July 4 and July 5 this year. This memorandum comes from you as the office manager

Think and Act Like a Healthcare Worker

1. For each of the following circumstances, decide what is wrong with the situation or how a healthcare worker should react to the situation. Apply the principles of effective communication you learned in this chapter.
   - A doctor says, "I think your problem is cholelithiasis."
   - The healthcare worker speaks in a very soft voice.
   - The clinic receptionist says to a patient, "I don't got any appointments at that time."
   - A patient with limited English nods his head, but still seems confused as the healthcare worker explains a procedure.

2. Add details as needed to make these oral reports complete, orderly, and concise.
   I think Mr. Crawford has a fever.
   Mrs. Krueger's blood pressure is pretty high.
   Mrs. Patel's leg hurts.

Go to the Source

1. Select a healthcare topic and list a few questions you have about the topic. Locate three research papers written about it. Read the abstract for each paper and explain which paper best fits your topic.

HOSA Event Prep: Prepared Speaking

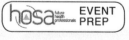

Imagine you have been asked to speak to junior high students about your healthcare career plans. Your speech should include descriptions of your health science classes and hands-on activities, ways HOSA can enhance your health science skills, and experiences that have influenced your healthcare career choices.

Think About It

1. What would you say in your speech?
2. Give two examples of situations where communication skills are important in health science.
3. Where are your communication skills strong? Where could they be improved?

Chapter 12 Healthcare Technology

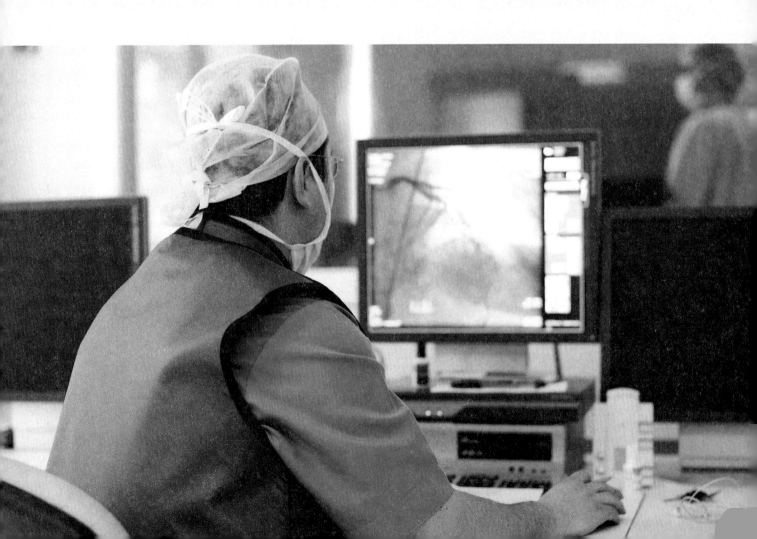

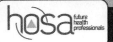

Great medical advances have been made because someone dared to create something better. Through medical innovations and inventions, medicine has evolved rapidly during the past 50 years. Being innovative and daring to create will make the future of medicine even brighter. However, medical inventors are not afraid to try and fail. Some medical innovations include laparoscopic surgery and even robotic surgery. *Medical Innovation* is a HOSA competitive event where teams can research and create new advances in health.

Go to the HOSA website to learn more about the HOSA *Medical Innovation* event. Find out the purpose of the event, what is involved in the event, and what knowledge is demonstrated in the event.

As you prepare for HOSA competitive events, be sure to check the website and talk with your HOSA advisor for the most up-to-date guidelines and procedures. Once you have learned about the *Medical Innovation* event, answer the following questions:

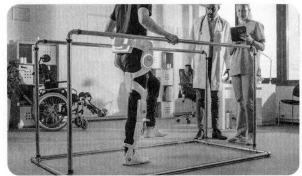

Gorodenkoff/Shutterstock.com

1. How might participating in this event benefit you personally and your future career? Explain.
2. Are you interested in participating in this event? Why or why not?

Connect with Your Reading

Think about your last visit to a healthcare facility such as a medical clinic, dental office, or hospital. What new equipment did you see? What procedures had changed from what you knew before? How was patient information recorded? Share your observations with your classmates and discuss what caused the changes or why the changes may have been made.

Map Your Reading

Make a four-door book using the image as a guide. Write *Healthcare Technology* in the center and label each door with the following categories: *Therapeutic, Diagnostic, Support Services*, and *Biotechnology Research and Development*. Open all four doors and label the left side *EHR History* and the right side *EHR Documentation*. As you read, list main points and important terms from the first lesson in the EHR History section and from the second lesson in the EHR Documentation section. For the third lesson, close the book and draw images on each door to represent technologies used in each healthcare pathway. Finally, open each door and write terms that describe the technologies.

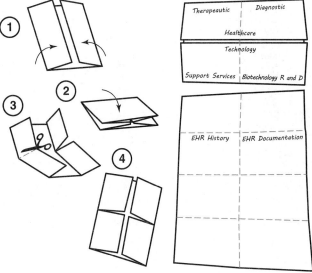

Goodheart-Willcox Publisher

Chapter opener image: U.Ozel.Images/E+ via Getty Images

Development of Electronic Health Records

ESSENTIAL QUESTION

How have electronic health records improved and presented new challenges in healthcare?

Learning Outcomes

After studying this lesson, you will be able to

12.1-1 differentiate between the electronic medical record and electronic health record.

12.1-2 state ways the US government has influenced the development of electronic health records.

12.1-3 explain how the 21st Century Cures Act promotes the interoperability of health information systems.

12.1-4 identify safety considerations for using a personal health record.

Professional Vocabulary

Essential Terms

breach access, use, or disclosure of protected health information that compromises the security or privacy of that information

de-identified information health documents from which specified personal data has been removed

electronic health record (EHR) a medical document that contains information from all the clinicians involved in a patient's care; and can be created and accessed by the patient and by providers across more than one healthcare organization

interoperability the ability of different health information systems to securely access, exchange, and use electronic health information within and across different healthcare organizations

personal health record (PHR) an electronic application through which patients can maintain and manage their health information from multiple providers in a private, secure, and confidential environment.

Important Terms

computerized patient records

electronic medical record (EMR)

Health Information Technology for Economic and Clinical Health (HITECH) Act

meaningful use

proprietary

Introduction

Technology is changing the way people communicate. Computers and personal devices such as smartphones, tablets, and smart speakers are at the heart of that change. People keep in touch by reading and responding to each other's posts and texts. They can apply for future jobs through online postings and video interviews. For personal communication, many people think emails are too slow.

Technology is also changing the way people communicate in the field of healthcare. All healthcare workers must have basic computer literacy skills. Computers have replaced paper in both healthcare documentation and facility operation. Even jobs with the smallest connection to direct patient care or medical records must interact with computers. A housekeeper updates an inventory of cleaning supplies. A central services technician barcodes supplies for billing purposes. A maintenance engineer runs computer diagnostics (dI-ag-NAHS-tihks) on the air-conditioning system to check for needed repairs. A hospital administrator uses a software presentation to communicate the growth plan for the facility.

12.1-1 From the Medical Record to the Electronic Health Record

Nowhere is technological change more far-reaching than in the development of the **electronic health record (EHR)**. The EHR has the potential to speed up the documentation process, improve the accuracy of patient records, and expand access to complete medical records for providers and their patients. The goal of improved care drives the efforts to implement effective electronic systems.

Medical providers have long realized the advantages that computerization brings to medical records. As early as the 1960s, efforts to develop **computerized patient records**—early versions of the EHR—were ongoing at the Mayo Clinic in Rochester, Minnesota; the Medical Center Hospital of Vermont; and El Camino Hospital in California. During the next two decades, many similar systems were developed. Computerized systems could quickly access information about drug dosages and drug interactions. They could communicate treatment plans to everyone caring for the patient. However, the size and processing power of a mainframe computer limited these systems.

During the 1990s, powerful new personal computers (PCs) and networking capabilities emerged. As the cost of computers decreased, several new companies entered the **electronic medical record (EMR)** market. EMRs were an earlier version of the current EHRs. Using EMRs, physicians' offices and outpatient clinics began to convert paper records to electronic formats. These less complex healthcare settings could use commercially available programs. However, the complexity of a hospital environment—with its many departments and services—delayed the adoption of electronic records systems. Many long-term care facilities and home health organizations also found the cost of computerization too high (**Figure 12.1**).

EMRs had a slow start when they were first introduced. Healthcare workers lacked confidence in their security and efficiency. Could someone alter these records without the physician's knowledge or consent? Would a power outage cause a computer "crash" and a loss of vital information? Was typing faster than writing? Many physicians who wrote all their records were reluctant to learn computer skills. Often, computers were not at the point of care, meaning staff had to leave patients to enter information on a computer keyboard.

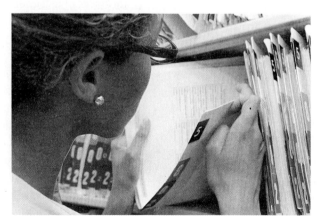

Figure 12.1 Before 2000, the medical records at many healthcare facilities looked like this.

Obstacles

As recently as 2010, fewer than 300 hospitals in the United States had fully implemented the use of EMRs. By comparison, most countries with national healthcare systems such as the Netherlands, Sweden, and New Zealand had fully implemented electronic records. Why did the process of converting to electronic records take more than 30 years when the benefit of improved patient care seemed so obvious?

First, converting to computerized programs is expensive. The cost of implementing an electronic record system falls on the healthcare facility. Some hospitals have mortgaged their facilities to provide capital for investing in a records system, but not all healthcare facilities can do this.

Additionally, electronic record systems can make sharing information more difficult. Healthcare in the United States is competitive. As a result, companies develop **proprietary** (pruh-PRI-uh-tair-ee), or *private*, systems that cannot communicate with other records systems. The record system from Company A cannot communicate with the record system from Company B. Proprietary systems limit the **interoperability** (ihn-ter-ah-per-uh-BIH-luh-tee) of the electronic record system. This means it cannot work with other systems in the healthcare provider network. A general practitioner using the latest system from one company cannot send a patient's record to a specialist down the hall who uses a product from a competing company. To exchange information, the general practitioner must print out the record and deliver it by hand. This reduces the electronic record system's advantages.

New Definitions and Broader Goals

In the early days of computerization, doctors were looking for a way to share patient treatment records with their peers. They wanted a system that would be easier to read than handwritten notes and easier to share than files filled with papers. They were developing the EMR, a system for computerizing clinical information in a patient chart. It included information such as patient demographics and medical history, progress notes and problem lists, vital signs, medications, lab and radiology reports, chief complaints, care alerts, and preventive care guidelines.

Soon, healthcare systems saw the advantages of incorporating other functions such as scheduling, transcription, e-prescribing, evaluation, and coding. Commercial companies developed these programs. Healthcare systems purchased their programs to deliver a more complete set of coordinated and computerized functions. This is the current electronic health record.

As healthcare systems implemented EHRs, sharing of information within a single healthcare network improved dramatically. Sharing information between differing healthcare systems remained a problem. However, one element was largely missing from the healthcare information picture: the patient. A patient could benefit from a complete **personal health record (PHR)**. With this, the patient could access personal medical history, lab reports, provider notes, and even insurance and cost information electronically. A true PHR would allow patients to access their combined information from all providers, even if the providers are from different healthcare systems. Government agencies are working to promote this goal.

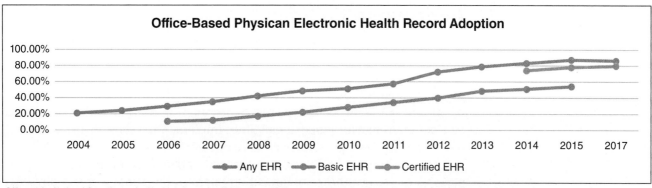

Office-Based Physican Electronic Health Record Adoption

Legend: Any EHR • Basic EHR • Certified EHR

X-axis: 2004, 2005, 2006, 2007, 2008, 2009, 2010, 2011, 2012, 2013, 2014, 2015, 2017
Y-axis: 0.00%, 20.00%, 40.00%, 60.00%, 80.00%, 100.00%

Office of the National Coordinator for Health Information Technology. "Office-based Physician Electronic Health Record Adoption," Health IT Quick-Stat #50. January 2019.

Figure 12.2   As of 2017, nearly 9 in 10 (86 percent) of office-based physicians had adopted any EHR, and nearly 4 in 5 (80 percent) had adopted a certified EHR.

12.1-2 Government Influences

In 2009, the **Health Information Technology for Economic and Clinical Health (HITECH) Act** was signed into law. This law encouraged more healthcare systems to use EHRs. To support this goal, the HITECH Act offered financial incentives to healthcare providers who demonstrated **meaningful use** of EHRs. This means the EHR improvements will benefit both the provider and the patient. The Centers for Medicare and Medicaid Services (CMS) and the Office of the National Coordinator for Health Information Technology (ONC) developed standards for records systems to achieve meaningful use. They offered certification for the systems that met the standards. They required that all systems working with Medicare and Medicaid must be certified to avoid payment penalties. These incentives dramatically increased the use of electronic records. By 2017, 96 percent of all nonfederal acute care hospitals used certified health information technology systems. In addition, 9 out of 10 physician offices used an EHR (**Figure 12.2**).

The HITECH Act made significant changes to HIPAA privacy and security regulations. For example, the law outlined penalties the US Department of Health and Human Services (HHS) could impose for violations of HIPAA rules. The HITECH Act also required business associates of healthcare providers to maintain the same level of security when accessing or exchanging health information between organizations. This means an independent medical transcriptionist or an accounting firm must have the same level of security as the healthcare provider when working with protected health information.

The new privacy and security requirements supported the federal government's plans to increase the use of health information technology (HIT) and health information exchange (HIE). The ultimate goals of nationwide EHR use are to reduce healthcare costs by avoiding duplication of medical tests and to improve patient outcomes through point-of-care access to a patient's complete medical history (**Figure 12.3**).

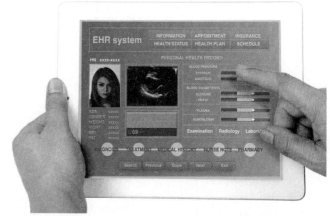

pandpstock001/Shutterstock.com

Figure 12.3   Most healthcare facilities have electronic health records systems. *What caused the rapid expansion in the use of electronic patient records?*

Anticipated Benefits

Physicians who use EHR systems are beginning to see improvements in care (**Figure 12.4**). One physician uses electronic patient data to identify patients with diabetes who are overdue for screening tests. Seconds later, the physician emails those patients a reminder or sends a letter. Two years ago, just 40 percent of the physician's patients with diabetes were in their target range on a standard test for blood sugar. Since implementing data checks and email reminders, that number has risen to 70 percent.

Consider how an EHR system improved patient care in the following scenario. A major healthcare organization operates the clinic where a physician works. The organization has installed a networked EHR system in every clinic and hospital it owns. The physician calls the emergency room (ER) at the hospital to ask if a patient with seizure-like symptoms should be sent to the neurology department or the emergency room. The ER physician checks the patient record, sees that the patient's symptoms are atypical for epilepsy, and has the patient transferred to emergency care. A cardiac monitor reveals an abnormal heartbeat that is corrected by implanting a pacemaker. Without the benefit of immediate access to an electronic record, this patient would likely have been referred to neurology, where a dangerous heart condition would not be diagnosed.

The HITECH Act identifies protected health information (PHI) and requires healthcare workers to keep this information confidential. Patients must authorize the release of PHI for other purposes such as marketing or medical research. However, **de-identified information** can be released because it is no longer considered PHI. The process of de-identifying health information removes all patient-specific information so there is no reasonable basis on which a person can be identified. Once information is certified as de-identified, it may be shared and used for marketing or research purposes. De-identified data provides a large pool of information for medical researchers to use in developing new treatment plans and improving patient outcomes.

Anticipated Benefits of the Electronic Health Record	
Benefit	**Effects**
Improved efficiency and reduced medical costs	• Reduce time spent on paperwork • Reduce duplication of medical tests
Improved care coordination	• Give every provider access to the same information about a patient • Up-to-date medication and allergy lists facilitate prescribing among physicians
Improved patient outcomes	• Improved patient compliance through automated reminders for routine screening • Reliable point-of-care information and reminders notifying providers of important health interventions
Improved quality and convenience	• Accurate coding and billing facilitated by legible documentation • E-prescriptions sent electronically to the pharmacy

Goodheart-Willcox Publisher

Figure 12.4 The goal of improved care drives the efforts to implement effective electronic health record systems.

Under the HITECH Act, healthcare providers must notify the Department of Health and Human Services (HHS) of any **breach** of privacy or security regarding patient information. Breaches can occur in many ways. For example, sending an email to the wrong person or letter to the wrong address is a breach (**Figure 12.5**). Losing a file that contains PHI is a breach. Sharing or posting passwords or letting a fellow worker use your login is a breach. Losing a laptop that is not encrypted is a breach. Accessing information you do not need to know for your job but are simply curious about is a breach.

The HHS Office of Civil Rights oversees the investigation of breaches and enforces privacy rules. HHS is authorized to fine healthcare businesses when a breach occurs. The publicity from a breach has a negative impact on a business. As a result, healthcare facilities carefully follow protocols that protect PHI and prevent breaches of confidential information.

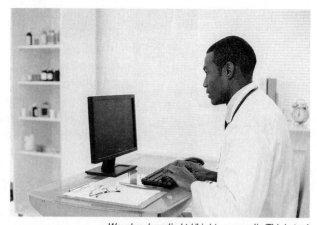

Wavebreakmedia Ltd/Lightwavemedia/Thinkstock
Figure 12.5 A simple mistake when sending an email can cause a breach of privacy or security. *What happens to a healthcare facility when it experiences a breach of privacy?*

Unintended Consequences

Electronic records systems still need improvement. Physician burnout is an unexpected consequence of electronic health records. According to a recent survey, 8 of 10 doctors report feelings of burnout, and almost one-half of physicians plan to change career paths. How could the promise of reduced paperwork backfire so dramatically? Physicians spend about two hours doing computer work for every hour spent face to face with a patient. In the examination room, physicians devote one-half of their patient time to facing a computer screen.

Programs were developed quickly to meet the HITECH Act requirements, so electronic programs have been combined to meet the needs of many different healthcare workers. For example, several different healthcare providers can add diagnoses to a patient problem list. However, they might describe the same diagnosis three different ways or use only a generic term that lacks relevant details needed by the next physician who sees the patient. The physician uses valuable time sorting through an overwhelming amount of information in what used to be a streamlined document updated by a single doctor. Physicians' handwritten notes were brief and to the point. Now the computer pastes large blocks of information, such as a two-page imaging report, into the record instead of selecting the important details. The next physician to see the patient has to hunt for those details.

In some cases, the data entry process is a burden. To document a test done during a patient exam, physicians will enter the current date, their name as the provider, the fact that the patient is present in the office, and so on. On paper records, these basic items did not have to be re-entered for each new procedure during an exam. It can take longer to use a computer for some documentation tasks. Searching through long lists of medication choices and countless clicks to document choices can be exhausting. Primary care physicians, who can see up to four patients per hour, will make as many as 4,000 clicks per day. That large number increases the chance for errors.

EHR systems are prone to problems such as software malfunctions that keep lab reports from being transmitted and patient records that get mixed up.

Medical coding guidelines change yearly, so coding software and electronic forms for code reporting must also be current. Sometimes software programs choose the wrong term. For example, an emergency room report may refer to a patient with morphine sulfate instead of multiple sclerosis.

Much work needs to be done to improve and perfect EHR programs. Meanwhile medical scribes assist some providers to reduce the burden of documentation. EHR companies continue to innovate and are exploring voice systems to streamline the documentation process.

12.1-3 Improving Interoperability

Healthcare systems have adopted EHR programs that communicate well with different facilities in the same system. However, when healthcare systems merge, communication between differing systems and different EHR software continues to present challenges (**Figure 12.6**). As a result, healthcare providers cannot always access patient records at the point of care. For example, a patient who is traveling enters a hospital emergency room far from home, and the physician cannot access electronic records from a different healthcare system. This lack of timely information means the patient may receive duplicate diagnostic tests. Sometimes incomplete transfer of information in a record, such as an allergy to a particular medication, results in treatment that can harm the patient.

As part of the 21st Century Cures Act, the Office of the National Coordinator (ONC) for Health Information Technology has published rules to improve healthcare interoperability. Interoperability means different health information systems can securely access, exchange, and use electronic health information within and across different healthcare organizations. Ideally, electronic health information could be shared safely worldwide. The goal of interoperability is to provide easy access to all of a patient's health information, regardless of location. This could improve the health of individuals and populations worldwide.

The rules focus on preventing information blocking. This occurs when one healthcare organization purposefully prevents another from obtaining patient health data. These rules apply to healthcare providers, companies that develop EHR programs, and established health information networks and exchanges that share medical information electronically. Why would these groups block information? From a business point of view, if a company makes a health record system interoperable with a competitor's system, it will be easier for a customer (such as a large healthcare provider organization) to switch to a different company. Why would a for-profit hospital spend money on a system that allows patients to take their health records and business to a new provider?

The rules also promote the use of application programming interfaces (APIs). APIs provide a method for disconnected applications and systems to communicate with each other. This will lead to more smartphone apps that provide new services and choices in care.

CMS certification standards are tied to these rules, and Medicare and Medicaid payments will depend upon the certification. That is a reason for healthcare providers to work toward interoperability.

Challenges to Interoperability

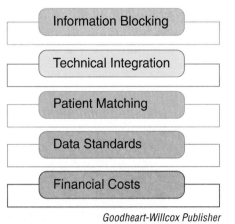

Information Blocking

Technical Integration

Patient Matching

Data Standards

Financial Costs

Goodheart-Willcox Publisher

Figure 12.6 There are several challenges to reaching full interoperability of electronic health records. *Which one can be the result of proprietary health records programs?*

One concern not addressed by the law is a standard patient identifier. When several systems combine health information, it is too easy for patient records to be mixed up. As you can imagine, incorrect matching of patient information leads to incorrect treatments. The opportunity for error is highest when different healthcare organizations exchange information. One research project contracted by the ONC found match rates as low as 50 percent, even between organizations that use the same EHR program. This remains an unresolved issue of interoperability.

12.1-4 Personal Health Records (PHRs)

Technology is changing the way people manage personal health. Health information technology (HIT) is not just for healthcare providers. Patients can use it to learn more about their personal health status and share information with healthcare providers. HIT allows patients to access health information more quickly and directly through online sources, communicate with healthcare providers electronically, and take actions to improve their personal health. It has the power to make the patient a key part of the healthcare team.

Advantages of PHRs

A personal health record (PHR) is similar to an EHR, but the patient controls the information that goes into it (**Figure 12.7**). The PHR helps you keep track of information from your doctor visits. It creates a digital storage center for important health information such as emergency contacts, health history, allergies and medications, lab test results, and immunization dates. Because you can import medical record information from different providers, the PHR can offer a more complete record of your health history.

The PHR can also reflect your personal health goals. Patients can use smartphone apps to track personal health indicators such as food intake, physical activity, or blood pressure readings. The PHR can provide additional information about healthcare outside the doctor's office by recording habits such as over-the-counter medication use or sleep patterns. In some cases, the PHR can link to the healthcare provider's EHR to share information electronically with a provider.

Ideally, patients can access EHRs from all the different providers they have seen. Under 21st Century Cures guidelines, this information should be provided free of charge. When full interoperability is achieved, patients will control their own health information. In the future, patients will be able to access the costs of procedures and treatments to become better consumers of healthcare.

Risks of PHRs

The HIPAA Privacy, Security, and Breach Notification Rules cover PHR systems offered by a healthcare provider or health insurance plan. Other companies that offer PHR systems must comply with the Federal Trade Commission's Health Breach Notification Rule. This means they will notify you if your protected information is released to or used by unauthorized third parties.

With a PHR you can . . .

> . . . have an informed discussion with your healthcare provider.

> . . . provide information to new caregivers.

> . . . access your health information while traveling or when your medical office is closed.

> . . . track your progress toward a personal health goal.

> . . . review physician instructions, medications, and insurance claims.

> . . . track appointments, vaccinations, and other healthcare services.

Goodheart-Willcox Publisher

Figure 12.7 The advantages of a personal health record (PHR).

Healthcare apps are not covered by these laws unless they are offered by your healthcare provider or insurance plan. How will you know that your information is secure? Have you evaluated each app's privacy policies? Are you comfortable with their security, and the ways your information may be shared? Many apps collect and sell data. When you enter your family medical history into a healthcare app, do you realize you are sharing your family's health information without their knowledge? When using independent healthcare apps, individuals are responsible for protecting their own health information. When you post information online—on a message board about a health condition, for example—it is not protected by HIPAA. Never post any private information online.

To protect your health information, secure your own computer files and use passwords for your email system. This will ensure your personal information has some protection if your computer or phone is lost or stolen. Strong passwords are hard to guess. They are at least eight characters long and include upper and lowercase letters, numbers, and symbols. Use two-step authentication wherever possible. Many devices and websites can add a second way to verify your identity. This can be a registered device, fingerprint scan, facial recognition, emailed code, QR code, or answer to a personal question. Update your device's antivirus protection, spam filters, and browser security weekly. For convenience, set this to update automatically.

Medical identity thieves try to steal personal and health insurance information to access medical treatments and get prescription drugs. Always verify your recipient's identity before sharing any personal or medical information. When discarding paper copies, be sure to shred health insurance forms, copies of prescriptions, and physician's statements.

Lesson 12.1 Review

 Complete the *Map Your Reading* graphic organizer for the section you just read.

1. More healthcare facilities are using _____ to provide a complete set of computerized patient information and health informatics functions. (12.1-1)
   A. computerized medical records
   B. electronic health records
   C. electronic medical records
   D. personal health records

2. Which Act encouraged healthcare facilities to implement electronic health records? (12.1-2)
   A. HITECH
   B. HIPAA
   C. 21st Century Cures
   D. OBRA

3. Which term means that different health information systems can securely exchange electronic health information within and between different healthcare organizations? (12.1-3)
   A. De-identification
   B. Stratification
   C. Accountability
   D. Interoperability

4. Which PHRs are protected by HIPAA privacy rules? (12.1-4)
   A. Healthcare apps from a healthcare provider or insurance plan
   B. Apps for tracking diet and physical activity
   C. Online personal health record programs for purchase
   D. Health condition message boards

Documentation in an Electronic Health Record

Learning Outcomes

After studying this lesson, you will be able to

12.2-1 identify components of an electronic health record.

12.2-2 demonstrate medical documentation that is accurate, complete, and timely.

12.2-3 explain the protocols for correcting errors in an electronic health record.

ESSENTIAL QUESTION

What are the elements of correct documentation in an EHR?

Professional Vocabulary

Essential Terms

e-prescribing   electronic generation, transmission, and filling of a medical prescription

medical documentation   written reports of observable, measurable, and reproducible findings from examinations, supporting laboratory or diagnostic tests, and assessments of a patient

Important Terms

addendum

assessment

authenticate

charting

clinical data

compliance

face sheet

problem-oriented medical record (POMR)

Introduction

In caring for patients, the smallest piece of information is potentially important. Healthcare workers learn to communicate and record patient information by documenting it in a patient's medical record. Healthcare workers appreciate the advantages of working with EHRs. However, EHR systems do not change the need for chart entries that are timely, complete, and accurate.

12.2-1 Components of an Electronic Health Record

A medical record is an important form of communication in the healthcare setting. All caregivers and support staff must be able to access a patient's record quickly and find information in it easily. This information is critical to providing consistent patient care and coordinating care and treatment between different caregivers and settings. High-quality medical records are vital to the smooth operation of any medical facility.

These records are the official documentation of

- the physician's **assessment**, or *evaluation*, of the patient's health;
- treatments the patient receives;
- changes in the patient's health; and
- communication between the patient and healthcare workers.

In the past, each patient had a paper folder with forms and reports from a visit to the healthcare provider. Each facility kept a record of every patient it saw, so individuals had several medical records if they visited multiple healthcare facilities. Though these paper folders still exist in a few offices, most healthcare facilities have converted to electronic records systems. Regardless of the system used, patient information must always be well organized, accurate, and complete.

Information in the Medical Record

While a patient's medical record contains both personal and clinical information, clinical information accounts for the largest amount of data. **Clinical data** is organized into several categories within a medical record (**Figure 12.8**). These categories include the history and physical, progress notes, narrative nurse's notes, reports, medication administration, correspondence, and additional forms.

History and Physical

- The chief complaint is the patient's reason for seeing the physician. Using the patient's own words in the form of a direct quote is most accurate.
- The medical history, also called the *family and personal history*, shows the patient's major illnesses and surgeries, as well as those of close relatives, including parents, grandparents, aunts and uncles, and siblings.
- The review of systems and physical examination includes the results of examining the patient's major body systems to look for undiagnosed conditions.
- The diagnosis, or *medical impression*, is the physician's opinion of the medical conditions experienced by the patient. A *differential diagnosis* includes all the possible conditions to be ruled out to identify the correct diagnosis.

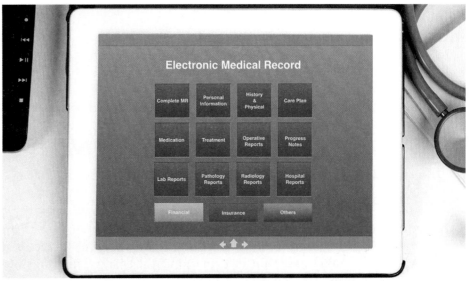

pandpstock001/Shutterstock.com

Figure 12.8 Both personal and clinical data are included in a patient's medical record. *Which data category is larger?*

Progress Notes

These notes describe what happens each time the patient sees a healthcare provider. The notes start with the history and physical information and include the active problem list and recommended tests and treatment plan, including new prescriptions or refills. They summarize each conversation with the patient, whether by phone, through email, or in person. Progress notes use an organized format, such as *SOAP*, so a healthcare provider can quickly understand the patient's situation and concerns (**Figure 12.9**).

Narrative Nurse's Notes

These notes describe the patient's complaints or symptoms and the actions of the nursing staff in response.

Reports

- Radiology reports contain information about X-rays, MRIs, CT scans, sonograms (SAH-nuh-grams), and other imaging studies completed in the office or another facility.
- The laboratory (including pathology) results section contains copies of the results of any blood tests, urine tests, or biopsies completed in the office or another facility.
- The results of specialized tests such as EKGs, stress tests, or colonoscopies are included.
- Consultation reports come from other physicians who have examined the patient at the request of the patient's primary physician. Therapists also submit consultation reports on the patient's progress.
- Operative reports and discharge summaries document hospital care and treatment.

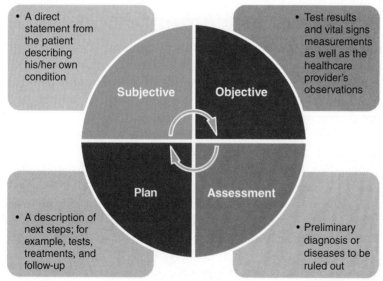

Goodheart-Willcox Publisher

Figure 12.9 The SOAP format is one communication technique used to document a patient visit. It was developed by Dr. Lawrence Weed, MD, in the 1960s as part of the problem-oriented medical record. SOAP notes provide a structured and uniform method for communicating information to other healthcare providers and for allowing providers to retrieve all patient records for a given medical condition.

Medication Administration

This section includes all the medicines administered or prescribed to the patient. Injections and vaccinations are included in this section.

Correspondence

Correspondence includes copies of all letters and memos involving the patient. Examples are letters sent to or received from the patient or letters received from or sent to other physicians.

Additional Forms

Additional forms include consent forms and the signed HIPAA privacy notice. These may also include copies of a living will, a healthcare power of attorney, or organ donation forms. All of these should be kept in the record. Health informatics workers scan all paper forms directly into the electronic health record of each patient.

Organization of Medical Record Information

All documents in a patient's medical record follow a specific system of organization. Today, electronic records software programs determine that system. Most electronic programs use a **problem-oriented medical record (POMR)** method of organization. Patient information is grouped according to the patient's problem.

In a POMR, the patient's medical problems appear on the first page of the record. A provider can quickly access all the information relating to a specific problem. This system works well in healthcare settings where the patient will see different providers due to rotating staff members. Each physician can quickly scan a POMR to review the patient's progress.

12.2-2 Medical Documentation

Medical documentation refers to the information healthcare workers add to a medical record by way of charting. **Charting** is the process of recording observations and information about patients. Many different healthcare workers complete the various aspects of charting. For example, a medical assistant may record demographic information about new patients or interview patients to complete a medical history form. Nurses routinely measure and record vital signs and specific care procedures they have performed, such as injections. Health information technicians code diagnoses and treatment procedures to facilitate payment from insurance companies.

While medical documentation promotes quality care, the medical record serves other purposes as well. For example, a medical record is a legal document that can serve as evidence in court to prove what care a patient received. When records are incomplete or illegible, there is no proof treatment was provided. The rule is, "If it wasn't documented, it wasn't done."

Careful documentation saves money by reducing duplicate tests and avoiding unnecessary procedures. By providing complete information, documentation promotes preventive steps and early intervention to reduce serious outcomes. For example, a complete record of rising blood pressure readings could prompt a physician to recommend lifestyle changes or medication to prevent blood vessel damage and an increased risk for a stroke.

Careful documentation follows the guidelines of regulatory agencies or government programs such as Medicare. **Compliance** with these guidelines is necessary for the healthcare facility to receive reimbursement of costs for treatment and reduce insurance denials of payment. Healthcare compliance means following the rules, regulations, and laws related to patient safety, the privacy of patient information, and billing practices.

Guidelines for Documentation

High-quality medical records meet three standards: they are accurate and complete; they are easy to read; and they are timely, meaning they are written when the procedure or treatment takes place. The following guidelines illustrate the steps for handwritten documentation, but many of the same principles apply to EHRs:

1. Use black or blue ink for handwritten notes.
2. Make sure your handwriting is neat and readable.
3. Verify the patient's name and identifying numbers before entering any information.
4. Since the patient's name is on every screen of the chart, you do not need to include it in each chart entry.
5. Chart your own observations and actions only. Never chart or sign for another healthcare worker. You are personally liable for the care you provide, and the chart is the legal record of your care.
6. Leave no blank or empty lines between entries in the record. This prevents others from making entries that will be mistaken for part of your documentation (**Figure 12.10**).
7. Record the correct date and time for each entry. Always use military time.

   Example: **06/16/23–0830.**

8. Do not erase, cover up, or cross out chart entries. If you make a mistake, draw a single line through the mistake, write "error," then date and initial the change.

   Example: **Ate 100% of ~~dinner~~ breakfast.**
   ————————error 06/16/23 TS

9. Record objective observations rather than your opinions. Record the patient's reactions using the patient's own words in quotation marks.

   Example: **Skin is red and moist to touch. States, "It itches like crazy!"**

10. Always record your verbal report to your supervisor.

    Example: **Temperature: 101.5—Reported to charge nurse.**

NURSE'S PROGRESS NOTES

DATE	TIME	NURSING CARE NOTES	SIGNATURE
06-16-23	0830	Refused breakfast ————————————	Tom Smith RN
06-16-23	0900	Complains of a sharp pain in shoulder ———	
		Skin appears red and warm to touch ———	Tom Smith RN

Goodheart-Willcox Publisher

Figure 12.10 Never leave blank lines in a chart entry. Draw a line through any empty spaces so coworkers do not use that space.

11. Use correct spelling, terminology, punctuation, and grammar. Use only facility-approved abbreviations. This avoids confusion that could lead to treatment errors.

For example, is "6IU of insulin" supposed to be *61 units* or *6 International Units*?

12. Write numbers and measurements in actual figures rather than using general terms such as "many" or "OK."

Example: **BP 120/80** is better than **BP *normal*.**

13. Complete the record as soon as possible after the activity being recorded has occurred. However, you should never record activity *before* it occurs. If you record treatment, begin to give the treatment, and are suddenly called to an emergency, the record will show the patient has already received treatment. This can lead to errors in procedures such as giving medication. Entries added later can result in dates or times that are out of order. These gaps between entries are confusing for anyone accessing the information (**Figure 12.11**). Timely entries provide greater accuracy since the event is still fresh in your mind.

14. Sign your name and title at the end of each entry.

Example: **Tom Smith, RN.**

All contact made with patients should be included in the medical record. Document all calls from patients, calls that give information to patients, and calls regarding prescriptions. These chart entries must contain the date and time of the call, what the patient said or asked for, your reply, and actions you took in response to the call.

Electronic Charting and e-Prescribing

Electronic records contain all the information found in a paper chart, but EHR software combines many additional medical office functions (**Figure 12.12**). For example, the EHR system can

- link to websites that show drug formularies (lists of prescription drugs covered by a health plan) and dosages;
- print patient education instructions;
- recommend codes for medical services;
- search charts to find patients due for routine health screenings;
- alert providers to a patient's drug and allergy interactions;
- streamline medical office communication using email, messaging, and templates for letters; and
- provide immediate access to a patient record from multiple facility locations.

NURSE'S PROGRESS NOTES

DATE	TIME	NURSING CARE NOTES	SIGNATURE
06-16-23	0900	Complains of a sharp pain in shoulder ———	
		Skin appears red and warm to touch ———	Tom Smith RN
06-16-23	0930	Late entry (06-16-23—0830) Refused	
		breakfast ————————————————	Tom Smith RN

Goodheart-Willcox Publisher

Figure 12.11 Notice how the out-of-order entry gives the impression that the patient's pain occurred before, rather than after, the patient refused breakfast.

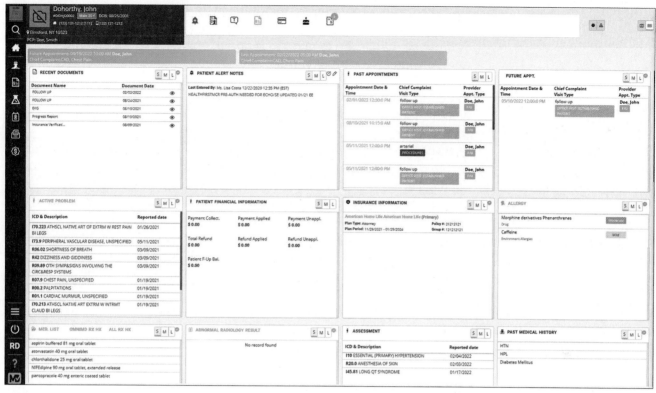

Courtesy of OmniMD

Figure 12.12 Electronic health records contain all the information of a paper medical record, but can also provide schedules, recommended codes for medical services, billing information, and much more.

In a paper record system, these functions require separate resources for looking up information, manually searching patient records, and repeatedly entering the same information for each new document.

 Healthcare Professions: Electronic Records

Maricela, who works as an LPN at a medical clinic, compares electronic records to paper records by asking if you would prefer a car (the electronic record) to a horse and buggy (the paper record). She vividly remembers

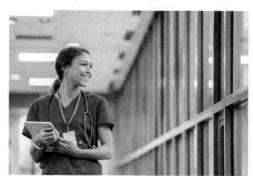

Courtney Hale/E+ via Getty Images

- trying to read handwriting;
- struggling to locate the exact information desired;
- damaging paper with a spill or tear;
- misplacing records; and
- being unable to keep paper records completely secure in a patient's room or file cabinet behind a desk.

Maricela also remembers the difficulty of sharing a patient's paper record with another facility. The record, which could contain as many as 100 pages, had to be located and photocopied by taking each page out and copying it individually. If a clinic called to request all records on a patient for the past year, you would need to flip through each section of the chart—including subcategories such as *Labs*, *Images*, and *Progress Notes*—look at the dates, pull out the correct pages, and photocopy them.

By comparison, reading an electronic record is far simpler. The requested record can be found with a click and shared with another clinic through a secure electronic data transfer. When you need to find a specific record—for instance, lab results for the past month—the computer finds exactly what you want.

Maricela believes electronic records are more secure. As long as each person accessing the information remembers to lock the computer after use, no one should gain unauthorized access to protected information.

The system of electronic prescribing, or **e-prescribing**, replaces handwritten prescriptions, faxed notes, or prescriptions called in by phone (**Figure 12.13**). A physician sends an e-prescription directly to the patient's preferred pharmacy over the internet. This process improves patient safety by automatically checking for drug and allergy interactions and eliminating medication errors due to poor handwriting.

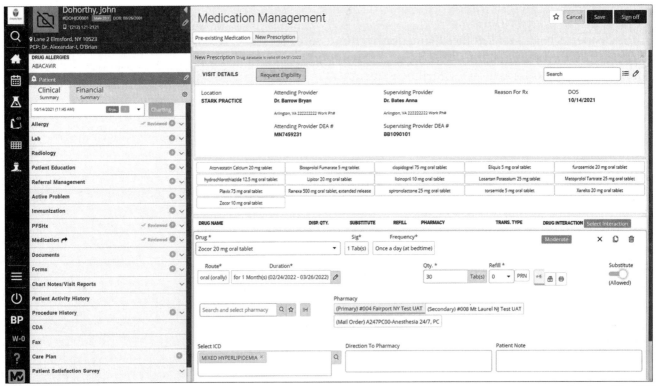

Courtesy of OmniMD

Figure 12.13 E-prescribing software automatically checks for drug and allergy interactions.

It might seem like a healthcare professional can quickly go into the record, check a few boxes, and be done with charting. However, a healthcare worker may need to access several screens, click on multiple tabs, and complete several entries. Using a computerized chart is like turning pages in a book; you do not see everything at once. When you chart tasks electronically, you access different screens and follow assigned tasks. There is a screen for pain management, another for vital signs, a third for intake and output, and so on.

The **face sheet**, or *dashboard*, on a patient's chart shows contact information, insurance information, and medical history. Healthcare workers edit the face sheet to record changes and additions such as a new insurance provider (**Figure 12.14**). Each office visit, or *encounter*, has a separate file showing progress notes for that visit. Information can be extracted or collected from different encounters to track specific services such as immunizations.

Thoroughly charting patient assessments, medications, treatments, education, changes in condition, care plans, and other patient information can take a long time. Even though electronic records have dramatically improved charting, it remains complex and can still be a time-consuming part of patient care.

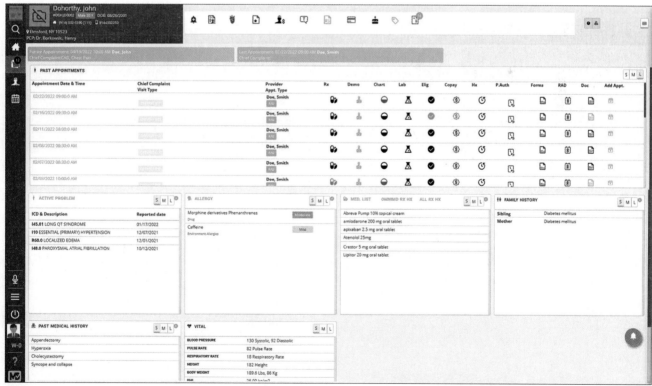

Courtesy of OmniMD

Figure 12.14 Healthcare workers use the patient's face sheet or dashboard to access specific records and add information to the chart.

12.2-3 Correcting Errors in the Electronic Record

Correcting errors in an electronic record can be a simple process, but it is important to never delete errors. Because the patient record is a legal document, you must be able to retrieve the original chart. This means you cannot remove parts of an active patient's medical record. If you correct an error, the original electronic document—including the error—must be stored and accessible. Keep these guidelines in mind as you correct errors in an electronic chart:

- If you find an error recorded by another healthcare worker, talk to that worker to verify it truly is an error. Ask that person to correct it. Remember you are responsible for charting only the care you provide. Never allow another worker to chart care under your username.
- To correct an error, note an **addendum** (uh-DEHN-duhm) on the electronic chart. This means new or corrected information is being added. Then type the reason for the addendum as well as the corrected information.
- Label information that was forgotten as *late entry*.
- **Authenticate** (aw-THEHN-tih-kayt), or give legal authority to, all addendums and late entries with your digital signature and healthcare credentials. Include the date and time with your signature.
- Follow your healthcare facility's specific protocols when correcting errors in electronic charts.

Lesson 12.2 Review

 Complete the *Map Your Reading* graphic organizer for the section you just read.

1. Which of the following is *not* part of an electronic health record? (12.2-1)
   A. Family health history
   B. Patient demographics
   C. Spouse's health history
   D. Medical test results

2. Which term describes the process of recording observations and information about patients? (12.2-2)
   A. Prescribing
   B. Recording
   C. Implementing
   D. Charting

3. High-quality medical records are accurate, complete, and (12.2-2)
   A. timely
   B. grammatically correct
   C. interesting
   D. biased

4. Because the original record must be stored for legal reasons, errors in electronic records must never be (12.2-3)
   A. changed
   B. deleted
   C. corrected
   D. revised

Technological Developments in Healthcare

Learning Outcomes

After studying this lesson, you will be able to

12.3-1 provide examples of computerized therapeutic equipment.

12.3-2 demonstrate appropriate use of digital communication and social media in healthcare settings.

12.3-3 distinguish telehealth from telemedicine.

12.3-4 provide examples of diagnostic applications of technology.

12.3-5 explain how support services workers use technology.

12.3-6 tell how to locate reliable online health information and research a scientific topic using valid resources.

12.3-7 describe the field of bioinformatics.

Professional Vocabulary

Essential Terms

bioinformatics a scientific discipline that combines the tools and techniques of mathematics, computer science, and biology to understand the biological significance of data

primary source a document that describes research in which the authors directly participated

secondary source a document that summarizes the results of several studies

telehealth the use of electronic information and telecommunications technologies to support long-distance clinical healthcare, health-related education, public health, and health administration

telemedicine the segment of telehealth that involves the remote diagnosis and treatment of patients using telecommunications technology

tertiary source a document compiled from primary and secondary sources that gives an overview of a specific topic

Important Terms

automated analyzer
barcode scanners
biorepositories
Digital Imaging Communications in Medicine (DICOM)
evidence-based practices
Human Genome Project

lab information system (LIS)
mHealth
near field communication (NFC)
peripheral devices
primary research articles

quick response (QR) codes
radio frequency identification (RFID)
regimens
review articles
simulate
social media
UV-C disinfection

> **?**
> **ESSENTIAL QUESTION**
>
> *What are some examples of technological developments in healthcare?*

Introduction

Modern technologies continuously change all aspects of healthcare. From new equipment to new systems for recording and organizing data, healthcare technology transforms the delivery of healthcare.

12.3-1 Computerized Therapeutic Equipment

Technology is changing therapeutic procedures (**Figure 12.15**). In the surgical suite, a physician can rotate a 3D image to practice the steps in a surgical procedure before performing surgery. Medical students play video games to learn how to use joystick technology for future surgeries. Computerized robotic hands guided by a physician may complete an actual surgical procedure when the surgeon's own hands are too large for the surgical site. Handheld robots help surgeons perform microsurgeries.

Patients receiving therapy use video games and virtual reality systems to improve balance and coordination. Work simulators and therapy robots restore patients' strength and mobility following injuries or joint replacement surgery. Speech pathologists use virtual reality and electronic stimulation to improve speech and swallowing for patients affected by stroke or Parkinson's disease. Tablet computers with applications that generate speech using buttons with symbols or eye movement restore communication for patients who cannot speak. Voice libraries allow these patients to select a human voice that matches their own age and gender.

A new dental crown used to require an initial visit for the placement of a temporary crown while the new crown was being made in an offsite dental laboratory. The permanent crown was installed a couple of weeks later during a second appointment. Now the dentist uses an electronic sensor to take a digital image of the original tooth and draws the crown on a computer screen right in the exam room. Dimensional data is sent electronically to the milling machine or a 3D printer located in the same office, and the new crown is created while the patient waits.

Patient monitoring systems help older adults stay in their own homes or apartments when health issues arise. You have probably seen advertisements for personal alert systems, which allow the user to press a button to summon help after a fall. However, a wide variety of sensors has increased the scope of patient monitoring. These sensors can monitor how often a person gets out of bed, flushes the toilet, or opens the refrigerator. No cameras or microphones are used, but family members and healthcare providers can receive alerts if typical patterns change. For example, an increase in toilet flushing could signal a urinary tract infection. These sensor-based monitoring systems are far less expensive than full-time assisted living or nursing home care. Combined with home health services, a sensor system allows older adults to continue living in their own homes or apartments.

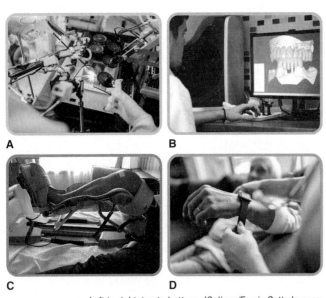

Left to right, top to bottom: JGalione/E+ via Getty Images, zoranm/E+ via Getty Images, NikNajmuddin Photography/Shutterstock.com, giuseppelombardo/Shutterstock.com

Figure 12.15 Technology such as surgery simulators (A), crown-designing software (B), continuous passive motion machines for rehabilitation following knee surgery (C), and wireless wearable devices for continuous vital sign monitoring (D) change and improve therapeutic procedures.

12.3-2 **Social Media**

Social media networks have changed the way people interact and communicate with each other. Should they also change the interactions and communication between healthcare providers and patients? As the worlds of social media and healthcare intersect, people are experiencing positive results but also finding areas of concern.

Advantages

Healthcare professionals embrace the use of social media to promote healthcare organizations. However, they emphasize that personal and professional communication must remain separate. One doctor maintains both a professional social media page, which anyone can view, and a personal page limited to friends and family. In this way, he complies with the American Medical Association (AMA) guidelines. The guidelines advise physicians to protect privacy and maintain appropriate boundaries when communicating with patients through social media (**Figure 12.16**).

Social media allows physicians to reach a wider audience. Physicians may post links to updated medical guidelines and patient-education resources. With patient permission, a cosmetic surgery center might post success stories with a description of treatment options, and an obstetrician might post photos of newborns. An orthopedist (or-thuh-PEE-dihst) promotes a fitness-challenge event on social media. Employees and patients respond by posting photos of themselves working to meet each week's new challenge. This creates a motivational competition.

Posts from physicians can send helpful alerts and reminders. One physician alerts patients when he is running late for appointments so they do not have to sit for a long time in the waiting room. Another sends a reminder about an upcoming immunization clinic.

While social media can enhance provider and patient communication, it cannot replace office visits. The use of social media and virtual communication for patient care is increasing. Healthcare workers must recognize that using social media does not remove their obligation to protect patient privacy and maintain professional relationships with patients.

Social Media Guidelines for Healthcare Professionals

Do not post individually identifying patient information online.

Use privacy settings to separate personal and professional online content.

Maintain professional boundaries.

Do not make disparaging remarks about patients, employers, or coworkers.

Do not take photos or videos of patients on personal devices, including cell phones.

Promptly report a breach of confidentiality or privacy.

Goodheart-Willcox Publisher

Figure 12.16 It is important for healthcare workers to use social media responsibly.

Concerns

Messages over social media can be useful for communicating information to patients, but they are not the best method for answering patient questions. The limited length of social media messages may require a physician to over-simplify a response.

Answering patient questions through social media also raises privacy concerns. For this reason, physicians use secure web portals for communication with patients to better answer their questions. Patients can use this same site to view their lab test results or schedule appointments. Physicians communicate with patients by email throughout the day to reduce the time needed to make phone calls to patients at the end of the day.

Healthcare workers must use common sense when posting information online. Violating patient confidentiality and making derogatory (dih-RAH-guh-tor-ee) remarks that disrespect patients are obvious errors in online communication. However, just the details of a diagnosis and treatment can identify a patient even if the information is posted without other identifiers.

Since anyone can post information online, medical advice on social media sites can be inaccurate. For this reason, patients should use links offered by healthcare providers.

12.3-3 Telehealth and Telemedicine

Telehealth and telemedicine offer new options for healthcare. The terms **telehealth** and **telemedicine** are often used interchangeably. They both refer to technology solutions that support long-distance clinical healthcare, patient and professional health-related education, public health, and health administration. More precisely, telehealth is a broad term that includes all health services. Telemedicine is a specific kind of telehealth that involves a healthcare professional providing medical services. An app that informs the public about a disease outbreak is telehealth. An app that lets physicians treat patients through video chat is telemedicine.

Telehealth and telemedicine are not exactly new. People used the telegraph to order medical supplies and report casualties during the Civil War. In the late 1800s, the telephone reduced unnecessary doctor's office visits. Today, telemedicine uses new therapeutic equipment, smartphones, computers, and other electronic devices.

Therapeutic Telemedicine

Personal devices and apps, short for *applications*, have fueled growth in mobile technology. Thousands of health-related apps are available. How are they making healthcare more mobile? What telehealth and telemedicine options do they provide?

Healthcare apps, which are sometimes called **mHealth** (mobile health) programs, can be divided into categories according to their purpose (**Figure 12.17**):

- **Electronic health records.** Healthcare professionals can access patient records and check lab results. With full access, physicians can dictate into the record, monitor a patient's vital signs, and e-prescribe from a smartphone.

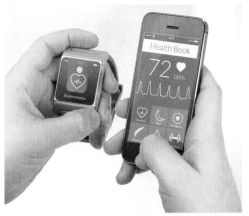

Alexey Boldin/Shutterstock.com

Figure 12.17 Mobile health (mHealth) programs provide health information on mobile devices such as tablets and smartphones. *Name two resources that mHealth programs offer.*

- **Point of care.** Providers can communicate with patients using images and videos to explain disorders and treatments. Some programs break down language barriers by providing medical phrases in languages other than English.
- **Medical reference and education.** These programs provide interactive images of human anatomy and disorders, drug interactions, procedure references, medical news updates, professional journal articles, and research case studies to enhance diagnosis.
- **Consumer health.** As you might expect, food and physical activity diaries, calorie trackers, and pedometer programs are widely available. Mobile pharmacy apps let you request a refill by scanning the barcode on your prescription. Practical apps for travelers can track medication schedules across time zones, send medication alerts, or locate the nearest emergency room.
- **Remote Patient Monitoring (RPM).** Some programs use devices that plug into the phone or tablet to measure and track health data. With these devices, you can monitor your blood pressure or blood glucose levels and send the data to your physician through your smartphone or tablet. Newer wireless systems use Bluetooth technology to transmit patient data to the healthcare provider.
- **Teletherapy.** Virtual visits for mental healthcare have become popular. It is a major convenience for the patient and improves access to care when there is a shortage of local care providers. Some patients report higher levels of satisfaction during therapy sessions because they are in the comfort of their own homes (**Figure 12.18**).

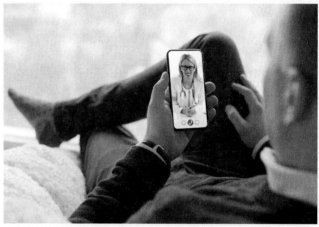

Kaspars Grinvalds/Shutterstock.com

Figure 12.18 Patients enjoy being at home when they access teletherapy appointments.

Older adults and their caregivers are using mobile health apps more often. Patients with chronic health conditions use apps to improve at-home monitoring. This reduces costs and improves patient outcomes by decreasing the number of patients readmitted to hospitals.

Linking EHR systems with apps for mobile devices is technologically challenging. However, medical facilities are developing apps that work with their electronic record systems to transfer patient data privately and securely. Regulations from the US Food and Drug Administration (FDA) may slow the approval of new mHealth programs, but they also remove apps that make false medical claims. Security and privacy remain a concern. Healthcare workers who carry their own smartphones for mHealth purposes must not check personal messages while working with patients. They should not record patient images or access social media on their personal devices while at work. Healthcare workers need to follow facility policies for phone use to preserve patient privacy and quality healthcare.

Diagnostic Telemedicine

Technology is expanding applications for patient diagnosis. Virtual visits let patients and doctors communicate in real time using video conferencing.

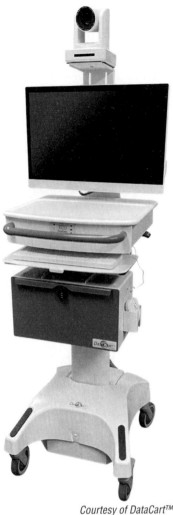

Courtesy of DataCart™

Figure 12.19 Using a media cart with an exam camera allows a patient in a local clinic to be examined by a specialist in a distant location.

These visits work well for conditions that do not require lab tests, an X-ray, or a hands-on exam. Virtual visits are especially useful during an outbreak of infectious illness. They keep vulnerable populations and people with infections from meeting each other in the waiting room. You can receive assessment and care for allergies, motion sickness, or other common conditions without visiting a health clinic. E-visits are non-video visits that let you communicate with your provider through the web portal of your healthcare system. You complete an online questionnaire. A physician reviews your responses and medical record and responds with appropriate treatment options. Telemedicine can replace a trip to your healthcare clinic depending upon your doctor's assessment.

Early telemedicine technology brought healthcare to patients with difficulty accessing healthcare. For patients in rural areas without specialty clinics, telemedicine can provide specialty diagnostics through local clinics. The US military also uses this technology and adopted telemedicine early for specialty care. For example, as a telemedicine technician, Tanya operates a mobile video cart (**Figure 12.19**). The cart includes **peripheral** (puh-RIH-fuh-ruhl) **devices** that attach to a computer, such as an exam camera, a video otoscope with an optic cable and light source, tongue depressor attachments, stethoscope, pulmonary function test equipment, and capture software for storing and forwarding data and images in the medical record. A separate cart contains audiology equipment with attachments for remote hearing aid programming.

Traditionally, a patient who needed hearing aids had to travel to a distant specialty clinic four different times. With telemedicine, the patient only travels to the specialty clinic for the initial hearing assessment. For the following three appointments, the patient sees Tanya, the telemedicine technician, at the local clinic. She connects the patient to the verification equipment and enters the patient's audiogram into the computer link. From there, the audiologist at the specialty clinic many miles away takes over and remotely adjusts hearing aid settings for the patient.

In addition to audiology, telemedicine is used for psychiatry, dermatology, ophthalmology, and even remote physical therapy. New applications continue to emerge. Patients who use telemedicine report improved satisfaction with healthcare services and appreciate reduced costs for specialty care.

Telemedicine no longer serves only rural patients. It provides convenient care for patients with mobility issues. Primary physicians may consult with specialists electronically by sharing a patient's medical data. Paramedics can send patient data to the emergency room doctor for assessment and begin treatment enroute. Today, patients might prefer telemedicine even when they can access clinic care. Telemedicine avoids fighting traffic to get to the clinic or sitting in a waiting room with other people who may have contagious illnesses. Telemedicine will continue to improve. It can provide a workable and even advantageous form of healthcare delivery for many medical situations.

12.3-4 Diagnostic Applications

New technologies continue to change diagnostic techniques. For example, Bailey, a medical technologist, says that information technology has become a part of everything done in a medical lab. The entire lab is automated, from specimen receiving and processing to running samples through analyzers linked to patient medical records. Automating lab functions increases lab testing volumes and reduces costs. A shortage of medical technologists also encourages automation.

Single specimens were traditionally handled three or four times during processing. Now they are handled only once when they are placed on an automated line that processes samples using an **automated analyzer** (**Figure 12.20**).

Software systems produce barcoded specimen labels. The analyzer scans the labels to read identification numbers and perform necessary lab tests. Test results are uploaded into the **lab information system (LIS)**. This system manages data about patients, lab test requests, and lab test results. Lab staff and the automated equipment can see what tests are pending. An LIS tracks every detail about patients, from the time they arrive until they leave, and stores the information for future reference. The system also directs test results to the appropriate hospital department or physician. Some labs use robotic sample handlers. This improves workflow and reduces the risk of pathogen exposure for lab workers.

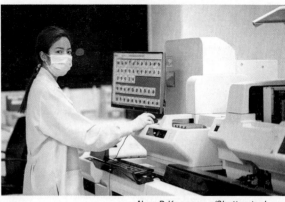

Near D Krasaesom/Shutterstock.com

Figure 12.20 Automated analyzing equipment like the machine shown here can quickly sort and prepare samples for analysis.

Medical equipment companies continue to develop new and improved imaging technologies. Meanwhile, the requirements for digitizing images have improved access for patients and medical providers. **Digital Imaging Communications in Medicine (DICOM)** is a standard for handling, storing, printing, and transmitting information. DICOM improves the distribution and viewing of medical images such as MRIs, CT scans, ultrasound images, and X-rays. Healthcare workers can access and transfer medical images between devices designed by different manufacturers when they use the DICOM standard format and communications protocol. This means images can be shared among medical staff at different locations. When healthcare facilities follow the DICOM standard, patients do not have to carry images from one doctor to another. Instead, the images can be sent electronically as part of the EHR.

12.3-5 Support Services Applications

Support services workers interact with technology daily. From programming mannequins to barcoding supplies, they maintain equipment and operate software that provides a secure environment for patient care.

Healthcare Professions: Support Services Technology

Kelvin was raising the hospital bed before changing the linens when the bed's alarm began to beep. He tried several buttons on the keypad with no luck. The constant beeping continued. He phoned maintenance, and a technician came in a few minutes to reprogram the bed controls. This made Kelvin consider all the ways that technology was transforming even simple pieces of equipment like hospital beds.

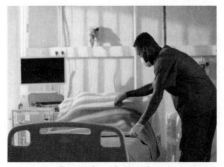

TommyStockProject/Shutterstock.com

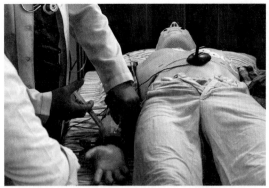

Michael Pervak/Shutterstock.com

Figure 12.21 Programmable mannequins simulate care situations and provide excellent training opportunities for healthcare workers. *Which healthcare worker maintains and facilitates use of these mannequins?*

Clinical Simulators

Healthcare facilities and educational programs use computerized clinical simulators. Simulators provide hands-on training for healthcare workers (**Figure 12.21**). These highly sophisticated mannequins can be programmed to **simulate**, or *imitate*, medical emergencies. They include speech capabilities and adjustable vital sign readings to make training realistic. The clinical simulator technician sets up simulation events and pre-programs the mannequin for care scenarios. Following a training session, the technician conducts technical debriefings. The technician also maintains and updates simulation software.

Barcode Technology

The central services department employs technology to improve inventory functions. **Barcode scanners** read the line codes on patient supplies. This system tracks inventory while assessing charges for patient care supplies. Check-in and check-out procedures track the location of reusable diagnostic tools and medical equipment. Healthcare facilities contain fixed inventory items such as chairs, televisions, and computers. Using a handheld computer, a worker can walk around scanning the barcodes on these objects. The worker can then run a report of all items in the facility. It will show which items are missing or have been moved.

Barcodes also play a role in patient identification. For example, nurses will scan a patient's barcoded wristband and the barcode on the patient's chart to verify they are talking to the right patient. Then they can view the patient's medical record on a computer screen and update charts by entering current vital signs and progress notes. Before administering medication, a nurse scans the patient's wristband, the medical record barcode, and the barcode on the medication. This verifies the nurse is with the right patient and has the right medication. Facilities also use barcode technology for lab specimens, radiology reports, and pharmacy labels. This reduces medical record errors and improves patient care.

QR Technology

Quick response (QR) codes, or *quick read codes*, are two-dimensional barcodes that can be displayed almost anywhere. They appear on print materials, such as magazines and brochures, or on a digital screen. They can appear on signs or products. You can use your smartphone to scan the code, which takes you to a website or video with more information. In healthcare settings, this technology can replace patient care videos and printed instructions. Instead of sending a patient with heart disease home with a DVD and binder of information, the patient can scan QR codes in a brochure to view videos with diet and physical activity recommendations, and postsurgical care guidelines. Healthcare marketing and public relations departments can use QR codes to provide information about healthcare services and clinic locations. Potential patients can scan physician QR codes to view physicians talking about their background, specialty, and willingness to accept new patients.

QR codes can connect you to your mobile pharmacy. By scanning the barcode on your prescription, you can quickly order a refill. You can also access an app that lets you manage prescriptions by showing expiration dates and remaining refills, providing a pharmacy locator, and sending medication reminders to your phone.

RFID Technology

Radio frequency identification (RFID) is a tracking technology. It uses electronic tags for storing data. Information moves only in one direction, from the tag to the reader. Like barcodes, RFID tags identify items. However, they do not require "line of sight" for reading because antennas on the RFID tag and reader use radio waves to exchange data. The tags on clothing and library books that prevent theft are common uses of RFID technology.

Another benefit of RFID technology is that each individual item can be tracked. For example, the Universal Product Code (UPC), a common example of a barcode, identifies a *type of item* such as a 16-ounce jar of peanut butter. However, an RFID code tracks *a specific jar* of peanut butter and can show jars in your inventory that have passed their expiration dates.

Hospitals use RFID systems to track inventory of medical devices such as stents and catheters. An employee must scan an RFID-tagged identification card before removing implants or other devices from a locked cabinet. The system automatically creates a digital record showing which items have been removed and who removed them. In addition, the system will use barcode scanning to track which items are used. When a worker selects an implant in three different sizes, the scanner can track which item is used and indicate the need for reordering. It can also track the return of the unused items and note which worker is responsible for the return. Once the surgery has concluded, the worker returns to the locked storage unit, scans their ID badge, and places any unused items back on the shelves. The system will automatically indicate those products were unused and returned.

NFC Technology

Near field communication (NFC) makes it possible to pay for merchandise with your phone. Like RFID, it uses an electronic chip in a device or sticker. It can transmit and exchange information wirelessly with the tap or swipe of a smartphone. The added security of NFC protects medical information. NFC can be used for ID cards that limit access to operating rooms or medical storage cabinets. In the same way, it can limit access to computers and protect patient data. NFC-enabled wrist bands can not only identify a patient, but also provide real-time information. For example, they can show when a medication was last given, or which procedure is scheduled.

NFC has advantages for tracking equipment and people. Swiping the tag on a piece of equipment shows the location of the equipment, when it was taken, and who took the equipment. If a piece of equipment is missing, it is easy to look it up in the online inventory, identify it, and locate it. In home healthcare, nurses swipe a tag on the mailbox when arriving and leaving a patient's home to create a log of provider visits. Swiping a patient ID card provides access to pertinent medical information.

Because smartphones and tablets have NFC capabilities, this technology is accessible to patients and providers. Medications and medical devices with an NFC tag can provide information and instructions for the patient. For home monitoring, an NFC-enabled wristband can track vital signs. When the patient taps the wristband to a smartphone, the data is sent to the doctor's office for review. This reduces the number of clinic visits (**Figure 12.22**).

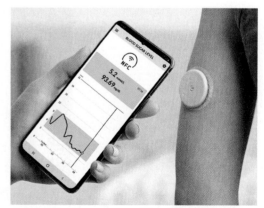

RSplaneta/Shutterstock.com

Figure 12.22 This sensor uses NFC technology to transfer blood-glucose readings to a phone.

UV-C Technology

Support services workers face the constant challenge of cleaning and disinfecting healthcare facilities. Using a **UV-C disinfection** device along with manual cleaning and disinfection keeps patients, visitors, and staff safer. These lightweight devices can be moved to any area, including small bathrooms. Each device has arms that emit UV-C rays. Housekeeping staff position the arms for best coverage and can begin working in another area while the device operates. The disinfecting energy emitted by the device eliminates organisms in a few minutes. This system wipes out pathogens and organisms that manual cleaning may miss. It also reduces exposure to the harmful chemicals used to fight resistant pathogens and organisms for housekeeping staff. UV-C technology disinfects patient rooms, surgery centers, staff offices, and patient reception areas.

Food Service Applications

A healthcare facility's dietary staff relies on technology to track and manage inventory and may employ barcode or RFID systems for that purpose. Computers are also essential for managing recipes, menus, and individual patient diets. When was the last time you used a cookbook? Even at home, online recipe access is commonplace. In a healthcare facility, software programs manage recipes and specify ingredients and amounts.

Dietitians and nutritionists use diet-analysis programs to manage diseases and conditions that require special diets. Using unique factors such as the patient's sex, age, height, and weight, software programs analyze food intake and physical activity. The results will show caloric needs and nutrient deficiencies or excesses. Then the program will make recommendations for changes to improve health (**Figure 12.23**). Using that information, the dietitian can plan menus and choose recipes to support improved health.

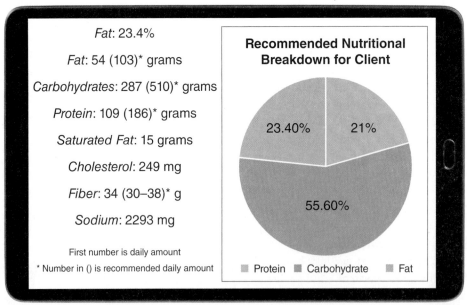

Yeti studio/Shutterstock.com

Figure 12.23 Dietitians use diet analysis programs to manage diseases that require special diets. *What features do these programs offer?*

12.3-6 Biotechnology Research and Development Applications

Advances in information technology have rapidly increased the amount of healthcare data and information generated. This means everyone must review online information carefully to find trustworthy sources. The field of bioinformatics develops methods for storing, accessing, and using research data to advance healthcare.

Reliable Sources for Health Information

When scientific information was printed on paper, you could easily see who wrote it and when. Today, people use electronic resources to access most of this information. Anyone can publish information online. How can you determine which information comes from a reliable source?

Look at the website address for basic clues. Addresses that end in .gov are most likely reliable government websites. They will offer statistics and objective reports. Site addresses ending in .edu are typically educational institutions. However, these sites may feature students posting personal opinions as well as university research publications. Remember that sites ending in .com are commercial sites trying to sell a product. While some .org sites contain excellent information, proceed with caution if they contain links to sites that sell products. These are general guidelines for narrowing your search.

When you research health information, remember that there is lots of health misinformation on the internet (**Figure 12.24**). Read all medical claims with skepticism. Be on the lookout for these common online scams:

- **Miracle cures.** If the claim seems miraculous, do not believe it. Remember, it is not true just because you see it in print. Be suspicious of "breakthroughs," "secret ingredients," and sites that use technical jargon to make the product sound impressive.
- **Celebrity endorsements.** Famous people, and especially medical experts, sell products. However, "celebrities" may be look-alike imposters.
- **Trial periods.** If the product is good, why do you have to buy it now? The words "act now" and "limited quantity" are red flags. When you do order, the sales agreement may be manipulated so you cannot change your mind about future deliveries and end up owing additional money.
- **Blogs.** Personal health stories help others facing similar challenges, but "fake blogs" exist as marketing tools to get you to buy a product. Again, be skeptical of a blog that talks about a secret ingredient, breakthrough, or the "only product that works."

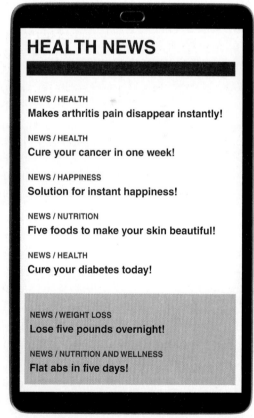

Yeti studio/Shutterstock.com

Figure 12.24 Remember that anyone can post information online. *Do you think these headlines are scams? Explain how you arrived at this answer.*

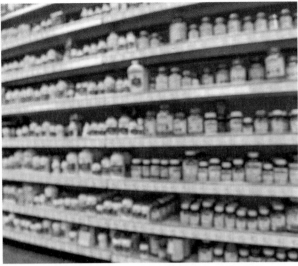
Trong Nguyen/Shutterstock.com

Figure 12.25 Store aisles are crowded with dietary supplements. *How can you know they contain what the label says?*

- **Phony testimonials.** When you see product endorsements written by customers, check if they are all written on the same or similar dates. If you cannot add your own comments, then the creators of the website posted those endorsements.
- **Missing contact information.** Check for the company name, address, and phone number before ordering. If you cannot find it on the website, do not order. You will not be able to resolve any problems with the product or the amount you are charged.
- **Seal of approval.** When you purchase supplements, look for the United States Pharmacopeia (far-muh-koh-PEE-uh) seal. This means the product has been tested and verified for quality. You can trust the product label regarding the purity and potency of a supplement. Without the USP seal, you truly have no idea what is in that bottle (**Figure 12.25**).

How can you know whether online health information is reliable? The National Library of Medicine offers solid guidelines to follow when evaluating online health information.

1. Find out who is responsible for the content.
   - Click on the "About Us" tab. Does the site belong to the federal government, a nonprofit or educational institution, a professional organization, a health system, a commercial organization, or an individual?
   - Look for a listing of professionals who reviewed the content of the website.
   - Valid websites have a way to contact the organization. Is there an email or a street address?
2. Check for funding sources.
   - Does the site use advertisements? If so, are they clearly labeled as ads, or do they look like health information with a link to an online store?
   - Is the site sponsored by a nonprofit organization and funded by donations? Is it an educational institution or government site funded by tax revenue, or does the information favor the sponsor of the site?
3. Evaluate the quality of the information.
   - Look for a description of the process for selecting and approving information, often called the *editorial, selection,* or *review policy.* Is the material reviewed before posting? Do the reviewers have expertise in the site's subject?
   - Look for the author of the information and the original source for the data and research. "Written by James Smith, MD," or "Copyright 2024, American Diabetes Association" are good examples.
   - Look for dates on documents to show information is current. Click on site links. If they are broken, the site may not be up to date.

4. Investigate privacy policies.
   - Does the site have a privacy policy, and does it tell you what information the site collects?
   - Does the site ask for your personal information, and does it tell you how that information will be used?
   - Are you comfortable with how your information will be used? Remember, health information should be confidential.

Take the time to evaluate your sources (**Figure 12.26**). Your knowledge and understanding of a healthcare topic will only be as good as the sources of information you use to learn about it.

Scientific Literature

Medical professionals read scientific literature to stay informed about healthcare advances and potential changes in diagnosis and treatment. Scientific communication appears in documentaries, news articles, professional journals, health-related websites, popular magazines, and government and university publications and presentations.

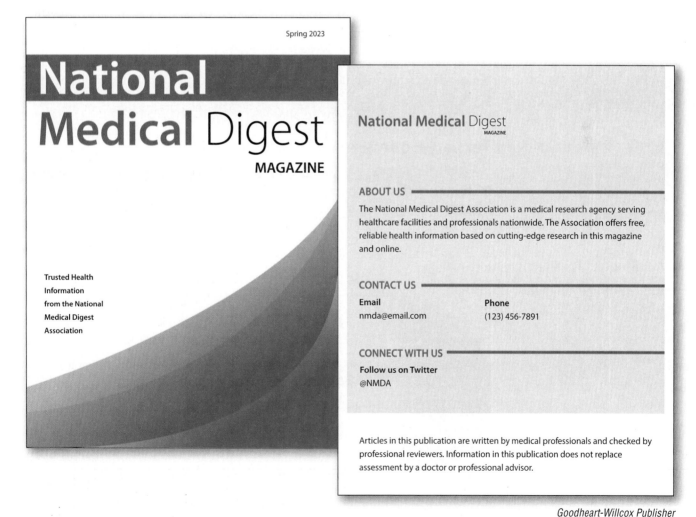

Goodheart-Willcox Publisher

Figure 12.26 What items indicate that this example magazine is a reliable source of online information?

Scientific communication's primary goal is to inform. Accuracy and validity are important components of scientific communication. Validity is achieved when a conclusion can be verified or proved to be true. Students studying health sciences must know how to select valid sources of information and learn how to read and evaluate scientific articles.

Primary Sources

Health science information can be primary, secondary, or tertiary (**Figure 12.27**). **Primary sources** are original research. Scientists complete research in the laboratory, then write about it and publish it in formal lab reports, case studies, or research articles. You will find primary research documents in health science journals. Primary sources contain detailed descriptions of experiments and references to experiments completed by other researchers. These sources tell you the latest findings about a topic, but they can be difficult to read unless you are an expert in the specific subject area of the research. This is because primary sources target people in the writer's field, who understand the common terminology.

Secondary Sources

Secondary sources talk about the original research of others. They summarize, analyze, and interpret information found in primary source documents. For example, you might read about research results in an article in the *Journal of the American Medical Association*, the health section of the *New York Times*, or on the Science Daily website. These articles will provide some facts and a summary of the research. They are written in easily understandable language but do not contain detailed descriptions of the experiments like the primary source. However, the articles do provide citations so you can locate and read the primary source for more details.

Tertiary Sources

Tertiary sources provide an overview of a topic. They sort and compile information from both primary and secondary sources. Almanacs, diagnostic and treatment manuals, dictionaries, and encyclopedias are tertiary sources.

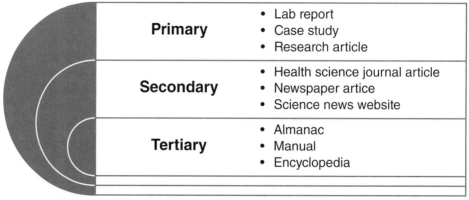

Sources of Health Science Information

Primary	• Lab report • Case study • Research article
Secondary	• Health science journal article • Newspaper artice • Science news website
Tertiary	• Almanac • Manual • Encyclopedia

Figure 12.27   *What type of source do you think this textbook is? Explain your reasoning.*

Researching a Science Topic

Imagine that you have just read a news article about sleep deprivation, which included the surprising statistic that 70 percent of adolescents are sleep deprived. Since you need to pick a topic for a science paper, you decide to do some research on this topic. You search for the work of the scientist quoted in the article and find a presentation the scientist gave to a professional association. You read the slides from the presentation, which are a primary source for information.

Next, you go to the Centers for Disease Control and Prevention (CDC) website, which is listed as a source in the article. You read results from a survey about adolescent lifestyles and find information about sleep habits. Finally, you log in to your school's media site and enter a database containing health science journal articles.

Your search locates a full-text article about the sleep habits of adolescents. It was recently published in a professional health science journal. This article looks great until you start reading. Unlike the previous sources, this one is written for other professionals in the field of health science. While you can read most of the words, you do not understand what they are saying. Since you want to pursue a career in health sciences, you decide to take on the challenge of understanding the content of this research article. Where do you begin?

First, determine which type of scientific paper you are reading. **Review articles** give an overview of a specific topic. They summarize the data and conclusions from several different studies. These articles provide a good starting point because they contain more background information about what has been happening in the field.

Primary research articles provide the original data and conclusions of researchers who conducted experiments. You will learn how the researchers organized their experiments and see charts of the resulting data. Primary research articles contain the following sections:

- **Abstract.** This is a summary of the paper. It highlights the research question, key results of experiments, and the researcher's conclusions. Abstracts are often available online at no cost. Reading the abstract helps you decide if the article presents the information you want to study (**Figure 12.28**).

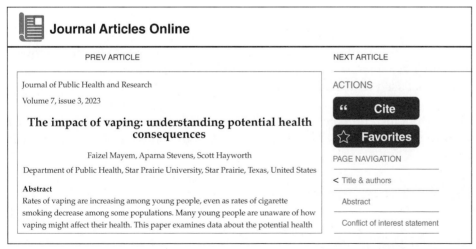

Alexander Lysenko/Shutterstock.com

Figure 12.28 *Is this information primary, secondary, or tertiary? What additional details will confirm your choice?*

- **Introduction.** The introduction provides background information about the research topic and identifies the specific questions addressed by the research. The footnote marker numbers found in the introduction link to resources listed in the references section. Use these to locate additional articles for your research. If you have difficulty understanding the introduction, the rest of the paper will frustrate you as well. In this situation, try reading other resources such as a textbook to learn more about the topic, or ask for the help of a mentor.
- **Materials and methods.** This section tells you exactly how the experiments were performed. Understanding the methods helps you determine the validity of the researcher's conclusions.
- **Results.** This section shows data from the experiments. Spend time looking at the figures, graphs, tables, and other visuals to understand the research findings. As you gain experience in reading scientific papers, you can begin to draw your own conclusions about different aspects of the research, including its accuracy, validity, and usefulness.
- **Discussion.** In this section, researchers give you their opinions about the results of their experiments and compare those results to previous findings or talk about a new direction for research. This provides a way for scientists to exchange ideas. Remember, you are reading opinions rather than facts in this section.
- **References.** This is a list of all the other papers referred to in the article. It contains enough information for you to locate a source in a library or online.

Reading a scientific article goes slowly. You must look up unfamiliar vocabulary and reread sections to gain understanding. Once you understand the content of the article, you can begin to analyze the value of the research. The best studies are clinical trials with control groups and several years of data. This type of research can show cause and effect. In some research studies, participants are surveyed, and the results of those surveys are analyzed to find connections or associations between behaviors. Other studies examine and compare information found in de-identified patient records.

Different studies can find the same behavior both beneficial and detrimental, and research results can contradict each other. For example, one study found an increased risk of breast cancer for females who drink even small amounts of alcohol. However, another study cited the cardiovascular benefits of moderate alcohol consumption. Other research disputed this claim, finding no health benefits associated with alcohol consumption. As a result, healthcare decisions become complex.

Healthcare professionals use **evidence-based practices** to guide diagnosis and treatment for a patient. This means they choose methods of diagnosis and treatment based on the best available current research, their clinical expertise, and the patient's needs and preferences. When there is conflicting research, the patient must ultimately make a choice. Healthcare providers who continue to learn the latest research findings can offer the best range of options to their patients.

Data Management

Handling data is a major task in biotechnology research and development. For example, mapping the human genome has created enormous amounts of data at increasingly faster speeds. The **Human Genome Project** completed the first DNA sequence over a period of 10 years at a cost of $3 billion.

Just a few years ago, people were paying $300,000 for their personal DNA sequence. Today, DNA sequencing technology uses semiconductor chips that "read chemistry" and digitize the information (**Figure 12.29**). Using this technology, an individual DNA sequence can be completed in as little as two hours and may cost less than $200.

By comparing DNA maps, healthcare professionals hope to target treatments to each person's specific needs. Scientists have already identified specific genes that increase risks for developing breast cancer, colon cancer, and Alzheimer's disease. Currently, researchers are studying the uses of genomic sequencing in pediatrics, cancer care, and clinical medicine to develop individualized gene therapies. Newly developed gene therapies have produced positive results toward curing sickle-cell disease and a blood disorder called beta thalassemia for two specific patients. In the next few years, the number of approved gene therapies is expected to increase dramatically.

In the meantime, the field of genomics is caught in an avalanche of data. The ability to determine DNA sequences is starting to outrun the ability of researchers to store, transmit, and especially analyze the data. The cost of analyzing a genome is greater than the cost of sequencing the genome. As a result of advances in genomics, the field of bioinformatics is expected to expand rapidly.

Computer skills are important for managing healthcare data. From the entry-level assistant to the lead researcher, biotechnology research workers use computers to record and analyze data.

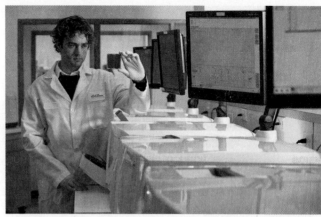
Volker Steger/Science Source

Figure 12.29 DNA sequencers are becoming faster and are producing large amounts of data that must be analyzed and stored.

 ## Healthcare Professions: Data Management

Nina is a clinical administrative assistant at a company that conducts medical research studies. She is responsible for supply inventory for inpatient clinical studies. Since her facility had no organized system for maintaining inventory, she developed a spreadsheet for ordering routine supplies. Spreadsheets store data in a grid of horizontal rows and vertical columns. Nina lists all the supplies along with container sizes and ordering information in her spreadsheet. Each week, she quickly checks the items and lists the amount needed for reorder. She sends the form to her company's central supply location by email.

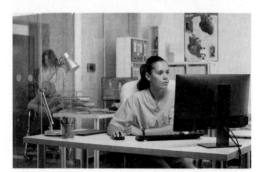
DC Studio/Shutterstock.com

Nina's simple form speeds up the ordering process and keeps her from forgetting items. The company recognized that her spreadsheet worked well, so now they use it at all their clinical sites across the United States. Nina knows how to use her computer to manage the data and information required for her job.

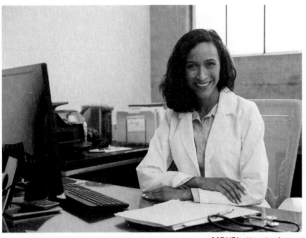

Figure 12.30 Bioinformaticians are in demand for their ability to analyze and extract pertinent information from large data sets. *What fields of study does this occupation include?*

MBI/Shutterstock.com

12.3-7 **Bioinformatics**

Bioinformatics combines biology, computer science, and information technology into a single field of study. Genome sequencing is creating massive databases of biological information. The field of bioinformatics develops tools that allow easy access to this information and make it possible to manage large amounts of genomic data. In addition, new mathematical formulas can analyze and extract information from large sets of data, such as locating a specific gene in a sequence (**Figure 12.30**).

Biology is becoming not only a lab-based science, but also an information science. Using a process called *database mining*, bioinformaticists can analyze and compare large amounts of data to find patterns. For example, you could compare the outcomes for patients treated with different drug **regimens** (REH-juh-mihns), or *plans*, for treating the same disease and determine which treatments work best.

The challenges of storing information include the additional challenges of securing and guarding that information. While researchers can benefit from sharing study results, information can be damaging in the hands of the wrong people. Recently, scientists altered a deadly flu virus to make it more contagious in order to assess the risk of a pandemic. They temporarily stopped their research because of fears that people could use the altered virus for terrorism. Researchers across the globe who were sharing their studies of the virus also voluntarily stopped publishing their detailed research. It was determined that the information could potentially be used to create a biological weapon.

Many research studies employ information technology specialists to develop data protection protocols. These protocols identify steps to prevent the theft or loss of important research data. They include methods for protecting access to data, the computer system itself, and the integrity of electronic data. Protecting the integrity of data involves recording the original date and time for all files, using encryption and electronic signatures to track changes, routinely creating backup files, and ensuring data that is no longer needed is properly destroyed.

Technology is also creating **biorepositories** (bI-oh-rih-PAH-zih-tor-ees), which act as libraries of biological information. When patients grant permission for the collection and storage of leftover blood or tissue samples, robots extract the DNA from each sample and match it with the patient's de-identified EHR. All the information is stored in a secure environment and may be accessed for medical research. This creates a large library of specimens from diverse populations and can significantly shorten research study times. A study may not have to recruit individual participants because the information it needs is in the biorepository. Using the biorepository, researchers may improve diagnostic procedures, enhance treatment therapies, or increase the ability to prevent disease.

Complete the *Map Your Reading* graphic organizer for the section you just read.

1. Which of the following is *not* an example of computerized therapeutic equipment? (12.3-1)
   A. Mobile video cart
   B. Surgical robot
   C. Patient monitoring system
   D. Therapy robot

2. Which of the following would be an appropriate use of social media for healthcare communication not delivered through a secure web portal? (12.3-2)
   A. Send patient test results
   B. Send appointment reminder
   C. Answer patient medical questions
   D. Post the details of a patient's injury

3. Which of the following is *not* an example of telemedicine? (12.3-3)
   A. Teletherapy
   B. Fitness tracker app
   C. Virtual appointment
   D. Remote patient monitoring

4. The _____ standard has improved access to digital medical images. (12.3-4)
   A. HITECH
   B. RFID
   C. DICOM
   D. LIS

5. Hospitals use _____ systems to track their inventory of medical devices. (12.3-5)
   A. UV-C
   B. RFID
   C. QR
   D. barcode

6. When doing research online, you should avoid searching site addresses that end in (12.3-6)
   A. .edu
   B. .gov
   C. .org
   D. .com

7. Which of the following describes a secondary source? (12.3-6)
   A. Reports on original research
   B. Provides a topic overview
   C. Is found in a treatment manual
   D. Summarizes the research of others

8. Which form of scientific communication will likely provide the most challenging reading? (12.3-6)
   A. Slides from a presentation
   B. Review article
   C. Primary research article
   D. Survey results

9. The field of _____ develops tools that allow easy access to information and help manage large amounts of genomic data. (12.3-7)
   A. biotechnology
   B. health informatics
   C. bioinformatics
   D. computer science

Chapter 12 Review and Assessment

Chapter Summary

12.1-1 Electronic medical records are the computerized version of paper medical records. They contain information about a patient's medical care and treatment from a single provider. Electronic health records contain the information from all the clinicians involved in a patient's care and can be shared across different healthcare systems. Patients can access their own healthcare information, pay bills, schedule appointments, and communicate with providers through a secure portal.

12.1-2 The HITECH Act increased the development and use of EHRs by providing financial incentives for achieving government certification. It established privacy and security requirements for the electronic exchange of healthcare information.

12.1-3 The 21st Century Cures Act improves interoperability between healthcare systems by preventing the blocking of information and promoting the use of application programming interfaces to improve communication between disconnected computer applications and systems.

12.1-4 Personal health records are protected by the HIPAA privacy and security rules only when offered by a healthcare provider or insurance plan. Patients must protect their personal health information by using secure passwords and shredding paper documents. Avoid sharing personal health information online.

12.2-1 The EHR contains both personal and clinical patient information such as health history, lab reports, and a record of medications and vaccinations. All correspondence is included, as well as other documents like a living will or healthcare power of attorney.

12.2-2 Medical documentation is accurate. Healthcare workers record only the care they personally provided and document objective observations rather than opinions.

Documentation is complete and uses actual measurements of signs rather than descriptions. Documentation is timely and recorded as soon as possible after care has been completed.

12.2-3 Healthcare workers correct only the errors they have personally recorded. They never delete errors but use an addendum to correct the error and authenticate entries with their signature, credentials, date, and time.

12.3-1 Computerized therapeutic equipment includes surgical and therapy robots, virtual reality simulations to improve balance or speech, 3D printing for dental crowns, and home monitoring systems.

12.3-2 Healthcare workers keep personal and professional online communications separate and are careful to protect patient confidentiality.

12.3-3 Telehealth includes all technology-based health services. Telemedicine involves a healthcare professional providing medical services.

12.3-4 Diagnostic applications of technology include automated analyzers for laboratory testing and lab information systems to manage test data. The DICOM standard for medical imaging allows images to be shared electronically.

12.3-5 Support services applications of technology include clinical simulators; barcode, RFID, and NFC systems for tracking supplies and equipment; and QR codes for accessing detailed information. UV-C technology for disinfection improves patient and worker safety by reducing exposure to harmful chemicals.

12.3-6 Finding reliable health information online begins with analyzing the website address. Sites ending in .gov, .edu, or .org are usually better than .com. Be alert to common medical scams like miracle cures or phony testimonials. Follow the guidelines from the National Library of Medicine to evaluate online health information.

Primary sources describe original research, while secondary sources summarize the research of others. Tertiary sources provide a topic overview. Primary research articles present a reading challenge. Read them slowly, look up unfamiliar vocabulary, and re-read sections to promote understanding.

12.3-7 Bioinformaticians develop methods for managing healthcare research data. They use data-base mining and biorepositories to advance medical research and develop protocols to protect data.

Maximize Your Professional Vocabulary

1. **Terms Categories.** In teams, create categories for the terms in this chapter. Then, classify as many of the terms as possible within the categories your team selected. Share your ideas with another team and discuss your categories.
2. **Picture It.** Select five professional vocabulary terms and draw a picture to represent each one. Trade pictures with a classmate and see if you can identify the terms used.

Reflect on Your Reading

1. Consider your last visit to a healthcare facility. Select one example of changing technology from your experience or from the chapter. How might this technology influence the field of healthcare and the quality of patient care? List both positive and negative effects of the change.

Review and Recall

1. Anya is sending test results to a patient through her facility's web portal. She is likely using a(n) (12.1-1)
   A. personal healthcare app
   B. electronic medical record
   C. electronic health record
   D. computerized patient record

2. Which of the following is *not* a provision of the HITECH Act? (12.1-2)
   A. Healthcare providers receive money to implement EHR systems.
   B. Healthcare providers who violate HIPAA privacy rules can be fined.
   C. Healthcare providers can freely share patients' personal health information for medical research purposes.
   D. Healthcare providers must notify the HHS if there is a breach of security that involves patient information.

3. The 21st Century Cures Act does all of the following *except* (12.1-3)
   A. promote interoperability between healthcare systems
   B. prevent blocking of information
   C. establish a standard patient identifier
   D. allow patients to access their online healthcare data free of charge

4. Which of the following meets the guidelines for a strong password? (12.1-4)
   A. PassWord!
   B. Strng4PW!
   C. Strg3r!
   D. #strOngest!

5. Which of the following is *not* part of the Reports section of a medical record? (12.2-1)
   A. Progress notes
   B. Lab test results
   C. Radiology reports
   D. Consultation reports from other physicians

6. All patient care must be _____ in the patient's medical record. (12.2-2)
   A. read   C. referenced
   B. mentioned   D. documented

7. Addendums and late entries in an EHR must contain a digital signature and credentials of the healthcare worker, along with the date and time of the entry. This process _____, or gives legal authority to, the entry. (12.2-3)
   A. originates   C. authenticates
   B. rectifies   D. invalidates

8. Home monitoring systems protect patient privacy by (12.3-1)
   A. allowing patients to remain in their homes
   B. recording videos of falls or other mishaps
   C. monitoring activities using sensors rather than video cameras
   D. frequently erasing video files

9. Which of these is an inappropriate use of technology in healthcare? (12.3-2)
   A. Text to confirm a medical appointment
   B. Publicizing a charity run on social media
   C. Praising a patient's hard work in rehab on social media
   D. Email reminder to check your online chart for a test result

10. Telemedicine could take care of which of these medical needs? (12.3-3)
    A. Blood test to determine cholesterol levels
    B. X-ray for injured wrist
    C. Physical examination
    D. Treatment for motion sickness

11. Which of the following is *not* a function of the diagnostic LIS? (12.3-4)
    A. Sending test results to the patient
    B. Tracking lab test results
    C. Displaying pending tests
    D. Storing test results

12. Which technology works well for providing educational information to patients? (12.3-5)
    A. RFID   C. UV-C
    B. QR   D. NFC

13. Which statements alert you to a possible online scam? Choose all that apply. (12.3-6)
    A. USP seal of approval
    B. Miracle cure
    C. Celebrity endorsements
    D. Trial periods

14. Which of these records the original research of scientists? (12.3-6)
    A. Primary source   C. Tertiary source
    B. Secondary source   D. None of these.

15. You would like to learn more about research studying Parkinson's disease. Which of the following resources would be a good place to begin your reading? (12.3-6)
    A. Primary research article
    B. Review article
    C. Online news article
    D. Interview with Michael J. Fox

16. Which bioinformatics system makes it possible to conduct some clinical trials without recruiting people? (12.3-7)
    A. Biomarker   C. Bioinventory
    B. Bioregimen   D. Biorepository

Build Core Skills

1. **Problem Solving.** Explain how the terms *proprietary* and *interoperability* relate to the implementation of the EHR.

2. **Writing.** Create a five-point chart to compare and contrast the features of electronic and paper medical records.

3. **Writing.** Review the Lesson 12.1 subheadings titled *Anticipated Benefits* and *Unintended Consequences*. Create a Benefits/Consequences chart. List at least five points in each section of the chart. Write one paragraph summarizing some of the positive and negative results of the rapid switch to EHRs.

4. **Reading.** Find an online article about telemedicine. What is telemedicine, and when is it used? Research your own healthcare provider. What telemedicine services are available to you? Write a two-paragraph summary of your findings.

5. **Speaking and Listening.** Survey healthcare workers about the records system used in the facilities where they work. Focus on the functionality, interoperability, and security of the system. Share your findings with the class.

6. **Critical Thinking.** Identify QR codes that you or your family currently use. How or why are they useful?

7. **Critical Thinking.** Relate the use of QR codes to healthcare. How are QR codes used in the following healthcare areas?
   - patient care
   - healthcare marketing and public relations
   - pharmacy

8. **Problem Solving.** Explain the differences between an EHR and a PHR. List elements that may be found in a PHR. Find out if your healthcare provider has a PHR program you can use.

9. **Problem Solving.** Develop a set of guidelines for healthcare workers to follow when they use social media to communicate with patients.

10. **Critical Thinking.** Using online resources, find the most outrageous and unbelievable medical claim possible. Share your findings with the class. Discuss why people would believe these claims and even spend money on the products.

11. **Problem Solving.** Identify which section of a primary research article would contain each of the following statements. If needed, review the information on primary research articles in the chapter. Do not use abstract, the summary of the article, as a choice.
    - The published data suggests a low rate (3/9,000) of malignancy in US white female population.
    - Systematic literature review was used as the data source.
    - Only studies reporting on the US population were included.
    - Further research is needed to include prevalence in additional ethnic populations.
    - The prevalence in the United States white population ranged from 4.7% to 8.2%.
    - To estimate the risk of malignant transformation in the white population.

12. **Critical Thinking.** Locate an article about bioinformatics or biorepositories. Briefly describe how you believe these concepts will influence healthcare.

Activate Your Learning

1. Review the following chart entry. Then rewrite the entry using the guidelines for documentation explained in the text.

12/16/23	1230	This crabby patient didn't eat any of her ~~breakfast~~ lunch.
12/16/23	1500	She is such a complainer—like her ankle is always hurting!
		Her vital signs are OK
		Susie Smith

2. Locate a healthcare-related QR code on a billboard, in a magazine, or in some other type of advertisement. How might you use this information in your role as a healthcare worker?

Think and Act Like a Healthcare Worker

1. The central services department has requested an inventory of equipment for a resident's room at your worksite. Imagine your classroom is that room. Identify and make a list of equipment and items that would have barcodes for tracking inventory. Then list 10 consumable items that could have barcodes for billing purposes. Compare your list with the lists your classmates created to see what barcodes you may have missed.

Go to the Source

1. Search online for an article about robotic surgery and document your source. Make sure the source is reliable and reputable. Highlight the key ideas presented in the article. Look for possible responses to the following questions:
   - What types of surgeries are typically done with robotics?
   - What are the advantages of robotic surgery versus manual surgery?
   - What is the success rate of robotic surgeries or a particular type of robotic surgery?
   - What skills does the person controlling the robot need?
   - What questions might a patient ask when considering robotic surgery?
   - What other questions need to be asked about robotic surgery?

2. Share your article about robotic surgery with the rest of the class. Mention five key things you learned about robotic surgery. Do your findings agree or disagree with those of other students?

3. Locate at least five different sources of information about a specific health-related topic. List the titles of these sources and label them as *primary*, *secondary*, or *tertiary*.

4. Visit a simulation lab to observe a simulation mannequin. How does the technician use this technology to create a realistic simulation? What are the advantages and disadvantages of this type of technology for someone training to be a healthcare worker?

HOSA Event Prep: Medical Innovation

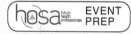

Jeff, a biomedical engineer, works with children who need prosthetic limbs. He is always trying to find ways to create limbs that will help children lead active lives. His specialty is prosthetics that let children and teens participate in sports. He has worked with sports medicine physicians and athletic trainers and even created a science and movement lab to study physical movement. He has spent hours looking at videos created in the movement lab to research aerodynamics of motions and angles. This helps him create a more stable limb that is lighter and bends more naturally. He also works with a colleague to ensure the limb is as comfortable as possible. All his research and study has allowed him to fit many children with limbs that are specific to them and allow them to be more active.

Think About It

1. Explain how the different steps Jeff has taken in the scenario further medical innovation.

2. What qualities do you think are most important in medical innovators? Why?

3. Is medical innovation a career area that interests you? Why or why not?

Chapter 13
Medical Math

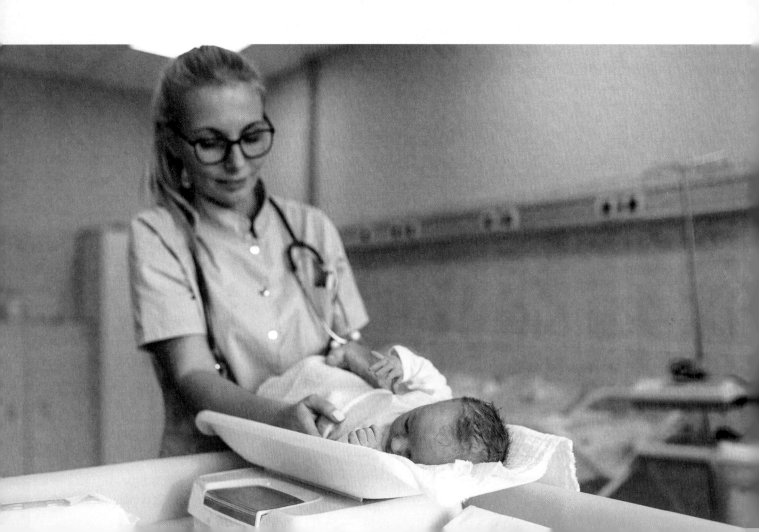

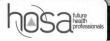
Taking math classes every year, you may have wondered why they were necessary. What real-life applications can math have? Math in medicine can help diagnose and treat patients, from finding precise measurements for radiology and proton therapy in treating cancer to basic dosage calculations. Having a good foundation in math is essential for health science education. Taking what you have learned in math and applying it to medicine is a HOSA—Future Health Professionals event.

Go to the HOSA website to learn more about the HOSA *Medical Math* event. Find out the purpose of the event, what is involved in the event, and what knowledge is demonstrated in the event.

As you prepare for HOSA competitive events, be sure to check the website and talk with your HOSA advisor for the most up-to-date guidelines and procedures. Once you have learned about the *Medical Math* event, answer the following questions:

1. How might participating in this event benefit you personally and your future career? Explain.
2. Are you interested in participating in this event? Why or why not?

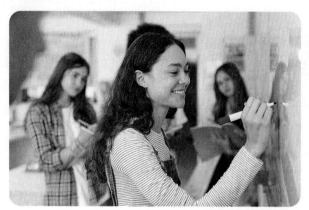

Rido/Shutterstock.com

 Connect with Your Reading

Think about the ways healthcare workers use math in their jobs. Predict which mathematical procedures and operations might be used in each of the following situations:

1. A medical assistant uses a mechanical scale to measure the height and weight of a patient.
2. A pharmacy technician fills a prescription for an oral medication.
3. A hospital housekeeper prepares a cleaning solution from a concentrate.
4. A nursing assistant records the amount of food consumed by a patient.
5. A data analyst prepares a chart showing the change in hospital admissions during the COVID-19 pandemic.

 Map Your Reading

As you read each lesson, list a healthcare task using the math operations and procedures described in the lesson. Write the specific formulas or equivalents used in your selected task. Then create a sample problem and show its solution.

Lesson	Healthcare Task	Formulas/Equivalents Used	Sample Problem and Solution
Lesson 1	*Write a healthcare task.*	*Write formulas/equivalents used.*	*Write a sample problem and solution.*
Lesson 2	*Write a healthcare task.*	*Write formulas/equivalents used.*	*Write a sample problem and solution.*
Lesson 3	*Write a healthcare task.*	*Write formulas/equivalents used.*	*Write a sample problem and solution.*
Lesson 4	*Write a healthcare task.*	*Write formulas/equivalents used.*	*Write a sample problem and solution.*

Goodheart-Willcox Publisher

Chapter opener image: sirtravelalot/Shutterstock.com

Measurement Systems and Conversions

ESSENTIAL QUESTION

How do healthcare workers use systems of measurement and conversions?

Learning Outcomes

After studying this lesson, you will be able to

13.1-1 identify systems of measurement, common units of measurement, and equivalent measurements healthcare workers may use.

13.1-2 convert within and between US Customary Units (household system) and the International System of Units (metric system).

13.1-3 convert between the 12-hour clock that uses a.m. and p.m. times and military time (24-hour clock).

Professional Vocabulary

Essential Terms

24-hour clock   a method of telling time that assigns a number to each hour of the day; also known as *military time*

metric system   the decimal measurement system based on the meter, liter, and gram as its primary units of length, volume, and weight or mass respectively

US customary units   the main system of weights and measures used in the United States based on the yard, pound, and gallon as units of length, weight, and liquid volume respectively; also known as *household measurements*

Important Terms

apothecary system
International Units (IU)
proportion

Introduction

From the most basic systems of measurement to the most complicated algorithms (AL-guh-rih-thuhmz) for calculating research data, healthcare workers use math skills every day. They typically use the metric system of measurement but must be able to convert to the household measurement system commonly used in the United States. They often use the 24-hour clock to prevent confusion between the a.m. and p.m. hours.

13.1-1 Systems of Measurement

Healthcare workers need to pay attention to systems of measurement when completing medical math calculations. To avoid serious mistakes, make sure you and your patients or fellow workers are using the same system of measurement. In healthcare settings, you are likely to encounter the metric system and the US customary system.

Consider the story of a British family whose vacation to the United States took a frightening turn. The family's young son had an asthma attack, so his mother took him to the emergency room to get a prescription for asthma medication. She gave her son the prescribed asthma medication, but there was no improvement in his breathing, so she took him back to the emergency room. As the physician reviewed the medication label, he asked the woman to confirm her son's weight. She said 40, meaning kilograms, but the label listed dosage amounts for a child weighing 40 pounds. Because 40 kilograms is closer to 88 pounds, her son was receiving only one-half the medication needed to alleviate his symptoms.

The United States is the only industrialized country that does not use the **metric system** as its official system of measurement. However, both the scientific and healthcare communities use metric measurement. Therefore, healthcare workers must know how to use this system. Yet most healthcare workers—and their patients—still think in pounds, ounces, inches, and feet.

As a result, healthcare workers frequently convert between household measurements and metric measurements. They typically measure in the metric system, but present information to patients in commonly used terms. A nurse might measure and record a newborn's weight as 3000 grams but tell the parents the baby weighs 6 pounds, 10 ounces.

Healthcare workers prefer to have patients use metric measurements for medicine. To promote this goal, some companies provide cups and syringes with measurements marked in metric along with the medicine. Their purpose is to increase the accuracy of doses. Many patients still use kitchen silverware to measure their medicine, which can result in inaccurate doses. The size of household teaspoons can vary significantly, and it is easy to misread *tbsp* (tablespoon) as *tsp* (teaspoon). Using kitchen silverware instead of an actual measuring spoon or other device that comes with a medicine can result in the wrong dosing—too much or too little of the medicine.

Apothecary System

While the metric system is the standard for healthcare measurement, you may see a prescription that looks like this: *Aspirin® gr xv.* Seeing the unit—grains, in this case—listed first and the amount listed second using lowercase Roman numerals tells you it is an **apothecary** (uh-PAH-thuh-kair-ee) **system** prescription. The apothecary system is an older system used by early pharmacists, or *apothecaries.* It may still be found in formulas for compounding older medications. Pharmacy workers need to recognize apothecary measurements to avoid serious errors in interpretation or measurement. When you see measurements listed as drams, grains, and minims, you are working with the apothecary system. These measurements will use lowercase Roman numerals and fractions rather than decimals.

Roman numerals are quite easy to interpret (**Figure 13.1**). They use letters to express numeric values:

I or *i* stands for 1
V or *v* stands for 5
X or *x* stands for 10
L or *l* stands for 50
C or *c* stands for 100
D or *d* stands for 500
M or *m* stands for 1,000

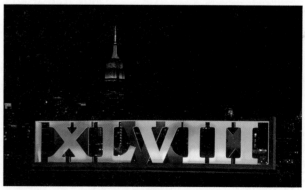

Figure 13.1 You may have seen Roman numerals while watching the Superbowl. *What do the Roman numerals here mean?*

Follow these guidelines for reading and writing Roman numerals:

- The letters should be arranged from largest to smallest.

  1,510 is written *MDX*, largest to smallest.

- When the same letter is repeated twice in a row, the two are added together. However, do not repeat a letter more than three times in a row.

  100 is written *LL*, not *XXXXXXXXXX*.

- When a letter with a smaller value comes before one with a larger value, the smaller number is subtracted from the larger number.

  4 is written *IV*, which literally means *5 minus 1*.

- When a letter with a smaller value follows one with a larger value, the smaller number is added to the larger number.

  6 is written *VI*, which literally means *5 plus 1*.

When you see *Aspirin® gr xv*, it means the prescription calls for Aspirin® at a strength of 15 grains. You will have to calculate how many tablets the patient must take to equal 15 grains of medication.

International Units (IU)

The word *units* commonly indicates a measure of insulin or heparin. These **International Units (IU)** measure the biological effect of manufactured medications and vitamins. For every substance to which an IU is assigned, there is an internationally accepted biological effect expected with a dose of 1 IU.

Because each substance is tested individually, there is no standard conversion from international units to metric equivalents. For example, 1 IU is equivalent to 0.0455 milligrams of insulin. However, 1 IU is equivalent to just 0.0003 milligrams of vitamin A and just 0.000025 milligrams of vitamin D.

Metric System

The metric system, or *International System of Units*, uses four basic units of measurement: the meter, gram, liter, and degree Celsius. The meter (m) measures length, the gram (g) measures weight, the liter (L) measures volume, and the degree Celsius (°C) identifies temperature. The L for liter is capitalized to avoid confusion with the numeral 1. Working within the metric system is mathematically easy because all units are based on multiples of 10. All conversions are calculated by multiplying by 10, 100, 1000, and so on (**Figure 13.2**).

Moving a decimal point easily converts units within the metric system. Suppose you need to convert an order for 1000 milligrams of medication to 1-gram tablets. Since *milli-* represents 0.001 of a gram, it is three places to the right of *gram*, as pictured in **Figure 13.2**. This means you will move the decimal point three spaces to the left to convert the measurement to grams. Thus, 1000 milligrams becomes 1 gram. The dose is 1 gram or one tablet.

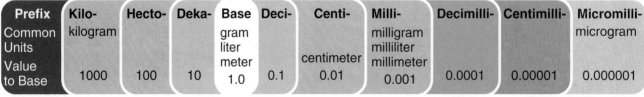

Prefix	Kilo-	Hecto-	Deka-	Base	Deci-	Centi-	Milli-	Decimilli-	Centimilli-	Micromilli-
Common Units	kilogram			gram liter meter		centimeter	milligram milliliter millimeter			microgram
Value to Base	1000	100	10	1.0	0.1	0.01	0.001	0.0001	0.00001	0.000001

Figure 13.2 Working within the metric system is mathematically easy since all the units are based on multiples of 10.

Follow these guidelines to reduce errors when recording metric measurements:

- Avoid using a comma as a separator (write 1000 mg rather than 1,000 mg).
- Avoid unnecessarily large numbers or trailing zeros (simplify 1000 mg to 1 gram).
- If possible, use whole numbers rather than decimals (write 25 mm rather than 2.5 cm).

United States Customary Units

US customary units, more commonly known as the *household system* of measurement, are familiar to students educated in the United States. The terms *inch* (in) and *foot* (ft) for length, *cup* (c) and *quart* (qt) for volume, and *ounce* (oz) or *pound* (lb) for weight are common. Converting between the units, however, may not be as familiar and requires knowledge of several *equivalents* (**Figure 13.3**).

When you know basic equivalents, you can convert to other units by using a **proportion**. A proportion shows that two ratios or fractions are equal. For example, you need to measure 4 tablespoons (T) of a liquid but have a measuring cup marked in ounces. You know the equivalent that states 2 tablespoons equals 1 ounce. If 2 tablespoons equals 1 ounce, then how many ounces does 4 tablespoons equal? Your proportion problem should look like this:

$$\frac{2T}{4T} \diagdown\diagup \frac{1\ oz}{x\ oz}$$

Solve the problem using the following steps:

1. Cross multiply to get $2x = 4$ oz
2. Divide each side of the equation by the number in front of x

$2x \div 2 = 1x$

$4 \div 2 = 2$

$x = 2$ oz

Thus, measuring 2 ounces will be equal to 4 tablespoons.

Common Household Measurements and Equivalents		
Type	**Name and Abbreviation**	**Equivalents**
Distance/length	inch (" or in) foot (' or ft) yard (yd) mile (mi)	12 in = 1 ft 3 ft = 1 yd 1760 yds = 1 mi
Capacity/volume	drop (gtt) teaspoon (t or tsp) tablespoon (T or tbsp) ounce (oz)* cup (c) pint (pt) quart (qt) gallon (gal)	60 gtts = 1 t 3 t = 1 T 2 T = 1 oz 8 oz = 1 c 2 c = 1 pt 2 pts = 1 qt 4 qts = 1 gal
Mass/weight	ounce (oz)* pound (lb)	16 oz = 1 lb

*Ounce is used for measures of volume and weight in household measurement.

Goodheart-Willcox Publisher

Figure 13.3 Healthcare workers in the US use these equivalents to convert within the household system and make measuring more practical and accurate. It is better to measure 1 cup rather than 16 tablespoons.

13.1-2 Converting Between Systems of Measurement

Remember the nurse who measured the infant at 3000 grams but told the new parents the baby weighed 6 pounds, 10 ounces? It is common for US healthcare workers to convert measurements like this from one system to another. Workers use equivalent measurements to make conversions (**Figure 13.4**). There are often no exact equivalents, so close approximations must be used. Memorizing the following equivalents will help you evaluate conversions from system to system:

1 fluid oz = 30 cc or mL = 6 teaspoons (t) or 2 T = 8 fluid drams

Using approximate equivalents, you can set up a proportion to convert measurements. For example, if you are the nurse weighing the newborn baby, you know the baby weighs 3000 grams, and you know that 30 grams = 1 ounce. So how many ounces is 3000 grams?

$$\frac{30\ g}{3000\ g} = \frac{1\ oz}{x\ oz}$$

1. Cross multiply to get $30x = 3000$
2. Divide each side of the equation by the number in front of x

$30x \div 30 = 1x$

$3000 \div 30 = 100\ oz$

The correct answer is $x = 100$ ounces, but that is not a typical measurement. Now you have to convert these ounces into pounds. You know that 16 ounces = 1 pound, so how many pounds is 100 ounces?

$$\frac{16\ oz}{100\ oz} = \frac{1\ lb}{x\ lb}$$

1. Cross multiply to get $16x = 100$
2. Divide each side of the equation by the number in front of x

$16x \div 16 = 1x$

$100 \div 16 = 6.25\ lbs$

Commonly Used Equivalents
Equivalents for Volume

Household System
- 1 tsp = 4–5 mL
- 3 tsp = 1 tbsp
- 1 tsp = 1/2 oz or 15 mL
- 2 tbsp = 1 oz or 30 mL
- 1 cup = 8 oz

Metric System
- 5 mL = 1 tsp
- 15 mL = 1 tbsp
- 30 mL = 2 tbsp
- 1 mL = 16 minims
- 500 mL = 0.5 liter
- 1000 mL = 1 liter

Apothecary System
- 1 fl dr = 4 mL or 1 tsp
- 4 drams = 1/2 oz
- 8 drams = 2 tbsp (1 oz)
- 16 minims = 1 mL
- 1 pint = 16 oz or 480 mL
- 1 quart = 32 oz or 960 mL

Equivalents for Weight

All Systems
- 1/60 grain = 1 mg
- 1 grain = 60 mg or 0.060 g
- 15 grains = 1 g or 1000 mg
- 2.2 lbs = 1 kg
- 1 mg = 1000 mcg

Goodheart-Willcox Publisher

Figure 13.4 These equivalents are used to convert between systems of measurement.

You know the baby weighs 6.25 pounds, but now you need to determine how many ounces are in 0.25 pounds. You know that 16 ounces = 1 pound, so how many ounces are in 0.25 pounds?

$$\frac{1\text{ lb}}{0.25\text{ lb}} = \frac{16\text{ oz}}{x\text{ oz}}$$

1. Cross multiply to get $1x = 4$
2. Divide each side of the equation by the number in front of x

   $1x \div 1 = 1x$

   $4 \div 1 = 4\text{ oz}$

So the answer is 6 pounds, 4 ounces. However, the nurse said the baby weighed 6 pounds, 10 ounces. This illustrates a problem with using equivalents—they are only approximately equal. In large numbers such as 3000 grams, the resulting conversion will be less accurate. A difference of 5 ounces may not be critical when recording a child's weight in a baby book. It would be very important, however, for calculating the amount of medicine a newborn infant needs. A more exact equivalent, such as 1 ounce = 28.34 grams, is needed. This equivalent will convert 3000 grams to 6 pounds, 10 ounces.

The more equivalents you know, the more accurate your converted measurements will be. You can also increase the speed at which you convert measurements. You can convert 3000 grams to kilograms by simply moving the decimal point three spaces to the left, giving you 3 kilograms.

To convert kilograms to pounds, remember that 2.2 kilograms = 1 pound, so you simply multiply 3 kilograms by 2.2 (3 kg × 2.2 = 6.6 lb). To convert 0.6 to ounces, multiply by the number of ounces in 1 pound (0.6 lb × 16 oz = 9.6 oz). Your answer is 6 pounds, 10 ounces (rounded to the nearest whole number). Using kilograms instead of grams was both faster and more accurate. Of course, the easiest conversions use equipment labeled with both metric and household measurements. **Figure 13.5** shows mathematical operations that will help you perform faster conversions.

Conversion Table: Metric to Household and Household to Metric				
Metric	Measures	US Customary (Household)	Convert from Metric to Household	Convert Household to Metric
2.5 centimeters	Length	1 inch	Divide by 2.5 (100 cm ÷ 2.5 = 40 in)	Multiply by 2.54
30 centimeters	Length	1 foot	Divide by 30 (100 cm ÷ 30 = 3.3 ft = 3 ft 4 in)	Multiply by 30.48
30 grams	Weight	1 ounce	Divide by 30 (1000 g ÷ 30 = 33 oz)	Multiply by 30
0.45 kilograms	Weight	1 pound	Multiply by 2.2 (50 kg × 2.2 = 110 lb)	Multiply by 0.45
30 milliliters	Volume	1 ounce	Divide by 30 (30 mL ÷ 30 = 1 oz)	Multiply by 30

Goodheart-Willcox Publisher

Figure 13.5 Memorizing these equivalents will make conversions faster and more accurate.

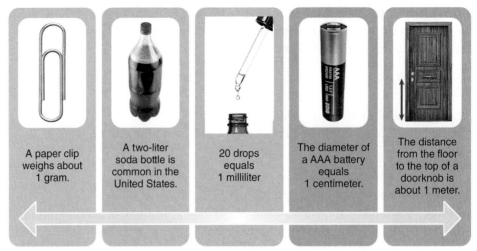

Left to right: ILYA AKINSHIN/Shutterstock.com, Givaga/iStock/Thinkstock, Layland Masuda/Shutterstock.com, Aigars Reinholds/Shutterstock.com, AlexKol Photography/Shutterstock.com

Figure 13.6 These household objects provide a visual reference for some common metric measurements.

If you are familiar with the household system, you can visualize its units of measurement. For example, you know what 1 pound of butter looks like and how heavy it feels when you hold it. So, if you read that a truck weighed 10 pounds, you would know that was an error. As you work with the metric system, try to develop a visual sense for basic units of metric measurement. This will improve your accuracy by helping you spot obvious errors (**Figure 13.6**).

13.1-3 **The 24-Hour Clock**

Many healthcare facilities use the **24-hour clock**, also called *military time* (**Figure 13.7**). Rather than 12 hours with an a.m. (before midday) or p.m. (after midday) designation, the 24-hour clock uses the numbers 1 through 24.

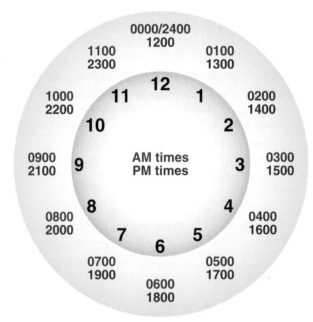

Goodheart-Willcox Publisher

Figure 13.7 Using the 24-hour clock helps healthcare workers avoid confusion between a.m. and p.m. times.

Each hour of the day has its own number. This avoids confusion between a.m. and p.m. and prevents medication or chart documentation errors when the a.m. or p.m. designation is omitted or misread.

Guidelines for using the 24-hour clock include the following:

- Always write the time using four digits with no colons to separate hours and minutes. For example, 9:00 a.m. is 0900, and 12:00 noon is 1200.
- Always state time in hundreds when speaking. For example, 2:00 a.m. is 0200 and is stated as "zero two hundred hours" or "oh two hundred hours." 7:00 p.m. is 1900 and is stated as "nineteen hundred hours."
- The last two numbers at the end of each time represent minutes after the hour. For example, 11:15 a.m. is 1115. This means it is fifteen minutes past eleven o'clock.
- If the time is between whole hours, drop the word *hundred* when speaking. Thus, 1115 is spoken as "eleven fifteen hours."
- Midnight (12:00 a.m.) is presented as 0000 or 2400 in military time, whereas 1200 is 12:00 noon.
- From midnight to noon, you can use the numbers on a standard clock (1 through 12) to tell military time. For example, 1:00 a.m. is 0100, and 10:00 a.m. is 1000.
- Convert p.m. hours to military time by adding 1200 to the time. For example, 1:00 p.m. plus 1200 is 1300, and 4:30 p.m. plus 1200 is 1630. Reverse the process and subtract 1200 when converting from military time to a.m./p.m. time.

Lesson 13.1 Review

 Complete the *Map Your Reading* graphic organizer for the section you just read.

1. The measurements 60 grains and 4 drams are part of which system? (13.1-1)
   A. Apothecary
   B. Household
   C. Metric
   D. International System of Units

2. Which of the following is *not* a metric unit of measurement? (13.1-1)
   A. Gram
   B. Grain
   C. Liter
   D. Meter

3. You can make conversions within and between systems of measurement using _____ . (13.1-1)
   A. auxiliaries
   B. parallels
   C. counterparts
   D. equivalents

4. When communicating with patients, US healthcare workers often make accurate conversions between metric and _____ systems of measurement. (13.1-2)
   A. International Unit
   B. household
   C. apothecary
   D. International System of Units

5. Which of the following illustrates a time using the 24-hour clock? (13.1-3)
   A. 1300
   B. 13:00
   C. 1300 p.m.
   D. 11:00 a.m.

Healthcare Tasks That Use Basic Math Skills

ESSENTIAL QUESTION

What are some healthcare tasks that use basic math skills?

Learning Outcomes

After studying this lesson, you will be able to

13.2-1 complete tasks that lead to reimbursement for medical services.

13.2-2 interpret a prescription and prepare an oral medication with patient instructions.

13.2-3 use a goniometer to measure range of motion.

13.2-4 prepare a designated amount of a solution using a dilution ratio.

Professional Vocabulary

Essential Terms

claims process   the procedure for submitting costs for medical services so payment can be collected or denial can be determined

goniometer   an instrument for measuring angles

solutions   uniform mixtures of two or more substances, which may be solids, liquids, gases, or a combination of these

Important Terms

assignment of benefits	Fowler's	Physician's Current Procedural Terminology (CPT)
concentration	fulcrum	
dilution ratio	high Fowler's	
dosage	International Classification of Diseases Clinical Modifications (ICD-CM)	semi-Fowler's
dose		solute
explanation of benefits (EOB)		solvent
	medications	third-party payers

Introduction

Healthcare workers complete tasks that provide reimbursement for medical care. They use the basic functions of addition, subtraction, multiplication, and division in many job settings. The following applications demonstrate a few ways healthcare workers use basic math skills to complete job tasks.

13.2-1 Reimbursement Tasks

Payment for healthcare services begins with medical coding. All diagnoses and procedures are given a numeric code. Workers use these codes when completing insurance claim forms so insurance companies will pay, or *reimburse*, the provider for the services the patient received. In addition, healthcare workers collect payments directly from patients at the time of service. They must be able to handle money, give correct change, and issue receipts for payment.

Coding Diagnoses and Procedures

Medical coding is the process of translating written medical documentation into a numeric form. Coding has several purposes:

- **Reimbursement.** Codes are printed on insurance claim forms. Insurance companies reimburse the facility or physician based on the codes for the diagnoses and procedures or services performed.
- **Research.** Physicians access medical records using coded information. For example, a physician might request medical records for all patients treated for appendicitis (codes 540–543) in one hospital or all hospitals within a system. Records with those diagnosis codes could be quickly identified in a computer listing.
- **Public health.** Government public health agencies use coded diagnostic information to track the occurrence of certain diseases. For example, they may want to know the number of new cases of *pertussis* (whooping cough), code 033.0, diagnosed in a particular part of the state.
- **Patient care.** Recently, a manufacturer of an artificial hip replacement recalled its product. The manufacturer alerted surgeons who had used this product. The surgeons or hospitals then retrieved the names of patients who had hip replacement surgery by searching for the procedure code 27130. The surgeons then contacted these patients to inform them of the product recall.

The World Health Organization (WHO) developed the coding system for diagnoses. Each year the Department of Health and Human Services (HHS) updates and publishes the **International Classification of Diseases Clinical Modifications (ICD-CM)**. Healthcare facilities use the 10th revision of ICD codes (ICD-10-CM). In this revision, the WHO uses alphanumeric (letters and numbers) codes to accommodate more diseases and specific information. For example, appendicitis codes range from K35 to K35.9. The 11th edition went into effect on January 1, 2022. This version increases the number of unique codes and includes more mental health conditions and built-in emergency pandemic codes. The US is expected to adopt this version in the next few years.

Each year, the American Medical Association (AMA) publishes the **Physician's Current Procedural Terminology (CPT)**. The numeric codes in this publication are used to report procedures and services to public and private insurance companies. There are additional codes for other topics such as dental services, injuries, and medical equipment.

Medical coding specialists use their expertise to identify a patient's specific diagnosis and procedure from the medical record (**Figure 13.8**). These specialists can distinguish between the smallest of differences in codes. For example, a 27660 code indicates closed treatment of *patellar* (kneecap) dislocation without anesthesia, but a 27562 code is the same treatment *with* anesthesia.

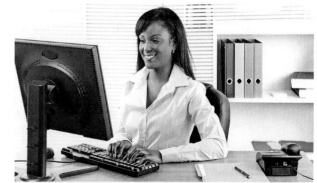

Elena Elisseeva/Shutterstock.com

Figure 13.8 The medical coding specialist assigns a code to each diagnosis, procedure, and service listed in the medical record. *How does this benefit healthcare facilities?*

In this example, the cost would be higher for the treatment that requires anesthesia. Medical coding specialists need to know these code differences because a misinterpretation of a code could mean more cost to the patient or reduced income for the provider.

Coders begin with the primary diagnosis and read for the specific details or location. The ICD codes are organized by disease or body system. When searching for appendicitis, coders begin by searching diseases of the digestive system.

Coders then move on to the specific treatments used for the primary diagnosis. This is where they use CPT codes. These codes are organized by the type of service given, such as anesthesia, surgery, radiology, or laboratory.

Errors in coding cost patients money when the insurance company denies a claim for a service that should be covered. Even bigger problems occur when a coding error causes a patient to be labeled incorrectly in an insurance database. For example, when the code for a "heart attack" is used instead of the code to "rule out a heart attack," a patient may be denied long-term care insurance or life insurance.

The complex process of accurate medical coding begins with the following steps:

- Use the latest edition of the ICD and CPT codes. Many errors result from using outdated editions.
- Always refer to the guidelines rather than relying on your memory.
- Check your codes to make sure the diagnosis and service codes support each other. For example, coding for an appendectomy is an obvious error when the diagnosis is an ear infection.
- Never hesitate to ask the physician to clarify a code, procedure, or documentation in the medical record.

Completing an Insurance Claim Form

Insurance companies, or **third-party payers**, provide a large portion of a medical practice's income. Therefore, health informatics workers must understand the **claims process** through which the medical practice receives payment. Following a patient visit, a health informatics worker completes a claim form and submits it to the insurance carrier, which is the company that insures a patient (**Figure 13.9**).

The top portion of a claim form lists all the patient's identifying information along with an address, name, and ID numbers for the insurance company. If the patient is not the person who carries the insurance, such as a child or spouse, the form will also show identifying information for the insured person. Because many people receive insurance benefits through an employer, the form may also ask for the name of the employer.

Adult patients sign the claim form, granting permission to release their medical information to the insurance company. The person carrying the insurance also signs the form, allowing payments to be made directly to the medical office. This process is called the **assignment of benefits**. Most offices have new patients sign a release form when they complete registration materials. Then the office can simply type in the words *Signature on File* when submitting claims. This can also be used for the physician's signature.

HEALTH INSURANCE CLAIM FORM

APPROVED BY NATIONAL UNIFORM CLAIM COMMITTEE (NUCC) 02/12

| | PICA | | | | | | | | PICA | |

1. MEDICARE (Medicare#) **MEDICAID** (Medicaid#) **TRICARE** (ID#/DoD#) **CHAMPVA** (Member ID#) **GROUP HEALTH PLAN** [X] (ID#) **FECA BLK LUNG** (ID#) **OTHER** (ID#)

1a. INSURED'S I.D. NUMBER (For Program in Item 1)
03654

2. PATIENT'S NAME (Last Name, First Name, Middle Initial)
Brown, Kathleen J.

3. PATIENT'S BIRTH DATE MM 06 DD 29 YY 1970 **SEX** M [ ] F [X]

4. INSURED'S NAME (Last Name, First Name, Middle Initial)
Brown, Kathleen J.

5. PATIENT'S ADDRESS (No., Street)
400 South Main Street

6. PATIENT RELATIONSHIP TO INSURED
Self [X] Spouse [ ] Child [ ] Other [ ]

7. INSURED'S ADDRESS (No., Street)

CITY Star Prairie **STATE** TX

8. RESERVED FOR NUCC USE

CITY **STATE**

ZIP CODE 74260 **TELEPHONE (Include Area Code)** (123) 701-0197

ZIP CODE **TELEPHONE (Include Area Code)** ( )

9. OTHER INSURED'S NAME (Last Name, First Name, Middle Initial)

10. IS PATIENT'S CONDITION RELATED TO:

11. INSURED'S POLICY GROUP OR FECA NUMBER
06172

a. OTHER INSURED'S POLICY OR GROUP NUMBER

a. EMPLOYMENT? (Current or Previous) YES [ ] NO [X]

a. INSURED'S DATE OF BIRTH MM DD YY **SEX** M [ ] F [ ]

b. RESERVED FOR NUCC USE

b. AUTO ACCIDENT? YES [ ] NO [X] **PLACE (State)**

b. OTHER CLAIM ID (Designated by NUCC)

c. RESERVED FOR NUCC USE

c. OTHER ACCIDENT? YES [ ] NO [X]

c. INSURANCE PLAN NAME OR PROGRAM NAME
DC Health Plan

d. INSURANCE PLAN NAME OR PROGRAM NAME

10d. CLAIM CODES (Designated by NUCC)

d. IS THERE ANOTHER HEALTH BENEFIT PLAN? YES [ ] NO [X] If yes, complete items 9, 9a, and 9d.

READ BACK OF FORM BEFORE COMPLETING & SIGNING THIS FORM.

12. PATIENT'S OR AUTHORIZED PERSON'S SIGNATURE I authorize the release of any medical or other information necessary to process this claim. I also request payment of government benefits either to myself or to the party who accepts assignment below.

SIGNED Signature on File DATE 11/12/2023

13. INSURED'S OR AUTHORIZED PERSON'S SIGNATURE I authorize payment of medical benefits to the undersigned physician or supplier for services described below.

SIGNED Signature on File

14. DATE OF CURRENT ILLNESS, INJURY, or PREGNANCY (LMP) MM 07 DD 30 YY 2023 QUAL.

15. OTHER DATE QUAL. MM DD YY

16. DATES PATIENT UNABLE TO WORK IN CURRENT OCCUPATION FROM MM DD YY TO MM DD YY

17. NAME OF REFERRING PROVIDER OR OTHER SOURCE 17a. 17b. NPI

18. HOSPITALIZATION DATES RELATED TO CURRENT SERVICES FROM MM DD YY TO MM DD YY

19. ADDITIONAL CLAIM INFORMATION (Designated by NUCC)

20. OUTSIDE LAB? YES [ ] NO [ ] **$ CHARGES**

21. DIAGNOSIS OR NATURE OF ILLNESS OR INJURY Relate A-L to service line below (24E) ICD Ind.

A. S93-439A B. E11.9 C. D.
E. F. G. H.
I. J. K. L.

22. RESUBMISSION CODE ORIGINAL REF. NO.

23. PRIOR AUTHORIZATION NUMBER

24. A. DATE(S) OF SERVICE From MM DD YY To MM DD YY | **B. PLACE OF SERVICE** | **C. EMG** | **D. PROCEDURES, SERVICES, OR SUPPLIES** (Explain Unusual Circumstances) CPT/HCPCS MODIFIER | **E. DIAGNOSIS POINTER** | **F. $ CHARGES** | **G. DAYS OR UNITS** | **H. EPSDT Family Plan** | **I. ID. QUAL** | **J. RENDERING PROVIDER ID. #**

#	From MM DD YY	To MM DD YY	B	C	CPT/HCPCS	E	$ CHARGES	Units		ID QUAL	
1	07 30 23	07 30 23	11		99213	1	200.00	1		NPI	
2	07 30 23	07 30 23	11		82947	2	50.00	1		NPI	
3										NPI	
4										NPI	
5										NPI	
6										NPI	

25. FEDERAL TAX I.D. NUMBER 54-0000000 SSN [ ] EIN [X]

26. PATIENT'S ACCOUNT NO. 0346

27. ACCEPT ASSIGNMENT? (For govt. claims, see back) YES [X] NO [ ]

28. TOTAL CHARGE $ 250.00

29. AMOUNT PAID $

30. Rsvd. for NUCC Use

31. SIGNATURE OF PHYSICIAN OR SUPPLIER INCLUDING DEGREES OR CREDENTIALS (I certify that the statements on the reverse apply to this bill and are made a part thereof.)
Signature on File
SIGNED DATE 11/12/2023

32. SERVICE FACILITY LOCATION INFORMATION
Sun View Medical
250 Brighter Lane
a. NPI b.

33. BILLING PROVIDER INFO & PH # (123) 701-3524
Sandra Black MD
Star Prairie, TX 74260
a. NPI b.

NUCC Instruction Manual available at: www.nucc.org   **PLEASE PRINT OR TYPE**   APPROVED OMB-0938-1197 FORM 1500 (02-12)

Courtesy of the Centers for Medicare & Medicaid Services

Figure 13.9 Health informatics workers fill out claim forms like this one so facilities can be paid for services rendered.

The bottom portion of the claim form lists the identifying and contact information for the provider and healthcare facility. It also lists the dates of service and specific ICD and CPT codes for diagnosis and treatment. You may see a number in the *Place of Service* column. Different facilities have different numbers, so 01 indicates a pharmacy, 11 is a medical office, and 21 is a hospital. In addition, charges for each service, as well as a total charge and balance due from the insurance company, are listed.

When the *Accept Assignment* section is marked *yes*, the provider will accept an agreed-upon amount as full payment. The costs of each service depend on the provider's contract with a particular insurance company. When the *Accept Assignment* section is marked *no*, the provider is free to charge any amount for services. If the charged amount is higher than the *insurance-allowed amount* (the amount the insurance company is willing to pay), the patient must pay the difference.

Accuracy of claims directly affects income for a medical practice. When a claim is returned because of incomplete or incorrect information, the claim must be resubmitted, and payment is delayed for several weeks. Taking the time to verify insurance coverage and double-check for accuracy before sending a claim will save time and money (**Figure 13.10**).

The electronic health record speeds up the claims process considerably. Software programs can extract required data from the patient's record and transfer it to the claim form. Electronic signatures complete the process, and the forms are submitted electronically.

When the claims administrator settles a claim, the medical provider and patient receive an **explanation of benefits (EOB)**. This report shows what, if anything, the insurance company is paying for; what it is not paying for; and why. The small numbers in the *Remarks* column align with a list of explanations. Always look at the bottom of the report to see the explanation of the charge (**Figure 13.11**).

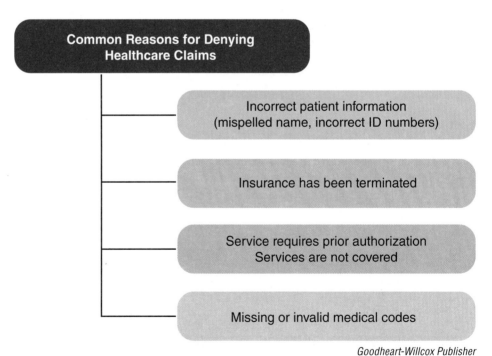

Goodheart-Willcox Publisher

Figure 13.10 Double-checking for accuracy before submitting claims can prevent claim denials that delay payments.

DC Health Plan

1600 Allen Blvd
Washington, DC 65432

Forwarding Service Requested

RITA JAMES

1234 ANYPLACE DRIVE **1**

STAR PRAIRIE, TX 74260

2

	7/20/2023
Patient Name:	RITA JAMES
Group Number:	06172
Claim Number:	102345678910 DENTAL
Patient ID Number:	03654

EXPLANATION OF BENEFITS

Below is an explanation of your benefits with DC Health Plan.
Please do not send money to DC Health Plan. Send any money owed to the provider of service.

THIS IS NOT A BILL 3

4 PROVIDER NAME: **SV ENDODONTICS**

Code	Description of Service	Date	Amount Charged	Amount Allowed	Deductible	Copay/ Coinsurance	Remark	Amount Paid
3330-03 **5**	Root canal **6**	6/20/23 **7**	$1,105.00 **8**	$1,066.32 **9**	**10**	$213.27 **11**	45 **12** 02	$853.05 **13**

13
Amount Paid by Plan: **$853.05**

14
Member Responsibility: **$251.95**

Remark Explanation(s):
45—Charge exceeds maximum allowable fee.   **12**
02—Coinsurance amount. Your 20% coinsurance is $213.27.

If you are covered by more than one health benefit plan, you should file all your claims with each plan.
If you have any questions about this claim, please call your Customer Service Team at (123) 456-7890 or 1-800-123-4567, or contact us at www.dchealthplans.org. Please see your member handbook or contract for claim appeal procedures. **15**

>>PLEASE KEEP A COPY OF THIS DOCUMENT FOR YOUR RECORDS<<

1. name of the main subscriber for your health insurance policy
2. summary of patient information
3. the EOB is **not** a bill or request of payment
4. the name of the provider or facility that provided healthcare services
5. medical code for the service or procedure required
6. general description of the services you requested
7. the date on which you received this healthcare service
8. the amount your provider has billed your health insurance for each service

9. the amount that your health insurance allows for each service billed
10. the amount applied to your deductible
11. the copay or coinsurance amount you must pay after your deductible is applied
12. additional messages that may explain how your claim was processed
13. the amount your health insurance will pay the provider for services you received
14. the amount you owe the provider. Your provider will bill you separately
15. information on how to contact Customer Service

Goodheart-Willcox Publisher

Figure 13.11 This EOB shows that the patient pays 20 percent of the total bill according to her insurance plan coverage. However, because the provider does not have a fee agreement with the health insurance plan, the provider has charged more than the amount allowed by the insurance plan. As a result, the patient owes $251.95 instead of $213.27.

On an EOB, the words *amount allowed* along with *network savings* means the medical provider has a contract with the insurance company. Under this contract, the medical provider accepts the insurance payment as full payment for a given service, even if the provider normally charges more for the service. This reduces costs for insurance companies and brings new patients to providers who have contracts with the patient's insurance company.

The EOB is *not* a bill, but it does include information about deductibles and coinsurance as they apply to the claim. Patients should review services, dates of services, and charges for services on each EOB to make sure this information is accurate. When claims are denied or payment is delayed, patients can contact the insurance company to get answers to their questions.

After the claims process has been completed, the medical provider bills the patient for any amount unpaid by the insurance company. A statement mailed to patients shows how much the physician's office billed the insurance company and how much the insurance company paid (**Figure 13.12**). After the insurance company's payment is deducted from the total cost for services, the patient pays the balance.

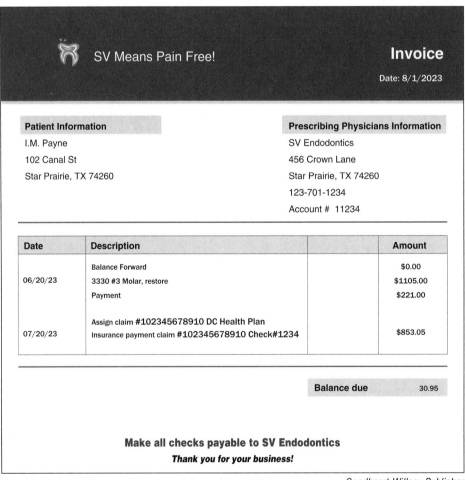

SV Means Pain Free!

Invoice

Date: 8/1/2023

Patient Information	**Prescribing Physicians Information**
I.M. Payne	SV Endodontics
102 Canal St	456 Crown Lane
Star Prairie, TX 74260	Star Prairie, TX 74260
	123-701-1234
	Account # 11234

Date	Description		Amount
	Balance Forward		$0.00
06/20/23	3330 #3 Molar, restore		$1105.00
	Payment		$221.00
07/20/23	Assign claim #102345678910 DC Health Plan Insurance payment claim #102345678910 Check#1234		$853.05

Balance due	30.95

Make all checks payable to SV Endodontics

Thank you for your business!

Goodheart-Willcox Publisher

Figure 13.12 This invoice shows how much the patient owes after the insurance company has paid its share.

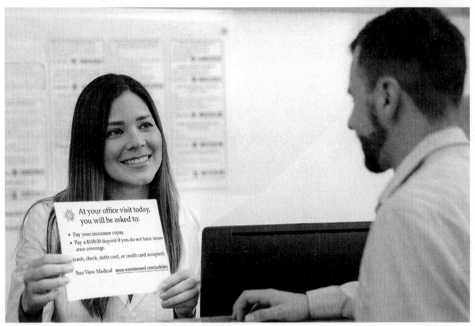

antoniodiaz/Shutterstock.com

Figure 13.13　A placard listing copay policies is usually displayed at the reception desk.

Receiving and Recording Office Payments

Medical providers often require copayments, or copays, before the patient sees the physician. This is an out-of-pocket fee paid by a person with health insurance at the time of a covered service, such as an office visit or prescription. Medical providers also have payment policies for individuals who do not have insurance coverage. The provider policy is typically displayed at the reception desk (**Figure 13.13**), and a brochure or the provider's website may explain it. Medical assistants or receptionists collect these payments at the patient registration desk and issue a receipt.

Patients pay at the time of service in one of three ways: cash, check, or credit/debit card. There are important procedures to follow for each of these payment methods.

- **Cash.** Secure the cash in a locked drawer and provide a printed receipt showing cash payment.
- **Check.** Get two forms of identification from new patients. Do not accept a third-party check unless it is from an insurance company. Inspect the check for the correct date, amount, and signature. Endorse the check with a stamp that says *for deposit only* (**Figure 13.14**). Provide a printed receipt showing payment by check.
- **Credit or debit card.** This is a more secure form of payment, but the provider pays a fee to the credit card company. Provide a printed receipt showing a credit payment.

All receipts should list the name of the medical provider, name and account number of the person paying, current date, amount of the payment, purpose for the payment, and form of payment. Record each payment received in the daily register of your EHR accounting management program (**Figure 13.15**).

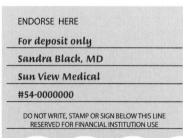

Goodheart-Willcox Publisher

Figure 13.14　This check has been endorsed properly.

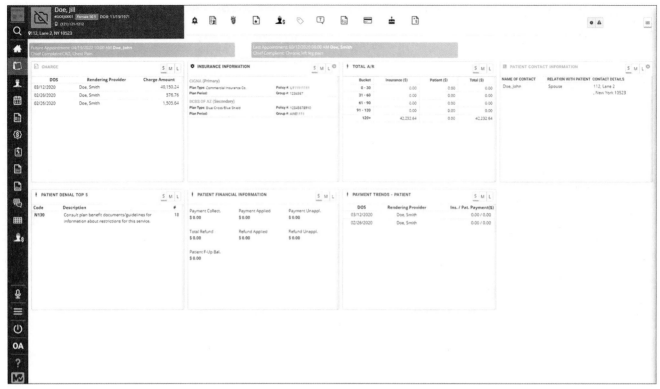

Courtesy of OmniMD

Figure 13.15 An electronic health record system can provide medical codes, record payments, and speed up the medical billing process.

13.2-2 Math and Medications

Suppose a prescription label gives instructions for a young child to receive 3.5 teaspoons of antibiotic liquid a day instead of the 3.5 milliliters the doctor ordered. Since 3.5 teaspoons equals 17.25 milliliters, the child will be receiving five times the amount of medicine prescribed if the label's instructions are followed. Because of this error, the child may experience severe diarrhea, a yeast infection, and a fungal infection.

Clearly, accuracy is critical when giving medicine to patients. For this reason, only authorized people with specialized training can prepare or administer medication. While some **medications** cure a disease, others help the body overcome a disease. In this section, you will learn some of the knowledge and skills needed to work with medications.

Forms of Medication

Medications can be liquid, solid, or semisolid. Liquid medications come in several different forms. These include an *aqueous suspension* (a mixture of water and undissolved particles of medicine), *suspension* (a liquid into which particles of medicine have been mixed but not dissolved), syrup, and *tincture* (an alcoholic base in which medicine has been dissolved).

Solid medications may come in capsules, caplets, tablets, or lozenges (LAH-zehnjs), which are small, flat pills that dissolve in the mouth. Semisolid medications may come as an ointment or *suppository* (suh-PAH-zuh-tor-ee), which is a small, firm mass of medicine that dissolves when inserted into a body cavity other than the mouth.

Administration of Medication

Medications can be administered in several ways or by different routes such as:

- **oral**: given by mouth; used for liquid and solid forms of medicine
- **rectal**: given in the rectum; used for liquids and suppositories
- **topical**: applied directly to the skin; used for ointments, liquids, and adhesive patches
- **sublingual**: given under the tongue; used for tablets, lozenges, or suspensions
- **injection**: given with a needle and syringe; used for liquids
- **inhalation**: medication that is inhaled or breathed in; used with sprays, inhalers, or other special machines

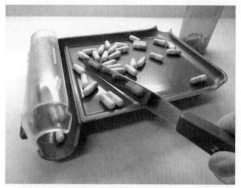

Figure 13.16 Medications must be calculated and counted carefully to ensure the correct dose and dosage.

When calculating amounts of medication, you will hear the terms **dose** and **dosage** (**Figure 13.16**). A dose is the portion of medicine administered at one time. The dosage is the total quantity of medicine that is to be administered. Dosage depends on the weight, sex, and age of the patient. It also considers the disease being treated, how the drug is to be administered, and the patient's tolerance of the drug. The following terms describe different types of doses:

- **initial dose**: the first dose
- **average dose**: the amount of medication proven most effective with minimal toxic effects
- **maximum dose**: the largest amount of medication that can safely be administered at one time
- **lethal dose**: the amount that could cause death

Preparing Medications

Oral administration of medications is the safest and most common route. Oral medications are produced at different strengths to meet individual patient needs. Therefore, you may have to calculate the amount of medication needed based on the strength you have available. For example, if the prescription calls for 200 mg, but your pharmacy only carries 100-mg tablets, you will have to double the number of tablets and adjust the prescription instructions accordingly.

Make sure your medication label and the prescribed medication are in the same measurement system or have been converted to the same system. Then follow this formula for calculating oral medication dosages:

$$\frac{\text{DA (dosage available)}}{\text{DF (dosage form)}} = \frac{\text{DO (dose ordered)}}{\text{DG (dose to be given)}}$$

Suppose you are a pharmacist, and a patient prescription calls for 500 mg of amoxicillin to be taken three times each day for three days. Your pharmacy has 250-mg amoxicillin tablets. You will use a proportion to determine the dose.

$$\frac{250 \text{ mg (DA)}}{1 \text{ tablet (DF)}} = \frac{500 \text{ mg (DO)}}{x \text{ (DG)}}$$

1. Cross multiply to get $250x = 500$
2. Divide each side by the number in front of x

$$250 \div 250 = 1x$$
$$500 \div 250 = 2 \text{ tablets}$$

Each dose will require two tablets, which means 2 tablets × 3 doses/day = 6 tablets × 3 days = 18 tablets in the entire dosage. Therefore, you will fill the pill bottle with 18 amoxicillin tablets. The prescription's label should direct the patient to take two tablets three times each day for three days.

Dosing syringes, dosing cups, or specially marked dosing spoons should be used to measure liquid medications (**Figure 13.17**). Medication dosages depend on the weight of the patient, so accuracy is especially important when giving liquid medicine to children. A small difference in the amount of medicine can have a serious negative effect on a young child. Measure liquid medicine at eye level, and never guess at the dose. Use the dose shown on the medication label.

When preparing liquid medications, calculate how many milliliters of medicine a patient should receive. For this calculation, you must know the **concentration** of the drug. The concentration describes how much of the drug is in a specific volume of liquid. Concentrations are normally given as a fraction, such as 20 mg/mL, which means there are 20 milligrams of medication in every milliliter of liquid.

Suppose the dose ordered (DO) from the physician is 30 mg of ketorolac liquid every six hours for 24 hours. The dose available (DA) is 15 mg/mL. How many milliliters of ketorolac liquid are needed in the 24-hour period?

$$\frac{15 \text{ mg (DA)}}{1 \text{ mL (DF)}} = \frac{30 \text{ mg (DO)}}{x \text{ mL (DG)}}$$

1. Cross multiply to get $15x = 30$, and then divide each side of the equation by 15. This means that $x = 2$ mL, which tells you the patient needs 2 mL of ketorolac per dose.
2. You know the patient receives a dose every six hours. In a 24-hour period, the patient will receive four doses of medication ($24 \div 6 = 4$).
3. Finally, multiply the total number of doses in a 24-hour period by the total number of milliliters per dose (4 doses/24 hr × 2mL/dose = 8 mL/24 hr).

Physicians commonly use abbreviations to indicate the route and times for administering medication. For example, *240 mg of Aspirin®, qd in am* means the patient will take 240 mg of Aspirin® every day in the morning. Technicians interpret the abbreviations and clarify the time and frequency for taking each medication. They print easy-to-understand instructions on the medication label. For *240 mg of Aspirin®, qd in am*, the label instructions might read, "Take one tablet by mouth each day in the morning" (**Figure 13.18**).

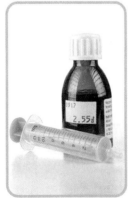 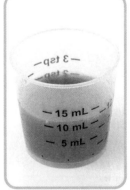 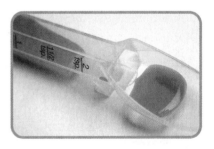

Figure 13.17   Dosing devices include the dosing syringe, dosing cup, and dosing spoon.

Prescription Abbreviations		
Question	**Abbreviation**	**Meaning**
How often should you take your medication?	ad lib	freely, as needed
	bid	twice a day
	prn	as needed
	q	every
	q3h	every 3 hours
	q4h	every 4 hours
	qd	every day
	qid	four times a day
	qod	every other day
	tid	three times a day
When should you take your medication?	ac	before meals
	hs	at bedtime
	int	between meals
	pc	after meals
Where should you get your medication?	Rx	prescription
	OTC	over the counter
How much medication should you take?	caps	capsule
	gtt	drops
	i, ii, iii, or iiii	the number of doses (1, 2, 3, or 4)
	mg	milligrams
	mL	milliliters
	ss	one half
	T̈, TT̈, TTT̈	the number of tabs/caps (1, 2, 3)
	tabs	tablets
	tbsp	tablespoon (15 mL)
	tsp	teaspoon (5 mL)
Where should you administer your medication?	ad	right ear
	al	left ear
	c̄	with
	od	right eye
	os	left eye
	ou	both eyes
	po	by mouth
	s or ø	without
	sl	sublingual
	top	apply topically
	IV	intravenously

Goodheart-Willcox Publisher

Figure 13.18 Prescription abbreviations are commonly used between healthcare workers to communicate dosage information.

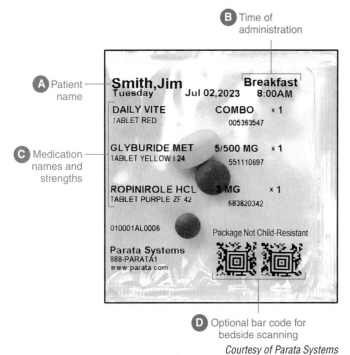

A Patient name

B Time of administration

C Medication names and strengths

D Optional bar code for bedside scanning

Smith,Jim
Tuesday   Jul 02,2023   8:00AM
Breakfast

DAILY VITE   COMBO   × 1
TABLET RED   005363547

GLYBURIDE MET   5/500 MG   × 1
TABLET YELLOW I 24   551110697

ROPINIROLE HCL   3 MG   × 1
TABLET PURPLE ZF 42   683820342

010001AL0006   Package Not Child-Resistant

Parata Systems
888-PARATA1
www.parata.com

Courtesy of Parata Systems

Figure 13.19 Medications can be prepackaged in pouches labeled with the following information: (A) patient name, (B) time of administration, (C) medication names and strengths, and (D) an optional bar code for bedside scanning. In addition, any special instructions—such as the need to take a medication with food—will be listed below the name of that medication.

Medication Safety

Some long-term care facilities receive residents' medications in prepackaged doses ready to be administered at timed intervals (**Figure 13.19**). This type of packaging can also be helpful when patients are away from home for long periods, such as children who go to summer camp or businesspeople who travel frequently. For patients who take several medications each day, this packaging can save time and prevent dosing errors. Each year, the US Food and Drug Administration (FDA) receives more than 100,000 reports about suspected medication errors. These errors can send individuals to a hospital, cause a disability, or even result in death.

The more medications a patient takes, the easier it is to make an error. A patient taking five different medications three times each day must open and select a correct dose from a medication container fifteen times each day. **Figure 13.20** shows the medication orders for a patient named Adrian Hartman, who lives in a long-term care facility. The pharmacy technician who receives these orders sees that the resident takes six different medications each day and a seventh only when needed.

The technician interprets the routes and times for each medication and groups the medicines taken at the same time into one package. Each package lists the date, time to administer, and name and dosage of each medication in the package. For Adrian Hartman, the pouch for 0800 (8:00 a.m.) will contain furosemide, Plavix®, Lipitor®, Aspirin®, and Toprol®. The pouch for 1130 (11:30 a.m.) will contain furosemide; and the pouch for 2200 (10:00 p.m.) will contain Tylenol®. Nitrostat® is delivered in a separate pouch to be administered as needed.

Medication Orders for Adrian Hartman		
Medication Orders	**Dosing Times**	**Interpretation of Medication Orders**
20 mg furosemide	bid in am hours	Twice each day, in the morning
75 mg Plavix®	qd in am	Every day in the morning
10 mg Lipitor®	qd in am	Every day in the morning
240 mg Aspirin®	qd in am	Every day in the morning
25 mg Toprol XL®	qd in am	Every day in the morning
650 mg Tylenol®	qd hs OTC	Every day at bedtime; not a prescription; purchase over the counter
0.4 mg Nitrostat®	prn sbl	Use as needed for chest pain; place under the tongue

Goodheart-Willcox Publisher

Figure 13.20 Shown here are the medication orders and interpretations for one patient.

Technicians follow medication safety practices that promote giving the right medication at the right time and in the right dose. Pharmacists check each package to ensure that medications, amounts, and times are correct. They pay attention to possible drug interactions and special instructions such as taking medicines before, with, or after meals.

13.2-3 Measuring Angles

Healthcare workers use angles to measure and describe joint movement, inject medications correctly, and position patients in bed. They measure angles in degrees from a *reference plane*. For example, when you lie flat on your back in bed, your body is the reference plane at 0 degrees. When you raise your arm straight toward the ceiling, you have created a 90-degree angle between your body and your arm. Raising your arm above your head and moving it all the way back down to the bed surface creates a 180-degree angle (**Figure 13.21**).

When injecting medications, healthcare workers vary the angle of the needle based on the type of medication they are administering or the procedure they are performing. The surface of the patient's skin is the reference plane at 0 degrees (**Figure 13.22**).

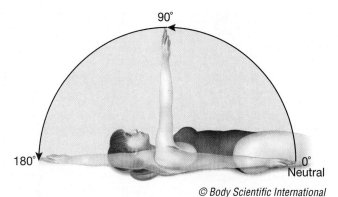

© Body Scientific International

Figure 13.21 Healthcare workers use angles to measure and describe joint movement. *If a patient can raise the arm straight up, what degree of movement would you record in the patient's chart?*

Angles are also important for positioning patients. Physicians may order the head of a patient's bed to be elevated 30 to 45 degrees. The purpose of this position is to help the patient breathe more easily or prevent aspiration of fluids into the lungs. Nurses will raise the bed from 60 to 90 degrees when feeding patients to help them swallow more easily. These are called *Fowler's positions* and include **semi-Fowler's** (30 degrees), **Fowler's** (45 degrees), and **high Fowler's** (90 degrees).

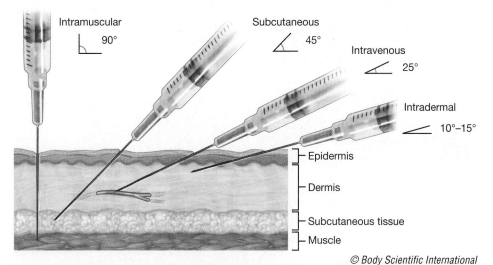

© Body Scientific International

Figure 13.22 Healthcare workers use specific angles for different types of injections. Intramuscular injections are given through the skin and into the muscle at a 90-degree angle. Subcutaneous injections go into the tissue layer between the skin and the muscle at a 45-degree angle. Intravenous injections are given into a vein at a 25-degree angle. Intradermal injections are given into the dermis layer of the skin at a 10- to 15-degree angle.

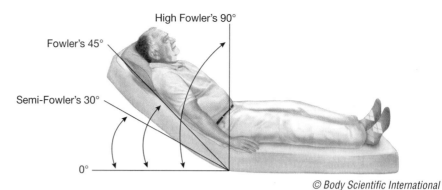

High Fowler's 90°

Fowler's 45°

Semi-Fowler's 30°

0°

© Body Scientific International

Figure 13.23 Fowler's positions allow the patient to breathe more easily and help prevent the aspiration of fluids.

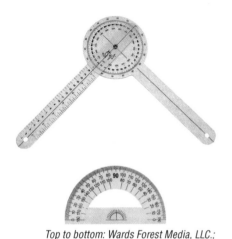

Top to bottom: Wards Forest Media, LLC.; exopixel/Shutterstock.com

Figure 13.24 A goniometer and a protractor both measure angles.

The terms indicate the number of degrees the patient is elevated from the 0-degree plane, which is lying flat on the bed in supine position (**Figure 13.23**).

Physical therapists use angles during patient rehabilitation. They measure the range of motion for an injured joint. As therapy progresses, measurements will document the improvements in range of motion. The therapist uses a tool called the **goniometer** (goh-nee-AH-meh-ter) to measure joint angles and records range of motion in degrees (**Figure 13.24**). While the most accurate measurements are taken from radiographs (X-ray images), the goniometer is a less expensive tool that works like a protractor to measure joint angles on the human body.

When taking a joint measurement with a goniometer, always stabilize the stationary part of the body (the part that does not move), which is proximal (close) to the joint you are testing (**Figure 13.25**). This isolates the joint movement and results in a more accurate measurement.

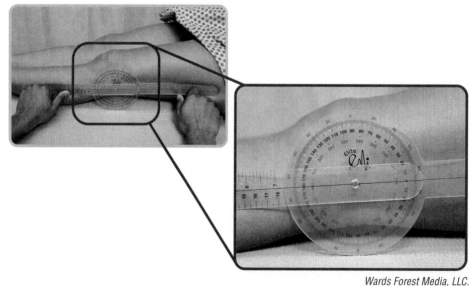

Wards Forest Media, LLC.

Figure 13.25 The arms of the goniometer must be positioned correctly for an accurate measurement. This image shows full knee extension of 0 degrees.

Follow these steps to measure the angle of a joint:

1. Align the **fulcrum** or pin of the goniometer with the fulcrum of the joint to be measured. This is the support point for the joint. Since the location of the fulcrum can vary, you will need to check the location for each specific joint. In the knee and elbow joints for example, place the pin of the goniometer over the lateral epicondyle (ehp-ih-KAHN-dihl).
2. Align one arm of the goniometer with the stationary limb.
3. Align the other arm of the goniometer with the limb that moves.
4. Read the goniometer by noting the degree measurement from the 0 point to the endpoint at the arrow or line before removing it from the patient's body. The degrees between the zero point and the endpoint represent the entire range of motion.
5. Record the range of motion for the joint.

A therapist will compare the patient's range of motion with previous records and the average range of motion. This will help with determining the patient's progress and developing therapy plans for continued improvement (**Figure 13.26**).

13.2-4 **Preparing Solutions**

Luciana needs a 1:10 bleach solution for disinfecting surfaces in patient rooms. Quinn needs to mix frozen juice concentrate with water in a ratio of one part concentrate to four parts water. A dermatologist wants his patient's wound treated with a 10-percent vinegar solution. From housekeeping to food service, from nursing to the medical laboratory and pharmacy, healthcare workers prepare solutions for a wide variety of uses.

Solutions are mixtures that contain two or more chemicals. The liquid that dissolves a chemical is called the **solvent**. The chemical to be dissolved is the **solute** (SAHL-yoot). All the previous examples use water, which is a common solvent. A 1:10 proportion, called the **dilution ratio**, for bleach solution uses one part bleach and nine parts water. A recipe for making bleach solution calls for ¼ cup of bleach and 2¼ cups of water. This represents the measurable amounts for a 1:10 solution.

What if you need a larger quantity of bleach solution? Follow these steps to calculate specific amounts of a solution:

1. Begin with the total volume; for example, 1 gallon of bleach solution.
2. Divide this total volume by the second number in your dilution ratio. This second number tells you how many total parts are in the dilution, so the answer will tell you the size of each part.

   Example: 1 gallon (16 cups) ÷ 10 = 1.6 cups

3. Multiply your answer by the first number in your dilution ratio to learn the amount of solute you need to measure. Since the first number is often 1, this calculation is easy. You will need 1.6 cups of bleach.
4. Subtract the amount of solute from the total volume of the solution to learn how much solvent will be needed (16 cups – 1.6 cups = 14.4 cups of water).
5. Note that 0.6 of a cup and 0.4 of a cup are difficult to measure. Convert these amounts to a combination of tablespoons, teaspoons, and fractions of a cup for accurate measurements because measuring cups aren't calibrated for tenths of a cup.

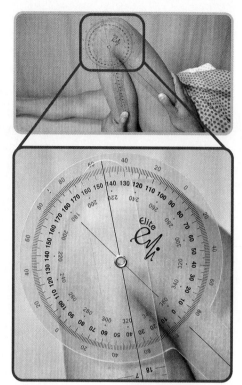

Wards Forest Media, LLC.

Figure 13.26 This angle shows that the patient has full range of motion. Read the measurement shown on the goniometer here.
What is the patient's range of motion for knee flexion?

Working in metric numbers makes calculations and measurements easier. For instance, follow these steps to make 4 liters of 1:10 bleach solution:

1. 4 L ÷ 10 = 0.4 L
2. 0.4 L × 1 = 0.4 L of bleach (0.4 L can be measured as 400 mL)
3. 4 L – 0.4 L = 3.6 L of water (0.6 L can be measured as 600 mL)

Mixing juice using one part juice concentrate and four parts water means you are making a 1:5 solution (1 + 4 = 5 total parts in the solution). You can calculate the amounts to make 1 liter of grape juice using the same steps you used for the bleach solution:

1. 1 L ÷ 5 = 0.2 L
2. 0.2 L × 1 = 0.2 L (200 mL) of juice concentrate
3. 1 L – 0.2 L = 0.8 L (800 mL) of water

Solutions are often expressed as percentages. Percent means *per hundred*, so a solution expressed as a percentage tells you how much solute is in every 100 mL of the solution. For example, a 10-percent vinegar solution contains 10 mL of vinegar in 100 mL of solution. Ten percent represents the ratio 10:100, which can also be expressed as 1:10 (**Figure 13.27**). Therefore, the vinegar solution uses the same dilution formula as the bleach solution. You can use the same steps to calculate the amounts of vinegar and water for the total volume of solution you will mix.

Because solutions contain chemicals, always be alert for possible hazards. Consult safety data sheets (SDS) and never mix solutions until you have verified the chemicals are compatible. Follow all safety guidelines for handling, storing, disposing of, and removing spills of chemical solutions.

Consider the effectiveness of the solutions you prepare and use. They may have a limited life. For example, bleach solutions lose their disinfectant power quickly when exposed to heat, sunlight, and evaporation. To keep a bleach solution strong enough to kill germs, mix a fresh solution each day and discard unused amounts at the end of the day.

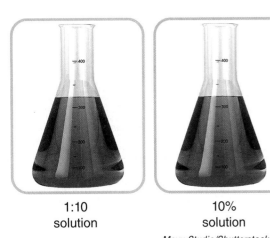

1:10 solution

10% solution

Maxx-Studio/Shutterstock.com

Figure 13.27 Solutions can be expressed as percentages or ratios. *Which solution is stronger?*

Lesson 13.2 Review

 Complete the *Map Your Reading* graphic organizer for the section you just read.

1. Which process changes written medical documentation into numeric form? (13.2-1)
   A. Coding
   B. Co-payment
   C. Conversion
   D. Claims process

2. The total amount of medication given to a patient is the _____ . (13.2-2)
   A. portion
   B. route
   C. dose
   D. dosage

3. To assess range of motion, a healthcare worker measures the _____ of a joint and records the range of motion in degrees. (13.2-3)
   A. tension
   B. depth
   C. angle
   D. flexibility

4. The liquid used to dissolve a chemical in a solution is called the _____. (13.2-4)
   A. solute
   B. solvent
   C. ratio
   D. proportion

Healthcare Tasks That Use Mathematical Conversions

Learning Outcomes

After studying this lesson, you will be able to

13.3-1 convert measurements between the Fahrenheit and Celsius scales.

13.3-2 list guidelines for measuring food accurately.

13.3-3 relate the value of using standardized recipes in healthcare settings.

13.3-4 estimate and record percentage of food intake by food item or meal total.

13.3-5 enumerate the components measured as part of fluid intake and output.

ESSENTIAL QUESTION

What are some healthcare tasks that use mathematical conversions?

Professional Vocabulary

Essential Terms

fluid balance a state in which the amount of fluid taken into the body equals the amount of fluid that leaves the body

intake and output (I&O) measurements of all the fluids that enter and leave the body

portion the amount of food in one serving

yield the number of portions a recipe will produce

Important Terms

Celsius scale	graduated cylinder	unit cost
commode hat	ingredient cost	urinals
conversion factor	recipe cost	
Fahrenheit scale	tare weight	

Introduction

Healthcare workers convert measurements for temperature between the Fahrenheit and Celsius scales and adjust measurements when preparing food. They estimate a patient's food intake and measure fluid intake and output to check for fluid imbalance.

13.3-1 Temperature Conversions

US temperature readings typically use the **Fahrenheit scale**. Some US facilities and most facilities in other countries use the **Celsius scale**, or *Centigrade scale*. Healthcare workers must understand temperature readings in both scales and be able to convert between the two scales. To avoid confusion, workers should communicate temperature using the scale familiar to the patient.

Two basic comparisons show that water boils at 212 degrees Fahrenheit (°F) and 100 degrees Celsius (°C), and water freezes at 32°F and 0°C. If you tell patients from another country their temperature is 100 degrees, do not be surprised if they think their blood is boiling. While 98.6 degrees is an average adult temperature in the Fahrenheit scale, 37 degrees is the average temperature in the Celsius scale (**Figure 13.28**). Temperatures are typically written as 98.6°F or 37°C and read as "ninety-eight point six degrees Fahrenheit" or "thirty-seven degrees Celsius."

To express degrees Fahrenheit in the Celsius scale, use this formula:

$$°C = \frac{5}{9}(°F - 32).$$

Example: To express 98°F in the Celsius scale:

1. Write the formula. $\qquad °C = \frac{5}{9}(°F - 32)$

2. Substitute the specific value. $\qquad °C = \frac{5}{9}(98 - 32)$

3. Calculate. $\qquad °C = \frac{5}{9}(66)$

$$5 \div 9 \times 66 = 36.7°C$$

To express degrees Celsius in the Fahrenheit scale, use this formula:

$$°F = \frac{9}{5}°C + 32.$$

Example: To express 36°C in the Fahrenheit scale:

1. Write the formula. $\qquad °F = \frac{9}{5}°C + 32$

2. Substitute the specific value. $\qquad °F = \frac{9}{5}36 + 32$

3. Calculate: $\qquad 9 \div 5 \times 36 + 32 = 96.8°F$

It may be easier for you to remember a conversion guide expressed in words. For °F to °C, subtract 32, then multiply by 5, then divide by 9.

Example: To express 98.6°F in the Celsius scale:

1. 98.6 − 32 = 66.6
2. 66.6 × 5 = 333
3. 333 ÷ 9 = 37°C

For °C to °F, multiply by 9, then divide by 5, then add 32.

Average Temperature Ranges		
Method Used to Obtain Temperature	**Fahrenheit (°F)**	**Celsius (°C)**
Oral	97.6 to 99.6	36.5 to 37.5
Rectal	98.6 to 100.6	37 to 38.1
Axillary	95.3 to 98.4	35.2 to 37
Tympanic	96.6 to 99.7	35.9 to 37.6
Temporal	98.2 to 100.2	36.7 to 37.8

Goodheart-Willcox Publisher

Figure 13.28 Healthcare workers must know average temperature ranges in both Fahrenheit and Celsius and make conversions between these temperature scales.

Example: To express 37°C in the Fahrenheit scale:

1. $37 \times 9 = 333$
2. $333 \div 5 = 66.6$
3. $66.6 + 32 = 98.6°F$

There are a few tips that can help you "think" in Celsius and recognize abnormal body temperatures. First, to compare Celsius to Fahrenheit, remember that 16°C is about 61°F, and 28°C is about 82°F. Second, use this rhyme to remember key temperatures on the Celsius scale:

39 is too hot

37 is nice

35 is too cold

Because 0 is ice

13.3-2 Measuring Food

Whenever possible, food service workers measure food by weight using a food scale. Food weight measurements are more accurate and consistent than volume measurements. For example, one-half cup of brown sugar that is not packed will weigh less than one-half cup that is packed or pressed firmly into the measuring cup. Food weights can be measured using ounces and pounds or grams and kilograms.

Healthcare Professions: Food Costs

Gerry is the dietary manager for a small hospital. He is responsible for meeting the dietary needs of patients, but he also manages the hospital cafeteria used by employees and visitors. To meet budget expectations, Gerry carefully tracks the costs of food purchased by the hospital and uses recipe costing to monitor prices charged for cafeteria meals. Food portions are carefully measured to meet patients' dietary requirements, but also to manage the cost of foods served in the hospital.

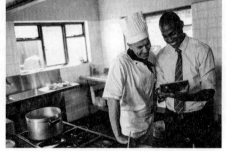

wavebreakmedia/Shutterstock.com

Workers must consider **tare weight** when using a food scale. This is the weight of the container that holds the food being measured. Place the empty container on the food scale and reset the weight indicator to zero. Then place the food in the container for an accurate reading of food weight. Most scales can be reset to account for tare weight. If your scale cannot be reset, simply subtract the weight of the empty container from the total weight of the food and the container. If the container weighs 1 ounce, and the total weight of the food and container is 8 ounces, the weight of the food alone is 7 ounces.

A fluid ounce is the basic unit of volume in the US system. Smaller units include the teaspoon, which is 1/6 ounce, and the tablespoon, which is 1/2 ounce. Larger units of volume include the cup, pint, quart, and gallon.

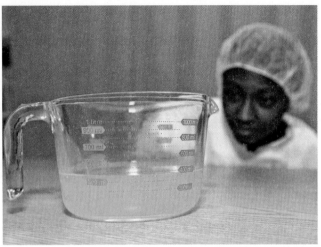

Wards Forest Media, LLC.

Figure 13.29 For accurate liquid measurements, place the measuring cup on a level surface and read the measurement at eye level.

The metric system uses the liter as the basic unit of volume. The milliliter, which is 1/1,000 liter, is also commonly used for volume measurements.

Knowing the correlation between the weight and volume of certain liquids can save measuring time. For water or other liquids with a similar density, such as broth, milk, or juice, 1 fluid ounce is equal to 1 ounce in weight. Similarly, in the metric system, 1 milliliter is equal to 1 gram, and 1 liter is equal to 1 kilogram. If your recipe calls for "16 oz milk," that will be the same as 16 fluid ounces. Since 1 cup equals 8 fluid ounces, you can simply measure 2 cups for 16 oz of milk. In the metric system, 480 grams of milk is the same as 480 milliliters and can be measured using a liquid measuring cup with mL markings.

Two additional measuring steps will ensure your individual measurements are accurate. When measuring dry ingredients, always level the measuring container. Begin by overfilling the cup or spoon and then use a spatula to scrape off ingredients above the rim of the measuring container. For liquid ingredients, set the container on a level surface, bend if necessary, and read the container at eye level (**Figure 13.29**).

13.3-3 Using Standardized Recipes

In a standardized recipe, the list of ingredients, amount of each ingredient, and preparation methods allow you to make the food item the same way each time. Standardization of food items is important to customers who expect the same food product each time they order it. For patients, standardization can be critical when a health condition depends on including or avoiding particular food items or ingredients. For this reason, healthcare food service workers carefully follow standardized recipes without making changes. Ingredient substitutions must be approved so therapeutic diets remain accurate and wholesome for each patient.

A standardized recipe has several distinct parts and includes more details than the typical home recipe (**Figure 13.30**):

1. The name of the recipe matches its listing on the hospital menu.
2. The **yield** section describes the quantity or number of servings the recipe will make. Yield can be adjusted to make more or fewer servings.
3. **Portion** size indicates the amount for each serving. Portion size can be listed by weight, volume, or count. For example, one portion could be 8 ounces, 1 cup, or 3 pieces of a food item such as chicken strips. Food service workers use specific ladles and scoops to serve individual portions. These tools have been selected because they will scoop an accurate portion of the food being served each time. Food scales may also be used to weigh individual portions. Accurate food portioning is important to the health of patients on specialized diets. It also satisfies customers who expect the same amount as the next person with the same order. Portioning also controls food costs.

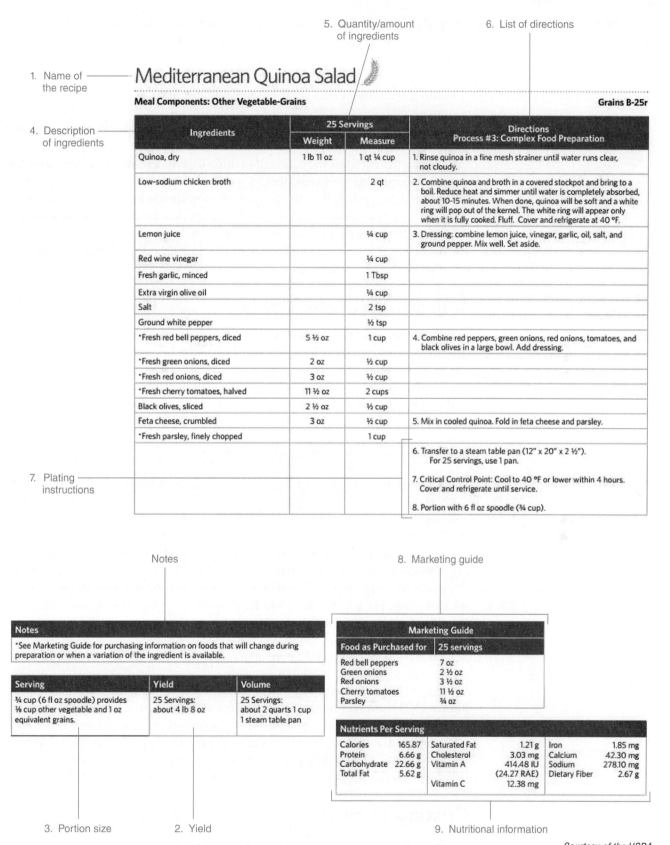

1. Name of the recipe

5. Quantity/amount of ingredients

6. List of directions

4. Description of ingredients

7. Plating instructions

Mediterranean Quinoa Salad

Meal Components: Other Vegetable-Grains

Grains B-25r

| Ingredients | 25 Servings | | Directions |
	Weight	Measure	Process #3: Complex Food Preparation
Quinoa, dry	1 lb 11 oz	1 qt ¼ cup	1. Rinse quinoa in a fine mesh strainer until water runs clear, not cloudy.
Low-sodium chicken broth		2 qt	2. Combine quinoa and broth in a covered stockpot and bring to a boil. Reduce heat and simmer until water is completely absorbed, about 10-15 minutes. When done, quinoa will be soft and a white ring will pop out of the kernel. The white ring will appear only when it is fully cooked. Fluff. Cover and refrigerate at 40 °F.
Lemon juice		¼ cup	3. Dressing: combine lemon juice, vinegar, garlic, oil, salt, and ground pepper. Mix well. Set aside.
Red wine vinegar		¼ cup	
Fresh garlic, minced		1 Tbsp	
Extra virgin olive oil		¼ cup	
Salt		2 tsp	
Ground white pepper		½ tsp	
*Fresh red bell peppers, diced	5 ½ oz	1 cup	4. Combine red peppers, green onions, red onions, tomatoes, and black olives in a large bowl. Add dressing.
*Fresh green onions, diced	2 oz	½ cup	
*Fresh red onions, diced	3 oz	½ cup	
*Fresh cherry tomatoes, halved	11 ½ oz	2 cups	
Black olives, sliced	2 ½ oz	½ cup	
Feta cheese, crumbled	3 oz	½ cup	5. Mix in cooled quinoa. Fold in feta cheese and parsley.
*Fresh parsley, finely chopped		1 cup	
			6. Transfer to a steam table pan (12" x 20" x 2 ½"). For 25 servings, use 1 pan.
			7. Critical Control Point: Cool to 40 °F or lower within 4 hours. Cover and refrigerate until service.
			8. Portion with 6 fl oz spoodle (¾ cup).

Notes

8. Marketing guide

Notes

*See Marketing Guide for purchasing information on foods that will change during preparation or when a variation of the ingredient is available.

Serving	Yield	Volume
¾ cup (6 fl oz spoodle) provides ⅛ cup other vegetable and 1 oz equivalent grains.	25 Servings: about 4 lb 8 oz	25 Servings: about 2 quarts 1 cup 1 steam table pan

Marketing Guide

Food as Purchased for	25 servings
Red bell peppers	7 oz
Green onions	2 ½ oz
Red onions	3 ½ oz
Cherry tomatoes	11 ½ oz
Parsley	¾ oz

Nutrients Per Serving

Calories	165.87	Saturated Fat	1.21 g	Iron	1.85 mg
Protein	6.66 g	Cholesterol	3.03 mg	Calcium	42.30 mg
Carbohydrate	22.66 g	Vitamin A	414.48 IU	Sodium	278.10 mg
Total Fat	5.62 g		(24.27 RAE)	Dietary Fiber	2.67 g
		Vitamin C	12.38 mg		

3. Portion size

2. Yield

9. Nutritional information

Courtesy of the USDA

Figure 13.30 This USDA recipe shows the distinct parts of a standardized recipe.

4. The recipe lists ingredients with descriptions or specifications. For example, the carrots are diced, the onion is chopped, the tomatoes are fresh, and the pork is boneless loin.
5. The quantity or amount of each ingredient is listed by weight. For small amounts of food items such as seasonings, teaspoon or tablespoon units are given.
6. The list of directions includes cooking times and temperatures to ensure food safety.
7. Plating instructions may indicate which dish to use when serving and the specific method for garnishing.
8. A marketing guide lists the amount of ingredients to purchase. For example, how many ounces of red peppers do you need to purchase to equal the 1 cup of diced peppers in a recipe?
9. Nutrition information is often listed to show amounts of major nutrients provided by the food item.

Adjusting Recipe Yields

Sometimes you will need to change the yield of a recipe to prepare more or fewer servings. To do this, you need to know how many portions the recipe makes and how many portions you need. Then you can determine the **conversion factor**. The conversion factor adjusts the amount of each ingredient from the original recipe to how much is needed in the revised recipe. Calculate a conversion factor using this formula:

new yield ÷ old yield = conversion factor

Now you can apply the conversion factor to each ingredient in the recipe:

original quantity × conversion factor = new quantity

Gerry, the dietary manager, would like to sample a new recipe before adding it to the hospital menu. While the standardized recipe for Mediterranean Quinoa Salad (**Figure 13.30**) makes 25 portions, he will need only five portions for sampling. He adjusts the yield by determining the conversion factor. For Gerry's recipe, the formula looks like this:

5 portions ÷ 25 portions = 0.2 conversion factor

Gerry now converts the ingredient measurements using the conversion factor. **Figure 13.31** shows the converted ingredient measurements. Note that for calculations of smaller amounts of an ingredient, the nearest measurable amount is used. For example, the measurement for salt in **Figure 13.31** is 2 tsp. When multiplied by the conversion factor of 0.2, the result is 0.4 tsp. The nearest measurable amount is 1/2 tsp because measuring spoons do not have markings in 1/10 increments.

Costing Recipes

Like most food service establishments, healthcare facilities purchase food in bulk amounts such as a case, bushel, or flat. To stay within budget guidelines, the manager must figure out the **unit cost**, meaning how much money is needed to make each food item. This process is called *costing*.

Recipe Ingredient Conversions		
Ingredient	25 servings	5 servings
Quinoa	1 lb, 10½ oz	5.3 oz
Chicken broth, low salt	2 quarts	12.8 oz
Lemon juice	¼ cup	0.4 oz
Vinegar, red wine	¼ cup	0.4 oz
Fresh garlic, minced	1 tbsp	½ tsp
Olive oil	¼ cup	0.4 oz
Salt	2 tsp	½ tsp
Pepper, white ground	½ tsp	⅒ tsp
Peppers, sweet red, fresh, chopped	5½ oz	1.1 oz
Parsley, raw, chopped	1 cup	0.2 cup
Green onions, diced	2 oz	0.4 oz
Red onion, chopped	3 oz	0.6 oz
Cherry tomatoes, halved	11½ oz	2.3 oz
Black olives, sliced	2½ oz	0.5 oz
Feta cheese, crumbled	3 oz	0.6 oz

Goodheart-Willcox Publisher

Figure 13.31 Food service workers use a conversion factor when adjusting recipe yields.

To cost a recipe, you must convert the bulk purchase units into the units used in the recipe, such as pounds, ounces, or pieces. When you know the unit cost of each item, you can calculate the total cost for each ingredient in a recipe. Use the following formulas to determine the unit cost of food items.

- **Per-pound unit cost:** divide the unit cost by the number of pounds in the unit.

  Example: $73.00 (per case of apples) ÷ 40 (pounds per case) = $1.83/pound

- **Per-ounce unit cost:** divide the price per pound by 16 to get the price per ounce.

  Example: $14.00 (per pound of blue cheese) ÷ 16 = $0.88/ounce

- **Per piece unit cost:** divide the cost of the unit by the number of pieces in the unit.

  Example: $40.00 (per box of oranges) ÷ 75 (oranges in each box) = $0.53/orange

When you know the unit cost of each ingredient, you can easily multiply the unit cost by the number of units used in the recipe to determine the **ingredient cost** of each item. For example, Gerry's recipe calls for feta cheese: 3 oz (in the recipe) × $1.00 (unit cost per ounce) = $3.00 (cost for feta cheese used in the recipe).

Add the cost for each ingredient to determine the total food costs for a recipe, or the **recipe cost**. Since recipe costing is repeated regularly to reflect changing food costs, most organizations use a software program that will automatically cost a recipe as new food prices are entered into the program.

Gerry follows a budget for the hospital food services department, so he tracks the costs of all foods purchased. In addition, he costs the recipes used in food preparation. Knowing the cost of each recipe, Gerry can make appropriate substitutions to save money. For example, he can save money by substituting canned tomatoes for fresh tomatoes in a chili recipe. In addition, he uses the cost of a recipe as a guide for pricing menu items sold in the hospital cafeteria. **Figure 13.32** shows how Gerry determines the recipe cost for his new recipe.

Note that standard equivalents, such as 1 cup equaling 8 ounces, work only for liquid ingredients. Measurements of dry ingredients like the parsley used in this recipe must be calculated based on the actual weight of each ingredient. For example, 1 cup of parsley does not weigh nearly as much as 1 cup of butter.

Recipe Cost Sheet			
Recipe: Mediterranean Quinoa Salad Yield: 25 servings Portion: ¾ cup			
Ingredient	**Amount**	**Unit Cost**	**Total Cost**
Quinoa	1 lb, 10½ oz	$0.43/oz	$11.40
Chicken broth, low salt	2 quarts = 64 oz	$0.10/oz	$6.40
Lemon juice	¼ cup = 2 oz	$0.07/oz	$0.14
Vinegar, red wine	¼ cup = 2 oz	$0.22/oz	$0.44
Olive oil	¼ cup = 2 oz	$0.31/oz	$0.62
Salt	2 tsp = 0.4 oz	$0.03/oz	$0.01
Pepper, white ground	½ tsp = 0.08 oz	$3.51/oz	$0.28
Peppers, sweet red, fresh, chopped	5½ oz	$0.16/oz	$0.88
Parsley, raw, chopped	1 cup = 0.9 oz	$0.35/oz	$0.32
Green onions, diced	2 oz	$0.30/oz	$0.60
Red onion, chopped	3 oz	$0.09/oz	$0.27
Cherry tomatoes, halved	11½ oz	$0.29/oz	$3.34
Black olives, sliced	2½ oz	$0.45/oz	$1.13
Feta cheese, crumbled	3 oz	$1.00/oz	$3.00
Total recipe cost: $28.83 Date costed: 11/19/2023 Portion cost: $1.15			

Figure 13.32 Food service workers use recipe cost sheets for tracking portion and total recipe costs.

13.3-4 Measuring and Recording Food Intake

Because healthcare workers use therapeutic diets to improve patients' medical conditions, workers pay attention to not only food service but also food intake. Serving the healthiest foods will not improve a patient's condition if the patient does not consume the food. For this reason, healthcare workers estimate and record food intake for residents in most long-term care facilities and for some patients in hospitals. Sometimes you will estimate the total percentage of a meal that was consumed, such as *ate 70% of breakfast, 80% of lunch, and 50% of dinner*. If a person eats less than 70 percent of a meal, record and report that information to the nurse.

In some facilities, you will record the percentage of each food eaten, such as *for dinner—ate 100% of rice, 50% of chicken breast, 80% of salad, and 100% of bread* (**Figure 13.33**). A dietitian converts these percentages into total calories consumed and records this information in the patient's chart. Using standardized recipes that include nutritional information simplifies this calculation.

13.3-5 Measuring and Recording Intake and Output

Fluid balance is a match between the amount of fluid entering and amount leaving the body. It is important to the healthy functioning of your body. It prevents heatstroke and helps maintain proper kidney and heart functions. A drop in fluid levels can result in hypotension and reduced kidney function. Healthcare workers must be alert for signs of fluid imbalance in all patients because it can result in dehydration (too little fluid) or edema (excess fluid). Patients with medical conditions such as heart or kidney disease, severe burns, or hemorrhaging require particular attention regarding fluid balance.

When the physician writes an order to "maintain intake and output measurements," healthcare workers will measure and record all fluids that enter and leave the body using an **intake and output (I&O)** sheet. In healthcare facilities, fluids are measured in milliliters (mL) or cubic centimeters (cc).

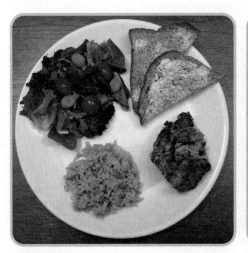 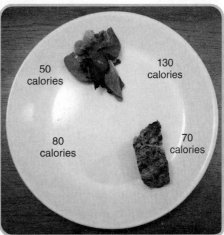

Photographs taken by Susan Blahnik

Figure 13.33 Using the nutritional information for each food item, a dietitian converts the percentages of each food eaten into total calories consumed. In this instance, the patient ate 100 percent of the rice, 50 percent of the chicken breast, 80 percent of the salad, and 100 percent of the bread.

One fluid ounce equals 30 mL or 30 cc. At the end of each shift and at the end of each 24-hour period, the amounts are totaled. Ideally, the intake amount will roughly equal the output amount to maintain fluid balance. Adults should consume 48 to 96 ounces (1440 to 2880 mL) of liquid each day to keep up with the fluids that normally leave the body as urine, feces, sweat, and air exhaled.

Fluid intake includes all the fluids you drink as well as foods that are liquid at room temperature. Gelatin, broth, ice cream, and sherbet are part of fluid intake. If a patient receives IV fluids or enteral (tube) nutrition, the nurse will record the amounts given.

Follow these steps to record fluid intake:

1. Begin by learning the amount of fluid held by the cups, glasses, and bowls used in your facility.

2. Be prepared to convert ounces to milliliters.

   Example: 8 oz glass × 30 mL = 240 mL

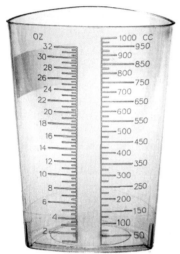

© Medline Industries, Inc., 2013

Figure 13.34 Liquid intake is measured in a graduated cylinder and recorded in milliliters.

3. Remember to record the amount consumed rather than the amount that remains.

   Example: If a patient leaves an 8-oz glass 3/4 full, he has consumed 1/4 of the 8 oz (1/4 × 8), which equals 2 oz. Multiply by 30 and record (2 oz × 30 mL = 60 mL).

4. Estimate the amount consumed unless the patient requires an exact intake measurement.

   Example: About 1/4 (25%) of an 8-oz glass of juice remains when the patient is finished. That means the patient has consumed 3/4, or 75%, of the 8 oz (3/4 *or* 0.75 × 8 oz = 6 oz). Multiply by 30 to convert and record (6 oz × 30 mL = 180 mL).

5. When an exact measurement of fluid intake is ordered, collect all remaining liquids at the end of a meal in a **graduated cylinder** (**Figure 13.34**). Place the cylinder on a flat surface and read the amount at eye level. Subtract this amount from the total amount of liquids offered at the meal to find the accurate fluid intake measurement.

   Example: The patient receives 4 oz of juice, 6 oz of coffee, and 8 oz of milk for a total of 18 oz or 540 mL (18 × 30) of liquid offered with breakfast. At the end of the meal, leftover liquids are poured into the graduated cylinder. They measure 120 mL (540 mL offered – 120 mL not consumed = 420 mL of fluid intake).

Measure fluid output the same way you measured fluid intake. Urine, vomit, blood, wound drainage, and diarrhea are all considered fluid output. Always wear gloves when measuring fluid output. A patient who uses the toilet will need to urinate into a measuring device called a **commode hat**. This container is placed under the toilet seat before the patient urinates. Commode hats and **urinals**, which are used by males confined to bed, have measurements marked on the container for easy reading (**Figure 13.35**).

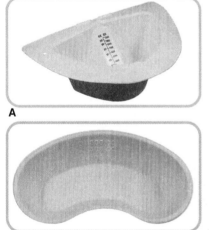

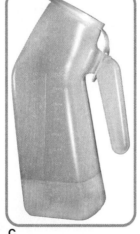

A

B

C

Rob Byron/Shutterstock.com, Rob Byron/Shutterstock.com, MARGRITHIRSCH/Shutterstock.com

Figure 13.35 Liquid output is frequently measured using a commode hat (A), emesis basin (B), or urinal (C).

Urine from a bedpan or urinary catheter drainage bag must be emptied into a graduated cylinder for measuring.

Vomit is measured using the markings on an emesis (EH-meh-sihs) basin. A nurse estimates amounts when a patient vomits on the floor or bedsheets. Amounts for diarrhea, blood, and wound drainage are also estimated unless there is a drainage device to collect wound fluids. Remember to record all output and tally the total amounts at the end of each shift and at the end of each 24-hour period (**Figure 13.36**). The physician will compare fluid intake and output numbers to assess the patient's fluid balance (**Figure 13.37**).

Intake and Output Record

Water glass 180 mL   Cup 120 mL

Patient's Name: Ben Jones   Juice glass 100 mL   Soup bowl 200 mL

Date: 10/14/2023   Small bowl 120 mL   Mug 240 mL

Time	Oral	IV	Irrigation	Remarks	BM	Emesis	Urine	Suction	Remarks
0715	50 mL						550 mL		
0800	240 mL								
0945	120 mL								
1000									
1115	80 mL								
1200 (noon)									
1300									
1430							400 mL		
1500									
TOTAL	490 mL			8 Hr Intake 490 mL			950 mL		8 Hr Output 950 mL
1600	240 mL								
1730	180 mL								
1800	300 mL						375 mL		
1900									
2000									
2130	50 mL					400 mL			
2200									
2300									
TOTAL	770 mL			8 Hr Intake 770 mL		400 mL	375 mL		8 Hr Output 775 mL
2400 (midnight)						200 mL			
0115						150 mL			
0230						80 mL			
0300									
0400									
0530		500 mL					300 mL		
0600									
TOTAL		500 mL		8 Hr Intake 500 mL		430 mL	300 mL		8 Hr Output 730 mL
TOTALS	1260 mL	500 mL		24 Hr Intake 1760 mL		830 mL	1625 mL		24 Hr Output 2455 mL

Figure 13.36 This record shows intake and output for one 24-hour period.

Patient Summary

Problem List

Order History

Vital Signs

I&O

Lab

JONES, BEN—65/M

6 ft 2 in 273 lb

Allergies/ADRS No Known Allergies

1 Hour	4 Hours	8 Hours	12 Hours	24 Hours

Date	Jun 26 07:00	Jun 25 07:00	Jun 24 07:00	Jun 23 07:00	Jun 22 07:00	Jun 21 07:00
Total Intake	1400				860	1000
Total Output	800				900	1100
Fluid Balance	600				-40	-100
I: Oral	100				360	0
I: IV	1300				500	1000
O: Urine	800				600	500
O: Emesis						600
# Bowel Movements					1	
Weight (lb)	273					273

Goodheart-Willcox Publisher

Figure 13.37 Once intake and output is entered, the physician can check daily totals in the electronic health record. *Why do you think it is important to track the patient's weight?*

Lesson 13.3 Review

 Complete the *Map Your Reading* graphic organizer for the section you just read.

1. Which of the following body temperatures is part of the Celsius scale? (13.3-1)
   A. 98.6 degrees
   B. 100 degrees
   C. 37 degrees
   D. 101.8 degrees

2. Which of the following is *not* a guideline for measuring food? (13.3-2)
   A. Weigh ingredients whenever possible
   B. Read liquid measurements at eye level
   C. Include container weight when weighing ingredients
   D. Level dry ingredients

3. Not _____ recipes may affect the health of patients with restricted diets. (13.3-3)
   A. measuring
   B. standardizing
   C. interesting
   D. costing

4. Food intake is estimated and recorded as a (13.3-4)
   A. fraction representing the food remaining on the plate
   B. percentage representing the food remaining on the plate
   C. fraction representing the food missing from the plate
   D. percentage representing the food missing from the plate

5. Healthcare workers measure and record intake and output to monitor (13.3-5)
   A. food balance
   B. fluid balance
   C. nutrients in food
   D. drug levels

Healthcare Tasks That Use Data Analysis and Interpretation

Learning Outcomes

After studying this lesson, you will be able to

13.4-1 describe and explain how to calculate the mean, median, and mode of a data set.

13.4-2 state the purpose for using a chart or graph to display data and demonstrate the steps for reading the information in a chart or graph.

13.4-3 calculate adult body mass index and chart height and weight measurements for a child.

13.4-4 relate several questions to consider as you analyze research study results.

13.4-5 explain ways to interpret risk assessments and healthcare research findings as they relate to relative risk, absolute risk, number needed to treat, and number needed to harm.

Professional Vocabulary

Essential Terms

absolute risk   ratio of the number of people who have a medical event to those who could have the event because of a medical condition

bias   a systematic error producing a research finding that deviates from a valid finding

body mass index (BMI)   a method of relating weight to height; used to define normal weight, overweight, and obesity

number needed to treat (NNT)   the number of patients who must be treated to prevent the occurrence of the condition under examination

relative risk   ratio of the chance of a disease developing among people who are exposed to a specific factor compared with those who are not exposed

risk assessments   methods used to calculate and describe a person's chance of becoming ill or dying of a specified condition

Important Terms

bar graph
base rates
benefits
circle graph
data
harms

line graph
mean
median
mode
number needed to
   harm (NNH)
percentiles

pictograph
probability
quantitative data
recurrence
statistics
table

ESSENTIAL QUESTION

What are some healthcare tasks related to data analysis and interpretation?

Introduction

Researchers, health informatics workers, and clinical workers assess and interpret data as part of their work. Their tasks are as varied as analyzing graphs and charts representing patient trends or recording and graphing height and weight to assess growth. They know how to analyze research results and can interpret statistical data to make accurate judgments about research findings.

13.4-1 Understanding Numerical Data

The healthcare industry relies on the collection and interpretation of large amounts of **data** to direct effective patient care. Data also guides the business operations of the healthcare facility. Data usually consists of a group of facts that reveal information about a specific topic. The science of **statistics** analyzes and interprets data. Healthcare workers handle numerical data daily and must be able to understand, analyze, and interpret this information.

Comparing the mean, median, and mode in a set of data is one method of analysis. The **mean** is the mathematical average of your data. To find it, add all the numbers in your data set and divide by how many numbers are in that set. **Median** describes the number found exactly in the middle when your data is listed in numerical order. In an even-numbered data set, you take the mean of the middle two numbers to determine the median. **Mode** is the number that occurs most frequently in your data set. If no number occurs more often than any other, then there is no mode. There can be zero, one, or multiple modes in a data set.

Healthcare Professions: Using Mean, Median, and Mode

Devon is collecting data to determine the average age of clients in his physical therapy practice. He records the ages of patients he sees on a given day. On the first day, he sees seven clients whose ages are 3, 13, 15, 45, 52, 57, and 75. The average, or *mean*, age of his clients on the first day is 37.

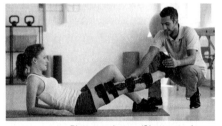

Photographee.eu/Shutterstock.com

Since interpretations rely on the data collected, statistics may vary when you collect sets of data in different circumstances. On the second day of data collection, Devon sees five clients whose ages are 17, 45, 48, 61, and 61. On this day, the average, or *mean*, age of his clients is 46.

Client Ages in PT Practice		
Category	**Day One**	**Day Two**
Patient ages	3, 13, 15, 45, 52, 57, 75	17, 45, 48, 61, 61
Mean	Sum (260) divided by the number of clients (7) = 37	Sum (232) divided by the number of clients (5) = 46
Median	45	48
Mode	Since there are no duplicate numbers, there is no mode.	61

Goodheart-Willcox Publisher

If Devon sees each client once a week, how many days of data should he collect to determine the average age of his current client group? Your first thought might be to collect seven days of data since there are seven days in a week. However, what piece of information or data do you need to know before you can answer accurately?

When interpreting data, people often refer to the *average*. Usually, but not always, they are talking about the mean of a data set. However, the term *average* can be confusing. Suppose 1,000 people live in your hometown, and all of them earn $50,000 per year. The mean and median of this data are both $50,000. A new resident moves into town and earns $1 billion this year. The median stays the same because the middle number is still $50,000. The mean becomes $1.04 million. However, the "average" resident is not earning more than a million dollars each year.

Healthcare Professions: Average Confusion

Tracy has several friends and family members who work in the field of nursing. As a newly graduated practical nurse, Tracy wants to figure out whether a potential job is paying an "average" wage. To do this, Tracy makes a chart of the wages earned by each of her friends and relatives.

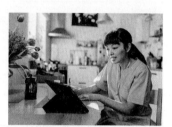

visualspace/E+ via Getty Images

Nursing Wages of Family and Friends	
Family Member/Friend	**Wage per Hour**
Aunt Sue, RN	$45
Barry, CNA	$15
Darien, CNA	$15
Uncle James, NP	$55
Mom, LPN	$25

Data Analysis	
Analysis	**Result**
Mean	$31
Median	$25
Mode	$15

Goodheart-Willcox Publisher

Her potential employer told her the average wage for a practical nurse is $19 per hour and offers to pay Tracy $17 per hour. That offer sounds reasonable. It is $2 above the mode. However, it is $8 below the median and $14 below the mean of the data she has collected and analyzed.

What might explain the differences in the wages of Tracy's acquaintances? Years of work experience, specialized training, or specialized skills might be influencing Tracy's data. It would be more helpful for her to compare the wages paid to nurses with abilities and years of experience similar to her own.

Tracy's next set of data compares entry-level wages for practical nurses at a variety of healthcare facilities. How does her wage offer compare to this new set of data? What additional piece of data would help you determine whether Tracy's potential employer is offering a reasonable wage?

Entry-Level Nursing Wages	
Healthcare Facility	**Hourly Wage for Entry-Level Practical Nurses**
Sun View Medical Clinic	$18
Angelic Skilled Nursing Facility	$19
Pine Acres Assisted Living	$17
Merciful Care Hospice	$20
Sun View Hospital	$20

Data Analysis	
Analysis	**Result**
Mean	$18.80
Median	$19
Mode	$20

Goodheart-Willcox Publisher

13.4-2 Reading and Interpreting Charts and Graphs

Charts and graphs display data visually. When constructed carefully, charts and graphs make data easier to comprehend, compare, and use. Five basic types of charts include

- a simple **table**, which arranges data in rows or columns;
- a **line graph**, which shows changes in data over time;
- a **bar graph**, which shows comparisons between categories of data;
- a **circle graph** (pie chart), which shows the relationship of parts of a data set to the whole; and
- a **pictograph**, which presents data using images.

The elements of a chart or graph must be created to scale to accurately represent the data. Using computer software makes this task much easier.

A graph has three main elements: the vertical axis (*y-axis*), horizontal axis (*x-axis*), and at least one line, set of bars, circle, or image. Follow these steps to read the information in a graph or chart:

1. Read the title of the graph.
2. Read the labels and range of numbers along the side (vertical axis) and the information on the bottom (horizontal axis).
3. Determine what units the graph uses. This information can be found on the axis or in the legend. In **Figure 13.38** for example, the y-axis uses occupational groups, and the x-axis uses percent changes in employment.
4. Look for patterns, groups, and differences.

For example, **Figure 13.39** shows the US labor force by age group for selected years. This graph tells you that the workforce is getting older. What might this trend mean for the workforce in future years?

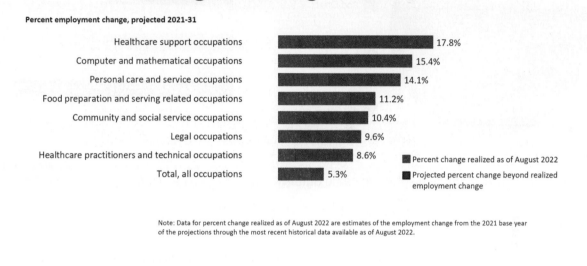

Projected Percent Change by Selected Occupational Groups, 2021–31, Including Realized Employment Change as of August 2022

Percent employment change, projected 2021-31

Occupational Group	Percent
Healthcare support occupations	17.8%
Computer and mathematical occupations	15.4%
Personal care and service occupations	14.1%
Food preparation and serving related occupations	11.2%
Community and social service occupations	10.4%
Legal occupations	9.6%
Healthcare practitioners and technical occupations	8.6%
Total, all occupations	5.3%

■ Percent change realized as of August 2022
■ Projected percent change beyond realized employment change

Note: Data for percent change realized as of August 2022 are estimates of the employment change from the 2021 base year of the projections through the most recent historical data available as of August 2022.

US Bureau of Labor Statistics

Figure 13.38 This chart uses a bar-graph format. The length of the bars provides a visual comparison of projected percent changes in employment. *Which occupational groups are projected to see the greatest increases in available jobs?*

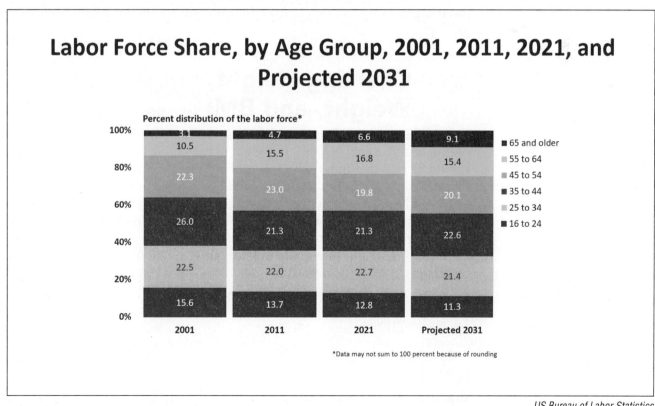

Labor Force Share, by Age Group, 2001, 2011, 2021, and Projected 2031

Percent distribution of the labor force*

*Data may not sum to 100 percent because of rounding

US Bureau of Labor Statistics

Figure 13.39 This graph uses blocks of color to make it easier to see the trends in labor force data about worker age groups.

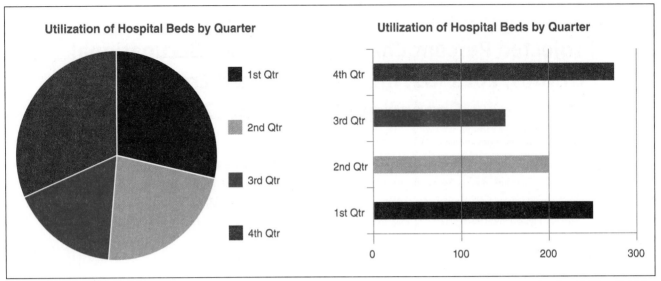

Figure 13.40 These charts display the same data. *Which chart gives a clearer picture of hospital bed utilization in each quarter of the year?*

When displaying data, carefully consider which type of chart will provide the clearest visual representation of your information. **Figure 13.40** shows two different ways of displaying data about the utilization of hospital beds per quarter. If you want to show which quarters have the highest utilization rates, the circle graph works better because it shows percentages of the whole. However, if you want to compare the actual utilization rates, the bar graph is the best choice because it shows the numerical value for each quarter.

13.4-3 Charting Height, Weight, and BMI

For adult patients, height and weight are recorded to better understand overall health. Rapid changes in weight may indicate a medical issue. Height should be recorded in feet and inches. For example, 5′3″ indicates a height of five feet and three inches. Weight should be recorded in pounds. For example, 130 lbs indicates a weight of one hundred thirty pounds. Be prepared to convert weight into kilograms, since a metric weight may be needed to calculate medication doses.

To convert weight in pounds to kilograms, divide the number of pounds by 2.2.

Example: To find the metric weight of 130 pounds:

$130 \div 2.2 = 59.09$ kg

To convert weight in kilograms to pounds, multiply the number of kilograms by 2.2.

Example: To find the pound equivalent of 60 kilograms:

$60 \times 2.2 = 132$ lbs

Calculating BMI

Healthcare providers currently use **body mass index (BMI)** to screen for weight measurements that may lead to health conditions. Body mass index is a number calculated from a person's weight and height (**Figure 13.41**). It provides an indicator of weight category for individuals. Since BMI is not a diagnostic tool, providers use additional assessments, such as skin-fold thickness measurements and evaluations of diet, physical activity, and family history, to determine health risks associated with a high BMI.

Standard categories showing underweight, normal, overweight, and obese BMI measurements are used for all adults beginning at 20 years of age (**Figure 13.42**). For children and teens (2 years of age to 19 years of age), the categories are interpreted using both age and sex. The BMI and age of a child are recorded on the CDC's "body mass index for age percentiles" chart for the child's sex to determine a percentile number. The percentile number is compared to a graph that assesses weight status for children. While BMI is an accurate health guide for most people, it can overestimate body fat in athletes and others who have a muscular build. It may also underestimate body fat in older persons and others who have lost muscle.

How to Calculate Body Mass Index	
Measurement Units	**Formula and Calculation**
Kilograms and meters (or centimeters)	**Formula:** weight (kg)/[height (m)]²
	In the metric system, the formula for BMI is weight in kilograms divided by height in meters squared. Since height is commonly measured in centimeters, divide height in centimeters by 100 to obtain height in meters.
	Example: Weight = 68 kg, Height = 165 cm (1.65 m)
	Calculation: 68 ÷ (1.65)² = 24.98
Pounds and inches	**Formula:** weight (lb)/[height (in)]² × 703
	Calculate BMI by dividing weight in pounds (lb) by height in inches (in) squared and multiplying by a conversion factor of 703.
	Example: Weight = 150 lbs, Height = 5′5″ (65″)
	Calculation: [150 ÷ (65)²] × 703 = 24.96

Courtesy of the Centers for Disease Control and Prevention

Figure 13.41 Shown here are formulas for calculating BMI.

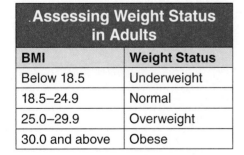

Assessing Weight Status in Adults	
BMI	**Weight Status**
Below 18.5	Underweight
18.5–24.9	Normal
25.0–29.9	Overweight
30.0 and above	Obese

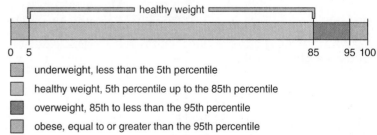

Weight Status by Percentile for Children and Teens

- underweight, less than the 5th percentile
- healthy weight, 5th percentile up to the 85th percentile
- overweight, 85th to less than the 95th percentile
- obese, equal to or greater than the 95th percentile

Courtesy of the Centers for Disease Control and Prevention

Figure 13.42 For adults, these standard categories of BMI indicate weight status. For children and teens, both age and sex are used along with the BMI to assess weight status. Comparisons to other children of the same age and gender provide a percentile ranking. BMIs between the 5th and 85th percentiles are considered healthy.

BMI and Disease Risk

Waist circumference measurements provide another method of screening for health risks associated with overweight and obesity. Patients have a higher risk for type 2 diabetes and heart disease when most of their body fat is located around the waist rather than the hips. Risk increases when the waist size is greater than 35 inches for females or greater than 40 inches for males (**Figure 13.43**). You can measure a patient's waist size while the patient is standing by placing a tape measure around the patient's middle, just above the hipbones. Have the patient breathe out and take the measurement.

When weight assessments indicate overweight or obesity, the following conditions increase the risks for heart disease and stroke:

- hypertension
- high LDL or low HDL cholesterol
- high triglycerides
- high blood glucose
- family history of early heart disease
- unhealthy diet
- lack of physical activity
- cigarette smoking

Patients whose weight assessments indicate overweight or obesity and who experience two of these risk factors can improve future health by getting more physical activity, and following a healthy diet.

Healthcare providers record and track patient BMIs over time the same way they track vital signs. BMI readings, just like blood pressure readings, provide signals for recommending lifestyle changes to improve the patient's future health. Electronic health record systems can automatically calculate a patient's BMI and will graph changes over time to illustrate an increased risk for disease development.

Classification of Overweight and Obesity by BMI, Waist Circumference, and Associated Disease Risks				
Weight Classification	BMI (kg/m²)	Obesity Class	Risk for Type 2 Diabetes, Hypertension, and Cardiovascular Disease Relative to Normal Weight and Waist Circumference: Males 102 cm (40 in) or Less, Females 88 cm (35 in) or Less	Risk for Type 2 Diabetes, Hypertension, and Cardiovascular Disease Relative to Normal Weight and Waist Circumference: Males Greater Than 102 cm (40 in), Females Greater Than 88 cm (35 in)
Underweight	<18.5	–	–	–
Normal	18.5–24.9	–	–	–
Overweight	25.0–29.9	–	Increased	High
Obesity	30.0–34.9	I	High	Very high
Obesity	35.0–39.9	II	Very high	Very high
Extreme Obesity	40.0	III	Extremely high	Extremely high

Courtesy of the National Heart, Lung, and Blood Institute

Figure 13.43 BMI classification of overweight, obesity, and waist circumference with the associated disease risks.

Measurements for Infants and Children

Height and weight measurements for infants and children are charted on graphs from the Centers for Disease Control and Prevention (CDC). The charts show the average height and weight of children based on age and sex (**Figure 13.44**).

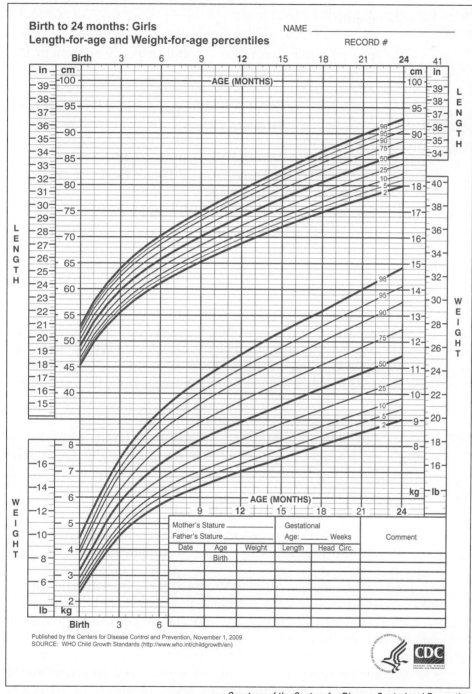

Birth to 24 months: Girls
Length-for-age and Weight-for-age percentiles

Courtesy of the Centers for Disease Control and Prevention

Figure 13.44 The CDC's National Center for Health Statistics provides charts for monitoring the growth of infants and children. The sample chart here tracks height and weight for girls from birth to two years of age. In addition to height and weight, charts are available for monitoring head circumference and BMI. Separate charts are developed for boys and girls, and they cover birth to two years of age and 2 to 20 years of age.

Ounces with Decimal Equivalents		
Ounces	**Fraction**	**Decimal**
2	1/8	0.125
4	1/4	0.25
6	3/8	0.375
8	1/2	0.5
10	5/8	0.625
12	3/4	0.75
14	7/8	0.875

Inches with Decimal Equivalents		
Inches	**Fraction**	**Decimal**
1	1/12	0.0833
2	1/6	0.1667
3	1/4	0.25
4	1/3	0.3333
5	5/12	0.4167
6	1/2	0.5
7	7/12	0.5833
8	2/3	0.6667
9	3/4	0.75
10	5/6	0.8333
11	11/12	0.9167

Figure 13.45 Measurements in ounces and inches with equivalent fractions and decimals.

Healthcare providers use these charts to compare growth in infants, children, and adolescents with a reference tool based on measurements of children of all ages and racial or ethnic groups. Follow these steps to chart height and weight for infants and children:

1. Select the correct growth chart based on the age and sex of the child. Enter the child's name and medical record number.
2. Record all historical data. This may include the height of the parents, child's birth date, and child's weight and length at birth.
3. Record current data, including today's date, the child's current age (to calculate current age, subtract birth date from the date of the measurement), and the height and weight measurements.
4. Convert the weight and height measurements to decimal values using the charts shown in **Figure 13.45**. For example, 25 lbs 4 oz = 25.25 lbs and 30½ in = 30.5 in.
5. Calculate the child's BMI using the appropriate formula.

   BMI = weight (kg) ÷ stature (cm) ÷ stature (cm) × 10,000

   or

   BMI = weight (lb) ÷ stature (in) ÷ stature (in) × 703

6. Record the BMI to one place after the decimal point (for example, 25.325 = 25.3). While this formula varies slightly from the method described in Figure 13.41, the results will be the same using either method. Note that BMI is not used for infants younger than two years.
7. Plot the measurements you have recorded in the data table.

   - Find the child's age on the horizontal axis. Use a straight edge to draw a vertical line up from that point.
   - Find the appropriate measurement on the vertical axis (weight, height, or BMI) and use a straightedge to draw a line from that point until it intersects the vertical line.
   - Make a small dot where the two lines intersect.

These measurements are recorded at each subsequent visit. Once again, electronic records can automatically graph measurements once you have entered the data.

The curved lines on the growth chart show selected **percentiles** that define the rank of the child's measurement. A dot that is plotted on the 50th percentile line for height by age means that 50 out of 100 (50 percent) of children of the same age and sex are taller.

Healthcare providers compare a child's measurements with percentile indicators to determine whether a health concern exists. They also compare the child's current percentile rank with the rank from previous visits to identify any major changes in the child's growth pattern that point to the need for further assessment (**Figure 13.46**).

WHO Growth Charts 2nd and 98th Percentiles (Birth to 2 Years)		
Anthropometric Index*	Percentile Cut-Off Values**	Nutritional Status Indicator
Length-for-age	< 2nd	Short stature
Weight-for-length	< 2nd	Low weight-for-length
Weight-for-length	> 98th	High weight-for-length

CDC Growth Charts 5th and 95th Percentile (2 to 20 Years)		
Anthropometric Index*	Percentile Cut-Off Values**	Nutritional Status Indicator
BMI-for-age	≥ 95th	Obesity
BMI-for-age	≥ 85th and < 95th	Overweight
BMI-for-age	< 5th	Underweight
Stature-for-age	< 5th	Short Stature

*This is an *Anthropometric Index*, which means that it pertains to human body measurements used for comparison.

**Cut-off value* means "a measurement that indicates a dividing line between average development and a health concern."

Courtesy of the Centers for Disease Control and Prevention

Figure 13.46 Healthcare providers compare a child's measurements with percentile indicators to identify health concerns.

13.4-4 Analyzing Research Results

High-quality research studies try to produce valid results, but research free of bias is nearly impossible to conduct. **Bias** is anything that produces a systematic yet unexpected change in the results of a study. Researchers want to know the true relationship between their prediction and the outcome of their research. They struggle, however, to separate the subjects of the study from other factors that influence them. As you analyze the results of a research study, consider whether bias may affect the data and your conclusions.

There are multiple sources of bias that researchers try to avoid as they design research studies. The following are examples of types of bias:

- **Selection bias.** If you run a survey online, only individuals with internet access can participate. If you select fewer participants, intentionally or unintentionally, your results can be biased because your participants may not represent all people who are affected.
- **Attrition bias.** Consider the effect of people who drop out of a study. If participants who are not losing weight drop out, then a weight-management study will appear successful because the only results reported will be for the people who lost weight.
- **Measurement bias.** If your equipment is faulty, your survey participants forget to include information, or your participants cannot read or understand your questions, then your results will not be valid.
- **Researcher bias.** If you or another researcher have a strong belief and try to prove that belief, the research methods may include "leading" questions that influence participants' responses.

Trial #1

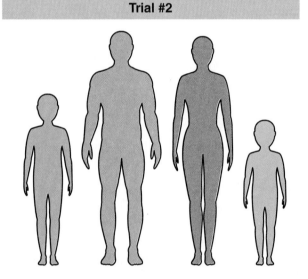

Trial #2

Trial #3

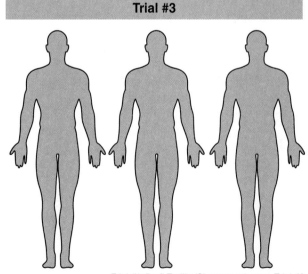

Trial #1: Profi Trollka/Shutterstock.com, Trial #2:
MaskaRad/Shutterstock.com, Trial #3: AV-Art/Shutterstock.com

Figure 13.47 *Which clinical trial is likely to yield the most useful results for an adult male?*

- **Publication bias.** Successful results are published more often than studies that show a treatment to be ineffective or even harmful. As a result, a treatment may be judged safe and effective because that is the only information available to healthcare providers.

When you read about a new medical research finding, the National Institutes of Health (NIH) recommends you consider several questions as you analyze the results of the research study:

- Was the study conducted with people in everyday situations rather than with animals or in a lab setting? Better yet, were the people similar to you in age, sex, ethnicity, health concerns, and lifestyle? If so, then the study results are more likely to apply to you (**Figure 13.47**).
- Was the research a randomized, controlled clinical trial that involved thousands of people? These studies provide the best information about whether a treatment or lifestyle change is effective.
- Where was the research conducted? Large hospitals and medical schools have the resources to lead complex experiments and can employ scientists who have more experience with a research topic.
- Do the reports agree with previous studies? Unexpected results must be verified in multiple studies before they are considered valid.
- Are the results presented in numbers that are easy to understand? Are the results statistically significant? This means the results are probably not due to chance, but they still might not be important to your own health decisions.
- What are the side effects? Side effects can sometimes be as negative as the condition being treated. The treatment may even cause another health condition to get worse.
- Who paid for the study? Does the funder have a financial interest in the outcome of the research? A nonprofit foundation may fund research because it believes the topic is important, but a company may fund research to develop a product for sale.
- Where did you find the results? News articles alert you to new research results, but you should study the research results and discuss them with your physician to determine whether the study results will affect your healthcare decisions.

While new research results are exciting, always remember that progress in medical research takes many years. The results of a single study must be considered along with the results of similar studies conducted in different locations and over a significant period of time before they can be accepted as general medical practice.

13.4-5 Interpreting Statistical Data

"One in Ten Chance," "40% Improvement," "Very Low Risk," or simply "It Worked for Me!" All these headlines grab your attention for the purpose of improving your healthcare knowledge or selling you a product. How do you know which claims are true or even what the statistics actually mean (**Figure 13.48**)?

Health news reports affect how you feel about a product or treatment and influence your healthcare decisions. Therefore, it is important to understand statistical data gathered through research. Interpreting healthcare **risk assessments** can help you draw valid conclusions about healthcare information (**Figure 13.49**).

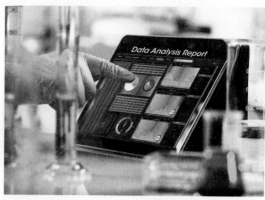

Figure 13.48 Research scientists understand and know how to interpret statistical data.

Percentages and Probability

Understanding statistical data begins with understanding percentages. You can convert a proportion into a percentage. If a person has a 1 in 1,000 chance of having an allergic reaction to a medication, this is a 0.1 percent chance.

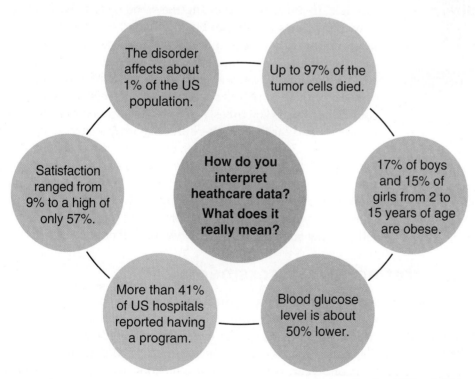

The disorder affects about 1% of the US population.

Up to 97% of the tumor cells died.

Satisfaction ranged from 9% to a high of only 57%.

How do you interpret heathcare data? What does it really mean?

17% of boys and 15% of girls from 2 to 15 years of age are obese.

More than 41% of US hospitals reported having a program.

Blood glucose level is about 50% lower.

Goodheart-Willcox Publisher

Figure 13.49 Understanding healthcare data begins with understanding percentages and types of risk assessment. *If the US population is 328 million, how many citizens are involved when a disorder affects 1 percent of the population?*

Example:

$$1 \text{ in } 1{,}000 = \frac{1}{1{,}000} = 1 \div 1{,}000 = 0.001$$

$0.001 \times 100 \text{ (to convert to percentage)} = 0.1\%$

Conversely, or working from the opposite data format, you can convert a percentage into a proportion. For example, a person has a 10 percent chance of having an allergic reaction to a medication. This is a 10 in 100 chance because percentage is the rate or proportion per 100. If 1,000 people take this drug, how many people do you expect to experience an allergic reaction? Set up a proportion equation to solve this problem:

$$\frac{10}{100} = \frac{x}{1{,}000}$$

1. Cross multiply to get $100x = 10{,}000$
2. Divide each side by the number in front of x

   $100x \div 100 = 1x$

   $10{,}000 \div 100 = 100$

3. $x = 100$

You would expect 100 people to experience an allergic reaction.

Risk is the chance that something bad will happen, such as getting a disease or being involved in an accident. However, risk is never 100 percent predictable. You can assess the level of a risk and use that information to make healthcare decisions, but you can never be certain about the outcome (**Figure 13.50**).

Mathematicians use the laws of **probability** to assess risk. For example, if you flip a coin using the same motion 1,000 times, how many times do you predict it will land on heads? Because there are two sides to a coin, you would expect heads to appear about one-half of the time. That does not mean, however, you will have exactly 500 flips showing heads.

Because there is a 50-50 chance for each coin toss, the results could show heads 200 times, 800 times, or any number of times between 1 and 1,000. Since there are so many possible outcomes, such as 450-550, 512-488, 900-100, and so on, the probability of getting exactly 500 each of heads and tails is low. Outcomes that are further and further from a 50-50 split become more and more unlikely. Probability tells you how likely or unlikely the chances are that something will or will not occur. It can never tell you that something *definitely* will or will not occur.

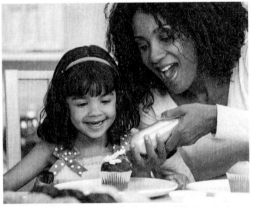

Spotmatik Ltd/Shutterstock.com

Figure 13.50 Tiana has been told by her physician that making some lifestyle changes could reduce her risk of developing diabetes by 60 percent. *Do you think it is worthwhile to make the changes? Why or why not?*

Interpreting Risk Assessments

When a magazine reports that a medication causes a 50 percent increase in heart attacks, it sounds alarming However, the actual number of patients affected is often quite small. For example, in a medication study of 1,000 patients, 500 patients took the medication, and 500 patients did not. Over the course of one year, three patients who took the medication had heart attacks. In the group not taking the medication, two patients had heart attacks. This increase of 1 patient, from 2 to 3, is the 50 percent increase reported by the magazine.

Relative Risk

This example involves comparing risk. Researchers use **relative risk** to compare the risks in two groups of people, or the same group of people over time. Relative risk can be expressed as a ratio, such as the following ratio for heart attack risk in the medication example:

$$RR = \frac{\text{risk to people taking the medication (3)}}{\text{risk to people not taking the medication (2)}} = \frac{3}{2} = 1.5$$

Another way of expressing this ratio is 3:2.

When the relative risk is greater than one (as it is above at 1.5), there is an increase in risk. When it is less than one, there is a reduction in risk. A ratio of exactly 1.0 would mean that there was no increase or decrease; both groups had the same risk.

So how did the magazine arrive at a 50 percent increase? The percentage increase describes the increase in heart attacks for people taking the medication (3 − 2 = 1) divided by the number of heart attacks among the people who did not take the medication (2).

Percentage of increased risk $= \frac{1}{2} = .50 \times 100$ (to convert to percentage) $= 50\%$

Absolute Risk

Absolute risk, which describes the incidence of a condition in a population, provides a clearer understanding of the difference in risk for the population as a whole. Suppose, for example, that the normal incidence of heart attack in a specific population is 2 heart attacks in 1,000 people. Among people who take the medication, a 50 percent increase is one more person, or 3 heart attacks in 1,000 people. Stated in this way, the additional risk does not seem so alarming (**Figure 13.51**).

Absolute risk is the percentage of people affected. As a percentage, the absolute risk of having a heart attack for people who do not take the medication is 2 heart attacks in 1,000 people.

$$AR = \frac{2}{1,000} = 0.002 \text{ or } 0.2\%$$

For the people who took the medication, the risk is 3 heart attacks in 1,000 people.

$$AR = \frac{3}{1,000} = 0.003 \text{ or } 0.3\%$$

The increased risk is the difference between the two groups.

0.3% − 0.2% = 0.1% increased risk

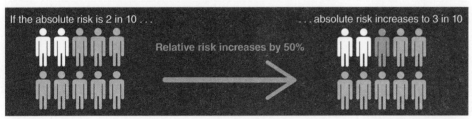

Figure 13.51 A relative-risk increase of 50 percent does not provide a clear picture. Absolute-risk numbers help you understand the difference in risk for the whole population.

Understanding health risks means learning to live with uncertainty. By reading the data in **Figure 13.52**, you can see that smoking increases your risk of dying from lung cancer. The risk of lung cancer for people who do not smoke is very low, but it is not zero. Some people who have never smoked die of lung cancer. Conversely, females with BRCA breast cancer genes have a high risk of developing that disease. But there are also females with those genes who never develop breast cancer.

While you may not have the statistical skills to calculate risk levels, considering the following questions will help you interpret health risk data:

- What is the risk outcome? If the data refers to dying from a disease, then it does not tell you about your risk of having symptoms or developing the disease. Having regular screenings for a disease does not prevent the disease. At best, screening detects a disease in its early stages when it is easier to treat effectively. However, it is also important to remember that screening tests are not 100 percent effective. False negative and false positive results do occur.
- What is the length of time? Data covering a period of 10 years is more meaningful than lifetime risk data. Risk changes over time, often increasing with age. A period of 10 years is long enough for you to make lifestyle and treatment changes to reduce your risk.
- How big is the risk? Look for data expressed in absolute terms, such as "1 out of 1,000 females who do not smoke and are 45 years of age die of lung disease within 10 years." Comparisons to other risks can also be helpful. For example, "A 50-year-old female who smokes is about 10 times more likely to die from lung cancer than from an accident."

Emotion and Risk Assessment

Emotion plays a role in healthcare decisions, and it may cloud your judgment about health risks. For instance, a recent study looked at a group of women affected by breast cancer who chose to have a double mastectomy to prevent getting cancer in the unaffected breast. Emotion played a role in their decision with varying consequences.

Risk of Death from Lung Cancer Among Women Who Smoke and Do Not Smoke													
Age	20	25	30	35	40	45	50	55	60	65	70	75	80
Women Who Smoke (number of deaths in 1,000 women in next 10 years)	Less than 1	Less than 1	1	2	4	10	21	36	65	85	124	137	136
Women Who Do Not Smoke (number of deaths in 1,000 women in next 10 years)	Less than 1	Less than 1	Less than 1	Less than 1	Less than 1	1	2	3	5	7	10	11	11

Goodheart-Willcox Publisher

Figure 13.52 Risk of death from lung cancer among women who do and do not smoke.

First, consider that risk means living with uncertainty. While removing a healthy breast reduces the risk of developing breast cancer, it does not eliminate the risk. Some breast tissue remains after a mastectomy, and it is still possible to develop cancer in this tissue.

Next, consider the size of the risk. About 30 percent of the women who chose a double mastectomy had a higher risk of **recurrence** (return of the cancer). This was caused by a family history of ovarian cancer, two or more close relatives with breast cancer, or the presence of the BRCA breast cancer genes.

However, the other 70 percent of women who chose a double mastectomy had a very low risk of recurrence of breast cancer—about 5 or 6 percent over the next 20 years. A larger percentage of women had a lower risk of recurrence. This means these women chose a major surgery and risked its complications even though they had a 95 percent chance of the breast cancer never returning.

When asked about their decision, 90 percent of the women said they were afraid the cancer would return. They used emotion rather than data to make the decision. If they had considered the question objectively, they might not have chosen the surgery. After all, their risk of getting breast cancer a second time was very low, and removing a healthy breast does not reduce the risk of recurrence in the tissue left from the cancerous breast that was removed.

When emotion clouds your ability to make healthcare decisions, consider stepping back and taking some time to look at the risks and benefits. Healthcare professionals suggest patients think about what they would recommend if they were helping another person make this decision. This technique may help patients weigh benefits and risks more objectively and less emotionally.

Comparing Harms and Benefits

Medical treatments can have **harms** as well as **benefits**. Reducing your risk of illness or death from a disease is a clear benefit. However, medications and surgical procedures may have inconvenient or even life-threatening risks. The value of any treatment is determined by comparing its benefits and risks (**Figure 13.53**).

Knowing the absolute risk numbers and expressing risks through a **number needed to treat (NNT)** makes your choices clearer. For example, imagine you are offered a medication that will reduce your risk of a heart attack. However, the medication will also increase your risk of developing colon cancer. You read the research and learn there was a clinical trial involving 200 patients. One hundred patients received the medication, and 100 received a placebo, which is a fake medicine that does not contain any of the medication to prevent heart attacks. People involved in the study did not know whether they were receiving the medication or the placebo. Three heart attacks occurred in the treated group and six in the placebo group. There were three cases of colon cancer in the treated group and one in the placebo group. The following shows what your evaluation of the medication's benefits and harms might look like:

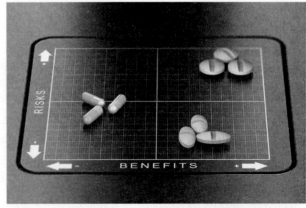

Olivier Le Moal/Shutterstock.com

Figure 13.53 The value of any treatment is determined by comparing its benefits and risks.

Benefits: Using relative risk, you can accurately say the new drug *reduces* heart attack risk by 50 percent or cuts the risk of heart attack in half:

$$RR = \frac{\text{risk to people taking the medication (3)}}{\text{risk to people not taking the medication (6)}}$$

or $3 \div 6 = 0.50 \times 100$ (to convert to percentage) = 50%

Using absolute risk, the heart attack risk is *reduced* by 3 percent. The change in absolute risk is the difference between the two groups:

$$\begin{array}{cc} \text{percentage of heart} & \text{percentage of heart} \\ \text{attacks in the placebo group} & \text{attacks in the treated group} \end{array}$$

(6 of 100) or 6% – (3 of 100) or 3% = 3%

Harms: Using relative risk, you can accurately say the risk of developing colon cancer *increased* by 200 percent:

$$RR = \begin{array}{ccc} \text{number of people} & \text{number of people} & \text{number of people} \\ \text{developing colon} - \text{developing colon} \div \text{developing colon} \\ \text{cancer in the} & \text{cancer in the} & \text{cancer without} \\ \text{treated group} & \text{placebo group} & \text{treatment} \end{array}$$

$3 - 1 = 2 \div 1 = 2 \times 100$ (to convert to percentage) = 200%

Using absolute risk, you can accurately say the risk of developing colon cancer *increased* by 2 percent:

$$AR = \begin{array}{cc} \text{percentage of people developing} & \text{percentage of people developing} \\ \text{cancer in the treated group} & \text{cancer in the placebo group} \end{array}$$

(3 of 100) or 3% – (1 of 100) or 1% = (2 of 100) or 2%

Note that relative risk makes the benefits or harms look larger, and absolute risk makes them look smaller. Understanding how a percentage increase or decrease affects actual numbers is beneficial. For a true comparison, the benefits and harms should be expressed in the same terms—relative risk or absolute risk. When studies report an increase or decrease of a given percentage, it is generally compared to the original number. Notice how percentage increases or decreases affect the final quantity (**Figure 13.54**).

Understanding Percentage Increase and Decrease				
Initial Quantity	Percentage Increase/Decrease	Final Amount Compared to Initial Amount	Calculation	Final Quantity
100	10% increase	110%	100% of initial + 10% of increase = 110% of initial	1.10 of the original
100	100% increase	200%	100% of initial + 100% of increase = 200% of initial	double the original
100	500% increase	600%	100% of initial + 500% of increase = 600% of initial	6 times the original
100	40% decrease	60%	100% of initial – 40% of decrease = 60% of initial	0.60 of the original

Goodheart-Willcox Publisher

Figure 13.54 Knowing how percentage increases and decreases affect actual numbers provides a clearer picture of study results.

Knowing the number needed to treat (NNT) to produce a benefit or the **number needed to harm (NNH)** helps you evaluate risk data. You calculate these numbers by dividing 100 by the absolute reduction or increase in percentage points in risk.

$$NNT \text{ or } NNH = \frac{100}{\text{absolute reduction or increase in percentage points of risk}}$$

Benefit: $NNT = \dfrac{100}{3} = 33.3$

This means that 33 people must be treated with the medication to prevent one heart attack.

Harm: $NNH = \dfrac{100}{2} = 50$

This means that, for every 50 people treated with the medication, you could expect to see one additional case of colon cancer. Therefore, one in every 33 people taking this medication will be spared a heart attack, but 1 in every 50 people will get colon cancer.

As you encounter news reports about healthcare research, look for **quantitative data** that can be measured rather than stories about the experiences of people. While personal stories make the material more interesting, they do not help you evaluate research data objectively. The clearest data shows absolute risk in numbers and provides a time frame such as "This medication reduced the risk of heart attack from 6 in 100 to 3 in 100 over 10 years."

Base rates, such as "reduced from 20% to 10% or 0.0002% to 0.0001%," help you see the significance of a change given in percentages. Both examples show a 50% reduction, but 20% to 10% is a far more significant change.

Media formats designed to sell a product typically list benefits in large print and harms in fine print or quickly read audio. Be aware that many news articles, which have limited space, will omit the study limitations. When you read about a 200 percent reduction in the symptoms of a disorder that affects you personally, remember to read the details. Yes, a 200 percent reduction is great, but if the study only looked at a small number of people over a short period of time, the chances the treatment will work for you are far less likely.

Lesson 13.4 Review

 Complete the *Map Your Reading* graphic organizer for the section you just read.

1. Which of the following is *not* part of a comparison for data analysis? (13.4-1)
   A. Mean   C. Mode
   B. Moderate   D. Median

2. Which of the following is not true of a chart or graph? (13.4-2)
   A. Makes a data set easier to understand
   B. Makes a data set easier to compare
   C. Displays a table of numbers
   D. Displays data in a visual form

3. Children's height and weight are plotted on specific charts based on which of the following? Choose all that apply. (13.4-3)
   A. Health status   C. Current BMI
   B. Age   D. Sex

4. Which of the following represent a type of research bias? Choose all that apply. (13.4-4)
   A. Acquisition bias
   B. Researcher bias
   C. Publication bias
   D. Selection bias

5. Which of the following make the results of research easier to understand and compare? Choose all that apply. (13.4-5)
   A. Qualitative data
   B. Base rates
   C. Absolute risk numbers
   D. Study limitations

Chapter 13 Review and Assessment

Chapter Summary

13.1-1 Healthcare workers complete and record measurements using the metric system. They often convert measurements into the household system.

13.1-2 Memorize basic equivalents to make conversions between metric and household measurements faster.

13.1-3 Using the 24-hour clock in healthcare settings avoids a.m. and p.m. errors. Each hour of the day has its own number.

13.2-1 Health informatics workers collect copays, code medical services, and submit claim forms to receive payment for services rendered.

13.2-2 Pharmacy workers interpret medical prescriptions and prepare medication in the correct form and dosage.

13.2-3 Therapeutic workers use different angles to position patients and give injections. They measure the angle of a joint to assess its range of motion.

13.2-4 Support services workers prepare solutions using a dilution ratio. They know how to adjust measurements to prepare the required amount of a solution.

13.3-1 To convert from °F to °C, subtract 32, then multiply by 5, then divide by 9. To convert from °C to °F, multiply by 9, then divide by 5, then add 32.

13.3-2 For accuracy, measure food ingredients by weight whenever possible and consider the tare weight in your measurement. Level dry ingredients and read liquid measurements at eye level.

13.3-3 Using standardized recipes results in a consistent food product.

13.3-4 Estimate food intake for a complete meal or each food item as your facility requires. Record food intake as a percentage of food eaten.

13.3-5 Fluid intake includes all the fluids you drink. Gelatin, broth, ice cream, sherbet, IV fluids, and enteral tube nutrition are also part of fluid intake. Fluid output includes urine, vomit, blood, wound drainage, and diarrhea.

13.4-1 The mean is the average of all numbers in a data set. The median is the number in the middle of a data set listed in numerical order. The mode is the number occurring most frequently in a data set.

13.4-2 Charts and graphs display data in a visual form so it is easier to understand and compare.

13.4-3 Healthcare providers currently use body mass index to screen for weight measurements that may lead to health conditions. They compare graphs of infant/child height and weight with average ranges to assess growth.

13.4-4 Look for signs of bias when considering the results of a research study. Then check to see if the study used participants like you, and if it was a large, randomized trial conducted by a major research facility.

13.4-5 Look for absolute risk numbers for a clearer picture of risk assessment results. Consider the outcome of a risk, length of time, and size of the risk. Use NNT and NNH to compare the benefits and risks of a treatment.

Maximize Your Professional Vocabulary

1. **Terms Flash.** Working in pairs, locate a small image online that visually describes each of the professional terms. Create flash cards by writing each term on a notecard and pasting the image on the opposite side. Take turns quizzing each other on the terms.

Reflect on Your Reading

1. Review the list of math operations and procedures you made for the *Connect with Your Reading* activity. How accurate were your predictions? In which math skills are you already proficient? Which skills do you need to improve to succeed in a healthcare setting?

Review and Recall

1. Which of the following systems measures the biological effect of manufactured medications and vitamins? (13.1-1)
   A. Metric system
   B. Roman numerals
   C. International Units
   D. Apothecary system

2. Which measurement is equivalent to 1/4 cup? (13.1-2)
   A. 1 T
   B. 3 tsp
   C. 6 tsp
   D. 4 T

3. Which of the following indicates midnight in military time? Choose all that apply. (13.1-3)
   A. 0000
   B. 1200
   C. 2400
   D. 12:00 a.m.

4. Healthcare reception workers often collect _____ before the patient sees the physician. (13.2-1)
   A. claims
   B. copays
   C. authorizations
   D. codes

5. Medication can be given (13.2-2)
   A. topically
   B. by inhalation
   C. by injection
   D. All of these.

6. Which are reference planes for measuring angles in the body? Choose all that apply. (13.2-3)
   A. Surface of the skin
   B. Lying flat on the back
   C. 90-degree angle
   D. 0-degree angle

7. You are preparing 1 liter of a 2:10 cleaning solution. Which statement is accurate? (13.2-4)
   A. You will measure 200 mL of solvent.
   B. You will measure 400 mL of solute.
   C. You will measure 600 mL of solute.
   D. You will measure 800 mL of solvent.

8. Which of these statements is incorrect in the Celsius scale? Choose all that apply. (13.3-1)
   A. 39 is too hot.
   B. 38 is nice.
   C. 37 is too cold.
   D. 32 is ice.

9. You are measuring milk for a pudding recipe and are doubling the recipe yield. The original recipe calls for 16 ounces of milk. Which measurement is accurate and easiest to measure? (13.3-2)
   A. 2 cups
   B. 32 ounces
   C. 4 cups
   D. 8 ounces

10. Which of the following is *not* a reason for portioning foods? (13.3-3)
    A. To save money
    B. To make plated foods more appealing
    C. To be fair to all diners
    D. To follow specialized diets

11. A nurse is estimating food intake as a percentage of a meal. The nurse notes that one-half of the potato, none of the meat, three-fourths of the vegetable, and one-half of the bread are left on the resident's plate. What percentage of the meal was eaten? (13.3-4)
    A. 32 percent
    B. 44 percent
    C. 65 percent
    D. 56 percent

12. Which of these is *not* part of fluid intake? (13.3-5)
    A. Ice cream
    B. Pudding
    C. Flavored gelatin
    D. Sherbet

13. What is the average or mean of this data set: 18, 46, 49, 62, 65? (13.4-1)
    A. 48
    B. 49
    C. 62
    D. 65

14. You want to compare the number of patients seen in your clinic each year. Which type of graph would show this most clearly? (13.4-2)
    A. Line graph
    B. Bar graph
    C. Circle graph
    D. Pictograph

15. For which group of patients might a BMI measurement provide an inaccurate indicator of weight status? Choose all that apply. (13.4-3)
    A. Teens
    B. Athletes
    C. Middle-age people
    D. Older people

16. Which research study has the best chance of leading to an effective treatment? (13.4-4)
    A. Animal research study
    B. Research showing a high incidence of side effects
    C. Clinical trial with 3,000 participants
    D. Research funded by a product manufacturer

17. Which data is the most important consideration when making healthcare decisions? (13.4-5)
    A. Relative risk
    B. Absolute risk
    C. Risk of recurrence
    D. Harms versus benefits

Build Core Skills

1. **Math.** Better Medical Clinic is comparing the number of morning and afternoon medical appointments to adjust staffing. For each set of data, find the mean, median, and mode.

   Morning: 17, 30, 25, 35, 28

   Afternoon: 13, 20, 20, 25, 10

2. **Math.** Create a chart or graph that compares estimated figures of rates for newly diagnosed cases of cancer in different states. Find a partner, share your data results, and discuss how your chart compares. Explain why you used a certain method to display the data.

MT: 5,550	VT: 4,060	NV: 13,780
WI: 31,920	TX: 110,470	MS: 15,190
CA: 165,810	KY: 25,160	

3. **Math.** Convert Fahrenheit temperatures to Celsius and Celsius temperatures to Fahrenheit.

   A. 98°F

   B. 102°F

   C. 83.8°F

   D. 44°C

   E. 33.9°C

   F. 15.5°C

4. **Math.** Convert each of the following weights from pounds (lb) to kilograms (kg).

   A. 185 lbs

   B. 248 lbs

   C. 34 lbs

   D. 194 lbs

   E. 215 lbs

   F. 62 lbs

   G. 150 lbs

   H. 26 lbs

5. **Math.** Convert the times to military time.

   A. 2:30 p.m.

   B. 1:15 a.m.

   C. 4:50 a.m.

   D. 12:00 a.m.

   E. 5:30 a.m.

6. **Math.** Move the decimal point to convert these metric measurements.

   A. 70,263 g = _____ kg   C. 1450 cm = _____ m

   B. 12.7 cm = _____ mm   D. 76.25 L = _____ mL

7. **Math.** Refer to Figure 13.3 and use equivalents to convert these household measurements.

   A. 67 oz = _____ lbs

   B. 63 in = _____ ft, _____ in

   C. 12 ft = _____ yd

   D. 6 T = _____ oz

   E. 18 oz = _____ c

   F. 3 gal = _____ qt

8. **Math.** Use Figures 13.4 and 13.5 to convert these measurements into units in a different measurement system.

   A. Mrs. Jergens' newborn baby weighs 7.5 lbs and is 20½ in long. How will you record this information in metric measurements for the baby's medical record?

   B. Mr. Castillo drank 6 oz of orange juice, 12 oz of lemonade, and 4 oz of water during your work shift. How many total ounces of liquid intake is this? How will you record this in metric measurements on his chart?

9. **Reading.** Refer to Figure 13.18 to translate these prescriptions. Then write easy-to-understand instructions for patients to follow when taking each prescription. Label the dose and dosage listed in each prescription.

   Example: Toradol 10 mg #20

   T· tab q6h for inflammation

   Answer: Take one 10 milligram Toradol tablet (dose) every 6 hours for inflammation. Dispense 20 tablets (dosage).

   A. Amoxicillin 500 mg #30, T· cap po tid x 10 days

   B. Motrin 800 mg #90, T· tab po tid c̄ food

   C. Colace 100 mg #30, T· tab po qhs

   D. Zofran 4 mg IV, q4h prn nausea

10. **Math.** For dinner, each patient in your care receives the following meal: a 4-oz chicken breast (186 calories), cup of green beans (44 calories), small dinner roll (87 calories), and cup of apple juice (110 calories). Calculate the total number of calories consumed by each patient using the percentages shown.

    A. Mabel ate 50% of chicken breast, 90% of green beans, 100% of dinner roll, and 100% of apple juice.

    B. Saul ate 80% of chicken breast, 20% of green beans, 100% of dinner roll, and 100% of apple juice.

11. **Critical Thinking.** Answer the following questions related to intake and output (I&O).

    A. Why or how is fluid balance critical to body functioning?

    B. Which items are considered intake, and which are included in output?

    C. Why are gelatins, ice cream, and sherbet considered part of fluid intake?

    D. How are I&O measurements taken and recorded?

    E. How does the physician use I&O data?

12. **Math.** Calculate the specific amounts of solute and solvent for solutions based on the percentages or dilution ratios listed.

    A. 1 liter of a 10% solution

    B. 100 mL of a 25% solution

    C. 5 mL of a 15% solution

    D. 2 gallons of a 50:100 solution

13. **Math.** Convert all proportions to percentages and percentages to proportions.
    A. 3 chances out of 50 that a stroke will occur
    B. 15% risk of an allergic reaction among 500 people
    C. 4 occurrences of cancer in 3,000 cases
    D. 7.6% chance that the medication will not be effective in a group of 600 people

14. **Math.** Review the following research results and reorder them from clearest and most useful to least useful for understanding benefit or harm.
    A. Eight out of 10 people who have cancer are below the dietary requirements for daily intake of vitamin D.
    B. Older people who exercised for at least 30 minutes at least three times a week over the course of five years were 15 times less likely to be diagnosed with depression.
    C. Women who are carriers of the arthritis gene were found to have reduced joint range of motion compared to women who were not carriers.
    D. Eating at least 1 cup of blueberries per week can reduce a woman's risk of heart attack by 25 percent.

Activate Your Learning

1. Chester is a 25-year-old male who weighs 175 lbs and is 6′ tall. Calculate his BMI. Once you know Chester's BMI, identify whether he has normal weight, overweight, underweight, or obesity.

2. Use a goniometer provided by your instructor for this exercise. With a partner, practice measuring joint angles for flexion and extension of the knee and elbow. Record your measurements.

3. Find a low-fat recipe that has at least six ingredients. Convert the recipe by doubling the yield. Then, visit a local grocery store or use the internet to find prices of the various ingredients. Cost the original recipe.

4. Assemble equipment and supplies provided by your instructor and practice weighing food items. Record the food weights, accounting for the tare weight of the container used.

5. Assemble supplies and equipment provided by your instructor. Prepare 500 mL of a 1:10 solution.

Think and Act Like a Healthcare Worker

1. As a pediatrician, you will have patients of varying ages, sexes, weights, heights, and BMIs. Imagine a young girl named Corina is one of your female patients. She is 6 years of age, her height is 4′10″, and she weighs 57 lbs. Calculate Corina's BMI.

Then go to the CDC website and print out the correct children's BMI for age percentiles chart for Corina's sex. Graph the data and refer to Figure 13.44 to determine whether the data indicates cause for concern about Corina's growth.

Go to the Source

1. Use Figure 13.9 and use the following information to complete a health insurance claim form. Use the internet to find the correct medical coding for this diagnosis and research realistic charges for these services.

A male patient named Robert Blake first went to his doctor, Roy Blanchard, at Better Medical Clinic on January 10, 2023, for an office visit. Robert had a unilateral chest X-ray, which revealed a broken rib due to a car accident on January 8, 2023. There was a follow-up office visit on March 15, 2023. Robert lives at 2400 East Highland Drive, Boland, MN 84672. His phone number is (123) 456-7891. His wife, Shelly, drove him to the clinic. She does not work outside the home. Robert is insured with a signature on file through the Benefit Health Plan, group number 02635. His I.D. number is 04635. Robert was born November 11, 1984. The patient account number is 0429 with an accepted assignment federal tax I.D. number 38-0000.000. The billing provider's phone number is (198) 765-4321. Robert has not paid for services yet.

HOSA Event Prep: Medical Math

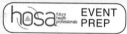

Chase, a three-year-old, was seen in the emergency room (ER) for fever and a possible respiratory infection. He weighs 37 pounds and has no allergies. His fever is currently 102.4 degrees Fahrenheit. The physician wants ibuprofen 10 mg/kg to be given now. Ibuprofen suspension comes in 100 mg/5 mL.

Test Your Knowledge

1. How many kilograms is 37 pounds? Round to the nearest whole number.
   A. 12 kg   C. 24 kg
   B. 17 kg   D. 37 kg

2. The physician ordered ibuprofen 10 mg per every kilogram of weight. Calculate the milligrams of ibuprofen desired.
   A. 10 mg   C. 100 mg
   B. 50 mg   D. 170 mg

3. Use the following formula: amount desired (mg)/amount available (mg) × quantity (mL) = dose (mL). Calculate the correct dose of ibuprofen for Chase.
   A. 5 mL   C. 8.5 mL
   B. 5 mg   D. 8.5 mg

Unit 4

Essential Knowledge and Skills for Health Science

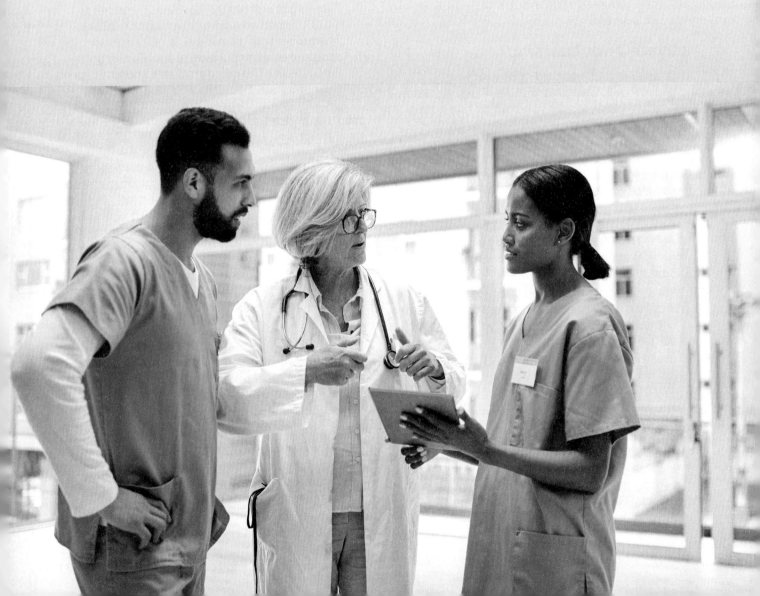

Healthcare Insider

Brett—Sales Representative

As a sales rep, my job is to effectively negotiate, sell, and service equipment and disposable products. This means that I make presentations, talk directly to customers, and help them when equipment and products need repairs. The products that I specifically work with are used for minimally invasive spinal procedures. It's my responsibility to foster a good relationship with my customers. I do that by providing quality service in a timely manner, handling all product complaints appropriately, training physicians and staff members on products, and assisting with product application during procedures.

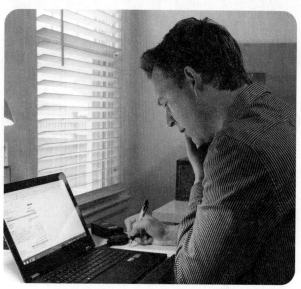

Photo by Leah Garczynski

Discussion Activity

Brett works independently. He must sell, deliver, repair, and educate customers about medical products and equipment. He has even entered operating rooms to train physicians to use products he sells. For him, providing quality service for his customers is primary.

1. What values are important for you?
2. What healthcare careers will make you feel you are doing valuable work?

Chapter 14 Systems

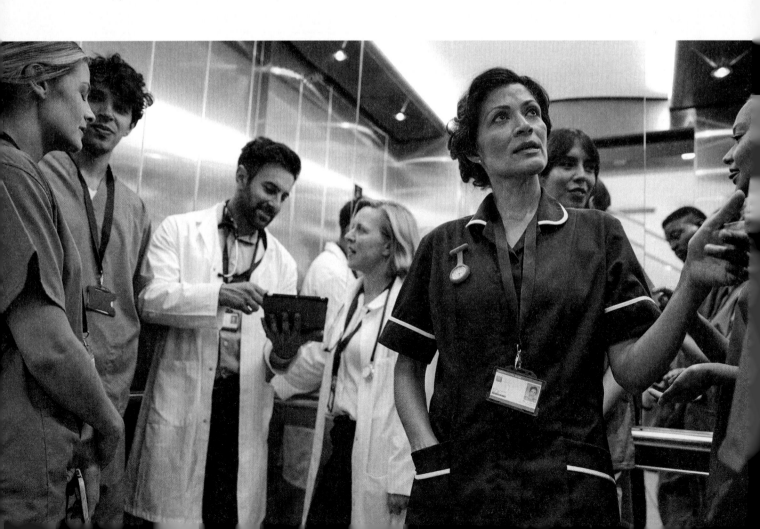

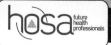

Public health focuses on how to improve health for the public. While you might think public health primarily works with communicable diseases, that is just part of the job. Public health professionals also study socioeconomics and how poverty affects health and access to care. They may study chronic diseases and how they relate to the public—for example, the number of people newly diagnosed with diabetes in a community and trends among them. Many times, public health involves educating the general public about prevention and ensuring all have adequate medical care. HOSA—Future Health Professionals has a team event called *Public Health*. Each year, HOSA provides an annual *Public Health* topic for teams to use as the basis for a dynamic and creative presentation.

Go to the HOSA website to learn more about the HOSA *Public Health* event. Find out the purpose of the event, what is involved in the event, and what knowledge is demonstrated in the event.

As you prepare for HOSA competitive events, be sure to check the website and talk with your HOSA advisor for the most up-to-date guidelines and procedures. Once you have learned about the *Public Health* event, answer the following questions:

1. How might participating in this event benefit you personally and your future career? Explain.
2. Are you interested in participating in this event? Why or why not?

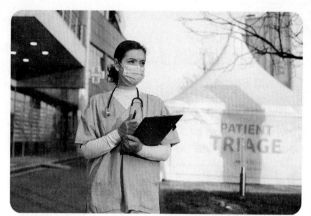

Cryptographer/Shutterstock.com

Connect with Your Reading

Think back to a time you were inside a healthcare facility. Do you remember the different types of workers who were there? How did they all seem to fit together? Would you say they were part of a larger system? How do you imagine this system works?

You may not realize it, but you have been interacting with systems all your life. Most people have a limited understanding of healthcare as a system, but it is an important concept for both healthcare workers and consumers. As you read, look for the many pieces of this broad system. How do they work together? What will your role be? How will your actions affect the functioning of the system?

Map Your Reading

People use systems theory to think about and prevent or solve problems. While reading the first lesson, identify a type of healthcare delivery system in which you might be interested in working. Write this at the top of your page.

Through the rest of the chapter, look for healthcare issues that may affect this system. Make three columns to record these as you read. In the first column, list the healthcare *issues* you identify. In the second column, list potential *causes* of these issues. In the third column, list potential *solutions* for the type of healthcare system you selected. Think broadly. Be prepared to discuss the parts of the system affected and possible changes to the system that might resolve one of these issues.

Chapter opener image: Monkey Business Images/Shutterstock.com

Healthcare Delivery Systems

ESSENTIAL QUESTION

How are healthcare delivery systems organized to provide for a wide range of healthcare needs?

Learning Outcomes

After studying this lesson, you will be able to

14.1-1 explain the use of systems theory.

14.1-2 differentiate between healthcare delivery systems and related agencies.

14.1-3 describe the purpose of an organizational chart in the healthcare delivery system.

Professional Vocabulary

Essential Terms

organizational chart a diagram that shows how departments in an organization relate to one another

system an organized structure composed of many parts that work together and depend on each other to carry out a set of functions

Important Terms

acute care
ambulatory care
Centers for Disease Control and Prevention (CDC)
Centers for Medicare & Medicaid Services (CMS)
Department of Health and Human Services (HHS)
emergency medical services (EMS)

environment
feedback loop
hierarchy
home healthcare
hospice care
hospitals
infrastructure
input
long-term care facilities
National Institutes of Health (NIH)
nonprofit organization

output
pharmaceutical company
throughput
US Department of Veterans Affairs (VA)
US Food and Drug Administration (FDA)
US Public Health Service (USPHS)
World Health Organization (WHO)

Introduction

Today's complex, technological world is composed of many **systems**. A system is an organized structure with many interdependent parts that work together to carry out a particular function. People who use cell phones rely on a system of cell towers to connect to friends. People who drive use the global positioning system (GPS) of satellites to find out how to get from their home to new restaurants. The US educational system is organized by state and local governments to prepare individuals for future careers and participation in society. Every problem or situation you face occurs within a larger system.

Two major systems are involved in the US healthcare system. One is the healthcare delivery system. The other is the healthcare payment system. Before examining these two systems, however, you will learn how to break down the parts of a system and consider how they interact. Analyzing complex systems helps you understand how they work and anticipate how they will react to changes.

14.1-1 Systems Theory

A system achieves its goals by maintaining balance between its many parts. Each system is made up of five factors: input, throughput, output, feedback loop, and environment (**Figure 14.1**).

- **Input** is everything coming into the system, including the population being served and their needs or wants that the system serves. Inputs also include the resources a system needs to function, such as workers, equipment, and money. In healthcare, inputs are patients, healthcare workers, and equipment, as well as insurance payments.

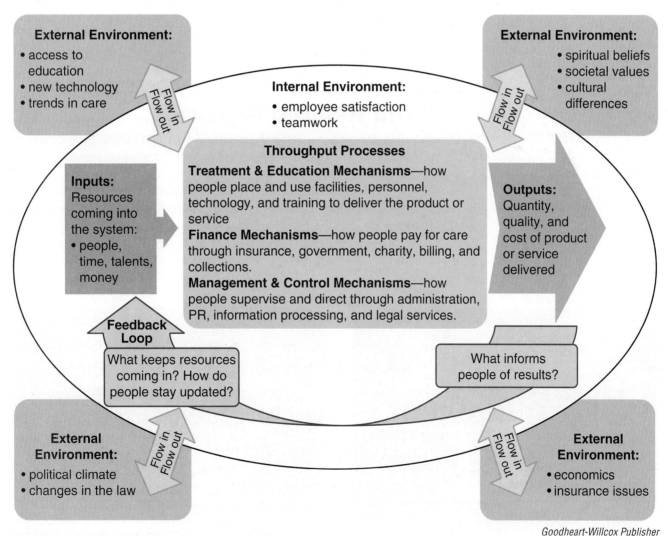

Goodheart-Willcox Publisher

Figure 14.1 A healthcare system must maintain a balance between input, throughput, output, feedback loop, and environment. *How do healthcare workers contribute to throughput?*

- **Throughput** refers to how the system processes or uses inputs to achieve its goals. Patient-care processes, purchasing decisions, staff management, and training are important throughputs for the healthcare system.
- **Output** is the result produced by the system's functioning. In healthcare, outputs include patient outcomes, costs, and gains in information and abilities.
- The **feedback loop** involves responses to the functions used to keep the system going. What can be done differently to provide greater satisfaction? What will bring customers and resources back into the system?
- Finally, **environment**, or surrounding conditions, affects every system. Internal factors, such as employee satisfaction, teamwork, equipment maintenance, and a good financial position, keep the system healthy. Changes in the external environment also affect the system. A change in resources, shift in demographics, creation of new laws, or development of new technology can have a huge impact on a healthcare system.

You can use the five factors that make up systems theory to analyze various systems. The parts of a system should work together in a balanced way toward a common purpose. Analyzing a system and the relationship among its parts can help anticipate and solve problems. Systems analysis can also help improve outcomes, reduce costs, or evaluate how peoples' actions contribute to achieving or delaying a system's goal.

14.1-2 Healthcare Delivery Systems and Related Agencies

Healthcare is one of the largest industries in the United States. The healthcare delivery system is a mix of individuals and organizations that provide healthcare products and services. Healthcare facilities provide services ranging from medication and consultation to surgery and around-the-clock care. They vary in size from private offices to national organizations. Some try to make a profit, while others are nonprofit. Most share the common goals of preventing, curing, or providing support for health issues (**Figure 14.2**). As you learn about the wide range of facilities, consider where you might be interested in working.

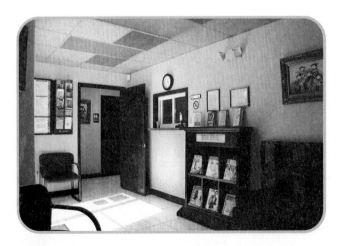 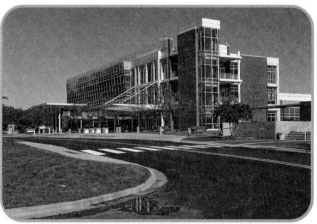

Samuel Acosta/Shutterstock.com, Konstantin L/Shutterstock.com

Figure 14.2 All healthcare facilities, whether one small office or a giant complex, operate as systems that can be analyzed through systems theory.

Government and Nonprofit Agencies

Government agencies fund research, support access to care, and create rules for the healthcare industry. For example, the **World Health Organization (WHO)** is an agency of the United Nations that works worldwide to promote public health. The WHO monitors disease epidemics such as coronaviruses, assists people affected by disasters like earthquakes, and sets international standards such as water quality for safe drinking.

In the US, the **Department of Health and Human Services (HHS)** has 12 divisions that oversee many programs focused on improving the health of people in the US. These programs include the following:

- The *Administration for Children and Families (ACF)* works to improve the well-being of children, families, and communities.
- The *Administration for Community Living (ACL)* provides older people and people with disabilities access to community support systems that help them live productive and satisfying lives.
- The *Administration for Strategic Preparedness and Response (ASPR)* coordinates efforts to prepare for and respond to natural disasters and public health emergencies.
- The *Agency for Healthcare Research and Quality (AHRQ)* conducts research to improve the safety, quality, and efficiency of healthcare.
- The *Agency for Toxic Substances and Disease Registry (ATSDR)* protects people from exposure to hazardous substances in the environment, waste sites, and chemical spills.
- The **Centers for Disease Control and Prevention (CDC)** focuses on disease outbreaks and prevention in the US.
- The **Centers for Medicare & Medicaid Services (CMS)** provides health insurance for 100 million people under its Medicare and Medicaid programs.
- The **US Food and Drug Administration (FDA)** regulates medical products, tobacco products, foods, dietary supplements, cosmetics, and radiation-producing electronic devices.
- The *Health Resources and Services Administration (HRSA)* oversees organ donations and improves access to healthcare for people who are uninsured, isolated, or medically vulnerable.
- The *Indian Health Service (IHS)* provides access to comprehensive and culturally acceptable healthcare for Native Americans and Alaska Natives.
- The **National Institutes of Health (NIH)** conducts research and provides information to improve public health through 27 different agencies.
- The *Substance Abuse & Mental Health Services Administration (SAMHSA)* offers resources to reduce the impact of substance use and mental health conditions on US communities.

The Department of Health at the state and county levels has many roles. They collect statistics, conduct research, promote health, oversee licensure of healthcare workers, and enforce regulations to prevent disease and injury. The US Department of Labor's Occupational Safety and Health Administration (OSHA) regulates the safety of workplaces, including healthcare facilities. The Veteran's Health Administration, a division of the **US Department of Veterans Affairs (VA)**, provides healthcare benefits, programs, and facilities to support the unique needs of those who have served in the military. Also, military

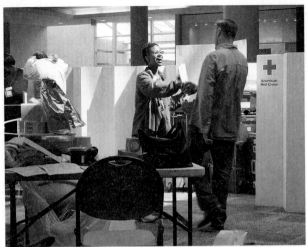

littleny/Shutterstock.com

Figure 14.3 The American Red Cross is a nonprofit organization that provides disaster relief, CPR certification, first aid classes, and blood donation services.

personnel in the Commissioned Corp of the **US Public Health Service (USPHS)** support public health during manmade and natural disasters. As government organizations, all these agencies and facilities are funded by tax dollars.

Many **nonprofit organizations** also support healthcare needs at national, state, and local levels. Funded by donations and grants, they have both paid staff and volunteers. They use profits to achieve charitable goals, such as research, education, and low-cost care. For example, March of Dimes focuses on preventing congenital conditions and premature birth. The American Red Cross (ARC) conducts health and safety training, disaster relief, and blood and supply collections (**Figure 14.3**). The American Heart Association (AHA) fights heart disease and strokes. The American Cancer Society (ACS) funds research, fights for policy changes, and supports those affected by cancer. These are just a few examples of the many nonprofit organizations dedicated to healthcare issues.

Healthcare Provider Settings

People with sudden and severe illness or injury need **acute care**. Hospitals are acute care facilities that use technical equipment to provide inpatient care, surgery, intensive care, physical therapy, radiology, and laboratory services. The size, focus, and funding of a hospital determine what technology and services it offers. Hospitals range in size from limited services and just a few beds to numerous large departments with hundreds of beds. They may provide general care or specialize in a particular age group or disease. A government agency, university, nonprofit, religious organization, or profit-making corporation may operate them.

Emergency medical services (EMS) provide rapid response care for those with a sudden illness or injury. Ambulance and flight-for-life services make medical care available from the point of injury to the emergency room (**Figure 14.4**). These services can extend life, but they come at a high cost that health insurance may not fully cover.

An urgent care center or acute care clinic can manage conditions that need immediate, short-term attention but are not life threatening. These facilities have diagnostics and medical workers to care for sprains, deep cuts, minor burns, infections, and flu symptoms. The cost for care is lower than a hospital emergency room.

An **ambulatory care** clinic offers ongoing outpatient care that does not require hospitalization. This is a walk-in clinic for nonemergency care. Many outpatient surgeries can be performed in a doctor's or dentist's private office. This avoids the high cost and stress of a hospital stay.

Medical and dental practices can save resources in a group practice that shares an office and support staff. These practices may be specialized.

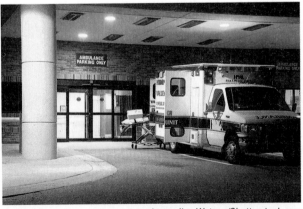

Jacqueline Watson/Shutterstock.com

Figure 14.4 Ambulances transport patients to the emergency room when injury or illness occurs suddenly.

Surgical centers perform a variety of outpatient surgeries. Cosmetic surgery clinics use medical and surgical techniques to enhance appearance. Pulmonology clinics provide respiratory therapy. Orthodontic care centers specialize in correcting bite issues and straightening teeth.

Behavioral and mental health services are a huge field. They include substance use disorder treatment, psychiatric evaluation, group therapy, eating disorder treatment, probation or parole services, and intimate partner violence programs. Care may be inpatient or outpatient and is often ongoing. Insurance provides the same coverage for mental health treatment as physical health.

Special support is available for people who are frail or have disabilities or dementia. This support allows them to live as independently as possible. Senior centers organize social activities and link older people to a support network. Adult day care can supervise daytime activities while family members are at work. Respite care programs can provide family members with a short-term, planned break from their role as caregiver. Community-based residential facilities include group homes for people with particular support needs due to conditions such as Down syndrome or Alzheimer's disease.

Some people who are older or have disabilities remain in their home with additional support from **home healthcare**. The home health team often includes nurses, home health aides, clergy, and rehabilitation professionals. Physical therapy, occupational therapy, speech therapy, and respiratory therapy are common rehabilitation services that help people adjust to or heal from serious injuries and health issues. A case manager can assess the client's needs and direct them to additional services, such as home medical equipment, transportation, and meal services. Without these services, many more people who are older or have disabilities would end up in expensive long-term care facilities.

A *continuum of care* can connect different facilities to provide easier movement between many levels of support. Independent living apartments are available for people who are older or have disabilities and are still able to take care of themselves. **Long-term care facilities** provide additional services for residents who are frail or cannot live independently. People who do not need nursing care may use an *assisted-living facility* (**Figure 14.5**). This apartment-like setting offers help with meals, laundry, medication, and housekeeping. Some people need a *skilled nursing facility* for nursing care or rehabilitation after an injury or surgery. Residents with dementia or physical disabilities who need help with their daily care, such as bathing and toileting, may live in a *nursing home*. Long-term care insurance can help cover costs that are not included in traditional healthcare insurance.

Hospice care is available for clients who have been diagnosed with a terminal illness and generally have fewer than six months to live. This type of care focuses on quality of life. Palliative care helps patients who are dying make their last days as pain free, meaningful, and dignified as possible. Hospice care also includes support for family members coping with their loved one's imminent death and grieving afterward.

Satellite facilities are a common way to bring healthcare to the public. For example, physical therapy clinics may be found in health clubs,

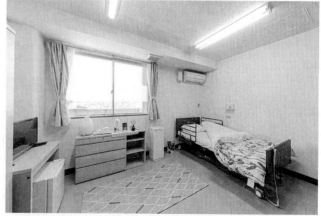

mapo_japan/Shutterstock.com

Figure 14.5 Long-term care facilities include assisted-living facilities, nursing homes, and skilled nursing facilities. *What are the differences between these long-term care settings?*

pharmacies are common in grocery stores, and optometrists have offices in department stores that sell glasses. Many day spas incorporate healthcare services such as light therapies and massage therapies. You may receive a vaccination at your local pharmacy rather than going to a doctor's office. Satellite facilities are a cost-effective way to make healthcare more accessible.

Many of the same facilities and services that exist for people are also available for animals. Animal hospitals, veterinary offices, and doggie day spas provide a variety of healthcare services. Animal care may also require laboratory and medical imaging services. Health insurance for pets can help cover the cost of this increasing array of services.

Research, Testing, and Technology Facilities

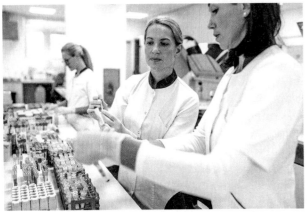

sanjeri/E+ via Getty Images

Figure 14.6 Healthcare workers in labs test blood, body fluids, and tissues to help diagnose illness.

Medical research has improved the safety of medications, advanced medical treatments, and increased longevity. Biomedical research and testing facilities include laboratories, engineering firms, and pharmaceutical (far-muh-SOO-tih-kuhl) companies. Computers and advanced technology support their work.

Laboratories perform tests on blood, body fluids, and tissues to help physicians diagnose disease (**Figure 14.6**). These labs may be freestanding or part of a healthcare facility such as a hospital or clinic. **Pharmaceutical companies** develop, test, and market new medications. Engineering firms make medical equipment for patient diagnosis and treatment, such as ultrasound and robotic surgical machines.

Medical software and computer technology firms have a growing role in healthcare. Wide ranges of wearable smart devices can track medical conditions, such as diabetes, glaucoma, and seizures. Electronic health records (EHR) can gather information from connected smart devices and share health information. Medical technology and robotics can increase precision and bring healthcare to remote areas. Electronic simulators can be programmed to help train healthcare workers. Although these facilities may not provide hands-on care, they are an important part of the healthcare system.

14.1-3 The Organization of Healthcare Systems

A healthcare system is a whole network of interconnected agencies, facilities, insurers, and providers working together to provide and finance healthcare services. The names of departments within large healthcare organizations are often unfamiliar. Healthcare workers may need to explain the system's organization to patients as they help them obtain services.

The **organizational chart** is an outline of the **hierarchy** (HI-er-ahr-kee), or levels of authority, within an organization. Within healthcare organizations, services are divided into separate departments. The number of departments depends on the size of the facility. **Figure 14.7** is an organizational chart for a large medical clinic. It shows how all the departments are connected to reach the organization's goals. Organizational structures in therapeutic and support services provide two examples of this.

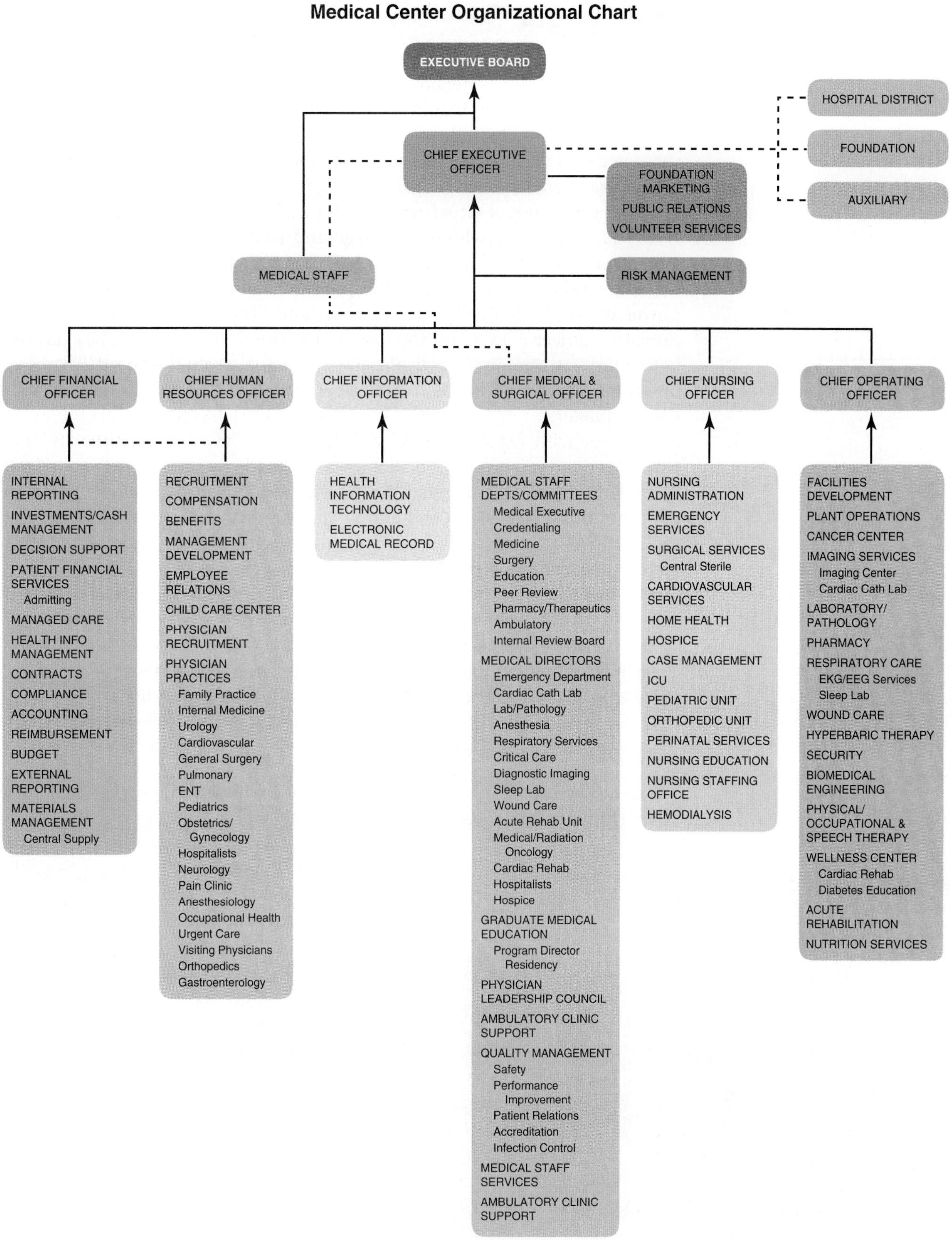

Medical Center Organizational Chart

EXECUTIVE BOARD

CHIEF EXECUTIVE OFFICER

HOSPITAL DISTRICT

FOUNDATION

AUXILIARY

FOUNDATION MARKETING
PUBLIC RELATIONS
VOLUNTEER SERVICES

MEDICAL STAFF

RISK MANAGEMENT

CHIEF FINANCIAL OFFICER

INTERNAL REPORTING
INVESTMENTS/CASH MANAGEMENT
DECISION SUPPORT
PATIENT FINANCIAL SERVICES
  Admitting
MANAGED CARE
HEALTH INFO MANAGEMENT
CONTRACTS
COMPLIANCE
ACCOUNTING
REIMBURSEMENT
BUDGET
EXTERNAL REPORTING
MATERIALS MANAGEMENT
  Central Supply

CHIEF HUMAN RESOURCES OFFICER

RECRUITMENT
COMPENSATION
BENEFITS
MANAGEMENT DEVELOPMENT
EMPLOYEE RELATIONS
CHILD CARE CENTER
PHYSICIAN RECRUITMENT
PHYSICIAN PRACTICES
  Family Practice
  Internal Medicine
  Urology
  Cardiovascular
  General Surgery
  Pulmonary
  ENT
  Pediatrics
  Obstetrics/
    Gynecology
  Hospitalists
  Neurology
  Pain Clinic
  Anesthesiology
  Occupational Health
  Urgent Care
  Visiting Physicians
  Orthopedics
  Gastroenterology

CHIEF INFORMATION OFFICER

HEALTH INFORMATION TECHNOLOGY
ELECTRONIC MEDICAL RECORD

CHIEF MEDICAL & SURGICAL OFFICER

MEDICAL STAFF DEPTS/COMMITTEES
  Medical Executive
  Credentialing
  Medicine
  Surgery
  Education
  Peer Review
  Pharmacy/Therapeutics
  Ambulatory
  Internal Review Board
MEDICAL DIRECTORS
  Emergency Department
  Cardiac Cath Lab
  Lab/Pathology
  Anesthesia
  Respiratory Services
  Critical Care
  Diagnostic Imaging
  Sleep Lab
  Wound Care
  Acute Rehab Unit
  Medical/Radiation
    Oncology
  Cardiac Rehab
  Hospitalists
  Hospice
GRADUATE MEDICAL EDUCATION
  Program Director
  Residency
PHYSICIAN LEADERSHIP COUNCIL
AMBULATORY CLINIC SUPPORT
QUALITY MANAGEMENT
  Safety
  Performance
    Improvement
  Patient Relations
  Accreditation
  Infection Control
MEDICAL STAFF SERVICES
AMBULATORY CLINIC SUPPORT

CHIEF NURSING OFFICER

NURSING ADMINISTRATION
EMERGENCY SERVICES
SURGICAL SERVICES
  Central Sterile
CARDIOVASCULAR SERVICES
HOME HEALTH
HOSPICE
CASE MANAGEMENT
ICU
PEDIATRIC UNIT
ORTHOPEDIC UNIT
PERINATAL SERVICES
NURSING EDUCATION
NURSING STAFFING OFFICE
HEMODIALYSIS

CHIEF OPERATING OFFICER

FACILITIES DEVELOPMENT
PLANT OPERATIONS
CANCER CENTER
IMAGING SERVICES
  Imaging Center
  Cardiac Cath Lab
LABORATORY/ PATHOLOGY
PHARMACY
RESPIRATORY CARE
  EKG/EEG Services
  Sleep Lab
WOUND CARE
HYPERBARIC THERAPY
SECURITY
BIOMEDICAL ENGINEERING
PHYSICAL/ OCCUPATIONAL & SPEECH THERAPY
WELLNESS CENTER
  Cardiac Rehab
  Diabetes Education
ACUTE REHABILITATION
NUTRITION SERVICES

Goodheart-Willcox Publisher

Figure 14.7 An organizational chart shows the lines of authority in an organization—in this case, a hospital. *According to this chart, who would be your immediate supervisor if you worked in the emergency services department?*

Therapeutic Services

Within the organizational chart, therapeutic services are usually grouped by medical specialty. For example, the emergency department, anesthesiology, and respiratory services would each have their own director. Each department serves a different role in the overall function of the facility. Although they are separated on the chart, specialists often work together as an interdisciplinary healthcare team.

The organizational structure provides a vertical line of authority, or *chain of command*, showing who is in charge and who reports to whom. This creates a smooth flow of information between the decision makers at the top and the workers below. A governing board has the most decision-making power within large healthcare organizations. The board includes the chief executive officer (CEO) and the heads of various committees. They address both administrative and medical issues. Decisions from the board are passed down to department heads. Smaller organizations may have fewer upper-level managers.

Workers with more training and experience have more authority than workers with fewer credentials. For instance, in the medical department, medical assistants work under the direction of a physician. Residents have more authority than interns, but less than a fellow or attending physician. In nursing, certified nursing assistants report to a licensed practical nurse or registered nurse, and the director of nursing oversees all nursing staff.

When you have concerns at work, be clear, honest, and respectful with your supervisor. If the concerns are not addressed, seek support from your supervisor and move up the chain of command until the issue is resolved. When everyone commits to following the chain of command, system throughput is more efficient. In healthcare, this can save time, money, and lives.

Support Services

The horizontal organization of the chart often includes support services. Most people in support services do not work directly with patients or provide healthcare. Even so, they are vital to a healthcare facility's ability to provide efficient, high-quality care. You will rely on these workers to create an environment that supports a smooth flow in the throughput and feedback mechanisms of the healthcare system (**Figure 14.8**).

Facilities managers ensure that a healthcare facility is in good repair and operates smoothly. They address issues concerning the facility's **infrastructure**, which includes all the internal systems a facility needs to function day-to-day. Facilities managers are responsible for regular operations, such as keeping water running and hallways lit and maintaining parking facilities and other areas used by outpatients and visitors. They must plan for emergencies, making sure there is a backup power supply in case of a power outage. They are also concerned with controlling costs and avoiding waste in all facility operations.

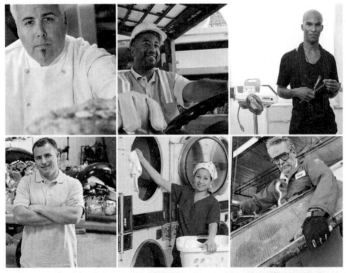

sirtravelalot/Shutterstock.com

Figure 14.8 Employees in support services create an environment that helps the facility run smoothly.

Housekeeping and other support services workers make sure the environment is clean, stocked, and ready to use. Biomedical equipment technicians ensure diagnostic equipment is working properly. Central services workers sterilize and stock linens and supplies so they are available for hands-on care providers (**Figure 14.9**). Support services are essential to maintaining a stable healthcare environment.

Health and safety workers ensure healthcare facilities follow all occupational health and safety laws and regulations. They examine conditions and equipment for potential hazards, conduct safety trainings, provide security, and investigate accidents. Their goal is to increase employee productivity and save money by reducing fines, insurance premiums, and workers' compensation costs. They use a systemic approach to finding and fixing hazards before people are injured.

Some healthcare facilities maintain their own pharmacies so they can provide both inpatients and outpatients with necessary medications. *Controlled substances* are powerful medicines with strict government rules for their use. Pharmacy workers must carefully maintain records, check labels, and prevent errors that could endanger health or allow illegal access to drugs.

Dietary services workers support patients by helping them follow the diet prescribed in their healthcare plans. They also serve employees and visitors through the cafeteria food service. Dietary workers need to manage their inventory and pay attention to special food-handling procedures so food does not spoil or cause issues for people with food allergies or special diets.

Interpreters communicate with patients who speak a different language. This supports informed consent for medical procedures. Interpreters also help healthcare providers gather information to diagnose, make treatment decisions, and avoid medical errors. Interpreters usually specialize in one or more languages, including American Sign Language (**Figure 14.10**).

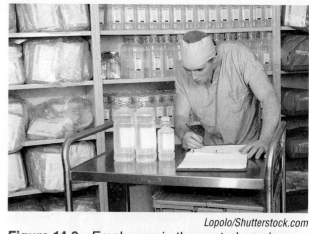

Lopolo/Shutterstock.com

Figure 14.9 Employees in the central services department help maintain a healthcare facility's inventory of equipment, instruments, linens, and uniforms.

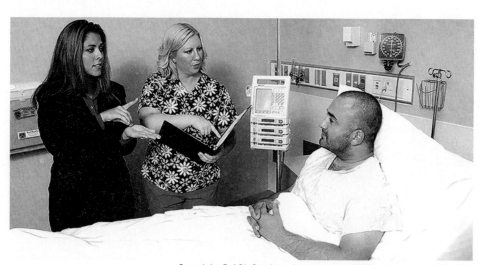

Copyright © ASL Services, Inc. and www.ASLServices.com, 2010–2014

Figure 14.10 Each state has its own requirements for certification or licensure of interpreters. The training for sign language interpreters is different from training for other language interpreters.

Hospitals, nursing homes, hospice facilities, and funeral homes have bereavement staff trained to support patients, family, and staff in dealing with end-of-life issues and emotions. Some facilities, such as hospitals, care centers, hospices, or nursing homes, also have a *morgue*. This is where dead bodies are kept in refrigerated chambers until viewing, identification, or autopsy can be completed, or until the bodies are taken to funeral homes.

Through your training and experience, you will learn whom to contact for different types of issues. All healthcare workers are important to the daily operations of a facility, regardless of their level of contact with patients. Be sure to show them your appreciation for their role.

Lesson 14.1 Review

 Complete the *Map Your Reading* graphic organizer for the section you just read.

1. Which of these can be used to think through the causes and effects of changes between related parts of healthcare delivery and payment systems? (14.1-1)
   A. Infrastructure
   B. Feedback loop
   C. Systems theory
   D. Hierarchy

2. Which type of healthcare facility provides acute care? Choose all that apply. (14.1-2)
   A. Hospitals
   B. Clinics
   C. Ambulances
   D. Home health

3. Which workers make sure supplies and equipment are available? (14.1-3)
   A. Health and safety workers
   B. Central supply
   C. Infrastructure
   D. Bereavement

4. The _____ shows the connections between departments and the hierarchy within a department. (14.1-3)
   A. input
   B. feedback loop
   C. NIH
   D. organizational chart

Healthcare Economic Systems and Related Terms

Learning Outcomes

After studying this lesson, you will be able to

14.2-1 define basic health insurance terms.

14.2-2 explain the origins of the US health insurance system.

14.2-3 compare common managed-care payment systems.

Professional Vocabulary

Essential Terms

insurance a purchased contract for shared financial protection against an unexpected loss

managed care a system that limits access to and use of healthcare to keep costs down

Important Terms

claim

coinsurance

copayment

deductible

exclusive provider organization (EPO)

health maintenance organizations (HMOs)

high-deductible health plan (HDHP)

Medicaid

Medicare

point-of-service (POS)

preferred provider organization (PPO)

premiums

primary care provider (PCP)

worker's compensation

> **? ESSENTIAL QUESTION**
>
> *How do healthcare economic systems impact delivery of care in the United States?*

Introduction

There are many ways to cover the cost of healthcare, and each system has its pros and cons. Great Britain, Spain, and Cuba use a single-payer system with healthcare organized by the government and funded through taxes. The government controls services and keeps costs low. In Germany, France, and Switzerland, employers and employees pay for a nonprofit insurance system for everyone. Government regulation keeps costs low. The national health insurance models of Canada, Taiwan, and South Korea use a government-run insurance system that controls costs by limiting payment for services and providers. Less industrialized countries have more limited medical systems and use an out-of-pocket payment model. Access to hospitals and doctors is limited to those who can afford to pay. What are your thoughts on access to healthcare? What should be provided, and who should pay for it?

In the US, a complex mixture of individuals, employers, insurance companies, and government agencies cover the cost of healthcare (**Figure 14.11**). Government tax dollars pay for healthcare for certain groups of citizens. Large grants and donations may fund healthcare focused on a specific goal, such as smoking cessation. Many employers offer private health insurance for employees and their families. Employers take advantage of group discounts to lower their cost for insurance. Individuals may also purchase private health insurance plans through an exchange market, use off-exchange plans, or pay for healthcare procedures out of their own pocket. All these payment systems bring money into the healthcare delivery system, which absorbs the cost for some people who cannot pay their medical bills.

Healthcare costs have risen significantly over the last few decades, from $62 billion in 1970 to $4.1 trillion in 2020 (**Figure 14.12**). Of that amount, the government paid $1.6 trillion from taxes. Healthcare costs are expected to nearly double in the next 10 years, and the government's portion will continue to grow. These rising costs are not sustainable and will affect the quantity and quality of care provided. Efforts to lower costs have not been effective, and access to care has not been equal. This has many people calling for changes in the healthcare payment, or **insurance**, system.

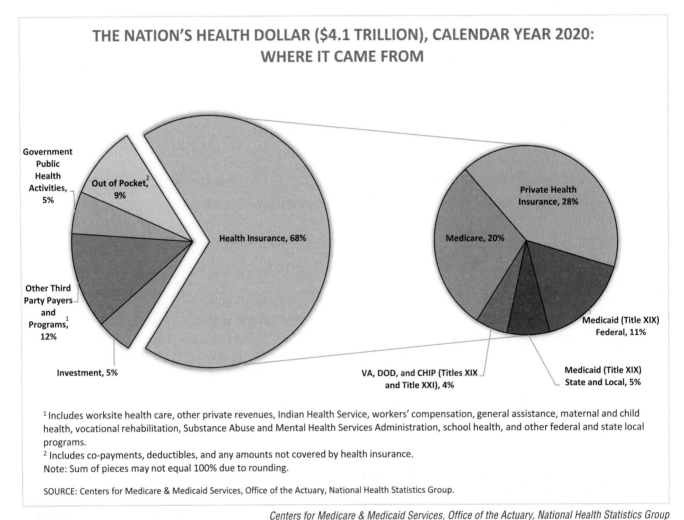

THE NATION'S HEALTH DOLLAR ($4.1 TRILLION), CALENDAR YEAR 2020: WHERE IT CAME FROM

Government Public Health Activities, 5%

Out of Pocket,[2] 9%

Health Insurance, 68%

Other Third Party Payers and Programs,[1] 12%

Investment, 5%

Private Health Insurance, 28%

Medicare, 20%

Medicaid (Title XIX) Federal, 11%

VA, DOD, and CHIP (Titles XIX and Title XXI), 4%

Medicaid (Title XIX) State and Local, 5%

[1] Includes worksite health care, other private revenues, Indian Health Service, workers' compensation, general assistance, maternal and child health, vocational rehabilitation, Substance Abuse and Mental Health Services Administration, school health, and other federal and state local programs.

[2] Includes co-payments, deductibles, and any amounts not covered by health insurance.

Note: Sum of pieces may not equal 100% due to rounding.

SOURCE: Centers for Medicare & Medicaid Services, Office of the Actuary, National Health Statistics Group.

Centers for Medicare & Medicaid Services, Office of the Actuary, National Health Statistics Group

Figure 14.11 A variety of payment systems cover the cost of healthcare in the US. In 2020, 31.2 million people did not have insurance, 200.3 million people had private insurance, and 159.3 million people had government insurance plans.

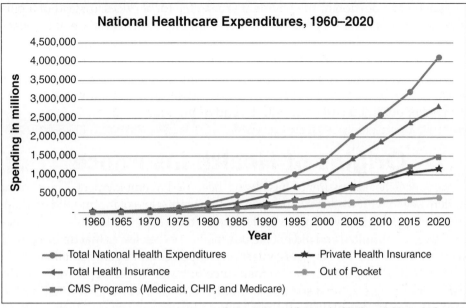

National Healthcare Expenditures, 1960–2020

Legend:
- Total National Health Expenditures
- Total Health Insurance
- CMS Programs (Medicaid, CHIP, and Medicare)
- Private Health Insurance
- Out of Pocket

Data courtesy of Centers for Medicare & Medicaid Services

Figure 14.12 Healthcare costs have risen significantly in the last few decades and are expected to continue rising. Hospital services, physician/clinical services, and prescription drugs have risen faster than other medical expenses. *What changes in the healthcare system might account for these increases?*

14.2-1 Insurance Basics

Insurance is a risk pool that groups together many people who face a risk. These individuals contribute money to the pooled funds, sharing the total cost. The monthly fees individuals pay into this money pool to receive insurance coverage are called **premiums**. Insurance helps pay for provider services, medications, hospital care, and special equipment when you are sick. It also helps pay for immunizations, annual check-ups, screening, and counseling. When insured people use healthcare services, they can submit a **claim**. This is a request for the insurance company to pay for the cost of care using the pooled funds. Then, the insurance policy determines how much is covered and what the patient owes. An *explanation of benefits (EOB)* for each claim will show the costs, deductibles, limits, payments, and amounts owed by the patient for each claim. Insurance may pay the healthcare provider directly or reimburse the patient.

Insurance plans differ in the providers you can see and how much you pay. Some plans require pre-authorization, or *referrals*, to see specialists. Most plans require individuals to pay some of their own healthcare costs to reduce overuse of healthcare and insurance. They set a minimum amount the patient must pay out-of-pocket, called a **deductible**, before the insurance company will pay its portion of healthcare claims. Some plans also set a maximum amount the insurance company will pay for services, such as home care or physical therapy visits in a year. These restrictions reduce overuse but may result in less effective healthcare if they cause patients to avoid going to the doctor.

An insured person's share of the costs compared to the insurance company's share is called **coinsurance**. Coinsurance is a percentage or ratio, such as 80/20, which means the insurance company pays 80 percent of qualified costs, and the patient pays 20 percent. If you need a cavity filled at the dentist, you may be asked to pay 20 percent of that bill. When these fees add up to your deductible, the insurance company will pay all these costs through the end of the year.

When your portion of the payment is a set fee for services, instead of a percentage, this is called a **copayment**. For example, patients may pay a copayment of $20 to see their primary care physician, and their insurance pays the rest of the bill. Copayments do not count toward the deductible. Insurance may set a maximum you will pay each year out of pocket. Once your coinsurance and copayments total that amount, the insurance company will pay 100 percent of qualified costs through the end of the year.

14.2-2 Origins of Health Insurance

In the US, health insurance has always been tied to employment. The current system began with workers wanting to protect against loss of income and employers wanting to reduce work time lost to illness. In the early 1900s, these "sick benefits" were very limited and did not include medical expenses. At that time, medical costs were low, and nonprofit organizations helped cover larger hospital bills.

People did not push for health insurance until the Great Depression. Medical societies were against socialized medicine, and funds were limited, so the Social Security Act of 1935 did not include health insurance. During World War II's wage freeze, employers offered health insurance benefits to attract workers. This became an expected part of an employee's benefits. The growing insurance industry increased profits by deciding whom to insure, what services to cover, and how much to charge for premiums. Early hospitalization insurance turned into a variety of private health insurance plans. Unfortunately, the growth of employment-based insurance left those with the least resources and greatest medical needs without healthcare coverage.

In the 1950s and 1960s, government-financed healthcare grew for people not covered by employers. **Medicare** coverage was designed for people 65 years of age and older (**Figure 14.13**). This program helps with the cost of healthcare, but it does not pay for all medical expenses or long-term care. Medicare is divided into parts that pay for different types of services. Part A covers inpatient hospital and skilled-nursing costs, Part B covers outpatient care, Part C is Medicare coverage offered through private insurance companies, and Part D covers prescription drugs. To control prescription costs, insurance plans issue a drug list, or *formulary,* organized into several levels, or *tiers,* of costs. Generic drugs may be substituted for brand names in the lowest tiers, and coverage may be limited in upper tiers. Private "Medigap" or "Medicare Advantage" policies cover costs not paid by Medicare. The cost of care for those eligible for Medicare is about three times higher than the average working adult. Why do you think healthcare for this age group is so expensive?

People with low incomes and those who have disabilities and cannot work may receive **Medicaid**. State governments manage this health insurance program, so eligibility and coverage vary. Many states also provide federal funds, or *subsidies*, to buy insurance from the Health Insurance Exchange Marketplace. Without this support, households with low income would have to choose between paying for food and housing or medical care. The *Children's Health Insurance Program (CHIP)* covers children in families with low incomes that do not qualify for Medicaid.

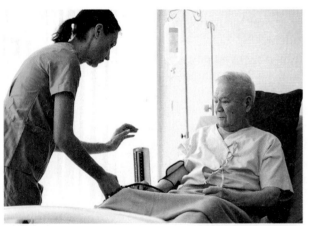

Rapeepat Pornsipak/Shutterstock.com

Figure 14.13 Medicare, a health insurance system funded by the government, provides coverage to people 65 years of age and older. *What does each part of Medicare cover?*

Federal, state, or employer-paid **worker's compensation** plans may cover people who are injured on the job. These plans pay for healthcare costs and loss of income due to injury. This includes disability compensation for workers who get a work-related illness, such as hearing loss from long-term exposure to loud equipment. *TRICARE* and *CHAMPVA* are government healthcare programs for uniformed service members, veterans, and their dependent families. Healthcare spending accounts for more than 25 percent of the federal budget. Approximately 35 percent of the US relies on the government for their healthcare insurance.

14.2-3 Development of Managed Care

The lack of a "free market" in healthcare has allowed costs to rise faster than for other purchases. Competition usually keeps prices balanced through supply and demand, but there is not fair competition in healthcare. People lack the medical knowledge to evaluate services, price information to compare value, and willingness to negotiate when health is involved. They usually follow a doctor's care plan and are not aware of the real cost of care contracted by health insurance companies. Healthcare providers set high prices with the assumption insurers will negotiate lower payments. There is currently no regulation on maximum pricing for healthcare services, prescriptions, medical devices, or insurance premiums, and they continue to rise.

When insurance began, healthcare facility payments were based on the actual cost to provide care. Insurance reimbursed the provider for any covered procedure. This encouraged providers to recommend more procedures to keep business flowing. At the same time, new treatments and technology encouraged people to demand more healthcare. Higher costs for patients and insurance companies resulted. Both the government and private insurers developed **managed care** systems to limit overuse and reduce rising costs. Managed care uses referrals, fees, and other methods to restrict access and discourage use of healthcare services.

The government reduced insurance costs through a diagnostic-related grouping (DRG) reimbursement system. DRGs are medical coding for medical conditions based on the diagnosis, procedure, and level of severity. The DRG code determines how much the insurance plan will pay the healthcare facility for treatment. If care is provided at a lower price than what is set for that DRG, the provider can keep the excess. If care costs more, the provider will have to pay any added costs. Most insurance providers adopted this predetermined payment, or *prospective payment system*, in the 1980s. A fixed price took away the incentive for healthcare providers to add more tests, treatments, or days in the hospital. It also encouraged better-quality care to avoid complications.

Insurers have created several managed care systems. These include health maintenance organizations (HMOs), preferred provider organizations (PPOs), point-of-service (POS) plans, and exclusive provider organizations (EPOs) (**Figure 14.14**).

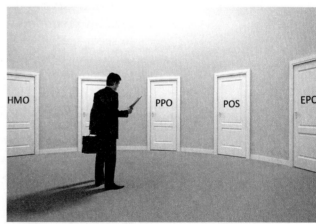

BPTU/Shutterstock.com

Figure 14.14 There are several different types of healthcare insurance plans for people in the United States. *What differences would a patient see in their choices and costs for each of these healthcare plans?*

Each type has different options and limits on healthcare services. Most use a specific network of healthcare providers who have agreed to reduce their fees in return for an increased number of patients. Insurance customers should know the differences to choose the best plan for their needs.

Health Maintenance Organizations (HMOs)

Health maintenance organizations (HMOs) employ doctors, pharmacists, dentists, laboratories, and hospitals in an integrated and patient-focused network. This type of insurance does not cover providers outside their network. The patient's main doctor is a **primary care provider (PCP)**. This may be a pediatrician for children, general practitioner or internist for adults, or geriatrician for older adults. Some plans use a nurse practitioner or physician assistant as the PCP. Specialists, such as a cardiologist, oncologist, or podiatrist, would require a referral from the PCP. Low deductibles and copayments allow patients to see their PCP more regularly for preventive care to maintain good health. A *capitation payment system* discourages overuse by the PCP. This means providers are paid by the number of patients enrolled in the plan instead of how much care they provide. They may also earn a bonus for keeping costs low (**Figure 14.15**). What do you like about this type of insurance? What potential problems do you see?

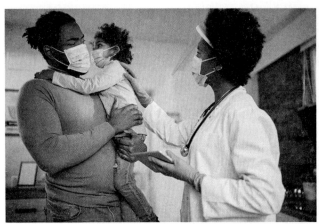

Drazen Zigic/Shutterstock.com

Figure 14.15 Having a healthcare plan like an HMO may mean that people see their doctors more often, leading to better health.

Preferred Provider Organizations (PPOs)

Some patients prefer the flexibility and wider choice of a **preferred provider organization (PPO)**. This type of insurance negotiates group discounts with a wide range of private physicians, specialists, and hospitals. The PPO only pays when providers actually provide care, so they have an incentive to offer more high-end services than an HMO. The insurance company may charge higher monthly premiums for a PPO than for an HMO but does not require a referral to see a specialist. They also use copayments for each service to discourage overuse by patients. What type of patient might prefer this type of insurance? What might cause this plan to become too expensive?

Point-of-Service (POS) Plans

A variation that combines elements of the HMO and PPO is a **point-of-service (POS)** plan. This plan uses a network of providers and requires you to see a PCP, like an HMO. Patients can be referred to a specialist outside the network for a higher fee, like a PPO.

Exclusive Provider Organizations (EPOs)

An **exclusive provider organization (EPO)** is similar to a PPO, but only network providers are covered, making the choice more limited. You do not have to see a PCP but may need permission to see a specialist. Providers are paid on a fee-for-service basis, and patients pay small copayments to reduce overuse of the services.

High-Deductible Health Plans (HDHPs)

Individuals may also have the option to use a **high-deductible health plan (HDHP)** along with a *health savings account (HSA)*. An HDHP has a lower monthly premium, but you will pay more healthcare costs before the insurance company begins to pay their portion. Your employer may set up an HSA to pay some of these expenses. Some of your earnings from each paycheck can go to this account before you pay income taxes. Depending on your tax bracket, this can save you 10 percent or more. However, it requires careful planning. The money placed in an HSA is taxed and penalized if used for other purposes before age 65. Any insurance plan may be offered as an HDHP, with or without an HSA.

Independent Practice Associations (IPAs)

Physicians with an independent or small group practice may join an Independent Practice Association (IPA) to stay competitive with larger practices and managed care prices. An IPA allows them to share resources, information, and business costs. IPA members still operate as independent businesses but gain some bargaining power to negotiate contracts as a group payer. Managed care organizations may contract with them as specialists.

There are many options, but health insurance remains expensive. Costs are rising, and the fragmented system does not provide high-quality or equitable care at an affordable price. Regulations have increased paperwork requirements and costs. The Health Insurance Portability and Accountability Act (HIPAA), for example, was supposed to make it easier for healthcare providers and insurance companies to share information. In the process, it actually added more layers of paperwork and security requirements. Many have suggested the US healthcare provider and payment systems need a complete overhaul. The difficult question is how to do this without interrupting care or causing more problems.

Lesson 14.2 Review

 Complete the *Map Your Reading* graphic organizer for the section you just read.

1. The amount paid by the patient before insurance pays the rest of a claim is the (14.2-1)
   A. referral
   B. penalty
   C. premium
   D. deductible
2. Government-financed _____ protects families with low incomes. (14.2-2)
   A. worker's compensation
   B. Medicare
   C. Medicaid
   D. *TRICARE*

3. What is the purpose of managed care? (14.2-3)
   A. To provide more healthcare
   B. To provide better quality of care
   C. To make healthcare more accessible
   D. To control the rising cost of healthcare
4. _____ plans focus on maintaining health through regular checkups to prevent costly disease. (14.2-3)
   A. HMO
   B. EPO
   C. POS
   D. PPO

Applying Systems Theory to Emerging Issues in Healthcare

Learning Outcomes

After studying this lesson, you will be able to

14.3-1 explain how quality improvement supports systemic changes in healthcare.

14.3-2 discuss the influence of changes to healthcare system inputs.

14.3-3 explain how changes in system throughput affect the healthcare delivery and payment systems.

14.3-4 analyze systemic changes caused by emerging issues in the external environment of healthcare systems.

Professional Vocabulary

Essential Terms

human testing controlled experiments performed on human beings in order to evaluate the safety and effectiveness of medical treatments

precision medicine using population data to customize medical care to an individual's genetic, biological, and lifestyle differences

quality improvement (QI) a systematic approach to analyzing practices and improving efficiency or success

Important Terms

Common Rule

compliance

emerging diseases

generic

medical error

off-label

patent

Patient Protection and Affordable Care Act (ACA)

self-advocate

Introduction

Systems theory brings a new way of looking at and anticipating the effects of change on healthcare. Change may come at any point in a healthcare system. The needs and wants of patients, available finances, technology, laws, and economic conditions continually change the environment within which healthcare delivery and payment systems operate. A change in one part of the system causes a ripple effect of changes in other parts of the system.

Systems thinking involves broadly viewing how a complex system of people and services are connected and interact. You must look for patterns of behavior and include information from every point of view. This helps you anticipate what will work best and avoid unintended consequences.

An outward sign of problems in a system is an increase in negative outcomes and feedback. When more patients are suffering or dying, something needs to change. As you examine a problem in healthcare, look at each part of the system and consider what effect a change would have. In this lesson, you will learn about quality-improvement measures and think through several systemic issues that affect healthcare.

14.3-1 Using Quality Improvement in a Healthcare System Feedback Loop

Quality improvement (QI) focuses on productivity and efficiency. In healthcare, QI helps monitor the quality of services, improve patient care, and support physicians' credential renewal requirements. QI is a systemic approach. It uses data to describe how the system is working and analyze what happens when changes are applied. Quantitative data, such as the number of medication errors or length of wait times, comes from lab reports, waiting room logs, and admissions forms. Qualitative data, or descriptions of things that cannot be measured, may include patient or employee satisfaction from surveys, interviews, or observations. Analyzing quantitative and qualitative data helps make decisions about healthcare services and opportunities for improvement.

You can look for opportunities to improve healthcare throughput by mapping out who performs each step in a healthcare process. This *process map* shows connections between people involved and who is affected by changes to the system (**Figure 14.16**). It may also reveal gaps, inefficiencies, or overlaps in service. Larger

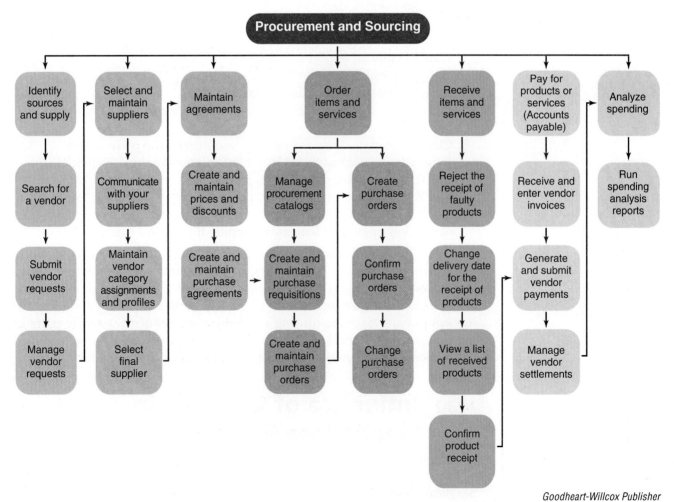

Goodheart-Willcox Publisher

Figure 14.16 Quality improvement might include the use of a process map, which shows connections between all people involved in a process or procedure. *How does a process map help with the task of quality improvement?*

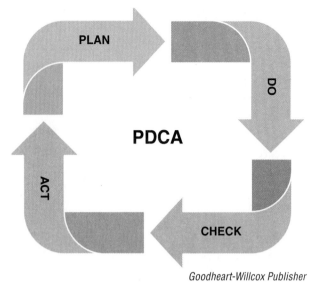

Goodheart-Willcox Publisher

Figure 14.17 In quality improvement projects, try following the PDCA cycle to determine changes you may need to make to a procedure or system.

healthcare facilities have dedicated staff to coordinate the QI process and help teams work on specific projects.

The QI team considers how changes will affect the larger healthcare system. QI teams are usually interdisciplinary. They should include someone who works with the process, someone who is affected by the process, and someone in authority who can assign resources and give permission to make changes. For example, if central services wanted to review cleaning procedures of diagnostic equipment, their QI team might include the following:

- a medical laboratory technician who uses the equipment daily
- a biomedical technician who evaluates the durability of equipment and identifies problems caused by specific cleaning methods
- a central supply worker who performs cleaning, disinfection, and sterilization tasks
- the central supply manager who oversees cleaning procedures and makes sure they meet OSHA guidelines

Quality improvement often uses a Plan-Do-Check-Act (PDCA) model (**Figure 14.17**). Each cycle can be *reactive*, responding to an identified problem, or *proactive*, showing an opportunity for improvement. This cyclic process includes the following steps:

1. **Plan.** Identify an opportunity for change. Suggest the root causes and design a possible solution. Gather baseline data and set a goal for improvement in performance measures.
2. **Do.** Begin making changes on a small scale in a controlled setting and collecting data on performance and outcomes.
3. **Check.** Compare data to your own baseline and the performance standards, or *benchmarks*, set by other facilities. Analyze feedback loop data for successes and additional problems.
4. **Act.** Begin using successful solutions as everyday practices. Continue monitoring data to show changes are working and identify additional needs. Solve new problems by beginning the process again.

The PDCA model teaches teams to monitor their own performance and take corrective action. The focus of QI is always on fixing system processes that allowed a problem to occur, not on blaming people who made mistakes. Solutions may include adding safeguards, retraining staff, replacing equipment, or streamlining procedures to reduce waste. Benefits of implementing QI include improved patient health outcomes, reduced costs, increased efficiency, and higher patient and staff satisfaction.

14.3-2 Influence of Changes in Healthcare System Input

Patients and their health are a major input in the healthcare delivery system. Some patients have difficulty accessing healthcare. Others have significantly higher healthcare needs. All patients have the right to a healthcare system that meets their needs, but they must use the system responsibly so it can function effectively for them. QI can help the system adjust to the changing needs of patients.

Patient Rights and Responsibilities

The American Hospital Association (AHA) developed the first Patient's Bill of Rights to improve patient care. It reminded healthcare workers of their responsibilities to the patient and encouraged patients to be more active in their own care. A US Advisory Commission adopted a Patient's Bill of Rights in 1998 to help patients feel more confident in the healthcare system. It stressed the importance of strong patient-provider relationships and the key role patients play in their own health. Many healthcare facilities now have a patient's bill of rights that includes these key ideas:

1. **Information disclosure.** Consumers have the right to receive accurate and understandable information about their diagnosis, prognosis, treatment options, costs, care providers, and facility so they can make informed healthcare decisions.
2. **Choice of providers and plans.** Consumers have the right to choose from a variety of high-quality healthcare providers and insurance options.
3. **Access to services.** Consumers have a right to continued access to medically necessary healthcare services as they move between healthcare facilities.
4. **Participation in treatment decisions.** Consumers or their representatives have the right to full participation in their healthcare decisions. This includes the right to refuse treatment and to choose whether to participate in experimental research.
5. **Respect and nondiscrimination.** Consumers have the right to receive respectful and equal treatment from all members of the healthcare team (**Figure 14.18**).
6. **Confidentiality of health information.** HIPAA laws protect the consumer's right to privacy of information. They also have the right to review, request corrections, and copy their medical records.
7. **Complaints and appeals.** Consumers have the right to a fair and efficient process for resolving problems with their healthcare plans, providers, and facilities.
8. **Consumer responsibilities.** Consumers are encouraged to be more involved in their care and support a cost-conscious environment.

Increasing emphasis is being placed on consumer responsibilities. Patients should maximize healthy habits, such as being physically active, eating a healthy diet, and not smoking. Most people who have healthy habits have fewer health conditions and require less healthcare.

In 2003, AHA materials shifted from the *Patient Bill of Rights* to the *Patient Care Partnership: Understanding Expectations, Rights and Responsibilities.* They now focus on patients sharing information about their health and asking questions when confused. **Compliance**, or following through on instructions, and keeping appointments are important for patient health. If patients cannot follow the treatment plan, they should let their care provider know to make adjustments. They should pay their bills on time and be considerate of the provider's business needs. These actions lead to a better relationship with the care provider and better healthcare at a lower cost.

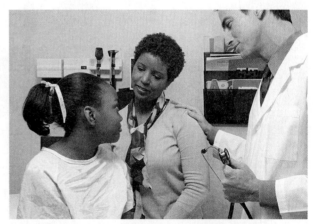

XiXinXing/Shutterstock.com

Figure 14.18 Consumers have the right to considerate, respectful care from healthcare workers. *What are some simple ways you can show respect for patients?*

Some people see healthcare providers as authority figures and have difficulty asserting themselves during an appointment. It is important for patients to **self-advocate**, or speak up for themselves. Patients can prepare for appointments by writing down questions and concerns. When they disagree with a treatment plan, they should say so and can ask for a second opinion. To avoid confusion about instructions and ensure concerns are addressed, people who are forgetful or easily confused can take notes or ask someone to attend appointments with them. Every state also has an *ombudsman* (ahm-BUDZ-muhn) program in the long-term care system. This is a person to address complaints and advocate for patient rights.

The **Patient Protection and Affordable Care Act (ACA)** of 2010 also specifies certain rights for all people legally in the US. These rights focus on health insurance, but also affect the healthcare people receive. The law sets minimum standards for insurance products and reduces barriers to gaining insurance coverage. Insurance companies can no longer deny coverage for preexisting conditions or cancel patients who become too expensive. Dependent children are covered until age 26. Preventive care must be included at no charge. Additional funds are provided to states that offer expanded access to Medicaid insurance benefits. The hope is this will lead to a healthier population.

Recent focus has shifted to the broader human right to health and universal access to healthcare. The four components of this movement are:

- access to affordable and complete care for all
- culturally appropriate and responsive care for diverse needs
- adequate healthcare in all geographic areas
- quality healthcare that is medically appropriate, timely, and guided by standards

How do you think this movement will affect the healthcare system?

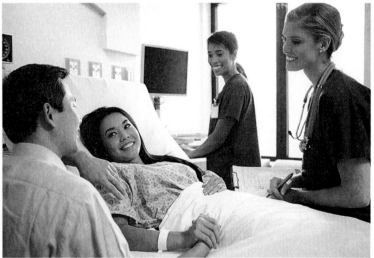

MBI/Shutterstock.com

Figure 14.19 Healthcare workers may encounter health disparities and language barriers when caring for patients from different cultures. *List some ways that this could affect all aspects of a system—input, throughput, output, and the feedback loop.*

Health Disparities

Differences in social and economic conditions can create health disparities, or unequal health outcomes for marginalized populations (**Figure 14.19**). Systemic racism or bias may be a root cause of health disparities, but it is difficult to identify or quantify. A system's pattern of procedures, practices, and policies can penalize and create disadvantages for some groups of people. The unconscious judging, or *implicit bias*, of healthcare providers may also play a role. This stems from *ethnocentrism*, or the assumption that your culture is the correct way. Through self-evaluation, you can recognize unintentional, unconscious biases about people different from yourself. These biases influence behavior, which may lead to unequal or inappropriate treatment.

The growth of ethnic diversity in the US means healthcare workers need to be aware of health disparities and more culturally responsive to healthcare needs. Patients may be less comfortable sharing their health concerns with providers different from themselves. They may mistrust a healthcare system with a history of exploiting them. These issues make access to care even more difficult and may result in poor outcomes and unsatisfied customers.

Health literacy is also a key factor in decreasing health disparities. Patients must be able to gather, understand, and use health information to participate in the healthcare system. Low health literacy affects more people who have low socioeconomic status, low education, low English proficiency, and old age. This can cause problems accessing healthcare and following healthcare instructions. It results in higher healthcare costs and death rates. What could you change in system throughput to become more patient-centered and improve outcomes for these patients?

Changing system throughput can address input concerns, such as diverse patient needs. Adding interpreters is a common response, but it only helps with language barriers. Adding information about social determinants of health to the EHR could increase awareness. Providers could familiarize themselves with a person's situation to be more culturally responsive, communicate openly, and share decision-making. Staff may need sensitivity training on the social issues and inequities their patients face. Many facilities are trying to increase staff diversity and project a more multicultural image. Patient advocates or navigators can also help patients understand how to use complex healthcare systems. These changes will further affect the system's input, throughput, output, and feedback loop.

Uninsured Populations

About 10 percent of US citizens lack health insurance, and another 20 percent have gaps in their insurance coverage. Those who are uninsured or underinsured are at risk for poor access to healthcare and high medical debt. This socioeconomic issue is of greatest concern for the unemployed, young adults shifting to their own insurance, and millions of children without enough coverage.

Systems theory helps people think about the effect large numbers of uninsured people have on healthcare delivery and payment systems. Socioeconomics affect the resources, or input, coming into the healthcare system. A large number of uninsured young adults keeps insurance costs high because young adults tend to be healthier than older adults. If young adults were paying into the insurance pool, their premiums would help cover the cost of services for older adults. People without insurance also tend to wait until their health conditions are advanced before seeing a doctor. This makes them more difficult and expensive to treat, which affects the system's throughput and output.

Children without health insurance may not go to the doctor for checkups or vaccines each year. This means they can spread a preventable illness, such as measles. Growing epidemics of whooping cough, or *pertussis*, and tuberculosis show this is a problem in system output. People without insurance are also not connected to a particular care provider, creating fragmented care. This affects the feedback loop.

The ACA tried to solve these problems by improving access to high-quality health insurance. It created the Health Insurance Exchange Marketplace (**Figure 14.20**) as one large risk pool to help reduce costs. It also required most employers to offer health insurance for employees. How do you think this increased input of insured patients would affect the throughput or output of the healthcare system?

Every change in a system causes changes to other parts of the system. After the ACA passed, the number of people without insurance went down to 10 percent, but premiums, copayments, and deductibles went up. Many people could not afford the copayments and deductibles to see their doctor. Rising costs were blamed on the high number of new patients, more insurance coverage requirements, and high costs of technology and medicine. More employers opted out of providing insurance, and the tax penalty for not having insurance was removed. Many people without health conditions dropped their insurance. This raised the proportion of people with health conditions in the risk pool, and costs went up again the next year. Insurance costs are now at an all-time high, and people are asking for more changes to the insurance system.

Mental and Behavioral Health Issues

Mental and behavioral health issues are a growing issue in healthcare system input. Rates of depression and burnout for patients and healthcare workers skyrocketed during the COVID-19 pandemic. The stigma attached to these conditions creates a barrier to those who need support.

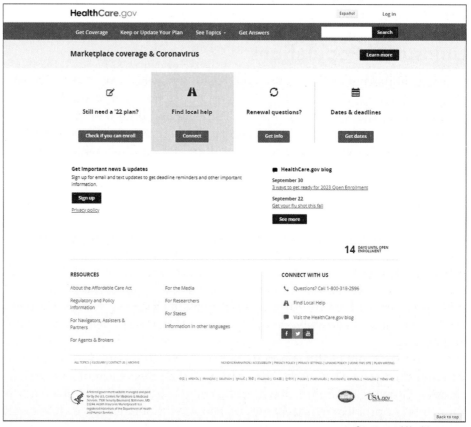

Courtesy of Healthcare.gov

Figure 14.20 The Affordable Care Act, signed in 2010, used health insurance exchanges to increase access to affordable insurance. This change in system input affected the entire healthcare system.

Society's labels and assumptions about people with mental and behavioral health issues can cause people to feel devalued, excluded from decision-making, or discriminated against. People may be reluctant to disclose or seek support for a mental or behavioral health condition, allowing these issues to affect their health and day-to day lives. Changes in healthcare throughput can help address these concerns.

Substance misuse is another aspect of behavioral health that has increased significantly in the last few decades. The US National Institute on Drug Abuse reports that tobacco, alcohol, and illegal drug use affect more than 20 million adults. Alcohol-related disorders are the most common, but opioid use disorders and marijuana vaping are the fastest growing. Some substance use disorders begin with medically prescribed painkillers. This indicates the need for better treatment options and prescribing practices.

Living with a substance use disorder can have long-term health effects and social consequences. The impact is lifelong for infants affected by drugs or alcohol before birth. Costly specialists are needed to manage these issues. In the past, the legal system handled many of these substance misuse and mental health conditions. Options were limited and not covered by most health insurance until the Mental Health Parity and Addiction Equity Act of 2008. A shift in thinking is needed to solve this systemic issue. How can people interrupt the cycle and reduce the number of people overdosing or needing treatment?

"Just say 'No'" education programs have had limited success, and adolescent use and addiction are increasing. **Figure 14.21** lists some of the many tools for treating substance use disorders. Early diagnosis and treatment of substance use disorders can limit health effects and keep costs down, but systematic coordination is needed. Primary care, mental health providers, treatment centers, emergency departments, hospitals, schools, community health centers, and others must work together. Healthcare providers need to know the signs and symptoms of mental health and substance use disorders. They should include screening questions as part of their standard care in system throughput. Early detection will result in a need for additional treatment facilities, but at a lower cost overall. There will also be better outcomes for patients.

Treating Substance Use Disorders

- Educate patients about the risks of using addictive substances.
- Make it harder to obtain addictive substances.
- Expand insurance coverage for treatment.
- Make Naloxone available to counteract effects of opioids on the body.
- Educate people about how to use Naloxone during an overdose.

Goodheart-Willcox Publisher

Figure 14.21 There are many tools available to help with the prevention and treatment of substance use disorders.

An Aging Population

An aging population is also straining the healthcare system. Financially, Medicare has fewer young people paying into the system as the number of older people using Medicare increases. A shortfall of Medicare Part A funds is predicted unless costs decrease or Medicare payroll taxes increase.

People are now living longer and with more serious health issues. This creates a need for more specialists to diagnose and treat complex health conditions. These services are mainly located in larger cities. As older family practice and general medicine doctors retire, and more medical students go into specialty fields, rural areas are seeing a shortage of primary care doctors.

The medical needs of aging baby boomers create increased demand for care and greater use of expensive technology. Insurance has responded to increased costs by reducing the number of days they will pay for hospital stays. Care is moved to cheaper outpatient, rehabilitation, and home health services.

As a result, these facilities are experiencing an overload of patients and staffing shortages. Long-term care staff must care for more complex needs, which they may not be trained to manage. This can lead to medical errors and poorer outcomes for patients.

The nursing shorting is also due to aging. Female baby boomers had fewer career options than today's youth, and many of them became nurses. Baby boomer nurses are now retiring at a faster rate than new nurses are entering the field. Those who became nurse instructors are also retiring, causing enrollment limits in nursing schools. As workloads increase, even more nurses are burning out and leaving the field. Duties of medical assistants and nursing assistants have increased to help cover for nursing shortages. This shift in the care model can affect quality of care. How does lower quality of care affect other parts of the system?

14.3-3 Effects of Changing System Throughput

Rising costs, medical errors, and constant changes in technology affect the healthcare system's throughput. This impacts patient-care processes, purchasing decisions, and training needs. QI studies look for new approaches to solve these systemic issues.

Rising Costs

Many people play a role in keeping healthcare costs down. For patients, a combination of lifestyle changes, preventive care, and following doctor's recommendations can help lower healthcare costs. Avoiding medical care due to the high cost has a negative impact on health. This affects the input side of the healthcare system, which increases the workload and complexity of care for healthcare workers on the throughput side.

Overuse of healthcare services also raises costs and stresses an already busy system. *Defensive medicine* is when healthcare professionals intentionally overuse healthcare services. They may recommend more diagnostic tests or perform a procedure just to protect against a possible malpractice lawsuit. The expectation that all illnesses can and should be cured, preventing death through any means possible, also drives overuse of healthcare. It is wasteful to spend money on healthcare services that do not produce a better health outcome. About $50 billion per year is spent on medical liability and defensive medicine in the US. What parts of a system—input, throughput, output, or feedback—do these practices increase?

Facilities have many ways to lower costs (**Figure 14.22**). Just like families saving money in their home, managers look for waste in system throughput activities. Insurance and government agencies try to reduce costs by promoting preventive care and healthy lifestyles. This includes regular physical exams, vaccines, physical activity, and a healthy diet. The goal is to prevent or catch conditions early before they become expensive to treat.

Facilities can lower costs by

- using motion-activated lights in offices and restrooms
- purchasing in bulk
- using more efficient electronic records
- cutting rarely used services
- reducing staff and hours of operation, as long as patient safety is not compromised
- cross-training workers to perform more than one job
- avoiding work injuries, hospital-acquired infections, and medical errors

Goodheart-Willcox Publisher

Figure 14.22 Good communication, accurate records, and careful use of supplies will also reduce the cost of care. *What other ways do you cut costs at home that might work in healthcare?*

On the other hand, increased screenings have also led to more *false positives*, or tests that suggest cancer or another condition is present when it is not. This results in more tests or procedures.

Because of rising prices, Medicare and many private insurers limit coverage for lab tests and medical imaging. They try to reduce the system's input and throughput to control costs. It is hard to know in advance how much a routine diagnostic test will cost. Published prices do not show the cost reductions each insurance company has agreed to. There are also regional differences. A blood test in Baltimore for $22 could cost $725 in Miami. Standardizing processes between different providers and insurance plans would reduce administrative costs and level out huge differences in price.

The No Surprises Act of 2020 and various healthcare payment reform laws at the state level protect patients from insurance passing on excessive medical costs. Further changes are needed to reverse the trend of rising healthcare costs.

Medical Errors

Healthcare workers can make throughput changes to reduce **medical errors**. These preventable mistakes are the third leading cause of death in the US. The cost in Massachusetts for one year was $617 million. On a national level, this is approximately $30 billion per year. You often hear about errors of commission, where a healthcare worker does something wrong, such as the wrong surgery site, medication, or dosage. However, errors of omission, or actions not taken, cause just as much harm. Following accepted practices during a procedure can help avoid complications, infections, and the need to readmit patients. A 2019 report showed the number is dropping, but preventable safety events still happen in about 11 percent of hospital cases.

Patient misidentification is a significant cause of medical errors. The wrong person may be billed for or receive the wrong medical care due to misidentification. It is important to match the correct patient to the correct treatment before beginning a procedure (**Figure 14.23**). Use at least two methods to identify them. Patients with names that sound almost the same may have a "name alert" and require extra caution so you do not confuse them.

Open communication is key to avoiding medical errors. Patients can reduce harmful, or *adverse*, reactions by telling you what medications they currently take and which have caused allergic reactions. Surgeons can avoid cutting in the wrong location by having patients mark the correct body part. Letting patients know what you are doing will allow them to ask questions and participate more effectively in their care.

Healthcare employers are working to create a culture of safety so medical errors will be reported and addressed. Surveys show that patients are less likely to file a lawsuit if you admit your error and apologize. Ten states have laws requiring that medical errors be made known. Two-thirds do not allow information from an apology to be used in a malpractice lawsuit. This removes one of the biggest reasons for not reporting or admitting to errors.

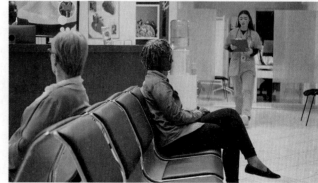

DC Studio/Shutterstock.com

Figure 14.23 You can ask for the patient's name, birth date, or address to check their identity.

Increasing Technology

New tests, treatments, and equipment can be expensive. Forbes estimates that new medical technology causes 40 to 50 percent of healthcare cost increases. Healthcare providers spent more than $40 million on information technology (IT) alone in 2019. In addition to the purchase price, changes create the need to retrain workers. Facilities may need new staff and more space for the equipment. There are also operating and maintenance costs. New technology may extend life, increasing the cost of extended care. It may also bring new side effects and their treatment costs. Many factors affect estimating the cost of technology.

Although technology has increased the cost of healthcare, recent investments in IT are lowering some costs by improving coordination of care and reducing inefficiency. Through the EHR, providers can share diagnostic test results and clinical information to avoid repeating tests. Electronic prescriptions reduce medication errors caused by messy handwriting and improve crosschecks for drug interactions and allergies. The database of patient information helps send patient reminders and track healthcare trends of large populations. These advances support system throughput and output.

Telehealth, virtual reality, and interconnected wearable devices improve access to healthcare, reduce the need for office visits, and save billions of dollars. Patients with dementia and brain damage can access virtual experiences that improve their well-being and provide motor therapy. Virtual reality can help with pain management, in place of medications. Computer simulations and robotics also support healthcare throughput. Providers plan complicated surgeries, practice new skills, and support treatments with virtual reality tools.

Artificial intelligence (AI) problem-solving models also save time and money. Biotechnology, DNA, and AI together improve the speed and accuracy of diagnostics and decision-making. Computer algorithms safely explore drug interactions and speed the process of developing and testing new drugs. Increased availability of AI-powered systems will bring many changes in throughput and output.

Robots assisted by artificial intelligence (AI) can support patient care (**Figure 14.24**). Their speed, accuracy, and ability to work without breaks has improved laboratory procedures, medication preparation, and many other repetitive tasks. They cut bone and position tools during surgery with greater precision than humans. They package medical devices and deliver supplies without contamination. They disinfect patient rooms, reducing the risk of infection for housekeeping. AI-controlled robots even serve as patient companions.

Unfortunately, adding these technologies increases the risk of data breaches and need for IT support. Some people do not trust the technology, feel that AI is too impersonal for healthcare, or worry that robots will displace people from their jobs. How do you feel about the use of robotics and AI in healthcare? What benefits and problems do you anticipate as technology increases?

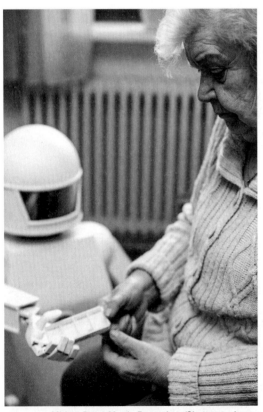

Miriam Doerr Martin Frommherz/Shutterstock.com

Figure 14.24 Autonomous medical robots can help lower costs for patient care.

Impact of the External Environment on Healthcare Systems

Healthcare adjusts to a constantly changing environment. Political influence, legal restrictions, public opinion, and funding are major influences on medical research and healthcare (**Figure 14.25**). Although these external issues are outside your control, being aware of them can help you prepare and adjust.

Biotechnology has gone through major changes in the past few decades. Since the cloning of Dolly the sheep, what biotechnology *can* do has created fear about what scientists *will* do. The power to clone humans and manipulate genetics could be misused or abused. There are also moral objections to tampering with natural selection or the creation of life. Public and political debates around these topics can affect research, legislation, and funding to resolve emerging issues.

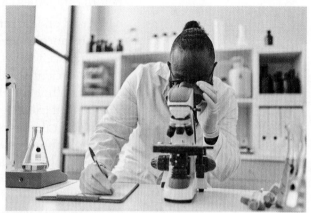

Krakenimages.com/Shutterstock.com

Figure 14.25 Although lab workers may feel isolated while performing their research, many outside factors can influence their work.

Government Regulation of Biotechnology Research and Development

Public policies control controversial issues in biotechnology research and development. There are strict rules for product development and human testing. These affect the development, availability, and safety of medications, medical devices, and procedures. When government grants fund research, politics can slow progress. Do you think the current public and political climate is favorable toward biotechnology research, or not?

Human Testing

Since the United Nations Declaration of Human Rights in 1948, the US government has tried to ensure the safety and dignity of human subjects during research. **Human testing** is research on people to show the safety and effectiveness of new treatments, as well as the nature and severity of side effects. However, the rights of a test subject must always come before the interests of a research group.

One government protection is the **Common Rule**. This regulation sets ethical standards for human subject research. It requires informed consent and gives special protection to vulnerable populations. As the name suggests, it applies to all research projects funded by the federal government and all research a federal agency regulates.

The Common Rule requires an *Institutional Review Board (IRB)* to review protections for physical safety, dignity, privacy, and informed consent of human subjects during testing. Researchers must report any adverse events that occur. Updated in 2017, the New Common Rule eases regulations on research of minimal risk, makes the review process less complex, and improves consent processes.

Product Approval

The FDA regulates the production and sale of drugs, vaccines, and other medical products based on effectiveness and safety. While it does not test drugs or medical devices itself, the FDA requires a strict approval process before companies can sell new treatments. They follow these general steps:

1. Based on laboratory studies or animal testing, a company decides a substance could be effective as a treatment (**Figure 14.26**). They submit evidence to the FDA, requesting approval for human testing.
2. FDA scientists review the application and order that further testing be put on hold or allow it to continue.
3. Clinical trials determine effectiveness and identify potential side effects in several phases of controlled clinical studies that take many years.
4. The company submits data from clinical trials and other sources to prove the drug is safe and effective and applies to the FDA for approval.
5. The FDA reviews the proposed label and inspects manufacturing facilities.
6. FDA scientists from different fields review the clinical trial data and recommend its approval if they find the drug both safe and effective.

The long process for product approval restricts the healthcare system's ability to treat patients. The 21st Century Cures Act speeds up the process for making new drugs and devices available. It emphasizes biologics, cancer treatments, products to combat the opioid crisis, and antibiotics to fight drug-resistant bacteria. The Cures Act tries to protect the patient's right to access new treatments while they are still in the development stage.

During the COVID-19 pandemic, the FDA granted *emergency-use authorization* to make new vaccines available sooner. This permission to use unapproved medical products, or use products in unapproved ways, is only allowed in public health emergencies where no other options exist. Basic safety criteria and scientific evidence of effectiveness still must be met. Manufacturers distributed COVID-19 vaccines with shorter clinical trials than usual. Their use was closely monitored and halted several times to investigate potential problems. This permission to change system throughput saved many lives.

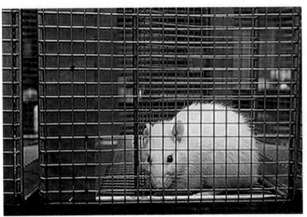

©iStock/Iculig

Figure 14.26 Medications are often tested on animals before they are tested on humans. *What is the purpose of animal testing?*

The long and rigorous approval process for drugs in the US has benefits. In the 1950s, German researchers developed the drug *thalidomide* as a sleeping pill. It also improved morning sickness in people who were pregnant. Thalidomide was sold over the counter in Germany and by prescription in the United Kingdom. The FDA refused to approve thalidomide for sale in the US until it completed the approval process showing it was safe and effective. Its use in Europe caused several thousand children to be born with limb deformities, while the impact on the US was limited to those in clinical trials.

The process is not foolproof, however. Sometimes problems from approved drugs and medical devices take years to show up. The FDA Adverse Event Reporting System (FAERS) collects data on negative effects of approved drugs. Reporting is mandatory for drug and biologic manufacturers and distributors.

The Sentinel Initiative, begun in 2008, uses EHR data to monitor the safety and effectiveness of drugs and medical devices. Those that are not safe can be *recalled*, or withdrawn from the market. In addition, the FDA alerts the public about major safety issues.

Public information can push the recall process forward. In 2010, the FDA cited the manufacturer of infant liquid forms of Tylenol®, Motrin®, Zyrtec®, and Benadryl® for manufacturing problems. The manufacturer voluntarily recalled 43 products. In 2020, the FDA requested that Zantac®, used for heartburn and acid reflux, be removed from the market due to reports of carcinogens and serious side effects. The number of drug recalls listed on the FDA website has been increasing as the system uses changes in throughput and output to improve safety.

Sale of Medical Products

The FDA regulates the marketing, labeling, and sale of medical products. Pharmaceutical companies spend an average of $21,000 per doctor per year on marketing, grant funding, conference attendance, and gifts. Doctors write more than four billion prescriptions per year in the US. They often participate in clinical trials or receive free samples (**Figure 14.27**). When a doctor benefits from recommending a particular medication or procedure, this creates a conflict of interest that can put patient health at risk.

Ethics guidelines of professional organizations serve as an external constraint, but updates in 2002 and 2009 did not end these influential practices. The cost of medications rose faster than all other medical expenses in the last 15 years. This led the Office of the Inspector General to restrict direct financial relationships between pharmaceutical companies and doctors. How would you change the system to reduce the influence of pharmaceutical companies?

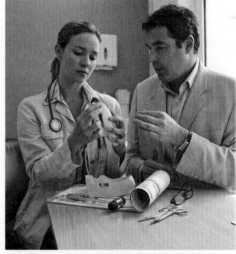

Image Point Fr/Shutterstock.com

Figure 14.27 Doctors receiving free samples or payments from pharmaceutical companies to push certain drugs can create a conflict of interest.

The FDA also regulates labels for prescription drugs and medical products sold in the US. Package labels and inserts must contain a summary of the approved safe and effective uses, dosing instructions, and warnings for known risks or contraindications. They give doctors the information they need to prescribe drugs appropriately. This information must be based on data from human clinical trials. The label cannot contain false or misleading advertising.

In off-label use, a doctor prescribes a medication in a way not specified in the product information. There may be evidence that off-label use is safe and beneficial, but it has not been through rigorous testing. Some off-label uses take advantage of known side effects, such as drowsiness. They may also be prescribed for an age group not listed in the drugs' information. Because the medical industry regulates prescribing practices, not the FDA, off-label use is legal but may be risky.

Negative side effects and dangerous outcomes increase with off-label use. For example, when children take adult psychiatric medications to treat attention-deficit disorders, there is a higher risk of suicide. Broader testing could avoid these risks, but would also slow new medications reaching the market. How do you feel about these external limitations on medical products? Would you consider taking a drug prescribed off-label if there were no other medications available?

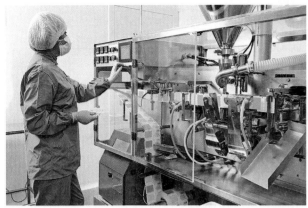

Dmitry Kalinovsky/Shutterstock.com

Figure 14.28 The lengthy development and approval process for new drugs can be expensive. *How does this relate to funding for biotechnology research?*

Biotechnology Research Funding

Funding priorities of government organizations, such as the National Science Foundation and NIH, are an external constraint that changes with political agendas and societal events. Funding affects which biotechnology research projects are completed. Funding for genetics, preventive care, infectious disease, and mental health has surpassed funding for individual diseases such as cancer and HIV.

Cooperative research agreements with government agencies encourage companies to invest in research that will benefit society. Funds may cover broad areas far removed from healthcare. However, advances in one industry, such as space science, can produce technology that advances the study of another area. Tools you use every day in homes and hospitals, such as infrared thermometers and water purification systems, were developed through space science research. The growth of biomedical research and scientific gains in the US keep the nation competitive in the global economy.

The development of new drugs is risky, costly, and time-consuming (**Figure 14.28**). It costs more than $1 billion to bring a new drug through the research and approval process before it starts to earn a profit. Products marketed to large numbers of people, such as new treatments for arthritis or high blood pressure, are usually most profitable. *Orphan drugs*, used by a very small number of people, would not be profitable without incentives such as biotechnology funding and tax credits.

Owning a **patent** restricts others' ability to copy a new invention and increases profitability. Other researchers must pay to use the patented product or technique. To qualify for a 20-year patent in the US, a research process or material must be unique or changed in some way to make it more useful. Researchers have patented recombinant DNA, synthesized sequencing of DNA, stem cell production lines, and specialized techniques for diagnostic testing. How do the constraints of patents affect the healthcare system?

A patent holder usually charges high prices for their product while it has patent protection. This helps them recover research and development costs but limits growth of related ideas. Once a patent expires, competitors can develop comparable products. **Generic** drugs are chemically identical to brand-name products and meet the same standards for quality and performance but usually cost less.

Follow-up patents can expand or block further research on a patented discovery. For-profit research companies worry patents will limit free exchange of research material and future innovation. Some have joined patent pools to make groups of related discoveries and research tools available with one licensing fee. This reduces profits but encourages collaboration. Patent pools have improved access for countries with lower incomes to develop AIDS medications.

Emerging Diseases and Epidemics

The cost and effort to control infections has a major impact on the healthcare system. Many infections, such as the seasonal flu virus, have been around for a long time and follow predictable patterns. Aseptic practices and vaccination help prevent outbreaks and reduce seasonal demands for healthcare services. Many healthcare facilities require their employees to be vaccinated each year.

Reemerging and **emerging diseases** are those that suddenly increase or threaten to increase. Since 1970, more than 1,500 new pathogens have been discovered. Many are emerging diseases. Some have become major epidemics that risk public health, and the number of outbreaks is becoming more frequent (**Figure 14.29**). The worst epidemics are infections that are easily spread and hard to kill. COVID-19, caused by the novel coronavirus (2019 nCoV), became a global pandemic in early 2020. In two years, it infected more than 500 million people and took more than 6 million lives. Although vaccines were developed, it mutated and spread easily. It is likely people will continue to live with a seasonal version of this virus and its variants.

One key to slowing the spread of epidemics has been testing and tracing close contacts of those infected. During an epidemic, this places an added strain on the healthcare delivery system. A rapid and effective test must be developed. Then, diagnostic workers must collect and analyze samples from a large number of people to locate and isolate the source.

Sometimes the source of infection is a creature, rather than another person. Hanta virus spreads by exposure to infected mice droppings. The Black Plague spreads by fleas on infected rats. Mosquitoes carry Zika virus, malaria, dengue, and yellow fever. These diseases hit countries with the lowest incomes and densest populations the hardest. The WHO and other health organizations play a large role in wiping out, or *eradicating*, these diseases by providing clean water, mosquito netting, and vaccination programs. Using a systems-thinking model, what ideas can you suggest to slow the number of emerging diseases and epidemics or their impact on people?

Drug-resistant bacteria are a growing concern. These strains of bacteria were once treatable but are slowly becoming immune to more and more antibiotics. Vancomycin is the strongest antibiotic for use against the worst intestinal infections, but it no longer works on more than 30 percent of *Enterococcus* bacterial infections. In 2020, the WHO called attention to the growing need to fund research for new antibiotics to fight drug-resistant bacteria.

Time Line of Epidemics (2000–2020)

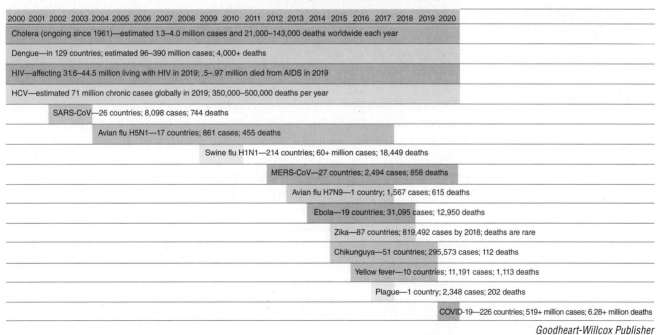

Goodheart-Willcox Publisher

Figure 14.29 This time line shows the increase in epidemics from 2000 to 2020.

Biotechnology can solve problems with epidemics and drug-resistant bacteria, but the external environment limits options. Regulations slow the development process, while pricing and reimbursement issues take away financial incentives. New classes of antibiotics have not reached the market since 1987, and there are few specialists remaining in the field to take on this complex research. Even if a new class of antibiotics is developed, it must be used sparingly to slow further resistance. Limited use increases the cost per dose and reduces potential profits. This requires a new economic model to make it cost effective. What changes to the external environment would support continued research on antibiotics?

Advances in Biotechnology

Advances in biotechnology affect the environment healthcare systems operate in and the way care is provided. These advances bring legal and ethical questions that challenge social norms. Those on the leading edge will face academic, political, and public scrutiny.

The ability to customize medical care to an individual patient promises better outcomes. Genomic medicine involves using information from a person's genetic markers to make decisions about healthcare. The high cost of processing individual DNA samples and tailoring each person's treatments limits this approach. There is no one to share the cost of developing each treatment. Lower-cost sequencing options exist, but they provide less accurate and useful data.

When the cost of genome sequencing becomes more affordable, genetic information may be added to the EHR at birth. This would help predict and prevent disease, identify drug sensitivities, and determine treatments. These are wonderful advances for healthcare, but will it be affordable? Will insurance cover it? How will this immense amount of data be stored and secured? Who will have access to the data, and for what purposes? People have begun to ask these important questions as the technology moves forward.

Pharmacogenomics is concerned with an individual's response to medications. Healthcare workers already test bacteria to know which antibiotics work best to treat specific types of infection (**Figure 14.30**). Having a genetic understanding of an individual's disease, such as cancer, allows even more precise treatment. Drug dosages are already calculated according to the height, weight, and age of a patient. They can also be adjusted for each person's genetic attributes to gain the most benefit with the smallest amount of unwanted side effects.

Precision medicine uses pharmacogenomics and other tools to choose targeted therapies. These are based on genetic, biological, and environmental data from a large population with similar patterns of disease, responses to treatment, and other characteristics. Computers predict which treatment and prevention strategies will work best for a large group of people or set of disease markers. Not all breast cancers should receive the same chemotherapy or radiation treatments. Treatments do not work the same for all populations.

The popularity of personal electronics and smartphones has led to the development of health-tracking devices that support precision medicine. Phone apps can monitor activity level, heart rate, and other data. Treatment devices, such as adjustable insulin pumps, can be individualized. New attachments for smartphones, such as an echocardiogram or real-time blood sugar monitor, bring lab testing right into the doctor's office for immediate action and discussion. Doctors can also monitor treatment from a distance and send a patient to the hospital before small changes become life threatening.

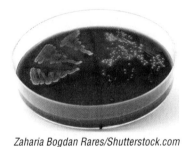

Zaharia Bogdan Rares/Shutterstock.com

Figure 14.30
Antibiotic-sensitivity tests determine how bacterial infections respond to different medications. Pharmacogenomics can predict how some people will respond to certain treatments.

Precision medicine will require changes in the healthcare system. Data-collection methods must be standardized to share research data across the country. Genetic information will need to be added to the EHR. The information overload will require AI to sort, analyze, and monitor the large data sets. Healthcare providers will need more training on molecular genetics and biochemistry to apply the information to clinical care and explain it to patients.

There are also concerns about equal access with the increasingly diverse population and expected high costs of these new treatments (**Figure 14.31**). The NIH launched the *All of Us* Research Program in 2018 to increase diversity in the biomedical data pool. Combining this biomedical data with data on social determinants of health may help identify, predict, and solve health issues for all populations. Will patients from different cultures be open to these new methods? Are healthcare providers prepared to talk about precision medicine with people who have historically had low health literacy? These issues may result in even wider gaps between socioeconomic groups. This affects nearly all areas of the healthcare system—input, throughput, output, and the feedback loop.

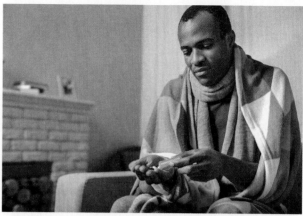

Dmitry Zinkevych/Shutterstock.com

Figure 14.31 The high cost of new treatments can mean that some people do not have equal access to healthcare.

Lesson 14.3 Review

 Complete the *Map Your Reading* graphic organizer for the section you just read.

1. Quality improvement tasks use a PDCA model that relies on quantitative and _____ data. (14.3-1)
   A. statistical
   B. benchmark
   C. qualitative
   D. reactive

2. Which of these is a preventable and treatable mental health condition best managed by coordinating healthcare provider systems? (14.3-2)
   A. Substance use disorder
   B. Health disparities
   C. Pertussis
   D. Tuberculosis

3. Baby boomer retirements and increased demand are causing a shortage of _____, as well as PCPs in rural areas. (14.3-2)
   A. medicine
   B. treatments
   C. nurses
   D. health insurance

4. Constantly changing technology has increased costs in healthcare, but _____, telehealth, and AI can lower costs and make care safer, more accessible, and efficient. (14.3-3)
   A. defensive medicine
   B. the EHR
   C. patents
   D. biotechnology

5. Which technology can help physicians practice new skills? (14.3-3)
   A. Virtual reality
   B. AI
   C. Robotics
   D. Telehealth

6. Cases of emerging diseases are increasing, and those that spread easily can become a(n) (14.3-4)
   A. epidemic
   B. vaccine
   C. infection
   D. flu

7. Outside influences in biotechnology include government regulation, _____, and funding. (14.3-4)
   A. organizational rules
   B. public opinion
   C. hospital rules
   D. CDC guidelines

Chapter 14 Review and Assessment

Chapter Summary

14.1-1 Healthcare delivery and payment both operate as systems. Systems theory can analyze the causes and effects of changes between related parts of a system. A change in input, throughput, output, feedback, or the environment will have a ripple effect on all other resources, structures, processes, and end results in a system.

14.1-2 There are many types of healthcare delivery facilities and services at the national, state, and local levels. Each has a different purpose or serves a different group of people.

14.1-3 An organizational chart shows the relationships between people in an organization. The lines of authority show who is in charge.

14.2-1 Health insurance pools together monthly premiums from many people to cover the cost of healthcare. It is important for healthcare workers and consumers to understand terms related to insurance coverage, claims, and fees.

14.2-2 Health insurance in the US was originally tied to employment. Government-financed healthcare grew for people not covered by employers. Insurance now covers many procedures and has become very expensive.

14.2-3 Managed care refers to a payment system that attempts to control healthcare costs. HMOs, PPOs, Medicare, and Medicaid are common forms of health insurance.

14.3-1 Quality improvement is a process teams use to make a systemic change. Aspects include setting goals for improving system processes, collecting quantitative or qualitative data, comparing results to benchmarks, and integrating successful solutions.

14.3-2 Poor patient health, lack of access to healthcare or insurance, increasing substance use, and the aging population make the healthcare system more expensive. Patients have the right to a healthcare system that meets their needs, but they must use the system responsibly.

14.3-3 Changes in system throughput, such as rising costs and increasing technology, impact system input and output. Some changes are beneficial, supporting healthcare professionals and patients and making healthcare safer and more efficient.

14.3-4 Emerging issues, such as the spread of infection and advances in biotechnology, have caused systemic changes. Government regulations, funding, public opinion, and political climate in the external environment may affect response to these issues.

Maximize Your Professional Vocabulary

1. **Storytelling.** Create a short story using a minimum of eight terms from the chapter in a realistic manner. Underline the terms you have used.

2. **Term Charades.** Make term cards using the professional vocabulary terms in this chapter. You can use these cards to play term charades in groups of four or more students.

   A. Use one deck of term cards for four or more players. Divide players into two teams. Play alternates between the two teams.

   B. The first person will draw a term card from the deck to act out for their team. They have one minute to nonverbally communicate the meaning of this term to their team through acting or drawing. They cannot use words or letters of any kind.

   C. After one minute, if the team has not guessed the word, the other team can join in to guess the term.

   D. The point goes to the team that correctly guesses the term. The team with the highest score at the end of the game is the winner. The game ends after a preset amount of time or when you run out of new term cards.

Reflect on Your Reading

1. Reconsider your last experience in a healthcare facility. Can you identify the type of healthcare system? What were the inputs, throughputs, outputs, and feedback loops for your experience? What is one internal or external environmental constraint that affected this facility and the way they function? Use your new professional vocabulary in your responses.

Review and Recall

1. Which of the following are factors of a system? Choose all that apply. (14.1-1)
   A. Analysis
   B. Input
   C. Throughput
   D. Environment

2. The healthcare delivery system is a mix of _____ and organizations that provide healthcare products and services. (14.1-2)
   A. clinics
   B. hospitals
   C. individuals
   D. doctors

3. The _____ is an outline of the levels of authority within an organization. (14.1-3)
   A. clinic chart
   B. department map
   C. support map
   D. organizational chart

4. What is the shared healthcare payment system of groups of people who face a risk? (14.2-1)
   A. Insurance
   B. Premium
   C. Coinsurance
   D. Copayment

5. During World War II's wage freeze, employers offered _____ to attract workers. (14.2-2)
   A. medical leave
   B. short-term disability
   C. health insurance
   D. Medicare

6. Which of these was developed to limit overuse and reduce rising costs of health insurance? (14.2-3)
   A. Free market
   B. Managed care
   C. Sick leave
   D. Payment systems

7. Which is *not* part of the PDCA model? (14.3-1)
   A. Identify opportunities for change
   B. Make changes and collect data on performance
   C. Analyze data for successes and failures
   D. Discipline employees for mistakes

8. Patient _____ include(s) receipt of accurate information, choice of providers, access to care, participation in treatment decisions, equal treatment, privacy of information, and the ability to appeal decisions. (14.3-2)
   A. rights
   B. care
   C. privacy
   D. consent

9. Which changes have a negative effect on healthcare system throughput? Choose all that apply. (14.3-3)
   A. Rising costs
   B. Medical errors
   C. Electronic health records
   D. Artificial intelligence

10. Which of the following statements about biotechnology is false? (14.3-4)
    A. Biotechnology research on individual diseases is a current funding priority.
    B. A long drug-approval process is required to test safety and effectiveness.
    C. External constraints have restricted the development of new antibiotics.
    D. Precision medicine could widen the gap between socioeconomic groups.

Build Core Skills

1. **Reading.** Review Lesson 14.1 about healthcare delivery systems. Use the internet or personal knowledge to identify providers in your community that fit the descriptions for five types of healthcare delivery systems.

2. **Critical Thinking.** Review the section on QI. How does this process support the healthcare system? Whom does it benefit? Whom could it negatively impact? What concerns do you have about the PDCA process? Would you get involved in a QI team? Why or why not?

3. **Critical Thinking.** Compare and contrast terms using a Venn diagram. What are the similarities and differences between *independent living* and *home health care*? *HMO* and *PPO*? *CDC* and *NIH*? *Medicare* and *Medicaid*?

4. **Speaking and Listening.** With a partner or small group, debate the pros and cons of practicing defensive medicine. Why do insurance companies focus on this issue?

5. **Reading.** Go to the Department of Health and Human Services website to learn more about the agencies that protect health. Write a summary of the duties and responsibilities of the Department of Health and Human Services.

6. **Writing.** If the government is responsible for healthcare, should government ensure you take care of yourself? Should government control which foods people can eat? How do your state and local governments affect health services in your community? Write brief answers to each question and discuss with a partner.

7. **Critical Thinking.** Visit two types of healthcare facilities. Use a Venn diagram to compare and contrast the two facilities you visited.

8. **Math.** Suppose a person who has health insurance has an 80/20 copayment. How much would this person pay if billed for $300 worth of care? What would the cost to the insured person be if there was a $500 deductible and the copayment did not take effect until the deductible was met?

9. **Math.** A family of four is trying to choose health insurance that will cost the least based on their typical care needs from the prior year. Explain which plan you would choose for them and why.

   Plan A has a monthly premium of $300 and charges a $10 copayment per prescription, but all office visits and dental care are included.

   Plan B has a monthly premium of $250 and charges a $15 copayment per prescription and 10 percent copayment per office visit. Two dental cleanings are included per person, but additional dental work requires a 20 percent copayment.

   The family visited the doctor's office 10 times last year at an actual cost before insurance averaging $120 per visit. They purchased 20 prescriptions during the year. Each family member had two cleanings, and there was one filling at an actual cost of $300.

10. **Speaking and Listening.** Suppose you have a toothache but are told the next available appointment is in two weeks. What should you do and say to self-advocate? Practice with a partner. Switch roles, listen, and give your partner feedback as well.

11. **Writing.** Research information about signs and symptoms of a substance use disorder. Create a poster to educate others about how to recognize the signs and symptoms and how they can get help.

12. **Reading.** Review Lesson 14.3 on patient rights and responsibilities. Why should healthcare professionals understand and honor patient rights? Why should patients be compliant? What happens to the quality of care when either of these is missing?

13. **Writing.** Write a five-sentence paragraph demonstrating your understanding of patient rights. Use terms and concepts from the chapter.

14. **Math.** A study of 780 Medicare patients discharged from hospitals revealed the following statistics related to medical errors:

    1.5% died due to medical error.

    14.3% experienced permanent medical harm.

    14.3% suffered temporary harm that was caught and reversed.

    Answer the following questions.

    A. How many patients died? How many experienced permanent harm?

    B. Now put these statistics in perspective. What is the ratio of your school population to this group of Medicare patients?

    C. If your school were that group of patients, how many students in your school would die, and how many would be personally affected by medical errors?

15. **Math.** Visit the Brookings.edu website. Use the search tool to find "A dozen facts about the economics of the US healthcare system." Analyze the graph(s) and explanation for one of the facts listed. Write three sentences summarizing the data provided in the graph(s).

16. **Reading.** Choose a political figure and research their views or voting record on a biotechnology issue such as genetic engineering, stem cell research, genomic medicine, FDA product approval guidelines, or antibiotic production. What types of biotechnology issues do they support? Which do they oppose?

17. **Critical Thinking.** Think of a healthcare delivery system in your community, such as a hospital, nursing home, or mental health facility. Identify or describe each aspect of this system:

    A. Input—who or what are the resources coming into the system?

    B. Throughput—how does this facility's location connect with its purpose? How do people who use this facility pay for their care? How do people learn about this facility?

    C. Output—what are the quantity, quality, or cost outcomes of this system's operation?

    D. Feedback loop—how does the facility keep a flow of people, information, and resources coming back into the system?

    E. Environmental constraints—identify a potential internal constraint (such as employee satisfaction or teamwork) and external constraint (such as changing cultural makeup of the community) that affect how this system functions.

18. **Critical Thinking.** In 2020, there were 200.3 million private insurance enrollees and 159.3 million government insurance enrollees. How can private insurance plans cover so many more people at a lower cost than government-based plans? Consider who is likely to need Medicare and Medicaid insurance plans.

Activate Your Learning

1. Imagine you are a public relations specialist for a local nonprofit organization. Search their website to gather information about the services they provide and the ways youth could support their mission. Develop a brochure, public service announcement, or other promotional material to encourage people to support them.

2. Patient responsibilities to "maximize healthy habits" include being physically active, eating a healthy diet, following your doctor's recommended diagnostic testing, and not smoking. Conduct a survey of at least 20 people. Which of these responsibilities are they willing to follow? Which are they not willing to do? Summarize your findings. What does this mean to you as a future healthcare worker?

Think and Act Like a Healthcare Worker

1. Using the systems theory model from Lesson 14.1, discuss how changes in technology would affect diagnostic workers' jobs, the cost of healthcare, and the safety of healthcare professionals and the public. What are the anticipated changes in input, throughput, output, and feedback loops in a healthcare facility?

2. Imagine you work in a large hospital with an organizational chart similar to the one in Figure 14.7. Several patient surveys show some dissatisfaction with the bedside manner of their orthopedic surgeons. Design a QI project to address this issue following the PDCA model. Whom would you include on your QI team? What would you suggest the team do to address the problem? What data would you use to monitor your progress?

3. Suppose you work as a dental hygienist. How will you call the patient from the waiting room? When you get the patient to the chair, how will you make sure you have the correct person before proceeding with care?

4. Imagine you are a biotechnology researcher for a new cure for a particular type of cancer. You are ready to begin clinical trials on patients who have this cancer. You must obtain informed consent from your research subjects to meet requirements of the Common Rule. Develop a written statement explaining the nature of the treatment, any risks or discomfort that may be involved, and any available alternatives to the treatment. End with a statement about what information will be collected and how it will be used and asking them to sign the voluntary informed consent form to participate.

Go to the Source

1. Review a summary of insurance benefits and coverage. You can find samples of this document for many health insurance plans online. Find an example of a limitation and an exclusion in a health insurance summary.

2. Visit the Grants.gov website. Use the "Search Grants" tab and enter an area of medical research to find possible funding sources. Examine the requirements for one grant. Summarize the purpose, who can apply, how much money is available, and who is providing the funds.

HOSA Event Prep: Public Health

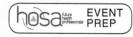

Tim is a public health nurse who works in a local community seeing an increase in type 2 diabetes among young adults. He has also noticed an increase in hypertension and early heart disease. Many people in the population use government assistance to purchase food. When considering ways to help with lifestyle changes and nutrition classes, Tim assesses the neighborhood. The nearest grocery store is 10 miles away, and many rely on public transportation. In the immediate area, there are many fast-food restaurants and a few gas stations. There is a community center with a big, open lot. Tim surveys people in the community about their needs and interests. Using this feedback, he schedules weekly nutrition classes and gets people together on Saturdays to grow a garden. During weekly classes, Tim gives heart-healthy food demonstrations and talks about healthier habits. He also sets up weekly blood pressure checks. Within a month, many have improved their blood sugar and blood pressure.

Think About It

1. Explain how Tim's actions support public health.

2. What environmental constraints are affecting this community?

3. What is another approach that could reduce the incidence of diabetes in this community?

Chapter 15

Ethical Issues

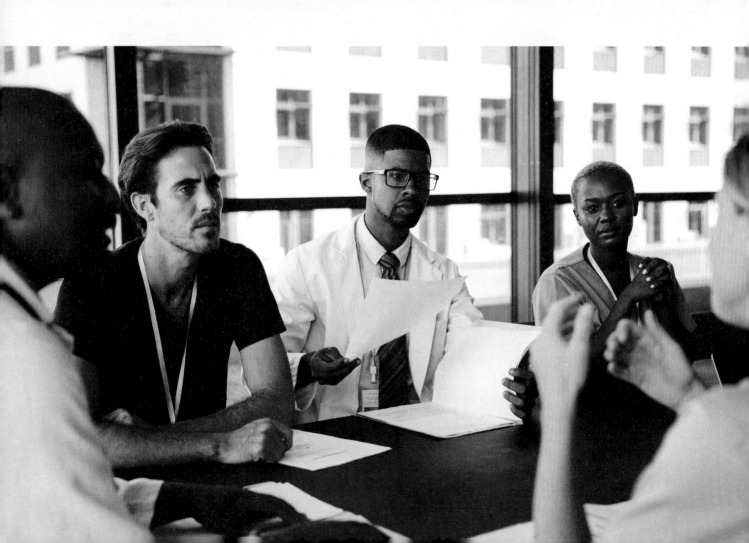

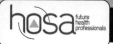

Issues in healthcare may not be black and white. There can be many sides or choices. Sometimes choices may have ethical implications, which can lead to debates about what to do. Debating is a way to discuss pros and cons of a topic. It is also a way to persuade people to understand your perspective or your beliefs. Ethics are an important part of the discussion of medical issues. Each year HOSA provides a topic for the *Biomedical Debate* competition. This is a team event, and teams prepare to debate the pros and cons of the annual health topic. This allows competitors to research both sides of the issue.

Go to the HOSA website to learn more about the HOSA *Biomedical Debate* event. Find out the purpose of the event, what is involved in the event, and what knowledge is demonstrated in the event.

As you prepare for HOSA competitive events, be sure to check the website and talk with your HOSA advisor for the most up-to-date guidelines and procedures. Once you have learned about the *Biomedical Debate* event, answer the following questions:

1. How might participating in this event benefit you personally and your future career? Explain.
2. Are you interested in participating in this event? Why or why not?

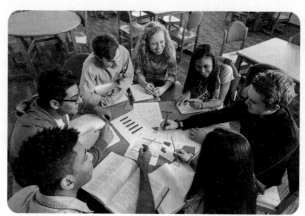

SDI Productions/E+ via Getty Images

 ## Connect with Your Reading

What is the most difficult decision you have had to make? How did you decide what to do? Decision-making in the field of medicine is complex. It may involve several people and competing points of view. When Dr. Braun was caring for Ann at the end of life, Ann said she wanted to try every possible treatment. She was in her 60s and already had multiple complications of heart failure, diabetes, and kidney failure. Dr. Braun knew her life could not be saved. What options should he present, knowing treatment would be difficult, expensive, and futile? If she asked for treatment anyhow, should he do it? Should he allow her to make poor decisions for herself? If she asked for medication to end her life, should he comply? These are some of the difficult questions the field of medical ethics can help people answer.

 ## Map Your Reading

Can you identify some of the ethical issues healthcare workers face in their career? What support is available to help with these decisions? Create a visual summary to record your ideas. Begin with a sheet of paper. Fold the top edge down and the bottom edge up to meet near the center of the page. Label the top flap *Ethical Issues* and the bottom flap *Decision-Making*. When you finish reading each section in the chapter, open the flaps and add key words or symbols to illustrate the main points. Finally, write a sentence on each flap to summarize these important topics.

Chapter opener image: Goodboy Picture Company/E+ via Getty Images

Ethical Principles in Healthcare

ESSENTIAL QUESTION

How do ethical principles and codes support a healthcare worker faced with an ethical decision?

Learning Outcomes

After studying this lesson, you will be able to

15.1-1 differentiate between legal and ethical principles impacting healthcare.

15.1-2 explain the purpose of a professional code of ethics.

15.1-3 describe ethical dilemmas in healthcare.

15.1-4 explain how to manage ethical decision-making.

Professional Vocabulary

Essential Terms

code of ethics   a set of guiding principles that tell professionals how they are expected to act

dilemma   a situation requiring you to make a difficult choice between two or more conflicting options

ethical   fitting with someone's personal morals or professional rules of conduct

Important Terms

ethics committee

morals

values

Introduction

You make many decisions every day. Easy decisions require little effort, and their outcomes may be unimportant. Other decisions can be more difficult and may have lasting consequences. A healthcare worker's decisions can impact many people. They cannot be made on a whim or with selfish intentions. Healthcare workers need guidelines for decision-making that can be applied to many situations for the good of all.

15.1-1 Defining Ethical Principles

Morals and values define **ethical** issues, while laws define legal issues. **Morals** are people's beliefs about right and wrong learned from family, friends, traditions, and experiences. **Values** express which principles are most important to a person. These two factors guide ethical decision-making and standards of appropriate behavior. For example, do you value honesty or success more?

When you need to pass a test, is cheating acceptable if it helps you succeed? Or will you risk failure to avoid cheating?

People justify their ethical decisions with specific theories and principles. In the medical field, four ethical principles form the basis for decision-making:

- *Autonomy* is the patient's right to make decisions for individual medical care, including the right to refuse care.
- *Beneficence* is the duty to do good or act in the best interest of the patient.
- *Non-malfeasance* is the duty to do no harm or cause the least harm possible to reach a beneficial outcome for the patient.
- *Justice* is the idea that all persons are equal and should receive fair and equal treatment.

15.1-2 Ethical Codes

Many careers have expected standards laid out by their professional organization. These may be written in a **code of ethics**, or formal statement of expected conduct for professionals in that field. Professional codes of ethics usually tell healthcare workers to put patients above all other interests and maintain professional standards. They often emphasize patient rights and personal responsibility.

One of the best-known ethical codes is the Hippocratic Oath for Physicians. Most doctors swear to some form of this oath when they graduate from medical school (**Figure 15.1**). The oath dates back to Hippocrates, an ancient Greek philosopher known as the "father of medicine." The words have changed over time to use more modern language and avoid controversial ethical topics in the original oath.

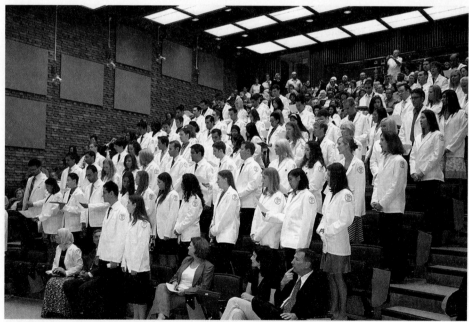

Wayne State University School of Medicine

Figure 15.1 These medical students at Wayne State University are swearing the Hippocratic Oath, now called the Physician's Pledge, as part of their graduation ceremony. *What questions or concerns would you have about swearing a professional oath?*

Adopted by the 2nd General Assembly of the World Medical Association, Geneva, Switzerland, September 1948 and amended by the 22nd World Medical Assembly, Sydney, Australia, August 1968 and the 35th World Medical Assembly, Venice, Italy, October 1983 and the 46th WMA General Assembly, Stockholm, Sweden, September 1994 and editorially revised by the 170th WMA Council Session, Divonne-les-Bains, France, May 2005 and the 173rd WMA Council Session, Divonne-les-Bains, France, May 2006 and amended by the 68th WMA General Assembly, Chicago, United States, October 2017

The Physician's Pledge

AS A MEMBER OF THE MEDICAL PROFESSION:

I SOLEMNLY PLEDGE to dedicate my life to the service of humanity;

THE HEALTH AND WELL-BEING OF MY PATIENT will be my first consideration;

I WILL RESPECT the autonomy and dignity of my patient;

I WILL MAINTAIN the utmost respect for human life;

I WILL NOT PERMIT considerations of age, disease or disability, creed, ethnic origin, gender, nationality, political affiliation, race, sexual orientation, social standing or any other factor to intervene between my duty and my patient;

I WILL RESPECT the secrets that are confided in me, even after the patient has died;

I WILL PRACTISE my profession with conscience and dignity and in accordance with good medical practice;

I WILL FOSTER the honour and noble traditions of the medical profession;

I WILL GIVE to my teachers, colleagues, and students the respect and gratitude that is their due;

I WILL SHARE my medical knowledge for the benefit of the patient and the advancement of healthcare;

I WILL ATTEND TO my own health, well-being, and abilities in order to provide care of the highest standard;

I WILL NOT USE my medical knowledge to violate human rights and civil liberties, even under threat;

I MAKE THESE PROMISES solemnly, freely, and upon my honour.

Courtesy of the World Medical Association (WMA)

Figure 15.2 The Physician's Pledge describes the standards of conduct expected of doctors.

The World Medical Association (WMA) adopted the most recent version of this oath in 2017 (**Figure 15.2**). Codes of ethics promote high standards of practice, spell out core values, and provide professionals with guidance to help them handle difficult choices. They encourage professionals to build a relationship of trust and respect with their patients, patients' families, and coworkers. They also require them to cooperate in any investigation of unethical behavior for themselves or others and report violations they see.

15.1-3 Ethical Dilemmas

All people face ethical **dilemmas** at some point in their lives. These are problems that require a difficult choice between two conflicting but morally or ethically correct options. Sometimes the choice is personal, such as which friend to support in a disagreement. Others may involve a conflict between work requirements and personal or religious beliefs. For example, some people may view medical procedures like organ donation, in vitro fertilization, or euthanasia as "playing God" or deciding who should live or die.

Laws guide some decisions, such as privacy and scope of practice. Scope of practice is a legal term that describes limits on the skills healthcare workers can perform within their training and certification. With current workforce shortages, healthcare workers may be tempted to complete tasks outside their scope of practice. They may feel they have watched a procedure often enough to do it themselves. They may have experience from working in a different state under different rules. They may even feel a moral obligation to help a patient when no one else is available. Remember that scope-of-practice laws were created to protect patients. Operating outside your scope of practice is unethical, especially when the patient is not aware of the limits of your training and scope of practice. Patients have the right to qualified care providers and safe healthcare practices.

In healthcare, two different principles in your code of conduct may also come into conflict. Consider the conflicting values of organ donation. Transplanting living tissue, such as bone marrow or a kidney, may cause pain or harm to a healthy donor. Is this acceptable to save someone else's life? How do you decide who should receive the available organs? The United Network for Organ Sharing (UNOS) maintains the nation's transplant waiting list and creates policies for best using the limited supply of organs. UNOS and the donor's physician can help donors think through possible complications and whether they want to do a direct donation, transplant exchange, or donation to a stranger (**Figure 15.3**).

No religion formally requires or bans organ donation or transplantation, but some people may prefer living donation or xenotransplantation (from animals). Organ transplantation increased to about 108 transplants per day by 2020. Still, a new person is added to the transplant waiting list about every 10 minutes, and about 20 people die each day while waiting. The majority of organ donors are deceased. The best way to have your organ-donation wishes followed, whether you want to donate or not, is to talk to your family about your wishes and complete a living will.

Another decision involving values is what to do with leftover embryos, eggs, or sperm after in vitro fertilization. Should a couple pay for cryopreservation (frozen storage), donate them to someone else, bury them, have them destroyed, or sign them over for medical research? Fertility centers will present the options as part of informed consent paperwork, but the couple may have a strong attachment to their embryos after completing the fertilization process. If the couple separates before their embryos are used, they may end up in court to decide the fate of their embryos. People with certain religious beliefs may consider an embryo an unborn child with a right to life and strongly oppose its destruction or use in research.

Likewise, should healthcare workers support their patient's right to die, or does this conflict with their code of ethics? As of 2021, either physician-assisted suicide or euthanasia was legal in California, Colorado, District of Columbia, Hawaii, Maine, Montana, New Jersey, Oregon, Vermont, and Washington. Seventeen more states were discussing laws. Each state sets its own rules, but physician-assisted suicide generally applies to patients with terminal illnesses and requires some level of medical professional involvement. These laws may bring conflict between the principles of autonomy and non-malfeasance. Physician-assisted suicide may also conflict with the values of a religion-based healthcare employer.

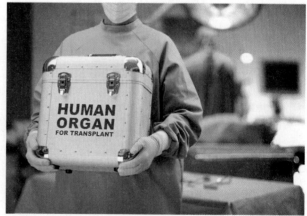

sturti/E+ via Getty Images

Figure 15.3 Organ transplantation may involve conflicting values. *Have you discussed this topic with your family?*

15.1-4 Ethical Decision-Making

Ethical decision-making has become more difficult as new advances change healthcare. New techniques, medications, and technology have extended life and redefined death. Healthcare providers and families face difficult decisions that did not exist a generation ago. Today, healthcare providers must ask what "quality of life" is and how they can preserve or improve it for patients. When should someone be resuscitated versus allowed to die a quick death? Should a doctor recommend painful treatments that might extend the life of a patient with a terminal illness who has just weeks to live? Should a doctor recommend supportive care for a patient to spend those last weeks pain-free at home? Should machines be used to keep alive a patient in a vegetative state who has no hope for recovering? To what extent, and expense, should healthcare go to save a "micro preemie" baby born at 22 weeks with a 10-percent chance of survival and 70-percent likelihood of lifelong disabilities?

Issues that are not defined by law may require the help of an **ethics committee** or board. This group meets to discuss unusual or controversial cases. They provide clarity, make sure all sides are represented, and give opinions, but they do not make final decisions.

When faced with a difficult decision, you can use a decision-making process to think through your options (**Figure 15.4**). First, determine what the problem is and which people are involved or affected. It is important to differentiate between assumptions and facts. Next, explore all the possible actions, including inaction. What are the effects or potential outcomes of each option? Look at the issue from different points of view, considering all the stakeholders involved. Then, clarify the values involved and establish what is most important in this situation. Finally, choose the best action for meeting everyone's needs while causing the least possible harm.

Steps for Ethical Decision-Making

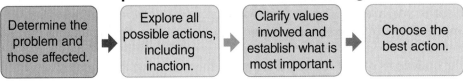

Determine the problem and those affected. → Explore all possible actions, including inaction. → Clarify values involved and establish what is most important. → Choose the best action.

Goodheart-Willcox Publisher

Figure 15.4 To use ethical decision-making, you can follow the steps shown here.

Lesson 15.1 Review

 Complete the *Map Your Reading* graphic organizer for the section you just read.

1. Morals guide _____ decisions about right and wrong. (15.1-1)
   A. legal
   B. ethical
   C. correct
   D. important

2. The Hippocratic Oath is a famous professional code of _____ outlining the principles of beneficence, non-malfeasance, autonomy, and justice. (15.1-2)
   A. laws
   B. conduct
   C. ethics
   D. morals

3. _____ can provide advice on how to handle ethical dilemmas that involve a conflict between two codes of ethics. (15.1-3)
   A. Moral committees
   B. Ethics committees
   C. Values committees
   D. Conduct committees

4. An ethical decision-making process requires you to consider which of the following? Choose all that apply. (15.1-4)
   A. The nature of the problem
   B. The effect on each of the stakeholders
   C. All possible options
   D. The effect of inaction

Ethical Work Practices

Learning Outcomes

After studying this lesson, you will be able to

15.2-1 discuss the benefits of a strong work ethic and soft skills.

15.2-2 explain how to provide patient-centered care.

15.2-3 make progress in your knowledge and respect for religious, social, and cultural values.

15.2-4 discuss ethical situations that challenge cultural norms.

15.2-5 explain the importance of equal access to healthcare.

15.2-6 describe ethical conflicts surrounding healthcare mandates.

ESSENTIAL QUESTION

How do ethics impact the way healthcare workers interact with their patients?

Professional Vocabulary

Essential Terms

cultural diversity   differences in age, gender, sex, physical and intellectual abilities, sexual orientation, nationality, or ethnicity that influence what people believe, think, and do

soft skills   employability skills related to communication, attitude, teamwork, and problem solving that are difficult to teach but critical to workplace success

Important Terms

ethnocentrism
work ethic

Introduction

In addition to obeying laws, healthcare workers need to behave ethically. Professional codes of ethics usually tell healthcare workers to put patients above all other interests and maintain standards of professional competence. Workers must follow codes of ethics developed by their employer. These codes often emphasize patient care and comfort, professional competence, and personal responsibility.

15.2-1 Soft Skills

Many employers say that young workers do not understand the importance of **soft skills**. These are subjective employability skills that create a successful work culture, such as communication, attitude, teamwork, and problem solving.

Employers want workers to dress appropriately, show up on time, solve problems through critical thinking, work collaboratively, and show good customer-service and communication skills. These nontechnical skills are difficult to teach, which makes them more important to an employer than technical skills.

Flexibility, attention to detail, and problem solving are important soft skills for healthcare workers who must make quick decisions. Healthcare workers must be on time, follow procedures rather than take shortcuts, be honest in admitting their mistakes, and show integrity by sticking to their principles about what is right and wrong. The ability to communicate clearly and collaborate with others is crucial for a healthcare team. Employers look for people who can demonstrate empathy and emotional stability when working under stress. These soft skills are shown in the way you present yourself during an interview and what your references say about your past conduct at school or on the job.

Work ethic is commonly mentioned when employers ask about an applicant's soft skills. This is described as your own value for working hard, being self-reliant and dependable, and not wasting time (**Figure 15.5**). Employers value a strong work ethic. This demonstration of accountability and professionalism is an important part of success in the workplace. It takes self-discipline and determination to choose work over social distractions. Employees who have the initiative to look for more to do when their regular duties are completed are an asset to an employer. Those who meet these high standards can feel a sense of accomplishment and pride in their work. They must also be careful to balance their work and personal lives so they do not burn out. At the end of an important project, take time to relax and remember to acknowledge those around you who were involved in your success.

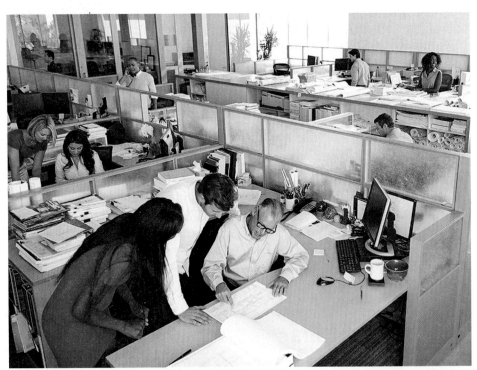

Monkey Business Images/Shutterstock.com

Figure 15.5 Part of a good work ethic is avoiding distractions, even in a busy work environment. *What are some distractions you have had to deal with in school or on the job?*

15.2-2 Providing Patient-Centered Care

Caring for people is at the forefront of healthcare. Patient-centered care should put the patient's, client's, or family's health needs, desired outcomes, and individual circumstances at the center of decision-making and care practices. This provides the best outcomes and highest level of satisfaction for patients. To achieve this, providers must determine what is important to their patients and demonstrate respect for patients' values or preferences. They must develop a good rapport (harmonious connection), learn about the patient, and seek the patient's opinion on care options. They need to keep them informed about their condition, prognosis, or treatment. They must be attentive to the patient's comfort, emotional needs, and desire for continuity of care. Research has shown that when patients feel their care providers are experienced, empathetic, and communicate well, then patients are more likely to follow through with care recommendations, require less extensive treatment, and have a better outcome.

Customer service provides support for patients and their family before, during, and after care. Speak politely, or with *civility*, in all situations. Be courteous and respectful, even if the patient is not. The patient may be feeling ill, scared, or confused and need your empathy. Illness affects individual patients and their families differently (**Figure 15.6**). Some react better to pain and disease than others. Patients have their own individual fears and concerns. One patient may be reacting to a negative healthcare experience from the past. Another may worry how their family will manage without them. The family of another may be stressed about paying the medical bills. Treat each person as an individual. Use your listening skills and be sympathetic to patients' needs.

In addition to the care team's empathetic treatment of patients, patient-centered care includes many other aspects of the healthcare system. The processes of finding a care provider, scheduling an appointment, paying for care, and accessing healthcare information should also be smooth and patient centered. Patients should be able to access information about procedures and processes on the healthcare or insurance system's website, as well as by phone. A real person, rather than an automated system, should be available. An efficient system reduces wait times. Well-trained staff should be able to answer questions and direct patients to the correct place or person. Frustration is a sign the system is not working and needs improvement.

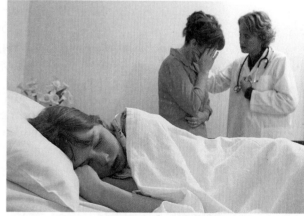

Hemera Technologies/AbleStock.com/Thinkstock

Figure 15.6 The stress of illness affects everyone differently. Some patients may be optimistic and focused on recovery, while others are focused on fears and concerns. *What concerns might this family be experiencing?*

15.2-3 Respecting Diversity

While customer service, flexibility, and communication skills help create a good work environment, today's world also requires workers to be comfortable around people of different cultural, social, and ethnic backgrounds. Culture is embedded in communication, but **cultural diversity** is much larger than communication differences (**Figure 15.7**).

Cultural Issues May Affect Healthcare Communication	
Cultural Element	**Selected Examples That May Affect Communication**
Language	Words and meanings can vary. Do you drink from a *water fountain* or a *bubbler*? When you pass out, do you *graduate* or *become unconscious*?
Names	Using first names can be seen either as friendliness or inappropriate and discourteous.
Pain	Some patients are expressive, while others are stoic. How do you know who needs pain relief?
Eye contact	Lack of eye contact can show disinterest or respect for the speaker.
Visitors and family	Large numbers of demanding family members may show respect for an ailing parent.
Gender and age	The patient may not have the authority to speak. A relative may control communication between the patient and the healthcare worker.

Goodheart-Willcox Publisher

Figure 15.7   Cultural issues may affect healthcare communication.

Differences in age, sex, gender, sexual orientation, religion, nationality, ethnicity, and physical and intellectual ability can all influence what people believe, think, and do. Do men and women see the world in the same way? Do young and old people make the same choices? Does your culture or ethnicity influence the way you dress, where you live, or who your friends are? How has your cultural, social, or ethnic background influenced your level of education, career, interests, or religious views? Culture plays a huge role in how people make decisions, including decisions about healthcare.

Your background influences both conscious and unconscious choices. Your choices provide visible clues to your culture, but they do not tell the whole story. Do you assume people who live near you, go to school with you, and have the same career interests will have the same beliefs about healthcare practices? This is an example of being ethnocentric, or expecting others to think and behave like you do. **Ethnocentrism** is the evaluation of other cultures using your own culture as the superior model. The assumption that your way is the correct way can lead to negative views of others' beliefs, values, and actions that result in biased care. Racism, classism, ageism, and other forms of prejudice or discrimination have no place in healthcare.

Cultural sensitivity begins with learning about possible cultural differences. You become culturally sensitive when you recognize, understand, and react appropriately to customs, beliefs, and values different from your own (**Figure 15.8**). For instance, when a patient refuses to look at you while you provide care instructions, do you assume the patient is not interested? This may be a sign of respect for your position. In some cultures, looking you in the eye is rude. Patients may also have different ideas about wellness, illness, and the parts of the body that can be discussed or touched. Culture can be a strong influence on how people think about health issues, whom they see for health conditions, and how they respond to healthcare recommendations.

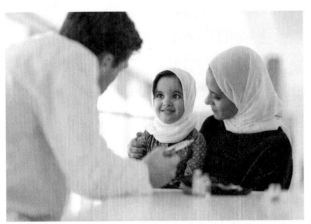

FatCamera/E+ via Getty Images

Figure 15.8   Cultural competence is an important skill for healthcare workers.

To meet the demands of increasing cultural diversity, the US needs a culturally competent workforce. Cultural competence requires some knowledge of possible cultural differences that might occur in the healthcare setting. This includes different beliefs, customs, and values of people from other ethnic and racial groups, as well as people with disabilities, different socioeconomic backgrounds, and members of the LGBT+ community. It also means learning not to make assumptions about the viewpoints and beliefs of others. Cultural humility requires people to acknowledge they will never know everything about another person or group of people.

Keep in mind that culture is learned, and individual differences are common. You cannot assume what someone's culture is based on their ethnicity. Through *acculturation*, people may learn and incorporate the culture of a new country. People may also belong to more than one cultural group, each with its own set of cultural norms. Culturally sensitive and competent healthcare workers are motivated to overcome any cultural barriers to serve their patients. They are sensitive to power imbalances and try to help others feel heard, seen, and included.

You may need to research cultures that are new to you and continually work to develop your cultural sensitivity and competence. Take the time to ask questions and develop a rapport with your patient. **Figure 15.9** provides some examples of cultural differences that may influence healthcare. A culturally competent healthcare worker is aware of and accounts for these differences by communicating culturally appropriate care options for the patient. Cultural competence involves building a relationship of trust and open communication with the patient to provide the best care and reduce health disparities.

Belief Systems May Influence Care Decisions	
Belief	**Selected Examples That May Influence Care**
Religion and spirituality	• Jehovah's Witnesses may not receive blood products or blood transfusions. • Orthodox Judaism forbids healthcare procedures on the Sabbath. • Christian Scientists may accept no medication or surgery.
Explaining health and disease	• People with a Native American background may believe an imbalance between the human spirit and nature causes illness. • Hispanic cultures may believe that fear, evil, or envy can lead to illness. • Several cultural groups view illness as a punishment from God.
Communicating "bad news" and death	• In some Asian cultures, it is proper to reveal a terminal diagnosis to the patient's family. The family will decide whether the patient is told. • Many cultural groups oppose removing life support for religious reasons. • Muslims and Hmong may refuse organ donation or autopsy.
Gender and family roles	• In African, Asian, and Hispanic cultures, families may want to help care for the patient. Family is valued over individual needs. • Several cultural groups view the eldest male as the spokesperson and decision maker for all family members.

Goodheart-Willcox Publisher

Figure 15.9 Belief systems may affect healthcare decisions.

15.2-4 Challenging Cultural Norms

Efforts to be more culturally competent may challenge cultural norms for what is right and wrong. It can be difficult for healthcare providers to watch patients make healthcare decisions that will shorten their lives, but this is a patient's right. Healthcare workers must carefully weigh the basic principles of autonomy, beneficence, non-malfeasance, and justice to keep the best interests of patients at the center of care provided.

Cultural differences can cloud the issue of patient autonomy. A culture's rules and expected behavior, or *cultural norms*, influence how a patient communicates within and uses Western healthcare. Some cultures give care decision-making to the eldest male family member, rather than the patient. It may be a cultural norm to withhold information from the patient about their diagnosis. Cultural norms may also push patients to request procedures that are not in their best interest. Patients have a right to choose their care, who makes their decisions, or who knows their diagnosis, even when their cultural practices do not match best practices for Western healthcare.

 ## Healthcare Professions: Ethical Principles

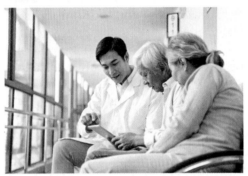

imtmphoto/Shutterstock.com

With an increasing number of patients of Korean ancestry in the area, Dr. White has been working on cultural competency skills. His newest patient was an older Korean woman with limited English language skills who wanted to be seen for chronic pain. The oldest male in her family brought her to the appointment and spoke for her. When asked, he said an interpreter was not needed. The woman gave permission for him to be present and looked to him whenever a response was needed. When tests showed she had cancer, Dr. White asked to use an interpreter to clearly communicate about the diagnosis and treatment options. He believed the patient had a right to know and be involved in the decisions for her care. Her spokesperson became angry. He believed telling her about the cancer diagnosis would cause a poor outcome. He did not bring her for the next appointment or return phone calls from Dr. White's office after that. What could Dr. White have done differently?

It is best practice to discuss patient preferences for communication as early as possible. When language is a barrier, recommend the use of an interpreter at the first interaction so the family can focus attention on their loved one. It may even be unethical to rely on family members to serve as interpreters. In addition to the emotional stress when a loved one is ill, there is the potential for interpretation errors, misunderstandings, and intentional withholding of information. A medical interpreter is trained in clinical terminology, facility procedures, cultural norms, and patient privacy. If the patient or family refuses an interpreter, it is a good idea to recheck this decision occasionally.

It is important not to overreact if the family asks you to withhold information from the patient. Never respond with, "This is how we do things." Instead, listen for their reasons. Show empathy and let them know you share their goal of protecting their family member from harm. Offer the support of other hospital services, such as a social worker or patient representative. Seek open communication that allows patients to voice their opinions about who should have their information for decision-making.

Changes in cultural norms also bring the ethics of some medical procedures into question. An increasing number of patients are requesting cosmetic surgeries to alter or enhance their physical beauty. You may find a patient's right to choose conflicts with other ethical principles. Should cosmetic surgery for minors be allowed? Should extreme transformations be performed, such as trying to look like a social icon or animal? Should procedures to mask someone's identity be performed? Cosmetic surgery may help improve someone's self-esteem, but the physical and psychological hazards must be weighed.

Ultimately, you must respect the cultural preferences of your patient. Once you have established a patient can make their own decisions, it is the patient's right to defer decision-making to others. It is also the patient's right to refuse care. If the patient asks for care you feel is medically inappropriate or goes against your code of ethics, you are not required to perform the procedure as long as you apply the same standards to all patients.

15.2-5 Providing Equal Access to Healthcare

Ethical codes require healthcare workers to provide services to any person without discrimination unless there is a justifiable reason. This makes sense, but environmental factors sometimes create limits. Equal access to healthcare is not available in all areas of the United States. People who live in large cities with up-to-date teaching hospitals that use current best practices will have more diagnostic and therapeutic options than those who live in rural areas. Mergers of smaller healthcare facilities to save money compound this issue. People with more money can also pay for more care, tests, medications, or insurance. These differences raise ethical questions. How can equal access to healthcare for everyone be assured?

During the COVID-19 pandemic, telehealth provided video access to physicians from anywhere a patient had a cell phone signal or internet. This improved access to doctors, but many medical tests still require physical access. Some government agencies, healthcare institutions, and nonprofit organizations are trying to improve access to medical tests for those who need them. The state of Arizona, for example, provides mobile mammography tests for females with low incomes who do not have health insurance. Mobile medical services in Boston bring a range of diagnostics to nursing homes, correctional facilities, and college campuses where patient travel is not practical. Many pharmacies have free blood-pressure monitoring stations (**Figure 15.10**).

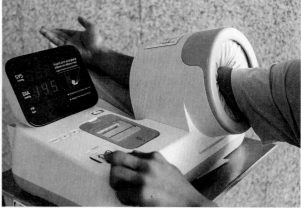

Chaikom/Shutterstock.com

Figure 15.10 Blood pressure monitors are often available in pharmacies for self-testing. *What other healthcare services do pharmacies offer?*

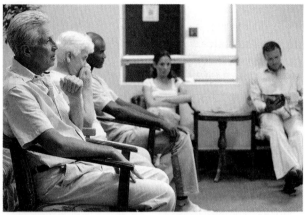

©iStock/monkeybusinessimages

Figure 15.11 In recent years, clinical trials and studies have used more diverse subjects. *What type of subject was used before the 1980s? What is the reason for the change?*

Some also offer free blood testing for diabetes. These programs improve access for people who cannot afford medical tests or live in rural areas.

Inequitable research practices are also changing. Clinical trial volunteers often do not represent the diversity of the US population. Before the 1980s, medical research was primarily conducted on white males in their mid-30s. Researchers assumed the medications and treatments that worked for them would work for other populations as well. Advocacy groups complained that this ignored the health of females and marginalized groups (**Figure 15.11**). Research showed differences in medication effectiveness and appropriate dosages for different populations. Researchers even discovered that males and females reported different symptoms for the same disease or condition. They could not assume results from studying white males in their mid-30s applied to females, people of different racial or ethnic backgrounds, children, or older adults.

Many drugs achieve different levels in the blood and different levels of effectiveness depending on factors such as body mass; the ratio of muscle to body fat; and other disease processes, reproductive hormones, or medications that are present. Females tend to weigh less than males, have a higher percentage of body fat, and process medicines differently. Only personalized medicine will truly adjust medication dosages to each individual's needs, but campaigns such as *All of Us* and *I'm In* have attempted to raise awareness among marginalized populations about the importance of diverse participation in clinical research.

Unfortunately, marginalized populations are less likely to trust healthcare providers or be involved in research studies. In addition to cultural differences and systemic racism, some knowledge of historical events will help you understand the origins of this mistrust. In the 1800s, some people who were enslaved were used for medical experiments and teaching demonstrations. This practice continued in exchange for medical services in charity wards after slavery was abolished. From the 1930s to 1970s, women who were black, Native American, or Puerto Rican were often sterilized without their consent after giving birth or having routine medical procedures. Thirty-one states took part in these state-run programs. The Tuskegee syphilis study from 1932 to 1972 withheld diagnosis and treatment from hundreds of men who were black so that doctors could learn more about the disease. People who are black are still undertreated for pain due to false beliefs that they have a higher pain tolerance. This history will help you understand why some marginalized populations were hesitant to receive the COVID-19 vaccine in 2021. Many worried they might be used as test subjects or given something other than a lifesaving treatment.

As you work to provide high-quality patient care, you will need to advocate for the rights of your patients. Equity and disparity issues are linked to access, quality, and cost of care. Get involved in quality-improvement projects. Focus on the shared goals of protecting people and improving healthcare. Develop your cultural competence. Encourage open communication and empower your patients to speak up about their care. These efforts will help improve patient access, equity, and health outcomes.

15.2-6 Following Healthcare Mandates

Healthcare has seen a variety of official requirements, or *mandates*, that attempt to fix problems in the healthcare system. Any decision that applies to everyone brings concerns about ethical issues such as autonomy, non-malfeasance, fairness, and equity.

Mandates can have unintended consequences. Medicare and Medicaid legislation of 1965 improved healthcare coverage for older people and those with low incomes. These laws shifted the financial burden of care to the government and onto all taxpayers. This helped people who could not afford their own care, but some older people began transferring an inheritance to their children rather than using the money to pay for healthcare. As a result, Medicare and Medicaid legislation ended up costing more than planned. Cost controls from new Medicare mandates in the 1980s limited everyone's access to healthcare rather than fixing the rising costs. The Affordable Care Act (ACA) of 2010 was intended to improve access and coverage for healthcare, but it caused even higher prices, and many people could not afford the copayments to use the insurance plans they were required to buy. These mandates have also been difficult for healthcare providers to follow.

People are often unaware of risks associated with healthcare mandates. For example, the 21st Century Cures Act included mandates for healthcare to stop blocking data exchanges and make healthcare information more accessible for patients. This was often done through phone apps, which are not regulated by the same privacy laws as healthcare. When patients accept app permissions, they may not realize the difference and unknowingly be sharing their personal health information with other apps or services.

Immunization programs illustrate additional ethical concerns and dilemmas related to mandates. The US began requiring vaccination of school children in the 1850s to prevent smallpox, a disease that is now eradicated. The CDC now recommends immunization against 15 different diseases before the age of 18. Some school-age immunizations are required in all 50 states. Vaccines reduce the spread of disease and prevent millions of deaths each year. Having a high rate of vaccination helps protect those who cannot be vaccinated and reduces the growth of virus mutations. However, vaccine mandates may violate your right to choose what to do with your body. There was strong resistance when the COVID-19 vaccine was required for some people to keep their jobs. Should the government be able to mandate a healthcare procedure, or should this be an individual decision?

Federal guidelines require healthcare workers to provide an information sheet before a vaccine is given, but workers are not required to make sure the information is understood (**Figure 15.12**). Although vaccines are tested for safety, side effects can range from mild discomfort to even death from a serious allergic reaction. A government fund compensates those affected by serious complications from vaccines, but most states only allow exemption from vaccination for health or religious reasons. This does not accommodate cultures that do not believe in the use of Western medicine or people who do not trust the government officials requiring them to be vaccinated.

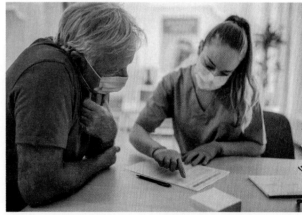

South_agency/E+ via Getty Images

Figure 15.12 Healthcare workers are required to provide information about a vaccine and its side effects, but they do not have to make sure the patient understands it.

Vaccine shortages, like those seen during the COVID-19 pandemic, also create concerns about fairness and equitable access. Even when vaccines are readily available, people with low income and those without health insurance are less likely to be vaccinated than others. There are also equity and ethics concerns surrounding research and testing of vaccines. Clinical trials have not traditionally matched the ethnic or racial diversity of the US population. This creates concerns about effectiveness and safety for these populations. The need to test vaccines for safety with vulnerable populations, such as children or people who are already ill, must be balanced with protecting their safety during the process.

Lesson 15.2 Review

 Complete the *Map Your Reading* graphic organizer for the section you just read.

1. Employers prefer to hire workers who demonstrate _____ skills at their interview because these skills are difficult to teach. (15.2-1)
   A. soft
   B. hard
   C. strong
   D. vague

2. The_____'s needs, desired outcomes, and individual circumstances should be the focus of decision-making and care practices. (15.2-2)
   A. physician
   B. client
   C. healthcare worker
   D. community

3. Culturally _____ healthcare workers recognize cultural differences and build open communication with the patient to provide culturally appropriate care. (15.2-3)
   A. compliant
   B. ethnocentric
   C. diverse
   D. competent

4. Cultural _____ may not match the practices of Western medicine, but it is the patient's right to choose. (15.2-4)
   A. ideas
   B. competence
   C. norms
   D. conflicts

5. Clinical trials have become more diverse in recent years because _____ people have with certain medications can be different for different populations. (15.2-5)
   A. reactions
   B. morals
   C. ethics
   D. ideas

6. Immunization programs create ethical conflicts for healthcare workers (15.2-6)
   A. because they have been around for a long time
   B. when religious exemptions are allowed
   C. when they are required by law
   D. when they are tested on diverse populations

Bioethics

Learning Outcomes

After studying this lesson, you will be able to

15.3-1 discuss bioethical concerns that result from biobanking.

15.3-2 discuss the use of genetic testing for prevention, diagnosis, and treatment of disease.

15.3-3 explain how people are protected from genetic discrimination.

15.3-4 discuss ethical concerns surrounding genetic engineering.

15.3-5 analyze ethical considerations for stem cell research.

15.3-6 explain the importance of reliability and validity in medical research.

Professional Vocabulary

Essential Terms

bioethics   the study of ethical practices in medical research and use of advanced technology to treat patients

genetic discrimination   the use of genetic information by employers and insurance companies to deny employment or insurance coverage or treat individuals differently because of a genetic condition

Important Terms

biobanking
eugenics
genetic engineering

> ❓ **ESSENTIAL QUESTION**
>
> *How do bioethical concerns influence healthcare?*

Introduction

As healthcare workers challenge the system to find new ways of providing care, they inevitably run into ethical issues. New technological advances can create difficult decisions balancing what is possible with what is appropriate. Since the first in vitro fertilization (IVF) in 1978, the idea of tampering with the creation of life has been controversial (**Figure 15.13**).

A fuller understanding of human genetics in the last few decades has made it possible to manipulate genes and create new cells. The possibilities of future discoveries continue to raise new legal and ethical concerns.

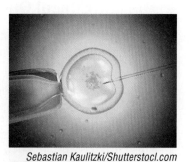

Sebastian Kaulitzki/Shutterstocl.com

Figure 15.13   The first in vitro fertilization, which was done in 1978, was just the beginning of ethical concerns related to biotechnology.

The field of **bioethics** addresses these serious questions. Bioethics focuses people's attention on the ethical implications of biological research and development. It questions what is considered good or moral in healthcare. Recent debates have centered on issues related to privacy, genetics, cloning, and equity.

15.3-1 Biobanking

Biobanking is the collection and storage of human tissue samples and related data for research purposes. These samples are cataloged and stored in a repository where the information and samples can be easily retrieved, shared, and analyzed. The name of the donor is generally changed to a cataloguing number to protect the donor's identity. These collections are usually focused on a particular disease, clinical trial, or group of people. This practice has been going on for more than 100 years, and the demand for samples is growing. The samples are used for medical testing, research, and product development.

After medical testing is completed, labs should have a policy for the storage, use, and disposal of remaining specimens. Patients should know this policy and be given the opportunity to refuse to participate in medical research using their tissues. The ethical concerns are privacy, ownership, and profits (**Figure 15.14**). Facility policies vary widely across the US. These issues will continue to be argued in court.

The story of Henrietta Lacks demonstrates this issue. Her cells were taken without consent during a biopsy in 1951. They were later used in experiments to grow cells that could be kept alive and used for medical testing. When the process was successful, those cells were donated and sold repeatedly from a biobank without her consent or compensation to her family. They are the *HeLa* cell line used in labs around the world for medical and biological research. They were used to develop the first polio vaccine and first successful cloning of a human cell. In 1990, courts finally ruled that discarded cells and tissues are not a person's property and can be used for commercial purposes. In 2015, NIH collaborated with the Lacks family to develop a controlled-access policy for genomic data from the HeLa cell line. Legal cases such as this show the need to balance commercial, academic, and ethical interests when patenting new cell lines. Medical facilities have also updated their informed-consent policies to avoid some of these legal issues.

Ethical Questions About Biobanking

? Can the patient's identity and PHI be protected, particularly when genome analysis may reveal information that can connect back to the donor?

? Who owns the samples left over from medical procedures, such as abortion, surgery, or biopsy?

? If a saleable product, such as a medical cure, is created from an individual's tissue, should the person receive any profits from its sale?

AditRachi/Shutterstock.com

Figure 15.14 These questions demonstrate some of the ethical concerns related to biobanking.

15.3-2 Genetic Testing

Genetic health-risk tests are available on pharmacy shelves and through family history research organizations without a doctor's order. These tests can provide important information about inheritable genetic risks. Knowing you may pass on a genetic disorder can be useful when making decisions about whether to have children. Tests confirming a diagnosis can help with planning lifestyle changes, choosing treatments, and preparing for health changes and end of life. The FDA limits the sale of diagnostic tests used for medical decisions. These must involve a doctor to order the test and interpret the results.

The ability to test for genetic health risks and conditions raises many questions about how results can or should be used. Testing does not change a person's risk for a genetic condition, but it may increase stress levels. What uses are appropriate? If expectant parents learn their unborn child has a genetic disorder or is not the desired sex, should they be able to terminate the pregnancy based on that information? Can children be forced to undergo genetic testing or have their genetic material used to benefit a sibling? If people's genetic profiles reveal they are more likely to develop breast cancer, should insurance pay for preventive mastectomies of healthy breasts? Should genetic testing for a terminal illness justify euthanasia before a patient has symptoms?

Medical testing also creates privacy and equity concerns. Who should have access to the results? If an employer pays for the insurance that covers testing, should the employer have access? Should society or the courts be concerned about intolerance of differences growing because of access to genetic testing? Many people have placed their DNA profile on family history websites to search for relatives. What are the rights of relatives who share a portion of that DNA? Should biotechnology companies or police be able to use this genetic information for other purposes, such as for-profit research or identification of criminals?

15.3-3 Genetic Discrimination

Genetic discrimination is the use of genetic information to treat individuals with certain genetic conditions differently. As genetic testing has become more common, people have reported many cases of such treatment. Some workers lost their jobs even though there were no complaints about their job performance. Others were denied health insurance because they had a genetic disorder, sometimes before they even showed symptoms of the disease.

Genetic discrimination led to public demand for protection. Some states passed laws to prevent genetic discrimination. The effort was boosted in 2008, when Congress passed the Genetic Information Nondiscrimination Act (GINA). That law banned health insurers from making decisions regarding enrollment, extent of coverage, or premium amounts based on genetic information. It also banned employers with more than 15 employees from basing decisions regarding hiring, firing, promotion, pay, or job tasks on genetic information (**Figure 15.15**). Employers cannot require genetic testing as a condition of employment or request the results of genetic tests taken by employees.

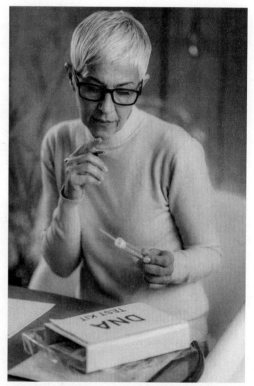

Microgen/Shutterstock.com

Figure 15.15 By law, employers and insurance companies cannot use genetic information to make decisions.

The Affordable Care Act (ACA) of 2009 also guarantees access to health insurance for people with a genetic condition and prevents insurers from increasing premiums based on an individual's diagnosis. This includes people identified to have a likelihood, or *predisposition*, to develop a genetic condition. Unfortunately, neither GINA nor the ACA protect against discrimination for other types of insurance, such as life, long-term care, or disability insurances.

15.3-4 Genetic Engineering

Increased knowledge about human genetics has also led to ethical concerns about **genetic engineering**. This process of editing genetic material is usually done using recombinant DNA. The goal is to remove harmful traits or insert desirable ones. Technicians duplicate and extract DNA from one or more desired genes, then recombine and insert the new genetic material into a cell where the original DNA has been removed. The cell then follows the instructions of the new DNA.

Agriculture uses genetic engineering to produce strains of crops, such as corn, tomatoes, and soybeans, that are more resistant to disease or insects (**Figure 15.16**). In healthcare, the major controversy over genetic engineering concerns modifying human genes. For instance, researchers have tried to introduce human genetic material into pigs so the modified animals can provide organs such as hearts and kidneys that are in short supply for human transplants. Athletes have used genetically modified cells or genes to increase how much hormones and protein their cells make. Three-parent IVF procedures take the DNA from a mother and father and then implant them into a healthy cell from a surrogate. Fetal gene therapy is still experimental in the United States, but it may allow treatment for life-threatening illnesses, such as muscular dystrophy, in the womb while the body is still developing.

Not everyone is in favor of genetic modifications. Modern science often conflicts with traditional values. Some people think combining human and animal genes is immoral or has the potential to spread animal diseases with devastating results. Others are concerned about the health conditions shown in clones and worry children born through recombinant techniques will not have normal or healthy life spans. Still others worry about the ethics of using human trials to determine the safety and effectiveness of genetic therapies.

There is also concern about the possibility of governments using genetic engineering in ways that harm specific populations. **Eugenics**, or the attempt to promote desirable genetic characteristics, arose in the late 19th century and gained considerable influence in the early 20th century. Eugenicists typically aimed to promote the reproduction of their own ethnic group or race and suppress others. In the United States, the eugenics movement led several states to pass laws in the early 1900s that mandated sterilization for those with mental health conditions. As a result, several thousand people were sterilized. These laws became models for Nazi Germany, which sterilized 300,000 to 400,000 people who were classified as having mental health conditions. The possibility of some future government using genetic engineering to promote racist ideology worries many people.

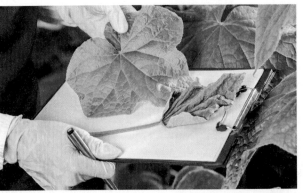

Vlad Teodor/Shutterstock.com

Figure 15.16 Genetic engineering has already been used in the world of agriculture. *What are the main concerns of those who are opposed to genetically modified organisms, or GMOs?*

The potential for genetic engineering to create "superhumans" who have physical abilities or intelligence beyond that of most people is also alarming. Could the government create an army of superhumans? It is already common for fertility clinics to selectively screen embryos before implanting them. Will couples be able to order "designer babies" by manipulating the genes in a fetus to match the qualities they want? Some groups have raised serious objections to such activities.

The long-term effects of some types of genetic engineering are unknown. Unintended mutations could occur, and edited genes could affect other health conditions in unpredictable ways. In 2018, there was strong backlash against the Chinese researcher He Jiankui, who modified the genes of human embryos to make them resistant to HIV. The WHO asked countries to stop experiments that would lead to the birth of altered humans. There is still concern that it is too easy to obtain the materials for underground embryo-editing clinics.

In the US, genetic-therapy research requires many layers of regulation and approval. It is regulated by the Office for Human Research Protections within the Department of Health and Human Services (HHS). The FDA regulates any drugs, medical devices, and biological products that are produced. They make sure these are safe and effective for use. Human gene therapies are a biologic, regulated by the FDA's Center for Biologics Evaluation and Research (CBER). They require extensive testing, which begins with a review and approval from the Institutional Review Board (IRB). These agencies are supported by a federal advisory committee, the Novel and Exceptional Technology and Research Advisory Committee (NExTRAC), which reports to the NIH.

15.3-5 Stem Cell Research

Stem cells are specialized cells that are easily replicated and can generate any type of cell. This is useful in research where testing requires large numbers of the same type of cell. There are two sources of stem cells (**Figure 15.17**).

The use of embryonic stem cells for research generates ethical debate because the process destroys an embryo. Although the cells are taken before the embryo develops a nervous system or is ready to implant in the uterus, those who believe life begins at conception view this procedure as murder.

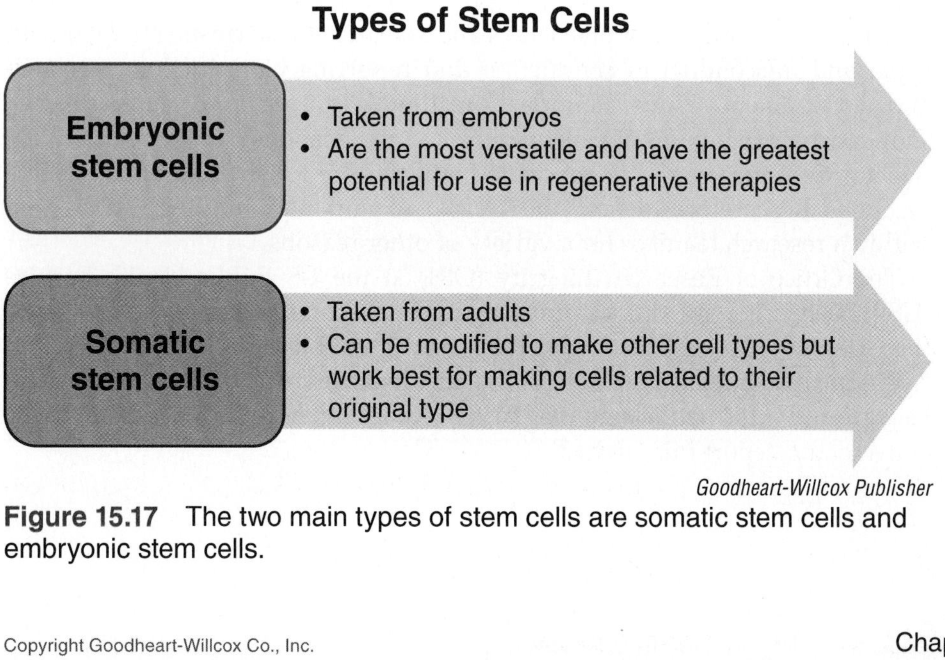

Types of Stem Cells

Embryonic stem cells
- Taken from embryos
- Are the most versatile and have the greatest potential for use in regenerative therapies

Somatic stem cells
- Taken from adults
- Can be modified to make other cell types but work best for making cells related to their original type

Goodheart-Willcox Publisher

Figure 15.17 The two main types of stem cells are somatic stem cells and embryonic stem cells.

Many people also object to creating embryos specifically for the purpose of harvesting stem cells. Others warn there is a potential for the abuse of women's rights in harvesting large numbers of egg cells to be fertilized for this use.

In 1994, President Clinton ordered that no federal money could be used for research on embryos created specifically for research. This did not ban privately funded stem cell research or the use of embryos left over from in vitro fertilization, abortion, or other procedures. In 2001, President G.W. Bush issued a partial ban on federal funding for stem cell research using new embryonic stem cell lines. This limited the number of cell lines available for research. This ban was lifted in 2009 by President Obama, but political and religious debate continues.

While research using somatic stem cells is less controversial, it is uncertain whether they work as well as embryonic stem cells. Somatic stem cells are also more difficult to obtain and reproduce in large quantities. In one respect, somatic stem cells may be more promising than embryonic stem cells. An adult's immune system may be less likely to reject stem cells that are taken from that person's body, modified to produce a desired treatment, and then placed back in the body. However, this has not been proven. As with much stem cell research, a huge amount of work still needs to be done before effective treatments are possible.

15.3-6 Research Reliability and Validity

Questions remain about the reliability and validity of biotechnology research. Several studies have shown that when private companies conduct clinical trials, the results are more likely to be positive than when nonprofit groups do the research. When biotechnology firms are responsible for testing and reporting to the FDA on the effectiveness of their own products, this creates a conflict of interest.

Test protocols describe how a test is done so the results can be replicated. The design of the test must measure what it says it is measuring and interpret the information correctly to produce *valid* results. A test that can be repeated and produce the same results is *reliable*. A genetic test or medication trial that produces the same results on many different occasions can be trusted.

An alarming number of physicians and researchers have been charged with fraud and misconduct in conducting and reporting biotechnology research and development results. Reports from the Government Accounting Office show participants being given unapproved medications, reports being falsified for tests that were not conducted, and failure to report serious adverse reactions. Research results may be falsified to gain more funding, gain tenure within a research team, or for a variety of other reasons.

The Office of Research Integrity (ORI) at the US Public Health Service (USPHS) has a legal duty to investigate research misconduct. USPHS and the National Science Foundation have a combined average of 18 findings of research misconduct per year. These incidents involve falsified data, false background information, and plagiarism. All researchers have a responsibility to avoid and report misconduct.

Researchers use scientific journals to study medical research and build their knowledge base. Researchers may repeat a study to show reliability. They may change a factor to test a similar theory. Each additional set of research results helps build a knowledge base that leads to further innovation. When the knowledge base is flawed and studies are based on invalid test results, more invalid science is produced.

Lesson 15.3 Review

 Complete the *Map Your Reading* graphic organizer for the section you just read.

1. Patients should be informed of _____ policies for the storage and use of tissue samples remaining after medical procedures. (15.3-1)
   A. research
   B. biobanking
   C. genetic
   D. bioethics

2. An important ethical concern in diagnostic medicine is equal _____ to testing and treatment facilities. (15.3-2)
   A. predisposition
   B. opportunity
   C. rights
   D. access

3. Unfair treatment of individuals based on their genetic makeup, called _____, has been banned by the Genetic Information Nondiscrimination Act. (15.3-3)
   A. genetic testing
   B. genetic discrimination
   C. eugenics
   D. biobanking

4. Genetic _____ has been used to modify agricultural crops, but concerns still exist about its use on humans. (15.3-4)
   A. testing
   B. biobanking
   C. engineering
   D. bioethics

5. Although the use of _____ stem cells is controversial, they are the most versatile. (15.3-5)
   A. embryonic
   B. live
   C. HeLa
   D. somatic

6. Tests should be repeated with similar results to show they are (15.3-6)
   A. usable
   B. reliable
   C. valid
   D. correct

Chapter 15 Review and Assessment

Chapter Summary

15.1-1 Appropriate behavior for healthcare workers is guided by both laws, defined by the legal system, and ethical principles, defined by personal morals and professional codes of ethics.

15.1-2 A professional code of ethics outlines the ethical behavior expected of healthcare workers. It serves as a reference point for decision-making.

15.1-3 Ethical dilemmas occur when two different ethical principles are in conflict.

15.1-4 An ethics committee can help healthcare professionals work through difficult issues. It is important to have a clear understanding of the issues, options, values, and stakeholders involved when seeking the best solution.

15.2-1 Employers look for workers with good soft skills and a strong work ethic because these skills are more difficult to teach than technical job skills.

15.2-2 Patient-centered care puts the patient's needs, wants, and circumstances at the center of decision-making and care practices. The goal is to provide the best outcomes and highest level of satisfaction for patients in all areas of the healthcare system.

15.2-3 Healthcare workers must become familiar and comfortable with diverse beliefs, customs, and values. This includes other ethnic and racial groups as well as people with disabilities, different socioeconomic backgrounds, and members of the LGBT+ community. Culturally competent healthcare workers are motivated to overcome these differences to provide culturally appropriate care options for their patients.

15.2-4 Cultural norms may not match best practices in Western medicine. Early and open communication is important to clarify and respect patient wishes.

15.2-5 Equal access to diagnostic tests is a concern in rural areas and for those who cannot afford the increasing costs of medical testing.

Telehealth and mobile testing services have increased access. It is important that the US population's diversity be represented in medical research and clinical trials.

15.2-6 Mandates can create ethical dilemmas. They remove the right to choice and may create inequities.

15.3-1 Bioethics explores questions that arise from biological research and development. Concerns focus on genetics, right to life, privacy, and equity issues. Patients should be informed of how any tissues remaining after a medical procedure will be used, stored, or sold.

15.3-2 Genetic testing raises many questions about how the results should be used and who should have access to the information.

15.3-3 The Genetic Information Nondiscrimination Act (GINA) bans employers and insurance companies from unfair treatment of individuals based on their genetic makeup.

15.3-4 Genetic engineering to remove a harmful trait or insert a desirable trait has been widely used in agriculture but is still controversial in medicine. There are concerns about combining human and animal DNA, the potential for superhumans through eugenics, and the unpredictability of heritable gene mutations.

15.3-5 Stem cells can duplicate many times and develop into many different types of cells and tissues. They can be used for regenerative therapy. There is some concern about the use of embryos or discarded patient tissues to create stem cells for sale or use without the patient's knowledge.

15.3-6 Falsified test results to hide errors or produce favorable results is a huge concern in research. Tests should be repeated and produce similar results to show they are reliable. Using a knowledge base built on flawed test results produces invalid science.

Maximize Your Professional Vocabulary

1. **Scrambled Vocab Terms.** Unscramble the following professional terms from the chapter. Then use them appropriately in a new sentence to show your understanding.
   A. ceehimnnorstt D. korw cehit
   B. ceeginsu E. bcehiiost
   C. adeilmm

2. **Find Your Match.** Your teacher will write this chapter's professional vocabulary terms on notecards and their definitions on separate cards. As you enter the classroom, you will select a term or definition from the shuffled notecards. When you find the person with your term's definition, sit down with that person and review your professional vocabulary. At the beginning of class, each student with a term will present the matching definition.

3. **Creating Sentences.** Select eight to 10 of the professional vocabulary terms in this chapter. Without using the actual term, create a sentence or two that explains the term and your understanding of the concept. Share your sentences with a partner and have them identify the term, then trade roles to identify their terms.

Reflect on Your Reading

1. Review the story about Ann and Dr. Braun at the beginning of the chapter. Using the notes in your *Map Your Reading* visual summary, identify what ethical dilemmas Dr. Braun is facing and which basic principles are involved. Act as a member of the ethics board and suggest what actions he can take to help with decision-making. If Ann belongs to a marginalized group, what additional challenges might she face? If genetic engineering offers any additional options that could extend Ann's life, what bioethical concerns might be involved? Try to use your professional vocabulary as you support your answer.

Review and Recall

1. What is the term for beliefs about right and wrong learned from family, friends, traditions, and experiences? (15.1-1)
   A. Ethics C. Values
   B. Morals D. Laws

2. Many careers have expected standards called (15.1-2)
   A. the Hippocratic Oath
   B. a code of ethics
   C. a code of behavior
   D. a code of conflicts

3. Problems that require a difficult choice between two conflicting but morally or ethically correct options are called (15.1-3)
   A. conflicts C. ethics committees
   B. ethical decisions D. dilemmas

4. Ethical decision-making is complicated by (15.1-4)
   A. ethics committees C. medical advances
   B. laws D. resuscitation

5. _____ create(s) a successful work culture through communication, attitude, teamwork, and problem solving. (15.2-1)
   A. Ethical codes C. Work ethic
   B. Soft skills D. Values

6. The processes of finding a care provider, scheduling an appointment, paying for care, and accessing healthcare information should be (15.2-2)
   A. civil C. physician-centered
   B. patient-centered D. service-centered

7. Which term refers to differences in age, gender, sex, sexual orientation, religion, race, ethnicity, and physical and intellectual ability? (15.2-3)
   A. Ethnocentrism C. Customs
   B. Acculturation D. Cultural diversity

8. A culture's rules and expected behavior, which influence how a patient communicates within and uses Western healthcare, are called (15.2-4)
   A. ethical decision-making
   B. cultural differences
   C. cultural norms
   D. cultural accommodations

9. Before the 1980s, medical research was primarily conducted on _____, and it was assumed that medications and treatments that worked for them would work the same for other populations. (15.2-5)
   A. white men in their mid-30s
   B. white women over 50
   C. diverse populations of all ages
   D. people in low-income areas

10. Which of the following statements is true about immunization programs? (15.2-6)
   A. A high rate of vaccination protects those who cannot be vaccinated.
   B. All populations have equitable access to immunization programs.
   C. Healthcare workers must make sure patients understand the virus information sheet.
   D. Most states allow exemptions from immunization programs for personal reasons.

11. Which of these helps focus peoples' attention on the ethical implications of biological research and development? (15.3-1)
   A. Ethical conduct   C. Bioethics
   B. Biobanking   D. Eugenics

12. Which of these can be used for planning lifestyle changes, choosing treatments, and preparing for health changes and end of life? (15.3-2)
   A. Genetic tests
   B. Eugenic tests
   C. Genetic engineering
   D. Biobanking

13. Which of these guarantees access to health insurance for people with a genetic condition and prevents insurers from increasing premiums based on an individual's diagnosis? (15.3-3)
   A. US Public Health Services
   B. Genetic Information Nondiscrimination Act
   C. The Office of Research Integrity
   D. The Affordable Care Act

14. Which of these is the process of editing genetic material using recombinant DNA? (15.3-4)
   A. Genetic testing
   B. Genetic engineering
   C. Biologics
   D. Eugenics

15. Which type of stem cell may an adult's immune system be less likely to reject? (15.3-5)
   A. Embryonic stem cell
   B. Somatic stem cell from someone else's body
   C. Somatic stem cell from the patient's own body
   D. None of these.

16. Tests that can be repeated and produce the same results are (15.3-6)
   A. effective   C. reliable
   B. valid   D. replicated

Build Core Skills

1. **Speaking and Listening.** Work with a partner or small group to develop a list of culturally appropriate questions you can ask patients to understand their culture and preferences within the healthcare system. Then, practice asking each other the questions and responding appropriately to them.

2. **Critical Thinking.** Consider the potential for ethical dilemmas associated with providing care for a culturally diverse population with different cultural norms. Identify a possible dilemma that might occur for each of the four ethical principles. Then, summarize the guidelines for resolving these dilemmas.

3. **Critical Thinking.** Review the ethical dilemmas presented in Lesson 15.1. Choose one and discuss both sides of the issue. Who are the people affected by this dilemma? What are the possible consequences for each of these people? If you sat on the board of ethics for this case, what recommendations would you make?

4. **Reading.** Find an article about biobanking, genetic testing, genetic engineering, or stem cell research. Read the article and answer the following questions:
   A. What is the purpose?
   B. What are the potential challenges and benefits?
   C. What are the relevant ethical issues?
   D. What new or unexpected findings did you encounter as you read the article?

5. **Speaking and Listening.** Share your findings from the article you read for the previous activity. Give a one- to two-minute oral report to the class. Plan so that you can pronounce any difficult terms. Be prepared to answer questions about your presentation. Listen to and ask at least one question during the presentations of your classmates.

6. **Speaking and Listening.** Customer service is an important soft skill that employers look for in employees. Work with a partner to create a conversation between a healthcare worker and a patient that demonstrates poor customer service and communication skills. Then revise the dialogue to show how the conversation should have gone if the worker was demonstrating good customer-service and communication skills.

7. **Speaking and Listening.** Create a response you could use during an interview when asked to give an example of how you have demonstrated a good work ethic. Practice the response with a partner until it comes out smoothly and sounds confident.

8. **Writing.** Imagine you are Henrietta Lacks. Write a letter to medical researchers regarding your feelings about the use of your stem cells.

9. **Speaking and Listening.** Explain the reasoning behind focusing early medical research and human testing primarily on white

males in their mid-30s. Discuss this concept with classmates in terms of pros and cons, results, assumptions, demographics, and implications for medications and treatments. Summarize the reasons you identified for more diverse testing.

10. **Math.** To reflect the diversity of the US today, which ethnic groups, and how many from each, would you seek for a medication trial of 1,000 subjects?

11. **Writing.** Chose a bioethics debate topic, such as "Should people with a genetic condition that causes significant disability be allowed to have children?" or "How should people determine who receives donated organs?" or "Should euthanasia be legal for patients with dementia who are not at the end of life?" Your teacher will assign you to either the affirmative or negative side of the debate. Research and prepare a four-minute persuasive speech for your constructive opening argument.

12. **Speaking and Listening.** Working in pairs, have a debate using the format in the HOSA competitive event guidelines for Biomedical Debate. Begin with the argument prepared for the previous activity. Listen to the other side's constructive speech and present your cross-examination. Follow up their cross-examination with a rebuttal.

13. **Math.** Mathematical models of risk are used for making medical decisions. If the risk of death for taking a new medication is 0.001 percent, what does that mean? Is there a situation in which you feel that is an acceptable level of risk?

Activate Your Learning

1. Suppose you are a medical researcher. Design a test to show a specific treatment can fight cancer. How many samples would you include? How many times would you repeat the test? How would you ensure it is effective for a diverse group of patients?

2. What cultures are represented in your community? Investigate how to greet people and ask how they are feeling for each of these cultures.

Think and Act Like a Healthcare Worker

1. Imagine you are a genetic counselor. How will you explain genetic testing to individuals who come to your organization to have a test performed? Write a script and act out the scene with a classmate.

2. Your new patient is pregnant, speaks a different language than you, and seems hesitant about being in your clinic. What will you do as part of your patient-centered care to create the best possible outcome? Consider how you can develop rapport and respect cultural norms.

Go to the Source

1. Find the AHIMA Code of Ethics on the internet. Compare it with the Physician's Pledge listed in Figure 15.2. What are three ethical expectations they have in common?

2. Visit the Bioethics.com website. Scroll down to choose one of the links to current articles on ethical issues. Read the article. Summarize the topic being presented. Identify the ethical issue involved. State your opinion on the subject.

3. View a brochure about childhood vaccinations from your local clinic. Why are vaccines recommended? At what ages should they be given? How many doses of each type of vaccine are recommended? What are the most common side effects noted?

HOSA Event Prep: Biomedical Debate

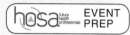

Mark and Heather were preparing for their first child. Heather was 23 weeks' pregnant when she began to have cramping. Her doctor told her to come immediately to the hospital. Heather was in labor, but her baby was just at the point of viability. Her doctor began medications to stop labor, gave steroids to help mature the baby's lungs, and consulted with the neonatologist. The neonatologist told Mark and Heather that if their baby survived, it would spend months in the hospital, possibly have severe lung and health conditions, and would need costly medical interventions. If born in the next 24 hours, they were given the choice to use heroic measures to save the baby or just let the baby pass away. Mark and Heather were devastated and conflicted on what to do. They asked for a second opinion, and this neonatologist agreed the baby could have significant health issues and would spend months in the hospital. He also told them the survival rate of an infant at 23 weeks would be around 55 percent, and there was a high chance of long-term health issues. Each week they could keep her pregnant improved their odds.

Think About It

1. At what point in a pregnancy should decision-making shift from autonomy of the pregnant person to balancing this with the best interests of the unborn child?

2. How much input should parents have on the doctor's decision to continue or withdraw treatment for a prematurely born infant?

3. If you wanted to argue the parents should allow their barely viable premature infant to pass away without heroic measures, what information would you use to support your argument?

4. What arguments could you make for using heroic measures to save a barely viable premature infant?

Chapter 16 Legal Issues

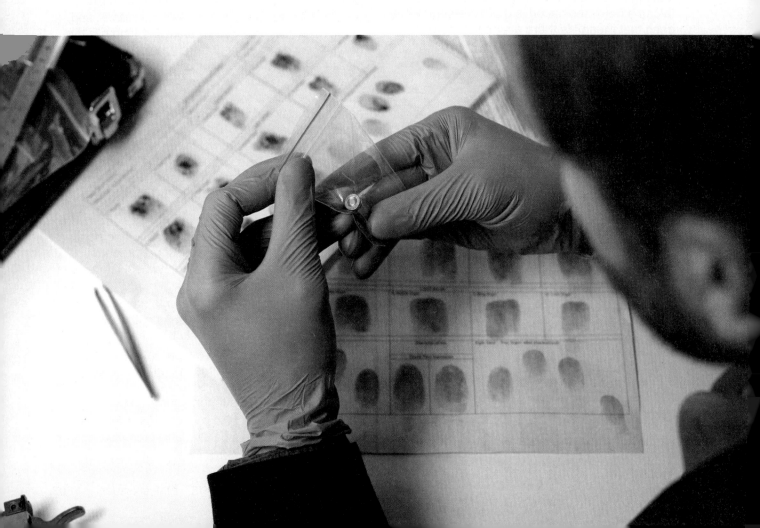

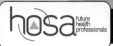
Did you know a patient can refuse care? This is part of a patient's rights. Patients also have the right to know about their diagnosis, treatment, risks and benefits to treatment, and what will happen if they do not have treatment. This is called *informed consent*. Healthcare professionals work within the limits of the license they hold and follow reasonable standards of care. Failing to obtain consent or practice in the current standards of care can be a criminal offense. Healthcare workers make many decisions that do not have definite answers and they may base their decisions on ethical standards. It is important for healthcare professionals to know how to solve ethical dilemmas in the realm of their license to best protect their patients and themselves. The HOSA event *Medical Law and Ethics* involves a test on these sometimes challenging topics, such as medical law, ethics, and bioethics.

Go to the HOSA website to learn more about the HOSA *Medical Law and Ethics* event. Find out the purpose of the event, what is involved in the event, and what knowledge is demonstrated in the event.

As you prepare for HOSA competitive events, be sure to check the website and talk with your HOSA advisor for the most up-to-date guidelines and procedures. Once you have learned about the *Medical Law and Ethics* event, answer the following questions:

1. How might participating in this event benefit you personally and your future career? Explain.
2. Are you interested in participating in this event? Why or why not?

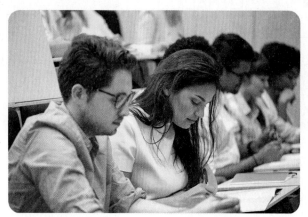
Ground Picture/Shutterstock.com

Connect with Your Reading

If you have not been involved in healthcare or the legal system, much of your knowledge is probably based on TV shows, movies, and the news. Your imagination has filled in the details. So, what do you think? What happens to healthcare workers when they do something harmful? What are patient's rights? Are there laws protecting your health and safety? Do healthcare workers have any legal protection?

Talk with a partner about each of these questions. Then, as you read this chapter, look for information to support or reject your answers.

Map Your Reading

Make a visual summary to record your understanding of legal issues. Begin with a square sheet of paper—an 8½-inch square works well. Fold each of the four points of the square to the center. You can break legal issues down into several areas. Label the four corner flaps with these topics: *Types of Law*, *Protecting Patient Rights*, *Regulating Health and Safety*, and *Employment Laws*. When you finish reading each of these sections in the chapter, open the appropriate flap and add pictures, symbols, or words to illustrate your understanding of the legal issues and how to avoid them. At the end of the chapter, use the back to summarize the potential consequences for violating legal requirements.

Chapter opener image: Motortion Films/Shutterstock.com

Legal Basics

Learning Outcomes

After studying this lesson, you will be able to

16.1-1 differentiate between criminal and civil law.

16.1-2 differentiate between implied, expressed, and informed consent in a contract.

Professional Vocabulary

Essential Terms

contract a legally binding agreement between two or more people or agencies

informed consent a patient's choice to accept or reject a procedure after receiving information about available options and possible consequences

legal related to laws made by the government

Important Terms

civil law
criminal law

expressed
implied

legal disability

Introduction

Laws enforced by the government define **legal** responsibilities. The US Congress, state legislatures, and local governments write laws. Laws may be used to enforce commonly held ethical principles. Where laws conflict, or where regulations are unclear, court decisions (case law) may clarify how to apply the law. This lesson provides an overview of two basic types of law and how they apply to healthcare.

16.1-1 Criminal Law Versus Civil Law

Many laws affect healthcare workers, whether they provide hands-on care or not. The Emergency Medical Treatment and Active Labor Act (EMTALA) says that hospitals with federal funding cannot turn away patients who cannot pay for emergency care (**Figure 16.1**). The Hill-Burton Act requires hospitals to meet the language needs of patients who do not speak English. AIDS legislation addresses fair treatment for patients with HIV or AIDS.

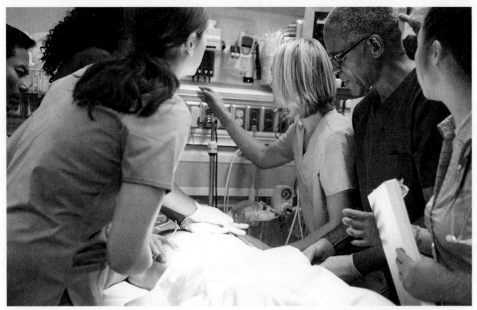

Monkey Business Images/Shutterstock.com

Figure 16.1 The EMTALA ensures that patients in emergency situations receive care even if they cannot pay.

Employment laws such as the Civil Rights Act, Americans with Disabilities Act, and Family Medical Leave Act (FMLA) affect both healthcare and other workplaces. Additional laws are passed and old laws can change each year, so it is important to stay informed.

The first step to being informed is understanding the difference between the two main types of law: criminal law and civil law. **Criminal law** regulates peoples' actions to protect society as a whole. Practicing healthcare without the proper credentials and misusing narcotics are crimes. In some cases, it is a crime *not* to perform an action. For instance, almost every state requires healthcare workers to report cases of suspected child abuse to state authorities. Failure to do so is a crime in most states. Some states may allow both criminal and civil charges for some crimes.

Federal, state, and local governments prosecute violations of criminal law. In criminal cases, the defendant accused of the crime has the right to an attorney. The government, acting through a prosecuting attorney, brings the charges. A jury usually decides the case. If found guilty, the defendant is sentenced to some form of punishment, such as a fine or time in prison. A defendant who is found not guilty beyond a reasonable doubt goes free.

Civil law establishes rules for contracts, personal injuries, and disagreements between individuals with a business relationship. Court cases involving civil law begin with a lawsuit, in which the person injured (the plaintiff) accuses the other person (the defendant) of causing some harm to the plaintiff's person, property, or rights. A judge or jury decides the case. If found guilty, the defendant may be ordered to pay the plaintiff a specific amount of money, called *damages*. If the defendant is found not guilty, no payment is required.

16.1-2 Contract Law and Informed Consent

There are many areas of civil law, but most civil cases in healthcare involve either contracts or torts. **Contract** law applies to the doctor-patient relationship. Contracts must have four elements to be legally enforceable:

- *Offer*, or promise to provide a service or product. Employees of a healthcare provider may create a contract when they schedule an appointment for a patient.
- *Consideration*, or transfer of something of value in exchange for the service provided. A healthcare provider may be paid for treatment as an "out-of-pocket" expense or through insurance.
- *Enforceability*, or a legal basis for the action. A contract to sell illegal drugs, for instance, is invalid because it is not allowed by law.
- *Consent*, or permission to act. This can be either **expressed**, meaning consent has been asked for and answered, or **implied**, meaning permission is assumed based on the actions of both people. When a care provider takes out a blood pressure cuff, and you put your arm on the desk without being asked, it is implied consent. When the provider asks to take your blood pressure and you say, "Yes," and offer your arm, there is expressed consent. Consent does not need to be written or detailed to form a contract.

You and your doctor usually have an implied contract for care that meets an accepted standard of quality. You schedule an appointment and show up. You may not always discuss the payment and course of treatment at the beginning of your appointment, but there is good faith both will occur. The doctor will usually have you or your guardian sign a general consent for treatment when you check in, but it contains no details about the treatment.

When treatment will be more extensive, such as surgery or cancer treatments, **informed consent** is needed. This consent for care will be expressed in great detail. It is usually discussed verbally and also provided in a written format. You must be given the information you need and be involved in the decision to receive the care being discussed. This communication shows respect for your patient rights. Before beginning treatment, the doctor must verify that you fully understand your condition and care options (**Figure 16.2**).

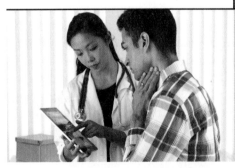

Informed Consent

The doctor must verify you understand:

- the *diagnosis*, or identification of the illness
- the purpose and nature of the treatment
- benefits and risks of the treatment
- possible treatment options and their benefits and risks
- risks of not receiving treatment

Rocketclips, Inc./Shutterstock.com

Figure 16.2 As part of informed consent, a doctor must verify a patient understands the diagnosis and treatment.

When you are providing care, your job will be to make sure your patient has enough information to make informed decisions. Always explain procedures in terms the patient can understand. Check for understanding and answer questions before you begin. Try asking, "Can you tell me what you expect will be done today?" If the response shows the patient does not understand the procedure or has incorrect information, explain further. A signature is not always required, but you should document the discussion as your evidence of informed consent. Do not perform a procedure if the patient refuses or is asking for more information.

For a contract to be valid, both people must be fully capable of entering into the agreement. For example, a person with a **legal disability** cannot enter into a contract. This includes minors who are under the age of consent, people ruled mentally incompetent, or anyone in an altered mental state due to drugs or semi-consciousness. In these cases, a parent or guardian must give consent. There are a few situations, such as treatment for sexually transmitted infections, where minors can give consent at age 16. Consent is assumed in emergency situations when the patient cannot give it and a guardian cannot be reached.

People who form a contract do not always provide the service or payment they promised. In these situations, the terms of the contract are broken, and a *breach of contract* takes place. For example, if a home health agency is paid to provide weekly nursing care, and the nurse does not show up, a breach of contract has occurred. A patient who refuses to pay for an operation has also committed a breach of contract. When this happens, the person affected by the breach—the home care patient in the first case or the surgeon in the second—can sue the other person, claiming injury.

Lesson 16.1 Review

 Complete the *Map Your Reading* graphic organizer for the section you just read.

1. Violations of _____ law, such as practicing without a license, may result in jail time. (16.1-1)
   A. criminal
   B. civil
   C. personal
   D. case

2. Which type of law covers contracts, personal injuries, and business disagreements? (16.1-1)
   A. Criminal law
   B. Civil law
   C. Personal law
   D. Case law

3. Therapeutic workers must provide information and check for understanding to obtain (16.1-2)
   A. implied consent
   B. informed consent
   C. implicit consent
   D. the care plan

4. Which of the following prevents a person from entering into a contract? (16.1-2)
   A. Implied consent
   B. Legal disability
   C. Visual impairment
   D. Hearing loss

Legal Responsibilities and Implications of Tort Law

Learning Outcomes

After studying this lesson, you will be able to:

16.2-1 identify legal limitations created by a professional's scope of practice.

16.2-2 avoid behaviors that would result in charges of misconduct.

16.2-3 demonstrate respect for patient privacy.

16.2-4 differentiate between privileged communication and mandatory reporting requirements.

Professional Vocabulary

Essential Terms

mandatory reporting   the legal requirement for certain health issues to be reported to authorities

misconduct   behavior at work that is unprofessional, unethical, and/or illegal

scope of practice   tasks an employee is legally allowed to perform based on their training and certification

tort   an action that harms another person's body or property or takes away freedom of action in some way

Important Terms

abandonment	false imprisonment	misappropriation
abuse	fraud	neglect
assault	invasion of privacy	negligence
battery	involuntary seclusion	privileged
caregiver laws	liable	communication
defamation	malpractice	standard of care

Introduction

Legal issues between healthcare providers and patients that are neither criminal nor a breach of contract may fall under tort law. A **tort** is a harmful action that causes injury, restricts someone's freedom, or damages someone's property or reputation. **Fraud**—a deceitful practice—is one example of a tort. A company that falsely and knowingly claims a product will cure a health condition may be found guilty of committing a tort against a person harmed by using that product. The injured person has a right to payment for the damages the product caused. Filing an insurance claim for a made-up injury, inflated expense, or person not included in the insurance policy are common forms of healthcare fraud. Fraud steals billions of dollars a year. The False Claims Act allows a person who provides information exposing fraud against Medicare or Medicaid to earn a portion of the money recovered.

16.2-1 Working Within Your Scope of Practice

Credentials and **scope of practice** place legal limits on the actions of healthcare workers. Credentials show that you have met the legal and professional requirements to practice your career. Some credentials, such as certification, may be voluntary, but licensure and registration are usually required by law. State and federal laws control, or *regulate*, the training and practice of many healthcare careers to protect public safety.

Most federal laws are very broad, while state laws have more specific and varying requirements. For instance, the federal Omnibus Budget Reconciliation Act (OBRA) defines minimum requirements for certified nursing assistants (CNAs). It requires at least 75 hours of training and passing written and skill tests. Individual states require between 75 to 200 hours of training for CNAs. Similarly, a psychologist in Alaska must have 1,500 hours of supervised experience to be licensed, but Florida requires 4,000 hours. Some healthcare careers have less rules than others. For example, medical assistants, medical coders, and phlebotomists do not need a license or certification to work in most states.

Scope of Practice and Liability

Your scope of practice includes all the skills from your training that you are allowed to use. It also defines the level of supervision needed. Scope of practice is different for each career and may vary from one place to another. Healthcare workers should never provide care outside their scope of practice.

 ## Healthcare Professions: Scope of Practice

Sarah learned her job as a pharmacy technician through on-the-job training at a local pharmacy. She prepares prescriptions written by a doctor. A pharmacist must always check them and answer any questions customers have about the medications.

As a physical therapy assistant, Debbie was trained to provide range-of-motion

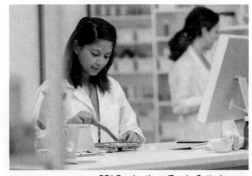

SDI Productions/E+ via Getty Images

exercises under the supervision of a physical therapist for patients needing rehabilitation. She knows she must tell her supervisor if a patient is not responding well. She is not allowed to change the prescribed exercises herself. That authority lies outside her scope of practice.

Patel works as a radiation therapist. He delivers radiation treatments to patients with cancer. He understands the importance of following the dosage prescribed by the oncologist.

As a nursing assistant, Claudio is trained to carry out the nursing plan set by a registered nurse. He knows he cannot perform sterile procedures. Although he may recognize and report common symptoms, he cannot tell the patient what diagnosis he suspects or recommend a treatment.

Each of these workers is legally and ethically limited by their scope of practice.

Healthcare workers can be held liable—legally responsible—for completing tasks within their scope of practice. They must perform the correct tests, use equipment properly, and read and report results carefully and accurately. This ensures doctors and patients are fully informed about patients' conditions and can make the best decisions. For example, if Patel does not deliver the ordered dosage of radiation or Claudio performs skills above his level of training, they could be liable for negative effects on a patient's health. If they provide the correct care, and their patients show no visible signs of distress *during* treatment, they are not responsible for any ill effects their patients experience *after* treatment.

Scope of practice places limits on what healthcare workers are allowed to do. Liability occurs if a worker goes beyond those limits. If Patel decides on his own that a particular patient should receive radiation for a longer period than ordered, he has exceeded his scope of practice. Working outside your scope of practice could be viewed as operating without a license, which is illegal.

To avoid liability, employers check credentials and work history. They may also limit your scope of practice. Before doctors can work at a hospital, they must apply to the hospital board for medical staff membership and hospital privileges. Doctors already on the medical staff at that hospital review the applicants' credentials and recommend whether the board should accept them (**Figure 16.3**). This review considers evidence of past training, experience, and competence. It also considers an applicant's character and judgment shown in past practice.

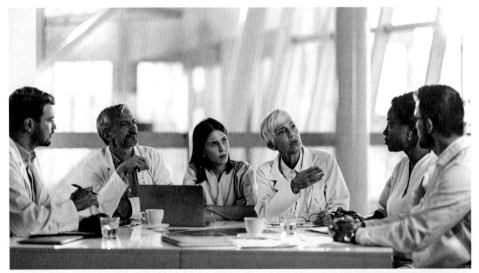

skynesher/E+ via Getty Images

Figure 16.3 A hospital board must approve a physician's application for membership in the hospital staff. *What kind of information does the hospital board review in these situations?*

If doctors are accepted, the hospital will list which procedures they can perform there. The hospital does not want staff members who are not well-qualified because they would put the facility's accreditation and reputation at risk.

Due to healthcare workforce shortages and high costs of care, many states have expanded the scope of practice for some healthcare workers. Nurse practitioners and physician assistants can prescribe medicine or practice without supervision in some states. This could increase the number of primary care providers available in rural communities and provide care at a lower cost. Some states are slow to make this change due to concerns about patient safety, but data from states with broader laws can help them understand the level of risk. During the COVID-19 pandemic, many states temporarily expanded scope-of-practice limits to increase healthcare workers' abilities to provide needed care in hospitals and clinics. Common scope-of-practice laws across the US would help reduce confusion between states and level out average salaries within the same profession.

Standard of Care and Malpractice

Within a healthcare professional's scope of practice, a certain **standard of care** is required. This is the level of care healthcare professionals are expected to provide based on their level of training and the patient's condition. For example, doctors are expected to respond to patients who have particular conditions with generally accepted treatments. When a trained professional knowingly provides care below this standard, and the patient suffers harm that could be reasonably expected, that professional is guilty of **malpractice**. This term literally means "bad practice." It is when professionals violate their scope of practice or standard of care and cause injury they should have known would occur.

Malpractice is usually a matter of civil law rather than criminal law. Patients who believe they have suffered injury can bring malpractice lawsuits. The plaintiff—the patient bringing the suit—must prove that the provider had a duty to provide care, that the provider did not meet that duty, and that the plaintiff suffered injury because of that failure. Failure to cure a disease or condition is not grounds for malpractice if the doctor treating the patient followed standards of care for that disease or condition. Treatments are not guaranteed to succeed.

Malpractice suits are typically brought against physicians, but other healthcare professionals can also face these charges. Healthcare professionals who face the possibility of malpractice charges can purchase insurance to protect themselves from the cost of losing a malpractice suit.

Negligence

Negligence is failing to do what a reasonable person should have known to do—or carelessness—that causes injury. In cases of medical negligence, unlike malpractice, you must show the error of the medical professional was not intentional. For example, dental hygienists know their dental tools must be sterilized between uses. If Calysta is in a hurry and just rinses the instruments off, she is *knowingly* taking the chance of transmitting a serious disease. This is malpractice. If Calysta removes the tools from the autoclave and does not realize they have not yet been sterilized, this is negligence (**Figure 16.4**). She can still be held legally responsible for the injury caused by her actions.

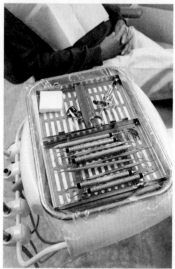

Mike Watson Images/moodboard/Thinkstock

Figure 16.4 Failing to properly sterilize medical instruments, such as these dental tools, is considered malpractice. *What could happen if unsterilized tools were used on a patient?*

16.2-2 **Avoiding Misconduct**

Providing high-quality care is the ultimate goal of all healthcare workers. The relationship between the healthcare worker and patient is based on trust. Behavior that breaks that trust or does not follow recognized standards of care can be considered **misconduct**. This includes a wide range of wrongful actions.

Many states have **caregiver laws** to protect children, older adults, and people with disabilities from misconduct by those who provide direct care, supervision, and protection. These laws cover topics such as neglect, abuse, and misappropriation of property. Violations of these laws can limit your ability to work in healthcare, childcare, and education.

Misappropriation

Misappropriation by employees is a special concern in the support services and therapeutic pathways. Workers in central supply, housekeeping, and the pharmacy, among others, have access to patient belongings, expensive medical supplies, and controlled medications. Taking these items is theft, whether the items belong to a patient, visitor, or the facility. This is more than just an ethical concern—theft is a crime.

You can avoid charges of misappropriation by conducting yourself properly. You should never touch patients' belongings without their permission. Never reach inside their bags, drawers, or pockets. If you must move a patient's belongings to clean around them, be sure the patient knows what you are doing. If you are asked to remove a patient's jewelry before transporting them to surgery or the morgue, have another employee witness your actions and fill out an inventory list of the patient's belongings.

In addition to legal issues, misappropriation also represents a betrayal of trust to the facility and its patients. The misappropriation of items meant for patient care could leave some patients without the supplies or medications they need. It also drives up the cost of healthcare. If you know of another worker's illegal or unethical behavior, report those actions to your supervisor or a higher-level authority.

Abuse, Neglect, and Other Torts

Abuse is an act that causes physical or emotional harm. There are many types of abuse. Slapping or pinching a patient are examples of physical abuse. Verbal abuse uses words to damage a patient's self-esteem. Sexual abuse includes any unwanted sexual contact. Physical and emotional **neglect** are passive forms of abuse in which the caregiver fails to provide the care needed.

Charges of abuse are based on the degree of harm. A felony is a serious crime punished by imprisonment or large fines. Misdemeanors, which are less serious than felonies, have shorter jail sentences and smaller fines. In some states, people with felony abuse or neglect convictions are permanently barred from caregiver jobs and facilities.

Some families have charged elder-care facilities with another form of abuse called **involuntary seclusion**. This is the practice of isolating a person to prevent interaction with others. You will work with many vulnerable populations in healthcare, so it is important to be aware of potential exploitation. Watch for unexplained injuries, fearfulness, or unusual behavior. Healthcare workers are required by law to report any signs of abuse.

False imprisonment is holding people against their will or limiting their movement without the right to do so. This includes the wrongful use of restraints or not allowing a patient to leave the hospital. Patients may sign a waiver form if they want to leave their care facility against medical advice. You can usually avoid restraints by adapting care to the patient's needs. For instance, residents with dementia are at high risk for falling. Long-term care staff can avoid restraining them in a wheelchair by distracting them with activities or a snack (**Figure 16.5**). Environmental safeguards include monitors to draw staff attention when residents get out of their chair or open a door.

Words or actions that lead a person to fear that you intend to harm them are considered **assault**. Assault is often charged along with **battery**, which is touching a person without their consent. Both assault and battery are crimes. Be careful in your choice of words and actions so your patients do not feel threatened. When you provide care, let your patients know what you are doing and get their permission before starting. Failing to get permission before removing a patient's clothing is battery. Telling your patient, "If you don't go to the bathroom on the toilet, I'll hang your dirty clothes out for everyone to see!" is assault. If you become frustrated with a patient, get help from a coworker rather than taking it out on the patient.

Even if you are tired, frustrated, or at the end of your shift, you cannot leave a patient who is dependent on your care. To avoid being guilty of **abandonment**, you must transfer care of the patient to someone else of equal or greater licensure. When there is a shortage of healthcare workers, this could mean working late until someone else is available.

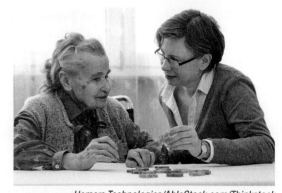
Hemera Technologies/AbleStock.com/Thinkstock
Figure 16.5 Older residents are at risk for falling, but do not necessarily need to be restrained. *What kinds of activities might engage a person and avoid the use of restraints?*

16.2-3 **Respecting Patient Privacy**

Lawsuits can even involve healthcare workers who do not provide hands-on care. For health informatics workers, tort cases most likely involve **invasion of privacy**. This means failing to keep an individual's details from being known by others. Privacy applies to both personal information and one's body. Any type of record or communication concerning your patient is private. You should only release it to the patient or guardian, care team, or others specifically authorized by the patient. You should never discuss patient information with people who are not involved in the patient's care (**Figure 16.6**). Healthcare workers must be careful never to discuss patients or their needs in a public area where people can overhear personal details. If an unauthorized person asks you for patient information, you can say, "I'm sorry, but I can't discuss that because it is private patient information."

Medical information can be released legally for a number of reasons. Patient information may be sent to someone involved in patient care or to file an insurance claim. In these cases, a signed patient authorization form must be on file before the information is released.

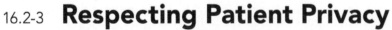
andresr/E+ via Getty Images
Figure 16.6 Personal information about patients must be kept private. *Does the scene here show an area in which healthcare workers can discuss sensitive information? Why or why not?*

A patient release is not required for a court order or government request for medical records. Reportable incidents and diseases, such as gunshot wounds and sexually transmitted infections, must be reported to protect public health.

For patients who receive medical testing, privacy and discrimination are very real concerns. Patients may worry about how family, friends, or employers will react if they hear of a positive test result for a disease. Patients may also worry about being overlooked for a promotion or turned down for a new job based on their test results. There are even cases of healthcare workers treating patients differently or refusing to provide care for patients who test positive for contagious diseases. This misuse of health information is both unethical and illegal.

Physical privacy must also be protected. If patients are in a public area, ask to move them to a more private area before discussing healthcare issues or beginning personal care. If a procedure requires the patient to change into a hospital gown, leave the room to provide privacy. Always knock before entering a patient's room, even if the door is open. This keeps you from overhearing private conversations. Use the privacy curtain before providing care, even when the door is closed. Announce yourself and pause before going behind a privacy curtain. This helps patients feel protected and prevents unintended bodily exposure. If visitors are in a patient's room, ask them to step into the waiting room until you are done. Most people do not want others watching when they receive personal care.

Different cultures may have different requirements for physical privacy. For example, people who are Muslim may prefer to receive care from someone of the same sex to fit with their rules of modesty. Showing concern for your patient's dignity and privacy helps build trust with the patient. Some facilities also have policies that require a female to be present when a male does a breast or vaginal exam on a female. These policies ensure the patient's comfort and protect the healthcare worker from false claims of inappropriate behavior. During procedures, keep the patient covered as much as possible. A robe or second gown worn backward will cover gown openings when the patient goes out into the hallway (**Figure 16.7**).

Exposing patients' personal information or bodies can harm their reputation and cause embarrassment. **Defamation** (deh-fuh-MAY-shuhn) of character means damaging someone's good name or reputation. Verbal defamation, such as gossip, is known as *slander*. When done in writing, defamation is called *libel*. You are guilty of libel if you post online or text a friend about a patient's stay in rehab. Defamation and invasion of privacy can affect someone's personal life, social life, and career. You may need to sign a confidentiality agreement before you begin working or volunteering in a healthcare facility.

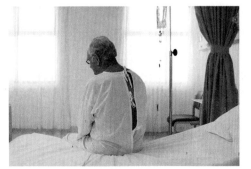

Sam Edwards/iStock/Getty Images Plus via Getty Images

Figure 16.7 Healthcare workers must always preserve the privacy of their patients. *If you saw a patient standing in the hallway with a loose hospital gown, how would you handle the situation?*

16.2-4 Privileged Communication and Mandatory Reporting

Healthcare providers have a special duty to maintain privacy of a patient's information. This duty goes beyond the rules of confidentiality that restrict sharing of patient information outside the care team. Patients must feel free to communicate openly with their care providers. This helps care providers make the proper diagnosis, design the best treatment, and ensure the treatment is followed. Therefore, private conversations between a healthcare professional and patient, known as **privileged communication**, cannot be testified about in court. The patient would have to give permission for this information to be shared.

How far does this right to privacy go when another person's health may be at risk? State laws grant this privilege, so the extent of protection may vary from one state to another. Generally, the only exception is when patients threaten to harm themselves or others and have a plan and means to do it. In situations that place a person in imminent danger, care providers must warn authorities and the person who is at risk. Suppose a patient has a communicable disease and does not want their life partner to know. What would you do?

While providing hands-on care, healthcare workers may see suspicious injuries or suspect abuse. An emergency medical technician may see that a knife or bullets made the wounds being treated. An emergency room nurse may smell alcohol on the breath of someone who was in a car accident. A patient may test positive for a communicable disease. A school nurse may hear stories that suggest a child has been sexually abused. Laws vary by state, but sharing this information is generally not a violation of confidentiality. These incidents and conditions involve people's safety, so they usually fall outside privileged communication rules. They must be reported as part of **mandatory reporting** laws.

Healthcare Professions: Mandatory Reporting

As a physician assistant (PA) in a hospital emergency room, Dyna often placed casts on broken bones. As she wrapped one young boy's arm, Dyna was shocked to see round scars that looked like cigarette burns on his arm. The boy's mother said he poked himself by accident.

Dyna knew this needed to be reported as a possible case of child abuse. She thought the mother seemed nice and she

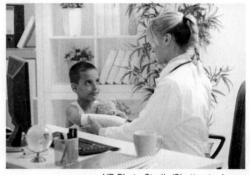

VP Photo Studio/Shutterstock.com

could see the woman's close bond with the child. She knew the process of investigating child abuse would probably involve removing the boy from his home until the situation could be investigated. Dyna did not want to cause the boy further distress. She also knew that people who have experienced abuse often know and protect those who abuse them. What would you do in Dyna's position?

Mandatory reporting helps protect people from abuse. This is more important than protecting the doctor-patient or parent-child relationship. Under the federal Child Abuse Prevention and Treatment Act (CAPTA), healthcare workers are required to report suspected physical, sexual, or emotional neglect or abuse to the state's child protective services (CPS). Reportable issues include apparent failure to provide for the basic needs of food, clothing, shelter, and medical care. Rules vary by state. It is your responsibility to know the rules in the facility and state where you work. Failure to report suspected abuse is usually classified as a misdemeanor. Knowingly making a false report of abuse is also punishable by law. People reporting suspicions of abuse "in good faith" cannot be held liable for a report that cannot be proven.

Many people who experience human trafficking will access healthcare during their captivity, so it is important to recognize and respond to this situation when it occurs (**Figure 16.8**). People who traffic others often target young and vulnerable women, such as those with disabilities, mental health conditions, and substance use concerns. Drugs, debts, or the offer of services are used to control them. Care is limited, and people who are being trafficked are closely watched during health visits to prevent them from talking about their situation.

As a healthcare professional, be empathetic and supportive. Congress passed the SOAR (Stop, Observe, Ask, and Respond) to Wellness Training Program in 2018 to provide training for healthcare and social service providers on human trafficking. The National Human Trafficking Resource Center offers a hotline in more than 200 languages to support both healthcare professionals and people who have experienced human trafficking.

Signs of Human Trafficking

Physical Signs	Behavioral Signs	Signs of Control
• Many injuries in various stages of healing • Exhaustion • Malnourishment • Delayed care • Frequent STI testing	• Overly nervous • Unaware of surroundings • Unwilling to answer questions • Using scripted answers • Refusing necessary care	• Controlling the patient's ID or money • Insisting on being present for exams • Claiming to be related but lacking personal knowledge of the patient

Goodheart-Willcox Publisher

Figure 16.8 Any signs of human trafficking should be reported.

Lesson 16.2 Review

 Complete the *Map Your Reading* graphic organizer for the section you just read.

1. Healthcare professionals can be held liable for harm caused when violating the law or practicing outside their (16.2-1)
   A. expertise
   B. delegated tasks
   C. scope of practice
   D. comfort zone

2. Intentionally providing care that is below accepted standards and causes harm is (16.2-1)
   A. negligence   C. abuse
   B. defamation   D. malpractice

3. Which of these are torts? Choose all that apply. (16.2-2)
   A. Involuntary seclusion
   B. Mandatory reporting
   C. False imprisonment
   D. Defamation

4. Threats to harm someone are considered verbal (16.2-2)
   A. battery   C. negligence
   B. assault   D. defamation

5. Which of these respects a patient's physical privacy? (16.2-3)
   A. Opening the door without knocking
   B. Staying in the room while a patient undresses
   C. Providing personal care around visitors
   D. Announcing yourself before going behind a privacy curtain

6. Unless a patient is planning to harm someone, a care provider cannot testify in court about _____ shared during patient care. (16.2-4)
   A. privileged communication
   B. any communication
   C. public communication
   D. threats

Laws Protecting Patient Rights

Learning Outcomes

After studying this lesson, you will be able to:

16.3-1 describe laws protecting basic patient rights.

16.3-2 describe advance directives and their implications for healthcare workers.

16.3-3 explain requirements for safety, privacy, and confidentiality of health information.

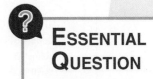

ESSENTIAL QUESTION

How do laws support patient rights?

Professional Vocabulary

Essential Terms

advance directive   a legal document prepared by patients before a health crisis occurs to guide healthcare decisions in situations when patients cannot speak for themselves

Health Insurance Portability and Accountability Act (HIPAA)   a federal law that makes it easier to obtain healthcare coverage and protects personal health information

Important Terms

Consolidated Omnibus Budget Reconciliation Act (COBRA)

do-not-resuscitate (DNR)
living will
Patient Self-Determination Act (PSDA)

power of attorney (POA)
protected health information (PHI)

Introduction

The first effort at defining and protecting patient rights was the Patient's Bill of Rights. This came from the American Hospital Association (AHA) rather than a law-making entity. Since then, Congress has passed several laws adding legal weight to patients' rights. A broad Patient Rights Act was introduced as a bill in 2019 but has not yet become law. The main purpose of these efforts was to guarantee patients' fair treatment, access to information, privacy of personal information, access to care options, and ability to take part in healthcare decisions.

While the *Patient Care Partnership* replaced the AHA *Patient's Bill of Rights* in 2003, healthcare facilities continue to enforce patient rights. These rights are embedded in many laws. You should be able to explain patient rights to your patient. Pay special attention to actions required or restricted by law. EMTALA provided the right to access care, so that an emergency room could not turn patients away if they could not pay for care. Changes to insurance laws expanded access to care. A multitude of tort laws protect against poor quality of care. A court decision provided the right to informed consent.

The Patient Protection and Affordable Care Act (ACA) added that insurers must explain benefits and claim denials using universal definitions. Additional laws protect your ability to make decisions and keep your information private. This lesson will expand your understanding of some of these laws.

16.3-1 Protecting Patient Access to Care

Many people see access to healthcare as a human right. Most people access and pay for healthcare through some form of health insurance. In the past, people with insurance benefits through their employer or spouse could lose healthcare coverage due to life events. A move, divorce, or change in employers could cut their connection to insurance. In 1985, the **Consolidated Omnibus Budget Reconciliation Act (COBRA)** was included in the Employee Retirement Income Security (ERISA) Act. This allowed employees leaving their job to continue their insurance for up to three years if they paid for it themselves. This was an important way to preserve access to care.

The ACA expanded access to care. It made insurance and healthcare more available and affordable by placing new restrictions on insurance companies (**Figure 16.9**). The ACA also allows people to purchase insurance from the exchange market within 60 days of a life event. In this way, the ACA further protects access to healthcare.

According to the ACA,

- Insurers cannot limit coverage of preexisting conditions or use lifetime coverage limits.
- Young adults can remain on their parents' insurance until age 26.
- People with insurance can choose their healthcare provider from their insurer's network
- All health insurance must include coverage for hospitalization, ambulatory care, emergency services, maternity and newborn care, mental health, brand-name prescription drugs, lab tests, preventive care, pediatric care, and rehabilitative services.

Goodheart-Willcox Publisher

Figure 16.9 The ACA placed limits on insurers and expanded healthcare coverage.

16.3-2 Patient's Right to Participate in Treatment Decisions

The **Patient Self-Determination Act (PSDA)**, passed in 1990, protects healthcare consumers' rights to make their own decisions. This act requires many healthcare institutions to provide information about decision-making rights and to ask patients if they have **advance directives**. These legal documents state a patient's wishes for care when they cannot make decisions, such as during a loss of consciousness. There are two main types of advance directives: a living will and a power of attorney. A physician or nurse practitioner may also write orders for the patient not to be resuscitated or intubated. The rules for these advance directives and physician orders vary from state to state.

A **living will** is a legal document that states what medical care patients do or do not want used to keep them alive. This may include a feeding tube, blood transfusion, resuscitation, or other procedures. Typically, the patient and a witness must sign these documents. A copy should be given to the primary care provider so the patient's wishes are known (**Figure 16.10**). In most states, a living will does not go into effect unless two doctors have certified you are *incapacitated*, or unable to make decisions for yourself. There may be other requirements, such as "terminal illness" or "permanent unconsciousness," in some states.

Some individuals have documents that state they are willing to donate usable organs when they die. Several states allow people to state this on their driver's license. Others have an organ donor card that can be carried in a wallet or purse. Organ-donation preferences can also be part of a living will.

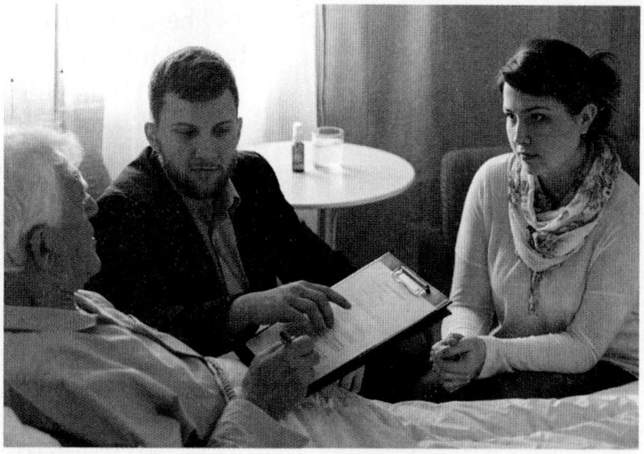

Some orders about life-sustaining treatments may be issued by hospital staff at a patient's request. **Do-not-resuscitate (DNR)** orders specifically state that a patient should not be revived with chest compressions or cardiac drugs if the patient stops breathing or the heart stops beating. Do-not-intubate (DNI) means that a breathing tube should not be used. Some hospitals use signs or give patients with DNR orders a special wristband to indicate their wishes.

Photographee.eu/Shutterstock.com

Figure 16.10 Living wills must be signed by the patient and witnessed by another person. *What information does a living will contain?*

Power of attorney (POA) for healthcare documents assign a legal representative, or *proxy*, to make healthcare decisions for people in the event they cannot make their own choices. Like a living will, these documents must be signed and witnessed to be legal. The POA generally becomes active when two doctors declare a patient incapacitated. It is important for the proxy of the POA to know what the patient would want or not want in different scenarios before the time comes to decide.

Rules differ from state to state, but family members may not be authorized to make decisions for adults without a POA document. This may place a doctor in charge of all healthcare decisions after a severe accident or stroke. If there are concerns, a guardian may be chosen by the court to decide what is in the best interest of the patient. Guardians may have less flexibility in decision-making than a proxy. This process can also be expensive, time-consuming, and emotionally draining for the family. The best way for patients to make sure their wishes are followed is to have advance directives in writing and discuss their wishes with their doctor, family, and proxy while they still can.

16.3-3 **Healthcare Privacy**

State laws and court decisions generally protect information shared between a patient and doctor as privileged information. The **Health Insurance Portability and Accountability Act (HIPAA)**, signed in 1996, was the first national health privacy law. HIPAA aimed to make it easier to share information for insurance coverage and payments while keeping healthcare records and personal health information safe. It required the Department of Health and Human Services to create privacy and security rules for storing and sharing health information. It also set civil and criminal fines for breaking privacy rules.

Goodheart-Willcox Publisher

Figure 16.11 Personal health information must be protected in all settings. *What are the consequences of breaching a patient's confidentiality?*

The 2003 HIPAA Privacy Rule gave patients some rights to access their health information and limited who could receive this information and how it could be used. It defined **protected health information (PHI)** as any information held by an organization concerned with health, healthcare, or payment for healthcare that can be linked to a person. This includes a patient's name, address, birth date, telephone number, email address, Social Security number, medical record number, and so on. PHI may come from personal contacts, messages, electronic files, computer displays, and many other forms of communication. Privacy notices must tell patients how their PHI will be used. This includes data used for treatment, billing, marketing, research, and reports to the Medical Information Bureau (MIB) for insurance purposes. Patients must sign a release for any other uses or sharing of their PHI, such as birth notices or posting a patient's name outside their hospital room. Healthcare workers have an obligation to know what PHI is and how to protect it (**Figure 16.11**).

The 2005 HIPAA Security Rule focused on electronically held PHI (ePHI). It required facilities to have clear HIPAA policies and procedures. Facilities were required to limit access to areas where data was stored. Any ePHI had to use encryption to protect online access. In 2009, a HIPAA Breach Notification Rule was added. Facilities must notify people when unsecure PHI is used or accessed without their permission. The HITECH Act of 2009 continued to build on these rules.

The first rule of confidentiality is to only share information with authorized people. Medical information should only be released to the patient or guardian, care team, or insurance company. PHI should not be provided unless the patient or proxy has signed a release form. When legitimate information requests are received, workers should only supply the specific information requested, never a patient's complete chart. Other uses would be both illegal and unethical. Report any accidental breaches to your supervisor immediately.

The penalties for breaking privacy rules can be severe. HIPAA is a federal law, so serious and willful violations, such as selling patient information, result in fines and jail time. Breach of confidentiality also violates professional ethics and can affect a healthcare worker's employability. Offenders may have a letter of reprimand placed in their personnel file or lose their job. Their actions also affect the reputation of their employer, leaving them open to lawsuits, penalties, bad publicity, and loss of business.

Lesson 16.3 Review

 Complete the *Map Your Reading* graphic organizer for the section you just read.

1. Which of the following is *not* a patient right? (16.3-1)
   A. Access to care
   B. Privacy of information
   C. Finality of decisions
   D. Participation in treatment decisions

2. Which of these are an advance directive? Choose all that apply. (16.3-2)
   A. Living will
   B. Power of attorney
   C. DNR order
   D. Court decision

3. A living will (16.3-2)
   A. says whom to give your possessions to
   B. says how to prepare your body at death
   C. appoints a person to make decisions for you
   D. says what medical care you do or do not want when incapacitated

4. Protected health information should only be shared with people who are (16.3-3)
   A. family members
   B. asking for information
   C. insistent
   D. authorized

Laws Regulating Health and Safety

Learning Outcomes

After studying this lesson, you will be able to:

16.4-1 explain when and how to use incident reports.

16.4-2 summarize laws protecting against biohazards.

16.4-3 explain how CLIA protects patients and lab workers.

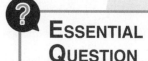

ESSENTIAL QUESTION

How do laws protect public and personal safety?

Professional Vocabulary

Essential Terms

Bloodborne Pathogens Standard prescribes safeguards to protect workers at risk of being exposed to blood and other potentially infectious materials

Hazard Communication Standard (HCS) requires employers to provide information and training for employees about handling potential health hazards in the workplace

incident report a form used to record the details of an unusual event, such as an accident or injury

Important Terms

Biohazard Prevention Act

Clinical Laboratory Improvement Act (CLIA)

Federal Needlestick Safety and Prevention Act

Medical Waste Tracking Act

Introduction

Health and safety laws protect both patients and workers in healthcare. Professionals in the diagnostic, therapeutic, and biomedical research pathways are more likely to work with body fluids, tissue samples, biomedical waste products, and other materials that increase the risk of infection. They are also more likely to be exposed to chemicals and radiation. As a result, their daily work is more tightly regulated by the Centers for Disease Control and Prevention (CDC) and the Occupational Safety and Health Administration (OSHA). The federal government has passed several laws that strictly regulate the handling of potentially dangerous substances.

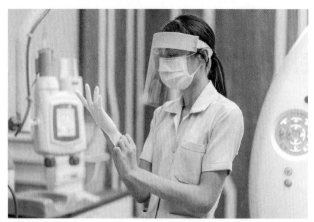
pang_oasis/Shutterstock.com

Figure 16.12 OSHA follows the recommendations of the CDC to create guidelines for healthcare worker safety.

16.4-1 Reporting Health and Safety Incidents

The CDC is a public health agency that does research to track and promote public health, respond to health issues, and support the creation and maintenance of safe and healthy workplaces. The CDC is also an excellent source of information about disease prevention and health promotion. OSHA creates rules to prevent work-related injuries, illnesses, and deaths. OSHA is also the main federal agency responsible for workplace safety. They are concerned about occupational exposure to hazardous substances on the job. OSHA closely follows CDC recommendations in these areas (**Figure 16.12**).

An **incident report** must be filed whenever a patient, employee, or visitor reports an injury, action, or behavior that affects someone's health or safety. This form collects factual information about who was involved, what happened, events leading up to the incident, harm caused, and actions taken. Each person involved or witnessing the event should complete their own report to include all points of view. The information is reviewed to determine how to avoid future events of this type through training, modifications to the care plan, and other systemic changes. It also serves as a legal record if there are criminal or civil charges.

Quality-improvement studies of incident reports can provide the push for changes in safety regulations. Before 2011, medications given by the wrong route harmed an alarming number of patients. Oral medications were given by IV, IV medications were given as an epidural, and so on. The problem was universal tubing connectors on the many different types of tubes used in patient care. In 2011, the Food and Drug Administration (FDA), which regulates the health and safety of food, drugs, and medical devices, began releasing new standards for tubing connections to help prevent misconnection errors. These connector standards currently apply to manufacturers, but healthcare facilities are transitioning to the new devices. In 2016, California was the first state to pass a law requiring healthcare facilities to use the new connectors.

16.4-2 Protecting Against Biohazards

Many hazardous chemicals and products are used in healthcare. The Environmental Protection Agency (EPA) controls the sale and use of hazardous chemicals; pesticides; nanotechnology; and asbestos-, lead-, and mercury-containing products. They work cooperatively with OSHA to enforce safety regulations. Their goal is to protect the health of workers, the public, and the environment.

OSHA's **Hazard Communication Standard (HCS)** requires employers to make employees aware of and ensure the safe handling of hazardous substances in the workplace. In addition to products regulated by the EPA, this includes blood and other body fluids, disinfectants, medications, chemicals, and compressed gases. Employers must provide proper training and have Safety Data Sheets (SDSs) readily accessible for each hazardous substance. Condensed SDS information must be placed on packages containing the hazardous substance.

OSHA designed the **Bloodborne Pathogens Standard** to protect workers at risk of being exposed to blood and other potentially infectious materials. The regulation is mainly aimed at the hepatitis B virus (HBV); the hepatitis C virus (HCV); and the human immunodeficiency virus (HIV), which can cause acquired immunodeficiency syndrome (AIDS). Employers must have a written exposure control plan; provide annual training for workers at risk for job-related exposure to bloodborne pathogens; and offer vaccinations, PPE, and other devices to decrease risk.

Needlesticks and sharps injuries are the most common ways healthcare workers are exposed to bloodborne pathogens. The **Federal Needlestick Safety and Prevention Act** of 2000 requires employers to regularly review their exposure control plan, maintain a sharps injury log, and seek safer medical devices to reduce their rate of injuries. This includes needleless systems and needles specially designed for safer injections and blood draws.

The **Medical Waste Tracking Act**, for OSHA, and the **Biohazard Prevention Act**, for the EPA, give state and federal agencies the power to investigate workplaces' storage and disposal methods for medical waste. These laws require workers to discard sharp objects, such as needles, in solid containers that cannot be punctured and to dispose of chemicals and blood products in secure containers (**Figure 16.13**). Biohazard signs must be posted to alert workers in areas that may contain medical waste. Healthcare facilities must be inspected regularly and contract with specialized disposal companies to handle, transport, treat, and dispose of biohazardous waste.

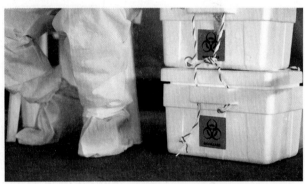

attakorn sanguanwong/Shutterstock.com

Figure 16.13 Biohazardous waste must be properly handled and disposed of to protect community health.

16.4-3 Protecting the Safety and Validity of Laboratory Tests

Diagnostic workers frequently use laboratory-developed tests. These tests are considered medical "devices" and must be approved by the FDA before being used to diagnose patients. This is to ensure each test's safety, effectiveness, reliability, and accuracy. The FDA evaluates the clinical validity of medical testing procedures to determine if they can actually find the diseases or injuries they claim to test.

Clinical laboratories and their workers must follow the **Clinical Laboratory Improvement Act (CLIA)** practices. CLIA applies to all laboratory facilities across the US. The federal government defines a *laboratory* as any facility that tests specimens derived from humans to give information for the assessment of health or prevention, diagnosis, or treatment of a disease or impairment.

CLIA regulates how a laboratory test is done and how test results are interpreted and reported. This assures the patient the lab results are accurate and reliable. **Figure 16.14** lists the requirements for labs under CLIA.

Laboratories must be certified and maintain compliance with CLIA regulations. Employers are required to provide training about the law and potential hazards for all employees. Facilities must keep detailed records of the training provided and document any accidents or incidents that violated CLIA regulations.

The CDC has been studying best practices for laboratory-quality improvement. They found blood culture samples are less likely to be contaminated if collected through a needle inserted in the vein by a dedicated phlebotomy worker. Electronic bar coding has been proven to reduce patient specimen and laboratory testing identification errors. Translating test results into common reporting formats allows faster automated reporting and follow-up on critical results. These best practices provide additional protection for the accuracy of patients' test results and may eventually become part of new regulations for diagnostic procedures.

Under CLIA, labs are required to

- use materials and equipment for testing that meet basic performance standards
- maintain equipment to meet the manufacturer's performance specifications
- create procedure manuals and quality-control procedures
- ensure employees are properly educated and trained to do their assigned work

Goodheart-Willcox Publisher

Figure 16.14 CLIA requires labs to follow certain safety guidelines.

Lesson 16.4 Review

 Complete the *Map Your Reading* graphic organizer for the section you just read.

1. A(n) _____ report must be filed when someone is injured. (16.4-1)
   A. breach
   B. incident
   C. accident
   D. correction

2. OSHA requires employers to have _____ readily available for each hazardous substance. (16.4-2)
   A. SDSs
   B. incident reports
   C. injury logs
   D. performance standards

3. The Bloodborne Pathogens Standard helps protect against exposure to which of the following? Choose all that apply. (16.4-2)
   A. Human immunodeficiency virus
   B. Tuberculosis
   C. Hepatitis C virus
   D. Hepatitis B virus

4. To protect patients from inaccurate diagnostic test results, the _____ regulates test procedures. (16.4-3)
   A. OSHA
   B. CLIA
   C. FDA
   D. CDC

Employment Laws

Learning Outcomes

After studying this lesson, you will be able to:

16.5-1 summarize laws that affect hiring and discharge.

16.5-2 identify employment laws that affect work hours and wages.

16.5-3 explain protection provided by the Civil Rights Act.

16.5-4 discuss legal protections against harassment.

16.5-5 describe other workplace laws.

ESSENTIAL QUESTION

How do laws protect employee rights?

Professional Vocabulary

Essential Terms

discrimination   unfair treatment of individuals on the basis of their membership in a specific group (i.e., age, race, color, nationality, citizenship, religion, sex, disability, veteran status, or genetic information)

Fair Labor Standards Act (FLSA)   a federal law that adopted an eight-hour workday, 40-hour work week, time-and-a-half overtime pay, and restricted employment of minors

harassment   unwelcome, offensive, and repeated language or actions, based on age, race, color, nationality, citizenship, religion, sex, disability, veteran status, or genetic information, that affect an employee's job performance or advancement opportunities or create an uncomfortable working environment

Important Terms

Age Discrimination in Employment Act (ADEA)

Americans with Disabilities Act (ADA)

Civil Rights Act

employment at will

Equal Employment Opportunity Commission (EEOC)

Equal Pay Act

Family and Medical Leave Act (FMLA)

Genetic Information Nondiscrimination Act (GINA)

Immigration Reform and Control Act

minimum wage

National Labor Relations Act (NLRA)

on-call

overtime

Rehabilitation Act

sexual harassment

union

wrongful discharge

Introduction

Many state and federal laws affect the employer-employee relationship. These laws cover a wide range of considerations, from how old you need to be before you can be legally employed, to how workers interact with one another. Some federal laws apply to all workplaces and involve workers' fundamental rights.

Other laws apply only to workplaces with a minimum number of workers or those with employees who work a minimum number of hours a week. Laws may be stricter at the state level. Whether you are in an entry-level job or have moved up the career ladder, you should know how employment laws and the protections they provide apply to you.

16.5-1 Laws That Affect Hiring and Discharge

The basic principle behind employment law is **employment at will**. This is the idea that employment is an equal agreement between employer and employee that either one can end whenever they want (**Figure 16.15**). An employee can choose to quit a job to take a new one. An organization can fire or lay off an employee. Generally, employers who end a worker's employment after their probationary period must have a valid reason for their action. They must show they have not violated a contract or broken any discrimination laws in deciding to fire someone.

The **National Labor Relations Act (NLRA)** of 1935 gives workers the right to unite and discuss ways of improving their working conditions. **Unions** bring together workers from the same company or region to bargain collectively. This collective voice of many employees negotiates with an employer for specific terms of employment, such as wages, hours, working conditions, or benefits. Employers cannot prohibit such discussions or punish workers who take part in them, but they can fire employees who take part in a *strike*, or refusal to work, unless it is to protest unfair labor practices.

When a work contract is formed, both the organization and the worker must follow its terms. These agreements usually specify the terms and conditions of employment, including grounds for dismissal. It may require the employer to document steps taken to fix the situation. Workers should be informed if their performance is not up to the desired standard. They may be given training or suggestions for improvement and a chance to fix the situation. If an organization fires a contracted worker without just cause, the worker may bring legal action. The worker might claim to be the victim of **wrongful discharge**, or being dismissed without cause.

State laws vary regarding union membership and dues. Many states have passed right-to-work laws that ban union-security agreements requiring all employees to become union members and pay dues. They will not be full union members but still benefit from union-bargained protections. In other states, the Beck Right says employees under a union-security agreement who object cannot be charged fees to support government-lobbying efforts.

Workers do not have to form a union to enjoy the benefits of collective bargaining. However, if they do, the employer cannot refuse to bargain in good faith with the union's elected representative. Some professional organizations, such as the American Nurses Association (ANA), function in similar ways to unions. These organizations also provide a collective voice and advocate for the needs and concerns of their members.

The **Immigration Reform and Control Act** of 1986 also set employment restrictions. Employers may not knowingly hire an undocumented immigrant. This law discourages

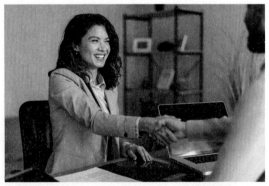

djile/Shutterstock.com

Figure 16.15 When employees are hired for a job, they must understand that an agreement has been created between them and their new employers. *What are the terms of this agreement?*

people from coming into the US illegally. Employers must check the identity and employment authorization of all new employees within three days of their hire. You may be asked to verify your citizenship with a US birth certificate, passport, driver's license, or Social Security card. A permanent resident (green) card allows an immigrant to legally live and work in the US. Some noncitizens have employment authorization. Others may need their employer to petition for them to work in the US temporarily or permanently.

Although it is not a law, many professional associations also require proof of identity and a Social Security number from anyone taking their certification exams. This avoids certifying an undocumented immigrant for work they could not be legally hired to perform. Employers who violate immigration reform laws may have to pay a fine or face other criminal penalties.

16.5-2 Laws That Affect Wages, Hours, and Minimum Age

The federal **Fair Labor Standards Act (FLSA)** affects wages, hours, and minimum age requirements for employment. FLSA restricts work settings and hours for workers younger than 18 years of age. The US Department of Labor monitors child labor to protect young people's health, safety, and educational opportunities. Sixteen is the minimum age to work in healthcare. Some cashiering, cleaning, lifeguarding, cafeteria, and office jobs are available to 14- and 15-year-olds (**Figure 16.16**). Workers younger than 16 years of age may not work during school hours, more than three hours on school days, or between the hours of 7:00 p.m. and 7:00 a.m.

Some jobs are more dangerous and require workers to be at least 18 years of age. Jobs using sharp tools, power-driven lifts, or mixing machines are among these hazardous occupations, so work for minors in kitchens, as nursing assistants, or as transport technicians may be restricted. State laws may also require a minor to obtain a work permit. Child labor laws no longer apply once a person reaches 18 years of age.

In addition to regulating child labor, FLSA sets minimum-wage and overtime rules. **Minimum wage** is the lowest hourly wage permitted by law. The minimum wage was set at $7.25 per hour in July 2009, but it has been raised in the past and could go up again. Some states have their own minimum-wage laws. When state and federal laws conflict, the employer must pay the higher of the two amounts. In 2023, for instance, the minimum wage was $15.00 or more per hour in California, Massachusetts, and Washington, DC.

FLSA also sets rules for payment of regular and **overtime** wages. Under federal law, employees who work more than 40 hours a week must be paid one and a half times their regular hourly rate for those extra hours. This is also known as *time-and-a-half* pay. Break times of fewer than 20 minutes are included as part of the hours worked. Meal periods of 30 minutes or longer, during which no work duties are required, are not counted in hours worked. FLSA does not specify a maximum number of hours that may be worked in one day.

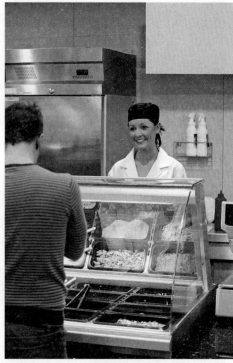

wavebreakmedia/Shutterstock.com
Figure 16.16 Workers who are 14 or 15 years of age can be hired for jobs such as food service in a hospital cafeteria.

These overtime pay rules do not apply to all workers. As of 2020, salaried "white collar" office or administrative professionals who earn at least $684 a week, traveling sales workers, and some computer employees may be exempt from the minimum wage and overtime provisions of FLSA. First responders, paramedics, licensed practical nurses, and other similar healthcare professionals are generally protected by FLSA because an advanced degree is not a standard requirement for their employment, and their salary may be less than the specified amount. Nurses and doctors, however, are considered exempt and are not entitled to overtime pay unless it is part of their employment contract.

The healthcare industry has some added exceptions to the normal overtime rules. Hospitals, nursing homes, and other healthcare facilities can form an agreement with their employees to calculate overtime based on work exceeding eight hours in a day or 80 hours in two weeks. This *8 and 80 system* allows an employee to work more than eight hours per day without receiving overtime as long as they do not exceed 80 hours in two weeks. Many nurses work three 12-hour shifts in a week and have four days off. How would you feel about a 12-hour workday?

Some emergency medical services (EMS) workers use *Garcia cycles* when calculating their standard pay and overtime (**Figure 16.17**). Some people call these *7K cycles* because they follow a maximum hour standard chart in statute 207(k) of the FLSA regulations. The chart is based on a repeating work schedule between 7 and 28 days in length. It is common for EMS workers to have a repeating shift of 24 hours on duty and 48 hours off duty. If employees are given a place to sleep for more than five hours during the 24 hours worked, their pay may be reduced for sleep time. Over a 28-day cycle, they may work as many as 240 hours. According to the FLSA schedule, anything over 212 hours is considered overtime.

Caregivers such as nurses and EMTs may have *mandatory overtime*. This means they cannot refuse to work overtime hours when requested. Refusing can result in penalties or termination unless those requests violate a contract, are unpaid, or would result in a health hazard. FLSA does not restrict the total number of hours employees may be required to work as long as they are properly compensated for overtime hours and the additional hours do not create a safety risk. This helps employers cover patient care needs when an employee calls in sick and a replacement has not been found to cover the shift. What concerns would you have about mandatory overtime at the end of your usual workday?

OSHA recognizes the risk that tired workers pose to themselves, their coworkers, and their patients. The agency recommends that employers provide extra breaks for workers whose shifts are longer than eight hours per day. They also suggest allowing at least eight hours of rest between shifts. These are guidelines for employers, but not part of any law. Some union contracts and states restrict the amount of overtime that can be requested of an employee.

FLSA also regulates **on-call** pay. Being "on call" means you must be available to answer calls at any time during that shift and may be required to come in to work on short notice. Doctors or EMS workers

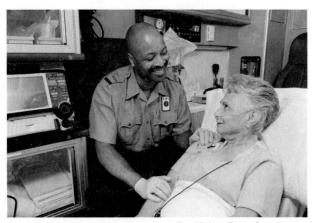

FangXiaNuo/E+ via Getty Images

Figure 16.17 EMS workers often need to work overtime. *What kind of shift do EMS workers commonly have?*

who are on-call may receive a weekly bonus for carrying a beeper. Workers who are required to remain on-site while waiting for a call to their next location must be paid an on-call wage for those hours. If they respond to a call outside their regular 40-hour workweek, they may be compensated by overtime pay in addition to their regular wage or bonus. If an employee is a professional exempted by FLSA, the employer may agree to compensation other than time-and-a-half pay. They may provide *compensation time*, allowing the employee to take an equivalent number of hours off instead of receiving more pay.

16.5-3 Antidiscrimination Laws

Discrimination, in legal terms, is the unfair treatment of people based on their membership in a specific group. In terms of employment, the main antidiscrimination law is the **Civil Rights Act** of 1964. This law bans employment discrimination based on a person's race, color, religion, sex (including pregnancy), or national origin. The law applies to workplace decisions such as hiring, starting salary, promotion, and firing. It is important to fight against systemic racism by notifying your employer when you see hiring, promotion, or disciplinary practices that favor one group of people over another.

Another important antidiscrimination law is the **Equal Pay Act** of 1963. It requires employers to pay males and females equally for performing the same job under the same conditions. If two maintenance engineers, one male and one female, have the same level of skill, responsibility, and effort required in their jobs, they should receive equal pay. However, if one job requires additional training and responsibilities, that employee may receive a higher rate of pay whether male or female.

The **Age Discrimination in Employment Act (ADEA)** of 1967 extended civil rights protection to workers 40 years of age or older. The **Rehabilitation Act** of 1973 and the **Americans with Disabilities Act (ADA)** of 1990 gave similar protection to workers with physical or mental disabilities. Under these laws, it is discrimination to refuse to make reasonable accommodations for a job applicant with a disability if the applicant is otherwise qualified for the job.

A person with a disability may request that an employer remove barriers created by rules or physical obstacles so they can perform their job duties and access the same benefits of employment as others. For example, people with visual impairments may require their employer to provide computer applications and equipment that allow them to listen as their computer reads text aloud. Those with diabetes may request specific break and meal times to take insulin and eat on a regular schedule. Employees in a wheelchair may request that break room appliances be moved to accessible heights so they can use them at lunch (**Figure 16.18**).

If you are protected by the ADA or Rehabilitation Act, your employer may be required to change your mandatory overtime schedule to accommodate a disability that causes fatigue, the need to change positions, or an inability to concentrate for long periods of time. The only limitation to reasonable accommodations is they should not cause significant hardship for the employer.

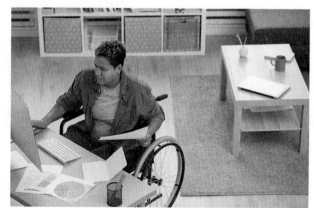

AnnaStills/Shutterstock.com

Figure 16.18 Workers with disabilities may make requests to modify their workspaces so they can better access files or other items necessary for their jobs.

Employers Covered by Federal Antidiscrimination Laws	
Law	Type of Employer Covered
Equal Pay Act of 1963	All employers
Civil Rights Act of 1964	Employers with 15 or more employees who work at least 20 weeks a year
Age Discrimination in Employment Act of 1967	Employers with 20 or more employees who work at least 20 weeks a year
Rehabilitation Act of 1973	Employers who have contracts with the federal government worth $2,500 or more
Americans with Disabilities Act of 1990	Employers with 15 or more employees who work at least 20 weeks a year

Goodheart-Willcox Publisher

Figure 16.19 Not all workplaces are required to follow all antidiscrimination laws. *What size of business has the most exemptions?*

Under the **Genetic Information Nondiscrimination Act (GINA)** of 2008, employers cannot discriminate against job applicants or employees based on their genetic information. This act puts strict limits on employers' ability to gather or disclose genetic information. Employers cannot refuse to hire or promote because of information about an inherited health condition that could affect job performance or the employer's health insurance costs.

In addition to banning discrimination, these laws prohibit employers from taking any negative action against a worker who files a complaint against them for violating workers' rights. For instance, an employee who files a lawsuit for age discrimination cannot be fired, have their pay cut, or be punished in any other way by the employer.

A federal agency known as the **Equal Employment Opportunity Commission (EEOC)** enforces these acts. The EEOC has the power to bring lawsuits on behalf of workers who believe they have experienced discrimination. Under the Lilly Ledbetter Fair Pay Act of 2009, compensation for wages lost can stretch back several years. While these antidiscrimination laws are meant to protect workers' rights, they do not necessarily apply to all workplaces. **Figure 16.19** shows which employers are covered by the different laws.

16.5-4 Antiharassment Laws

Title VII of the Civil Rights Act protects workers from all types of **harassment**. The EEOC defines harassment as "unwelcome conduct that is based on race, color, religion, sex (including pregnancy), national origin, age (40 or older), disability, or genetic information." They define **sexual harassment** as "unwelcome sexual advances; requests for sexual favors; and other verbal, nonverbal, or physical conduct of a sexual nature." Both male and female workers can experience sexual harassment. You do not have to be the direct recipient of harassment. The law applies to anyone the offensive conduct affects.

Harassment does not include simple teasing or single off-hand comments, but it can include unintentional actions, such as repeated off-color jokes or pictures displayed in a work locker. Harassment is illegal if:

1. enduring the harassment is a condition for continued employment;
2. a benefit or detriment, such as a raise or job loss, is directly linked to complying with the harassment; or
3. the harassment creates an intimidating or hostile environment.

If you experience harassment, tell the person to stop. If the behavior continues, make a formal complaint to your supervisor or the human resources office. Documenting harassment in a journal will help you make your case. A person who commits harassment may be tried under civil law. In organizations with 15 or more employees, employers are liable if they know about harassment and do not take immediate corrective action to prevent it. Employers should work to prevent harassment through training and zero-tolerance policies.

16.5-5 Other Workplace Laws

The **Family and Medical Leave Act (FMLA)** of 1991 grants workers the right to up to 12 weeks off work in a 12-month period to give birth to a child, care for a newborn or newly adopted child, care for a family member with a serious illness, or recover from a personal illness or injury (**Figure 16.20**). This is taken as *leave*, meaning unpaid time off. While the employer is not required to pay the worker or pay for their benefits during this time, the employee has a right to an equivalent job on their return to work. FMLA applies only to workers hired by employers with 50 or more employees who work 20 or more workweeks in a year.

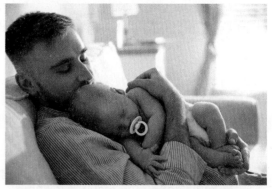

New Africa/Shutterstock.com

Figure 16.20 The Family and Medical Leave Act allows employees time away from work to care for a newborn child. *What other circumstances are covered under this law?*

The EEOC also prevents employers from enforcing English-only rules in the workplace. Problems can occur when people assume that a conversation in another language is about them. Employers have only a limited ability to require that English be spoken in work situations. For example, English may be required when communicating with customers, coworkers, or supervisors who only speak English. In emergencies, English may be required as a common language to promote safety. It is not legal to require English for casual conversations between employees.

Similarly, an employer has only limited ability to control an employee's use of social media. NLRA protects an employee's right to post and comment online, as long as the postings do not violate other laws such as privacy and libel. Employers may restrict use of social media during work hours or the use of the company's name or logo in postings. They cannot discriminate against employees, or potential employees, for their personal use of social media.

Lesson 16.5 Review

 Complete the *Map Your Reading* graphic organizer for the section you just read.

1. Under the principle of _____, either an employer or worker may end a job at any time. (16.5-1)
   A. wrongful discharge
   B. equal opportunity
   C. employment at will
   D. overtime

2. Workers younger than _____ may have limits on the number of hours they may work in a day or settings where they are allowed to work. (16.5-2)
   A. 21   C. 16
   B. 40   D. 12

3. The Civil Rights Act prohibits discrimination in workplace decisions based on which of the following? Choose all that apply. (16.5-3)
   A. Race   C. Age
   B. National origin   D. Disability

4. What should you do if you experience harassment at work? (16.5-4)
   A. Harass the person back
   B. Make a formal complaint to your supervisor
   C. Stay quiet
   D. Post about it online

5. Employers can restrict all of the following *except* (16.5-5)
   A. social media use during work hours
   B. use of the company's logo
   C. use of the company's name
   D. social media use outside work hours

Chapter 16 Review and Assessment

Chapter Summary

16.1-1 Committing a crime, breaking civil laws, or violating your professional code of ethics may result in financial penalties or loss of a job. Violating criminal laws puts society at risk and may result in jail time.

16.1-2 The doctor-patient relationship forms a contract that has an offer, consideration, enforceability, and consent. Informed consent requires enough information about the diagnosis, prognosis, and treatment for the patient to decide on care.

16.2-1 A healthcare professional's scope of practice is limited by state and federal credentialing laws and facility rules. Healthcare workers are legally liable for the care they provide.

16.2-2 Misconduct includes behaviors that do not follow recognized standards of care. Abuse causes physical or emotional harm. Caregivers need the patient's consent and choose their words and actions carefully to avoid assault or battery.

16.2-3 To protect privacy, keep the patient covered, knock before entering, and do not discuss patient care outside the care team.

16.2-4 Most patient information is privileged and cannot be testified about in court. Healthcare workers must follow mandatory reporting laws when they suspect abuse, neglect, or certain types of violence or communicable disease.

16.3-1 Laws protect patient access to care, the right to fair treatment, privacy, access to information, and the ability to take part in healthcare decisions.

16.3-2 Patients are encouraged to be involved in healthcare decisions and plan ahead through advance directives.

16.3-3 HIPAA laws help protect the privacy of patient information. Healthcare workers need to know what PHI includes and how to protect it.

16.4-1 OSHA requires an incident report be filed for any injury, action, or behavior that affects someone's health or safety.

16.4-2 OSHA's Bloodborne Pathogen Standard minimizes exposure to certain pathogens. The Medical Waste Tracking Act allows OSHA to make sure infectious waste and sharp objects are disposed of correctly.

16.4-3 The FDA evaluates laboratory developed tests for safety, effectiveness, reliability, and accuracy. CLIA regulates test procedures and how results are interpreted and reported.

16.5-1 Employment at will allows an employer or worker to end the employment at any time, though employers must have a legitimate reason after the probationary period. Workers have a right to form unions and create employment contracts.

16.5-2 FLSA restricts work hours and the types of jobs for minors, and sets federal minimum wage and overtime requirements.

16.5-3 Employers may not discriminate in employment decisions on the basis of race, color, religion, sex, national origin, age, or physical or mental disability.

16.5-4 If workers are being harassed, they should tell the person to stop and to let their supervisors know there is a problem.

16.5-5 Other workplace laws influence family and medical leave, languages spoken in the workplace, and use of social media.

Maximize Your Professional Vocabulary

1. **Remembering Terms.** Select five of the vocabulary words from this chapter that you are least likely to remember. Without using the term itself, develop a silly phrase or play on words to help you remember the term. For example, "assault—Having a salty attitude can get you in trouble!" or "scope of practice—See the work details with a microscope!" Draw a simple picture to go with it.

2. **Venn Diagrams.** Draw four Venn diagrams. Compare and contrast the following pairs of terms, writing their common qualities in the overlapping space and differences next to the individual terms: civil law and common law; malpractice and negligence; involuntary seclusion and false imprisonment; libel and slander.

Reflect on Your Reading

1. Review your responses from Connect with Your Reading at the beginning of the chapter. Summarize your conclusions using these questions. What happens to healthcare workers when they do something harmful? What are patient's rights? Is the health and safety of healthcare workers protected? Do healthcare workers have any legal protection?

Review and Recall

1. Not reporting a case of suspected child abuse is a violation of (16.1-1)
   A. civil law
   B. contract law
   C. criminal law
   D. None of these.
2. Offering your arm for a nurse to take your blood pressure is an example of (16.1-2)
   A. damages
   B. consideration
   C. expressed consent
   D. implied consent
3. If healthcare professionals work competently within their scope of practice, they are not responsible for ill effects that occur (16.2-1)
   A. after treatment
   B. during treatment
   C. due to malpractice
   D. because of negligence
4. Which of the following helps avoid charges of misappropriation? (16.2-2)
   A. Moving belongings without patient's knowing
   B. Reaching into a patient's pockets
   C. Touching a patient's belongings without permission
   D. Filling out an inventory list

5. What is the term for written defamation? (16.2-3)
   A. Slander
   B. Libel
   C. Abuse
   D. Neglect
6. Which of the following are signs of human trafficking? Choose all that apply. (16.2-4)
   A. Being overly nervous
   B. Being unaware of surroundings
   C. Willingness to answer questions
   D. Another person insisting on being present for exams
7. According to the ACA, health insurance must include coverage for (16.3-1)
   A. ambulatory care
   B. mental health
   C. preventive care
   D. All of these.
8. Which advance directive assigns a legal representative to make healthcare decisions when a patient cannot? (16.3-2)
   A. DNR order
   B. Power of attorney
   C. DNI order
   D. Organ donation card
9. Which are PHI? Choose all that apply. (16.3-3)
   A. Patient name
   B. Email address
   C. Birth date
   D. Social Security number
10. The purpose of an incident report is to (16.4-1)
    A. assign blame for an accident
    B. prevent future accidents
    C. punish healthcare workers
    D. exclude other points of view
11. Which law requires employers to educate employees about hazardous substances in the workplace? (16.4-2)
    A. Hazard Communication Standard (HCS)
    B. Federal Needlestick Safety and Prevention Act
    C. Medical Waste Tracking Act
    D. Biohazard Prevention Act
12. Under CLIA, labs must do which of the following? Choose all that apply. (16.4-3)
    A. Maintain equipment
    B. Create procedure manuals
    C. Document accidents
    D. Tell employees to seek training elsewhere

13. Workers that come together to bargain collectively are called (16.5-1)
    A. unions
    B. dependents
    C. contractors
    D. probationary workers

14. In the 8 and 80 system, healthcare workers cannot work more than 80 hours in (16.5-2)
    A. one month
    B. one facility
    C. two weeks
    D. eight weeks

15. Refusing to make reasonable accommodations for a job applicant with a disability is (16.5-3)
    A. rehabilitation
    B. discrimination
    C. sexual harassment
    D. negligence

16. Harassment is illegal if (16.5-4)
    A. enduring it is a condition of employment
    B. complying has a direct benefit or detriment
    C. it creates a hostile environment
    D. All of these.

17. Which law prevents English-only rules in the workplace? (16.5-5)
    A. NLRA
    B. FMLA
    C. EEOC
    D. HCS

Build Core Skills

1. **Problem Solving.** Research a recent biomedical lab safety event that put people in danger. Describe the circumstances of the event. What were the immediate and long-term dangers to health or safety? What steps were, or should have been, taken to protect people? Were any laws broken?

2. **Critical Thinking.** Imagine you work as a supervisor in a hospital's emergency room. What are three potential situations or actions of employees that would be valid and legal reasons for dismissal? Classify each as a criminal offense, civil offense, or legal action.

3. **Critical Thinking.** A swab from a Pap smear is sent to the lab to check for cervical cancer. How does CLIA protect the lab worker while analyzing the sample? How does CLIA protect patients when they receive their test results?

4. **Speaking and Listening.** Imagine a coworker has been making comments about your ability to do your job because of your age and gender. You feel harassed. What will you do to handle this situation appropriately? Practice aloud, telling a partner to stop, then trade roles.

5. **Critical Thinking.** Track the collection and disposal of waste in this scenario. Identify the laws that required these actions. EMTs bring a bleeding patient to the emergency room. You put on PPE before starting the exam. After giving an injection to numb the area, you clean the wound. You place the used needle in the sharps container, then dispose of your PPE in the hazardous waste hamper. Housekeeping replaces the full sharps container and double-bags the hazardous waste. It is moved to the dirty utility room to be packaged for disposal. A contractor picks up the labeled containers for incineration.

6. **Critical Thinking.** Which groups of workers are exempt from overtime pay provisions? Identify the laws involved. Why do you think mandatory overtime is common in healthcare?

7. **Math.** Ana is a support services worker. Last week, Ana worked 16 hours overtime in addition to her scheduled 40 hours. Calculate how much pre-tax money Ana earned last week if her regular hourly rate is $14.50/hour. Assume her overtime rate is time-and-a-half pay.

8. **Critical Thinking.** Which employment law applies to each of the following scenarios?
   A. Jessa and Karl started working as central services technicians at the same time. They both earn the same hourly wage.
   B. Andrew and his partner just adopted a child. He will be taking 12 weeks off work to stay home and care for the child.
   C. The housekeepers belong to a union.
   D. Luca's father has Huntington's disease, an inherited disease that affects the brain.

9. **Critical Thinking.** Suppose you are the medical assistant for Dr. Smith. Ms. Perez calls, complaining that she feels awful most of the time. You say, "Don't worry, Dr. Smith will make you feel better in no time," and you help her schedule an appointment for tomorrow. What are the terms of the contract you just created between Dr. Smith and Ms. Perez? On what basis can Dr. Smith be sued if the terms are not met?

10. **Critical Thinking.** Think of a crime show you watched in the past where the case was solved by asking a psychologist or doctor for information about the patient. Would this really happen? Under what circumstances?

11. **Critical Thinking.** Review the definitions of *scope of practice* and *liability*. Would a healthcare worker be liable if they used a new lift without training and dropped a patient during its use? What if they were trained and had experience in transfers, but forgot to lock the wheels? What if the patient shifted their weight unexpectedly and caused the fall? What would you need to do to report this incident?

12. **Problem Solving.** Imagine you are an emergency room physician. When a patient comes in with a deep cut and asks if there is anyone who can look at it, how was consent implied? What might you say to gain expressed consent? What additional information would you add to make it informed consent?

Activate Your Learning

1. Suppose you are a medical records technician. A parent is demanding a copy of the medical records for his 18-year-old daughter's recent visit to the doctor. The daughter is still in high school, and her parent pays for the insurance. As a result, the parent feels he has the right to know what is in the medical records. Role-play how you will handle this situation.
2. Role-play a better response to Ms. Perez from Build Core Skills question 9.

Think and Act Like a Healthcare Worker

1. Mario has come in with chest pains, difficulty breathing, and pain down his left arm. He needs to be evaluated and may need treatment for a possible heart attack. What are you obligated to tell Mario? How does your answer change, depending on your credentials? How will you protect Mario's privacy? Consider both his physical privacy and privacy of his information.
2. Imagine a patient who is preparing for surgery calls your healthcare facility with a question about the advance directives paperwork in the information packet. How will you explain the patient's rights and choices?

Go to the Source

1. Go to the website for the Equal Employment Opportunity Commission. Read about one aspect of employment the EEOC addresses. Use the menu's search box and enter "Challenge Yourself" to view scenarios, then check your understanding and write a paragraph about what you learned.
2. Use the internet to research an actual healthcare malpractice or negligence suit. What was the claim? Was the case settled in or out of court? Was there monetary compensation? If so, how much? Do you agree or disagree with the results? Why? Do you think the settlement was fair? Why or why not? What did you learn that could help you avoid a future malpractice suit?
3. Go to the website for the Department of Health and Human Services' National Practitioner Data Bank. Use the search bar to locate the "Data Analysis Tool." Explore both the data analysis and practitioner tabs. Build a table showing data for medical doctors in all states, in the most recent year available, and in the malpractice payment range of $1,000,000–$1,999,999. Answer these questions: How many payments were made by physicians in your state last year? Which state made the most payments? least? Change the table to show all types of practitioners in just your state. Which type of practitioner has made the most payments?
4. Use the internet to look at the state statutes for licensure of healthcare workers in your state. Search for the words "scope of practice." List the medical career you looked up and two things allowed or limited for their scope of practice.

HOSA Event Prep: Medical Law and Ethics

hosa future health professionals | EVENT PREP

Isabella was a 44-year-old patient who came to the emergency room (ER) with pain just over the sternum. The pain was so severe she said it was "taking her breath away," and she had noticeable shortness of breath. The ER physician noted Isabella had severe obesity and was Hispanic, then decided the problem was her gallbladder. He ordered a gallbladder scan and told the patient she should stop eating greasy, fried foods. Isabella's symptoms worsened. She became panicked and diaphoretic (sweating heavily), and her chest pain continued in spite of the medication given for gallstones. Ten minutes later, Isabella was found unresponsive with no heartbeat. After receiving cardiopulmonary resuscitation (CPR) and advanced life support, Isabella died. The coroner report showed that Isabella had a myocardial infarction (MI), or heart attack. If the ER physician had performed the standards of care for chest pain and shortness of breath, Isabella might be alive today.

Test Your Knowledge

1. What type of contract is the physician acting within?
   A. Expressed   C. Informed
   B. Implied   D. None
2. What legal concept should guide the doctor's required actions in this situation?
   A. Advance directives   C. Privacy
   B. Contracts   D. Standards of care
3. Which of the following legal issues best describes this doctor's conduct?
   A. Assault
   B. Criminal malpractice
   C. Neglect
   D. Negligence

Unit 5

Medical Terminology and the Human Body

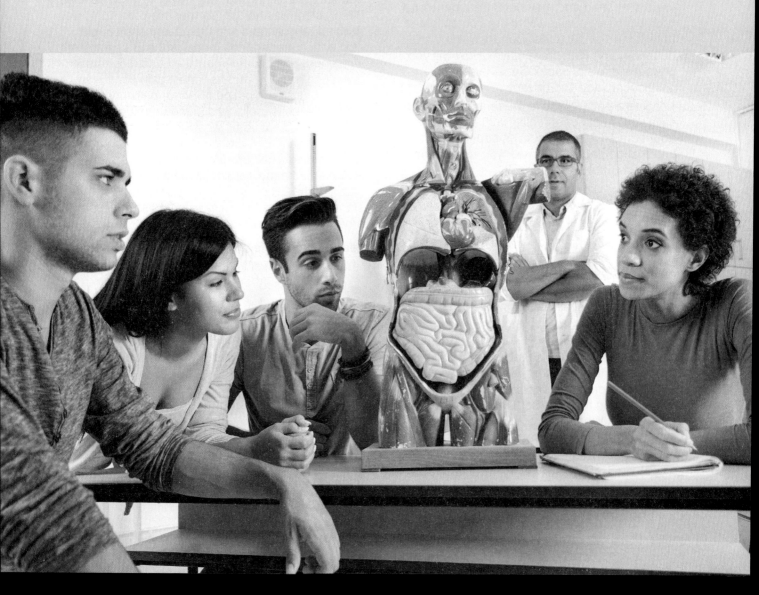

Healthcare Insider

Mindy, BS, ARDMS (ABD, OB/GYN, RVT), Ultrasonographer

I chose sonography as a career because I like anatomy, physiology, pathology, and imaging. As an ultrasonographer, I take images for the radiologist using an ultrasound scanner. I also find the pathology that goes along with each patient's signs and symptoms. I enjoy sonography because I have direct patient contact every day, but every interaction is different. I have to be creative when taking images for the radiologist, making sure they include all the information the radiologist needs to make a diagnosis. I am able to work independently as well as with a team of other sonographers and radiologists.

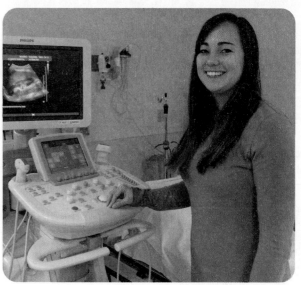

Photograph taken by Susan Blahnik

Discussion Activity

Mindy enjoys studying anatomy, physiology, and pathology. Her sonography career relies on her detailed knowledge of these subjects.

1. What do you enjoy studying?
2. What healthcare careers focus on the subjects that you enjoy?

Chapter 17

Medical Terminology and Body Organization

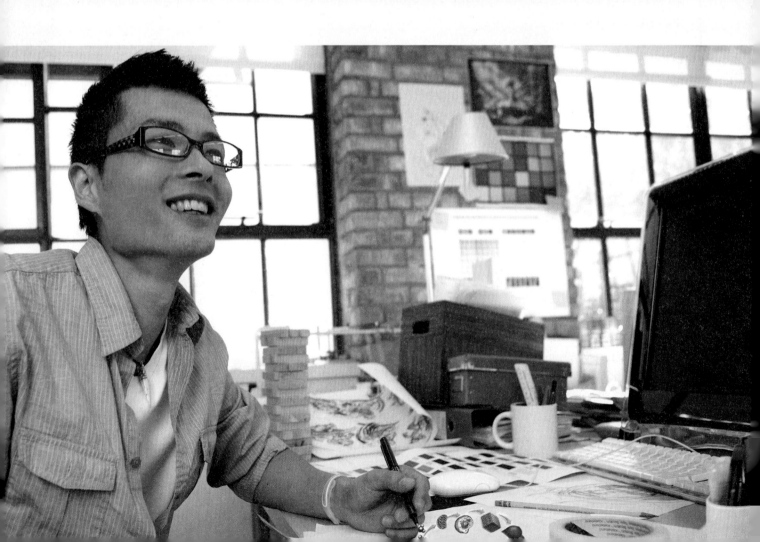

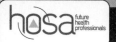

HOSA Event Prep: Medical Terminology

Did you know that medical terminology is used in all health science professions? Healthcare professionals must understand the terminology used so they can accurately diagnose and treat their patients. Most terminology comes from word parts, including prefixes, root words, and suffixes. That means if you know the definitions of the word parts, you can define the word. Descriptive terminology can describe locations, positions, and directions related to the body. Knowing body planes, regions, quadrants, and directional terms is crucial when assessing a patient and their symptoms. You can also use these skills in one of the largest HOSA events called *Medical Terminology*.

Go to the HOSA website to learn more about the HOSA *Medical Terminology* event. Find out the purpose of the event, what is involved in the event, and what knowledge is demonstrated in the event.

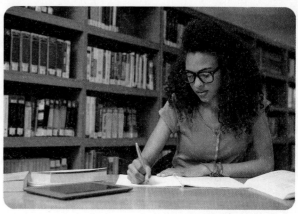

wavebreakmedia/Shutterstock.com

As you prepare for HOSA competitive events, be sure to check the website and talk with your HOSA advisor for the most up-to-date guidelines and procedures. Once you have learned about the *Medical Terminology* event, answer the following questions:

1. How might participating in this event benefit you personally and in your future career? Explain.
2. Are you interested in participating in this event? Why or why not?

Connect with Your Reading

Before you read this chapter, organize the terms in the list of *Professional Vocabulary* at the start of each lesson into logical categories based on your current knowledge. Use arrows or circles to show connections between related terms as needed. Share your newly organized list with a partner and discuss the differences in how you organized the terms.

Map Your Reading

Make a tablet organizer with four sheets of paper using the example shown. Stack the sheets, keeping the sides even, but move each sheet of paper up so that its bottom edge is ½ inch to 1 inch above the bottom edge of the sheet below it. Holding the center of the stack, fold all the sheets down so the top edge of the top sheet is ½ inch to 1 inch above the bottom edge of the top sheet. Crease all the layers and staple at the folded edge. Write *Understanding Body Organization* on the outside flap and list what you know about the organization levels in the body. Label the edges of the flaps below the top one with the headings *The Cell*, *Body Tissues*, *Organs*, *Body Systems*, *Body Directions*, *Body Regions and Quadrants*, and *Body Cavities and Planes*. On the back, write *Medical Terminology*. As you read, add visual cues, definitions of new terms, and notes on important concepts to each page of the booklet.

Understanding Body Organization
The Cell
Body Tissues
Organs
Body Systems
Body Directions
Body Regions & Quadrants
Body Cavities & Planes

Goodheart-Willcox Publisher

Chapter opener image: Ciaran Griffin/Photodisc/Thinkstock

Medical Terminology

ESSENTIAL QUESTION

How is medical terminology useful in the healthcare workplace?

Learning Outcomes

After studying this lesson, you will be able to

17.1-1 apply the basic rules of medical terminology to analyze new terms.

17.1-2 identify common Greek and Latin prefixes, roots, and suffixes that can be used to interpret new words.

17.1-3 apply rules for forming plural medical terms.

17.1-4 use accepted abbreviations for medical terms.

17.1-5 pronounce and spell medical terms.

Professional Vocabulary

Essential Terms

medical terminology special vocabulary that is used in healthcare and is often formed from Latin and Greek word parts

prefix letters in front of a root word that change the meaning of the word

root word the foundation of a term, giving the term its main meaning

suffix letters after a root word that identify the part of speech, if it is singular or plural, or add to the meaning of the word

Important Terms

abbreviation	combining vowel	plural
acronym	eponym	

Introduction

Knowledge of the body is important for all healthcare workers. Information about how the body is organized is the foundation on which all other academic knowledge for healthcare workers is based. As you study, you will be learning many new terms. This may seem overwhelming, and you may need some new strategies for studying this large volume of new information.

In this lesson, you will be introduced to the language of medicine and encouraged to apply techniques to help you break down and learn this new terminology more quickly.

17.1-1 Medical Terminology

Healthcare workers use a special language called **medical terminology** to communicate clearly about their patients. Understanding and using medical terminology is like speaking a different language. It takes effort and practice to speak a language besides your own. You will find the same is true as you study medical terminology. Most medical terms come from Greek and Latin root words. Learning these origins may help you understand and remember terms. Terms named after a person, called **eponyms**, may tell you who discovered a disorder or invented a medical tool.

All healthcare workers must be able to read, write, and understand medical terminology so they can communicate clearly with other professionals about their patients or research. Some healthcare workers, such as medical transcriptionists and scribes, will spend most of their day reading, writing, and listening to medical terms. Understanding written and spoken medical terminology is essential to preventing errors at all stages of care and treatment.

17.1-2 Understanding Word Parts

Every language has rules that determine how it is properly written and spoken. The rules are different for each language. Medical terminology, like any other language, follows specific rules for how words are formed, spelled, and pronounced.

A medical term is usually a combination of several word parts, like a train with many types of connected boxcars (**Figure 17.1**). Breaking down medical terms into their word parts will allow you to define many more terms than you could possibly memorize by studying them as whole words. **Figure 17.2** provides examples of all word parts.

A **root word** is the foundation of a medical term. It carries the term's main meaning, just as a train's boxcars hold the cargo to be delivered. It is usually a noun, such as a body part. For example, the root word *cardi* means "heart," and the root word *pulmon* means "lung."

Several root words may be combined in one word, like a compound word. They need a **combining vowel** to connect them when the next root or suffix does not begin with a vowel. Think of combining vowels like couplers that hold a train's boxcars together. The most common combining vowel is *o*, but *a, e, i,* or *u* may sometimes be used. The root is usually written with the combining vowel in a combining form, such as *cardi/o*. A combining vowel makes the complete term easier to pronounce. The word *cardiopulmonary* sounds smoother than *cardipulmonary* because of the letter *o* between the root words.

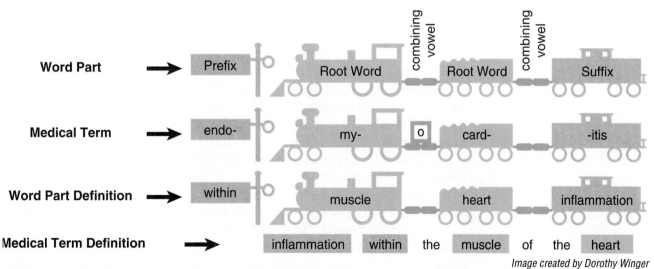

Image created by Dorothy Winger

Figure 17.1 "Word trains" like these provide visuals to help you understand how word parts are put together and defined.

Word Parts					
Word Part	**Purpose**	**Location**	**Use of Combining Vowel**	**Example**	**Explanation**
Prefix	Changes, adds to, or limits the meaning of the root; may tell you size, shape, color, position, or amount; is frequently a preposition or an adverb (Not all words have a prefix)	Beginning of the word	No combining vowel is needed between the prefix and root word.	bi-	bi- = two bifocals = eyeglasses with two portions in each lens to adjust for both near and far vision
Root word	Main meaning of the word; usually a noun, such as a body part	Middle of the word (or beginning of the word if there is not a prefix)	Drop the combining vowel if the next word part begins with a vowel.	dent- or dent/o-	dent/o- = tooth dentist = a doctor who examines teeth and treats teeth-related health issues
Suffix	Changes the meaning of the root; makes the term a noun, adjective, or verb and tells if a noun is singular or plural	End of the word	Use a combining vowel if the suffix begins with a consonant.	-logy	-logy = the study of physiology = the study of nature
Combining vowel	Makes it easier to pronounce the term	Between word parts	When there is more than one root word, use a combining vowel between the root words. When the suffix begins with a consonant, use a combining vowel between the root and suffix.	-o-	musculoskeletal = muscul-**o**-skelet-al

Goodheart-Willcox Publisher

Figure 17.2 Understanding the purpose, location, and examples of word parts can help you break down and interpret medical terms.

pre- = before, in front of

A **prefix** appears at the beginning of a word, like a signal light in front of a train. The light tells the engineer whether to change the train's route or speed, just as the prefix can change, add to, or limit the meaning of the root word. The prefix may tell you the size, shape, color, position, or amount of the root. A combining vowel is not needed between a prefix and a root word. Not all words have a prefix.

A **suffix** appears at the end of a word, like the caboose of a train. It tells you what is being done to the root word, just as a brakeman used to ride in the train caboose to watch how the train and brakes were operating. The suffix can change the root into an adjective, noun, or verb, and it can show if a word is singular or plural. It can also add to the meaning of the root. It may identify size or describe a condition or procedure. If a suffix begins with a vowel (*a, e, i, o, u*, and sometimes *y*), it attaches directly to the root. If a suffix begins with a consonant (*b, c, d, f,* and so on), a combining vowel is needed between the root and the suffix.

Medical terms usually contain at least two word parts. These are usually one or more roots and a suffix. There are some exceptions. When a term breaks down into just two word parts, you may find combinations of a prefix and root rather than a root and suffix. Some words cannot be broken down. Eponyms and some words taken directly from other languages must be memorized as whole terms.

17.1-3 Forming Plural Medical Terms

Creating a **plural** word in medical terminology does not follow the same rules as Standard English. In Standard English, the suffix *-s* or *-es* is added to show there is more than one. This is often not appropriate in medical terminology. Different Latin and Greek suffixes use different plural endings. Use the information in **Figure 17.3** to change medical terms to their plural forms and plurals to singular. How would you say more than one *nucleus*?

Defining medical terms is like solving a puzzle. To discover the meaning of a term, you will break it down into its individual parts and define each part. Define the suffix first, and then define the remaining word parts from left to right. Combine the definitions of the word parts to discover the meaning of the whole term. For example, *cardiopulmonary* can be broken into *cardi* (which means "heart"), *o* (the combining vowel), *pulmon* (which means "lung"), and *ary* (which means "pertaining to"). Together they mean *pertaining to the heart and lung*.

Practice analyzing medical words that you see and hear. A medical dictionary will be an important tool when a term comes from a proper name, cannot be broken down, or has an unclear meaning. However, you can understand the general meanings of most medical terms quickly by interpreting the word parts.

17.1-4 Abbreviations

Abbreviations provide a shortened way to write or say medical words and phrases. You are already familiar with many abbreviations used in everyday language, such as *a.m.* and *p.m.* for morning and afternoon. Abbreviations are an important part of medical terminology. They can save time, space, and effort.

An abbreviation can be a shortened form of a word. For instance, *chemo* is a shortened way of saying *chemotherapy*. Some abbreviations are **acronyms**, meaning that each letter in the abbreviation stands for a word. For example, *MRI* is an acronym for "magnetic resonance imaging." Sometimes each letter of an abbreviation represents a Greek or Latin word part, as in *ECG*, which is an abbreviation for "electrocardiography." These abbreviations may not make sense until you understand their Latin and Greek origins.

Plural Forms of Common Latin and Greek Suffixes				
Ending	**Singular Forms**	**Drop**	**Add**	**Plural Forms**
-y	deformity, family	-y	-ies	deformities, families
-is	diagnosis, fibrosis	-is	-es	diagnoses, fibroses
-us	alveolus, stimulus	-us	-i	alveoli, stimuli
-um	ileum, bacterium	-um	-a	ilea, bacteria
-a	vertebra, ruga	-a	-ae	vertebrae, rugae
-ma	sarcoma, melanoma	-ma	-mata	sarcomata, melanomata
-ax	thorax, anthrax	-ax	-aces	thoraces, anthraces
-ex	cortex, index	-ex	-ices	cortices, indices
-ix	appendix, matrix	-ix	-ices	appendices, matrices
-on	spermatozoon, protozoon	-on	-a	spermatozoa, protozoa
-en	foramen, lumen	-en	-ina	foramina, lumina
-nx	larynx, pharynx	-nx	-nges	larynges, pharynges
-yx	calyx	-yx	-yces	calyces

Goodheart-Willcox Publisher

Figure 17.3 Medical terms with Latin and Greek suffixes follow different rules for plural forms.

Different medical facilities in different parts of the US may write abbreviations in different ways. Some use a period to separate lowercase letters, as in *b.i.d.* for "twice in a day." Some use all capital letters, as in *BID.* Facilities may or may not have lines over certain abbreviations. The abbreviation for "after" may be written as either $\bar{p}$ or *p*, depending on the facility in which you work.

Messy writing and misread letters and numbers that look alike can cause preventable medical errors. Although the use of electronic charting has reduced problems with messy handwriting, healthcare workers should be aware of and only use abbreviations on the approved list for their facility. Note the "Do Not Use" list of abbreviations from The Joint Commission shown in **Figure 17.4**. Never make up your own abbreviations. Use your best judgment about when abbreviations are helpful and when to avoid them to prevent additional confusion. Always write neatly and check spelling when necessary. Medical charts are a legal record and must be understandable for everyone who uses them.

17.1-5 **Pronunciation and Spelling**

Healthcare workers must become comfortable reading and saying medical terms. These terms may seem hard to pronounce, especially if you have not already heard them spoken. Many medical words have similar and sometimes confusing sounds. They may also look long and difficult. These tips will help with pronunciation. First, break each term into its word parts. Then pronounce each word part separately. **Figure 17.5** provides some basic pronunciation rules. You should emphasize the part of the word in capital letters when you speak. Some pronunciations vary in different parts of the US and in other countries. If you are unsure about the commonly used pronunciation where you work, listen to others or ask a trusted coworker.

Error-Prone Abbreviations and Symbols			
Error-Prone Abbreviation or Symbol	**Intended Meaning**	**Misinterpretation**	**Solution**
U, u	unit	numeral 0, numeral 4, or cc	Write *unit.*
IU	International Unit	IV (intravenous) or numeral 10	Write *International Unit.*
Q.D., QD, q.d., qd	daily	Q.O.D., QOD, q.o.d., qod (every other day)	Write *daily.*
Q.O.D., QOD, q.o.d., qod	every other day	Q.D., QD, q.d., qd (every day) *or* Q.I.D., QID, q.i.d., qid (four times a day)	Write *every other day.*
Trailing zero after decimal point	5.0 mg	50 mg (if the decimal is missed)	Omit the trailing zero (5 mg).
No leading zero before a decimal point	.5 mg	5 mg (if the decimal is missed)	Write a zero to the left of the decimal when a number is less than a whole unit (0.5 mg).
MS	morphine sulfate *or* magnesium sulfate	magnesium sulfate *or* morphine sulfate	Write *morphine sulfate* or write *magnesium sulfate.*
MSO$_4$	morphine sulfate	MgSO$_4$ (magnesium sulfate)	Write *morphine sulfate.*
MgSO$_4$	magnesium sulfate	MSO$_4$ (morphine sulfate)	Write *magnesium sulfate.*

Goodheart-Willcox Publisher

Figure 17.4 The list of "Do Not Use" abbreviations at your facility will help to avoid errors.

Pronunciation Rules

Rule	Examples
c and *g* have a soft sound (like *s* and *j*) when they appear before the letters *e, i,* and *y*.	cycle (SI-kuhl)
	gender (JEHN-der)
	giant (JI-ant)
c and *g* have a hard sound (like *k* and *guh*) when they appear before other letters.	cranium (KRAY-nee-um)
	cut (KUHT)
	gonad (GOH-nad)
ch sounds like *k* when it appears before consonants.	chlorine (KLOHR-een)
	chronic (KRAHN-ik)
p is silent at the beginning of a word when followed by the letters *s* and *n*.	psychic (SI-kik)
	pneumonia (noo-MOH-nyuh)
i sounds like *eye* when added to the end of a word to form a plural.	stimuli (STIM-yool-eye)
	alveoli (al-VEE-ohl-eye)
ae and *oe* generally sound like *ee* in the middle of a word.	amoeba (uh-MEE-buh)
ae and *oe* pronunciation at the end of a word varies regionally; you may hear *ee, ay,* or *eye*.	coxae (kahk-SEE, kahk-SAY, kahk-SI)
es is often pronounced as a separate syllable when found at the end of a word.	nares (NAR-eez)
	stases (STAYS-eez)

Goodheart-Willcox Publisher

Figure 17.5 The rules in this table will help you pronounce medical terms correctly. You can also find pronunciations for medical terms in a medical dictionary.

Although these rules will help you pronounce new terms, you should not spell medical words by sounding them out. Some terms sound alike but are spelled differently. One letter can change the entire meaning of a body part or drug name. Misspelling a medical term can create confusion and result in an incorrect diagnosis or procedure. You cannot rely on technology to find your errors because spell-checkers may not recognize medical terminology. When you are unsure of a term's spelling or meaning, you should look up the term in a medical dictionary.

Lesson 17.1 Review

 Complete the *Map Your Reading* graphic organizer for the section you just read.

1. People who work in medical careers must understand, speak, spell, and use _____ correctly. (17.1-1)
   A. acronyms
   B. combining vowels
   C. eponyms
   D. medical terminology

2. Most medical terms have one or more _____, but they may not have a prefix. (17.1-2)
   A. root words
   B. acronyms
   C. eponyms
   D. suffixes

3. _____ medical terms may not be formed by adding *-s* or *-es* to the end, as in common English words. (17.1-3)
   A. Latin
   B. Greek
   C. Standard English
   D. Plural

4. It is important that you use only the _____ accepted by your facility. (17.1-4)
   A. plural forms
   B. combining vowels
   C. abbreviations
   D. medical terminology

5. _____ rules can be used to sound out medical terms, but there may be more than one spelling for a particular sound. (17.1-5)
   A. Pronunciation
   B. Acronym
   C. Plural
   D. Medical terminology

Body Organization and Related Medical Terms

ESSENTIAL QUESTION

How is the human body organized?

Learning Outcomes

After studying this lesson, you will be able to

17.2-1 differentiate between anatomy and physiology.

17.2-2 categorize body structures by their level of organization within the body.

Professional Vocabulary

Essential Terms

anatomy   the physical structures or parts of the body

body system   a group of organs working together to perform a vital function in the body

cell   a small group of organelles that fulfill a specific purpose and are held together by a membrane

physiology   the functions or inner workings of the body

Important Terms

atom	Golgi apparatus	organ
cell membrane	lysosomes	organelle
cytoplasm	mitochondria	ribosomes
DNA (deoxyribonucleic acid)	molecule	tissue
endoplasmic reticulum	nucleolus	vacuole
	nucleus	

Introduction

All healthcare workers must understand anatomy and physiology so they can recognize and communicate effectively about a patient's health condition. A medical coder's knowledge of anatomy will help them identify the correct code for a procedure or body part mentioned in the record. Many discoveries and treatments are developed by studying the body and its functions.

In this lesson, you will learn about the organization of the human body. You will also learn about the anatomy and physiology of the cell.

17.2-1 Anatomy and Physiology

When healthcare workers discuss body systems, the parts of the body are its **anatomy**, and how the body works is its **physiology** (fih-zee-AH-luh-jee). Anatomy and physiology work together. The shape and location of a body part tell you a lot about what it does.

The anatomists who drew and studied the parts of the body hundreds of years ago spoke Greek and Latin, which explains the origins of terms for anatomy and physiology. Today, pathophysiologists (path-oh-fihz-ee-AHL-uh-jihsts) study *pathologies*, or diseases and disorders that occur when the body is not functioning properly. We study normal anatomy and physiology so that we can recognize when a problem exists.

physi/o = nature
-logy = the study of

17.2-2 Levels of Organization

Your body structures are put together in a very organized way. Each level of organization builds on the next to form a larger structure (**Figure 17.6**).

Atoms and Molecules

Beginning at the chemical level, **atoms** are the smallest organizational unit of the body. Hydrogen, oxygen, carbon, and nitrogen are the most common atoms in the human body. Atoms bond together to form **molecules** (MAHL-uh-kyoolz). For example, hydrogen (H) and oxygen (O) atoms form a molecule of water (H_2O). Water and protein are the most abundant molecules in the body. At the cellular level, different molecules combine to form **organelles**, which are the structures within cells. Cells join to form tissues. Different types of tissues work together as a body organ. A body system is a group of organs that perform a vital function in the body. All these parts function together to form a living organism.

Molecular biologists study life at the chemical and cellular levels. The information they discover about how genes, DNA, bacteria, and viruses work in a cell helps healthcare professionals diagnose, prevent, and treat diseases. Biotechnology uses information about how microorganisms work to stay on the cutting edge of these discoveries.

bi/o = life
-logist = specialist in the study of

The Cell and Its Organelles

A **cell** is considered the smallest living thing. It is so small it usually cannot be seen without a microscope. Even though it is small, a cell performs all the activities that define life. Biologists say something is living if it can take care of its own structures, interact with its environment, grow, and reproduce. Cellular biologists study how to support or manipulate the chemical reactions of cells. Therefore, chemistry is very important in healthcare careers that require understanding how the body works.

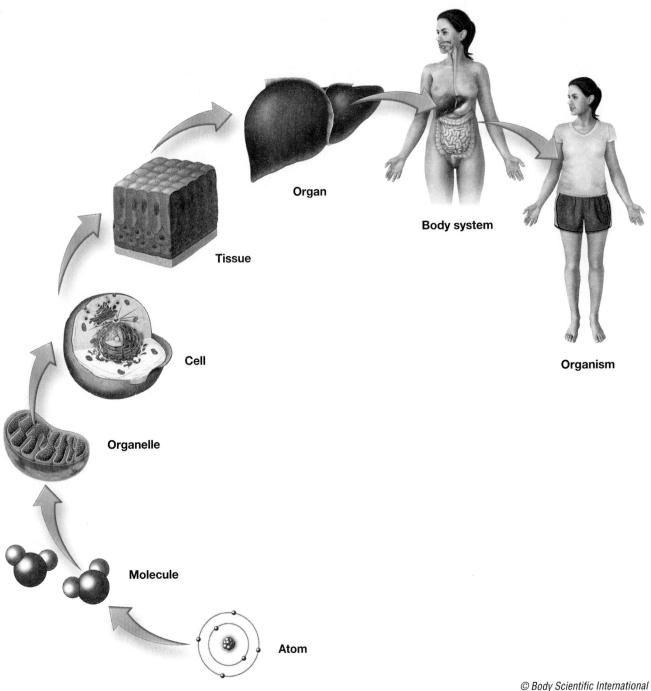

Organ

Body system

Tissue

Cell

Organism

Organelle

Molecule

Atom

Figure 17.6 The organizational hierarchy of the body, from chemicals to organism, is shown here. *What are some examples of organelles, organs, and body systems?*

The word *cell* comes from the Latin word *cellula*, which means "small room." You can think of each cell in your body as a room in a factory, creating a product or doing a job for that factory. Cells may have specialized roles as nerve, bone, blood, epithelial, or muscle cells. Although each room in your factory has the same basic structure and furniture, different rooms need special equipment for their specific jobs. Different types of cells also have the same basic organelles, but contain different amounts and kinds of organelles depending on the cell's purpose. The anatomy or structure of a cell is closely related to its physiology, or function.

You can picture the cell's organelles as the furnishings and equipment in a factory (**Figure 17.7**). Every factory room needs walls for structure and protection from the environment outside, but also windows and doors to allow some things in and out. Similarly, the **cell membrane** is a semipermeable (sehm-ee-PER-mee-uh-buhl) outer covering with holes, or *pores*, that act as its doors and windows. Some molecules can easily pass through the "security guards" at these pores. Other molecules require cell energy to be actively carried through the membrane. **Vacuoles** (VAK-yu-wohlz) are like the doors of the loading dock. They allow larger enzymes and waste molecule packages to pass through the cell membrane. Fat cells have large vacuoles and not many other organelles. Cells use chemical messages to communicate about which materials to allow through the membrane.

semi- = half

The cell membrane may have other structures that fulfill special needs. If a cell must be able to move, as with sperm, then it may have a tail, or *flagellum* (fluh-JEHL-uhm), as part of its cell membrane. This is like having a scooter to get around your factory. Some cells, like those of the intestines, need to absorb fluids or nutrients from the environment like a sponge. These cells have tiny hairs called *cilia* (SIHL-ee-ah) to increase the available surface area of their outer membrane. Just as air is contained within the walls of a factory, a semifluid **cytoplasm** (SI-toh-plaz-uhm) is contained within the walls of a cell. Chemical reactions take place in the cytoplasm as parts of the cell communicate and complete their work.

cyt/o = cell
-plasm = formation, structure

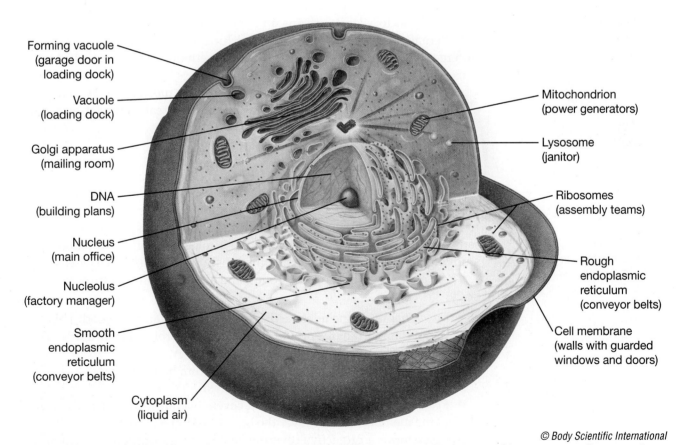

© *Body Scientific International*

Figure 17.7   The parts of a cell can be compared to different parts of a factory. *Choose one cell part and compare it to its corresponding factory component.*

The **nucleus** is the factory's main office. It controls the cell's activity. The **nucleolus** (noo-KLEE-oh-luhs), located at the center of the nucleus, is the factory manager. It uses assembly teams called **ribosomes** (RI-buh-sohmz) to build proteins following the **DNA (deoxyribonucleic acid)** plans for items the cell builds. Sections of DNA form genetic material that builds inherited characteristics. The nucleus interprets these directions and tells the cell what to build and when to build it. It also makes copies and produces its own new cells when needed.

gen/o = origin
-tic = pertaining to

Factories often use a conveyer belt to sort and transport materials for production. **Endoplasmic reticulum** (ehn-doh-PLAZ-mihk rih-TIHK-yuh-luhm), or *ER*, in the cell is like a conveyor belt on the production floor, moving construction materials (ribosomes) in and out of the nucleus as they are assembled. Rough ER is covered with ribosomes from the nucleus for building proteins. Smooth ER builds and stores fats and carbohydrates and detoxifies harmful substances. The **Golgi apparatus** (GOHL-jee ap-uh-RAT-uhs) is made up of layers of membranes in the cytoplasm that function like a mailing room. This organelle inspects, sorts, and packages proteins for use within or removal from the cell.

endo- = within
plasm/o = structure
-ic = pertaining to
reticul/o = network
-um = structure

Cells and factories require energy to operate. Power stations provide energy to factories. **Mitochondria** (mI-toh-KAHN-dree-a) are power stations for cells. They produce adenosine triphosphate (ATP) from carbohydrates, fats, and proteins. Breaking the bonds of ATP creates energy for the cell. Muscle cells have more mitochondria than other cells because their work requires a lot of energy. After cells have used the available energy, digestive enzymes in the **lysosomes** (LI-suh-sohmz) destroy used, dead, and foreign materials that are left behind, much like a factory janitor cleans up after workers.

lys/o = destruction
-some = body

Different types of cells have different functions, and each organelle has a different task within the cell. A cell may have more or fewer specific organelles, such as mitochondria, lysosomes, ribosomes, or cilia, depending on its job. Which organelles would you expect to find in a muscle cell? Which organelles would the liver's cells need to clean the blood, break down fat, and detoxify alcohol?

Body Tissues and Membranes

Tissues are groups of cells with the same function. Analysis of tissue samples provides important information to healthcare professionals. When doctors suspect a disease such as cancer, they may do a biopsy, obtaining a tissue sample to examine under a microscope. Histologists work with pathologists, studying these tissues to determine the cause and treatment of a disease.

hist/o = tissue
-logist = specialist in the study of

There are four main types of tissues, and all four are found throughout the body:

- *Connective tissue* includes cartilage, bones, body fat, and blood. This tissue is important for providing support, absorbing shock, and storing and transporting nutrients.
- *Nervous tissue* conducts impulses to and from body organs.
- *Muscular tissue* is important for movement.
- *Epithelial tissue* forms the skin that covers the outside of the body, as well as the membranes that cover the organs and line body cavities. This tissue forms a protective covering, allows the absorption of nutrients, helps filter harmful substances out of the blood, and forms secretions.

Body Organs and Systems

Groups of tissues working together form **organs**. Each organ performs specific bodily functions. For example, the heart pumps blood, and the vessels carry blood to all parts of the body. Groups of organs work together as **body systems**, such as the circulatory system. Different medical professions may specialize in the study of specific organs and systems. A cardiologist studies the heart and cardiovascular system. An oncologist studies cancers of the blood and other tissues. Internal medicine doctors study multiple body systems and their interaction. In health informatics, a medical coder looks up surgical procedures by body system and subcategorizes them by the specific organ.

Body systems work together as part of a complete organism (the human body) to control, move, support, protect, and reproduce. **Figure 17.8** lists the human body systems with their major organs and functions. The acronym *SLIC MEN R RED* will help you remember the names of the systems.

The tasks of the body systems often overlap, and some organs belong to more than one system. For example, the pancreas is part of both the digestive and endocrine systems. Some systems share similar functions and may be studied together. For example, the urinary system and integumentary system both secrete waste and can be studied together in the excretory system. All cells, organs, and body systems work together to keep your body healthy and maintain a constant state of balance, or homeostasis (hoh-mee-oh-STAY-sihs). Diseases and disorders disturb this delicate balance.

home/o = same
-stasis = stopping, controlling

Body Systems		
Body System	**Major Organs**	**Major Functions**
Skeletal	Bones, ligaments	Support, protection
Lymphatic (immune)	Lymph nodes, tonsils, thymus, spleen	Fluid return, immunity
Integumentary	Skin, hair, nails	Protection
Cardiovascular	Heart, vessels	Transportation
Muscular	Muscles, tendons	Movement
Endocrine	Glands	Body communication and control
Nervous and Sensory	Brain, spinal cord, nerves, nose, mouth, ears, eyes, skin	Body communication and control
Respiratory	Pharynx, trachea, bronchi, lungs, alveoli, diaphragm	Gas exchange
Reproductive	(Female:) ovaries, uterus, fallopian tubes (Male:) testes, vas deferens, prostate	Offspring production
Excretory (urinary)	Kidneys, ureters, bladder, urethra	Waste filtration
Digestive	Stomach, liver, pancreas, intestines, colon	Nutrient breakdown and absorption

Goodheart-Willcox Publisher

Figure 17.8 Each body system contains multiple organs that work together to perform a specific function.

Comparisons are a good learning tool because they help you organize and combine new information with ideas already familiar to you. You can compare the organizational structure of the human body, for example, to building a house (**Figure 17.9**). When constructing a house, you need to begin with some basic building materials. The wood and fiberglass you use to build the walls of a house are like the cells that make up body tissues.

Comparing House Structure to Body Structure			
House Diagram	**House Structure Examples**	**Body Structure Examples**	**Body Diagram**
	Building Elements	**Molecules**	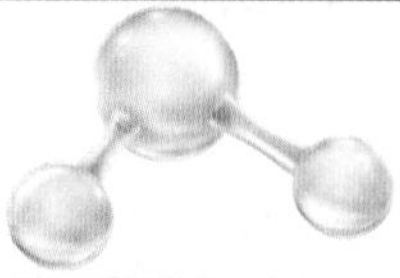
	iron wood fiber carbon	carbohydrates amino acids water	
	Building Materials	**Cells**	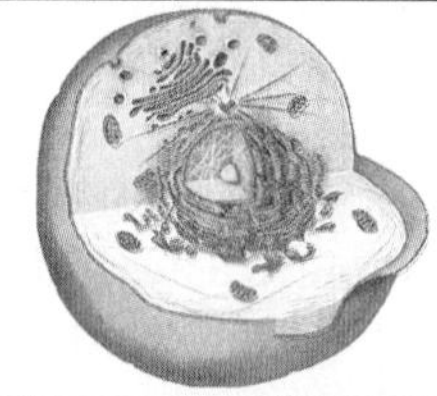
	fiberglass wood nails brick wire	fat cell bone cell muscle cell skin cell neuron	
	Groups of Materials	**Tissues**	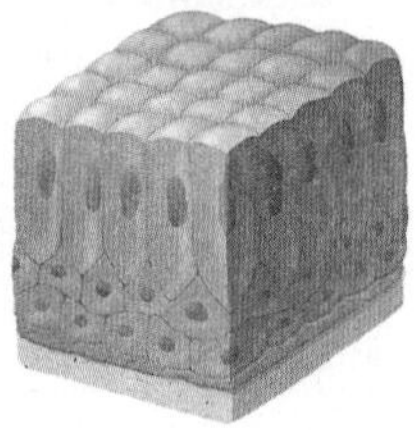
	insulation wood rafters wood studs tile flooring brick siding electrical circuits	connective tissue muscular tissue epithelial tissue nervous tissue	
	Basic Structures	**Organs**	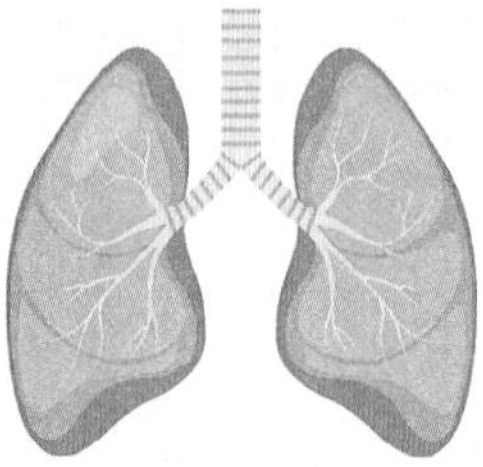
	roof walls chimney floors water pipes air conditioner electric meter	skin bones bronchi blood vessels brain	
	Structural System	**Body System**	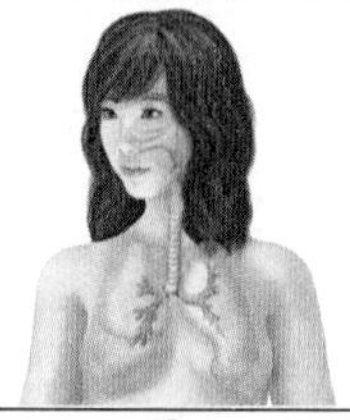
	roofing system plumbing system air conditioning system electrical system	integumentary system circulatory system respiratory system nervous system	
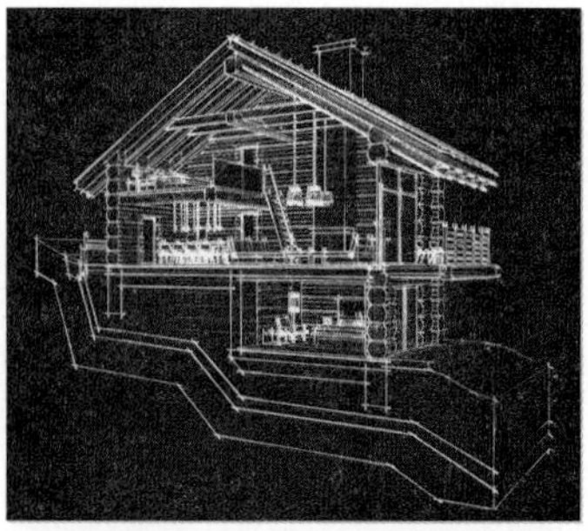	**Structure**	**Organism**	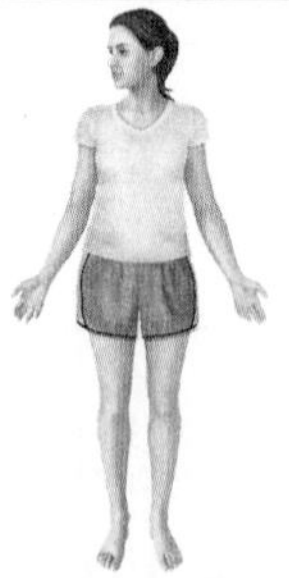
	house	human being	

Goodheart-Willcox Publisher, House: korisbo/Shutterstock.com, Molecule: Kindlena/Shutterstock.com, Cell: © Body Scientific International, Tissue: © Body Scientific International, Lungs: Katalin Macevics/Shutterstock.com, Respiratory system: © Body Scientific International, Organism: © Body Scientific International

Figure 17.9 The structure of the body can be compared to the structure of a house.

You need different types of body tissues to make body organs, just as the builder needs different groupings of wood and insulation to build the roof and walls. The fireplace, chimney, and vent of a house's heating system are like the lungs, bronchi, and trachea of your respiratory system. Just as the parts of the heating system work together for a common purpose, so do the organs of each body system.

You can compare the structural, plumbing, air-conditioning, and electrical systems in a house to the skeletal, circulatory, respiratory, and nervous systems of the human body. Both a house and the human body need all their systems to work together to provide a comfortable living environment. What other connections can you see between the organization of the body and the structures that form a house? Can you think of a different comparison?

Lesson 17.2 Review

 Complete the *Map Your Reading* graphic organizer for the section you just read.

1. Anatomy includes all the structures of the body, while _____ describe(s) how they work together. (17.2-1)
   A. body systems
   B. physiology
   C. DNA (deoxyribonucleic acid)
   D. organization levels
2. Molecules are made of bonded (17.2-2)
   A. tissues
   B. atoms
   C. organs
   D. cells
3. The nucleus contains the cell's DNA, which provides instructions for the cell's _____ to build materials such as proteins. (17.2-2)
   A. molecules
   B. ribosomes
   C. tissues
   D. cellula

4. Which of the following are main types of tissues in the body? Choose all that apply. (17.2-2)
   A. connective
   B. nervous
   C. epithelial
   D. muscular
5. *SLIC MEN R RED* is an acronym to help you remember the names of (17.2-2)
   A. atoms
   B. body systems
   C. organs
   D. tissues

Anatomical Terminology

ESSENTIAL QUESTION

How does anatomical terminology help with describing body locations?

Learning Outcomes

After studying this lesson, you will be able to

17.3-1 demonstrate anatomical position.

17.3-2 use directional terms to describe the locations of body structures.

17.3-3 use regional terms to describe the locations of body structures.

17.3-4 identify the major organs of each abdominal quadrant.

17.3-5 identify the body cavities and their major organs.

17.3-6 identify body planes used to study anatomy.

Professional Vocabulary

Essential Terms

abdominal region   one of nine equal areas of the abdomen that are named and used as reference points

body cavity   a hollow space within the body that is lined by a membrane and contains body organs

body plane   a flat surface seen by cutting away part of the body through surgery or medical imaging; serves as a point of reference when discussing anatomy

body region   an area of the body with a specific name, which is used as a reference point when discussing location on the body

standard anatomical position   the agreed-upon reference for body position when studying anatomy; standing erect, facing frontward, with the arms at the sides and palms facing forward

Important Terms

abdominal cavity	dorsal cavity	sagittal plane
abdominal quadrants	frontal plane	spinal cavity
abdominopelvic cavity	inferior	superficial
anterior	lateral	superior
caudal	medial	supine
cranial	midsagittal plane	thoracic cavity
cranial cavity	pelvic cavity	transverse plane
deep	posterior	ventral
distal	prone	ventral cavity
dorsal	proximal	

Introduction

In this lesson, you will learn about the directions and regions used to describe anatomy. Whether looking at a patient's body, writing about it in a medical chart, or coding patient information for the insurance company, all healthcare workers must use the same terms and points of reference. After this lesson, you will be prepared to look at each body system in more depth.

17.3-1 Anatomical Position

Medical examiners, surgeons, and medical illustrators all study the human body from the **standard anatomical position**. This is when the person is standing erect, facing forward, with the arms at the sides and palms facing forward. Try standing in this position. This provides a standard point of reference for other anatomical terms.

When a cadaver (kuh-DAV-er)—a dead body—lies on the examination table for anatomical study, it is usually in **supine** position, or face up with the arms out to the sides and palms facing up. You can remember that "supine is on your spine." **Prone** position would be facedown. You could think of this as being left "prone to attack."

17.3-2 Body Directions

Directional terms are used to describe parts of the body or their position in reference to standard anatomical position. These terms usually occur in pairs with opposite meanings:

- **Anterior** is the front side of the body. **Posterior** is the back. You can see the anterior view by looking in the mirror, but you need the reflection of another mirror to see the posterior.
- **Medial** refers to a point closer to the center of the body, while **lateral** is toward the side. Men's clothing usually buttons and zips at the midline, but some women's clothing zips laterally at the hip.
- **Superior** means "above" or higher up on the body. **Inferior** means lower down. The shoulders are superior to the hips but inferior to the ears.

anter/o = front
-ior = more toward
poster/o = back, behind, after
medi/o = middle
-al = pertaining to
later/o = side
super/o = above, upon
infer/o = below

Sometimes healthcare professionals use more specific terms, such as **cranial** or cephalic to talk about a point closer to the head and **caudal** for a point closer to the tailbone.

crani/o = skull
cephal/o = head
-ic = pertaining to
caud/o = tail

- **Superficial** refers to the outside surface of the body, as opposed to **deep** tissues, which are farther below the surface. The heart is deep in the chest, and the ribs are more superficial.
- Left and right are labeled from the patient's perspective. The patient's right side is on your left when you are facing them.

Consider the differences and similarities of these directional terms for a two-legged creature compared to a four-legged creature (**Figure 17.10**). Which directional terms best describe the spine of a dog?

Proximal Versus Distal

proxim/o = near
-al = pertaining to
dist/o = apart
-al = pertaining to

Descriptions of appendages (limbs) are based on their point of attachment to the body. For example, your arm is attached to your body at the shoulder, your hand is attached at the wrist, and your lower leg is attached at the knee. **Proximal** indicates a part is closer to the point of attachment, while **distal** refers to a part farther away from the attachment site. As shown in **Figure 17.11**, the proximal end of the humerus (a bone in your upper arm) is near the shoulder, and the distal end is at the elbow. The terms *proximal* and *distal* can also describe internal organs. Like other terms based on standard anatomical position, these descriptions remain the same regardless of movement or repositioning of the body.

Anterior, Ventral, Posterior, and Dorsal

ventr/o = belly
-al = pertaining to
dors/o = back
-al = pertaining to

While the terms *anterior* and *ventral* as well as *posterior* and *dorsal* are frequently used interchangeably, there are specific differences in their meanings and uses. The terms *anterior* and *posterior* describe the front and back of the body. The terms *ventral* and *dorsal* describe body surfaces according to the way joints flex.

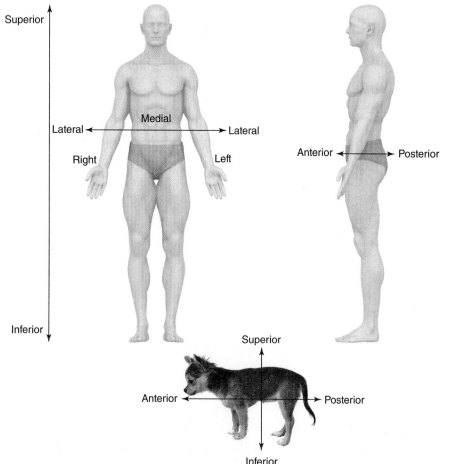

Human figure: CLIPAREA | Custom media/Shutterstock.com, Dog: Vitaly Titov & Maria Sidelnikova/Shutterstock.com

Figure 17.10 Directional terms usually come in pairs that have opposite meanings. *What pairs of terms do you see in this figure? How are they opposite?*

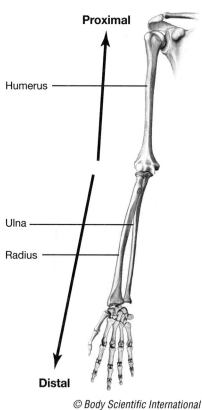

© Body Scientific International

Figure 17.11 *Proximal* means "closer to the site of attachment." *Distal* means "farther away from the site of attachment." *What is found at the proximal end of the radius? at the distal end of the ulna?*

Ventral (VEHN-truhl) surfaces move closer together when you bend a joint. They are generally lighter in color than dorsal surfaces and are often on the front side of the body. Try bending your arm at the elbow, and you will see that the lighter-colored, ventral surfaces of your inner arm move toward each other. **Dorsal** (DOR-suhl) surfaces are generally located on the back of the body. They often receive the most sun, so are more likely to be tanned (**Figure 17.12**). The backside of the upper and lower arm is dorsal. These surfaces move away from each other as the elbow is bent.

The legs on the person in Figure 17.12 illustrate the differences between the terms *ventral* and *dorsal* as opposed to *anterior* and *posterior*. When the knee is bent, the two lighter, ventral surfaces pulled toward each other are on the backsides of the legs. The backs of the legs are posterior by position, but they are ventral based on the way they move. The hip joints of a human rotate the dorsal side of the legs toward the front to provide support in a standing position. The surfaces of the legs turned to the front in standard anatomical position are anterior by position, but they are dorsal based on the way they move.

You can also see the difference between humans and four-legged animals in Figure 17.12. If you rub the belly of a dog, you will notice the light coloring of its ventral underbelly carries over onto the ventral inside of its legs. If people lie on their backs like dogs and lets their legs relax and roll out to the sides, the lighter (ventral) surface of the legs will also rotate more toward the front side of their body. When people stand on two legs, these ventral surfaces will rotate in toward the back of the body.

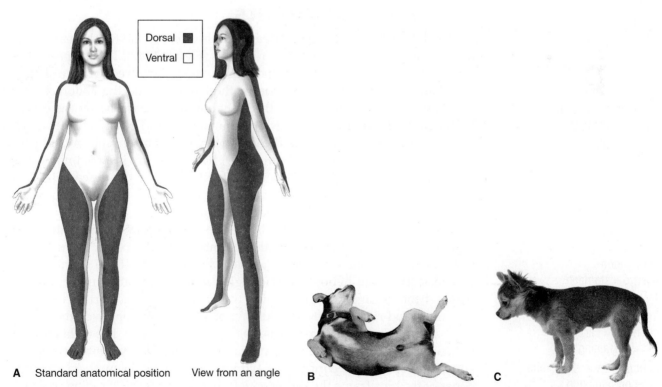

A Standard anatomical position   View from an angle   B   C

Human figure: © Body Scientific International, Dog (left): Annette Shaff/Shutterstock.com, Dog (right): Vitaly Titov & Maria Sidelnikova/Shutterstock.com

Figure 17.12 In standard anatomical position, the fronts of the legs are anterior by position but dorsal based on how they move. The backs of the legs are posterior by position but ventral based on movement. The view from an angle shows the division between dorsal and ventral surfaces. Compare the ventral and dorsal surfaces on a four-legged animal to a two-legged human.

17.3-3 Body Regions and Sections

When a patient complains of pain, healthcare workers need an easy way to communicate with each other about the different areas where the pain may be. This is why the medical community has given names to different **body regions**. These names provide a common language so you can easily refer to different areas on the surface of the body.

Many terms come from the names of the bones under the skin that act as landmarks and give the areas their shape. For example, the head may be called the *cranial region*, the thigh the *femoral region*, and the shoulder blade area the *scapular region*. The *cervical region* in the neck, *thoracic region* on the chest, and *lumbar region* of the lower back are named for their types of vertebrae. The *gluteal region* is named for the muscles of the buttocks.

Some body region terms, such as *abdomen* and *calf*, are part of everyday language. Other regional terms are used more specifically in the medical field. For example, a nurse wraps the blood pressure cuff around the part of the upper arm called the *brachial* (BRAY-kee-uhl) *region*. Blood is usually drawn from the *antecubital* (an-tee-KYU-bih-tuhl) *region* on the inside of the elbow. The *axillary* (AK-suh-lair-ee) *region* is the term a medical assistant uses when taking a temperature under the arm. Males may experience a hernia in their groin, or *inguinal* region. Understanding these regional terms helps you communicate without additional explanation.

cervic/o = neck
-al = pertaining to

brachi/o = arm
-al = pertaining to
axill/a = armpit
-ary = pertaining to
inguin/o = groin
-al = pertaining to

17.3-4 Abdominal Regions and Quadrants

The abdomen is such a large area that it is often divided into smaller sections, which are either quadrants or regions (**Figure 17.13**). This helps healthcare professionals focus on the abdominal organs involved when a patient complains of abdominal pain. One method is to divide the abdomen into four **abdominal quadrants** with the belly button, or *umbilicus*, at the center. Each quadrant contains just a few abdominal organs. The right upper quadrant (RUQ) contains the liver and gallbladder. The stomach, spleen, and pancreas lie in the left upper quadrant (LUQ). The appendix is a common cause of complaint in the right lower quadrant (RLQ), while the descending and sigmoid colon are in the left lower quadrant (LLQ). The small intestines are spread across the right and left lower quadrants.

A more detailed method is to divide the abdomen into nine **abdominal regions**, like a tic-tac-toe board, with the umbilicus at the center of the umbilical region. The epigastric region above it houses most of the stomach and pancreas. The right hypochondriac region refers to the area under the cartilage of the ribcage, which contains the gallbladder and part of the liver, intestines, and right kidney. The left hypochondriac region holds the spleen and parts of the stomach, pancreas, colon, and left kidney. The right and left lumbar regions below the ribcage are named for the nearby lumbar vertebrae and contain parts of the intestines, kidneys, and colon. Below them, the iliac bones of the hips frame the right and left iliac regions. These regions contain the intestines, the appendix on the right, and the sigmoid colon on the left.

abdomin/o = abdomen
-al = pertaining to
quadri- = four

epi- = upon
gastr/o = stomach
-ic = pertaining to
hypo- = below, under
chondr/o = cartilage
-ac = pertaining to
lumb/o = lower back, loins
-ar = pertaining to

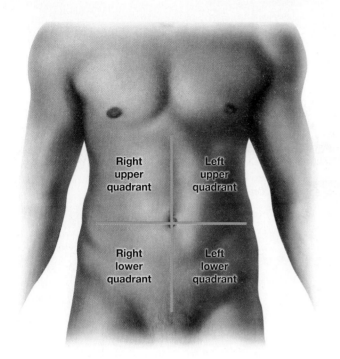
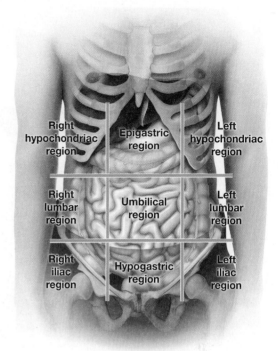

© Body Scientific International

Figure 17.13 The abdomen can be divided into quadrants or regions. *How might healthcare professionals use these quadrants and regions?*

Keep in mind, the patient's right is your left. The hypogastric region is well below the stomach and includes the bladder, uterus (in females), and part of the small intestines.

These points of reference are helpful when a patient complains of abdominal pain. What organs would you expect to be coding treatments for if progress notes indicated sharp pains in the patient's right iliac region?

hypo- = below, under
gastr/o = stomach
-ic = pertaining to

17.3-5 **Body Cavities**

The interior of the body is divided into **body cavities**, or spaces that contain the vital organs (**Figure 17.14**). Each body cavity is separated by a membrane that covers and protects the organs within. Bones also protect these organs. The ribs and pelvic bones surround the **ventral cavity** in the front. The bones of the skull and vertebrae protect the **dorsal cavity** in the back. There are also smaller sinus, orbital, oral, and nasal cavities in the head.

The diaphragm muscle separates the ventral cavity into the **thoracic cavity** above and the **abdominopelvic cavity** below. This separation helps prevent infections from moving between parts of the body. The thoracic cavity includes the pericardial cavity for the heart, surrounded by two pleural (PLOOR-uhl) cavities for the lungs. The abdominopelvic cavity includes the **abdominal cavity** for the digestive organs and the **pelvic cavity** that houses the reproductive organs, bladder, and rectum.

orbit/o = wheel track, circle
-al = pertaining to
or/o = mouth
nas/o = nose
thorac/o = chest

peri- = around
cardi/o = heart
pleur/o = side, rib
abdomin/o = abdomen
pelv/o = pelvis, hip region

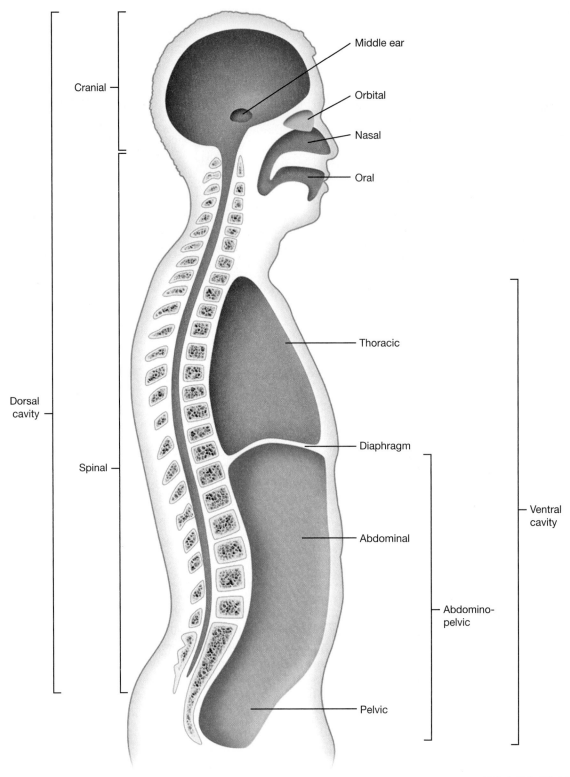

Middle ear

Orbital

Nasal

Oral

Cranial

Thoracic

Dorsal
cavity

Diaphragm

Spinal

Ventral
cavity

Abdominal

Abdomino-
pelvic

Pelvic

Figure 17.14 The interior of the body is divided into cavities that are separated by membranes. *Which cavities are included in the head?*

The *peritoneum* (pair-ih-toh-NEE-um) is a membrane that lines the abdominal cavity. It separates the abdominal and pelvic cavities along an imaginary line from the top of the iliac bones of the hips down to the pubic bones in front.

The dorsal cavity contains the **cranial cavity** for the brain and the **spinal cavity** for the spinal cord. In addition to the bony protection provided by the skull and vertebrae, membranes called the *meninges* (meh-NIHN-jeez) line these cavities.

spin/a = spinal cord
-al = pertaining to

17.3-6 Body Planes

Some medical professionals cut into the body with scalpels for surgery or dissection. Others use imaging technology to see inside the body without cutting it open. Body dissection and imaging technology both allow professionals to see the inside of the body in flat sections, or **body planes**. Naming these imaginary flat slices through the body gives professionals a common language to describe these views of structures within the body.

dis- = apart
sect/o = to cut
-ion = action, process, condition

If you look at an apple from the outside, you can only see the peel and overall shape. If you slice the apple from the top down through the core, you will see the inside, with the core down the middle and the seeds and flesh on each side of the core. If you had sliced the apple horizontally across the middle, you would have seen the core at the center, encircled by its seeds, and the apple flesh around that—a very different view.

Just as you can get a different view of the inside of an apple by cutting it in different directions, you can view the inside of a body along different planes, depending on what you want to see (**Figure 17.15**). The direction of the cut determines the name of the body plane:

- The **frontal plane**, also called the *coronal plane*, divides the body (or organ) into its front and back sections.
- The **sagittal** (SAJ-iht-uhl) **plane** divides the body, organ, or appendage into right and left sections. You can make a sagittal cut at various points along the width of the body. When the body is divided exactly down the center, or *midline*, this is called the **midsagittal plane**. Zippers and buttons often appear on the midsagittal line. A midsagittal view of the head shows the different lobes of the brain.
- The **transverse plane**, also called the *horizontal plane*, divides the body into top and bottom sections. It cuts across the body, perpendicular to the frontal and sagittal planes.

trans- = across

Each section, or *plane*, shows different angles through different organs. Medical imaging technicians must recognize the organs from different directions. These workers also know how superficial or deep in the body organs are located.

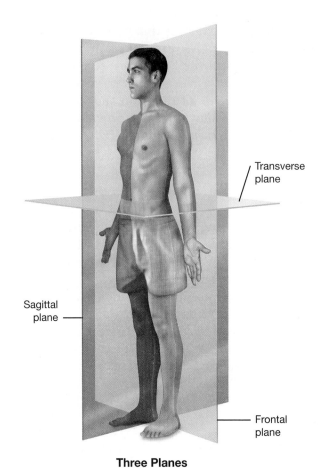

Three Planes

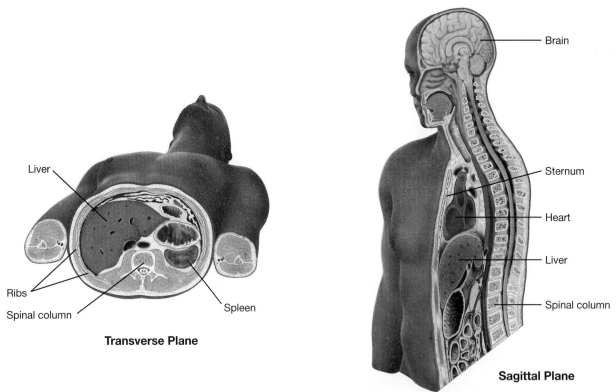

Liver

Ribs

Spinal column

Spleen

Transverse Plane

Brain

Sternum

Heart

Liver

Spinal column

Sagittal Plane

© Body Scientific International

Figure 17.15 The three planes divide the body from three different directions. Each creates a different cross-section to view different organs and internal matter. *What would you expect to see in the frontal cross-section of the top figure?*

Lesson 17.3 Review

 Complete the *Map Your Reading* graphic organizer for the section you just read.

1. Terms for body directions are based on standard _____ position, in which a person stands erect, facing forward, with the arms at the sides and palms facing forward. (17.3-1)
   A. anterior
   B. anatomical
   C. prone
   D. supine

2. The scapular region is _____ to the hips and lateral to the spine. (17.3-2)
   A. superior
   B. anterior
   C. medial
   D. inferior

3. The upper arm, where a nurse wraps a blood pressure cuff, is called the (17.3-3)
   A. cervical region
   B. thoracic region
   C. brachial region
   D. antecubital region

4. Abdominal _____ divide the abdomen into four sections. (17.3-4)
   A. regions
   B. cavities
   C. quadrants
   D. grids

5. The appendix is located in the right lower quadrant or _____ region. (17.3-4)
   A. right iliac
   B. left hypochondriac
   C. right hypogastric
   D. right lumbar

6. Vital organs are protected inside _____ by membranes and bones. (17.3-5)
   A. body cavities
   B. body planes
   C. body regions
   D. body directions

7. The _____ cavity contains the brain and spinal cord. (17.3-5)
   A. dorsal
   B. ventral
   C. thoracic
   D. abdominopelvic

8. Which body plane divides the body into equal left and right sections? (17.3-6)
   A. Transverse plane
   B. Sagittal plane
   C. Frontal plane
   D. Midsagittal plane

Chapter 17 Review and Assessment

Chapter Summary

17.1-1 It is important to understand, speak, spell, and use medical terminology correctly in all medical careers.

17.1-2 Medical terms are formed from Latin and Greek word parts. Learning these word parts can help you break down and interpret new words.

17.1-3 Plural forms of medical terms may not be formed in the same way as the plurals of common English words.

17.1-4 Abbreviations are a shortened way of writing medical terms. Only use abbreviations approved by your facility.

17.1-5 Phonetic rules of pronunciation are helpful for sounding out medical terms, but you should not spell medical terms based on how they sound.

17.2-1 Anatomy refers to the parts of the body, while physiology refers to how the body works.

17.2-2 Body structures are built in an organized way, from atoms up to a complete organism. Different types of cells contain different amounts of organelles, based on their purpose. Four main types of tissues build all the body organs.

17.3-1 In standard anatomical position, a person stands erect, facing forward, with the arms at the sides and palms facing forward.

17.3-2 Terms for body directions are based on standard anatomical position and are used to describe the location of a body structure.

17.3-3 Body regions provide a common set of terms for referring to areas on the surface of the body.

17.3-4 Abdominal quadrants divide the abdomen into four sections for investigating conditions of abdominal organs, while abdominal regions divide the abdomen into nine areas.

17.3-5 Body cavities are spaces in the body that contain vital organs and are protected by membranes and bones.

17.3-6 Body planes are imaginary flat slices through the body to give different views of the structures within.

Maximize Your Professional Vocabulary

1. **Word Train Game.** Each player makes flash cards for each of the medical word parts in the list that follows, placing the word part on one side of the card and its definition and a visual aid on the other side. Follow these directions with the completed cards:

   A. The first player chooses a root word and a suffix and/or prefix card to form a medical term. The player lays the cards down with the word parts facing up, says the medical term that was created, and defines it.

   B. The next player must place a word part card on top of a word part that is already showing, then read the new term and define it.

   C. If a definition is challenged by other players, the cards are turned over, and a definition is formed. If the definition was wrong, all the cards on the table go to the hand of the person who defined the term incorrectly. If the definition is correct, all cards go to the challenger's hand.

   D. Play begins again with the next player placing a root word, suffix, and/or prefix card on the table and defining the new term. Players may not place an identical card on top of a card that is already displayed.

   E. The object of the game is to get rid of as many cards as possible. Players may only "pass" if they are unable to make a word with their current cards, or if they only have cards identical to those on the table. The game ends when no more words can be made. The player with the fewest cards left is the winner.

   Prefixes

dis-	hypo-	quadri-
endo-	peri-	semi-
epi-	pre-	trans-

Root Words

abdomin/o	dors/o	physi/o
anter/o	gastr/o	plasm/o
axill/a	gen/o	pleur/o
bi/o	hist/o	poster/o
brachi/o	home/o	proxim/o
cardi/o	infer/o	pulmon/o
caud/o	inguin/o	reticul/o
cervic/o	later/o	sect/o
chondr/o	lumb/o	spin/a
crani/o	lys/o	super/o
cyt/o	medi/o	thorac/o
dist/o	pelv/o	ventr/o

Suffixes

-ac	-ion	-some
-al	-ior	-stasis
-ar	-logist	-tic
-ary	-logy	-um
-ic	-plasm	

2. **Poster.** Choose one term in this chapter to study. Create a poster for the term that includes its definition, a synonym, an antonym, another term with the same root, a sentence using the term, and a picture that helps you understand the term. If there is not a true antonym for the term, substitute a term that might be confused with the term you chose.

Reflect on Your Reading

1. Review your sorted word list from the *Connect with Your Reading* activity at the beginning of the chapter. Make changes to your organization based on what you learned and remember from your reading of the chapter.

Review and Recall

1. Most medical root words come from which languages? Choose all that apply. (17.1-1)
   A. Latin
   B. Greek
   C. Standard English
   D. Spanish

2. In the word *cardiovascular*, *cardi* is an example of a (17.1-2)
   A. prefix
   B. combining vowel
   C. root word
   D. suffix

3. What is the plural form of the word *vertebra*? (17.1-3)
   A. Vertebras
   B. Vertebraes
   C. Vertebrata
   D. Vertebrae

4. Which of these abbreviations is an acronym? (17.1-4)
   A. cell
   B. chemo
   C. p
   D. MRI

5. If you are unsure about the spelling of a medical term, you should (17.1-5)
   A. look it up in a medical dictionary
   B. use a spell-checker
   C. sound out the word
   D. use your best guess

6. Diseases and disorders are also called (17.2-1)
   A. anatomies
   B. physiologies
   C. pathologies
   D. etiologies

7. Which of these is the power station of a cell? (17.2-2)
   A. Golgi apparatus
   B. Endoplasmic reticulum
   C. Nucleus
   D. Mitochondria

8. Groups of tissues that work together are called a(n) (17.2-2)
   A. atom
   B. body system
   C. organ
   D. organism

9. In anatomical position, the palms are facing (17.3-1)
   A. forward
   B. to the side
   C. back
   D. upward

10. The elbow is at the _____ end of the humerus bone in the upper arm. (17.3-2)

    A. distal   C. proximal

    B. superficial   D. inferior

11. Which term refers to the groin region? (17.3-3)

    A. Scapular   C. Inguinal

    B. Femoral   D. Axillary

12. Which abdominal quadrant contains the liver and gallbladder? (17.3-4)

    A. RUQ   C. RLQ

    B. LUQ   D. LLQ

13. Which of the following is part of the ventral cavity? (17.3-5)

    A. Spinal cavity

    B. Cranial cavity

    C. Thoracic cavity

    D. All of these.

14. Which body plane divides the body into top and bottom sections? (17.3-6)

    A. Frontal plane

    B. Sagittal plane

    C. Midsagittal plane

    D. Transverse plane

Build Core Skills

1. **Critical Thinking.** Explain how nonstandard abbreviations could have a negative effect on a patient, the workers in your healthcare facility, and the workers in other healthcare facilities who receive your records.

2. **Critical Thinking.** Review the requirements in Lesson 17.2 that a biologist uses to define a living thing. What evidence did you find to support the fact that a cell is alive?

3. **Reading.** Research the work of three of the following people who made important discoveries about the human cell. What were their roles in forming the current understanding of the cell? Be prepared to share your information with the class.

    A. Robert Hooke

    B. Anton Van Leeuwenhoek

    C. Rudolf Virchow

    D. Theodor Schwann

    E. Camillo Golgi

    F. James Watson and Francis Crick

4. **Writing.** Type the following paragraph into a word processor. Correct any errors found by the spell-check feature.

> All patience complained of stomach pane. The gastrenterologist noted stomach distention in every patient examined. The CNA reported that the patients complained of nawzea. Lab tests were ordered to confirm a diagnosis.

    A. What problems were corrected?

    B. What problems were missed?

    C. What problems were created?

Activate Your Learning

1. Using Figure 17.7 as a reference, build the following "edible cell" model or create a model using different edible materials. Then answer the questions.

    • cell membrane—slice of bread with crust

    • cytoplasm—honey

    • nucleus and nucleolus—sucker or lollipop with the stick cut off

    • vacuoles—small pretzel twists

    • lysosomes—black jellybeans

    • mitochondria—gummy bears

    • endoplasmic reticulum—fruit leather cut and unrolled into long, thin strips

    • ribosomes—sprinkles

    • Golgi apparatus—gummy worms

    A. Explain how each of the edible cell parts looks like or represents the organelles of a cell.

    B. If you add a few more gummy bears, what type of cell would this be?

    C. If you add a few more black jellybeans, how does the cell's function change?

2. Use masking tape to place dorsal and ventral labels on your arms, legs, and torso. Stand in anatomical position and have a partner check the labels. If there is any question, simply bend the nearest joint and check the label against the descriptions in Lesson 17.3.

3. Examine Figure 17.1. How would this figure, which shows how different word parts form a medical term, need to be modified for the following terms: *dorsal, epigastric, lysosome,* and *quadrant*?

4. Create a model of a person using a pickle or cream-filled snack cake for the body, a marshmallow for the head, and toothpicks for arms and legs. Perform the following steps of an autopsy. Use the professional vocabulary you learned in this chapter to describe the body regions, directions, and planes as you write up the death report.

A. For the gross assessment, examine the body surface. Note the location, size, shape, and color of any unusual markings. Draw an anterior and posterior view of the body and mark the locations of your findings.

B. Weigh and measure the body.

C. Open the ventral body cavity with a deep, Y-shaped incision. The arms of the Y should start at the anterior surface of the shoulders (A) and join at the inferior point of the sternum (B) to form a single cut that extends to the pubic area (C). Perform medial-to-lateral incisions from the umbilical area and down both sides (D) to open the abdominal cavity.

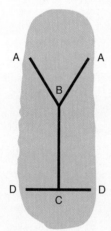

D. Open the thoracic cavity to examine the "internal organs." Weigh and measure them. Describe your findings, noting any abnormalities.

E. Decide on a cause of death and describe how your findings support that conclusion.

Think and Act Like a Healthcare Worker

1. Suppose you are an internal medicine doctor. Your patient complains of a stomachache. What locations would you examine based on your patient's complaint? Use professional vocabulary from this chapter in your description.

2. Suppose you hear or see a new term at work. List three different steps you can take to increase your understanding of this term.

Go to the Source

1. Watch a medical show and listen for medical terminology. Write down a minimum of 10 abbreviations or medical terms you hear. For each term, check your spelling using a medical dictionary, attempt to break the term into its word parts (prefix, root(s), suffix), and define the term.

2. Visit the Crime Scene website. Choose one of the "Previous Cases," and select "Case Files." View the coroner's report or autopsy for the case. Write *SLICMENRRED* vertically down the left side of your paper and match the abbreviations to each body system in the report. List the organs examined for each system in the report.

HOSA Event Prep: Medical Terminology

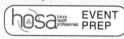

Sam was riding his bike when he was struck by a car. He felt severe pain in his left leg distal to his knee. He also had a hematoma (*hemat*, meaning "blood"; *-oma*, meaning "tumor") on his frontal lobe superior and lateral to his right eye. Upon assessment at the Emergency Department (ED), the physician noticed ecchymosis (*ecchym*, meaning "blood in the tissues"; *-osis*, meaning "abnormal condition") in the left upper quadrant with bruising. He also noticed when palpating (examining), Sam would guard the left upper quadrant of his abdomen. X-ray of his left leg showed a complete medial fracture of the left tibia and fibula. The computed tomography (CT) scan of his head showed a mild concussion. He is awaiting a CT of the abdomen.

Test Your Knowledge

1. Where is the severe leg pain?
   A. Closer to the patient's knee
   B. Closer to the patient's ankle
   C. Closer to the patient's hip

2. Where is the hematoma?
   A. At the back of the head
   B. Close to the nose
   C. Toward the ear

3. How many sections did the physician divide the abdomen into for this examination?
   A. One   C. Four
   B. Two   D. Nine

Body Systems for Support and Movement

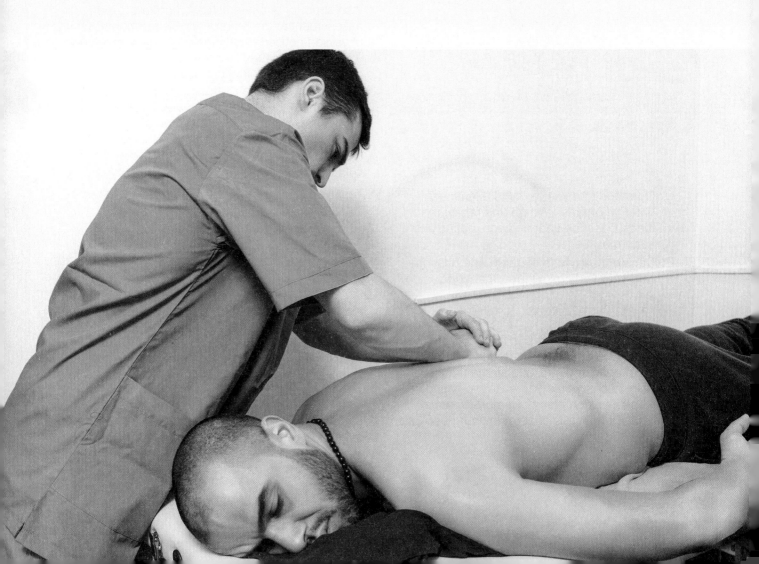

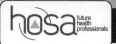
A simple definition of *disease* is an illness or sickness characterized by specific signs or symptoms. Pathophysiology is the study of the function of disease. Studying diseases can be interesting and challenging. Diseases do not always present with clear clues, and sometimes symptoms can be general and may not lead to a clear picture. When deciding on a diagnosis, healthcare professionals can use many diagnostic tools such as labs and radiology. They plug in these pieces of information with the patient's complaints and symptoms. There are times healthcare professionals do not find a diagnosis. Understanding anatomy and physiology helps healthcare professionals understand pathophysiology. HOSA has a health science event to help sharpen your diagnosing skills. If you like to dig deeper and find answers, then *Pathophysiology* may be a great event for you.

Go to the HOSA website to learn more about the HOSA *Pathophysiology* event. Find out the purpose of the event, what is involved in the event, and what knowledge is demonstrated in the event.

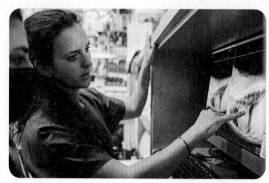

As you prepare for HOSA competitive events, be sure to check the website and talk with your HOSA advisor for the most up-to-date guidelines and procedures. Once you have learned about the *Pathophysiology* event, answer the following questions:

1. How might participating in this event benefit you personally and your future career? Explain.
2. Are you interested in participating in this event? Why or why not?

xavierarnau/E+ via Getty Images

 ## Connect with Your Reading

Connecting what you read to what you already know is an important part of learning. As you read this chapter, use sticky notes or your online comments tool to mark information in the chapter that makes you think of things you have observed before or already know. When the chapter reminds you of something you have read somewhere else, such as a book or newspaper, label the sticky note *TT* for *text to text*. If something in the chapter connects to something you have experienced in your own life, label it *TS* for *text to self*. If information in the chapter sounds like something you have seen or heard about happening somewhere in the world, such as on the news, label it *TW* for *text to world*. Be prepared to share at least one of your connections with the class.

 ## Map Your Reading

Make a tablet organizer with two sheets of paper using the example shown here. Stack the sheets, keeping the sides even, but move the top sheet up so its bottom edge is ½ inch to 1 inch above the bottom edge of the sheet below it. Holding both sheets of paper, fold both sheets down so the top edge of the top sheet is ½ inch to 1 inch above the bottom edge of the top sheet. Crease both layers and staple at the folded edge. Write the title *Systems for Support and Movement* on the top flap. Label the edges of the flaps below it with the headings *Integumentary System*, *Skeletal System*, and *Muscular System*. On the top flap, summarize what you know about the role of collagen in these systems. As you read, add a picture, the main functions, a related career, and related diseases to each system's page.

> *System for Support and Movement*
> Collagen adds strength, structure, and elasticity to the skin, bones, and muscles...
>
> INTEGUMENTARY SYSTEM (the skin)
>
> SKELETAL SYSTEM
>
> MUSCULAR SYSTEM

Goodheart-Willcox Publisher

Chapter opener image: Viacheslav Nikolaenko/Shutterstock.com

The Integumentary System

Learning Outcomes

After studying this lesson, you will be able to

18.1-1 explain the role of collagen in body systems for support and movement.

18.1-2 identify functions of the skin and label the layers.

18.1-3 explain the structure and functions of the epidermis, as well as associated diseases, disorders, and ways to prevent common conditions.

18.1-4 explain the structure and functions of the dermis, as well as associated diseases, disorders, and ways to prevent common conditions.

18.1-5 explain the structure and functions of the hypodermis, as well as associated diseases, disorders, and ways to prevent common conditions.

Professional Vocabulary

Essential Terms

collagen   a protein fiber that connects, supports, and gives strength to body tissues such as the skin, muscle tendons, and bone ligaments

dermis   the middle layer of the skin, which contains most of the skin's structures

epidermis   the thin, outer layer of the skin

hypodermis   the innermost layer of the skin, which stores fat

integumentary   related to the skin

Important Terms

hair follicle	pigment	subcutaneous fat
melanin	root	sudoriferous gland
nail bed	sebaceous gland	

Introduction

The integumentary system includes the skin, hair, and nails. The skin is mostly connective tissue, attaching it to the muscles and bones below. Connections between these systems and their related diseases and disorders will be discussed, beginning with their common connection to collagen.

18.1-1 The Role of Collagen

Your integumentary (ihn-tehg-yoo-MEHN-tuh-ree), muscular, and skeletal systems work together to support and move your body (**Figure 18.1**). Connective tissue gives these systems protection, support, and structure, while muscular tissue provides movement. Muscular tissue needs connective tissue to attach to skin and bones.

Most types of connective tissue contain **collagen** (KAH-luh-jehn) fibers to add strength. Collagen is found in the skin and hair of your integumentary system, tendons and muscle coverings of your muscular system, and bones and ligaments of your skeletal system. Collagen is the "glue" that keeps your skin firm, muscles flexible, and bones strong.

Vitamin C is important for producing collagen. Sailors used to develop a disease called *scurvy* because they did not have access to fresh fruits and vegetables—good sources of vitamin C—on long voyages. Sailors with scurvy experienced bleeding gums, weakness, bone pain, and tooth loss. Their bodies could not build the collagen needed for healthy skin, muscles, and bones because they did not have the correct nutrients. In the 1700s, James Lind proved that citrus fruits, such as oranges and limes, were an effective treatment for scurvy. The missing nutrient was later identified as vitamin C.

integument/o = skin
-ary = pertaining to

coll/a = glue
-gen = origin, formation, producing

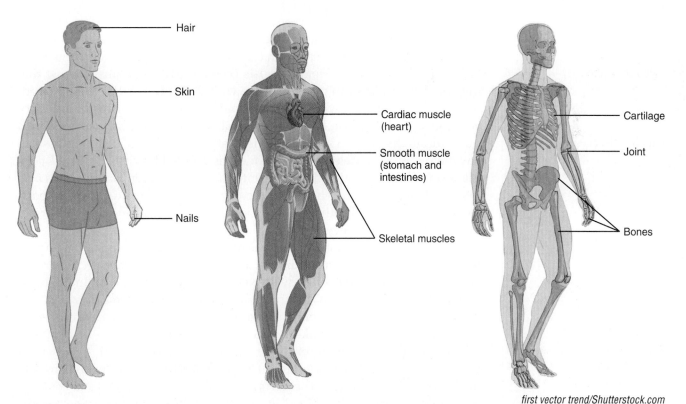

first vector trend/Shutterstock.com

Figure 18.1 Support and movement are provided by the integumentary, muscular, and skeletal systems. *How is collagen important to each of these systems?*

Different types of collagen serve different purposes. In tendons and muscle coverings, collagen fibers are lined up to provide strength for muscles pulling in one direction. In the skin and bones, collagen fibers run in different directions; they are not organized. This gives your body's structures extra protection.

In addition to collagen, there are many other factors that can lead to diseases and disorders of your integumentary, skeletal, and muscular systems. **Figure 18.2** shows the cause, or *etiology*; disease process, or *pathology*; diagnosis; treatment; and prevention of several common diseases of the systems for support and movement. Perhaps your future career will involve new ways to prevent or treat one of these conditions.

18.1-2 Understanding the Integumentary System

dermat/o = skin
-logist = specialist in the study of

If you have an interest in diseases and disorders of the skin, or **integumentary** system, you might want to become a dermatologist. To do so, you must earn a medical degree, then complete another year of medical or surgical internship and three years of residency in dermatology. Once you have finished this training, you may decide to specialize in immune disorders, laser medicine, cosmetic surgery, or diseases of the skin. Dermatology appeals to people who are both social and investigative but who want work that provides independence and a sense of accomplishment.

hemat/o = blood

path/o = disease

Many other healthcare workers also observe the skin, hair, and nails for early signs of serious medical conditions. For instance, emergency medical technicians look for color changes in the nails and skin that show an issue with breathing or blood flow. Hematologists (hee-muh-TAH-luh-jihsts) know that unusual skin bruises can mean an issue with the body's ability to stop bleeding. Very dry skin or excess sweating could be reasons to consult an endocrinologist (ehn-doh-krih-NAH-luh-jihst) about a hormone imbalance. A rash can indicate the need to see an allergist. Pathologists know that hair loss can have many causes. Male pattern baldness is a hereditary condition. *Alopecia* is a form of hair loss often due to an autoimmune disorder. Hair loss can also indicate poisoning. Any change in the condition of your skin, hair, or nails could be important. Healthcare professionals must understand what is normal for skin structures so they can recognize an abnormal change.

The integumentary system forms the outside surface of your body. Skin protects and supports the bones, muscles, and internal organs beneath its surface. Your skin works with other body systems to sense touch and maintain body temperature. It also plays a role in producing and storing some nutrients and getting rid of body waste. Compare the siding on a house to the skin covering your body. What do you think they have in common?

epi- = upon
derm/o = skin
-is = pertaining to
ex- = out, away from
-crine = to secrete
hypo- = below, under

Your skin has three layers—the epidermis, dermis, and hypodermis (**Figure 18.3**. The **epidermis** (eh-puh-DER-muhs) is the thin, outer layer mostly made up of dead skin cells. The **dermis** lies below the epidermis and contains the skin's sensory organs, blood vessels, hair follicles, and exocrine glands. The **hypodermis** (hI-puh-DER-muhs) lies beneath the dermis and contains a layer of fat and connective tissue that attaches the skin to muscle tissue and provides padding for underlying structures. Each layer of the skin has a different role in covering and protecting the body.

Common Diseases and Disorders for Systems of Support and Movement

Characteristics	Arthritis	Melanoma	Muscular Dystrophy
Etiology	Osteoarthritis—excess weight, overuse, or bacterial infection Rheumatoid—autoimmune disorder Gout—ureic acid buildup Fibromyalgia—unknown Childhood arthritis—unknown	UVA rays from the sun damage the skin's DNA, causing melanocytes to grow and multiply, then spread to nearby tissues.	A group of disorders caused by a genetic mutation on the X chromosome, so males are most commonly affected.
Pathology	Chronic wearing on the articular surface of joints causes pain and stiffness. Joints may become warm, red, and swollen. Occurs in 1 in 4 adults. More common in females (except gout).	Least common type of skin cancer, but most likely to become malignant. There are 100,000 cases and 6,000 deaths per year. 93% survival rate. More likely for those with light skin, blue eyes, blond or red hair, and a family history of skin cancer.	Results in muscle weakness that worsens over time and can affect the ability to walk, breathe, swallow, or speak. Nine types, each affecting different groups of muscles with different levels of severity, appearing at different ages, with differing life spans. Affects more than 50,000 people in US.
Diagnosis	Medical history, physical examination, X-rays, and blood tests distinguish between types and level of disease progress.	Report any unusual moles or skin changes so a dermatologist can complete a skin cancer screening. Biopsy to confirm diagnosis. If spread, then X-ray, CT scan, or PET scan will look for more cancer.	Parents report developmental delays, observe signs of muscle weakness, evaluate motor development. Confirm and identify type with muscle biopsy, DNA test, electromyography, enzyme test, heart monitoring, MRI, and/or ultrasound.
Treatment	Pain relievers, gentle movement to maintain function while minimizing joint damage, and possible joint replacement surgery can improve function and quality of life.	Thinner melanomas only require excision with a border of healthy tissue. A sentinel node biopsy determines whether the cancer has spread beyond the mole. Chemotherapy, radiation, and surgery.	No cure, but treatment can manage symptoms and improve quality of life. Medications, physical therapy to stay flexible, respiratory care if lungs are affected, mobility and positioning aids, speech therapy, and/or surgery to manage or correct complications.
Prevention	Maintain a healthy weight. Eat a balanced diet that includes calcium. Get regular physical activity. Avoid repetitive movements with the joint under stress. Avoid smoking.	Avoid sunburn and excess sun exposure, use sun protection clothing and lotions, monitor the UV index. Avoid sunlamps and tanning booths. Perform regular self-exams of your skin to watch for changes.	Genetic testing to identify if either parent carries the gene and choosing not to have children.

Goodheart-Willcox Publisher

Figure 18.2 Common diseases and disorders of the systems for support and movement.

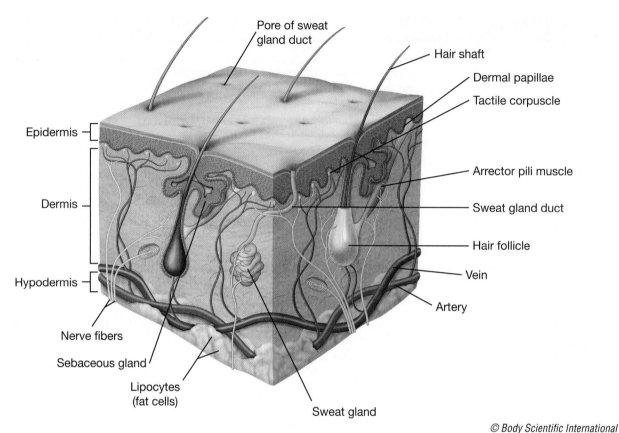

Figure 18.3 The epidermis is the outermost layer of skin, followed by the dermis and hypodermis. *Which layer contains most of the skin's structures?*

Labels on figure:
- Pore of sweat gland duct
- Hair shaft
- Dermal papillae
- Tactile corpuscle
- Epidermis
- Dermis
- Hypodermis
- Arrector pili muscle
- Sweat gland duct
- Hair follicle
- Vein
- Artery
- Nerve fibers
- Sebaceous gland
- Lipocytes (fat cells)
- Sweat gland

© Body Scientific International

18.1-3 The Epidermis

The epidermis is the thin, outer layer of your skin. It is actually made of four or five layers, or *strata*, of epithelial cells. New skin cells are constantly being pushed up to the surface of your skin. The epidermis contains no blood vessels, so as cells move away from their blood supply, they become dehydrated. As the cells dry out, their cytoplasm changes to keratin (KAIR-uh-tihn), a tough, orange-colored protein. This dried outer layer of keratin-filled skin cells makes it difficult for germs to get through your skin and holds in moisture to prevent dehydration.

Many kinds of skin irritation can occur, from acne and chicken pox to insect bites and blisters. **Figure 18.4** describes some common skin conditions. Aging brings an increase in skin tabs, moles, infections, and other skin irregularities. These conditions may cause pain, itching, and embarrassment. Some skin conditions, like crusts, may clear up on their own. Others, like scales, polyps, and infections, may require treatment.

It is important to keep the skin clean and dry. Bacteria penetrating your epidermis can cause *impetigo*, a highly contagious skin infection that is common in children. It usually appears as yellowish-brown crusts or blisters. Common viral skin conditions include warts and herpes. These are also contagious. Herpes appears as a collection of small blisters. Herpes simplex virus (HSV) causes cold sores and genital herpes. Herpes zoster, or *shingles*, is caused by the same virus as chicken pox. Fungal, or *mycotic*, skin infections are itchy but not usually serious. Ringworm, also known as *tinea*, is a common fungal infection that causes intense itching. Different forms of tinea affect different areas of the body.

de- = lack of, away from
hydr/o = water
-ate = pertaining to, composed of, process

myc/o = fungus
-tic = pertaining to

Common Skin Conditions

Condition	Drawing	Appearance	Description
Crusts	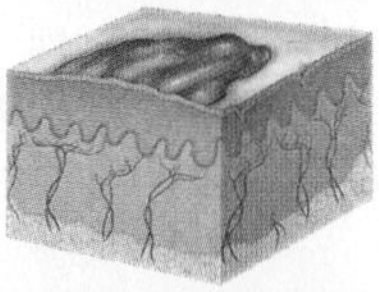	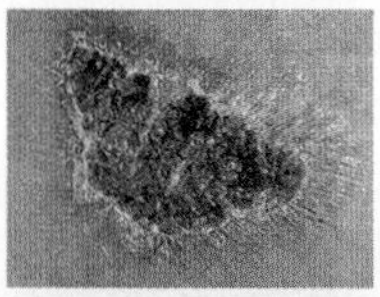	**Crusts** are dried blood and body fluid that scab over on the skin surface.
Scales	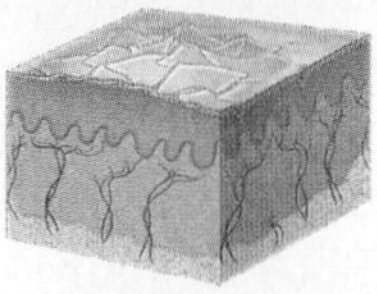	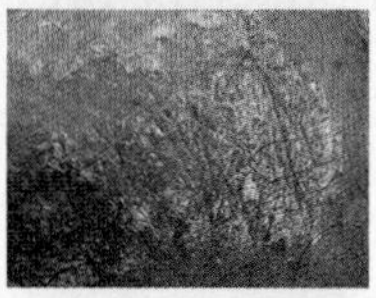	**Scales** are dry skin flakes that remain attached to the skin surface, as with eczema and psoriasis.
Seborrhea	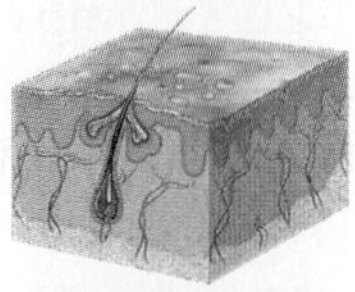	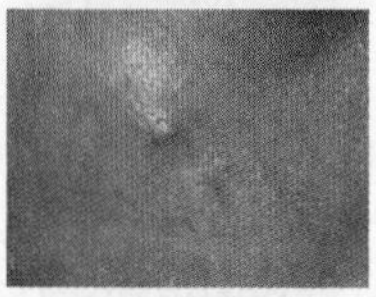	**Seborrhea** is the problem of oily skin, often seen during puberty when the sebaceous glands produce too much sebum.
Polyps	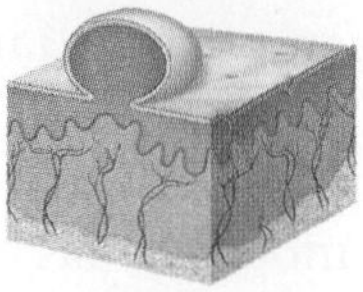	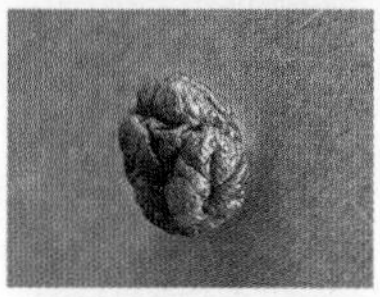	**Polyps**, or *skin tabs*, are small flaps of skin attached to the epidermis by a thin stalk. They are common on the neck, chest, armpits, and eyelids.
Macules	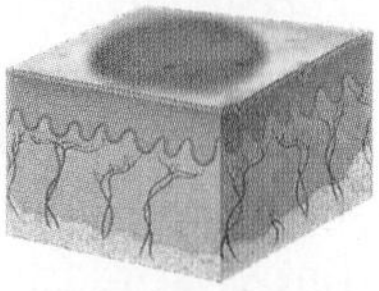		**Macules** are flat, colored spots on the skin surface, such as freckles.
Wheals	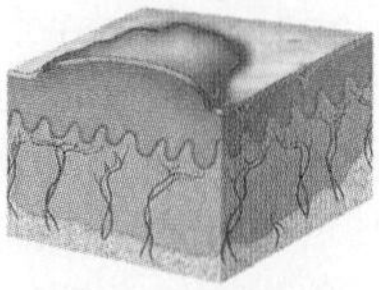		**Wheals**, or *welts*, are large, red, raised, itchy bumps, often seen in an allergic reaction called *hives*.
Papules	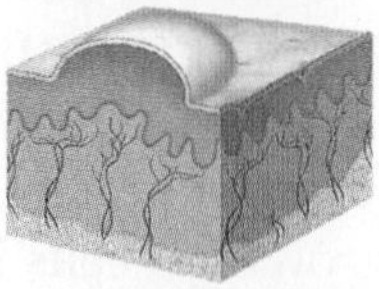	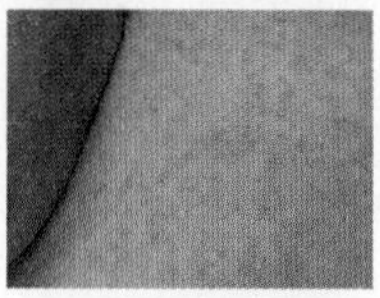	**Papules** are small, solid, raised bumps on the surface of the skin, like those seen with heat rash.
Pustules	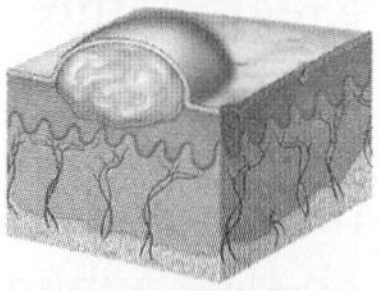	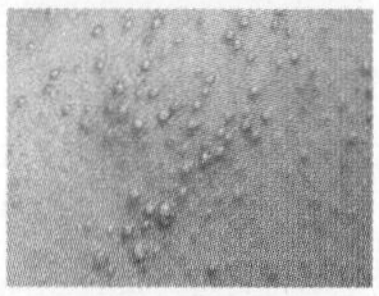	**Pustules**, or *pus-filled pimples*, like acne, are most common on the face, neck, and back.
Vesicles	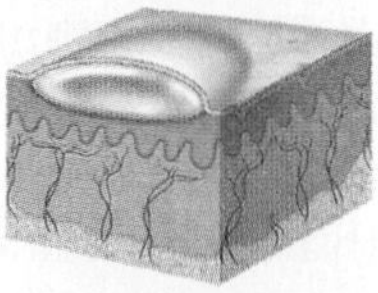	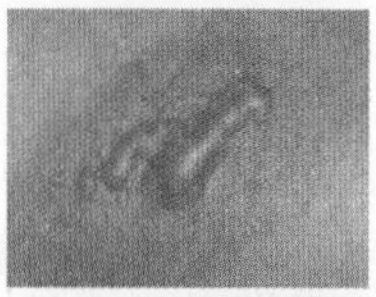	**Vesicles** are blisters filled with clear fluid that can burst and ooze.
Nodules	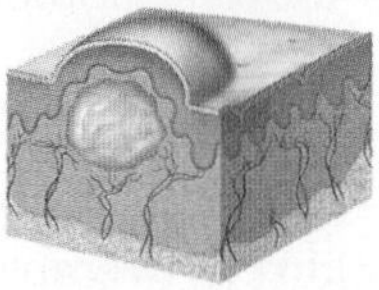	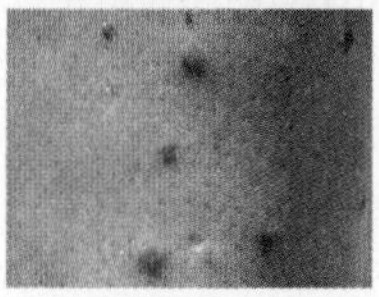	**Nodules** are filled sacs, or *cysts*, that form a firm bump going down into the dermis.

Goodheart-Willcox Publisher, Drawings: © Body Scientific International; Appearance (top to bottom): Roblan/Shutterstock.com, Sergey 77700/Shutterstock.com, Zay Nyi Nyi/Shutterstock.com, Evan Lorne/Shutterstock.com, rj lerich/Shutterstock.com, KuLouKu/Shutterstock.com, Glamorous Images/Shutterstock.com, Anton Gvozdikov/Shutterstock.com, Chutchawarn/Shutterstock.com, OlegD/Shutterstock.com

Figure 18.4 These common skin conditions have many causes and can affect anyone.

albin/o = white
-ism = condition

melan/o = black
-in = substance, chemical

Your skin color is determined by the amount and type of **pigment** in your epidermis. Skin, hair, and eye colors normally vary from very light to very dark (**Figure 18.5**). *Albinism* is a genetic condition that prevents the skin from making its dark pigment. As a result, the skin of a person with albinism is fair, the hair is whitish-blonde, and the eyes appear pale blue to pink. *Vitiligo* (vit-ih-LI-go) is a patchy loss of color when just some pigment-producing cells stop functioning.

Melanin (MEL-uh-nihn) is the brownish-black pigment produced by melanocytes (MUH-la-nuh-sItz), which are special cells in your epidermis. When your skin is exposed to ultraviolet radiation, these cells make more melanin. Think of a tan as a big melanin umbrella that comes out to protect the DNA in your skin cells from the sun's radiation. A *mole* is a clump of melanocyte pigment cells that can become cancerous and spread through the skin layers. You can protect yourself from skin cancer by spending less time in the sun between 10:00 a.m. and 4:00 p.m., covering up, and reapplying sunscreen often. A tan or sunburn are signs of damage to your skin.

Regular skin checks can help detect skin cancer. You can remember the signs of skin cancer with the acronym *ABCDE* (**Figure 18.6**). The deadliest skin cancer is malignant melanoma (muh-LIHG-nuhnt meh-luh-NOH-muh). It usually appears dark and asymmetrical and grows rapidly. The fact that it spreads easily makes it very dangerous. Basal cell carcinoma (BAY-suhl sehl kahr-sih-NOH-muh) is the most common type of skin cancer. It typically appears as a raised bump with an indentation in the center and is most often found on the face or neck. If you have a suspicious skin growth that fits any of the ABCDE symptoms, see a dermatologist.

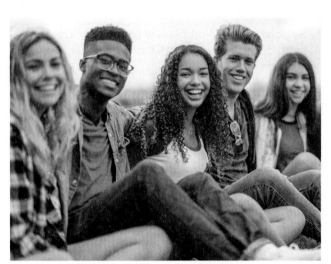

Figure 18.5 The amount of melanin produced by your skin cells determines your skin color.

FatCamera/E+ via Getty Images

cry/o = cold

Warts can also form lumps on the skin, but most are not cancerous. They result from an infection that causes an overgrowth of cells in the epidermis. Cryosurgery (krI-oh-SER-jeh-ree) uses freezing temperatures to destroy warts, moles, and other diseased tissues.

Dead cells are constantly being scraped off your skin's surface and make up the majority of household dust. Dead skin cells that fall from the scalp in clumps are called dandruff. An *abrasion* (uh-BRAY-zhuhn) is a scrape on the skin's surface, and dermabrasion (der-muh-BRAY-zhuhn) is the process of scraping off the top layers of the skin. Dermabrasion can help remove superficial scars, wrinkles, hair, or unwanted tattoos from the epidermis. An abrasion of the epidermal layer will heal well with no scar, but a cut, or *laceration* (la-suh-RAY-shuhn), into the layers below is more serious and will usually cause scarring.

trans- = across
derm/o = skin
-al = pertaining to

Skin characteristics vary on different areas of your body. Skin cells can specialize in absorption, protection, or secretion. The skin's ability to absorb chemicals through thin areas makes certain medications deliverable through a patch instead of a pill or injection. The medication in the patch, such as nicotine to help a person stop smoking, can be absorbed through the skin, or *transdermally*.

Normal and Cancerous Skin Growths

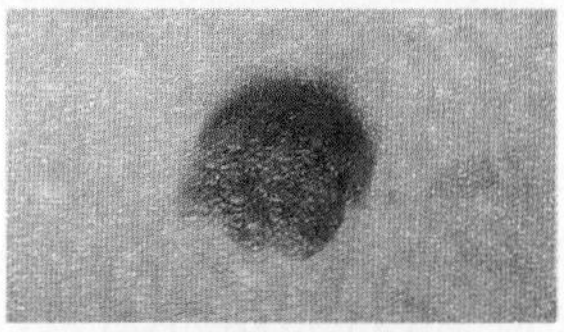

Normal mole

Cancerous Skin Growth	Sign	Characteristic
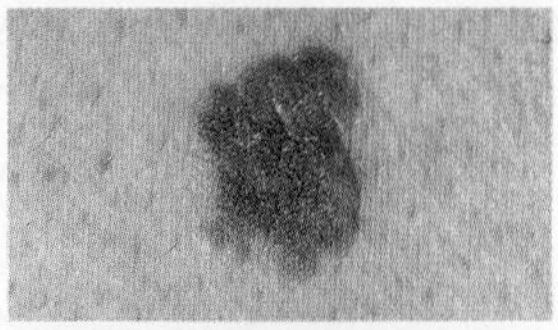	**A**symmetry	If you draw a line down the center of the marking, the two sides are different shapes.
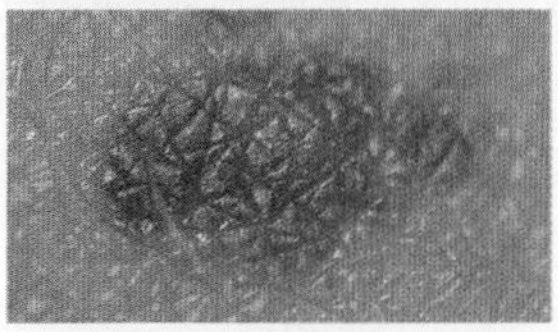	**B**order irregularity	The borders (edges) of the marking are blurry or uneven in shape rather than smooth.
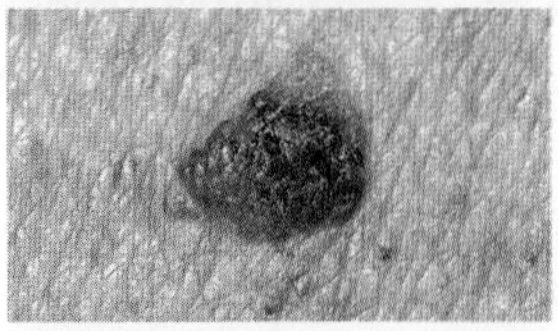	**C**olor changes	The marking changes color from one area to another (tan, brown, black, pink, blue, or white).
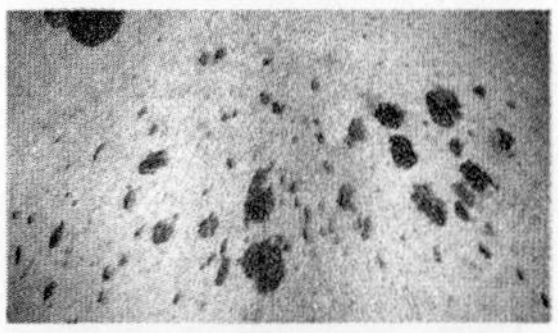	**D**iameter	The marking is larger across than a pencil's eraser (¼ inch).
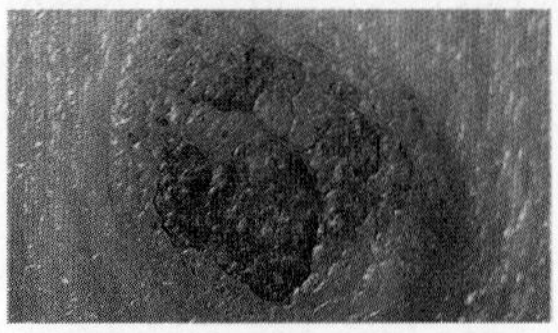	**E**volving	The marking changes over time in size, shape, color, bleeding, or other symptoms.

Goodheart-Willcox Publisher, Images top to bottom: Nathalie Speliers Ufermann/Shutterstock.com, LYphoto/Shutterstock.com, D. Kucharski K. Kucharska/Shutterstock.com, Nathalie Speliers Ufermann/Shutterstock.com, Oscar C. Williams/Shutterstock.com, D. Kucharski K. Kucharska/Shutterstock.com

Figure 18.6 It is important for people to know and understand the differences between a normal mole and a malignant one.

Skin on the soles of your feet lacks hair and forms thick calluses to cushion your bones as you walk. Skin on the palms of your hands produces sweat more quickly than other areas of your body. What differences do you see between the skin on your face and the skin on your arms?

18.1-4 **The Dermis**

The dermis is the second layer of your skin, just beneath the epidermis. It is made of connective tissue and contains most of your skin's structures, including sensory organs, blood vessels, hair follicles, and exocrine glands. *Dermal papillae* (puh-PIH-lee) are small bumps that connect your epidermis to the dermis.

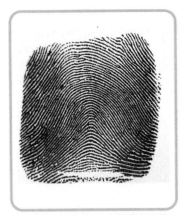

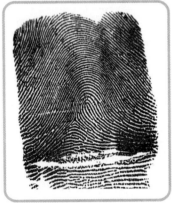

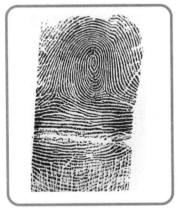

Kevin L Chesson/Shutterstock.com

Figure 18.7 Though everyone's fingerprints are unique, they all contain the basic shapes of the arch (top), loop (middle), and whorl (bottom). *Which shapes do you see in your own fingerprints?*

These papillae group together on your fingertips and feet to form ridges that make the patterns of your fingerprints and footprints. Three basic shapes—arch, loop, and whorl—in different combinations make each person's prints unique (**Figure 18.7**). This uniqueness is important in many ways. For example, babies' footprints are recorded at birth for identification, and forensic investigators use fingerprints to help solve crimes. Take a minute to examine your own fingerprints. What shapes and patterns do you see? Is the print on each finger different?

There are many nerve endings in your dermis. These sensors are more concentrated in some areas than in others. Different types of nerve endings sense different things, including light touch, heavy pressure, vibration, temperature, and pain. The base of each hair, fingernail, and toenail contains many nerve endings.

Hair and nails both grow from living roots in your dermis, but dead keratinized cells make up the hair and nails seen on the outside of your body, like your skin's surface (**Figure 18.8**). Your hair's growth begins in a **root** at the bottom of a tube called the **hair follicle**. The shaft of dead cells pushes up through your epidermis where you see it as hair. Similarly, your nail root produces a hard, dead "shell" called the *nail plate* as protection for the sensitive **nail bed** at the tips of your fingers and toes. The phrase "you cut me to the quick" means that someone has hurt you deeply—like when you cut your nail too close and the sensitive nail bed is exposed. There are no nerve endings in hair shafts or nail plates themselves so there is no pain when you cut them. Tiny *arrector pili* muscles connected to each hair follicle raise your body hair and cause goosebumps when you are cold or scared.

Two types of exocrine glands in the dermis produce substances that are excreted through ducts onto your skin's surface. **Sebaceous** (sih-BAY-shuhs) **glands** provide sebum, an oily secretion that coats your hair and skin with a softening, waterproof film. These glands are usually found in the hair follicle. As you grow from a baby to a teen and adult, your sebaceous glands become more active, providing more moisture and protection to your skin so it is less sensitive. When sebum traps dead skin cells in a pore, it can form a plug that becomes infected. This pus-filled pore is called *acne*. An infected hair follicle or sebaceous gland is called a *boil*. Keep your skin clean to help avoid these conditions. In old age, your sebaceous glands will become less active, and you may need moisturizers to prevent dry skin.

The second type of exocrine gland allows your skin to get rid of waste. Sweat, or *perspiration*, comes from **sudoriferous** (soo-duh-RIH-fuh-ruhs) **glands** in your dermis that empty through sweat pores onto your skin's surface. You can remember the difference between sebaceous and sudoriferous glands by remembering that sudoriferous can be "*odor*-iferous!" During puberty, the sudoriferous glands begin to produce perspiration, and body odor increases. Perspiration helps cool your body through evaporation, drawing warmth out of your skin. An active person can produce as much as 1 quart of perspiration per hour. Perspiration also helps get rid of body waste such as excess salt and other minerals. This waste provides food for bacteria and fungi that live on your skin's surface. In turn, these microorganisms produce lactic acid that discourages the growth of harmful bacteria such as *Staphylococcus*.

Unfortunately, an infestation of lice, called *pediculosis*, can affect anyone, whether they are sweaty, dirty, or clean. These tiny insects feed on blood and attach their eggs to the hair shaft. Head lice spread by close contact but do not carry other diseases. Other insect-like organisms, such as ticks, fleas, mites, and mosquitos, also pierce the skin to feed on human blood. Some do spread harmful infections and cause skin irritation and allergic reactions. The rate of mosquito-and tick-borne illnesses in the US has increased significantly in the last 10 years.

Blood vessels running through the dermis affect your skin's color. Although their purpose is to deliver nutrients and carry away waste, these vessels show through the skin in areas with less pigment and cause a variety of skin color changes. The term *pallor* describes skin that is a pale color due to a lack of blood and is sometimes seen on the face before a person faints. *Cyanosis* (sI-uh-NOH-sihs) is the blue color seen in the lips, skin, or nails when the blood is low in oxygen. Redness, or *erythema* (ehr-uh-THEE-muh), occurs with increased blood flow to the skin when you are embarrassed, ill, or exercising. *Petechiae* (puh-TEE-kee-I) are tiny red or purple spots caused by broken blood vessels in the skin. A bruise, or *hematoma* (hee-muh-TOH-muh), gets its color from bleeding under the skin, not from the blood vessels themselves. *Jaundice* (JAWN-dihs) is the yellow color caused by liver disease. Black spots are a common symptom of *necrosis*, which is tissue death. This occurs with gangrene, when tissue dies due to infection or lack of blood supply. Skin color is an important factor when assessing a person's condition.

cyan/o = blue
-osis = condition, process, state
erythr/o = red

hemat/o = blood

necr/o = death

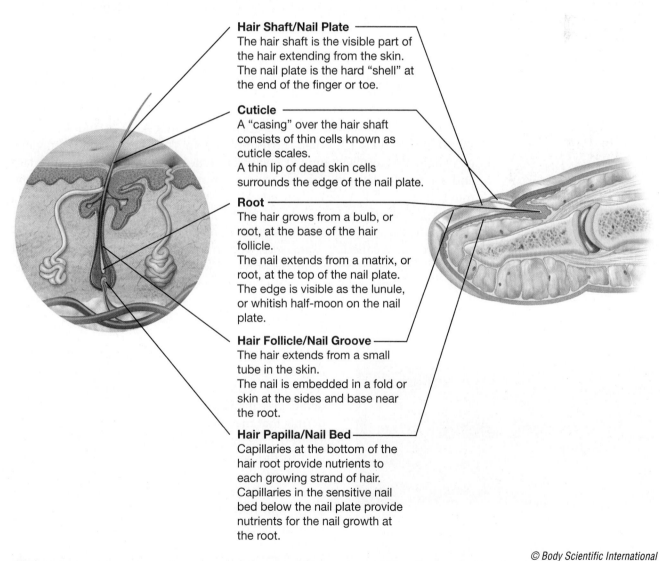

Hair Shaft/Nail Plate
The hair shaft is the visible part of the hair extending from the skin.
The nail plate is the hard "shell" at the end of the finger or toe.

Cuticle
A "casing" over the hair shaft consists of thin cells known as cuticle scales.
A thin lip of dead skin cells surrounds the edge of the nail plate.

Root
The hair grows from a bulb, or root, at the base of the hair follicle.
The nail extends from a matrix, or root, at the top of the nail plate. The edge is visible as the lunule, or whitish half-moon on the nail plate.

Hair Follicle/Nail Groove
The hair extends from a small tube in the skin.
The nail is embedded in a fold or skin at the sides and base near the root.

Hair Papilla/Nail Bed
Capillaries at the bottom of the hair root provide nutrients to each growing strand of hair. Capillaries in the sensitive nail bed below the nail plate provide nutrients for the nail growth at the root.

© *Body Scientific International*

Figure 18.8 Hair and nails have a similar structural makeup. *Are your nails and hair alive or dead? Explain your answer.*

The skin also helps keep your body's temperature at 98.6°F. Body fat and *vasoconstriction* (vay-soh-kuhn-STRIHK-shuhn) hold in body heat. The blood vessels in the dermis get smaller when you are cold, preventing heat loss. In Raynaud phenomenon, the hands or feet may turn bluish or white in response to narrowed blood vessels when cold or stressed. *Vasodilation* makes blood vessels wider so they can carry more warm blood to the body's surface where heat can be released. Babies have less body fat and more surface area for their body weight than adults, so babies are more likely to experience *hypothermia*, or low body temperature. How does your skin look and feel after exercising?

18.1-5 The Hypodermis

The hypodermis lies beneath your dermis and contains a layer of connective tissue that attaches your skin to the muscle below. Your hypodermis is mostly made of **subcutaneous fat**. It provides padding to absorb shock, holds in your body heat, and stores energy and nutrients. Fat cells have large vacuoles for fat storage. They shrink when you have a calorie deficit and expand when you have a calorie excess. Each additional pound of fat on your body requires an extra mile of blood vessels to supply that area with nutrients. This layer of fat will build up as you grow into adulthood but decrease again in old age, when the loss of fat and elasticity causes the skin to sag and wrinkle. Body-fat distribution, which describes where fat is stored on your body, is important. Having more fat around the abdomen, for example, is related to a higher risk for diabetes, heart disease, and cancer.

Some fat is required for normal body functions. Sex hormones are stored in your body fat. Fat-soluble vitamins such as vitamins A, D, E, and K are also stored in your body fat. When cholesterol in your skin is exposed to ultraviolet (UV) light, this forms vitamin D. Just five minutes of sun exposure on your face and arms each day will provide your recommended daily allowance of vitamin D (**Figure 18.9**). Your body needs some fat to store hormones, nutrients, and energy, as well as provide insulation from cold and pad other body structures.

Both pressure ulcers and burns cause damage to all layers of the skin. Pressure sores, also called *decubitus ulcers*, occur when something presses against the skin long and hard enough to prevent blood from reaching the skin cells. This causes those cells to die. Patients who are in wheelchairs or confined to bed should be repositioned or reminded to shift their weight regularly to increase circulation and prevent these sores.

Heat, electricity, or chemicals can cause burns (**Figure 18.10**). Both first-degree burns and pressure sores cause redness and affect only the epidermis. Second-degree injuries result in blisters and damage to the dermis that may take several weeks or longer to heal. Third-degree injuries damage the full thickness of the skin, including the hypodermis. Fourth-degree injuries extend into the muscle, tendons, and bone. Third- and fourth-degree injuries are serious enough to require surgery to remove dead skin, place skin grafts, and manage the scars and skin tightening that occur.

The size of a burn is estimated using the "rule of nines" (**Figure 18.11**). This rule divides the total body surface into sections representing multiples of nine.

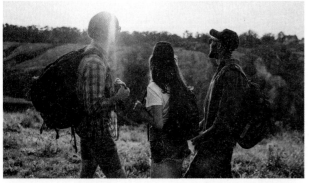

Master1305/Shutterstock.com

Figure 18.9 Some daily sun exposure can be healthy, but too much sun can damage the skin. *What are the benefits of sun exposure? How can you protect your skin from overexposure?*

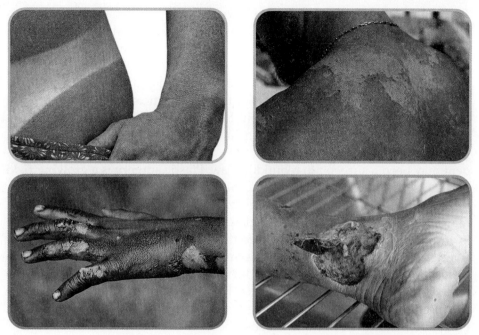

Left to right, top to bottom: Amy Walters/Shutterstock.com, sutulastock/Shutterstock.com, Naiyyer/Shutterstock.com, chatuphot/Shutterstock.com

Figure 18.10 Pressure, heat, electricity, and chemicals can all damage the skin layers. *What degree of damage does each of these images represent—first, second, third, or fourth?*

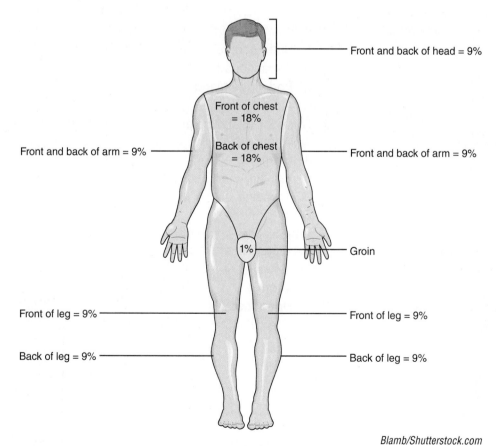

Blamb/Shutterstock.com

Figure 18.11 The rule of nines divides the body as shown here to determine what percentage of the body was damaged by a burn.

The larger the area affected, the more likely a patient is to have complications such as infection or dehydration. Always seek medical attention for a burn if your skin is broken, the injury covers an area larger than the palm of your hand, or the burn does not heal within a week.

Plastic surgery repairs, reshapes, or rebuilds skin and the structures below it. Cosmetic surgery is the best-known form of plastic surgery. However, not all forms of plastic surgery are about beauty-related enhancements. Reconstructive surgery helps repair damage and improve function after accidents, tissue damage, and disease. For example, someone who has been in an accident may need a surgeon to rebuild his jaw. Plastic surgery is a growing field for employment, research, and new technology.

When medical treatment requires an injection, healthcare professionals may insert the needle at different angles. This controls how fast the medication is absorbed. Intradermal injections go through the epidermis to deliver solutions, such as an allergy test, to the dermis for slow absorption. Subcutaneous injections, such as insulin, must go through the epidermis and dermis to the hypodermis for slightly faster uptake. Intramuscular injections, such as the flu vaccine, go through all three layers of the skin and into the muscle tissue below. There, they will be quickly absorbed.

intra- = within
derm/o = skin
-al = pertaining to

sub- = below, under
cutane/o = skin
-ous = pertaining to, having

muscul/o = muscle
-ar = pertaining to

Lesson 18.1 Review

 Complete the *Map Your Reading* graphic organizer for the section you just read.

1. Which of the following parts of connective tissue provides structure and support for the body? (18.1-1)
   A. Collagen
   B. Keratin
   C. Melanin
   D. Sudoriferous gland

2. Which of the following is *not* a layer of the integumentary system? (18.1-2)
   A. Epidermis
   B. Dermis
   C. Subcutaneous
   D. Hypodermis

3. Dead skin cells protect the surface of the (18.1-3)
   A. dermis
   B. hypodermis
   C. connective tissue
   D. epidermis

4. Which type of gland provides an oily secretion that softens skin? (18.1-4)
   A. Sudoriferous gland
   B. Sebaceous gland
   C. Endocrine gland
   D. All of these.

5. Changes in skin color can indicate which of the following conditions? (18.1-4)
   A. Cyanosis
   B. Fainting
   C. Jaundice
   D. All of these.

6. Which of the following are stored in subcutaneous fat? Choose all that apply. (18.1-5)
   A. Melanin
   B. Vitamin C
   C. Hormones
   D. Energy

The Skeletal System

Learning Outcomes

After studying this lesson, you will be able to

18.2-1 identify the basic functions of the skeletal system.

18.2-2 describe the structure and function of the different parts of a long bone.

18.2-3 explain the process of bone development and ways to prevent common bone diseases.

18.2-4 identify bones on a diagram and classify them by type.

18.2-5 describe different types of bone markings.

18.2-6 compare the functions of the axial skeleton and appendicular skeleton.

18.2-7 identify different types of joints.

18.2-8 describe different types of dislocations and fractures.

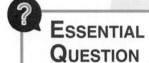

ESSENTIAL QUESTION

What are the structures, functions, and diseases associated with the skeletal system?

Professional Vocabulary

Essential Terms

appendicular skeleton   the bones of the arms and legs, including the shoulder and hip bones where they are attached

axial skeleton   the skull, spine, and rib cage bones, which surround an imaginary center line of the body

compact bone   the hard, dense, outer layer of bone tissue made to withstand stress

ligament   a tough, fibrous tissue that connects bones to other bones and holds organs in place

spongy bone   the lighter, less dense inner layer of bone tissue that contains red bone marrow

Important Terms

ball-and-socket joints	foramen	osteoclast
cartilage	gliding joint	pivot joint
condylar joints	hinge joints	saddle joint
diaphysis	irregular bones	sesamoid bones
epiphysis	long bones	short bones
flat bones	ossification	sutured
fontanel	osteoblasts	

Introduction

Although you cannot actually see your bones, you can see their outline and feel them through their covering of skin, muscle, and fat. You will understand the skeletal system better if you use your own body as a model. As you read this lesson, try to find the bones on your own body and feel how they move together.

18.2-1 Understanding the Skeletal System

Your skeletal system includes bones, joints, and cartilage named for their shape and function. Bones work with your muscular, circulatory, and digestive systems. Together, they provide structure, support, protection, muscle attachment sites, blood cell production, and mineral storage. Collagen provides structure, support, and strength for your skeletal system.

orth/o = to straighten
ped/o = foot
-ic = pertaining to

arthr/o = joint
-scopy = process of viewing, examination
-plasty = surgical repair

Orthopedic surgeons work closely with bones. The name for this field comes from early procedures that focused on straightening the feet. Orthopedic surgeons now correct a wide variety of misshaped bones and complicated breaks. The field of orthopedics is constantly developing new techniques to relieve pain and improve function. For example, in arthroscopy (ahr-THRAHS-kuh-pee), surgical tools are inserted through several small openings in the skin instead of one large cut. This allows faster healing and less exposure to infection. Joint replacement, or *arthroplasty* (AHR-thruh-plas-tee), is a major surgery to improve movement and relieve joint pain. Orthopedic surgeons must complete a five-year residency and will work an average of 50 to 55 hours per week for their $400,000 annual salary. These doctors may also specialize in sports medicine or hand, spine, or microsurgery.

ped/o = foot
orth/o = to straighten
-ist = specialist, agent
con- = with, together
gen/o = origin

If you do not see yourself as a future surgeon but are interested in working with bone structure, you may want to think about more creative therapeutic careers. A prosthetist (PRAHS-theht-ihst) makes custom-built artificial limbs, or *prostheses* (prahs-THEE-seez), for patients who are missing body parts (**Figure 18.12**). Orthotists (OR-thah-tihsts) make a variety of braces, or *orthotics*, to support weak bones or correct physical conditions. Pedorthists (PEHD-orth-ihsts) specialize in devices that relieve foot conditions caused by disease, *congenital* (present at birth) conditions, overuse, or injury. People in these careers are caring, social, and detail-oriented. They like to work with their hands and have a strong background in science and technology. They may work in a clinic, hospital, or rehabilitation center. A master's degree and one year of residency are required for certification in orthotics, prosthetics, and pedorthics.

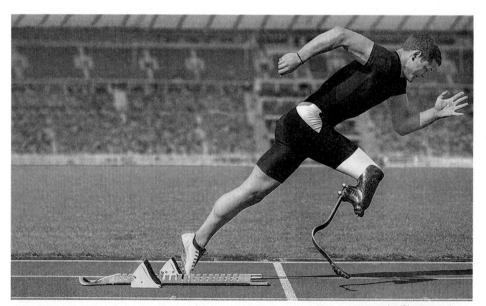

mezzotint/Shutterstock.com

Figure 18.12 Artificial limbs made by prosthetists can help people walk, lift objects, or even compete in sports. *What injuries or diseases might cause someone to lose a limb?*

18.2-2 Parts of a Bone

Your bones have many parts, each with a different function (**Figure 18.13**). Your bones provide mineral and fat storage and enable red and white blood cell production. Each of these jobs takes place in a different part of your bone.

Each end of a long bone forms a knob called the **epiphysis** (eh-PIHF-uh-sihs). The epiphysis is mostly **spongy bone**, a lighter and less dense structure than compact bone. Your blood cells are made in the red bone marrow of the epiphysis. This process is called *hematopoiesis*.

epi- = upon
-physis = to grow

hemat/o = blood
-poiesis = to make

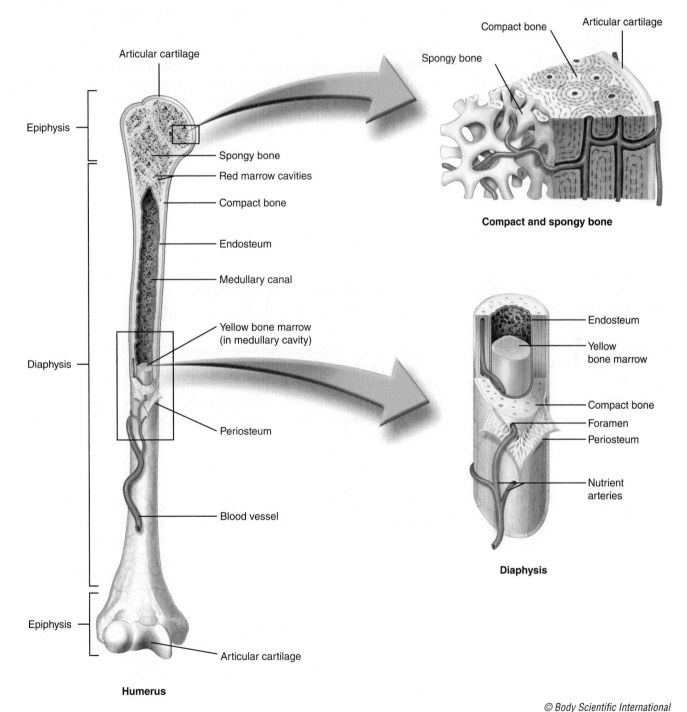

Compact and spongy bone

Diaphysis

Humerus

© Body Scientific International

Figure 18.13 Bones, which appear very simple on the outside, contain important structures and materials such as bone marrow and blood vessels. *Can you identify the functions of each part of the bone structure?*

Bone marrow transplants can help cure diseases like leukemia (loo-KEE-mee-uh), a blood disorder. Your epiphysis is covered with articular **cartilage**, which is found where two bones meet to form a movable joint. This strong but flexible substance allows your bone ends to slide smoothly across each other.

dia- = through, complete
-physis = to grow
epi- = upon
-eal = pertaining to
medull/o = middle
-ary = pertaining to

The **diaphysis** (dI-AHF-uh-sihs) is the long shaft of your bone between the two epiphyses. It is surrounded by **compact bone**, made of bone cells lined up close together to withstand stress. Bone growth occurs in the epiphyseal (ehp-ih-FIHZ-ee-ahl) plate where your epiphysis and diaphysis meet.

A hollow tube called the *medullary cavity* runs down the center of the diaphysis and stores your fat-rich yellow bone marrow. This soft center is what dogs like to lick out of a bone. Blood vessels and nerves run through this cavity, and an opening or hole called the **foramen** (fuh-RAY-mehn) allows them to pass through the compact bone.

Try to find one of your supraorbital foramina. Press a fingertip against the inner third of one of your eyebrows (the end near your nose). When you press on the foramen, you should feel a tingling sensation because you are compressing the nerve that runs through it.

peri- = around
oste/o = bone
-um = structure
lig/a = to tie

The diaphysis is wrapped in a thin membrane called the *periosteum* (pair-ee-AHS-tee-uhm). This is where ligaments and tendons attach to your bone. **Ligaments** (LIHG-uh-mehnts) are straps of connective tissue that hold your bones together at the joints and keep joints from moving the wrong way. Tendons are also connective tissues, but they connect muscle to bone for movement at your joints. Powerful muscles get their strongest attachment on the large, flat areas of a bone's surface.

18.2-3 Bone Development

Bones begin as tough, rubbery cartilage in the first few weeks of a fetus' development. Collagen fibers in the cartilage give it strength and provide the structure for making bones. Osteogenesis (ahs-tee-oh-JEHN-uh-sihs) imperfecta, commonly known as *brittle bone disease*, is a genetic mutation that causes abnormal or insufficient collagen so the bones break easily.

oste/o = bone
-genesis = origin, formation, producing
-blast = immature cell
oss/i = bone
-fic = making, causing
-ation = action of, process of
a- = without
chondr/o = cartilage
-plasia = development, formation

Osteoblasts are specialized bone-forming cells that begin the mineralization process. **Ossification** (ahs-uh-fuh-KAY-shuhn) is the process of taking calcium from what you eat or drink and depositing it into your cartilage to form bone. In *achondroplasia* (ay-kahn-droh-PLAY-zhee-uh) , the most common type of short-limbed dwarfism, the issue is not in forming cartilage, but in ossification to form bone.

Bones need vitamin D for calcium to deposit into the bones as they grow. Children with a poor diet or lack of exposure to the sun may develop *rickets* because they do not get enough vitamin D. Rickets causes bowed legs, softer bones, delayed growth, and weaker muscles. Fortifying milk with vitamin D to provide the vitamins and minerals needed for healthy bones helps prevent this condition in the United States.

oste/o = bone
-clast = break down

Your bones continue to change as you grow older. **Osteoclast** cells break down your bone during physical activity, so bone can be remodeled into new bone cells. Stress on your bones, such as jogging, helps your bones deposit more calcium where it is needed to become stronger. You will reach your maximum bone density by 25 years of age. After about 40 years of age, you will likely begin to lose more bone mass than you gain through diet and physical activity. Hormone changes during pregnancy and menopause also pull calcium out of the bones.

Osteoporosis is a loss of bone mass, which weakens the bones so they break easily. Osteoporosis affects spongy bone more severely than compact bone because spongy bone is less dense. Absorptiometry (ab-sorp-shee-AHM-eh-tree) uses X-ray beams to measure bone mineral density. Elderly white women, especially those with a petite build, have the greatest risk for osteoporosis (**Figure 18.14**).

oste/o = bone
por/o = opening
-osis = condition, process, state

At birth, you have about 300 soft bones that ossify and fuse together to become about 206 hard and permanent bones as you grow. The major bones are depicted in **Figure 18.15**, and all 206 bones can be seen in Appendix B: Bones of the Human Body. Some bones, such as your *cranium*, become **sutured** (SU-churd), growing together like interlaced fingers to form a strong and immovable joint. The frontal bone at the forehead, parietal bones on the top of the head, temporal bones above the ears, and occipital bone at the back of the head begin as separate bones in a fetus (**Figure 18.16**). This allows a baby's head to flex as it goes through the birth canal. The soft spot, or **fontanel**, on an infant's head is where the bones have not yet grown together.

crani/o = skull
-um = structure

Twenty-one facial and cranial bones become sutured and ossified to create the adult skull. This skull forms a protective shield around your brain, eyes, nose, and mouth, including the *maxilla* of your upper jaw. Your lower jaw, or *mandible*, is the only bone in your skull that moves freely. Your *hyoid* bone, just below your mandible, is the only bone in your body that does not attach to another bone.

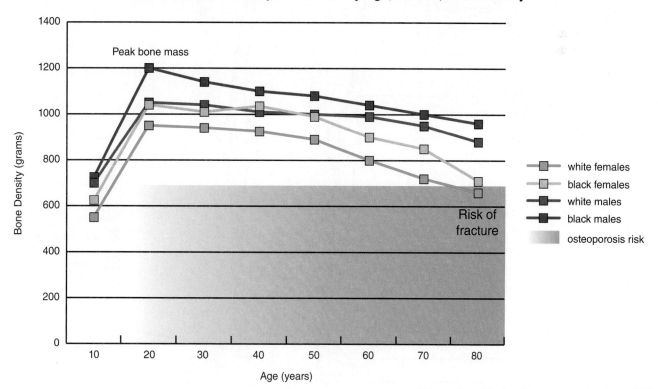

Bone Mass and Osteoporosis Risk by Age, Gender, and Ethnicity

Data courtesy of Looker, Osteoporosis International 1998

Figure 18.14 Risk for osteoporosis depends on age and ethnicity. *According to this chart, which group of people is most at risk for developing osteoporosis?*

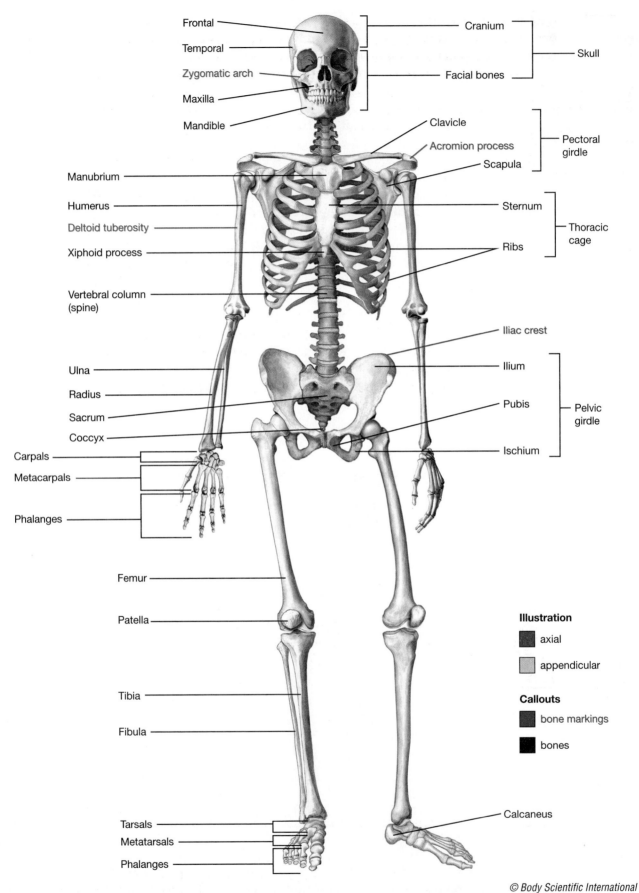

Figure 18.15 A fully grown adult has approximately 206 bones, while a baby has 300 bones. *Why do babies have more bones in their bodies than adults?*

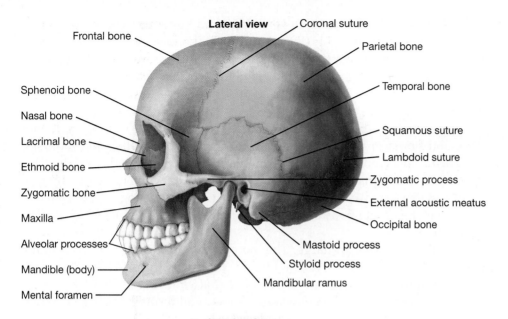

Lateral view

Frontal bone
Coronal suture
Parietal bone
Temporal bone
Sphenoid bone
Nasal bone
Lacrimal bone
Ethmoid bone
Zygomatic bone
Maxilla
Alveolar processes
Mandible (body)
Mental foramen
Squamous suture
Lambdoid suture
Zygomatic process
External acoustic meatus
Occipital bone
Mastoid process
Styloid process
Mandibular ramus

Anterior view

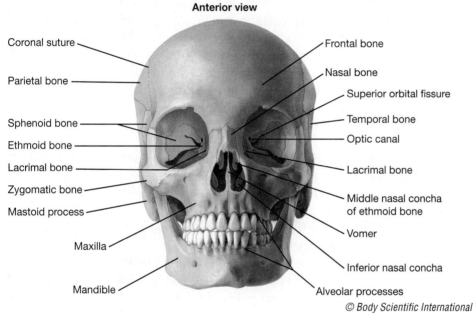

Coronal suture
Parietal bone
Sphenoid bone
Ethmoid bone
Lacrimal bone
Zygomatic bone
Mastoid process
Maxilla
Mandible
Frontal bone
Nasal bone
Superior orbital fissure
Temporal bone
Optic canal
Lacrimal bone
Middle nasal concha of ethmoid bone
Vomer
Inferior nasal concha
Alveolar processes

© Body Scientific International

Figure 18.16   Cranium and facial bones of the skull.

18.2-4   Types of Bones

Bones provide structure and support for your body, with different types of bones performing different roles. The **flat bones** of your cranium, sternum, scapula, ribs, and ilium sandwich a layer of spongy bone between two layers of compact bone (**Figure 18.17**). These bones are thin, flat, and effective as protective shells. As a large flat bone, the ilium (IHL-ee-uhm) in your hip is an ideal site for performing osteocentesis (ahs-tee-oh-sehn-TEE-sihs). This procedure uses a special needle to remove bone marrow for biopsy or transplants. The thin layer of compact bone on the ilium is more easily penetrated than in long bones, and there is more red marrow available.

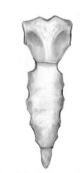

© Body Scientific International

Figure 18.17   Flat bone.

oste/o = bone
-centesis = surgical puncture

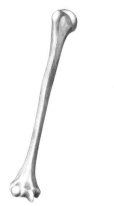

© Body Scientific International

Figure 18.18 Long bone.

meta- = beyond
carp/o = wrist
-al = pertaining to
tars/o = ankle, sole, flat surface
proxim/o = near
medi/o = middle
dist/o = apart

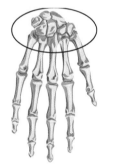

Katrin44/Shutterstock.com

Figure 18.19 Short bones.

oss/i = bone
-icle = tiny

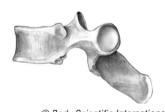

© Body Scientific International

Figure 18.20 Irregular bone.

Long bones, like the femur in your thigh and humerus in your upper arm, are longer than they are wide (**Figure 18.18**). The hollow design of a long bone's diaphysis provides strength without excess weight. If your skeleton was built out of steel to an equivalent strength, it would weigh five times as much. Long bones act as levers for your muscles to raise and lower different parts of your body.

Larger, stronger bones also bear weight. Compare the size of the femur, tibia, and fibula in your leg to the size of the humerus, ulna, and radius in your arm. These bones have the same basic structure, but the stronger leg bones have more mass than the arm bones to carry your body's weight. In Figure 18.15, compare the tibia and fibula in the lower leg of the skeleton. Which one bears the body's weight, and which one is only used for muscle attachments?

Not all long bones are large. The metacarpals in the palm of your hand, metatarsals in the arch of your foot, and phalanges (fuh-LAN-jeez) of your fingers and toes are all long bones. Notice that your fingers and toes have a similar structure and the same name. Directional terms name the different segments: proximal phalanges are closer to your palm or sole, medial phalanges are in the middle, and distal phalanges are at the ends of your fingers and toes. Although they are small, phalanges are still longer than they are wide and act as levers for muscles that move your body.

Short bones, such as the carpals and tarsals of the wrists and ankles, are useful for support (**Figure 18.19**). They are as long as they are wide and generally cube-shaped. They are made of spongy bone covered by a thin layer of compact bone. Notice again that your tarsals are larger than your carpals because they are weight bearing.

People can develop different numbers of **sesamoid** (SEHS-uh-moyd) **bones.** These are small, flat, sesame seed-shaped bones embedded within tendons or joint capsules to withstand friction. Most people have two patella (puh-TEHL-uh) bones, which form the two kneecaps. Sometimes additional sesamoid bones form in the feet or hands or fail to fuse together in the knee, so an adult has "about" 206 bones.

Irregular bones, like the vertebrae (VERT-uh-bray) of your spine; the sphenoid and facial bones of your skull; the ossicles of your ears; the hyoid in your neck; and the ischium and pubis of your pelvis, are complex shapes that do not fit in the other categories (**Figure 18.20**). When your ilium fuses with your ischium and pubis to become the coxal bone, it is also considered an irregular bone. These bones provide many surfaces to which your tendons and ligaments can attach. Irregular bones contain mostly spongy bone with a thin covering of compact bone. This higher proportion of spongy bone makes irregular bones more prone to osteoporosis. People with osteoporosis may develop a hunched back and lose an inch or more in height as their vertebrae lose mass and compact together. The ossicles (*malleus, incus,* and *stapes*) of your ear are also susceptible to this loss of bone density, which is linked to hearing loss.

18.2-5 **Bone Markings**

Healthcare professionals use a variety of markings—usually bumps and grooves—to describe locations on bones (**Figure 18.21**). *Condyles* (KAHN-dIlz) are the rounded knobs at the ends of your bones, where two bones meet to form a joint, such as where your tibia and femur meet at your knee (**Figure 18.22**).

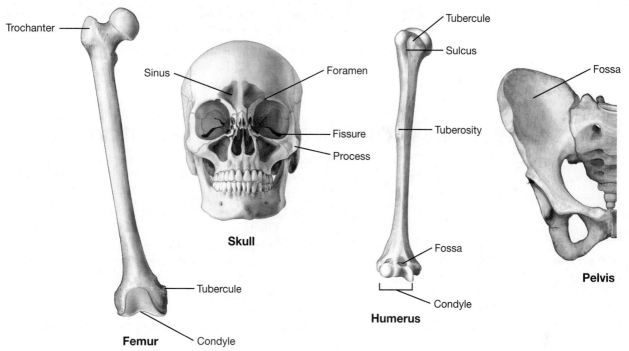

Trochanter

Sinus

Foramen

Fissure

Process

Skull

Tubercule

Condyle

Femur

Tubercule

Sulcus

Tuberosity

Fossa

Condyle

Humerus

Fossa

Pelvis

© Body Scientific International

Figure 18.21 Bone markings are attachment points for ligaments and tendons.

These condyles are named for their anatomical positions. Your medial condyle is located toward the midline of your body, and your lateral condyle is located on the outer side of your knee. Your elbow has similar but smaller bumps, called *epicondyles* (ehp-ih-KAHN-dIlz), where your ulna and humerus meet. Your medial and lateral *malleoli* (mah-LEE-oh-lI) are bumps that form your ankle where your tibia and fibula connect to your tarsals. These bumps provide attachment sites for your ligaments and tendons.

A *process* is a part of the bone that projects out like a bridge. For example, your acromion (ay-KROH-mee-ahn) process, shown in Figure 18.15, connects your scapula and clavicle in your shoulder. You can feel the process forming your cheekbone at your zygomatic (zI-goh-MAT-ihk) arch. A *tuberosity* (too-buh-RAHS-uht-ee) is a long bump, but it does not project out as far as a process, so it is more difficult to see or feel. A *crest* is a raised ridge at the edge of a bone. The iliac crest is the ridge you feel when you rest your hand on your hip. It is thicker and more prominent than a tuberosity, but it does not stand out as far as a process.

These bumps and ridges form as attachment sites for skeletal muscles. Wolff's Law says that a bone is shaped by the forces that put stress on it. This means that the greater the impact or stress, the more calcium your bone stores through the actions of osteoclasts and osteoblasts. This is why physical activity is important for forming and maintaining strong

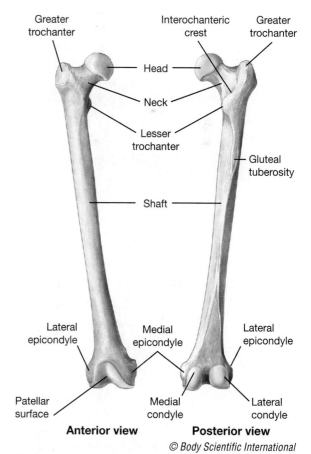

Greater trochanter

Interochanteric crest

Greater trochanter

Head

Neck

Lesser trochanter

Gluteal tuberosity

Shaft

Lateral epicondyle

Medial epicondyle

Lateral epicondyle

Patellar surface

Medial condyle

Lateral condyle

Anterior view

Posterior view

© Body Scientific International

Figure 18.22 Bone markings such as condyles and tuberosities are used to describe locations on bones, as shown on the femur in this illustration. *How does Wolff's Law explain the development of these markings?*

bones. The areas where your muscles pull on your bones to create movement will form bumps over time. The stronger your muscles, the larger the bumps formed. Anthropologists (an-thruh-PAHL-uh-jihsts) use these bumps found on skeletons—and other signs such as bone breaks and the weight or length of bones—to gather information about how people lived.

18.2-6 Divisions of the Skeleton

Your skeleton is divided into two parts called the axial (AK-see-uhl) skeleton and the appendicular (ap-ehn-DIHK-yuh-luhr) skeleton. Your **axial skeleton**, or center "axis" of your body, is formed by your skull, spine, and rib cage. Your arms and legs, or *appendages*, are part of your **appendicular skeleton**. The bones of the appendicular skeleton attach to the axial skeleton at the shoulders and hips. The shading in Figure 18.15 shows these two divisions.

Axial Skeleton

Your axial skeleton forms a line down the center of your body. Your vertebral column, or *spine*, supports your skull and ribs. Your spine is made of 33 bones divided into five groups (**Figure 18.23**). There are seven small cervical bones in your neck that connect your skull to your chest. The first two are named the *atlas* (C1) and *axis* (C2). Your chest is attached in the back to 12 slightly larger thoracic vertebrae. Five large lumbar vertebrae make up your lower back. Just above your buttocks, five bones are fused together into your *sacrum*, a flat triangular bone. Your tailbone, or *coccyx* (KAHK-sihks), is made up of four more tiny bones fused together below your sacrum. Many small muscles stabilize the bones of your vertebral column to keep you upright.

Your vertebral column has natural curves that help it support the weight of your body. Congenital conditions, poor posture, weak abdominal muscles, or a breakdown of the vertebrae can cause more extreme curves (**Figure 18.24**). *Lordosis* is an inward swayback, which causes the buttocks to stick out and the hips to tilt too far forward. *Kyphosis* (kI-FOH-sihs) is an outward hunchback, which causes the shoulders to slump forward and makes it difficult to raise the head. *Scoliosis* (skoh-lee-OH-sihs) is a sideways (lateral) curve that may require a brace to stabilize the spine. These conditions can require surgery when they limit movement, compress internal organs, or cause pain.

Your axial skeleton protects your body. Three different types of ribs form a protective cage around your internal organs. The first seven on each side are *true ribs* because they attach directly to your sternum in front and to your thoracic vertebrae in back. The next three are called *false ribs* because they attach to thoracic vertebrae in the back but only to cartilage in the front. There are also two *floating ribs* on each side that attach only to your last two thoracic vertebrae in back.

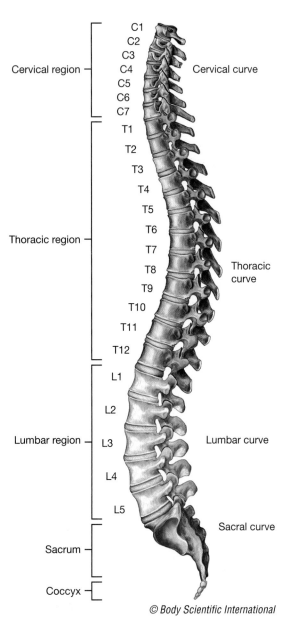

Cervical region

C1
C2
C3
C4 — Cervical curve
C5
C6
C7

Thoracic region

T1
T2
T3
T4
T5
T6
T7
T8 — Thoracic curve
T9
T10
T11
T12

Lumbar region

L1
L2
L3 — Lumbar curve
L4
L5

Sacrum — Sacral curve

Coccyx

© Body Scientific International

Figure 18.23 The 33 bones of the spine are divided into five regions. Within these regions, each bone is assigned a number. *Which section of the spine would you expect to be the most flexible? Why?*

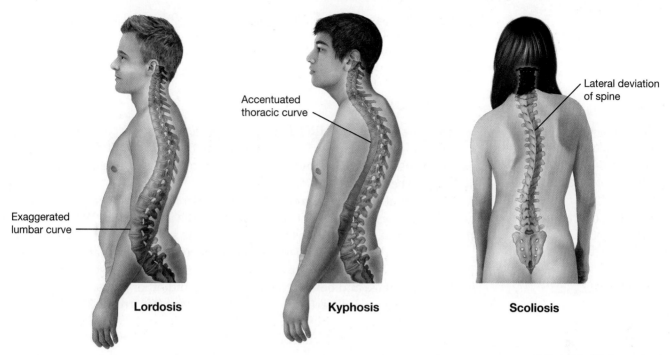

Exaggerated
lumbar curve

Accentuated
thoracic curve

Lateral deviation
of spine

Lordosis

Kyphosis

Scoliosis

© *Body Scientific International*

Figure 18.24 The three conditions illustrated here change the shape of the spine. *What can cause these conditions to occur?*

Your ribs are strong enough to protect your heart and lungs, but they flex and spring back when someone presses on your chest, such as during cardiopulmonary resuscitation (CPR).

The breastbone, or *sternum,* is where your ribs connect by ligaments and cartilage to complete the cage around your chest. Your sternum also has three interconnected parts. The upper section near your neck looks like the knot of a necktie and is called the *manubrium* (muh-NOO-bree-uhm). This is fused to the long, tie-shaped middle section called the *body.* The *xiphoid* (ZI-foyd) *process* is a small point at the bottom of your sternum that can sometimes break off under pressure, such as during CPR.

Appendicular Skeleton

While your axial skeleton provides protection, your appendicular skeleton allows you to move your appendages. In addition to the bones of your arms and legs, the appendicular skeleton includes your shoulder and hip bones. These bones attach your arms and legs to your axial skeleton.

Your shoulder, or *pectoral girdle,* is made up of three bones that connect your arm to your axial skeleton. Your collarbone, or *clavicle,* supports your arm from the front. Your shoulder blade, or *scapula,* provides extra surface area for attaching powerful shoulder muscles in your back. The acromion process forms a bridge between your clavicle and your scapula for extra stability. Your clavicle, acromion process, and scapula are fused together to make a "cup" for your shoulder joint.

pector/o = chest
-al = pertaining to

Your hip, or *pelvic girdle,* is also a combination of three bones fused together. Put your hands on your hips. The large, rounded top of each side of your pelvis is the *ilium.* The *ischia* (IHS-kee-uh) are the bony rings below your buttocks. A ligament between the two *pubis* bones connects your left and right hip structures in the pubic region. This bowl-shaped shell of your pelvic girdle protects your intestines, bladder, rectum, and—in females—reproductive organs.

pelv/o = pelvis, hip region
-ic = pertaining to

18.2-7 Types of Joints

The connection of two of your bones creates a joint. Different types of joints allow you to make different types of movements.

Diarthroses

dia- = through, complete
arthr/o = joint
-osis = condition, process, state
burs/o = fluid-filled sac

dys- = bad, difficult, painful
arthr/o = joint
-itis = inflammation

Diarthroses (dI-ahr-THROH-seez), or *synovial joints*, are your most freely movable joints. Cartilage covers the ends of these joints, and a capsule, or *bursa*, encloses them. The bursa contains synovial fluid to help your bones slide against each other smoothly without pain.

A variety of problems can occur in your joints. Excess weight, infection, and immune system dysfunction can damage the joint tissues. When the cartilage wears out, as in arthritis, the joints become swollen, and movement can be painful. Bursitis is an inflammation of the joint capsule that causes pain. Joint replacements made from a combination of metals and plastics can replace worn-out cartilage and bone in the hips, knees, and other joints.

There are several different types of diarthroses (**Figure 18.25**). **Ball-and-socket joints**, like your hip and shoulder, have a rounded head of bone that fits into a cup-shaped cavity of bone. This allows you the widest range of motion in many directions. **Condylar** (KAHN-dih-lahr), or *ellipsoidal* (ih-lihp-SOY-duhl), **joints** like your wrist and fingers can bend, straighten, and move side to side, but they move in the shape of an ellipse rather than a full circle. The first metacarpal bone of your thumb forms a **saddle joint**, which allows your opposable thumb to touch the other fingers and grasp things.

Gliding joint (intercarpal)

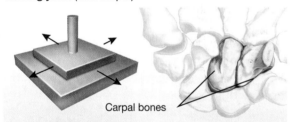

Carpal bones

Hinge joint (humeroulnar)

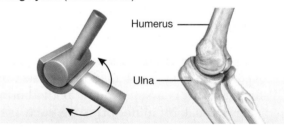

Humerus

Ulna

Pivot joint (radioulnar)

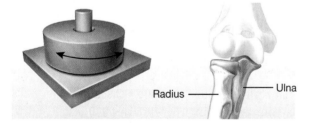

Radius

Ulna

Condylar joint (metacarpophalangeal)

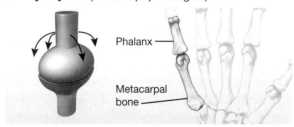

Phalanx

Metacarpal bone

Saddle joint (trapeziometacarpal)

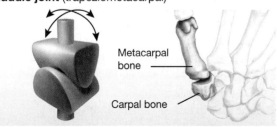

Metacarpal bone

Carpal bone

Ball-and-socket joint (humeroscapular)

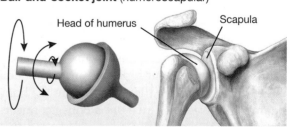

Head of humerus

Scapula

© Body Scientific International

Figure 18.25 Diarthroses are joints that can move freely. *Test out the range of motion for each of these joints yourself.*

Hinge joints, like your elbow or jaw, only bend and straighten or open and close with no side-to-side motion. Your flat wrist and anklebone surfaces slide over each other in a **gliding joint**, but strong ligaments limit their movement. The **pivot joint** formed by your top two cervical vertebrae allows you to turn your head from side to side to say no. At your elbow, your radius pivots in the notch at the base of your humerus. Bend your fingers—what type of joint allows you to do this?

Amphiarthroses

Amphiarthroses (am-fee-ahr-THROH-seez) are slightly movable joints. Your 7 cervical, 12 thoracic, and 5 lumbar vertebrae can all move a little bit backward, forward, and to each side. Disks made of cartilage separate them and pad the joints. Although each individual joint moves only slightly, these many small movements allow you to bend comfortably. A herniated (HER-nee-ayt-ed) disk, which occurs when the soft center of the disk bulges out between the vertebrae, puts pressure on the nerves running through the spine. This causes pain up and down the back and along the shoulder or thigh. Treatments include injections to reduce inflammation, removal of the damaged tissue, or surgery that fuses the vertebrae together. A chiropractor (KI-roh-prak-ter) adjusts the alignment of the vertebrae to help the muscles and joints function better and relieve pain.

amphi- = around
arthr/o = joint
-osis = condition, process, state

chir/o = hand
pract/o= practice
-or = one who does

Synarthroses

Synarthroses (sihn-ahr-THROH-seez) are fused in an immovable joint. For instance, your sacrum is made up of five bones located below your lumbar vertebrae that are fused into a flat triangle at the small of your back. Your tailbone is four fused bones located at the end of your vertebral column. Your skull is another example of a synarthrosis. A cleft palate occurs when the hard palate bones in the roof of the mouth fail to fuse into their synarthrosis during embryonic development. On the other hand, orthodontists sometimes use an expander to spread the synarthrosis of the hard palate to provide more space for growing teeth.

syn- = same, together

18.2-8 **Dislocations and Fractures**

When a bone "jumps out" of its normal location in a joint, damage to bones, ligaments, nerves, and blood vessels may occur. A dislocated joint is a separation of two bones that are normally held together by ligaments and muscles. A break in the bone, or *fracture*, may occur with or without dislocation (**Figure 18.26**).

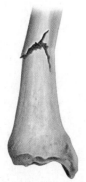
A *greenstick fracture* is incomplete. The break occurs on the convex surface of the bend in the bone.

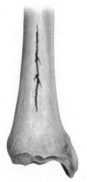
A *stress fracture* involves an incomplete break.

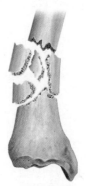
A *comminuted fracture* is complete and splinters the bone.

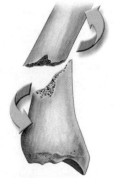
A *spiral fracture* is caused by twisting a bone.

© Body Scientific International

Figure 18.26 Some fractures are more serious than others. *Which of these types of fractures is common in children?*

Simple fractures leave the bone in its original position, while compound fractures break through the surrounding tissues and skin. The geometry of a fracture is often used to describe the direction of the break. Transverse fractures break straight across the bone, oblique fractures break at an angle, and spiral fractures twist around the bone. Comminuted fractures break into many small pieces, while stress fractures are cracks in bones that stay in one piece. Greenstick fractures, in which only one side of the bone breaks, are common in young children because they have more cartilage in their bones.

Both dislocations and fractures must be repositioned and immobilized until healed. Surgery may be required to realign, stabilize, or reattach tissues that have been damaged. Your body heals fractures by filling the gap with a temporary cartilage "callus," then bringing in osteoclasts to make new bone. After the injury has healed, strengthening exercises may help reduce your chance of another injury by ensuring the surrounding muscles support the bones.

Lesson 18.2 Review

 Complete the *Map Your Reading* graphic organizer for the section you just read.

1. Which of the following is *not* a function of the skeletal system? (18.2-1)
   A. Getting rid of body waste
   B. Mineral storage
   C. Blood cell production
   D. Structure and support

2. Which part of a long bone is composed mostly of spongy bone? (18.2-2)
   A. Diaphysis
   B. Epiphysis
   C. Medullary cavity
   D. Bursa

3. What is the name for a cell that breaks down bone? (18.2-3)
   A. Osteoblast
   B. Osteocyte
   C. Osteoma
   D. Osteoclast

4. What type of bone is the scapula? (18.2-4)
   A. Short bone
   B. Flat bone
   C. Long bone
   D. Sesamoid bone

5. Rounded knobs at the ends of your bones are called (18.2-5)
   A. tuberosities
   B. crests
   C. condyles
   D. processes

6. Which of the following are functions of the axial skeleton? Choose all that apply. (18.2-6)
   A. Connecting the appendages
   B. Protecting vital organs
   C. Supporting the body
   D. Moving the body

7. Which type of joint does *not* move? (18.2-7)
   A. Diarthrosis
   B. Amphiarthrosis
   C. Synarthrosis
   D. All of these.

8. Which type of fracture breaks straight across the bone? (18.2-8)
   A. Transverse fracture
   B. Greenstick fracture
   C. Spiral fracture
   D. Stress fracture

The Muscular System

Learning Outcomes

After studying this lesson, you will be able to

18.3-1 describe the basic functions of the muscular system.

18.3-2 identify muscle tissue types, functions, characteristics, control, and common diseases, injuries, and prevention.

18.3-3 explain the structures and functions of different muscle shapes and attachments.

18.3-4 identify muscle movements allowed by different types of joints.

18.3-5 use clues in a muscle name to identify its size, location, shape, or movement.

> **? ESSENTIAL QUESTION**
>
> *What are the structures, functions, and diseases associated with the muscular system?*

Professional Vocabulary

Essential Terms

cardiac muscle an involuntary, striated muscle tissue located in the walls of the heart

involuntary not under conscious control

skeletal muscle voluntary, striated muscle that connects to bones and is responsible for movement

smooth muscle involuntary, nonstriated muscle tissue located in the body's visceral organs and blood vessels; also known as *visceral muscle*

tendon a tough, fibrous tissue that connects muscles to bones

voluntary under conscious control

Important Terms

abduction	extension	muscle tone
adduction	fascicles	rotation
circumduction	flexion	striated

Introduction

Nearly all movement in your body is the result of the muscular system. You become more aware of your muscles during exercises and poses where you contract and relax specific parts of your body. Use your body as the model in this lesson to locate and remember the muscles you read about.

18.3-1 Understanding the Muscular System

Your muscles interact with your skeletal, nervous, digestive, and circulatory systems to maintain posture and produce stability, body movement, breathing, body heat, and digestive and cardiovascular functions. Your muscles also protect the internal organs of your torso, absorb shock, and reduce stress and friction on your joints. Collagen surrounds each muscle fiber and gives it strength. Collagen is also the main component of your **tendons**, the tough, fibrous tissue that connects your muscles to bones to allow movement. Many different healthcare professionals focus on building and maintaining the health and function of the muscular system.

Healthcare Professions: Athletic Training

Pat is a certified athletic trainer. He works nights and weekends, educating high school athletes on injury prevention, assessing sports injuries, and providing appropriate treatment and rehabilitation for bone and muscle injuries. He also works as a physical education and health teacher during the day. He completed his bachelor's degree in education and obtained his certification in athletic training through an internship program. The certification test was challenging but is required for this job in most states. Today, many states also require a degree in athletic training.

Pat works under the direction of a licensed physician and coordinates the care of his athletes with other healthcare providers. He likes the variety of work settings and personal interactions in his job, but he finds the variable schedule and long hours on his feet a challenge.

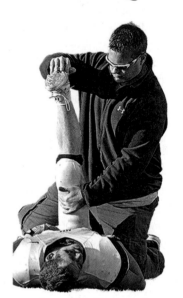

Aspen Photo/Shutterstock.com

He knows that athletic trainers for professional athletes may earn a little more than his $40 per hour, but those jobs are difficult to get. Many of the new jobs in this growing profession will be in healthcare facilities as a cost-effective way to increase healthcare and injury prevention services. Pat, however, prefers to work with high school students on the playing field and in the locker room.

A physical therapist assistant can obtain employment after just two years of education, but physical therapist (PT) training programs now require a doctoral degree. Most physical therapists work in a hospital or healthcare office, but some also work in home health, nursing homes, schools, and industrial settings. They provide therapy treatments to patients with physical disabilities and those recovering from surgery or injuries.

They teach these patients proper exercise techniques and use a variety of exercise equipment and activities to help strengthen muscles, improve mobility, restore function, and relieve pain.

Healthcare Professions: Recreational Therapy

As a recreational therapist in a nursing home, Kim uses a variety of activities, such as crafts, sports, dance, and interaction with animals. She aims to reduce residents' stress, stimulate their minds, help them recover basic motor functions, and build their socialization skills. She previously worked in a hospital and rehabilitation center, but she really enjoys working with older adults.

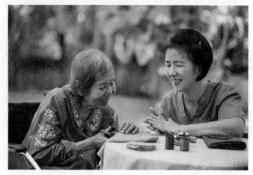

Toa55/Shutterstock.com

Jobs in nursing care facilities and outpatient settings have been increasing as the aging population requires more services. Kim completed a bachelor's degree in therapeutic recreation and would like to specialize in art therapy. Her state requires certification, but not all states do.

18.3-2 Types of Muscle Tissue

There are three types of muscle tissue in your body: cardiac, smooth, and skeletal muscle. Each muscle type has a different function. **Cardiac muscle** makes up the walls of your heart that pump blood throughout your body. You will learn more about cardiac muscle in relation to the circulatory system. **Smooth muscle**, or *visceral muscle*, moves food along your alimentary canal, moves blood through your blood vessels, and squeezes secretions out of your hollow organs. The main focus in this section is **skeletal muscle**, which attaches to bones to produce movement and provide stability to your body (**Figure 18.27** and **Figure 18.28**).

cardi/o = heart
-ac = pertaining to
viscer/o = internal organ
-al = pertaining to

Characteristics

Muscles share several characteristics. All muscles are *excitable*, meaning they respond to signals from the nervous system. They are *contractible*, shortening to create movement when stimulated, and *extensible*, so they can be lengthened through stretching. They also have *elasticity* to return to their normal size.

Your muscles depend on stimulation from your nervous system. Just as your bones are shaped by the forces placed on them, your muscles also remodel to fit their tasks. The more a muscle is used, or *stimulated*, the stronger and larger it grows, like the muscles of a bodybuilder. In contrast, a muscle that is not used will shrink, or *atrophy*.

a- = without
-trophy = development

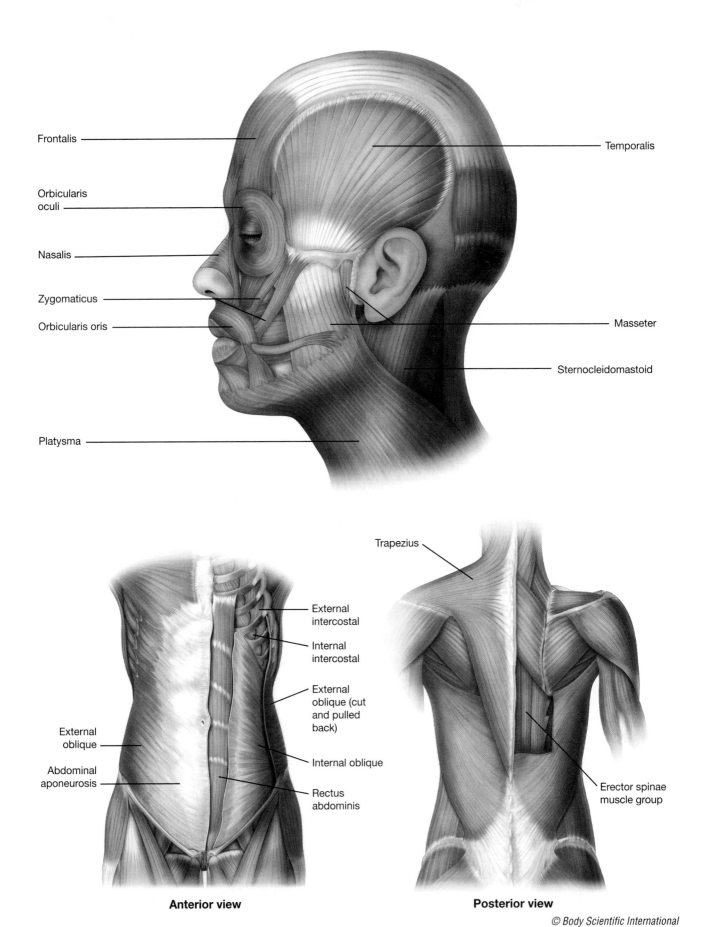

Figure 18.27 Skeletal muscles of the head and torso. *Which word parts can you identify in these muscle names that help you to understand their location, shape, size, or function?*

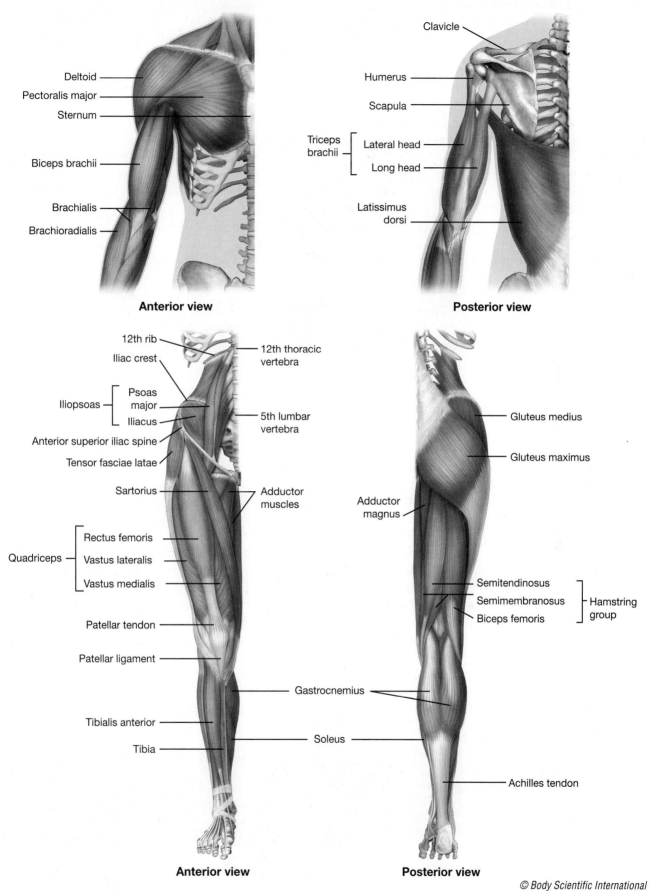

Anterior view

- Deltoid
- Pectoralis major
- Sternum
- Biceps brachii
- Brachialis
- Brachioradialis

Posterior view

- Clavicle
- Humerus
- Scapula
- Triceps brachii
  - Lateral head
  - Long head
- Latissimus dorsi

Anterior view

- 12th rib
- Iliac crest
- Iliopsoas
  - Psoas major
  - Iliacus
- Anterior superior iliac spine
- Tensor fasciae latae
- Sartorius
- Quadriceps
  - Rectus femoris
  - Vastus lateralis
  - Vastus medialis
- Patellar tendon
- Patellar ligament
- Tibialis anterior
- Tibia
- 12th thoracic vertebra
- 5th lumbar vertebra
- Adductor muscles

Posterior view

- Gluteus medius
- Gluteus maximus
- Adductor magnus
- Semitendinosus
- Semimembranosus
- Biceps femoris
- Hamstring group
- Gastrocnemius
- Soleus
- Achilles tendon

© *Body Scientific International*

Figure 18.28 Skeletal muscles of the arms and legs. *Which word parts can you identify in these muscle names that help you to understand their location, shape, size, or function?*

my/o = muscle
-cyte = cell
micro- = small
scop/e = to view
-ic = pertaining to

A nerve and blood vessel accompany each of your muscles. The nerve carries electrical impulses from your brain to stimulate the muscle and cause it to move. The blood vessel brings your muscle protein and other nutrients needed for growth and energy and carries away waste products. If your muscle loses the nerve connection that provides its stimulus or the blood supply that carries its nutrients, it will atrophy within a few weeks.

Muscles are also described as striated or smooth. Each muscle cell is a muscle fiber, called a *myocyte*. Both cardiac and skeletal myocytes are **striated** muscle. They have many microscopic protein fibrils arranged in a striped pattern. Striated muscle produces a single, short, "twitch" contraction, like the beating of your heart. Visceral muscle is called smooth muscle because it does not have a striped appearance when viewed under a microscope. It gives a long, sustained contraction when stimulated. Skeletal muscle is capable of both sustained and twitch contractions (**Figure 18.29**).

Control

The source of control for your muscle contractions varies. Both cardiac and smooth muscle are **involuntary**. This means they respond to signals from your nervous and endocrine systems, but you cannot consciously control them. These muscles are always working, even when you are asleep. In contrast, skeletal muscles are **voluntary** and under your conscious control, unless excited by a "reflex." You have practiced some of your voluntary muscle movements, such as walking, for such a long time that they become automatic and seem to occur without thought. You can choose to move the muscles attached to your bones, but not the muscle that makes up your heart or the insides of your organs and blood vessels.

Control of your skeletal muscles develops in an organized pattern. Your body contains more than 600 skeletal muscles, which account for about one-half of your body weight. When you were a child, you first learned to control your large motor muscles and then gained fine-motor skills that required more control. This control developed from your head down and from the center of your body outward. Babies hold up their head and control the muscles used to eat before they learn to coordinate the fine muscle movements used for speech. Babies reach with their arms before learning to grasp with their hands and will later learn the finger coordination necessary to write. They also sit before standing and walk before skipping or riding a bike. After about 30 years of age, the amount, size, and tone of muscle tissues begin to decrease again, resulting in a gradual loss of strength.

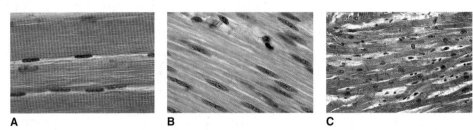

A   B   C

Left to right: Jose Luis Calvo/Shutterstock.com, Jose Luis Calvo/Shutterstock.com, Jose Luis Calvo/Shutterstock.com

Figure 18.29 There are three types of muscle tissue: (A) skeletal, (B) smooth, and (C) cardiac. *What is the function of each type?*

Disease and Injury

Muscular dystrophy, described in Figure 18.2, is the name for a group of diseases that cause atrophy and weakness in skeletal muscles (**Figure 18.30**). A defect in the structural protein—collagen—that gives muscles their strength causes some forms of muscular dystrophy. These diseases are more common in young males than females. Many forms also affect cardiac muscles, which may result in an early death. Muscular dystrophy is treated with physical therapy. There have been promising advances in medications and gene therapy, but there is currently no cure.

dys- = bad, difficult, painful
-trophy = development

Muscle injury, which is often due to overexertion, repetitive movement, or sudden movement, is more common than muscle disease. *Tendinitis* is an inflammation of the tendon due to stretching, stress, or repeated friction that irritates either the lining of the sheath enclosing the tendon or the tendon itself. This condition may cause pain, swelling, and reduced range of motion. Treatment usually includes eliminating the cause to prevent recurrence.

-itis = inflammation

Muscle strain can cause a moderate amount of damage to a muscle or tendon. *RICE*—an acronym that means "Rest," "Ice," "Compression," and "Elevation"—treats symptoms of tenderness and swelling. Muscle tears are more severe than strains and can include detachment from the bone. Surgery may be required to repair these injuries. Collagen is generated first after an injury, and then myofibers are regenerated to rebuild the muscle. Understanding how muscles are structured and how they work is important to understanding muscular disorders.

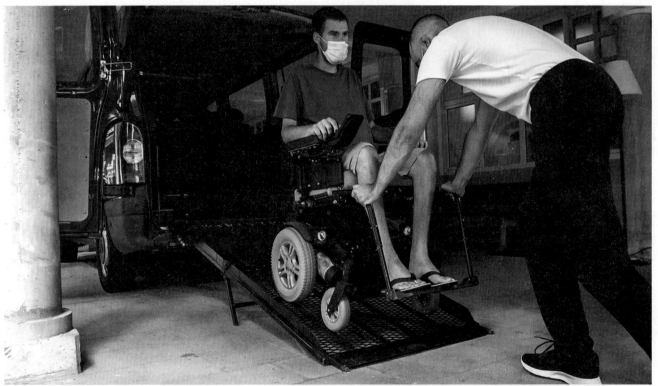

24K-Production/Shutterstock.com

Figure 18.30 Muscular dystrophy can occur in childhood or adulthood. The disease often requires that a person use a wheelchair.

18.3-3 Muscle Shape and Attachment

peri- = around
my/o = muscle
-ium = structure

epi- = upon

Muscle fibers gathered together in bundles, or **fascicles**, make up each of your muscles (**Figure 18.31**). Perimysium (pair-uh-MIHZ-ee-uhm), a thin layer of collagen-based connective tissue, wraps each fascicle. Epimysium surrounds groups of fascicles. Fascia is an additional layer of thick connective tissue that covers the muscle. These connective tissues extend beyond your muscle into cord-like tendons to attach the muscle to your bone.

carp/o = wrist
-al = pertaining to

Tendons have less bulk than muscle fibers, but their collagen base makes them very strong. They attach your skeletal muscles to the periosteum that covers your bones. Some of the best-known tendons are in your ankles and wrists. The large Achilles tendon on the back of the lower leg attaches your *soleus* and *gastrocnemius* (gas-trahk-NEE-mee-uhs) muscles to your heel (Figure 18.29). Many separate tendons in your lower arm attach to muscles for your fingers. These long tendons pass through a tunnel in your wrist bones. Carpal tunnel syndrome is a painful inflammation that squeezes the tendons, blood vessels, and nerves in your wrist. This interrupts the movement of tendons and muscles, as well as their nerve connection and blood supply.

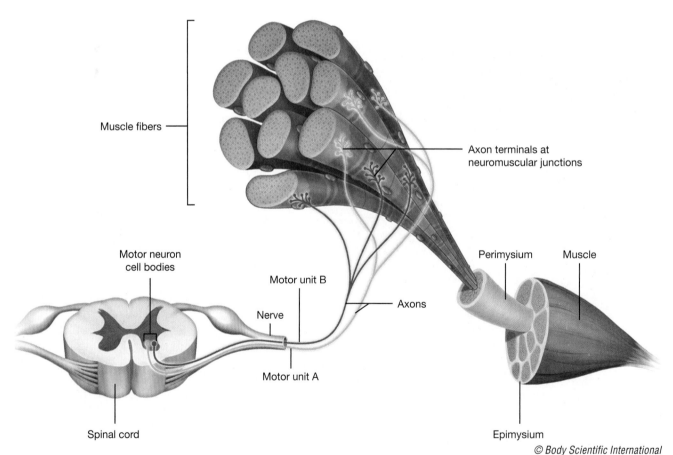

© Body Scientific International

Figure 18.31 A fascicle is a bundle of muscle fibers wrapped with perimysium. The epimysium encloses a group of fascicles to make a muscle. Motor neurons stimulate skeletal muscles.

Differently shaped muscles have different attachments. Muscle fibers form lines that point to your muscle attachments and show the direction in which your muscle will move (**Figure 18.32**).

A bundled muscle, such as your *rectus abdominus* in your abdomen, has flat sections of parallel fibers with tendons between them. It is supported by a flat sheet of fibrous connective tissue, or an *aponeurosis*, which is similar to a tendon but much wider (Figure 18.29). It can attach muscle to muscle, bone, or other tissues such as skin. The parallel fibers allow these muscles to contract quickly.

abdomin/o = abdomen

Fusiform muscles also have parallel muscle fibers, but they form a wide "belly" in the middle and taper down to tendons at both ends. This belly is the meaty bulk of muscle tissue. You can feel this when the muscle contracts, as in the *biceps brachii* of your upper arm.

brachi/o = arm

Convergent muscles are triangular. The muscle bundles spread over a broad attachment area on one end and come to a point on the other end. This allows muscles like the *pectoralis major* on your chest to produce motion in different directions by contracting different portions of the muscle set. Because they are spread over a larger area, there are also more muscle fibers for more power.

pector/o = chest

Circular muscles, or *sphincters*, such as the *orbicularis oculi* (or-bihk-yuh-LAIR-uhs AHK-yuh-lI) around the eye, have many short attachments around their outer edge. They form a circle and pull together to close an opening.

Muscle fibers in pennate muscles are parallel, but a tendon runs the full length of the muscle. Muscle fibers attach to long sections of it at an angle. This allows more muscle fiber attachments for more strength and power than fusiform muscles. Pennate muscles can be unipennate, like the *vastus lateralis* on the outer side of the thigh. All muscle fibers in a unipennate muscle are parallel and attach to one tendon that runs the length of the muscle. Pennate muscles may be bipennate, like the *rectus femoris* on the front of the thigh. Bipennate muscles are shaped like a feather, with the tendon running through the center of the muscle and parallel fibers grouped on both sides of the tendon. Muscles may even be multipennate, like the *deltoid* in the shoulder, with several sets of parallel fibers attached to several tendons that meet on one end. Compare the shape and attachments of the fusiform *biceps femoris* in the back of the thigh with the triangular *gluteus maximus* in the buttocks or the multipennate *rectus femoris* in the front of the thigh. Which muscles do you think are more powerful? Why?

later/o = side

Parallel fiber arrangements

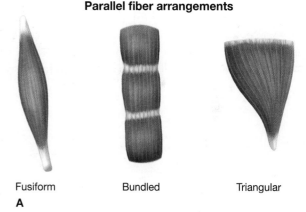

Fusiform   Bundled   Triangular

A

Pennate fiber arrangements

Skeletal muscles must have at least two points of attachment and must cross at least one joint for you to move. These muscle attachments are called the *point of origin* and the *point of insertion*. The point of origin is on the stationary bone. The point of insertion is on the bone that moves. For example, when you contract the *biceps brachii*, the humerus in the upper arm remains still, and the radius in the lower arm moves toward it. The point of origin for the *biceps brachii* is the attachment at the humerus, the point of insertion is the attachment on the radius, and the muscle crosses over the elbow joint to flex the arm. You can predict this direction of movement by following the direction of the muscle fibers.

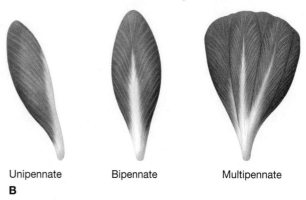

Unipennate   Bipennate   Multipennate

B

© *Body Scientific International*

Figure 18.32 Different muscle shapes and points of attachment allow movement in different directions.

18.3-4 Muscle Movements

Muscles always pull and get shorter to create movement; they cannot push. Muscle fibers contain protein filaments that pull together during a muscle contraction. This makes the muscle belly shorter and wider. After the contraction is complete, the muscle relaxes back to its normal shape.

If muscles always pull, then how do your joints unbend? Your muscles work together in opposing pairs to create movement and maintain posture. The biceps and triceps are an opposing muscle pair: the bicep bends the arm at the elbow, and the tricep straightens it (**Figure 18.33**). In concentric contraction, the muscle doing the work is called the prime mover, or *agonist*, while the relaxed muscle is called the *antagonist*. The skeletal muscles of the trunk and limbs usually remain in a partly contracted state known as **muscle tone** that helps maintain the body's balance and posture.

syn- = same, together

Most of your body movements require the support of more than one muscle. These functional groups of muscles are called *synergists*. The body has several layers of muscles. You are probably most familiar with the superficial muscles near the surface, but there are also layers of deep muscles below this, closer to the bone. Each layer attaches at a slightly different angle to add stability. When they pull together, each muscle gets some help from the other muscles in the group. This work uses energy that creates heat in the body. The harder the body works, the more energy is used, and the more heat is created. For example, the body burns about 200 calories per hour walking but about 500 calories per hour running. You need to burn about 3,500 calories of energy to work off 1 pound of body weight.

flex/o = bend
-ion = action, process, condition

Joint movements are most easily understood as pairs of opposing actions (**Figure 18.34**). These are movements you might help your patients perform so they maintain their full range of motion. **Flexion** moves a ventral surface toward a ventral surface, decreasing the angle of a joint.

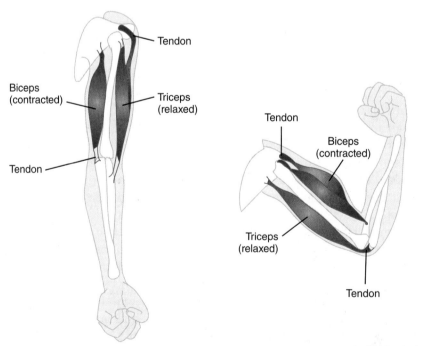

grayjay/Shutterstock.com

Figure 18.33 Flexion and extension, shown here, are opposing actions of this agonist and antagonist that result in joint movement.

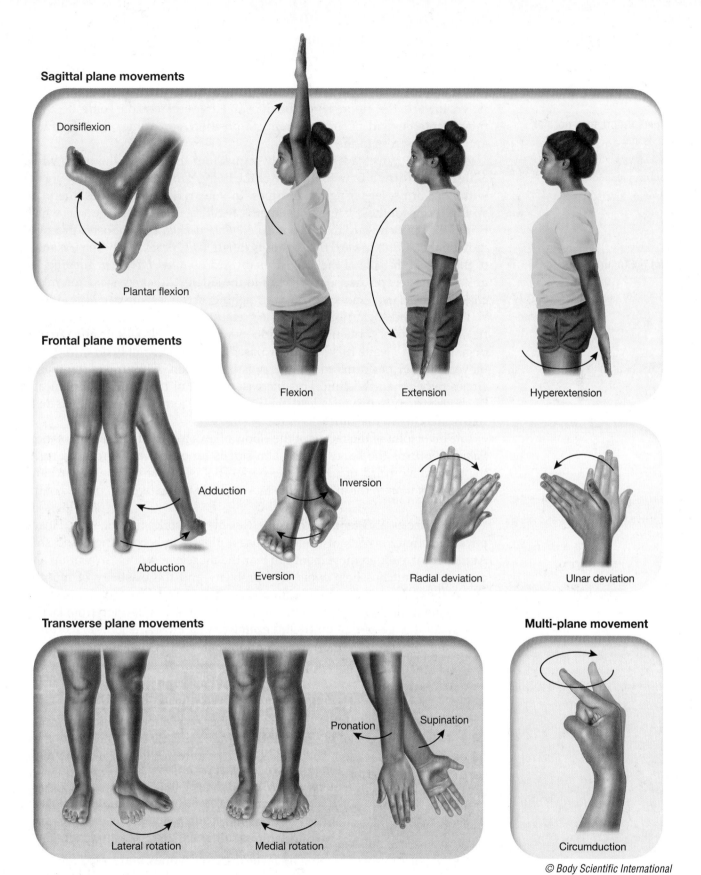

Sagittal plane movements

Dorsiflexion

Plantar flexion

Flexion

Extension

Hyperextension

Frontal plane movements

Adduction

Abduction

Inversion

Eversion

Radial deviation

Ulnar deviation

Transverse plane movements

Lateral rotation

Medial rotation

Pronation

Supination

Multi-plane movement

Circumduction

© *Body Scientific International*

Figure 18.34 Muscle movement terminology.

ex- = out, away from
tens/o = stretch
-ion = action, process, condition
dors/i = back
flex/o = bend
hyper- = more than normal, excessive
ab- = away
duct/o = to lead
ad- = to, toward

vers/o = to turn

circum- = around

Extension moves a dorsal surface toward a dorsal surface and increases the angle of the ventral surfaces of a joint. Most joints can flex and extend. In the ankle, there are special terms for these movements. Dorsiflexion brings the foot up toward the front of the shin, and plantar flexion brings the foot down toward the floor. Hyperflexion and hyperextension continue these movements beyond normal anatomical position, sometimes through force, and can add stress to the joint.

Abduction moves a limb laterally away from the side of the body, while **adduction** returns a limb to the side of the body. You can do these movements with your arms, legs, fingers, and toes. In your wrists and ankles, there are special terms for these lateral movements. Bending the wrist to the side, which brings the pinky toward the ulna, is called *ulnar flexion*. The opposite direction, moving the thumb toward the radius, is called *radial flexion*. Bending the ankle to the side so the sole of the foot turns inward is called *inversion*. Turning the ankle so the sole of the foot turns out to the side is called *eversion*. You might complete these movements through stretching, activities, or specific exercises.

Your ball-and-socket joints have the greatest range of motion. In addition to flexion, extension, abduction, and adduction, they can also rotate and circumduct. **Rotation** means turning on an axis. The limb does not bend during this movement, but performs more of a twisting motion. **Circumduction** makes circles rather than twisting. This increased range of motion in a joint means the bone structure provides less stability, so these joints have more muscle to return stability to the joint.

The pivot joint of the radius at the elbow allows for another type of rotation. *Supination* turns the hand so the palm side is up or forward. *Pronation* turns the palm downward or toward the back. This is similar to the inward and outward rotation of the arm, but the movement is in the forearm instead of the shoulder.

Your muscles and tendons must be flexible to work well together. Heavy physical activity or lack of use can cause a muscle to become tight and stiff. At that point, sudden movement can tear the muscle or tendon. Warm-up and cool-down stretches help avoid this problem, and the elasticity of muscles allows them to return to their original shape after stretching. *Contractures* are a permanent shortening of muscles and tendons that can develop from lack of movement. Range-of-motion (ROM) exercises that move the joint to its fullest extent are important for those who are immobile.

18.3-5 The Logic of Muscle Names

Not all muscle names are easy to remember or pronounce, but they make sense when you apply a few simple rules. Many muscle names indicate their action, structure, location, shape, or size. The adductor *longus* is a *long* muscle in the thigh that brings the leg toward the body. The *extensor* digitorum straightens, or *extends*, the fingers. The *inter*costals run *between* the ribs. The *tibialis anterior* is located on the *front* of the *tibia*. The *triceps* brachii has *three* attachments on the upper arm. The *trapezius* is a *trapezoid* shape. The gluteus *maximus* is a *large* muscle. When faced with a muscle name you do not know, look for descriptive words, directional terms, bone names, and words referring to muscle actions. These clues will help you find, understand, and remember muscle names.

Lesson 18.3 Review

 Complete the *Map Your Reading* graphic organizer for the section you just read.

1. Which of the following are functions of the muscular system? Choose all that apply. (18.3-1)
   A. Produce stability
   B. Produce heat
   C. Enable breathing
   D. Remove waste

2. Which types of muscle tissue are involuntary? Choose all that apply. (18.3-2)
   A. Cardiac muscle
   B. Skeletal muscle
   C. Smooth muscle
   D. Striated muscle

3. What is the recommended treatment for the tenderness and swelling associated with muscle strain? (18.3-2)
   A. Surgery
   B. Heat
   C. RICE
   D. Stretching

4. What is the name for a circular muscle that closes an opening? (18.3-3)
   A. Convergent muscle
   B. Bundled muscle
   C. Pennate muscle
   D. Sphincter

5. Which muscle movement describes moving a limb laterally away from the side of the body? (18.3-4)
   A. Abduction
   B. Flexion
   C. Adduction
   D. Extension

6. The term *maximus* can help you identify that a muscle is (18.3-5)
   A. triangular
   B. large
   C. long
   D. between two bones

Chapter 18 Review and Assessment

Chapter Summary

18.1-1 The collagen in connective tissue is important for the integumentary, skeletal, and muscular systems. It helps provide structure and support for the body.

18.1-2 The integumentary system, or *skin*, has three layers that cover the body. The structures of the skin provide protection, maintain body temperature, produce and store nutrients, and get rid of body waste.

18.1-3 The epidermis is the outermost layer of the skin. Observing changes in the skin is important for detecting many different disorders of the body. Keep the skin clean and protected from excess UV light to reduce the chance of infections and cancer.

18.1-4 The dermis, which is the middle layer of skin, contains sensory organs, blood vessels, hair follicles, and exocrine glands. Blood vessels affect skin color and body temperature. Sebum from sebaceous glands moisturizes the skin, while perspiration from sudoriferous glands cools the skin.

18.1-5 The hypodermis is the deepest skin layer and attaches skin to the muscle below. Subcutaneous fat pads the body and stores energy, hormones, and nutrients.

18.2-1 The bones of the skeletal system provide structure, support, protection, muscle attachment sites, blood cell production, and mineral storage. Bones, joints, and cartilage form the skeletal system. They provide structure, support, protection, blood cell production, attachments for muscles, and mineral storage.

18.2-2 Different parts of a bone have different functions such as providing storage of nutrients, withstanding stress, and producing blood cells.

18.2-3 Bones ossify and fuse together from about 300 soft and separated bones that are mostly cartilage at birth to about 206 hard calcified bones in adulthood. Calcium, vitamin D, and physical activity help to prevent osteoporosis.

18.2-4 The shape and structure of long bones, short bones, flat bones, irregular bones, and sesamoid bones all work in different ways to create movement and provide support.

18.2-5 Bone markings help healthcare professionals describe locations on bones.

18.2-6 The two divisions of the skeleton show the different roles of bones. Axial bones are for protection and support while appendicular bones are for support and movement.

18.2-7 At the joints, ligaments connect bone to bone for stability and tendons connect muscle to bone for movement. Different types of joints allow different types and amounts of movement. Diarthroses are freely movable, amphiarthroses are slightly movable, and synarthroses are immovable.

18.2-8 Bones can be injured through dislocation or fracture. Dislocations and fractures require different treatments.

18.3-1 The muscular system is involved in posture and stability, body movement, breathing, body heat, and digestive and cardiovascular functions. Muscles also protect internal organs, absorb shock, and reduce joint stress.

18.3-2 The three types of muscle tissue—cardiac, smooth, and skeletal—each have a different structure and purpose. Muscles are excitable, contracting in response to nerve stimulus. They must remain elastic in order to relax and extend. Skeletal muscles are voluntary, while cardiac and smooth muscles are not under your control. Stimulation from the nervous system and nutrients from the blood keep muscles from atrophying. Muscle injuries are often treated with rest, ice, compression, elevation, and eliminating the cause of the injury.

18.3-3 Muscles always have at least two points of attachment and cross at least one joint to create movement. The muscle fibers and tendons show the direction of movement. Broader, larger muscles have more attachments to provide more strength.

18.3-4 Agonist and antagonist muscles pull in opposite directions to create muscle tone, movement, and maintain posture. Synergistic muscle groups work together. Different types of joints allow different types of movement. Muscle movements such as flexion and extension occur as opposing actions. Contractures can be avoided with range-of-motion exercises.

18.3-5 Muscle names describe the action, structure, location, shape, or size of muscles.

Maximize Your Professional Vocabulary

1. **Term Snap.** Make flash cards for each word part in the following list. Sit in circles of three to five students and shuffle your cards, keeping them all facing the same direction. The first player places a card in the center, "term side" facing up. Other players go around the circle, taking turns to discard one card at a time with the definition side facing up. When the definition matching the term card in the center of the circle is discarded, the first to notice must slap the matching card. That player takes all the cards in the middle and draws the next term card. Play continues until the time is up or players run out of cards. The player with the most term cards at the end of play is the winner.

Prefixes

a-	circum-	dys-	meta-
ab-	con-	ex-	micro-
ad-	de-	hyper-	sub-
amphi-	dia-	intra-	syn-

Root Words

albin/o	dermat/o	melan/o	ped/o
arthr/o	dilat/o	muscul/o	por/o
burs/o	duct/o	my/o	pract/o
carp/o	erythr/o	myc/o	scop/e
chir/o	flex/o	necr/o	strict/o
coll/a	hemat/o	orth/o	tars/o
cry/o	hydr/o	oss/i	tens/o
cutane/o	integument/o	oste/o	vas/o
cyan/o	lig/a	path/o	vers/o
derm/o	medull/o	pector/o	viscer/o

Suffixes

-ate	-eal	-ism	-physis
-ation	-fic	-ist	-plasia
-blast	-gen	-itis	-plasty
-centesis	-genesis	-ium	-poiesis
-clast	-icle	-or	-scopy
-crine	-in	-osis	-trophy
-cyte	-is	-ous	

Reflect on Your Reading

1. Revisit the answers you gave for the *Connect with Your Reading* activity at the beginning of this chapter. Share one of the *text to self*, *text to text*, or *text to world* connections you made to your reading. Discuss how your reading of the chapter deepened, strengthened, or made you rethink your understanding of one of the connections you made.

Review and Recall

1. What type of tissue is collagen? (18.1-1)
   - A. Epithelial tissue
   - B. Stratified tissue
   - C. Connective tissue
   - D. Cardiac tissue

2. Which of the following is *not* a role of the skin? (18.1-2)
   - A. Protect and pad body structures
   - B. Maintain body temperature
   - C. Filter body waste
   - D. Produce vitamin D

3. Which of the following is *not* a sign of skin cancer? (18.1-3)
   - A. Symmetry
   - B. Border irregularity
   - C. Color changes
   - D. Evolution

4. Which of the following helps release body heat through the skin? (18.1-4)
   - A. Vasoconstriction
   - B. Vasorelease
   - C. Vasotransport
   - D. Vasodilation

5. Which skin layers does a third-degree injury damage? Choose all that apply. (18.1-5)
   - A. Epidermis
   - B. Dermis
   - C. Hypodermis
   - D. None of these.

6. What skeletal function does arthroplasty support? (18.2-1)
   - A. Providing structure for the body
   - B. Protecting internal organs
   - C. Producing blood cells
   - D. Moving the body

7. Which structure helps bones glide smoothly at the joints? (18.2-2)
   A. Compact bone
   C. Periosteum
   B. Cartilage
   D. Spongy bone

8. Rickets results from a lack of (18.2-3)
   A. vitamin D
   C. vitamin A
   B. vitamin C
   D. calcium

9. The femur in your thigh is a (18.2-4)
   A. sesamoid bone
   C. flat bone
   B. short bone
   D. long bone

10. Where your clavicle and scapula connect in your shoulder is a(n) (18.2-5)
    A. epicondyle
    C. tuberosity
    B. process
    D. malleolus

11. Which comparison of the axial and appendicular skeleton is true? (18.2-6)
    A. The appendicular skeleton protects vital organs, and the axial skeleton protects nonvital organs.
    B. Both the long bones of the axial skeleton and spine of the appendicular skeleton support the weight of the body.
    C. The axial skeleton protects the body, while the appendicular skeleton moves it.
    D. The axial and appendicular skeleton have an equal number of bones.

12. What type of joint allows you to bend your knee without sideways movement? (18.2-7)
    A. Condylar joint
    C. Pivot joint
    B. Hinge joint
    D. Gliding joint

13. A condition in which two bones held together by ligaments and muscles are separated is a (18.2-8)
    A. simple fracture
    C. dislocation
    B. spiral fracture
    D. stress fracture

14. Which function of the muscular system is *not* supported by collagen? (18.3-1)
    A. Maintaining posture
    B. Providing stability
    C. Producing body heat
    D. Moving the body

15. Muscles grow stronger and larger when they (18.3-2)
    A. atrophy
    C. are stimulated
    B. are not used
    D. are compressed

16. Muscle attachment to a stationary bone is called the point of (18.3-3)
    A. origin
    C. insertion
    B. anchor
    D. movement

17. Increasing the angle of a joint beyond normal anatomical position is called (18.3-4)
    A. hyperflexion
    C. hyperextension
    B. hypoflexion
    D. hypoextension

18. The prefix *inter-* tells you that intercostal muscles are located (18.3-5)
    A. above the ribs
    C. over the ribs
    B. below the ribs
    D. between the ribs

Build Core Skills

1. **Reading.** Go to the Get Body Smart website and view the section of skeletal bones you need the most practice to understand. Use the diagrams and your knowledge of body directions and bone terminology to help as you read. Check your understanding at the end with the quiz. Repeat this activity for practice with a section of the muscular system.

2. **Writing.** Find the human skeleton on the eSkeletons website. View the skull from the posterior angle. Draw the suture lines as shown and describe how they were formed.

3. **Math.** Suppose you are a doctor. You have a male patient who is 19 years of age and weighs 170 pounds (77 kg). He slipped and fell onto a hot grill with his arms outstretched, resulting in second-degree burns down the insides of both his arms and on his face. Use the rule of nines and the Parkland Formula that follows to calculate how much fluid to give him to prevent dehydration from his wounds.
   Parkland Formula: V (fluid volume) = % TBSA (% total body surface area) × body weight (kg) × 4 mL

4. **Math.** Examine Figure 18.14, which shows bone mass density and osteoporosis risk by age, sex, and ethnicity. Use the graph to answer the following questions:
   A. Who is at the lowest risk for osteoporosis?
   B. At what age does risk of fracture begin?
   C. Approximately how many years sooner would you expect a white female to develop osteoporosis than a black female?

5. **Critical Thinking.** Combine what you learned about skin layers with what you learned about burns to explain why a third- or fourth-degree burn is more likely to cause dehydration and infection than a first- or second-degree burn.

6. **Writing.** Imagine you are a bone. Write a love note to a muscle, telling it why you love it and how empty your life would be without it. Alternatively, imagine you are a muscle. Write a thank-you note to a bone, explaining why you appreciate it and how its existence has improved your life.

7. **Critical Thinking.** Use the suggestions from the section titled *The Logic of Muscle Names* in Lesson 18.3 to analyze a muscle name you do not already know from Figure 18.28.

8. **Critical Thinking.** Name a part of your body that contains more than one type of muscle tissue. Which types does it contain, and what do they do?

Activate Your Learning

1. Find objects to represent the structures of the skin. Explain your choices.

2. Make a model of a pair of opposing muscles using four wooden craft sticks, two pieces of duct tape, and two rubber bands. Tape two of the wooden sticks together, end to end, to represent bones at a bendable joint. Attach the rubber bands to represent opposing muscles. Demonstrate and explain your model.

3. Collect your fingerprints by rubbing pencil lead onto a scrap of paper, then rubbing each finger over the penciled area. Press each pencil-soiled finger onto a piece of cellophane tape and tape it down to a piece of paper. Label each print as the type of fingerprint it is—arch, whorl, or loop. Compare your own prints to each other, then compare them to other students' prints. How are they similar? different? How might this information be used?

4. Place a disposable vinyl glove on your nondominant hand and use makeup, art, or food items to make an area of the skin look like one of the skin lesions shown in Figure 18.4 or a burn shown in Figure 18.10. Prepare an index card describing the symptoms of this skin condition. Take turns with classmates playing the role of a patient wearing the glove of the skin condition and their dermatologist diagnosing the condition.

5. Attach a length of bulletin board paper to a wall or floor. Have someone trace around you on the paper. Inside the tracing, draw the outline of the major bones with a dark marker. Tape on lengths of yarn to represent muscle fibers for major muscles. Notice how the fibers build up at joints, then explain how tendons save space.

6. Review Figure 18.4. With a partner, practice naming and demonstrating each of the muscle movements for each joint. Repeat until you can name them without looking.

Think and Act Like a Healthcare Worker

1. Imagine you are a dermatologist. Your 15-year-old patient has neglected his skin care and has severe acne. You are concerned he will not follow the recommended treatment plan and is just looking for an easy solution. Your treatment will include washing the face with a medicated soap twice a day, applying a medicated cream, and avoiding contact with the pimples. How will you tactfully explain the treatment program and the importance of washing the face twice a day?

Go to the Source

1. Search the internet for "Gray's Anatomy osteology." Print and survey the section. The purpose for your reading is to compare different shapes of bone. Create a question to guide your reading. Underline main ideas and circle key terms as you read. Take notes in Cornell style. On the left side of your notes, compare this passage to the chapter's information on bone shapes. In the summary section of your notes, state what you learned in your own words.

2. Go to the Centers for Disease Control and Prevention website. Use the search tool's A-Z index to look up one of these skin disorders: pediculosis, skin cancer, mycotic diseases, jaundice, or tinea. Identify the etiology, pathology, diagnosis, treatment, and prevention.

HOSA Event Prep: Pathophysiology

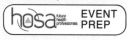

Mark came into Dr. Smith's office today with a chief complaint of joint pain and swelling. Pain is dull, aching, increases with use, and is somewhat relieved with NSAIDs. Sometimes he hears a grinding noise in his right knee while climbing stairs. His vital signs today are temperature—98.8 degrees, pulse—84 bpm, respirations—16 breaths per minute, blood pressure—124/88 mmHg, and oxygen saturation—98 percent. Weight is 230 lbs. Height is 5 feet 10 inches. A physical exam shows a calm patient in no immediate distress. There are no apparent injuries. Reflex responses are normal. No evidence of gross-motor or neural deficits. Strength of hands, shoulders, and hips is equal bilaterally. Range of motion (ROM) in fingers, neck, shoulders, and hips are slightly reduced. Knuckles of the hands are slightly enlarged, and patient complains of mild pain with pressure. Edema present in right knee. Comparison to last year's chart shows patient has lost 1/2 inch in height. Dr. Smith orders a CBC, bone scan, and X-rays of the hands and knees. The CBC is normal, the X-rays show osteoarthritis, and the bone scan shows osteoporosis in the spine. He refers Mark to a physical therapist for strengthening and stretching exercises. He recommends Mark increase his calcium intake, get at least 30 minutes of weight-bearing activity per day, and continue the NSAIDs as needed for pain.

Think About It

1. Explain how each of the doctor's orders makes sense given Mark's symptoms and results.

2. Imagine you are the physical therapist treating Mark. Using reliable and valid online resources, research your responsibilities and what skills you would need.

3. What qualities do you think are most important in a physical therapist? Why?

Chapter 19

Body Systems for Transportation and Exchange

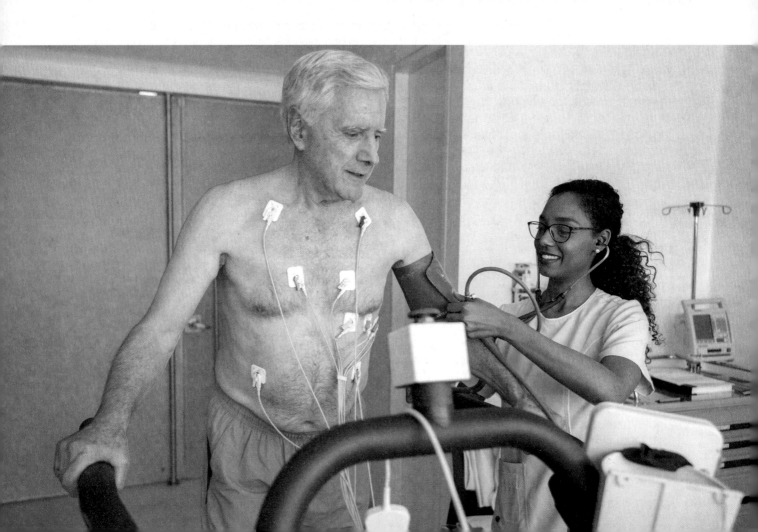

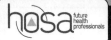

What have you learned so far about health science? What about HOSA? Could you take three of your friends and win a game of trivia about health science, parliamentary procedure, and all things HOSA? One of the most competitive events is *HOSA Bowl*. It is a team of four students who compete against another team to answer questions about health science, parliamentary procedure, and HOSA. Spectators can watch the final round.

Go to the HOSA website to learn more about the *HOSA Bowl* event. Find out the purpose of the event, what is involved, and what knowledge is demonstrated.

As you prepare for HOSA competitive events, be sure to check the website and talk with your HOSA advisor for the most up-to-date guidelines and procedures. Once you have learned about the *HOSA Bowl* event, answer the following questions:

1. How might participating in this event benefit you personally and your future career? Explain.
2. Are you interested in participating in this event? Why or why not?

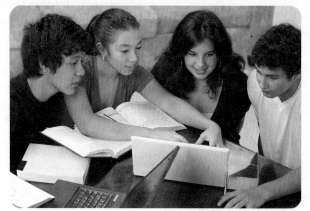

otnaydur/Shutterstock.com

 ## Connect with Your Reading

There are many new terms to learn when you study the body systems. Some terms will require more effort to remember than others. Using the steps listed here, create a study aid to help you organize and focus your attention on these important terms. Be prepared to share your work with classmates and learn from theirs.

1. Create a Vocabulary Sorting Organizer.
2. Fold a piece of paper lengthwise to create three columns.
   A. Unfold the paper and label the three columns as *New Terms*, *Terms I've Heard Of*, and *Terms I Know Well*.
   B. Sort the terms from the Professional Vocabulary list at the beginning of each lesson into the columns you have created.
3. On the back of your organizer, write one new term from your list in the center of the page along with the definition given in the chapter.
4. Divide the page into four sections and complete a "clinical diagnosis" of the new term.
   A. In one section of the page, explain how the word is used in the text. What topic is it related to? What does the context tell you about the meaning of the term?
   B. In the next section, list three or more related words that have a similar meaning or share a word part with this term.
   C. In the third section, use the word in a meaningful sentence or draw a picture of the concept described by the term.
   D. In the last section, explain the opposite of this term, or what it is not. Avoid using the word *not* or the prefix *un-*.

New Terms	Terms I've Heard Of	Terms I Know Well

How was the term used? What is the topic? What does the context tell you?	Opposites or non-examples of the term (what it isn't); don't use *not* or *un-*
Other words that relate to this term (shared word part, similar meaning)	Draw a picture to represent this term or use the word in a *meaningful* sentence.

(center: Term and Definition)

Goodheart-Willcox Publisher

Chapter opener image: andresr/E+ via Getty Images

Map Your Reading

Make a tablet organizer with two sheets of paper using the example shown. Stack the sheets, keeping the edges even, but move the top sheet of paper up so that its bottom edge is ½ inch to 1 inch above the bottom edge of the sheet below it. Holding both sheets of paper, fold them down so the top edge of the top sheet is ½ inch to 1 inch above the bottom edge of the top sheet. Crease both layers and staple at the folded edge. Write *Systems for Transportation and Exchange* on the outside flap and list things you know need to be moved around the body and in and out of cells. Label the edges of the flaps below it with the headings *Cardiovascular System*, *Lymphatic (Immune) System*, and *Respiratory System*. As you read, add visual cues, definitions of new terms, and notes on important concepts to each page of the booklet.

Systems for Transportation and Exchange
nutrients   hormones   heat oxygen   carbon   fluid waste   dioxide   WBC
(Circulatory System) CARDIOVASCULAR SYSTEM
(Immune System) LYMPHATIC SYSTEM
RESPIRATORY SYSTEM

Goodheart-Willcox Publisher

Lesson 19.1

The Cardiovascular System

Learning Outcomes

After studying this lesson, you will be able to:

19.1-1 identify the function and related disorders of components of blood.

19.1-2 describe the structures, functions, circulation pattern, and related disorders of blood vessels.

19.1-3 identify the structures, functions, circulation pattern, and related disorders of the heart.

19.1-4 explain the role of the cardiac cycle and vital signs in assessing patient health.

Professional Vocabulary

Essential Terms

artery   a blood vessel that moves blood from the heart out to the body tissues

capillary bed   a network of very fine, thin-walled blood vessels (capillaries) located in body tissues

cardiovascular   related to the heart and blood vessels

pulmonary loop   the flow of blood from the heart to the lungs and back to pick up oxygen and drop off carbon dioxide

systemic loop   the flow of blood from the heart to the body systems and back to drop off nutrients and pick up waste

vein   a blood vessel that moves blood from body tissues toward the heart

Important Terms

antibodies	hemoglobin	valves
antigen	leukocytes	ventricle
atrium	plasma	
erythrocytes	thrombocytes	

Introduction

Three major systems move and distribute substances within the body. These include the cardiovascular system, the lymphatic system, and the respiratory system. Your systems for transportation and exchange are involved in many disease processes. Their work impacts all other systems of the body. In this lesson, you will learn about the cardiovascular system. **Figure 19.1** introduces a few of the most common, yet serious, diseases and disorders of the cardiovascular system. In this lesson, you will learn more about risk factors and prevention for these and other conditions.

Common Diseases and Disorders for the Cardiovascular System			
Characteristics	**Hypertension**	**Myocardial Infarction**	**Cerebrovascular Accident**
Etiology	Cause is often unknown but may be lifestyle- or hormone-related. Risk factors include diet high in salt and fat, sedentary lifestyle, obesity, age 60+, African-American ethnicity, menopause, chronic kidney disease, diabetes, Cushing syndrome, hyperthyroidism, hyperparathyroidism, pregnancy, and sleep apnea.	Often caused by a buildup of fat and cholesterol as plaque that narrows the inside of arteries and reduces blood flow to the heart muscle; can also be due to an abnormal heart rhythm. Risk factors include high blood pressure, high blood cholesterol, smoking, sedentary lifestyle, obesity, diabetes, and family history of heart disease.	A blocked artery or leaking or burst blood vessel interrupts blood flow to the brain. Risk factors include high blood pressure, smoking, high blood cholesterol, diabetes, sleep apnea, sedentary lifestyle, obesity, a history of TIAs, COVID-19 infection, and a family history of stroke.
Pathology	Force of blood against the walls of the blood vessels damages the heart, blood vessels, and vascular organs. Correlated to atherosclerosis. Can increase the risk of heart attack, stroke, aneurysm, and shortened life span.	Damage or death of part of the heart muscle occurs due to lack of oxygen to the heart muscle. This affects the heart's strength and rhythm, which reduces the ability to pump blood.	When blood supply to the brain is interrupted, brain cells are deprived of oxygen and begin to die. Can cause paralysis, difficulty talking or swallowing, memory loss, thinking difficulties, emotional issues, pain, and changes in behavior and abilities.
Diagnosis	Monitor for blood pressure that is consistently higher than 130/80 mmHg. Known as the silent killer, there are often no noticeable symptoms. During a hypertensive crisis (over 180/120 mmHg), a person may experience headaches and nosebleeds.	Common symptoms include chest pain; difficulty breathing; dizziness; discomfort in the jaw, neck, or shoulder; and a cold sweat. An EEG can diagnose an abnormal rhythm. Blood tests will confirm that heart muscle has died.	Symptoms include trouble speaking or understanding speech, paralysis or numbness of the face or limbs, problems seeing, headache, and trouble walking or balancing. A physical exam and medical imaging tests will help diagnose and rule out other causes of symptoms.

Goodheart-Willcox Publisher

Figure 19.1 Common diseases and disorders of the cardiovascular system. (continued)

Common Diseases and Disorders for the Cardiovascular System (continued)			
Characteristics	Hypertension	Myocardial Infarction	Cerebrovascular Accident
Treatment	Control blood pressure through lifestyle changes (DASH diet, exercise, weight management, and reducing stress) and medication. Avoid salt, alcohol, and tobacco.	Call 911. CPR can maintain blood flow to vital organs until medical care can begin. Take nitroglycerin if prescribed. An AED can shock the heart back into rhythm. A stent, bypass, or transplant may be required.	Call 911. IV medications may break up blood clots. Emergency endovascular procedures can remove clots in the brain. Carotid endarterectomy or stent can open the artery. Surgery may relieve pressure on the brain and close off an aneurysm or malformation. Rehabilitation may help recover function.
Prevention	Limit salt intake, eat a healthy diet, get regular physical activity, maintain a healthy weight, avoid smoking, and learn to manage stress.	Daily aspirin regimen can thin the blood to prevent clots. Medications may help the heart function better or reduce blood pressure. Maintain a healthy weight, eat a heart-healthy diet that is low in salt and fat, get regular physical activity, and do not smoke.	Take prescribed medicines to prevent clotting. Treat the causes of stroke, including heart disease, high blood pressure, irregular heartbeat, high cholesterol, and diabetes. Change diet and physical activity or adopt other healthy lifestyle habits. Surgery may also be helpful.

phleb/o = vein
-tomy = to cut into, surgical incision
-ist = specialist, agent

intra- = within
ven/o = vein
-ous = pertaining to, having
endo- = within
trache/o = trachea, windpipe
-al = pertaining to

Working with the cardiovascular system is a career option at all levels of training. At the entry level, a phlebotomist (flih-BAHT-uh-mihst) draws blood for medical tests or donations. An emergency medical technician–basic (EMT-B) receives 200 hours or more of classroom training in basic life support. These workers handle cardiac, respiratory, and trauma emergencies (**Figure 19.2**).

Additional hours of classroom training, hands-on practice, and testing are required for paramedics. Certification requirements for paramedics vary in each state. Paramedics provide more invasive medical support. They may put in intravenous (IV) tubes for medications and endotracheal (ehn-doh-TRAY-kee-uhl) tubes for breathing. All these healthcare workers need a basic knowledge of the cardiovascular system's role in transporting materials throughout the body.

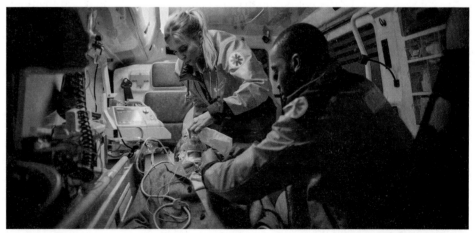

Gorodenkoff/Shutterstock.com

Figure 19.2   EMTs and paramedics respond to emergency health situations. *Who requires more training—EMTs or paramedics? What procedures are paramedics able to perform in your state?*

If you are willing to put in 13 to 15 years of study, job openings for cardiologists are increasing. Cardiologists make life-or-death decisions, pay attention to details, have good hand-eye coordination, and are sensitive to patient concerns. They combine their knowledge of body system interactions with information from other specialists to perform diagnostic tests, transplants, and surgeries.

Modern technology can help solve many heart and vascular conditions in the aging population. An electrocardiograph (EKG) technician uses an instrument to measure electrical signals from the heart. The technician then provides the cardiologist with this data about possible heart conditions. A perfusionist (per-FYU-zhuhn-ihst) operates the heart-lung machine during open-heart surgeries. A hematologist (hee-muh-TAH-luh-jihst) diagnoses blood-related diseases. All these professionals must communicate with each other to diagnose and treat cardiovascular illnesses. An increasing number of smart devices, such as wearable sensors for blood chemistry and heart activity, may assist them.

electr/o = electric
cardi/o = heart
-graph = instrument to record
per- = through
-fusion = to pour
-ist = specialist, agent
hemat/o = blood
-logist = specialist in the study of

19.1-1 The Role of Blood in the Cardiovascular System

Your **cardiovascular** system is a transportation route within your body. When your blood uses this system to move through your body tissues, it brings many nutrients and gases from other body systems to trade with your body's cells (**Figure 19.3**). Your blood also carries away waste so your cells do not die due to toxic buildup. Transportation and exchange are so important that your cardiovascular system is the first body system to begin functioning, and death occurs shortly after it stops.

cardi/o = heart
vascul/o = vessel
-ar = pertaining to

tox/i = poison
-ic = pertaining to

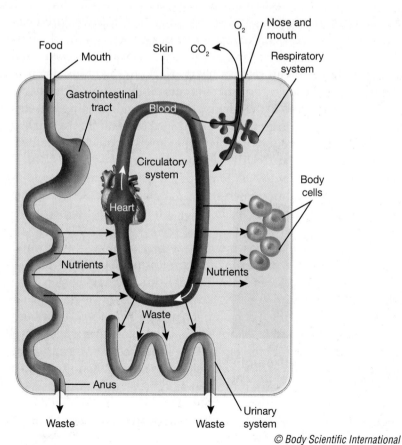

© Body Scientific International

Figure 19.3 Transportation and exchange of nutrients and gases in the body.

Because of its role in circulating blood and other materials throughout your body, the cardiovascular system is also called the *circulatory system*. Your heart, blood vessels, and blood are the key players in this delivery service. Your heart is the pump that keeps blood flowing. Your blood vessels are the route that blood follows from one place to another in your body. Different elements of your blood act together as a team of delivery people, carrying "packages" of water, oxygen, nutrients, hormones, and heat to all areas of your body. Each structure of your cardiovascular system has its own role and related diseases.

Blood Composition

The average adult's body contains about 4 to 6 liters of blood, depending on body size. More than one-half of your blood volume consists of a yellowish liquid called **plasma** (**Figure 19.4**). Your plasma is mostly water, but it also carries nutrients, hormones, and waste for your other body systems. Plasma maintains blood pressure. Shock occurs when blood volume decreases so much that major organs do not receive enough blood flow. Symptoms include tachycardia (ta-kee-KAHR-dee-uh); weak pulse; shallow breathing; blue lips; and cold, clammy skin. Shock can be life threatening and requires emergency medical attention.

tachy- = fast
cardi/o = heart
-ia = abnormal condition

Three types of blood cells make up the remainder of your blood's total volume. Blood products do not have to be present in large quantities to be important. **Leukocytes** (LOO-kuh-sIts), or *white blood cells* (WBCs), compose just 0.5 percent of your blood. These blood cells are important to the function of your immune or lymphatic system. Leukemia is a blood cancer that causes an increased number of underdeveloped white blood cells.

leuk/o = white
-cyte = cell
-emia = abnormal blood condition

Thrombocytes, also called *platelets*, compose another 0.5 percent of your blood. These cell fragments form blood clots to repair injured blood vessels. A *thrombus* is a blood clot that forms in a blood vessel. If the clot breaks loose and travels to another part of the body, it is called an *embolus*. An embolus in a blood vessel of the heart can cause a heart attack. In the brain, it can cause a stroke. The blockage caused by an embolus cuts off the supply of nutrients and oxygen, which causes tissues to die. Hemophilia is a condition that presents the opposite problem. People with hemophilia can bleed to death from a small injury because their cells do not produce a protein that holds blood clots together.

thromb/o = clot

-us = structure
embol/o = plug, stopper

Your **erythrocytes** (ih-RIHTH-ruh-sIts), or *red blood cells* (RBCs), are shaped like donuts with dented centers. Your RBCs contain the protein **hemoglobin** (HEE-muh-gloh-bihn), which helps them carry oxygen and gives them their red color. A hematocrit is a lab test that determines the percentage of RBCs in your total blood volume.

erythr/o = red
hem/o = blood
-globin = protein
hemat/o = blood
-crit = to judge, to separate
an- = without
-emia = abnormal blood condition

Anemia is a condition characterized by a lower-than-normal level of red blood cells in the blood, or lower-than-normal level of hemoglobin in the red blood cells. This reduces the ability of RBCs to carry oxygen. Anemia causes a person to look pale, tire easily, have a rapid heartbeat, and feel faint. There are many types of anemia. For example, in *sickle-cell anemia*, an inherited condition that is most common in people who are African-American, erythrocytes can become an abnormal crescent shape. These red blood cells carry less oxygen and clot more easily in blood vessels. People with anemia may need to increase their iron intake to make more hemoglobin.

trans- = across
-fusion = to pour

Some people with anemia receive a transfusion of donated blood to increase their RBC count. Although the life span of an erythrocyte is only four months, healthy people can donate blood every other month. This is because 140 million new red blood cells are manufactured every minute in bone marrow.

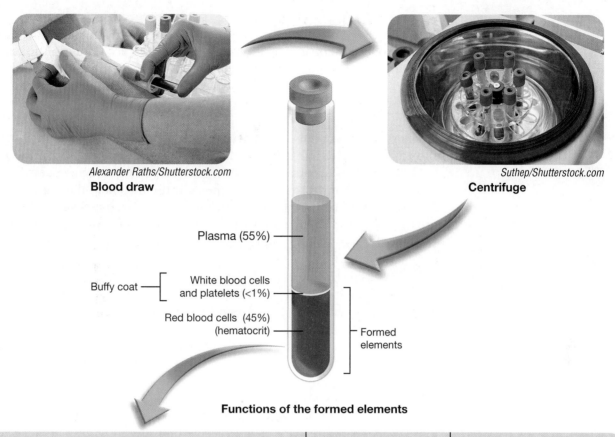

Alexander Raths/Shutterstock.com
Blood draw

Suthep/Shutterstock.com
Centrifuge

Plasma (55%)

Buffy coat — White blood cells
and platelets (<1%)

Red blood cells (45%)
(hematocrit)

Formed
elements

Functions of the formed elements

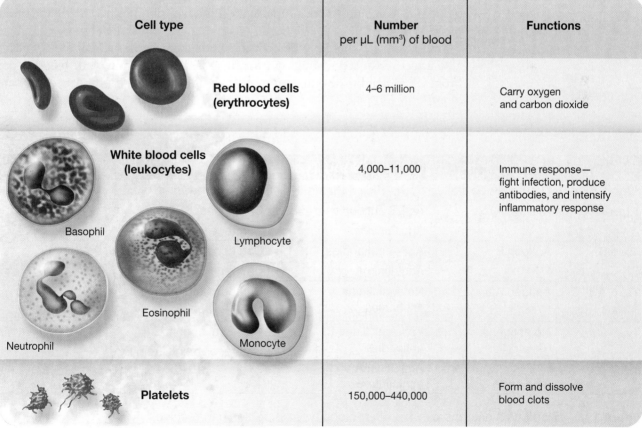

Cell type	Number per μL (mm³) of blood	Functions
Red blood cells (erythrocytes)	4–6 million	Carry oxygen and carbon dioxide
White blood cells (leukocytes) Basophil, Lymphocyte, Eosinophil, Neutrophil, Monocyte	4,000–11,000	Immune response—fight infection, produce antibodies, and intensify inflammatory response
Platelets	150,000–440,000	Form and dissolve blood clots

© Body Scientific International

Figure 19.4 Blood consists of plasma and formed elements, which are red blood cells, white blood cells, and platelets.

Blood Types

glutin/o = glue
-ation = action of, process of

anti- = against
-gen = origin, formation,
producing

Your blood is categorized as type A, B, AB, or O according to the protein molecules present on the surfaces of red blood cells (**Figure 19.5**). If the wrong blood types are mixed, blood cells stick together in clumps. This agglutination reaction can be fatal, so it is important to match blood types before a blood transfusion.

Type A red blood cells have **antigen** (AN-tih-juhn) A on their surface and produce **antibodies** in the blood plasma against antigen B. Your antibodies attach themselves to foreign antigens, such as pathogens, chemicals, or pollen, and disable or destroy them. Type A antibodies help the body destroy any type B blood cells that might enter the cardiovascular system. A person with type A blood can donate blood only to someone with type A or AB. A person with type A blood can receive blood only from someone with type A or O.

Similarly, type B red blood cells have antigen B on their surface and produce antibodies against antigen A. This means that people with type B blood can donate to those with type B or AB and receive blood from those with type B or O.

Type AB blood has both A and B antigens and no antibodies in the blood plasma. Type AB is known as a *universal receiver* because people with this blood type may receive type A, B, AB, or O blood without agglutination.

Type O blood is known as a *universal donor* because it does not have A or B antigens on the RBCs to cause agglutination and so can be donated to anyone. However, people with type O can receive only type O blood because their blood plasma contains both type A and type B antibodies to destroy the other blood types.

In addition to the ABO blood types, other antigens such as the *Rh factor* also affect the success of blood transfusions. Do you know your blood type? From what blood types can you receive blood? To which types can you donate blood?

Blood Types				
Blood Type	**On the Blood Cell**	**In the Blood Plasma**	**Blood Donation Notes**	**US Prevalence**
Type A	Antigen A	Anti-B antibodies Agglutinin B	Can donate to A or AB Can receive A or O	41%
Type B	Antigen B	Anti-A antibodies Agglutinin A	Can donate to B or AB Can receive B or O	9%
Type AB	Antigen A and B	No agglutinins or antibodies	Can donate only to AB Universal receiver	3%
Type O	No antigens	Anti-A and anti-B antibodies Agglutinin A and agglutinin B	Universal donor Can receive only from O	47%

Goodheart-Willcox Publisher

Figure 19.5 Blood type determines what other blood types a person can receive.

19.1-2 **Blood Vessels**

Blood vessels are parallel networks of tubes that allow blood to flow from your heart out to every cell in your body and then back to your heart (**Figure 19.6**). There are three types of blood vessels: arteries, capillaries, and veins.

Arteries

Arteries usually carry oxygenated blood away from your heart. The layers of connective tissue, smooth muscle, and endothelium in the thick artery walls expand and contract as they receive blood under high pressure from your heart. The *aorta* is your largest artery, carrying blood from your heart out to your body. Arterioles (ahr-TEER-ee-ohls) are small arteries that branch out into capillaries. Arterial bleeds are the most difficult to control because of the pressure from the beating heart. Apply pressure to avoid a serious loss of blood, or *hemorrhage*.

arteri/o = artery
-ole = small
hem/o = blood
-rrhage = to flow profusely

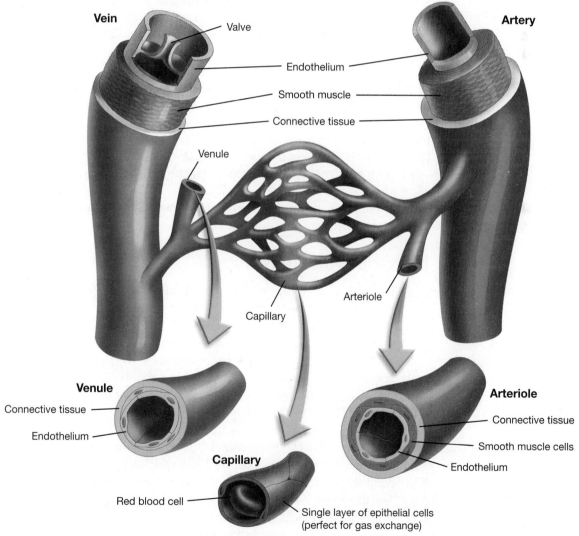

© Body Scientific International

Figure 19.6 Networks of blood vessels—consisting of arteries, capillaries, and veins—transport blood throughout the body. *What parts do these types of blood vessels have in common? What are their differences?*

Capillaries

Capillary beds contain many thin-walled blood vessels (capillaries) where gases, nutrients, waste, hormones, and heat can move in and out of your blood vessels. Blood plasma leaks out from your capillaries to carry nutrients to your cells. Once it soaks into the spaces between the cells of your tissues, it is called interstitial (ihn-ter-STIH-shuhl) fluid. Excess fluid returns to your capillaries, carrying waste products from your cells. As blood flows through capillaries close to your skin, it also gets rid of excess heat to help your body maintain a consistent temperature.

inter- = between

Veins

Except for the blood in your pulmonary veins going to your lungs, the blood in veins is oxygen-poor, or *deoxygenated*. Blood leaves its nutrients in your capillary beds, picks up waste, and flows into gradually larger venules. Your venules join to form **veins** (VAYNZ). The *vena cava* (vee-nuh KAH-vuh) is your body's largest vein. These blood vessels carry deoxygenated blood back to your heart. Intravenous infusions take advantage of this pathway. A needle placed in a blood vessel of your hand or arm can deliver medications and fluids to your body.

Your veins have less smooth muscle than your arteries and are farther from the pumping force of your heart. Veins use **valves** to prevent backflow as your blood moves against gravity toward your heart. You can identify venous valves on your inner wrist or the back of your hand by running your finger against the flow of blood. Varicose veins have defective valves that allow blood to leak backward and collect in swollen blue "knots" near the skin surface. Veins also depend on nearby skeletal muscle contractions to help move blood. When people with poor circulation are less active, elevating the legs and wearing elastic anti-embolism stockings help keep blood moving so varicose veins and blood clots do not form.

pulmon/o = lung
-ary = pertaining to
de- = lack of, away from
ox/y = oxygen
gen/o = origin
-ate = pertaining to, composed of, process
ven/o = vein
-ule = small

Major Blood Vessels

Your blood vessel locations and names follow a pattern (**Figure 19.7**). Blood vessels going out to your extremities can be divided into deep and superficial blood vessels. Large, deep veins and arteries usually run parallel to your major nerves and lymph vessels. Their names change depending on their location. Your *descending aorta* from your heart becomes your *abdominal aorta* in your belly. It then divides into your *left* and *right common iliac* (IH-lee-ak) *arteries* at your hips before running down each leg as your *femoral artery* and your *popliteal* (pah-plih-TEE-uhl) *artery* behind each knee.

Your aortic arch has three branches that become your *subclavian artery* running under your clavicle, your *carotid artery* going to your neck, and your *brachiocephalic* (bray-kee-oh-seh-FA-lihk) *artery* leading to your arm and head. Your deep veins typically have the same names as the arteries they accompany. For example, your brachial, ulnar, and radial veins run alongside your brachial, ulnar, and radial arteries in your arm.

Smaller superficial vessels run closer to the surface of your skin. You can sometimes see your *basilic* and *cephalic* veins through your skin, running from your wrist to your armpit. These superficial blood vessel names do not change from one location to another.

brachi/o = arm
cephal/o = head
-ic = pertaining to

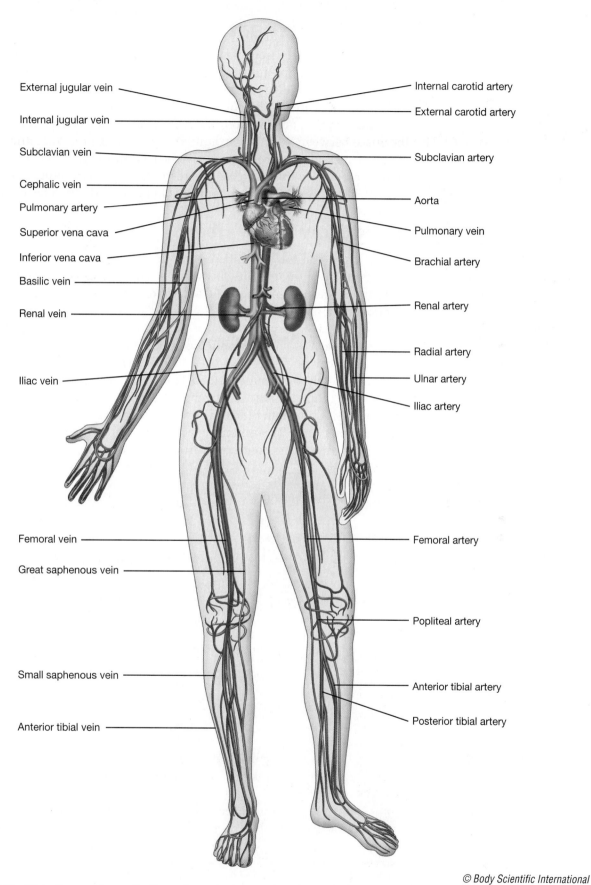

External jugular vein

Internal jugular vein

Subclavian vein

Cephalic vein

Pulmonary artery

Superior vena cava

Inferior vena cava

Basilic vein

Renal vein

Iliac vein

Femoral vein

Great saphenous vein

Small saphenous vein

Anterior tibial vein

Internal carotid artery

External carotid artery

Subclavian artery

Aorta

Pulmonary vein

Brachial artery

Renal artery

Radial artery

Ulnar artery

Iliac artery

Femoral artery

Popliteal artery

Anterior tibial artery

Posterior tibial artery

© *Body Scientific International*

Figure 19.7   This figure shows both major arteries and major veins. *What patterns do you see in the placement and naming of blood vessels?*

19.1-3 **The Heart**

endo- = within
cardi/o = heart
-um = structure
epi- = upon
peri- = around

Like your blood vessels, your heart is formed from three layers of tissue. The endocardium gives the inside of your heart a smooth surface that promotes blood flow. It also produces hormones that help with heart contractions. The epicardium forms the outside surface of your heart. The pericardium is a second covering around your heart's surface. A small amount of fluid fills the space between your epicardium and pericardium to keep these two layers from sticking together. Congestive heart failure occurs when excess fluid builds up between these layers. This restricts the heart's ability to expand and fill with blood, reducing the amount of blood pushed out to the body.

Blood Flow in the Heart

pulmon/o = lung
-ary = pertaining to

Your heart is a four-chambered pump for your cardiovascular system. It consists of involuntary muscle that is *striated* (striped) for twitch contractions, not sustained contractions. Each short, hard squeeze pushes 5 liters of blood along a one-way path through your body. Your blood travels through two loops to bring oxygen, nutrients, and hormones to your body's cells and remove waste. The short **pulmonary loop** carries deoxygenated blood from your heart to your lungs and back to the heart. The longer **systemic loop** takes this newly oxygenated blood from your heart to cells in all areas of your body, then returns deoxygenated blood to your heart (**Figure 19.8**). The double-loop system is an efficient way to keep oxygenated blood flowing through your body. This pumping action begins in the fifth week of embryonic development and continues throughout your life.

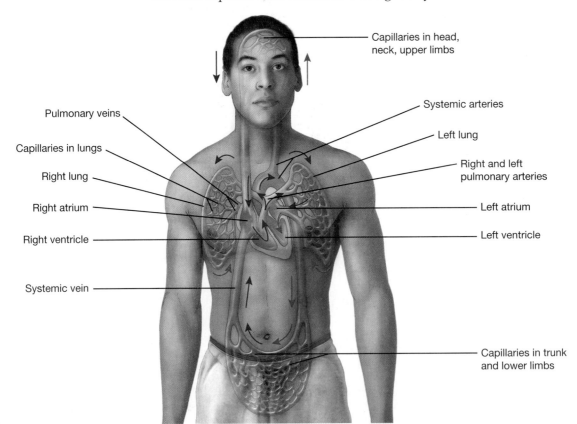

© Body Scientific International

Figure 19.8 The heart pumps blood through two loops—the pulmonary loop and the systemic loop. *Which loop transports oxygenated blood to the cells in the body? deoxygenated blood to the lungs?*

Heart Valves

Just as valves prevent blood from flowing backward in your veins, valves also prevent backward flow between the chambers of your heart. You can use **Figure 19.9** to trace the flow of blood through your heart. Deoxygenated blood from your vena cava enters your right **atrium**, the chamber at the top of your heart. The blood then flows through your tricuspid atrioventricular (ay-tree-oh-vehn-TRIH-kyuh-luhr) valve, or *AV valve*, and down to your right **ventricle**. Ventricles are the lower chambers of your heart. When the pressure in your right ventricle is higher than in your right atrium, your AV valve closes to prevent backward flow, and your *semilunar* pulmonary valve opens. The semilunar valves control blood flow coming out of your heart.

The act of the valves closing when your heart contracts produces the characteristic "lubb-dupp" sound associated with a heartbeat. The first sound ("lubb") is your AV valves sweeping closed, and the second, louder sound ("dupp") is your semilunar valves snapping shut after the strong push of blood out of your heart.

atri/o = entrance
-um = structure
tri- = three
cusp/o = point
-id = having a particular quality
ventr/o = belly
-ic = pertaining to
-ule = small
-ar = pertaining to
-icle = tiny
semi- = half
lun/o = moon

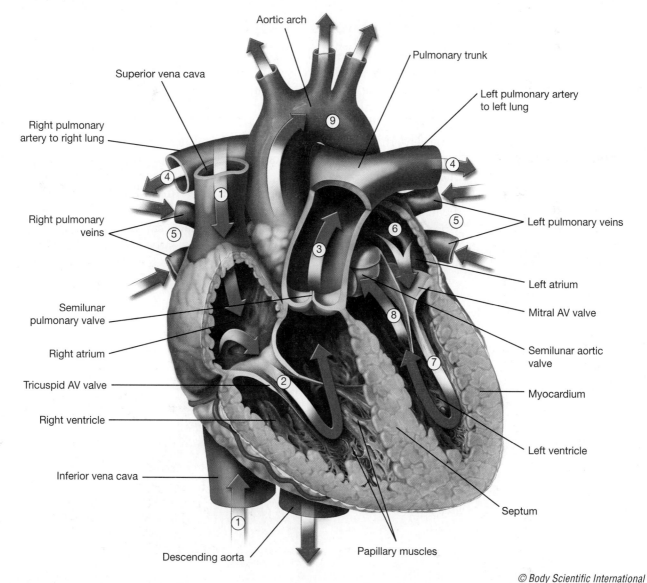

© *Body Scientific International*

Figure 19.9 The arrows and numbers on this diagram of the heart show where blood travels with each heartbeat. *Can you describe the flow of blood through the heart by naming the structures in order along the route?*

When a heart valve does not close properly, you can use a stethoscope to hear leaking blood flow. A structural condition present at birth or other diseases can cause this heart murmur. An artificial heart valve or pig's heart valve may be implanted to correct a heart murmur.

Your heart ventricles are more muscular than your atria. Blood is squeezed out of your right ventricle to your lungs through your pulmonary artery. This is the only artery that carries deoxygenated blood away from your heart. In the pulmonary loop, your blood will release its carbon dioxide (CO_2) in exchange for oxygen (O_2). Oxygenated blood returns from your lungs through your pulmonary veins to your left atrium. These are the only veins that carry oxygenated blood to your heart. The left atrium of your heart, like the right, has little muscle tone for the short push down to your left ventricle. When pressure in your ventricle is greater than in your atrium, your mitral AV valve closes, and your semilunar aortic valve opens. Your left ventricle is even more muscular than your right ventricle, so it can pump oxygenated blood out to your entire body. During heart surgery, blood flows through a heart-lung machine that temporarily takes over this work of warming, oxygenating, and circulating blood.

Coronary Blood Vessels

Your heart muscle requires a constant supply of oxygen and nutrients. This tireless muscle is fed by coronary arteries surrounding the outside of your heart, not by the blood within (**Figure 19.10**). If these arteries are blocked or damaged in some way, the heart cannot get nutrients, and the heart muscle dies. Atherosclerosis (a-thuh-roh-skluh-ROH-suhs) is caused by a buildup of cholesterol that forms a plaque and narrows the inside diameter of the artery. A narrow artery allows less blood to pass through. Think of this as trying to drink through a narrow stir-stick straw instead of a regular-sized straw.

A partial blockage in the coronary arteries limits the flow of nutrients to the heart muscle. Limiting the oxygen supply causes chest pain, called *angina*. More complete blockage can cause a heart attack, called a *myocardial infarction* (MI). Coronary bypass surgery replaces arteries of the heart with veins or arteries from another area of the body. This improves the blood supply bringing

pulmon/o = lung
-ary = pertaining to

coron/o = crown
-ary = pertaining to

ather/o = fatty substance
scler/o = hard
-osis = condition, process, state

angi/o = blood vessel
my/o = muscle
cardi/o = heart
-al = pertaining to

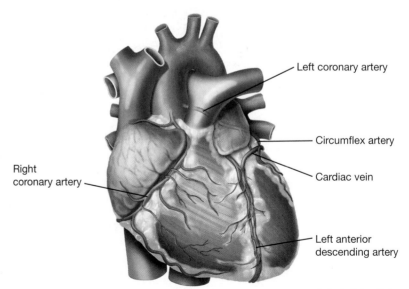

© Body Scientific International

Figure 19.10 Coronary arteries are essential to the healthy functioning of the heart. *What happens if these arteries are damaged?*

nutrients to the heart muscle. A double bypass replaces two coronary arteries, a triple bypass replaces three, and so on.

If the heart muscle is seriously damaged, a heart transplant may be required. Heart disease and coronary artery disease are the leading causes of death in the United States. These diseases currently begin as early as the teen years due to poor diet and physical activity habits as well as genetics. You should have your cholesterol levels checked every five years, ideally starting at 20 years of age. The latest thinking is that even slightly high cholesterol should be treated with lifestyle changes or medication.

19.1-4 The Cardiac Cycle and Vital Signs

Vital signs measure temperature, pulse (heartbeat), respiration (breathing), and blood pressure. The cardiovascular system controls several of these. When you measure a person's pulse, you are feeling or listening to the rhythm of the cardiac cycle.

Cardiac Cycle

The cardiac cycle has two parts: a contraction of the heart muscle followed by a relaxation of the heart muscle. Unlike skeletal muscle, which is voluntary, contractions of your heart muscle are involuntary. This means your heart muscle contracts without you thinking about it.

The cardiac cycle starts with an electrical signal from your sinoatrial node (SA node) telling your left and right atria to contract. When the signal reaches your atrioventricular node (AV node), it slows briefly, then continues down the conduction pathway through your bundle of His. It then divides into your left and right bundle branches to tell your ventricles to contract (**Figure 19.11**).

sin/o = sinus, cavity
atri/o = entrance
-al = pertaining to

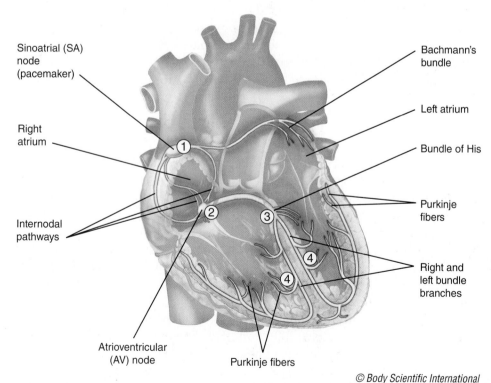

Sinoatrial (SA) node (pacemaker)

Right atrium

Internodal pathways

Atrioventricular (AV) node

Purkinje fibers

Bachmann's bundle

Left atrium

Bundle of His

Purkinje fibers

Right and left bundle branches

© Body Scientific International

Figure 19.11 Electrical centers of heart activity. *Which chambers of the heart contract first?*

Systole is the contraction of your heart's ventricles, and diastole is the relaxation of your ventricles as they refill with blood. These terms are also used for measuring blood pressure.

Pulse

Your pulse is felt in beats. These beats are caused by your heart pumping waves of blood through your arteries. The heart beats an average of 60 to 100 times per minute in a healthy adult. The average heart rate for an infant or child is much faster because the heart is smaller.

You can feel your pulse where your arteries run close to your body's surface. There are many different pulse points in your body. Your carotid pulse at your neck is easy to locate in an emergency. The brachial pulse at your inner elbow is typically used for measuring blood pressure. Your radial pulse at the thumb-side of your wrist is the most common site where pulse is measured.

A pulse oximeter measures heart rate through an artery in your finger. It also estimates the amount of oxygen in your blood by analyzing changes in the color of your blood vessels behind your fingernail (**Figure 19.12**). Sleep cycles, physical activity, stress, fever, drug use, and heart disease affect your heart rate. An unexplained change in heart rate may indicate a change in health status and should be closely monitored.

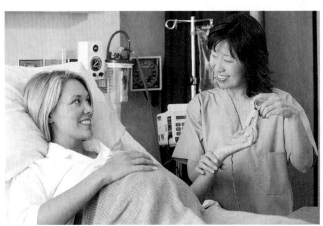

Monkey Business Images/Shutterstock.com

Figure 19.12 This nurse is using a pulse oximeter to measure her patient's pulse. *How does a pulse oximeter work?*

An arrhythmia is an irregular heart rhythm treatable with a pacemaker or medication. An ineffective flutter of the atrium or ventricle means the heart is unable to rest and fill with blood or is too weak to pump blood. This fibrillation can lead to cardiac arrest, in which the heart stops beating. An electrical shock from an automated external defibrillator (AED) can correct this. This lifesaving machine has become as common as a fire extinguisher in public buildings.

a- = without
rrhythm/o = rhythm
-ia = abnormal condition

Blood Pressure

Blood pressure (BP) is the force of your blood against the walls of your arteries, measured in millimeters of mercury (mmHg). It is another vital sign that should be monitored for changes. Systolic pressure measures the force of your blood against your artery walls when your heart is contracting. Diastolic pressure measures the force of your blood against your artery walls when your heart relaxes. Healthy young adults usually have a systolic pressure of about 100 to 120 mmHg and a diastolic pressure of about 60 to 90 mmHg. Blood pressure is usually recorded as a fraction with the systolic pressure written over the diastolic pressure.

High blood pressure, also called *hypertension,* is a condition in which blood pressure is consistently above 130/80 mmHg. This used to be 140/90 mmHg but has been revised to a lower number to avoid more damage to the blood vessels. Hypertension is an important predictor of strokes and aneurysms (AN-yuh-rih-zuhms). If a weak and bulging aneurysm of an artery bursts like a balloon, the affected person could quickly bleed to death. People who are

hyper- = more than normal, excessive
tens/o = stretch
-ion = action, process, condition

African-American have a higher risk for hypertension than others. Lifestyle changes such as physical activity, stress reduction, and dietary changes can reduce high blood pressure (**Figure 19.13**).

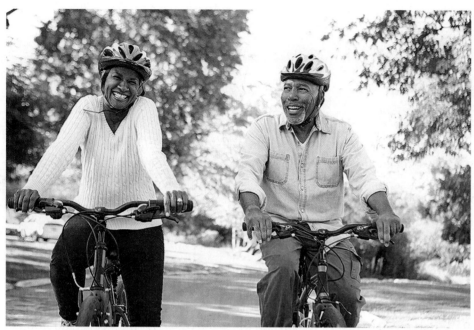

MBI/Shutterstock.com

Figure 19.13 Hypertension is a preventable health condition. Regular physical activity can lower your blood pressure and reduce your risk for hypertension.

Lesson 19.1 Review

 Complete the *Map Your Reading* graphic organizer for the section you just read.

1. The cardiovascular system functions as a _____ within the body. (19.1-1)
   A. paramedic
   B. filter
   C. transportation route
   D. waste disposal

2. The average adult's body contains about _____ liters of blood, depending on body size. (19.1-1)
   A. 2–4   C. 5–7
   B. 4–6   D. 6–8

3. Red blood cells carry oxygen, white blood cells fight infection, and the _____ carries nutrients, gases, hormones, and waste in the blood. (19.1-1)
   A. plasma   C. antigen
   B. platelet   D. hemoglobin

4. Which of the following are types of blood vessels? Choose all that apply. (19.1-2)
   A. Valves   C. Capillaries
   B. Veins   D. Arteries

5. Which are the names of the tissue layers that make up the heart? Choose all that apply. (19.1-3)
   A. Endocardium   C. Epicardium
   B. Atrium   D. Pericardium

6. Vital signs such as temperature, _____, respiration, and blood pressure are affected by the cardiovascular system. (19.1-4)
   A. arrhythmia   C. breathing
   B. circulation   D. pulse

7. High _____ can lead to a stroke or aneurysm. (19.1-4)
   A. oxygen levels   C. pulse rate
   B. blood pressure   D. respiration

The Lymphatic System

Learning Outcomes

After studying this lesson, you will be able to

19.2-1 explain the role of the lymphatic system in immune response.

19.2-2 describe the structures, functions, and related disorders of the lymphatic system.

Professional Vocabulary

Essential Terms

immune response the lymphatic system makes antibodies to protect against foreign substances in the body

lymphatic related to or containing the watery fluid (lymph) collected from body tissues

lymphocyte a type of white blood cell that determines how the body responds to foreign substances

Important Terms

adenoids	localized	spleen
appendix	lymph	systemic
cancer	lymph nodes	thoracic duct
cisterna chyli	lymphatic vessels	thymus
inflammation	mucous membranes	tonsils
lacteals	right lymphatic duct	vaccinations

Introduction

onc/o = tumor
-logist = specialist in the study of

The **lymphatic** system provides another type of circulation in your body, involved with a unique set of careers. Immunologists are medical doctors who focus on infections and allergies that affect the body. Oncologists manage the diagnosis, treatment, and prevention of different types of cancer. Both specialties are supported by biotechnology and pharmaceutical careers that research and develop new treatments, as well as medical imaging and laboratory technicians who help diagnose and provide treatments. Some common conditions affecting the lymphatic system are shown in **Figure 19.14**.

Immunologists and oncologists treat a system made up of lymphatic vessels, specialized blood cells, and several lymphoid organs and tissues. This network of vessels and organs returns excess fluid from your body tissues to your cardiovascular system, destroys invading microorganisms, and recycles dead blood cells. The lymphatic system is your body's main defense against infection, so it is important to the health of all your other body systems.

Common Diseases and Disorders for the Lymphatic System

Characteristics	Cancer	Lupus
Etiology	There are many carcinogens and many possible causes for this group of diseases. Most common are smoking, poor diet, obesity, hormones, sun, radiation, and viruses. Genetics also play a role.	Chronic, systemic lupus may result from a combination of hormones, genetics, and environment. Triggers may include sunlight, infections, or medications. Most commonly diagnosed in African-American, Hispanic, and Asian-American females ages 15–45.
Pathology	A group of diseases with abnormal cell growth that can invade or spread to other parts of the body. Most common types are breast, lung, prostate, colorectal, and skin cancer.	An autoimmune disease that attacks healthy tissue in the body. Inflammation often affects the kidneys, skin, joints, and heart. There is increased risk of infections, cancer, bone breaks, and miscarriage.
Diagnosis	Watch for warning signs. Confirm with imaging tests and biopsy.	Common signs and symptoms include fatigue, fever, joint pain, butterfly-shaped rash on the face, illness from sun exposure, and poor circulation to fingers or toes. Diagnosis supported with antinuclear antibodies test, anti-double stranded DNA test, and biopsy.
Treatment	Combination of surgery, radiation, chemotherapy, hormone therapy, or immunotherapy may destroy or slow growth of tumor. Medication and complementary therapies can treat pain and symptoms. Supportive therapy is provided when terminal.	No cure. Treatment includes avoiding triggers. Some medications can slow progress and treat individual symptoms.
Prevention	Eat a healthy diet, maintain a healthy weight, get regular physical activity, protect against the sun and exposure to radiation, get vaccinated, avoid tobacco and risky behaviors, and get regular checkups to catch cancer early.	Not preventable, but flare-ups can be reduced by avoiding triggers.

Goodheart-Willcox Publisher

Figure 19.14 Common diseases and disorders of the lymphatic system.

19.2-1 Lymphatic Support for the Immune Response

Your lymphatic system is part of your immune system. They share many structures that work together to fight infections. Many bacteria and fungi live on and in the human body. Some of these, called *normal body flora*, help your body digest food and maintain health. Microorganisms that cause disease are called *pathogens*. An overgrowth of normal body flora, the growth of microorganisms in the wrong place, or the growth of pathogens can cause illness or infection. Some infections, such as athlete's foot, are **localized** infections and affect only a small area of the body. Others are **systemic** infections, with generalized body symptoms, like influenza or sepsis.

immun/o = protection

path/o = disease
-gen = origin, formation, producing

leuk/o = white
-cyte = cell

lymph/o = lymph, watery fluid

hist/o = tissue
-ine = substance, chemical

phag/o = to eat

mono- = single

macro- = large

Your lymphatic system produces specialized blood cells for the immune system to defend against pathogens. Leukocytes are white blood cells that fight infections and diseases. Several types of leukocytes are made in your bone marrow (**Figure 19.15**). These include lymphocytes, eosinophils, basophils, neutrophils, and monocytes.

Lymphocytes are white blood cells that make antibodies to mark and destroy foreign substances. Eosinophils (ee-oh-SIHN-uh-fihls) help destroy the marked substances. Basophils release histamines that cause tissue swelling to cushion an injury. High counts of eosinophils or basophils occur during allergic reactions, such as those caused by food allergies or asthma. Neutrophils are also called *phagocytes*. They fight infection by attacking, surrounding, and eating pathogens in your blood. High numbers of neutrophils are common in a bacterial infection. Monocytes are phagocytes that surround and destroy foreign bodies and old red blood cells. Monocytes travel through your blood vessels to your lungs, liver, and other lymphatic tissue, where they develop into *macrophages*, which are large phagocytes. High numbers of monocytes indicate a chronic infection. A complete blood count (CBC) is a diagnostic test that measures the number of each type of blood cell present.

Natural Barriers

When pathogens enter the body, your immune system has several layers of defense against infections. Initially, your skin and **mucous membranes** provide a natural barrier that acts as your body's first line of defense against infection. Small hairs and mucus in these moist tissues at body openings trap invading microbes and foreign particles so they can be coughed or sneezed out. Tears, saliva, urine, and stomach acid have antimicrobial properties that help break down and flush out pathogens and irritants that enter your body.

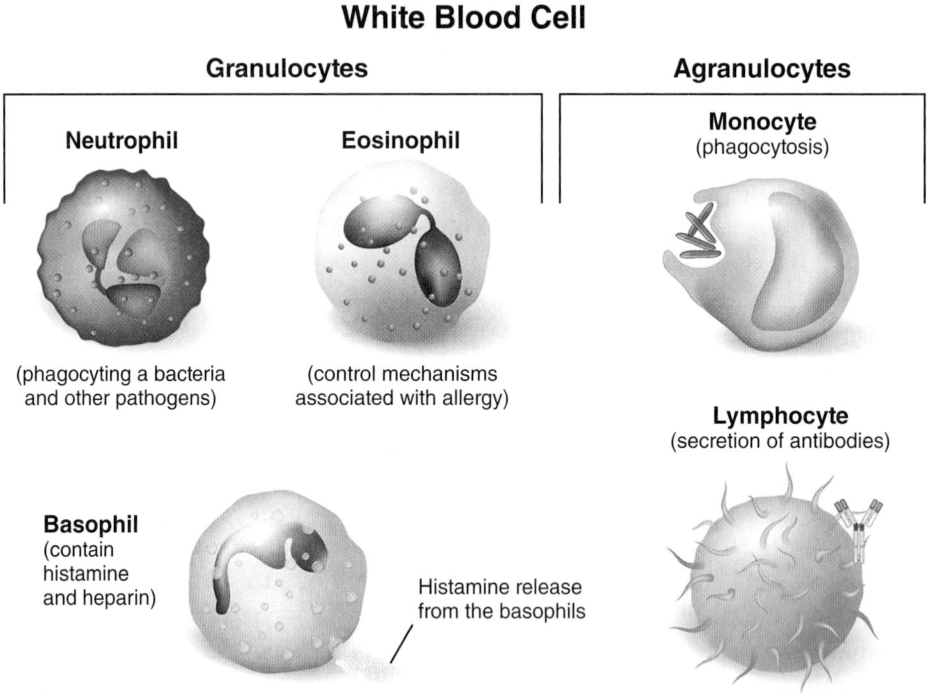

White Blood Cell

Granulocytes	Agranulocytes

Neutrophil

Eosinophil

Monocyte
(phagocytosis)

(phagocyting a bacteria and other pathogens)

(control mechanisms associated with allergy)

Lymphocyte
(secretion of antibodies)

Basophil
(contain histamine and heparin)

Histamine release from the basophils

Designua/Shutterstock.com

Figure 19.15 Each different type of leukocyte plays a unique role in fighting infections and diseases. *Which type would increase during an infection?*

Inflammation

Once a pathogen invades your body, your immune system provides a second line of defense. When cells are damaged by injuries, pathogens, toxins, excess heat, or other causes, they release chemicals, such as histamines, that cause **inflammation**. This swelling attracts white blood cells to trap and break down the pathogens. Pus is a collection of the dead tissue, bacteria, and white blood cells from this process.

hist/o = tissue
-ine = substance, chemical

An overactive immune system that attacks the body's own healthy cells can cause allergies and autoimmune diseases. Anaphylaxis (an-uh-fuh-LAK-suhs) is a severe allergic reaction that may cause death. Common triggers for anaphylaxis include insect stings, foods such as peanuts, or medications like penicillin. The first exposure to an allergen sensitizes the body and creates memory cells for the allergen's antigen. A future exposure to the allergen triggers a hypersensitive allergic reaction. The body releases large amounts of histamines that can cause a sudden drop in blood pressure and difficulty breathing. The restricted airways caused by this response require advanced medical help. Death can occur within minutes or hours without treatment. Epinephrine is a fast-acting prescription commonly used to treat anaphylactic shock (**Figure 19.16**). Immunologists can also treat allergic response by desensitizing the immune system. Immunotherapy uses a series of shots that provide limited exposure to an allergen so the body can build up a tolerance for it and reduce the hypersensitive allergic response.

auto- = self
immun/o = protection

Adaptive Immune Response

As a third line of defense, your **immune response** to antigens causes your body to make antibodies. Antibodies disable foreign substances and mark them for destruction. Lymphatic tissue traps microbes, destroys them, and then produces antibody memory cells against future invasions.

People do not often catch the same disease more than once. This is because memory cells created during the immune response allow for a faster reaction to that pathogen if it invades again. Your immune system adapts its defense system to new invaders.

Vaccinations take advantage of your immune system's ability to adapt. A vaccination, or *immunization,* stimulates your immune system to build protection against a particular disease. It contains a weakened or inactive pathogen or substance that is injected into the body. Most children are vaccinated against many diseases before they reach school age. This immunity prevents epidemics of serious infectious diseases such as polio and measles. Why do you think some vaccines are required every year?

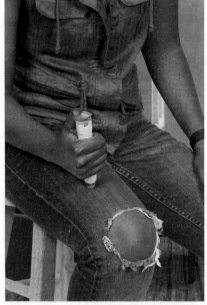

Rob Byron/Shutterstock.com

Figure 19.16 Epinephrine, which can be delivered through an *EpiPen*®, stimulates the heart to beat strongly so blood pressure can be restored. *When might this medication be required?*

immun/i = protection
-ty = quality, state

B-Cells

Leukocytes from your bone marrow, called *B-cells,* make antibodies to fight foreign invaders in the body. When B-cells attach to the surface of an antigen or pathogen, they release an army of antibodies into the bloodstream. The antibodies look for additional invaders of this type, then coat and trap them. This deactivates the invaders and marks them for destruction by macrophages.

T-Cells

cyt/o = cell
tox/i = poison
-ic = pertaining to

A butterfly-shaped lymphatic organ in your chest called the **thymus** grows during childhood as it helps program lymphocytes called *T-cells*. Your thymus shrinks after puberty when its T-cells have learned to tell the difference between your body cells and invaders. T-cells respond to antigens on the outside of infected cells. They mark them for destruction, then create memory cells for the pathogen and its antibody. Special killer T-cells are cytotoxic. They can be grown in a lab and used to fight cancer and viruses. For an organ transplant, this immune response must be suppressed with medications, such as cyclosporine. Otherwise, T-cells will identify antigens on the transplanted organ or tissue as foreign and direct the immune system to destroy it. This causes the body to reject the new organ.

pro- = before, in front
phylax/o = guard, preserve, protect
-is = pertaining to

The human immunodeficiency virus (HIV) attacks T-cells and reprograms them to make new HIV cells. Symptoms of HIV are similar to the flu, with fever or chills, muscle aches, sore throat, and swollen lymph nodes. People can live with latent HIV for 10 to 15 years, or even longer with antiviral treatment. The Department of Health and Human Services (HHS) is working to reduce the number of new HIV infections by linking people to medical care and increasing the use of pre-exposure prophylaxis (PrEP) among those most likely to be exposed to HIV. HIV infection can progress to acquired immunodeficiency syndrome (AIDS) if the number of T-cells in the body drops below 200 per microliter (µL) of blood. This low number of T-cells reduces the body's ability to fight infections. At this stage, people with AIDS may experience weight loss, night sweats, diarrhea, body sores, Kaposi sarcoma, pneumonia, and memory loss. People with AIDS can die from opportunistic infections, such as yeast and bacterial infections of the lungs. These infections are called *opportunistic* because they would not normally cause serious disease, but take advantage of the weakened immune system.

19.2-2 Structures and Functions of the Lymphatic System

lymph/o = lymph, watery fluid
-tic = pertaining to

inter- = between
intra- = within

Your lymphatic system shares an important role with your cardiovascular system in transporting fluids. In the blood, this fluid is called plasma. When it leaves the capillaries to deliver its oxygen, nutrients, and hormones, it becomes interstitial fluid. Any fluid that crosses the cell membrane becomes intracellular fluid. Lymphatic vessels pick up remaining fluid from your body tissues that did not seep back into capillaries, then return it to your cardiovascular system to maintain fluid balance. Once the fluid is in the lymphatic vessels, it is called **lymph.**

Fluid Collection

-edema = swelling

The lymphatic system has a network of **lymphatic vessels** similar to veins. Both have valves to prevent backflow. However, your lymphatic vessels form an open-ended, one-way system rather than a circular loop. Your lymphatic system also lacks a pump like the heart. Instead, your skeletal muscles press against your lymphatic vessels to squeeze fluid along as your body moves. Surgery that cuts through lymphatic vessels can interrupt the flow of lymph. This can cause lymphedema, or swelling with excess lymph fluid.

Unfortunately, lymph vessels also provide a route for some diseases to spread. **Cancer** is uncontrolled cell growth. Cancer can occur in any area of the body. It is the second leading cause of death in the United States. *Benign* growths are not cancerous. They may need to be removed if they press on another organ, but are not likely to spread or recur. A hemangioma is a tumor of the blood vessels that grows during infancy but usually shrinks or disappears by 10 years of age without causing harm (**Figure 19.17**).

hem/o = blood
angi/o = blood vessel
-oma = tumor

Malignant growths are cancerous. They are more harmful and tend to spread, or *metastasize,* to new areas in the body. Types of cancer are named for the part of the body where they begin. Metastatic breast cancer, for example, often travels to the bones, brain, liver, or lungs. Cancerous growth of these cells in the bones are still called breast cancer.

meta- = beyond
-stasis = stopping, controlling

Tests, such as a mammogram or colonoscopy, can help detect cancer early, when it is most treatable. The early warning signs of cancer indicate a need for a more complete medical exam. The acronym *CAUTION* will help you remember what to look for:

mamm/o = breast
-gram = record

Change in bowel or bladder habits

A sore that does not heal

Unusual bleeding or discharge

Thickening or a lump in the breast or elsewhere

Indigestion or swallowing difficulties

Obvious change in a wart or mole

Nagging cough or hoarseness

A variety of treatments have been developed for different types of cancer. A mastectomy is a surgical treatment for breast cancer that cuts out part of the breast and nearby lymph nodes, which are examined for cancer cells. This helps determine the best type of treatment. Controlled doses of radiation to damage the cancer cells' DNA treat some tumors. Chemotherapy uses chemicals to destroy fast-growing malignant cells and tissues. Unfortunately, these treatments damage healthy tissues in the process. In addition to searching for a cure, research has focused on avoiding cancer through a healthy lifestyle and vaccinations to prevent some types of cancer.

mast/o = breast
-ectomy = to cut out, surgical removal
chem/o = chemical

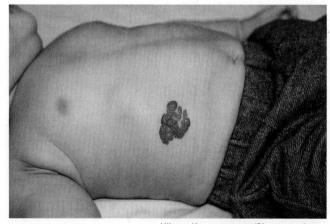

Hilman Kamaruzzaman/Shutterstock.com

Figure 19.17   A hemangioma is one example of a benign growth. *What are some other examples?*

Fat Absorption

Figure 19.18 shows the lymphatic system has many lymphatic vessels. **Lacteals** are specialized lymphatic vessels that pick up digested fats and fat-soluble vitamins in the villi of your small intestine. Vitamins A, E, D, and K are absorbed into the bloodstream through fat. When the fats mix with your lymph, the result is a milky-colored fluid called *chyle* (KI-ihl). This fat- and protein-packed fluid flows into the **cisterna chyli**. This is a large vessel near your midline that collects lymph in the abdomen.

Lymph from your cisterna chyli, lower body, left arm, and chest flows up your **thoracic duct**. This long collection vessel travels from the abdomen to the upper chest, just left of the midline. Your **right lymphatic duct** only collects fluid from your head and right side of your upper body. Both ducts empty lymph into your *subclavian veins* above your heart. In this way, the lymphatic system returns excess fluid and nutrients to your cardiovascular system.

sub- = below, under
clav/o = clavicle
-ian = relating to, one who does

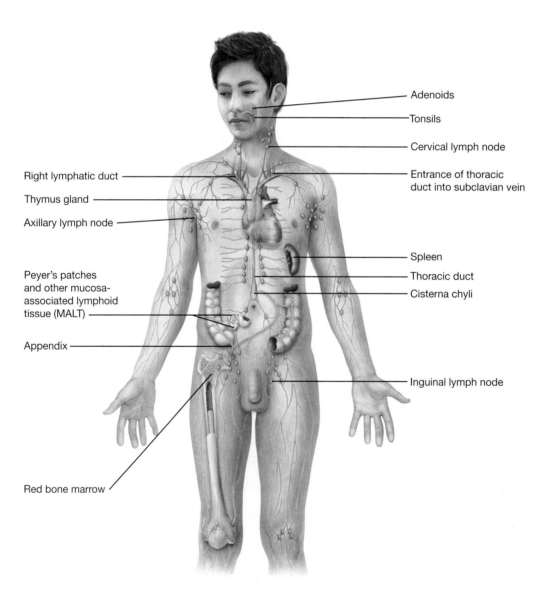

Right lymphatic duct

Thymus gland

Axillary lymph node

Peyer's patches and other mucosa-associated lymphoid tissue (MALT)

Appendix

Red bone marrow

Adenoids

Tonsils

Cervical lymph node

Entrance of thoracic duct into subclavian vein

Spleen

Thoracic duct

Cisterna chyli

Inguinal lymph node

© *Body Scientific International*

Figure 19.18 The organs of the lymphatic system. *What are the functions of the tonsils, thymus gland, and spleen?*

Lymph Filtration

Lymphatic tissues filter and clean interstitial fluid on its way to your cardiovascular system. **Lymph nodes** are small capsules where lymphocytes collect to remove dead cells, destroy pathogens, and create antibodies against infection. These nodes are located in clusters around your body. Cervical lymph nodes cluster along lymph vessels in your neck. You can feel axillary lymph nodes in your armpits. Inguinal (ING-gwuhn-uhl) lymph nodes filter fluid from your legs and pubic region. Swollen lymph nodes are a common sign of infection (**Figure 19.19**). Lymph moves through one or more lymph nodes on its way back to your cardiovascular system.

Some lymphatic tissues are located in mucous membranes. They are not surrounded by a capsule, but have similar functions to lymph nodes. Mucosa-associated lymphoid tissue (MALT) occurs in patches along your intestines. Your **tonsils** and **adenoids** are lymphatic tissues located in the back of your throat and behind your nose, respectively. When these tissues catch invaders, leukocytes rush in, and the tissue becomes enlarged. Some people with repeated infections may have their tonsils removed or adenoids scraped.

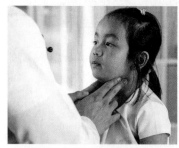

Photographee.eu/Shutterstock.com

Figure 19.19 A doctor might examine your lymph nodes to determine whether you have an infection. *Which three areas of the body have clusters of lymph nodes that can be felt?*

aden/o = gland
-oid = like

Removal and Destruction

Your **spleen** is a lymphatic organ just below your diaphragm on the left side of the stomach. It makes lymphocytes, filters your blood, and removes old and damaged red blood cells. Many macrophages are found in the spleen. In the process of breaking down old cells, the spleen saves iron to be reused in making bilirubin and hemoglobin. Because it can store up to a liter of blood, a ruptured spleen can cause uncontrolled internal bleeding.

Like MALT, your **appendix** also contains lymphoid tissue that can destroy bacteria in the intestines. People used to think this structure attached to the large intestine was a useless digestive organ, but now realize it assists with B-cell and antibody development. It may also play a role in maintaining the population of normal body flora that aid in digestion. There are likely connections between a defective appendix and the development of some inflammatory bowel diseases.

Lesson 19.2 Review

 Complete the *Map Your Reading* graphic organizer for the section you just read.

1. _____ manage the diagnosis, treatment, and prevention of different types of cancer in the body. (19.2-1)
   A. Biotechnologists
   B. Laboratory technicians
   C. Oncologists
   D. Immunologists

2. The body is protected against infection by the _____ system. (19.2-1)
   A. cardiovascular
   B. lymphatic
   C. circulatory
   D. lymphocyte

3. The body's three lines of defense against infection include natural barriers such as mucous membranes, inflammation that brings in leukocytes, and the _____ response that makes antibodies. (19.2-1)
   A. anaphylaxis   C. B-cell
   B. autoimmune   D. immune

4. An important function of the lymphatic organs is to return _____ to the cardiovascular system. (19.2-2)
   A. fluid   C. oxygen
   B. red blood cells   D. carbon dioxide

5. Uncontrolled cell growth is known as (19.2-2)
   A. T-cells   C. inflammation
   B. cancer   D. HIV/AIDS

The Respiratory System

ESSENTIAL QUESTION

What are the structures, functions, and diseases associated with the respiratory system?

Learning Outcomes

After studying this lesson, you will be able to

19.3-1 identify the structures, functions, and diseases of the respiratory system.

19.3-2 explain the two-stage process of respiration.

19.3-3 identify factors that affect respiration rate.

Professional Vocabulary

Essential Terms

respiratory   related to the act of, or organs involved in, breathing

respiration   the movement of oxygen from air to the cells

Important Terms

alveoli	external respiration	sinus cavities
bronchi	internal respiration	total lung capacity
bronchioles	larynx	trachea
cilia	pharynx	
epiglottis	pleurae	

spir/o = breathing, respiration

thorac/o = chest
-ic = pertaining to

ot/o = ear
rhin/o = nose
laryng/o = larynx, voice box
-logist = specialist in the study of

pulmon/o = lung

Introduction

Your **respiratory** system uses your cardiovascular system's network of blood vessels to exchange carbon dioxide (CO_2) for oxygen (O_2) in cells all over your body. For this reason, medical professionals who focus on the respiratory system will often work closely with those in cardiovascular careers. A respiratory therapist provides education, treatment, and rehabilitation for patients with breathing conditions caused by both heart and lung disorders. A thoracic surgeon, also called a *cardiothoracic surgeon*, can diagnose and operate on conditions of the heart, lungs, and esophagus. Both jobs frequently involve consulting with pulmonologists and cardiologists about treatments. They may also use new technology for robotic surgeries to increase precision, remote patient monitoring of oxygen levels, and smart spirometers to track lung function.

The organs of your respiratory system are located in your head and chest. An otorhinolaryngologist (oht-oh-rI-noh-lair-uhn-GAHL-uh-jihst) is a physician who specializes in the diagnosis and treatment of diseases of the ears, nose, and throat (ENT). A pulmonologist specializes in the diagnosis and treatment of lung disorders. Breathing difficulties can be life threatening, which makes their treatment stressful for both patients and caregivers. **Figure 19.20** describes some common diseases of the respiratory system.

Common Diseases and Disorders for the Respiratory System

Characteristics	Asthma	Cystic Fibrosis	Tuberculosis
Etiology	Allergies, physical activity, cold air, stress, or lung irritants may trigger attacks. Origins are unknown, but risk factors include excess weight, exposure to smoke or fumes, having a relative with asthma, or other allergies.	Recessive genetic condition with more than 1,500 known gene mutations that affect the flow of salt and water out of cells. When both parents are carriers, there is a 25% chance child will have CF, and 50% chance the child will be a carrier.	Bacterial infection. Many strains are antibiotic resistant. Risk is higher for people who live in or travel to areas with high rates of TB.
Pathology	Airways narrow and produce mucus, causing wheezing, difficulty breathing, and coughing. Can cause permanent lung damage over time. About 16% of children who are Black and 7% of children who are White have asthma. May be mild to severe and intermittent or persistent.	Lungs and digestive system produce thick and sticky mucus that can clog the lungs and pancreas, causing lung infections and blocking pancreatic enzymes. Shortens the life span, usually ending in respiratory failure by age 30–40. Approximately 1,000 new cases per year, usually under age 2.	Airborne contagious infection, usually affecting the lungs. Latent TB is asymptomatic because the immune system keeps it under control. Active TB causes coughing, blood in sputum, weight loss, fatigue, fever, chills, and loss of appetite.
Diagnosis	Physical exam and lung function test with a spirometer and/or peak flow meter. May also include a methacholine challenge, imaging tests, allergy testing, nitric oxide test, sputum eosinophil test, and/or stress test.	All newborns in the US are screened for CF. Common symptoms are salty skin, persistent cough, shortness of breath, wheezing, nasal polyps, poor weight gain, and mucus in stools.	TB skin test, blood test, or lung X-ray.
Treatment	No cure, but medication and inhaler can control symptoms. Emergency treatment may be needed if symptoms do not improve with inhaler.	No cure, but good nutrition and treatments to thin and remove mucus can extend and improve quality of life. Airway clearance techniques and inhaled medications support lung function. Frequent handwashing, a flu shot, and avoiding smoke and respiratory illnesses are recommended.	Strong antibiotics must be taken for several months to kill all the TB bacteria.
Prevention	The condition cannot be prevented, but attacks can be reduced by taking medication, asthma action plan, getting vaccinated for the flu and pneumonia, avoiding asthma triggers, and monitoring breathing for warning signs.	Genetic testing to identify if either parent carries the gene and choosing whether to have children.	Vaccines are available in some countries. Medications can reduce risk of active TB for those with latent TB. Wear an N95 mask to reduce risk of transmission. If you have active TB, stay home, ventilate the room, and wear a surgical mask to reduce risk for others.

Goodheart-Willcox Publisher

Figure 19.20 Common diseases and disorders of the respiratory system.

19.3-1 Structures, Functions, and Diseases of the Respiratory System

As oxygen moves through your respiratory system, it encounters many different organs (**Figure 19.21**). Oxygen moves from your nose and mouth, down your pharynx. It passes your epiglottis, larynx, and trachea to get to your bronchi, then your bronchioles, and finally your alveoli, which connect with the cardiovascular system to reach every cell in the body. This section will discuss each of these steps in more detail, but this is the basic route.

Mouth and Nose

Air first enters your respiratory system through your mouth and nostrils, also known as the *nares* of the nose. Your nasal septum is a cartilage and bone structure that divides your nasal cavity into right and left chambers. The air from your nasal cavity is funneled through nasal *conchae* (KAHN-kee), which are shaped like spiraled seashells, and into **sinus cavities** within your skull bones. The cavities' mucous membrane linings help warm, filter, and moisten the air you breathe.

Sinus infections cause inflammation of these mucous membranes, which results in congestion, pressure, and pain. Tiny **cilia**, or *hairs*, in your mucous membranes filter out dirt and foreign material, sweeping it toward your throat. A cough or sneeze will eliminate small particles before they can enter your lungs. The common cold is a viral infection of the upper respiratory system that produces symptoms such as coughing, sneezing, and a runny nose.

nas/o = nose
-al = pertaining to
sept/o = wall
-um = structure

sin/o = sinus, cavity
-us = structure

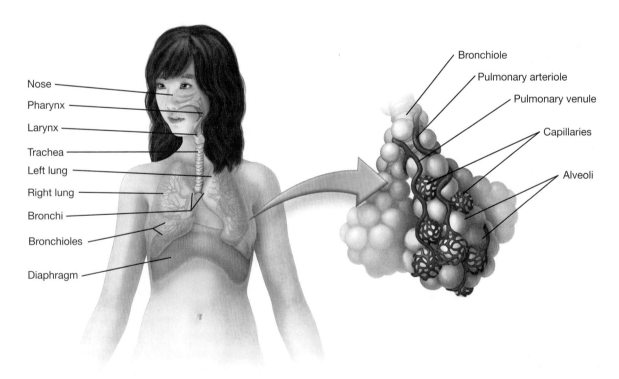

© Body Scientific International

Figure 19.21   The respiratory organs move oxygen to the cells when you take a breath. *Can you name the respiratory organs in the order oxygen passes through them along the route?*

Pharynx

Your **pharynx**, commonly referred to as your *throat*, is divided into three sections (**Figure 19.22**). These include your nasopharynx, oropharynx, and laryngopharynx. Your nasopharynx is located behind your nose and above your uvula, which dangles at the back of your throat. Your oropharynx is located at the back of your oral cavity, below your nasopharynx. Your laryngopharynx is the lower section of your pharynx, located behind your larynx. Lymphatic tissues trap and destroy microbes that make it to your pharynx. These tissues include your adenoids, located at the bottom of your nasopharynx, and your tonsils, located in your oropharynx. Your adenoids and tonsils usually shrink by the time you reach your teens, but they may be removed during childhood if they become too enlarged.

pharyng/o = pharynx, throat
nas/o = nose

or/o = mouth
laryng/o = larynx, voice box

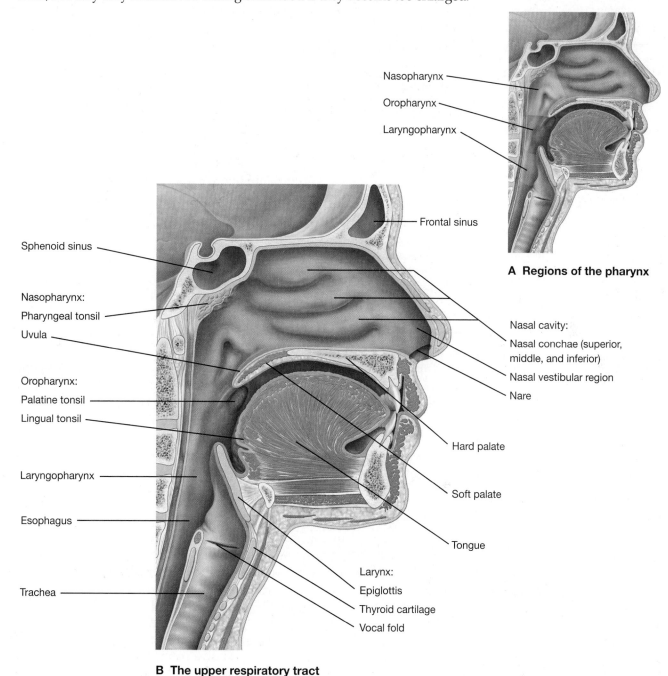

A Regions of the pharynx

B The upper respiratory tract

© *Body Scientific International*

Figure 19.22 The pharynx has three separate sections, each with a different purpose.

Air traveling down to your pharynx shares some of its route with food headed to your esophagus. Food should only use the oropharynx and laryngopharynx. The nasopharynx is intended for air. Sometimes, if you sneeze or laugh while drinking, it may come out your nose rather than go down your throat.

Epiglottis

epi- = upon
glott/o = tongue
-is = pertaining to

Located at the bottom of your pharynx, your **epiglottis** is a flap of cartilage that helps direct food and air down the correct tubes. The tube that leads to your stomach lies behind the trachea that leads to your lungs. Your epiglottis covers the opening to your trachea when you swallow food. If you swallow too quickly, your epiglottis may not have time to close your airway, resulting in food going "down the wrong tube." *Aspiration*, which occurs when food or fluid enters your lungs, can be very serious. An involuntary cough will help clear your trachea or lungs.

a- = without
spir/o = breathing, respiration
-ation = action of, process of

Larynx

Your **larynx**, also known as your *voice box*, contains vocal cords that vibrate to create sounds. When your vocal cords tighten and air flows through your laryngopharynx, your larynx produces sound. Your larynx connects your pharynx in the upper respiratory system with your trachea in the lower respiratory system. Laryngitis is an inflammation of the larynx that causes hoarseness, coughing, and difficulty swallowing. An upper respiratory infection (URI) is any infection of the trachea, larynx, throat, or nose.

laryng/o = larynx, voice box
-itis = inflammation

Trachea

Your **trachea** (TRAY-kee-uh), or *windpipe*, is the tube that leads to your lungs. Air travels from your upper respiratory system through your trachea to reach your lungs. C-shaped cartilage rings in your trachea keep your airway open during pressure changes caused by breathing. Mucous membranes similar to those of your nose and pharynx line your trachea.

Children younger than five years of age have a short, narrow trachea that makes them more susceptible to choking. When the throat swells or the trachea is blocked, a surgical opening can be created in the trachea to allow breathing. This operation is known as a *tracheotomy* (tray-kee-AHT-uh-mee). A tracheostomy tube is inserted between the cartilage rings below the larynx and can connect to a ventilator if breathing support is needed. Because air enters below the larynx and does not pass over the vocal cords, speech is not possible with a tracheotomy.

trache/o = trachea, windpipe
-tomy = to cut into, surgical incision
-stomy = to create an opening

Bronchi and Bronchioles

At the bottom of your trachea, tubes called **bronchi** (BRAHNG-kI) branch out to your left and right lungs. Your bronchi divide into smaller **bronchioles** that lead down to the air sacs in your lungs. A bronchoscope is a flexible, lighted tube that can be equipped with a camera, forceps, and other special tools to examine the inside of your bronchi. Bronchitis is a sudden inflammation of the bronchi that can result from a URI or exposure to irritants in the air. *Asthma*, a chronic allergic disorder, involves a combination of smooth muscle contractions and mucus buildup in the bronchi (**Figure 19.23**). The narrowed airways characteristic of asthma attacks cause coughing, wheezing, and breathlessness. Treatments include medications and avoiding triggers that cause flare-ups.

bronchi/o = bronchus
-ole = small
scop/e = to view
-e = instrument
-itis = inflammation

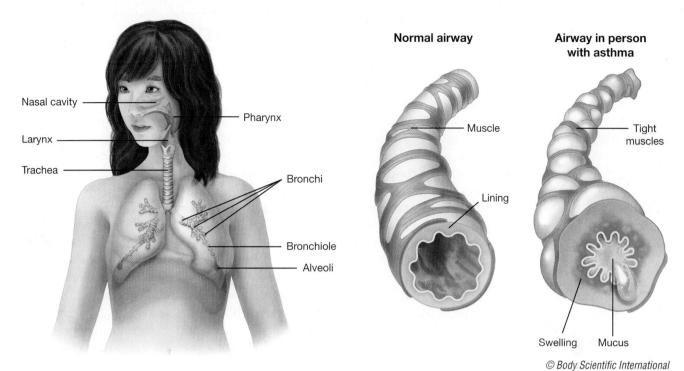

Normal airway

Nasal cavity

Pharynx

Larynx

Trachea

Bronchi

Bronchiole

Alveoli

Muscle

Lining

Airway in person with asthma

Tight muscles

Swelling   Mucus

© Body Scientific International

Figure 19.23   When a person has an asthma attack, the bronchi become swollen and mucus builds up, blocking the airways.

Alveoli

alveol/o = cavity, socket

Oxygen and carbon dioxide are exchanged in capillaries surrounding your **alveoli**. These are tiny, hollow air sacs clustered like bunches of grapes at the ends of your bronchioles. Your alveoli have elastic membranes that can expand and return to their regular size as air moves in and out. Infection and disease can destroy alveoli, making it difficult to exchange oxygen and carbon dioxide.

Chronic obstructive pulmonary disease (COPD) is a category of long-term lung disorders that reduce airflow. Two of the most common forms of COPD are emphysema and chronic bronchitis. People who have long-term exposure to airborne irritants, such as tobacco smoke, can develop emphysema. This causes the alveoli to lose their elasticity and rupture, leaving holes in the lung tissue. People with this condition take shallow breaths and have little room in their lungs for exchanging fresh air. Tuberculosis (TB) is a contagious disease caused by tiny, airborne bacteria that most often infect the lungs. It destroys alveoli and leaves scar tissue in their place. Pressurized oxygen flowing from a tank can help relieve the feeling of breathlessness for people with COPD (**Figure 19.24**).

Alveoli provide more surface area for gas exchange than one large, hollow lung. If all your air sacs were spread out flat, they would cover an area the size of a tennis court. Infants have fewer and much smaller alveoli, resulting in a faster breathing rate and less lung volume than adults. Pneumonia (noo-MOH-nyuh) also causes a faster breathing rate, because a buildup of fluid in the lungs reduces the surface area available for air exchange. A bubbling or rattling sound in the lungs, called *rales*, can be heard with a stethoscope when fluid or secretions are present. Pneumonia can be life threatening in infants and older adults.

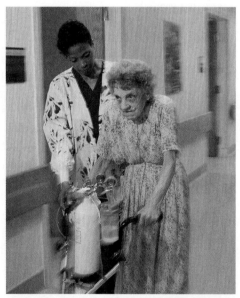

Stockbyte/Stockbyte/Thinkstock

Figure 19.24   Patients who have COPD sometimes use an oxygen tank to help them breathe.

pneumon/o = lung, air
-ia = abnormal condition

19.3-2 The Two-Stage Process of Respiration

re- = back, again
spir/o = breathing, respiration
-ation = action of, process of
ex- = out, away from
alveol/o = cavity, socket

The movement of oxygen from air to your cells, or **respiration**, occurs in two stages. **External respiration** happens in your lungs. This is when capillaries surrounding your alveoli absorb oxygen from the air in your lungs and release carbon dioxide from your blood. Your heart transports this oxygen from your lungs to other areas of your body. **Internal respiration** happens in capillary beds throughout your body. In this stage, carbon dioxide in your cells is exchanged for oxygen from your blood. External respiration happens during the pulmonary loop of your cardiovascular system. Internal respiration happens during the systemic loop of your cardiovascular system.

pulmon/o = lung
-ary = pertaining to

Oxygen and carbon dioxide are exchanged with your cardiovascular system during respiration. The thin walls of your capillaries allow gases to move in and out of your blood vessels. Carbon dioxide is released from your blood to the alveoli in your lungs, and new oxygen is taken in through the alveoli to blood in your capillaries. Then, your cardiovascular system transports this oxygen to your cells. Finally, your cardiovascular system collects carbon dioxide produced in your cells and sends it back to your lungs to be released from your body. A full cycle of respiration includes one inhalation and one exhalation (**Figure 19.25**).

During inhalation, oxygen-rich air is sucked into your lungs. Your lungs are a pressurized system surrounded by membranes, or **pleurae**. A visceral pleura covers each lung's surface. A parietal pleura lines your chest wall inside each pleural cavity. A lubricating fluid fills the pleural space between the two membranes to prevent friction as they slide against each other during respiration.

viscer/o = internal organ
-al = pertaining to
pleur/o = side, rib
pariet/o = wall
inter- = between
cost/o = rib

Contraction of your diaphragm, intercostal muscles, and abdominal muscles pull and expand your parietal pleurae. This pressure pulls and expands your visceral pleurae, which in turn pull and expand your alveoli to suck air into your lungs. A hiccup is a sudden contraction of the diaphragm that causes you to suck air in quickly. During exhalation, your diaphragm relaxes, and your ribcage compresses to force carbon dioxide out of your alveoli and complete the respiratory cycle.

pneum/o = lung, air
thorac/o = chest

Your lungs would collapse without the pressurized system created by your pleural membranes. A collapsed lung, or *pneumothorax* (noo-muh-THOR-aks), occurs when a pleural membrane is punctured or the space between the membranes fills with fluid. Without the negative pressure in this lined pleural cavity, the inner surfaces of the lungs would stick to themselves and cause difficulty breathing, or *dyspnea* (DISP-nee-uh). Fluid in the pleural cavity presses on the lungs and takes up space that would have been filled by air. Thoracentesis (thoh-ruh-sehn-TEE-suhs) uses a needle or tube to drain the air or fluid from the pleural cavity so the collapsed lung can expand again.

dys- = bad, difficult, painful
-pnea = breathing
thorac/o = chest
-centesis = surgical puncture

19.3-3 Variation in Respiratory Rate and Volume

Your respiratory rate is involuntarily controlled by your brain stem. Although you can consciously change your breathing rate, your body cannot store extra oxygen and requires a certain amount to continue functioning. Adults need to continue breathing an average of 1 pint of air about 12 to 20 times per minute. Infants have less surface area in the lungs and may breathe as many as 30 to 60 times per minute. Your respiratory rate naturally increases during exercise and illness and may decrease slightly during sleep.

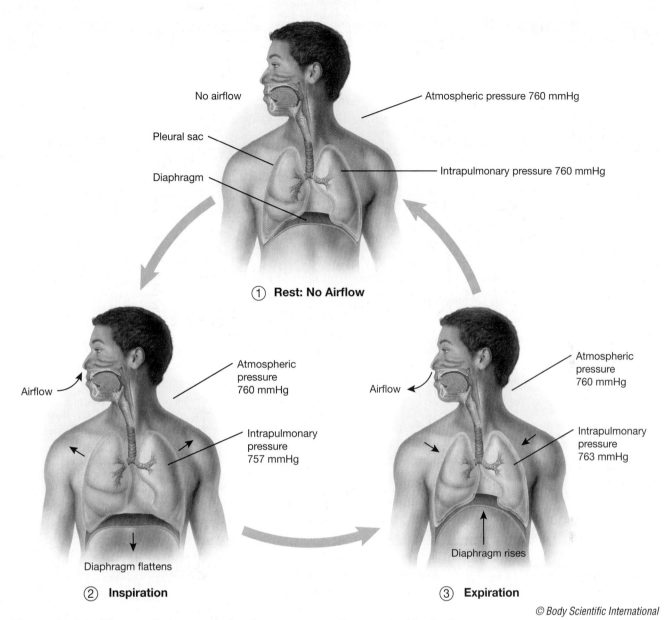

No airflow

Pleural sac

Diaphragm

Atmospheric pressure 760 mmHg

Intrapulmonary pressure 760 mmHg

① **Rest: No Airflow**

Airflow

Atmospheric pressure 760 mmHg

Intrapulmonary pressure 757 mmHg

Diaphragm flattens

② **Inspiration**

Airflow

Atmospheric pressure 760 mmHg

Intrapulmonary pressure 763 mmHg

Diaphragm rises

③ **Expiration**

© Body Scientific International

Figure 19.25 The respiratory cycle involves pressure changes inside the lungs.

Abnormal Breathing

Bradypnea (bray-DIP-nee-uh), an abnormally slow breathing rate, may result from damage to the heart. Apnea, when breathing stops temporarily, is often present in premature babies and adults who have obesity or are near the end of life. Hypoxia is a lack of oxygen. During hypoxia, a buildup of carbon dioxide in the blood triggers the brain to increase respiratory rate and volume.

brady- = slow
-pnea = breathing
a- = without

hypo- = below, under
ox/y = oxygen
-ia = abnormal condition

Lung Volume

Each breath moves air in and out of your lungs, but your lungs are never completely empty. **Total lung capacity** is the amount of air your lungs can hold when you take your deepest possible breath. This includes your *vital lung capacity* that can be exhaled after your deepest breath, plus your *residual volume* that remains in your lungs and airways after your strongest exhalation (**Figure 19.26**).

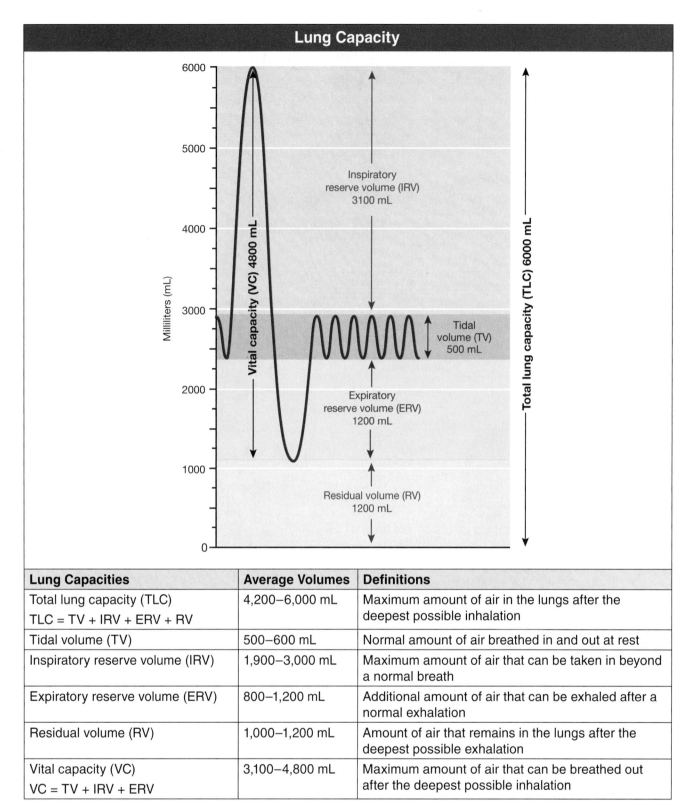

Lung Capacity

Lung Capacities	Average Volumes	Definitions
Total lung capacity (TLC) TLC = TV + IRV + ERV + RV	4,200–6,000 mL	Maximum amount of air in the lungs after the deepest possible inhalation
Tidal volume (TV)	500–600 mL	Normal amount of air breathed in and out at rest
Inspiratory reserve volume (IRV)	1,900–3,000 mL	Maximum amount of air that can be taken in beyond a normal breath
Expiratory reserve volume (ERV)	800–1,200 mL	Additional amount of air that can be exhaled after a normal exhalation
Residual volume (RV)	1,000–1,200 mL	Amount of air that remains in the lungs after the deepest possible exhalation
Vital capacity (VC) VC = TV + IRV + ERV	3,100–4,800 mL	Maximum amount of air that can be breathed out after the deepest possible inhalation

Goodheart-Willcox Publisher

Figure 19.26 This table shows lung capacities, as well as their average volumes and descriptions.

spir/o = breathing, respiration
-meter = measure

Tidal volume is the amount of air breathed in and out during light breathing while your body is at rest. This is a very small exchange of air in comparison to total lung volume, because resting does not require a lot of oxygen. A *spirometer* can measure respiratory rates and volumes.

Although residual volume cannot be exhaled, that air is important to the function of your lungs. It helps keep the inner surfaces of your lungs from sticking to each other, so it is easy for them to refill with the next breath. Just think how much easier it is to add air to a balloon that is half full than blow that first breath into a brand-new balloon that is not yet inflated. Residual volume also provides enough air for the Heimlich maneuver to force an object out of the throat when a person is choking.

Factors Affecting Lung Volume

Age, sex, body size, and physical condition affect lung volume. Your right lung is shorter, broader, and has greater volume than your left. It is also divided into three lobes. Your left lung has only two lobes to allow room for your heart. The surface area of your lungs decreases with age, which raises the respiratory rate in older adults. The number of cilia that protect your lungs from irritants declines with age at the same time mucus production increases. These changes, in addition to reduced mobility and immune status, leave older adults more susceptible to respiratory infections and aspiration.

Adults and those physically fit will have greater lung volume than infants, older adults, or those who are out of shape. Regular physical activity increases your total lung capacity and vital capacity, but body size is the main factor in determining residual volume. In old age, the lungs become stiffer, and respiratory muscle strength decreases (**Figure 19.27**). This decreases the vital capacity and expiratory reserve volume. Lungs usually reach their maximum capacity in early adulthood and then decline with age.

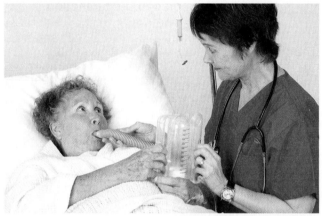
Lisa F. Young/Shutterstock.com

Figure 19.27 A manual incentive spirometer can be used to exercise and strengthen the lungs.

Lesson 19.3 Review

 Complete the *Map Your Reading* graphic organizer for the section you just read.

1. The respiratory system uses the _____ to exchange gases with cells all around your body. (19.3-1)
   A. lymphatic system
   B. cardiovascular system
   C. muscular system
   D. skeletal system

2. Which of the following is *not* part of the path oxygen takes to get to the cells? (19.3-1)
   A. Pharynx   C. Alveoli
   B. Bronchi   D. Esophagus

3. The process of respiration exchanges oxygen for (19.3-2)
   A. hydrogen   C. carbon dioxide
   B. liquid   D. fluids and gases

4. _____ respiration occurs in the systemic loop. (19.3-2)
   A. Internal   C. Upper
   B. External   D. Lower

5. During _____, the diaphragm muscles contract to expand the lungs and pull air in. (19.3-3)
   A. hypoxia
   B. aspiration
   C. exhalation
   D. inspiration

6. Factors that affect respiratory rate include age, sex, body size, and (19.3-3)
   A. exercise   C. diet
   B. location   D. ethnicity

Chapter 19 Review and Assessment

Chapter Summary

19.1-1 The cardiovascular, respiratory, and lymphatic systems work with other body systems to transport and exchange materials in the body. The heart, blood vessels, and blood cells are the main organs of the cardiovascular system. Blood follows the ABO blood typing system. Hemoglobin in the red blood cells carries oxygen. White blood cells provide antibodies to fight infection. Plasma carries nutrients, gases, hormones, and waste. Platelets help blood clot.

19.1-2 Oxygenated blood flows out of the heart under pressure through arteries. Gas exchange occurs through the thin walls of capillaries. Deoxygenated blood returns to the heart through veins, using valves to prevent backward flow.

19.1-3 Valves within the heart help control the flow of blood. Coronary blood vessels provide oxygen and nutrients for the heart muscle.

19.1-4 The heart's electrical system triggers pumping of the heart. The rhythm of the blood flow is pulse. The pressure created in the blood vessels is blood pressure. Blood flow also affects temperature and rate of respirations.

19.2-1 The lymphatic system has several defenses against infections. Natural barriers are the first line of defense. Inflammation and leukocytes provide a second line of defense. The immune response helps the body adapt to fighting new infections as a third line of defense.

19.2-2 The lymphatic system provides another type of circulation in your body. Lymphatic vessels return interstitial fluid to the cardiovascular system. Lymph nodes and lymphatic tissues filter this fluid along the way.

19.3-1 The respiratory system uses the cardiovascular system's network of blood vessels to exchange carbon dioxide for oxygen in the lungs. These gases flow through the nose and mouth, pharynx, larynx, trachea, bronchi, bronchioles, and alveoli to blood vessels that transport them to cells all over the body.

19.3-2 Respiration and circulation occur in two stages: external respiration in the lungs and internal respiration in body cells.

19.3-3 When the diaphragm and ribcage muscles contract during inspiration, air is sucked into the lungs. When the muscles relax or the ribs are forced downward, air is exhaled.

19.3-3 Breathing is both voluntarily and involuntarily controlled. Respiratory rate and volume are affected by age, sex, body size, and health status.

Maximize Your Professional Vocabulary

1. **Body Labels.** Attach a length of bulletin board paper to a wall or floor. Have someone trace around you on the paper. Inside the tracing, draw the outline of the major cardiovascular, lymphatic, and respiratory organs. Place as many of the professional vocabulary terms on the drawing as possible. Be prepared to explain why the unused terms cannot be shown on the drawing.

2. **Term Bingo.** Make flash cards for each word part listed. Shuffle your cards and pull out 25 at random. Arrange them in a 5x5 grid with the term side up. Have one person shuffle their set of flash cards, then draw one at a time and call out the definition. If you have the matching term on your grid, turn the card over. When you have five in a row (horizontally, vertically, or diagonally) or four corners and the center, call out "BINGO." Verify your matching definitions to show you have won.

Prefixes

an-	brady-	mono-	re-
anti-	inter-	per-	tachy-
auto-	macro-	pro-	tri-

Root Words

aden/o	cusp/o	mast/o	pneumon/o
alveol/o	electr/o	nas/o	rhin/o
angi/o	embol/o	onc/o	rrhythm/o
arteri/o	glott/o	or/o	scler/o
ather/o	glutin/o	ot/o	sept/o
atri/o	hem/o	ox/y	sin/o
bronchi/o	immun/o	pariet/o	spir/o
cephal/o	laryng/o	phag/o	thromb/o
chem/o	leuk/o	pharyng/o	tox/i
clav/o	lun/o	phleb/o	trache/o
coron/o	lymph/o	phylax/o	vascul/o
cost/o	mamm/o	pneum/o	ven/o

Suffixes

-crit	-globin	-ine	-rrhage
-e	-gram	-meter	-stomy
-ectomy	-graph	-oid	-tomy
-edema	-ia	-ole	-ty
-emia	-ian	-oma	-ule
-fusion	-id	-pnea	-us

Reflect on Your Reading

1. Review the vocabulary organizer you created for the *Connect with Your Reading* activity. Now that you have read the chapter, do you feel you better understand the terms in your *New Terms* column? Explain each of those terms in your own words and share with a classmate.

Review and Recall

1. Hemoglobin on _____ is essential for transporting oxygen in the blood. (19.1-1)
   A. erythrocytes
   B. hemocytes
   C. leukocytes
   D. thrombocytes

2. The _____ is your largest artery, carrying blood from your heart out to your body. (19.1-2)
   A. vena cava
   B. capillary
   C. aorta
   D. arteriole

3. Your heart is a pump with how many chambers? (19.1-3)
   A. Two
   B. Three
   C. Four
   D. Five

4. The cardiac cycle has two parts: a contraction of the heart muscle followed by a _____ of the heart muscle. (19.1-4)
   A. stiffening
   B. palpitation
   C. pulse
   D. relaxation

5. The lymphatic system is your body's main defense against _____, so it is important to the health of all your other body systems. (19.2-1)
   A. pathogens
   B. immunity
   C. flora
   D. inflammation

6. Blood plasma that remains between your cells after delivering its oxygen, nutrients, and hormones is called _____ fluid. (19.2-2)
   A. lymph
   B. vessel
   C. intracellular
   D. interstitial

7. You can remember general cancer warning signs by using the acronym (19.2-2)
   A. *BEWARE*
   B. *CAUTION*
   C. *DANGER*
   D. *WARNING*

8. Tiny _____ in your mucous membranes filter out dirt and foreign material, sweeping it toward your throat. (19.3-1)
   A. cilia
   B. nares
   C. conchae
   D. septum

9. The organs of your respiratory system are located in your (19.3-1)
   A. torso and abdomen
   B. mouth and throat
   C. ears and nose
   D. head and chest

10. _____ respiration is when capillaries surrounding your alveoli absorb oxygen from the air in your lungs and release carbon dioxide from your blood. (19.3-2)
    A. Internal
    B. External
    C. Lower
    D. Upper

11. What does the prefix *brady-* mean in the word *bradypnea*? (19.3-3)
    A. Breathing
    B. Oxygen
    C. Below normal
    D. Slow

Build Core Skills

1. **Problem Solving.** On a separate sheet of paper or document, create a three-column chart. Label the columns: *Problem*, *Cause*, and *Effect*. Then research three diseases—one each from the respiratory, cardiovascular, and lymphatic systems—and fill in the chart with the information you find.

2. **Reading.** Search the internet for the American Cancer Society's Tools and Calculators. Take one of the cancer quizzes and read the feedback. With this information, write a paragraph explaining the risks and what lifestyle changes you can make to decrease your risk of this type of cancer.

3. **Writing.** Imagine that you are a lung. Write a letter of complaint to a cigarette that focuses on the effects of smoking.

4. **Math.** Calculate your maximum heart rate during exercise by subtracting your age from 220. Then, calculate your target running heart rate by counting your pulse for one minute while your body is at rest and subtract that from your maximum heart rate. The next time you are exercising, stop and check your pulse to see if your workout is at an appropriate level of intensity.

5. **Critical Thinking.** Although 1 pound of fat does not look like much on the outside, it adds a mile of new blood vessels. Explain why a person with severe obesity is more likely to die from a sudden heart attack. Why would you expect the heart of a person with severe obesity to be enlarged when examined in an autopsy?

Activate Your Learning

1. To simulate what happens in the body of a person with anemia, create two lines of students—one to represent a person with anemia and one to represent a person with normal levels of hemoglobin. Each line will have a basket of tennis balls (oxygen) that must be carried from their baskets (lungs) on one side of the room to another set of baskets on the other side of the room (body cells). Students in the anemia line may carry one tennis ball at a time. Students in the other line can each carry up to four tennis balls at once. When all the tennis balls have been transported, discuss your observations. How much longer did it take the anemia line to get the oxygen to the cells? Oxygen is used in the cellular process of creating energy. Which line was more tired at the end of the activity? Discuss the effects of anemia on the body.

2. Using painter's tape, create a large outline of a heart on the floor. Add the heart chambers, valves, and vessels using Figure 19.9 as a guide. Practice walking the path of blood through your heart and naming the structures as you pass them. Add baskets at the pulmonary artery, pulmonary vein, aorta, and vena cava. Use red and blue balls to show where you pick up and drop off oxygen and carbon dioxide.

3. Use the following items to create a model of the lymphatic system, then explain what each item represents and why: straws, funnel, coffee filter, marshmallows, and assorted candies or jellybeans.

4. Use these instructions to create a model of a lung that inflates through negative pressure. You will need a 2-liter soda bottle, 8-inch piece of plastic wrap, large rubber band, small rubber band, round balloon, and 4-inch strip of tape.
   • Cut the soda bottle in half and keep the top half of the bottle.
   • Blow up the balloon and let the air out once or twice to stretch it out a little, then insert the bottom of the balloon into the mouth of the soda bottle and turn the balloon's lip over onto the top of the soda bottle opening.

- Hold the balloon edge in place with the small rubber band. Place the plastic wrap over the cut bottom of the soda bottle to cover the large opening and secure it in place with the large rubber band.
- Fold the tape in half and stick the center together but leave the two ends separated. Stick these two ends to the center of the plastic wrap, allowing the center of the tape to stick out like a small handle.
- Now, gently pull on the tape handle and watch the balloon expand. Release or press in and watch the balloon deflate. Label each part of the model with the respiratory system organ that it represents.

5. Go to the American Lung Association's website for breathing exercises in the lung health and wellness section. Read the information and try the breathing exercises. Explain which structures of the respiratory system are affected by the exercises and how this helps with breathing.

Think and Act Like a Healthcare Worker

1. You are working at a healthcare clinic when a man walks in from the parking lot. He is pulling at the collar of his shirt and sweating. He says he cannot catch his breath. He stumbles and grabs for the counter to steady himself. What are some logical assumptions about his health condition? What vital signs would assist in assessing his condition? What should you do?

2. You are working in a nursing home. A resident has taken his socks off because his foot was itchy. Now he wants help putting his socks and shoes back on. You notice that one foot has some odor and feels warmer to the touch than the other foot. It is also a little harder to fit the shoe on this foot. What are you suspecting may be wrong? What should you do?

3. You are in the hospital cafeteria eating lunch. A person at the next table is grasping their throat area and coughing. You recognize the signs of choking, call for help, and go to assist. You encourage the person to stay calm and keep coughing. How do you know when the airway is completely blocked and you should begin abdominal thrusts or chest compressions?

Go to the Source

1. Go to the American Heart Association's website on Congenital Heart Defects. On the "learn more" link you will find a review of normal heart function and a list of congenital heart defects. Select one of the conditions and review the information. Draw and describe how the anatomy of the heart for this condition varies from a normal heart.

2. Go to the American Lung Association's website for Lung Disease Lookup. Select one of the respiratory conditions to study. Create a poster showing the disease's symptoms, causes, and treatment options.

3. Go to the website for the National Institute of Allergy and Infectious Diseases. Use the dropdown menu on the left to view the list of Diseases & Conditions. Select a disease or condition and read one of the articles. Summarize the main point and list three important facts you learned.

HOSA Event Prep: HOSA Bowl

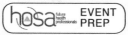

Susy is a 50-year-old female who began to experience severe right upper quadrant and epigastric pain. It started three months ago when she ate greasy or spicy food. Now it seems to be with every meal, and she experiences pain and nausea. One night as she was ready to go to bed, she began to have severe chest pain and epigastric pain. Fearing she was having a heart attack, she called 911 and was rushed to the ER. Upon arrival, her pain was an 8 on a pain scale from 1-10. Her EKG (electrocardiogram) and cardiac enzymes were normal; however, her amylase and lipase were elevated significantly. She also had an elevated white blood cell count. Due to her pain over the last three months, the ER doctor admits her and makes her NPO ("nothing by mouth") and schedules a gallbladder scan. Her scan showed significant sludge and cholelithiasis. They schedule Susy for a laparoscopic cholecystectomy.

Think About It

1. Which test determined that Susy was not having a heart attack?
2. Which abbreviation indicates a diet restriction?
3. Name an organ located in the right upper quadrant.
4. What is the meaning of the root word in *cardiac*?
5. What is the medical term that means "white blood cell"?

Chapter 20
Body Systems for Regulation and Communication

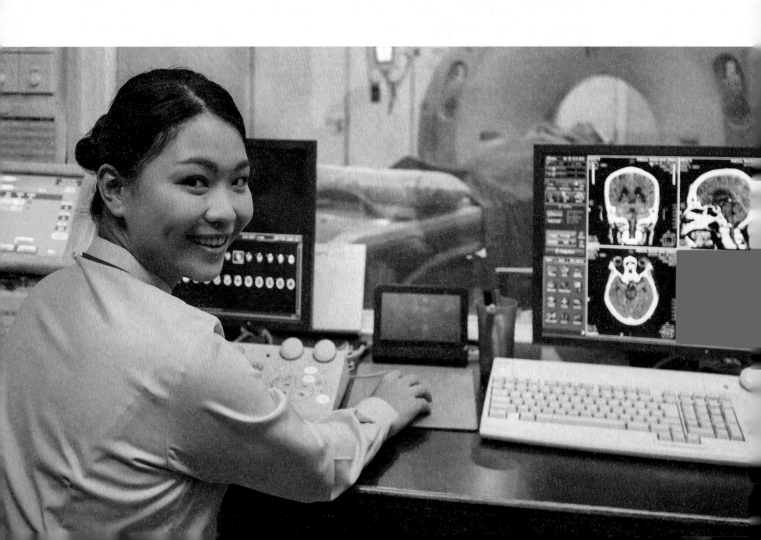

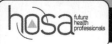

HOSA Event Prep: Behavioral Health

Holistic health is an approach to medicine that treats the whole person. To be truly healthy, one must look at the whole self. According to the Centers for Disease Control and Prevention (CDC), mental and physical health are equal components of overall health. Mental health is recognized in the HOSA—Future Health Professionals *Behavioral Health* event. This event tests your knowledge of the mind, psychology, behavioral health, related disorders, and their treatment and prevention.

Go to the HOSA website to learn more about the HOSA *Behavioral Health* event. Find out the purpose of the event, what is involved in the event, and what knowledge is demonstrated in the event.

As you prepare for HOSA competitive events, be sure to check the website and talk with your HOSA advisor for the most up-to-date guidelines and procedures. Once you have learned about the *Behavioral Health* event, answer the following questions:

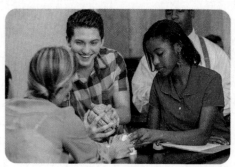

1. How might participating in this event benefit you personally and your future career? Explain.
2. Are you interested in participating in this event? Why or why not?

SDI Productions/E+ via Getty Images

Connect with Your Reading

Content about body systems is typically dense with new terms and information. As you read, questions may occur to you, but you may not have someone available to answer them. At other times, you may be so confused or overwhelmed you find yourself just reading without thinking. Asking questions as you read is a helpful tool to understand what you are reading.

Place a sticky note next to each main heading in the text or use comments if you read online. Before you read a section, create a question that prepares you for reading. These are commonly "who, what, when, why, or how" questions. You will find their answers in the text as you read, and the questions will serve as a review.

Leave space for at least one deeper question from the chapter as well. This is a question not answered by reading the text. It requires you to think about the information in a different way or add information from another source. It may be a good question to research further or ask in class to gain deeper understanding.

Map Your Reading

Make a tablet organizer with two sheets of paper using the example shown. Stack the sheets, keeping the side edges even, but move the top sheet of paper up so its bottom edge is ½ inch to 1 inch above the bottom edge of the sheet below it. Holding both sheets of paper, fold them down so the top edge of the top sheet is ½ to 1 inch above the bottom edge of the top sheet. Crease both layers and staple at the top folded edge. Write *Systems for Regulation and Communication* on the outside flap and list ways that body systems communicate with each other and the outside environment to control body functions. Label the edges of the flaps below it with the headings *Nervous System*, *Special Senses*, and *Endocrine System*. As you read, add visual cues, definitions of new terms, and notes on the main functions, careers, and diseases related to each system.

Systems for Regulation and Communication
hearing   touch   hormones
vision   smell   taste
speech/words
body language/actions
NERVOUS SYSTEM
SPECIAL SENSES
ENDOCRINE SYSTEM

Goodheart-Willcox Publisher

Chapter opener image: xavierarnau/iStock/Getty Images Plus via Getty Images

The Nervous System

Learning Outcomes

After studying this lesson, you will be able to

20.1-1 explain how the nervous system communicates with and regulates other body systems.

20.1-2 describe the structure of a neuron and how neurons transmit signals.

20.1-3 summarize the structures and functions of the central nervous system, including associated diseases and disorders.

20.1-4 analyze the roles of structures that protect the central nervous system, including associated diseases and disorders.

20.1-5 explain the purpose of the glymphatic system in supporting the brain.

20.1-6 summarize the structures and functions of the peripheral nervous system, including associated diseases and disorders.

Professional Vocabulary

Essential Terms

central nervous system (CNS)   the brain and spinal cord

cerebrum   the largest part of the brain, which is formed by the four lobes of the cerebral cortex

homeostasis   a state of balance between interdependent elements

neuron   a nerve cell

neurotransmitter   a chemical used to carry a signal from an axon to a receptor cell to pass along a message

peripheral nervous system (PNS)   the sensory and motor nerves that go out to the body's extremities

Important Terms

axon
brainstem
cell body
cerebellum
cerebral cortex
cranial nerves
dendrites
frontal lobes
ganglion
glial cells

hypothalamus
innervate
limbic system
meninges
myelin
occipital lobes
parietal lobes
plexus
primary motor cortex
spinal nerve

synapse
temporal lobes
terminal branches
thalamus

Introduction

The nervous system, special senses, and endocrine system support your body's regulation and communication mechanisms. Their interconnections are complex, and these systems connect to the functions of many other body systems. **Figure 20.1** presents a few of the diseases and disorders related to these systems. You will explore many other conditions as you learn the structures and functions of each system.

Common Diseases and Disorders for Body Systems of Regulation and Communication				
Characteristics	Cataracts	Concussion/ Traumatic Brain Injury	Diabetes Mellitus	Dementia
Etiology	Can occur at any age because of a variety of causes, including genetics, past eye injury, infection, radiation exposure, UV light, or use of corticosteroids or diuretics. Risks increase with old age, diabetes, smoking, and excessive drinking. The exact reason cataracts form is unknown.	Caused by a bump, blow, or jolt to the head or a hit to the body that causes the head and brain to move rapidly back and forth, damaging brain cells and releasing chemicals that affect brain function. One-half are due to falls. More than 170,000 are sports- or recreation-related.	A metabolic disease with genetic and environmental factors. Affects ability to move sugar from the blood into cells for energy or storage. Type 1 is an autoimmune disorder that destroys insulin-producing cells in the pancreas. Type 2 involves resistance to insulin. In gestational diabetes the placenta produces insulin-blocking hormones.	A group of symptoms, including cognitive decline and impaired memory associated with a variety of disease processes. Caused by brain cell death and neurodegenerative disease. It most commonly affects older adults.
Pathology	Painless, progressive clouding of the lens in the eye where proteins have broken down and clumped together. Over time, the cataract gets more severe, interfering with everyday activities. Causes blurry vision, faded colors, sensitivity to light, trouble seeing at night, double vision, and a halo around lights. Leading cause of vision loss in the US and of blindness worldwide.	Possible loss of consciousness, dizziness, clumsy movement, confusion, forgetfulness, slowed thinking, inability to concentrate, changes in vision, sensitivity to light or noise, depressed mood, headaches, nausea, or vomiting for a few days to weeks. Repeated TBIs increase chances of further damage.	Causes increased hunger and thirst, unexplained weight loss, frequent urination, blurred vision, extreme fatigue, sores that are slow to heal, recurring infections. Symptoms are often not noticed. High blood sugar can damage nerves, eyes, kidneys, and other organs.	Progresses in stages from mild cognitive impairment and forgetfulness, to mild dementia that impacts daily life, to moderate dementia that affects mood and activities of daily living, then severe dementia that affects communication, bladder and body control. Some types are terminal, while others can be resolved by curing the cause.

Goodheart-Willcox Publisher

Figure 20.1   Common diseases and disorders of the systems for regulation and communication. (continued)

Characteristics	Cataracts	Concussion/ Traumatic Brain Injury	Diabetes Mellitus	Dementia
Diagnosis	Slit-lamp microscopy to view the lens. Dilated eye exam to view the back of the eye.	Cognitive tests for verbal and visual memory, brain processing speed, and reaction time. Neurovestibular exam for balance, hearing or vision conditions. Brain imaging tests for bruising or bleeding.	Fasting plasma glucose test, A1C test, glucose challenge test, or oral glucose tolerance test.	Cognitive dementia tests or mini-mental state examination, observations of relatives or caregivers, routine blood tests, and a CT brain scan to rule out other causes.
Treatment	Initially able to use magnifying lenses and brighter lights for reading and other activities. Cataract surgery to replace the cloudy lens with an artificial intraocular lens improves vision for 9 out of 10 people.	Rest often, limiting physical and thinking activities. When symptoms are mild and nearly gone, gradually return to most regular activities with breaks if symptoms worsen. See a doctor before returning to competitive sports.	No cure, but can be managed with proper diet and physical activity to control blood sugar levels and insulin or medication. Effects of diabetes will need to be managed through medical care. Regular testing of blood sugar determines the amount of insulin needed.	Drugs may slow the progress of degenerative dementia. Brain training and memory aids may improve cognitive function in early stages. If the underlying cause is untreatable, the focus becomes managing care and symptoms.
Prevention	Use sunglasses with UV protection. Block sun with a hat brim. Quit smoking. Eat plenty of fruits and vegetables, especially dark, leafy greens. Keep diabetes under control. Limit alcohol. Get a dilated eye exam at least once every two years to watch for issues.	Use gates at the top and bottom of stairs to prevent serious falls, correct car seats for a child's age and weight, soft landing surfaces on playgrounds, right type and size of helmet for sports, and follow guidelines for sports restrictions after a brain injury.	Type 1 is not preventable, but some causes of type 2 and gestational diabetes can be controlled through physical activity and a diet low in fat and refined carbohydrates and high in fiber. Eat smaller portions and try to lose weight if overweight.	Some risk factors can be controlled: smoking, alcohol use, atherosclerosis, high cholesterol, and diabetes. Maintain a healthy weight, eat a healthy diet, get regular physical activity, and engage in regular mental and social activity.

20.1-1 Regulation and Communication in the Body

Your body has two main systems of communication—your nervous system and endocrine system. Your nervous system gathers information through your five senses, processes and stores that information, and responds to it. Your nervous system also provides centralized control for rapid and coordinated responses. It gathers information through your sensory system and carries messages back to your body through electrochemical impulses. Your endocrine system uses chemical messengers to control your body systems. The response of your endocrine system is generally slower and longer acting. Both systems work together to regulate your body functions and maintain balance, or **homeostasis**, within your body.

sensor/i = sensation
-y = process

home/o = same
-stasis = stopping, controlling

The nervous system serves as your body's main control system. It connects and directs all other body systems. Neurosurgery, which deals with structures of the nervous system, is one of the most specialized areas of medicine. Neurosurgeons benefit from advances such as microsurgery and functional brain imaging. Microsurgery makes it possible to repair small nerves and blood vessels. Functional magnetic resonance imaging (fMRI) can show which areas of the brain are active in different situations, as well as the anatomy of brain growth and tumors (**Figure 20.2**). Biotechnology and genetic engineering promise new advances for repairing vertebrae and regrowing spinal nerves.

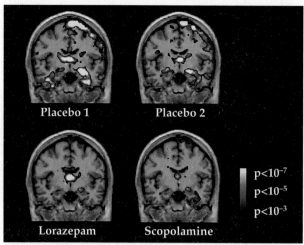

Sperling, R., D. Greve, A. Dale, R. Killiany, J. Holmes, H. Rosas, A. Cocchiarella, P. Firth, B. Rosen, S. Lake, N. Lange, C. Routledge, and M. Albert. "Functional MRI Detection of Pharmacologically Induced Memory Impairment." Proceedings of the National Academy of Sciences 99.1 (2002): 455-60. Web. Copyright 2002 National Academy of Sciences, U.S.A.

Figure 20.2 Functional magnetic resonance imaging (fMRI) shows activity in the brain under different conditions. *What might fMRI technology be used to diagnose?*

20.1-2 The Neuron

Nerve cells, called **neurons**, connect the structures of your nervous system. These cells grow and multiply in the brain as an infant develops. This development begins in the third week of embryonic growth and continues into early adulthood.

Different types of neurons have similar structures, but different purposes (**Figure 20.3**). Sensory neurons gather information from your body. Motor neurons stimulate your muscles to respond to information. Interneurons form connections between other neurons in your brain and spinal cord. Movement, thinking, and memory use these connections. Your neurons can reach lengths of several feet as they grow toward their target.

neur/o = nerve

inter- = between

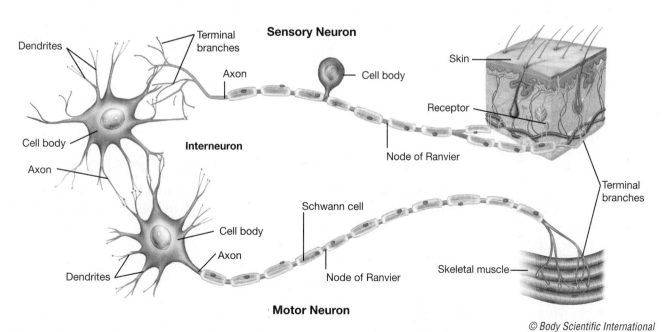

© Body Scientific International

Figure 20.3 Different types of neurons may have similar structures, but they have different purposes. *What are the purposes of sensory neurons, motor neurons, and interneurons?*

dendr/o = branching
-ite = resembling

termin/o = boundary, limit, end
-al = pertaining to

Think of your hand as a model for a neuron. Your palm would represent the **cell body**, where the nucleus is found. Your fingers are like **dendrites** that branch off the cell body to bring in information from other cells they touch. Your arm is like the **axon** that takes information out from the cell body to be processed. **Terminal branches** at the end of the axon connect to other cells like your shoulder connects your arm to your body. Nerve cells reach out to new areas to **innervate** them or provide them with a nerve connection to the brain. Your brain contains its greatest number of neurons in childhood. Unused and duplicate connections are reabsorbed to make processing more efficient. This *pruning* of unnecessary pathways occurs again in the late teen years, ending in early adulthood. Research shows there may be a link between autism spectrum disorders and a lack of pruning in some parts of the brain. This would help to explain the oversensitivity to stimuli seen with these conditions.

Development of motor neuron control in infants moves from the center of the body out to the limbs. Large muscle groups are connected first, followed by small muscles for fine-motor control. An axon must connect your brain to each muscle so it can receive the signal to contract. Your neurons communicate by creating electrochemical signals that travel along the axon. The signal is passed to connecting axons through a synapse. A **synapse** is a tiny gap between an axon and a receptor cell. When a pulse of electricity reaches the synapse, it releases a **neurotransmitter**. This chemical carries the signal across the synapse and triggers a chemical response in the receptor cell. An electroencephalogram (EEG) can measure this electrochemical activity. The absence of brain waves on an EEG is sometimes used as a legal definition of brain death.

electr/o = electric
chem/o = chemical
neur/o = nerve
trans/i = to pass, to go over
encephal/o = brain
-gram = record

Cell bodies and dendrites lying on the surface of your brain form *gray matter*. Gray matter's color comes from the dark nuclei in the cell bodies. Axons have a waxy coating that gives them a light color. They form *white matter* in your brain. This waxy sheath, called **myelin**, protects axons from "cross-connections" that slow or interrupt signals in your brain. Your hand is like a neuron, and your arm is like its axon. You can think of the myelin sheath as a sleeve covering the axon of your arm. Schwann cells along the myelin sheath produce the myelin.

myel/o = spinal cord
-in = substance, chemical

Defects in the myelin sheath can cause diseases such as schizophrenia spectrum disorder and multiple sclerosis (MS). Schizophrenia spectrum disorder is a group of mental illnesses characterized by a breakdown of thought processes, while MS often appears as muscle weakness. In these cases, the nerves do not communicate properly with each other because electrical signals are lost along the unmyelinated pathway.

ment/o = mind
-al = pertaining to

20.1-3 The Central Nervous System

Your nervous system can be divided into two main parts: your **central nervous system (CNS)** and your **peripheral nervous system (PNS)**, as shown in **Figure 20.4**. Your CNS includes the spinal cord and brain. Your PNS includes the sensory and motor nerves that carry communication between your CNS and your body. All parts of your nervous system work together to communicate sensations and control your body's responses.

peripher/o = outer edge
-al = pertaining to

The Brain

Your brain is the control center of your nervous system. Your brain, spinal cord, and nerves are formed from the ectoderm during embryonic development.

ecto- = outside
-derm = skin

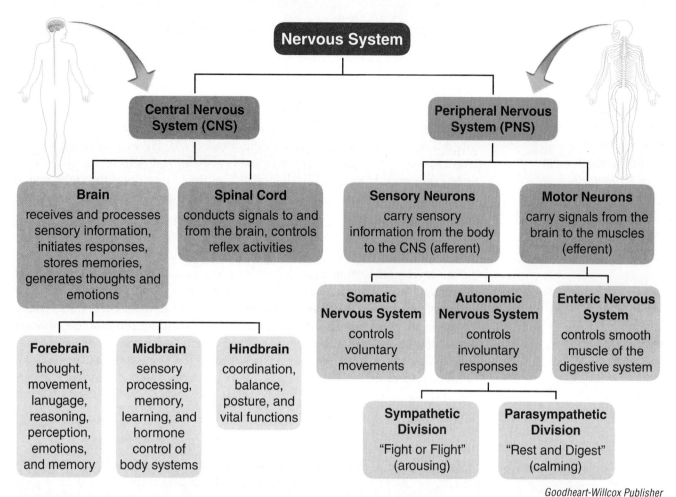

Figure 20.4 The nervous system can be divided into the central nervous system and the peripheral nervous system, each of which has its own components and purposes.

The ectoderm curls to form a neural tube (**Figure 20.5**). The top of the tube swells and folds forward to become the *forebrain*. The middle section folds in on itself to become the *hindbrain*. The forebrain grows large enough to cover the *midbrain* beneath it. As the brain grows and pushes for room, more wrinkles form until it looks like a large walnut without its shell.

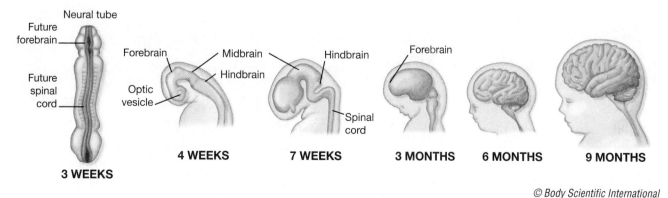

© Body Scientific International

Figure 20.5 In an embryo, the brain starts off as a neural tube, which then curls and folds to form the forebrain, midbrain, hindbrain, and spinal cord.

cerebr/o = brain
-al = pertaining to
hemi- = half
-sphere = ball, globe

corp/o = body
-us = structure
callos/o = hard, callous
-um = structure

vascul/o = blood vessel
-ar = pertaining to

trans/i = to pass, to go over
isch/o = to keep back, hold
-emic = pertaining to blood

gangli/o = swelling, tumor

fiss/i = split, cleft
-ure = result of

Your brain can be divided into two halves, called your *cerebral hemispheres*. Your left hemisphere controls the right side of your body and vice versa. A large bundle of nerves called your *corpus callosum* connects the two hemispheres at the center. Each hemisphere is made up of several distinct sections, each with a different function.

A stroke, or *cerebrovascular accident* (CVA), is caused by a blood clot or aneurysm that interrupts blood flow to the brain. A short-term interruption is called a ministroke, or *transient ischemic attack (TIA)*. TIAs can be a sign that a larger stroke is coming. The area of the brain affected determines the symptoms experienced. A stroke on the left side of the brain affects the right side of the body. Use the acronym BE FAST in **Figure 20.6** to recognize the symptoms of a stroke and get help.

The Forebrain

The forebrain is the largest part of your brain. It is made up of your **cerebrum**, basal ganglia, and limbic system. Your cerebrum sorts and classifies information. The outer surface, called your **cerebral cortex**, has many bumps and grooves. The deepest grooves, which separate some of your brain structures, are called *fissures*. These form when the embryo's neural tube folds during development. Fissures form the same basic patterns in all brains, suggesting that the folding pattern is controlled by genetics rather than randomly created.

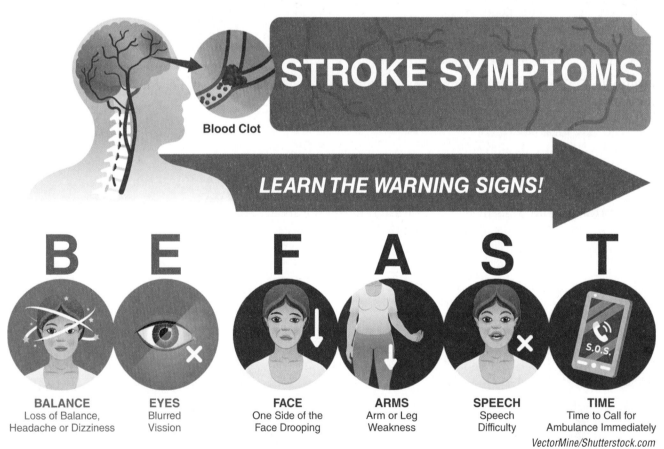

STROKE SYMPTOMS

Blood Clot

LEARN THE WARNING SIGNS!

B **E** **F** **A** **S** **T**

BALANCE
Loss of Balance, Headache or Dizziness

EYES
Blurred Vission

FACE
One Side of the Face Drooping

ARMS
Arm or Leg Weakness

SPEECH
Speech Difficulty

TIME
Time to Call for Ambulance Immediately

VectorMine/Shutterstock.com

Figure 20.6 Learn to recognize the signs of a stroke. Clot-busting medication is most effective within the first hour of symptoms starting.

The surface bumps of your brain are called *gyri* (JI-rI), and the small folds between them are called *sulci* (SUHL-kI). They form individually unique patterns during the last trimester of fetal development. This suggests that environment plays a large role in their development. These folds increase the total surface area that can fit into a small space. More surface area on your cerebral cortex means more gray matter is available for you to process information.

The fissures, sulci, and gyri serve as landmarks for identifying major structures of your brain (**Figure 20.7**). The longitudinal fissure divides your cerebrum into the left and right hemispheres. Each hemisphere is divided into four lobes. The central sulcus divides your frontal and parietal lobes. The parieto-occipital fissure separates your parietal and occipital lobes. The lateral fissure separates your temporal lobe. Each lobe has a different function.

hemi- = half
-sphere = ball, globe
pariet/o = wall
occipit/o = back of the head
-al = pertaining to
later/o = side
tempor/o = temple, side of the head, time

Lobes of the Brain

Your **frontal lobes**, located at your forehead, are responsible for voluntary muscle control, thinking, memory, language, judgment, creativity, and personality. The central sulcus separates them from your parietal lobes. Your precentral gyrus is a narrow strip along this groove that contains your **primary motor cortex**. It sends planned motor responses from your frontal lobes out to the muscles of your body.

pre- = before, in front of

Different parts of your primary motor cortex control muscles in different areas of your body. More neurons are needed to direct fine-motor control, so more space on your motor cortex is devoted to the connections for your fingers, eyes, lips, and tongue than to those for your torso or legs.

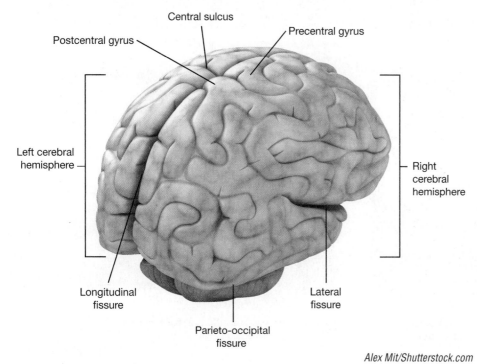

Alex Mit/Shutterstock.com

Figure 20.7 The fissures, sulci, and gyri found on the brain help identify major structures.

homin/o = human
-ule = small
-us = structure

pariet/o = wall
-al = pertaining to
somat/o = body
sensor/i = sensation
-y = process
post- = after

occipit/o = back of the head

tempor/o = temple, side of the
head, time

The motor homunculus is an exaggerated drawing that emphasizes this point (**Figure 20.8**). The frontal lobe also contains one of the Broca areas, which aids in speech production.

Your **parietal lobes** lie behind your frontal lobes, on the back of the central sulcus. Your somatosensory cortex, or *primary sensory cortex*, located on the postcentral gyrus, brings in information from your senses. The Wernicke area, which is located in these lobes, helps you understand written and spoken language. Similar to your primary motor cortex, different amounts of space on your primary sensory cortex are devoted to different areas of your body (Figure 20.8). The number of sensory nerves connected to each area determines the space dedicated to it. Damage to your parietal lobes can result in issues with sensation, perception, and spatial coordination.

Your **occipital lobes** are the smallest of the four pairs of lobes. They sit in the back of your skull behind your parietal lobes and under your occipital bone. They control your sight, visual-spatial processes, memory, and storage. Your primary visual cortex is located in this area. Damage to your occipital lobe can cause hallucinations, distorted vision, and issues with reading and writing.

Your **temporal lobes** lie on the outer side of the other lobes, near your ears. The lateral fissures separate them from your parietal lobes. These lobes control your hearing, balance, emotions, speech planning, and memory associations.

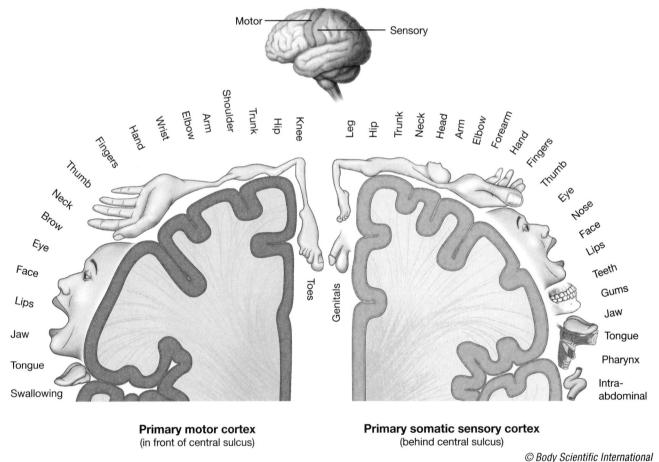

Primary motor cortex
(in front of central sulcus)

Primary somatic sensory cortex
(behind central sulcus)

© Body Scientific International

Figure 20.8 The motor homunculus demonstrates how areas of the body that require fine motor control take up more space in the precentral gyrus. Areas that are mainly gross motor control take up less space. The sensory homunculus shows space in the postcentral gyrus for parts of the body bringing in information.

Your primary auditory cortex, which processes sound, is located in your temporal lobes. Your temporal lobes are the last area of your brain to finish developing, so your frontal lobes help process emotions until temporal lobe development is completed around 20 years of age. This helps explain why children react physically to strong emotions.

audi/o = sound, to hear
-or = one who does
-y = process

Basal Ganglia and Limbic System

The basal ganglia and parts of your limbic system connect your cerebral cortex to your midbrain below (**Figure 20.9**). Basal ganglia, also called *basal nuclei*, are areas of gray matter that relay information between your midbrain and cerebral cortex. Your basal ganglia are involved in motor control, body position, and your sense of direction and distance. Defects in the basal ganglia's loop can result in tremors, tic movements, and Huntington's disease. Degeneration of these neurons results in the rhythmic contractions and relaxations of certain muscle groups. This is seen in Parkinson's disease and essential tremors.

gangli/o = swelling, tumor

Your **limbic system** is a horseshoe-shaped set of structures that includes the cingulate gyrus, hippocampus, and amygdala (uh-MIHG-duh-luh). These structures lie between your cerebral cortex and midbrain, surrounding your thalamus.

Your cingulate gyrus is an arched band that lies between your cerebral lobes and corpus callosum. It is involved with your emotions, attention, and social behavior. The front portion is related to depression, a mood disorder that includes periods of sadness, sleep disturbances, memory issues, and sometimes suicidal tendencies.

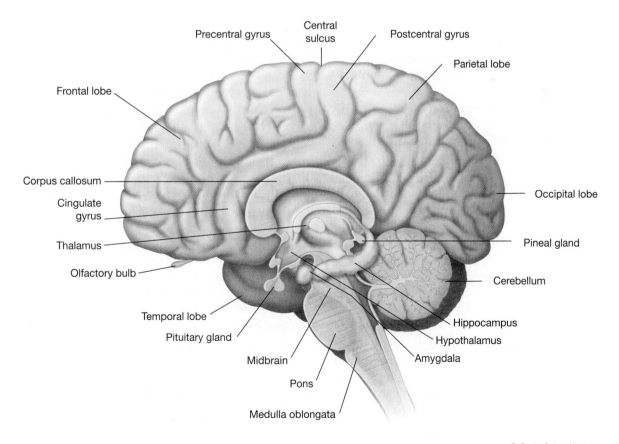

© Body Scientific International

Figure 20.9 A midsagittal section shows many of the brain's structures.

Bipolar disorder is characterized by extreme mood swings, from depression (low) to mania (high), that affect energy, judgment, and behavior. Depression responds well to antidepressant medications. More information on these disorders can be found in **Figure 20.10**.

hippocamp/o = seahorse
-us = structure

Your hippocampus is an arched group of nerve cells shaped like a sea horse. It connects your thalamus and amygdala, ending near your temporal lobe. It also relates to emotions, as well as navigation, spatial memory, and learning. Stress releases a hormone that slows the function of your hippocampus and activates your amygdala. This explains why you may not remember things under stress.

Common Disorders Affecting Mental Health			
Characteristics	**Depression**	**Bipolar Disorder**	**Anxiety Disorders**
Etiology	A mood disorder that causes persistent feelings of sadness, sleep disturbances, loss of energy, changes in eating patterns, difficulty concentrating, and loss of interest that may affect the ability to do normal daily activities or cause suicidal thoughts. Symptoms last for a long period of time.	A lifelong mental health condition that causes extreme mood swings from emotional highs (mania) to extreme lows (depression). There are several types with varying levels, lengths, and frequencies of highs and lows. Mania can trigger a break from reality.	Repeated episodes of intense, excessive, and persistent worry and fear that are out of proportion to the actual danger and interfere with daily activities. There are many types.
Pathology	A variety of factors may cause depression, including physical changes in the brain or an imbalance of neurotransmitters or hormones. There may be a genetic component. Traumatic or stressful events, drug use, medications, or serious illness can be triggers.	Physical changes in the brain and genetics appear to play a role, but the exact mechanism is unknown. Periods of high stress or drug or alcohol use may trigger the first episode.	May be linked to medication use or underlying health issues, such as heart disease, respiratory disorders, endocrine imbalances, drug use, chronic pain, or brain tumors. Trauma, stress, mental health conditions, and heredity may play a role. Symptoms may start during childhood and continue through adulthood.
Diagnosis	Psychological evaluation.	Psychological evaluation.	Psychological evaluation.
Treatment	Psychotherapy and medications such as antidepressants or anti-anxiety medications can reduce symptoms. Physical activity, stress management, and social interaction may help manage symptoms.	Psychotherapy and medications such as antidepressants or anti-anxiety medications can reduce symptoms. Physical activity and stress management may help manage symptoms.	Psychotherapy and medications such as antidepressants or anti-anxiety medications can reduce symptoms. Physical activity, stress management, and relaxation techniques may help manage symptoms.
Prevention	Participation in activities that involve physical activity and social interaction can increase resilience. Avoid drugs and alcohol, which can trigger episodes of depression.	May not be preventable, but early treatment can reduce severity. Pay attention to warning signs and patterns that need to be addressed. Avoid drugs and alcohol. Stay on prescribed medications.	Participation in activities that involve physical activity and social interaction can help reduce the buildup of anxiety. Avoid drugs and alcohol, which can worsen symptoms.

Goodheart-Willcox Publisher

Figure 20.10 Common diseases and disorders affecting mental health.

Sensory information is initially stored in your hippocampus just long enough to be recognized. If you pay attention longer by repeating the information and making connections, that information may be transferred to your long-term memory. The hippocampus is also the first area of the brain affected by mental health conditions such as post-traumatic stress disorder (PTSD), Alzheimer's disease (AD), and depression (**Figure 20.11**). What common symptoms of these conditions can you connect to malfunctions of the hippocampus?

ment/o = mind
-al = pertaining to

post- = after
traum/a = wound, injury
-tic = pertaining to

Your amygdala is an almond-shaped structure located near your temporal lobe. It is involved in strong emotions such as fear, anxiety, defensiveness, sexual arousal, and aggression. An anxiety attack is an overwhelming sense of fear or apprehension with symptoms of increased heart rate, shortness of breath, sweating, and tension. A balance of neurotransmitters in your brain normally keep these emotions under control. In obsessive-compulsive disorder (OCD), these controls do not work, and the amygdala takes over with obsessive thinking and compulsive rituals. Completion of OCD behaviors feels rewarding and perpetuates the cycle of behavior.

Drug use affects your limbic system. Drugs can block or trigger the transmission of neuron impulses in the synapse between two neurons. This is a good thing when you have a headache and take aspirin to relieve pain. It is not so good when drugs or alcohol prevent you from responding effectively to a stimulus, such as a traffic light changing to red.

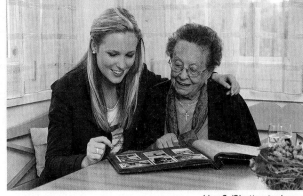

Lisa S./Shutterstock.com

Figure 20.11 The hippocampus, which is related to memory function, is affected in those who have Alzheimer's disease. *What are some things you can do to help improve your memory?*

The Midbrain

Your midbrain includes your thalamus, hypothalamus, pituitary gland (also called the *hypophysis*), and pineal gland (also called the *epiphysis*). Most sensory information comes through your **thalamus**. This area acts as a relay station for sorting, interpreting, and directing sensory signals to the appropriate area of your cerebral cortex. It also plays a role in attentiveness.

sensor/i = sensation
-y = process
sym- = together
pathet/a = suffering
-ic = pertaining to

Your thalamus controls the hormones for your sympathetic nervous system's fight-or-flight response to stressful situations. When you get nervous, your sympathetic system reacts by increasing your respiration and heart rate, raising your blood pressure, and sending hormone messengers to prepare your body to respond. A panic attack is an exaggerated example of this response mechanism. After the stressful situation has passed, the parasympathetic system reverses this physical response so your body returns to normal.

para- = near, beside, abnormal

Your **hypothalamus**, located just below your thalamus and behind your frontal lobe, is your brain's center for emotions and instincts. The hypothalamus stimulates your pituitary gland, located below, to release hormones that control your growth, body temperature, water balance, and sleep cycles. In this way, it helps to keep your body in homeostasis. It also controls pleasure, sleep, hunger, and thirst.

hypo- = below, under
thalam/o = thalamus
-us = structure

Your pineal gland lies near the center of your brain. It controls sleep cycles and your biological clock. It secretes melatonin to make you feel sleepy when it is dark. In the winter, when people are less exposed to natural light, they may develop seasonal affective disorder (SAD). This causes depression, sleepiness, and weight gain. Full-spectrum light therapy helps reduce symptoms of SAD. Have you experienced this difference in energy levels with winter blues or spring fever?

The Hindbrain

cerebell/o = little brain
-um = structure

Your hindbrain includes your cerebellum and brainstem. Your **cerebellum**, located below your occipital lobe, is the second-largest area of your brain. It coordinates incoming and outgoing messages to produce smooth skeletal movements. Without it, your actions would appear hesitant and clumsy. The cerebellum contributes to movement planning, motor memory, and error recognition. It looks like neatly folded layers, so you might think of it as the secretary of your brain that neatly organizes and smooths your daily functions. Tremors, decreased muscle tone, and an inability to control movements may indicate an issue with the cerebellum.

medull/a- = middle
oblong/o = elongated
-ata = place

Your **brainstem** is known as the *vital functions center* of your brain. It controls the smooth muscles of your heart and lungs that are essential for breathing, heart rate, blood pressure, and sleep cycles. It also controls digestion and some reflexes like swallowing and vomiting. Your brainstem has three parts: the midbrain, pons, and medulla oblongata (meh-DOO-luh ah-blawn-GAH-tuh). This is the midpoint where your sympathetic and parasympathetic nervous systems connect. Your medulla oblongata becomes your spinal cord when it exits your skull. The brainstem is generally not involved in mental health conditions, but injury to it can cause seizures, coma, or death.

Spinal Cord

sensor/i = sensation
-y = process
peripher/o = outer edge
-al = pertaining to
-esthesia = sensation, feeling
an- = without
alges/i = sense of pain
-ic = pertaining to

Your spinal cord acts as a highway, carrying information to and from your brain. Like a highway, your spinal cord is clearly divided into two directions of travel. *Afferent* (think "add") nerves travel from your body into the brain. *Efferent* (think "exit") nerves travel out of your brain to your body. Afferent neurons carry sensory information to your brain. After this information is processed, efferent neurons carry the appropriate motor response from your brain back to your body along peripheral nerves.

Anesthesiologists administer analgesic drugs that block these signals. If the afferent signals are blocked, then you do not experience pain. General anesthesia includes additional drugs to block motor responses. Can you think of other ways to block pain or muscle responses?

20.1-4 Structures Protecting the Central Nervous System

A variety of infections and physical injuries can affect your central nervous system. Bone, cerebrospinal fluid, a blood-brain barrier, and three layers of meninges protect your brain and spinal cord.

Meninges

mening/o = membrane
dur/a = hard
arachn/o = spider
-oid = like
pi/a = tender
-itis = inflammation

The **meninges** (meh-NIHN-jeez) are tough layers of tissue covering your brain and spinal cord (**Figure 20.12**). The three layers include the dura mater (the outer layer), arachnoid mater (the middle layer), and pia mater (the layer closest to your brain and spinal cord).

Like the skin, the meninges keep viruses and bacteria out of your brain. Bacterial meningitis is a serious inflammation of the meninges. It spreads through respiratory secretions during close contact. This illness affects more than 2,000 people each year. Symptoms include headaches, fever, neck stiffness, and nausea. These symptoms may be mistaken for a mild flu, but meningitis can cause convulsions, brain damage, or death in just a few hours.

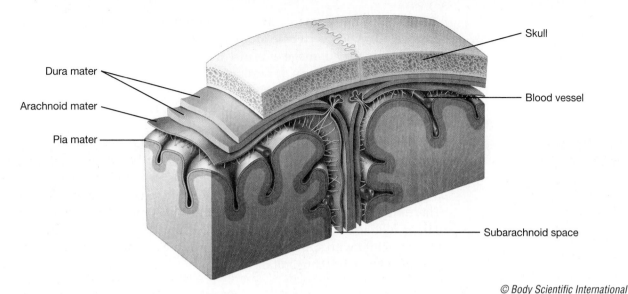

Dura mater

Arachnoid mater

Pia mater

Skull

Blood vessel

Subarachnoid space

© Body Scientific International

Figure 20.12   Three layers of meninges cover the brain and spinal cord to provide protection. *What are the symptoms of meningitis?*

The meningococcal vaccine is recommended for teens with a booster given before college.

Blood-Brain Barrier

The blood-brain barrier sounds like a lining that covers your brain, but it actually exists in the blood vessels of your CNS. Capillaries in your CNS have smaller gaps between their cells compared to other parts of your body. These blood vessels are very selective. They do not allow large, highly charged, or fat-soluble molecules to pass through the barrier.

This barrier protects your CNS from common bacterial infections, the influence of outside hormones or neurotransmitters, and other foreign substances that could cause harm. Active transport is required to move glucose across the barrier. Unfortunately, this barrier also makes it difficult to deliver antibiotics or other helpful drugs to your brain. Research is trying to develop new techniques for delivering materials such as medications and contrast dyes to brain tissues.

Bones

Bones also protect your brain and spinal cord. Your skull shields your brain, and vertebrae surround your spinal cord. These bones protect against the force of a blow to your head or back, but they do not offer cushioning. A concussion is bleeding and swelling on the surface of the brain. This can happen when the head whips back and forth quickly, bouncing the brain against the inside of the skull. See Figure 20.1 at the beginning of the chapter for more information on this condition.

If infants are shaken, their soft brains may be damaged even more easily than the developed brains of adults. Infants' neck bones also have less support from muscle and may allow the spinal cord to stretch enough to cause damage. This results in a condition known as *shaken baby syndrome*, which can cause permanent brain damage or death.

quadri- = four
-plegia = weakness
para- = near, beside, abnormal
-lysis = destruction
cervic/o = neck
thorac/o = chest
lumb/o = lower back, loins
spin/a = spinal cord
bi- = two
fid/a = split

Spinal injuries demonstrate the importance of vertebrae protecting your spinal cord. When vertebrae are fractured or dislocated, such as during a car accident, this may damage or bruise the spinal cord. Quadriplegia (kwa-druh-PLEE-jee-uh) is paralysis or weakness in all four limbs, most often caused by damage to the cervical vertebrae. Paraplegia is impaired motor or sensory function of the legs. It is usually caused by damage to the thoracic, lumbar, or sacral regions of the spine.

Spina bifida (spI-nuh BIH-fih-duh) is a congenital condition in which some vertebrae do not fully form around the spinal cord (**Figure 20.13**). This leaves the spinal cord exposed to injury and results in weakness or *paralysis* below the point of the defect. This limits the ability to move certain parts of the body. There may also be complications from infection or swelling in the spinal cord. Taking folic acid supplements before becoming pregnant can reduce the risk of having a child with spina bifida. Breakfast cereals are often fortified with folic acid to prevent this congenital condition.

Cerebrospinal Fluid (CSF)

cerebr/o = brain
spin/o = spinal cord
-al = pertaining to
sub- = below, under
arachn/o = spider
-oid = like

Cerebrospinal fluid (CSF) "floats" your brain inside your skull and cushions it to protect against concussions. Additional CSF also fills the ventricles inside your brain, the central canal of your spinal cord, and the subarachnoid space between the meninges of your spinal cord. The fluid provides glucose and other nutrients for your brain and spinal cord. It may also play a role in removing waste from the brain.

hem/o = blood
-rrhage = to flow profusely

A spinal tap, or *lumbar puncture*, uses a needle to draw CSF out of your spinal column for testing. A medical technologist examines the fluid for red and white blood cells, cultures it for bacteria, and measures levels of protein and other substances that do not belong. These tests will reveal hemorrhaging, infections, syphilis, and cancers affecting the brain or spinal cord.

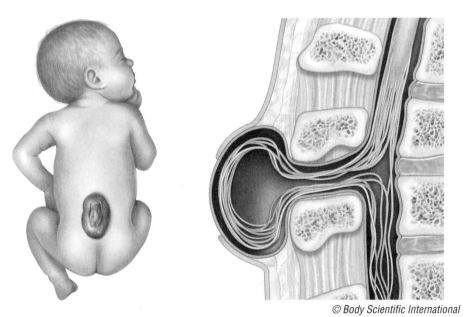

© Body Scientific International

Figure 20.13 The condition known as *spina bifida* can lead to spinal cord injury. *In which limbs would you expect this child to experience weakness or paralysis?*

20.1-5 The Glymphatic System

Researchers have been studying the idea that people may have another body system that supports the transport and cleaning of fluids and waste in the brain. It is named the "glymphatic system" because the CSF and interstitial fluid in brain tissues act as lymph for your glial cells. **Glial cells** are not neurons. Rather, they play an important role in supporting neuron development, structure, communication, nourishment, and protection. Most brain tumors are associated with mutations of glial cells.

Astrocytes are specialized glial cells that control the concentration of neurotransmitters, ions, nutrients, and water in your CNS. Together with lymphatic-like vessels in the meninges and blood vessels in your CNS, this fluid control system may help maintain homeostasis in your brain (**Figure 20.14**). This combination of lymphatic vessels, blood vessels, and interstitial spaces filtered by astrocytes seems to carry some CSF to and from your brain tissue. This helps clear waste products too large to cross over the blood-brain barrier. It is possible that issues with this system may allow the buildup of waste and large protein molecules in the brain. This may be the cause of some neurological conditions, such as Alzheimer's disease.

Interestingly, the glymphatic system is most active when you sleep. Sleep deprivation, aging, stroke, and traumatic brain injury can all disrupt the exchange of fluid along this transport system. This explains the connection between these factors, memory issues, and decreased brain function. Physical activity appears to maintain glymphatic function. Further study of the glymphatic system hypothesis may help with the development of new treatments for many brain disorders.

traum/a = wound, injury
-tic = pertaining to

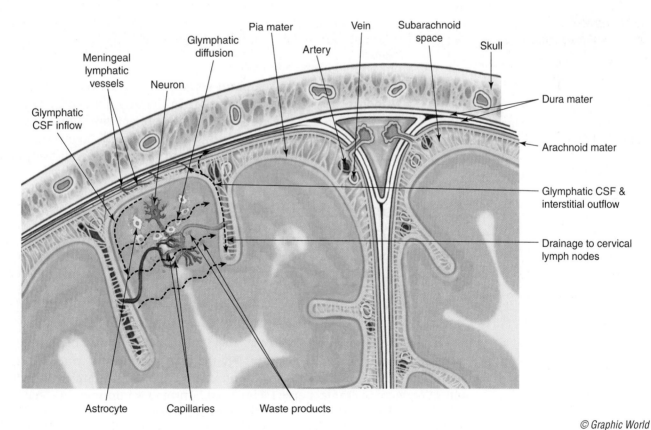

© Graphic World

Figure 20.14 The glymphatic system may filter large proteins and waste from the brain's interstitial and cerebrospinal fluid.

Chapter 20   Body Systems for Regulation and Communication   **773**

20.1-6 The Peripheral Nervous System

somat/o = body
auto- = self
enter/o = intestine

Your PNS uses neurons to connect your CNS to the rest of your body. As shown in Figure 20.4, your PNS can be further divided into the somatic, autonomic, and enteric nervous systems.

All divisions of your PNS can produce involuntary responses. Your enteric nervous system controls the smooth muscles of the digestive system. Enteric responses are all involuntary. You do not think about moving food through your digestive system or changing the speed at which it moves. Similarly, you do not think about your heart rate or blood pressure, which are autonomic responses. Your autonomic nervous system (ANS) provides involuntary control over smooth muscles of your circulatory and endocrine systems. This includes the "fight-or-flight" response of your sympathetic nerves, as well as the opposite "rest-and-digest" response of your parasympathetic nerves. You can, however, consciously control some autonomic responses, such as your breathing.

The somatic nervous system provides voluntary control of your skeletal muscles. You can remember that motor neurons are efferent. They *exit* your brain, and it takes *effort* to move your muscles. Sensory neurons are afferent. They *add* information to your brain, so you will *feel* the *ache* after working your muscles. Somatic responses are usually voluntary, but an involuntary response can also be produced. *Reflexes* are involuntary responses of your nervous system (**Figure 20.15**). They are predictable and will produce the same response each time. What reflex responses are familiar to you?

The purpose of a reflex is to maintain homeostasis and protect your body from harm. Reflexes use a shortcut to produce a faster response in your body. When a sensory neuron gathers information from your body, it typically sends it up your spinal cord to your brain for processing. The brain sorts the information and returns a response via a motor neuron, through your spinal cord, to your body. In an emergency, a reflex arc will connect your sensory message directly to a motor neuron in your spinal cord. Your brain may not process the pain sensation of an injury until after your body has already reacted.

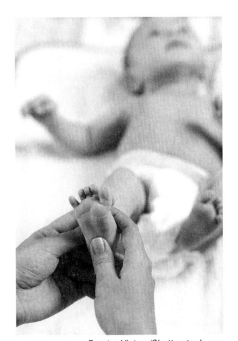

Dmytro Vietrov/Shutterstock.com

Figure 20.15 If you stroke the bottom of an infant's foot, the toes will fan outward. This is an example of a reflex.

Cranial and Spinal Nerves

There are 12 pairs of **cranial nerves** (**Figure 20.16**). They provide connections from your brain to your head and neck. Most of these pathways contain motor neurons, but some contain sensory neurons or a combination of both. The cranial nerves exit your skull through *foramina*, which are holes in the bones. Several nerves may use the same foramina, and blood vessels may travel with them.

Nerves are generally named for their location or function, much like muscles. Roman numerals also number the cranial nerves. If you view the underside of the brain, the nerves are numbered in order, beginning with the olfactory nerve as cranial nerve I. **Figure 20.17** provides information about the names, locations, and functions of the cranial nerves.

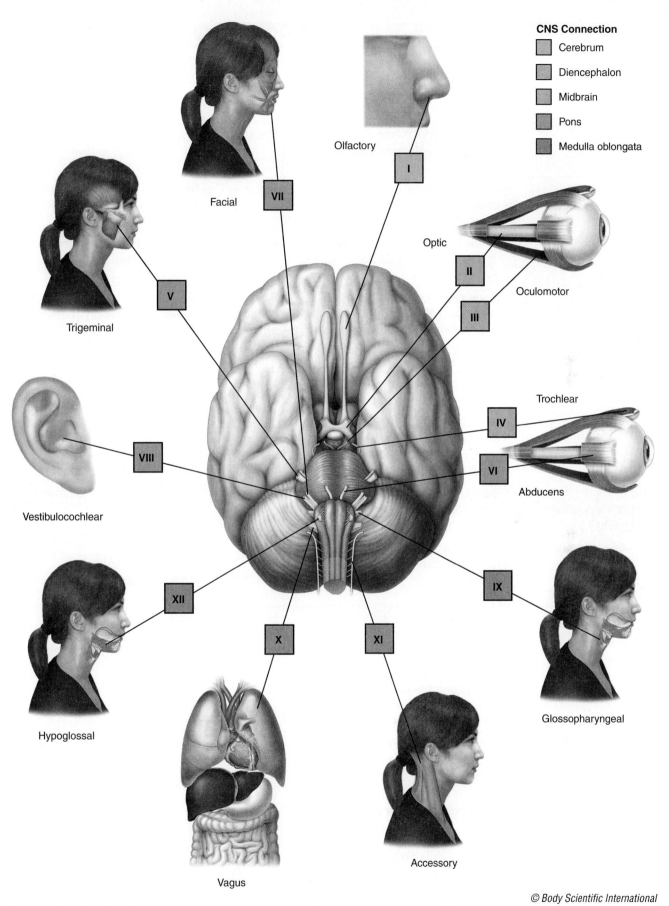

CNS Connection

- Cerebrum
- Diencephalon
- Midbrain
- Pons
- Medulla oblongata

Olfactory — I

Optic — II

Oculomotor — III

Trochlear — IV

Abducens — VI

Glossopharyngeal — IX

Accessory — XI

Vagus — X

Hypoglossal — XII

Vestibulocochlear — VIII

Trigeminal — V

Facial — VII

© Body Scientific International

Figure 20.16 The 12 cranial nerves and the parts of the body they control. *Where do cranial nerves exit the skull?*

Name, Location, and Function of the Cranial Nerves

Nerve Name	Location	Type	Function
I—Olfactory	Below the frontal lobe, exiting through the ethmoid bone into the nasal cavity	Sensory	Sense of smell
II—Optic	Below the frontal lobe, exiting through the sphenoid bone into the eye socket	Sensory	Visual signals
III—Oculomotor	Below the frontal lobe, exiting through the sphenoid bone into the eye socket	Motor	Muscle innervation to move and focus the eyes
IV—Trochlear	Below the frontal lobe, exiting through the sphenoid bone into the eye socket	Motor	Muscle innervation to move the eyes up, down, and inward
V—Trigeminal: V1—ophthalmic V2—maxillary V3—mandibular	In the pons, exiting in three locations: sphenoid bone into the eye socket, sphenoid wing behind the maxilla, sphenoid wing behind the zygomatic arch	Both sensory and motor	Muscle innervation for chewing; sensory innervation of the face
VI—Abducens	Below the frontal lobe, exiting through the sphenoid bone into the eye socket	Motor	Muscle innervation to move the eyes outward (abduction)
VII—Facial	Brainstem, between the pons and medulla, exiting through the auditory canal of the temporal bone	Both sensory and motor	Sense of taste; muscle innervation of the face, salivary glands, and tear ducts
VIII—Vestibulocochlear (Acoustic)	Brainstem, between the pons and medulla, exiting through the auditory canal of the temporal bone	Sensory	Sense of hearing and balance
IX—Glossopharyngeal	Medulla, exiting through the jugular foramen between the temporal and occipital bones	Both sensory and motor	Sense of taste from the back of the tongue; muscle innervation of salivary glands and tonsils; swallowing
X—Vagus	Medulla, exiting through the jugular foramen between the temporal and occipital bones	Both sensory and motor	Some sense of taste from epiglottis; muscle innervation of larynx and pharynx for speech and swallowing
XI—Accessory (Spinal Accessory)	Cranial and spinal roots, exiting through the jugular foramen between the temporal and occipital bones	Motor	Muscle innervation of neck
XII—Hypoglossal	Medulla, exiting below the tongue through the hypoglossal canal to the neck	Motor	Muscle innervation of tongue

Goodheart-Willcox Publisher

Figure 20.17 The types and functions of the cranial nerves.

Similar to the cranial nerves, 31 pairs of **spinal nerve** roots connect your spinal cord to the rest of your body (**Figure 20.18**). They are named with a letter and number according to the vertebrae where they exit. For example, the nerve exiting above your first cervical vertebra is C1, C2 exits your spinal canal between your first and second cervical vertebrae, and so on.

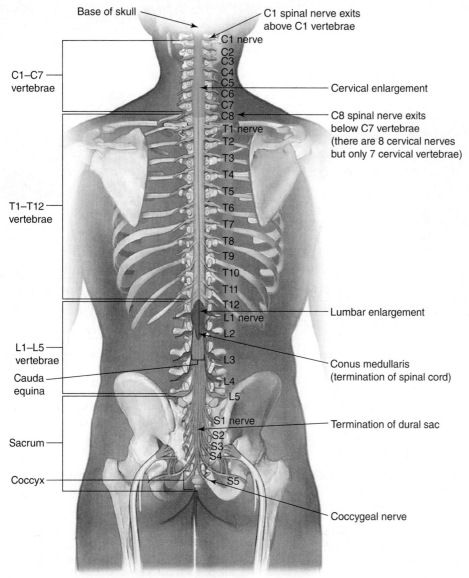

Base of skull

C1 spinal nerve exits above C1 vertebrae

C1 nerve
C2
C3
C4
C5
C6
C7
C8
T1 nerve
T2
T3
T4
T5
T6
T7
T8
T9
T10
T11
T12
L1 nerve
L2
L3
L4
L5
S1 nerve
S2
S3
S4
S5

C1–C7 vertebrae

T1–T12 vertebrae

L1–L5 vertebrae

Cauda equina

Sacrum

Coccyx

Cervical enlargement

C8 spinal nerve exits below C7 vertebrae (there are 8 cervical nerves but only 7 cervical vertebrae)

Lumbar enlargement

Conus medullaris (termination of spinal cord)

Termination of dural sac

Coccygeal nerve

© Graphic World

Figure 20.18   The 31 spinal nerve roots that connect the spinal cord to the rest of the body. *How are spinal nerves named?*

Your sacral nerves exit through holes in your sacrum bone. Your spinal cord and its meninges extend down to a swelling at your second lumbar vertebra. At this end of your spinal cord, the nerves separate into the cauda equina (kaw-duh ee-KWI-nuh), which looks like a horse's tail.

caud/o = tail
equin/o = horse

Nerve Pathways and Message Relays

Spinal nerves help direct messages entering and leaving your spinal cord (**Figure 20.19**). Your ANS requires two neurons to connect your brain to your body. The connection between the two neurons forms a **ganglion**, or *swelling*. Chains of these ganglia run down both sides of your spinal cord. The preganglionic neuron starts in your brain, runs down your spinal cord, and ends at the sympathetic ganglion. The postganglionic neuron runs from the ganglion out to the target organ in your body. All ANS neurons are part of a network connected by ganglia.

pre- = before, in front of
gangli/o = swelling, tumor
sym- = together
pathet/a = suffering
post- = after

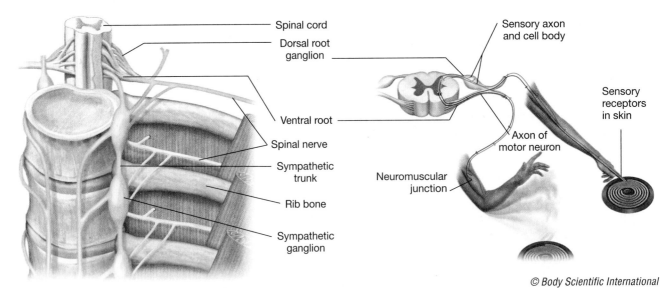

Spinal cord

Dorsal root
ganglion

Ventral root

Spinal nerve

Sympathetic
trunk

Rib bone

Sympathetic
ganglion

Sensory axon
and cell body

Sensory
receptors
in skin

Axon of
motor neuron

Neuromuscular
junction

© Body Scientific International

Figure 20.19   When a sensory receptor is stimulated by a hot surface, it sends an afferent signal through a sensory axon to the spinal cord. In a reflex, the signal is transferred by an interneuron directly to a motor neuron, stimulating quick removal of the hand. These neurons are connected at a ganglion.

Your spinal nerves are a collection of many separate axons gathered together. Their messages pass through a **plexus**, or *braid*, of interwoven spinal nerve roots. The cervical, lumbar, and sacral nerve plexuses continue to divide into trunks, divisions, and cords (**Figure 20.20**). These pathways become smaller as they spread out to their separate body regions. Then neurons separate from the nerve tract to connect nerves to body parts in that region.

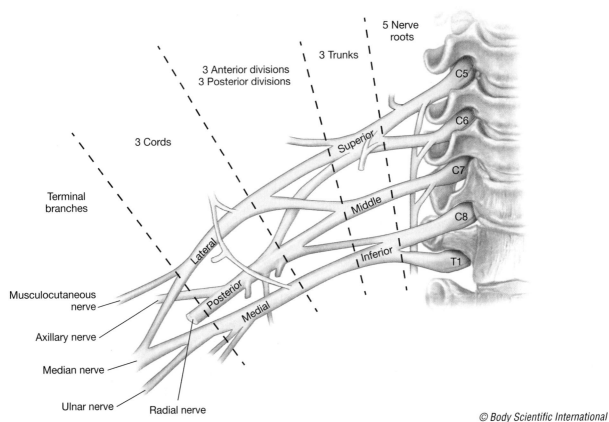

5 Nerve roots

3 Trunks

3 Anterior divisions
3 Posterior divisions

C5

C6

3 Cords

Superior

C7

Terminal
branches

Middle

C8

Lateral

Inferior

T1

Musculocutaneous
nerve

Posterior

Axillary nerve

Medial

Median nerve

Ulnar nerve   Radial nerve

© Body Scientific International

Figure 20.20   Spinal nerve plexuses begin as roots and then branch out into trunks, divisions, and cords. *Which nerve roots connect the ulnar nerve to the spinal cord?*

Your brachial plexus is an example of how nerve trunks divide into anterior and posterior divisions. Anterior nerves generally innervate flexor muscles, while posterior nerves innervate extensors. In your shoulders, the cervical plexus and brachial plexus are formed by cervical and thoracic nerve roots. Down the front of your arm, anterior divisions form the musculocutaneous, median, and ulnar nerves that flex your upper arm, wrist, and finger muscles. Down the back of your arm, posterior divisions form the axillary and radial nerves that innervate your upper arm, forearm, wrist, and finger extensor muscles.

Your thoracic spinal nerves connect directly to the muscles of your ribs, back, and abdomen. These nerves do not travel through plexuses. Their roots branch directly off your spinal cord to their target organs. Thoracic spinal nerves are important to muscles that support your breathing and balance.

Major nerves travel along the same pathways as major blood vessels (**Figure 20.21**). This provides a constant supply of oxygen and glucose to transmit nerve impulses. The lumbar and sacral plexuses serve your pelvis, legs, and feet. The lumbar plexus branches into the femoral nerve.

anter/o = front
poster/o = back, behind, after
cervic/o = neck
brachi/o = arm
thorac/o = chest
muscul/o = muscle
cutane/o = skin
-ous = pertaining to, having
medi/o = middle
axill/a = armpit

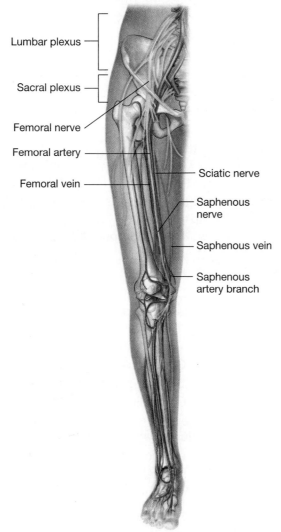

Lumbar plexus

Sacral plexus

Femoral nerve

Femoral artery

Femoral vein

Sciatic nerve

Saphenous nerve

Saphenous vein

Saphenous artery branch

© *Body Scientific International*

Figure 20.21 Major nerves require a constant supply of oxygen and glucose to transmit their impulses, so they travel along the same pathways as major blood vessels.

saphen/o = plain, visible
-ous = pertaining to, having

gluc/o = insulin, sugar

peripher/o = outer edge
-al = pertaining to
neur/o = nerve
path/o = disease
-y = process

The femoral nerve, artery, and vein run together in a sheath through the inguinal region. The saphenous nerve and artery branch off from the femoral nerve and artery, traveling together down the inner side of your knee to your ankle and foot. The sacral plexus branches into the sciatic nerve through your buttocks and down your legs. You have probably experienced numb legs from sitting too long in a position that cuts off the blood supply to this nerve.

The fact that blood provides glucose for nerve impulses helps explain why patients with diabetes have increased nerve pain and numbness. Their high blood sugar level increases the potential for those nerves to send impulses, even when there is no true pain demanding a response. This is one cause of peripheral neuropathy, or nerve damage.

Your nervous system serves all the other body systems. It gathers and directs the sensory and motor information that connects their functions. No system operates in isolation. The body systems are another example of this interconnectedness. A change in one system impacts the others.

Healthcare professionals need to be aware of connections between the body systems. With the trend toward specialization, medical professionals need to connect with specialists in other fields to solve many medical challenges. If a patient has very low blood pressure, there may be a connection to cardiovascular, kidney, or lung function. The patient may be dehydrated or taking a medication that lowers blood pressure as a side effect. Making a change to medications for organs of one system, such as the heart, may affect other body systems. General practitioners have a broad view of all body systems. Newer medical careers, such as hospitalists, also focus on coordinating care among a variety of different specialists.

Lesson 20.1 Review

 Complete the *Map Your Reading* graphic organizer for the section you just read.

1. What is the term for maintaining balance inside the body? (20.1-1)
   A. Homeostasis
   C. Endocrine
   B. Synapse
   D. Reflex
2. Which part of the neuron brings in information from other cells? (20.1-2)
   A. Axon
   B. Terminal branches
   C. Dendrites
   D. Cell body
3. Which brain lobe controls hearing, balance, emotions, speech planning, and memory associations? (20.1-3)
   A. Parietal lobe
   C. Temporal lobe
   B. Frontal lobe
   D. Occipital lobe
4. The part of the brain that controls sleep cycles and the biological clock is the (20.1-3)
   A. cerebellum
   B. hippocampus
   C. medulla oblongata
   D. pineal gland

5. The tough layers of tissue covering the brain and spinal cord are (20.1-4)
   A. the blood-brain barrier
   B. meninges
   C. bones
   D. CSF
6. What is the function of the glymphatic system? (20.1-5)
   A. Transmitting signals
   B. Clearing waste from the brain
   C. Supplying blood to the brain
   D. Controlling reflexes
7. The _____ nervous system produces voluntary movement of skeletal muscles. (20.1-6)
   A. enteric
   B. sympathetic
   C. autonomic
   D. somatic

The Special Senses

Learning Outcomes

After studying this lesson, you will be able to

20.2-1 describe the anatomy and physiology of structures involved in the sense of touch, including associated diseases and disorders.

20.2-2 summarize the anatomy and physiology of structures involved in the sense of taste, including associated diseases and disorders.

20.2-3 analyze the anatomy and physiology of structures involved in the sense of smell, including associated diseases and disorders.

20.2-4 explain how the anatomy and physiology of the ear enables hearing and identify types of hearing loss.

20.2-5 explain how the anatomy and physiology of the eye enables vision and identify vision conditions.

ESSENTIAL QUESTION

What are the structures, functions, and diseases associated with the special senses?

Professional Vocabulary

Essential Terms

primary sensory cortex   an area of the parietal lobe dedicated to gathering and interpreting information from afferent neurons regarding the five senses of the body

receptor   a nerve cell that receives stimuli

Important Terms

aqueous humor	olfactory bulb	tympanic membrane
choroid	ossicles	vestibular canals
cochlea	papillae	vitreous humor
cornea	sclera	
lens	taste bud	

Introduction

The special senses are part of your nervous system, but are sometimes studied separately as the sensory system. There are five senses: touch, taste, smell, vision, and hearing. Each special sense has many afferent, or *sensory*, **receptors**. These specialized neurons respond to different types of stimuli and gather different types of information. They allow you to explore the world around you.

Touch

sensor/i = sensation
-y = process
recept/o = receive
-or = one who does

hypo- = below, under
derm/o = skin
-is = pertaining to

There are many types of sensory receptors in your skin. These neurons can detect light touch, firm pressure, pain, vibration, temperature, and position. Each receptor is responsible for a specific area of skin. Some areas, such as your fingertips and lips, are more sensitive. They have more receptors per square inch of skin than other areas, such as your thigh.

Different areas of your skin have different types of receptors (**Figure 20.22**). For instance, hairy skin has nerve fibers wrapped around the hair follicles to sense when hairs move. *Ruffini endings* detect pressure in the dermis, while *Pacinian corpuscles* sense deep pressure and vibration in the hypodermis of both hairy and non-hairy skin. *Merkel disks* sense continuous touch, and *Meissner corpuscles* feel light touch in non-hairy skin. *Krause corpuscles* sense cold, pressure, and low vibrations in mucous membranes. *Free nerve endings* in the epidermis detect pain, touch, and temperature in many different skin types. Without a variety of receptors, you would not be able to distinguish between touch, vibration, and pain. It would be difficult to carry out everyday tasks, such as typing or picking up an object.

Information from your skin receptors travels to your spinal cord and up to your brain for interpretation. This sensory information is sorted in your thalamus, then passed on to the postcentral gyrus in your parietal lobe. This is the location of your **primary sensory cortex**, which interprets your senses. Your lips, face, fingers, and feet are the most sensitive parts of your body. These areas have the most cell bodies in the postcentral gyrus (Figure 20.8).

Infection, disease, or damage to your neurons or spinal cord can reduce your sense of touch. Touch, pain, and temperature sensations also decrease in old age because the number of receptors per square inch declines.

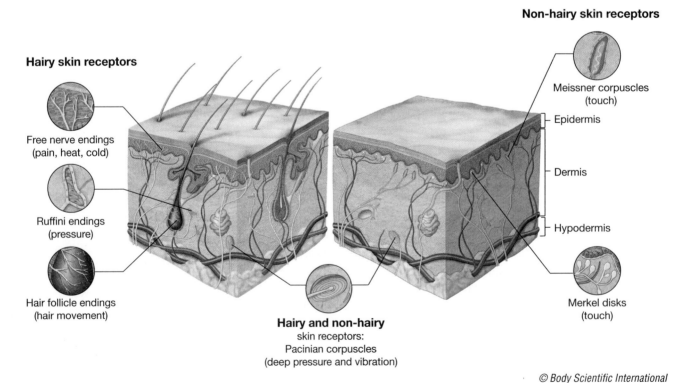

Non-hairy skin receptors

Hairy skin receptors

Free nerve endings
(pain, heat, cold)

Ruffini endings
(pressure)

Hair follicle endings
(hair movement)

Hairy and non-hairy
skin receptors:
Pacinian corpuscles
(deep pressure and vibration)

Meissner corpuscles
(touch)

Epidermis

Dermis

Hypodermis

Merkel disks
(touch)

© Body Scientific International

Figure 20.22 Hairy and non-hairy skin have some different types of skin receptors. *Choose one type of skin receptor shown here and use an example to explain what it senses.*

20.2-2 Taste

Your sense of taste, called *gustation*, is a combination of several different sensory inputs. Both flavor and smell molecules activate taste receptors in your tongue and mouth (**Figure 20.23**). These receptors can identify many different combinations of sweet, salty, sour, bitter, and umami (savory) flavors. Moisture, temperature, and "mouth feel" are also important to your taste perception. These inputs trigger memories and emotions. Taste can be enjoyable, unpleasant, or nostalgic.

As you bite into food, escaping molecules activate odor receptors in your nose. Smell and food memories help trigger saliva production. Saliva is important because food molecules must dissolve in fluid to access your taste sensory cells. Saliva and food molecules flow across your tongue and down your throat. Bumps called **papillae** (puh-PIH-lee) on the sides, tip, and back of your tongue become coated with saliva (**Figure 20.24**). A groove, or *moat*, around each papilla brings food molecules in with saliva to microvilli at the tip of each **taste bud**. Your tongue contains thousands of taste buds. These sensory cells convert flavors into electrical signals. Your limbic system interprets their messages, and your frontal cerebral cortex decides on a response.

Current research shows that there are five basic tastes: sweet, salty, sour, bitter, and umami. Umami is the newest flavor discovery. Its name is taken from the Japanese word for *delicious*. Umami is described as a rich and savory flavor found in meat and monosodium glutamate (MSG). Its chemical structure suggests it is a combination of sweet, salty, and sour flavors. Researchers are also investigating whether fat qualifies as a separate taste.

gust/o = taste
-ation = action of, process of

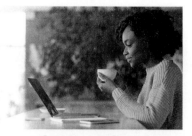

Prostock-studio/Shutterstock.com

Figure 20.23 As you eat, escaping molecules activate both taste and odor receptors. Smell enhances taste. *What food odors make your mouth water?*

papill/o = nipple-like

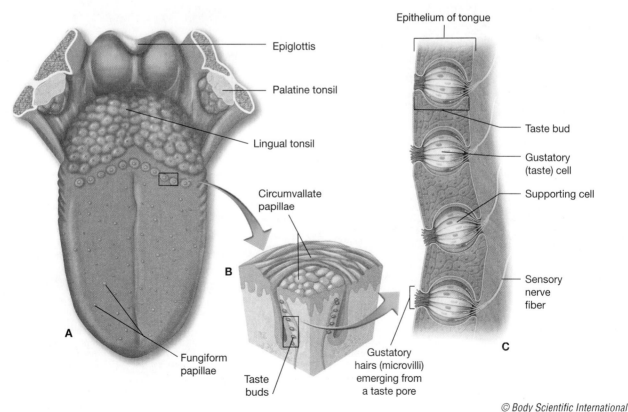

© *Body Scientific International*

Figure 20.24 The taste sensory organs include papillae and taste buds. *Why is it difficult to taste food when your mouth is dry?*

Old theories about certain areas of your tongue sensing different tastes have been proven wrong. Although some areas may have higher quantities of specific receptors, each taste bud may contain a variety of taste receptors.

Damage to taste cells can affect your sense of taste. Extreme heat, which might come from eating food that is too hot, can damage taste buds. Drugs, such as cancer treatments, may also destroy taste cells. Although new taste buds develop every 7 to 10 days, people gradually produce fewer taste buds. You have about 10,000 at birth and only about 4,000 as an adult. In old age, a reduced sense of taste may lead to a lack of appetite or a desire for more seasoning in your food.

Anything that affects molecules' ability to reach their receptors will affect your ability to smell or taste. Smoking, a dry mouth, or thick mucus caused by a cold can all reduce your sense of taste and smell. The business of creating new taste enhancers and ingredient substitutes for sugar, salt, and fat continues to be an area for research.

20.2-3 **Smell**

olfact/o = smell
-ion = action, process, condition

Your sense of smell is called *olfaction*. It is a chemical sensory system that works in a similar way to taste, but it is much more sensitive (**Figure 20.25**).

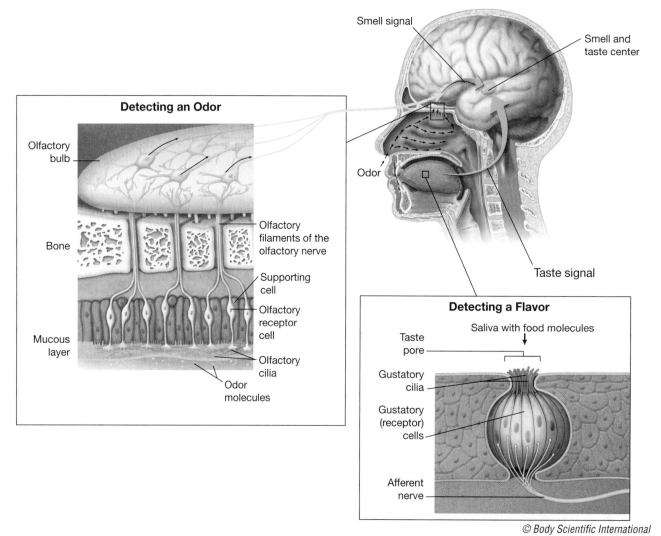

Figure 20.25 The chemoreceptors for smell and taste both share information with memory and emotion areas of the brain. *What taste or smell is connected to strong memories for you?*

You have about two dozen different kinds of olfactory receptors. Most odors are a combination of chemicals, so thousands of unique smells are possible.

When you inhale, scent molecules travel to the back of your nasal passage. Once there, the molecules dissolve into a small area of mucus covering your olfactory receptor cells. The sense of smell enhances taste, and some scent molecules may pass down your pharynx to taste receptors in the back of your mouth. A cold may cause thick mucus to block access to the receptor cells. This can reduce both taste and smell.

When scent chemicals trigger chemoreceptors in your olfactory cilia, the messages are passed to your brain. The chemoreceptors' axons pass through small holes in your skull to your **olfactory bulb**. Scent messages begin the sorting process with hundreds of glomeruli in your olfactory bulb. Neurons link your olfactory tract to your limbic system. This explains the strong connection between odors, memories, emotions, and compulsive behaviors such as overeating.

olfact/o = smell
-or = one who does
-y = process

chem/o = chemical
recept/o = receive
-or = one who does

20.2-4 **Hearing**

Your ear is an instrument for detecting sound waves. Sounds are actually waves of molecular vibrations picked up by the ear and converted to electrical impulses that are sent to your brain.

The Ear

Your ear can be divided into three sections: the outer ear, inner ear, and middle ear (**Figure 20.26**). Your outer ear includes the pinna and ear canal. Your *pinna* is the flap of cartilage on the side of your head that you recognize as an ear. It funnels sound waves into your auditory canal. Your **tympanic membrane**, or *eardrum*, divides your outer and middle ear. This thin membrane changes sound waves into vibrations.

Your **ossicles** are bones that transfer vibrations from your middle ear to your inner ear. Your largest ossicle, the *malleus*, sits against your tympanic membrane. Its vibrations move your other ossicles, the *incus* and *stapes* (STAY-pehz). Your stapes, in turn, pushes against the oval window of the vestibule. This is the entrance to the two fluid-filled chambers of your inner ear. These chambers are your **cochlea**, used for hearing, and your **vestibular canals**, used for maintaining balance. Inside your snail-shaped cochlea, the *organ of Corti* holds tiny hair receptor cells. The fluid waves created as your stapes vibrates move these nerve receptors. Different receptor cells wave in response to different pitches of sound. Your cochlear nerve transmits receptor movement and location to your brain's temporal lobe so the sounds can be identified, remembered, or responded to.

oss/o = bone
-icle = tiny

Balance and position are also sensed by your inner ear. Your vestibular canals sense movement of fluid. This gives you information about the position of your head. You can detect movements up and down, side-to-side, and tilting. Vertigo is the sensation that everything is spinning. It may also include dizziness, nausea, and a loss of balance.

vert/o = to turn

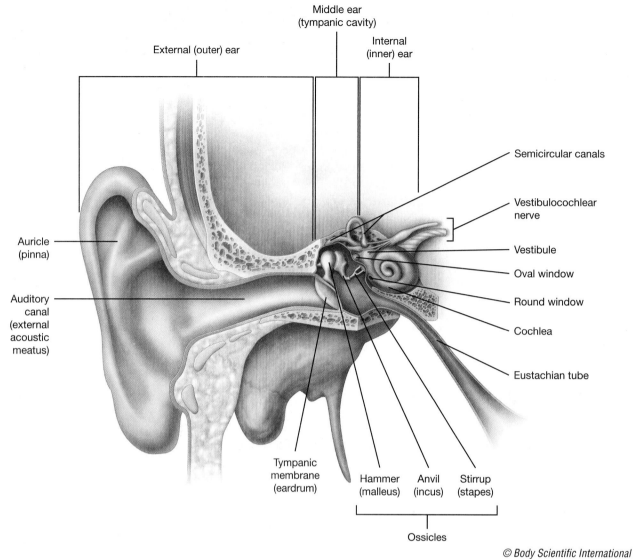

Middle ear
(tympanic cavity)

External (outer) ear

Internal
(inner) ear

Semicircular canals

Vestibulocochlear
nerve

Auricle
(pinna)

Vestibule

Oval window

Auditory
canal
(external
acoustic
meatus)

Round window

Cochlea

Eustachian tube

Tympanic
membrane
(eardrum)

Hammer
(malleus)

Anvil
(incus)

Stirrup
(stapes)

Ossicles

© *Body Scientific International*

Figure 20.26   The structures of the outer ear funnel sound waves from the air to vibrate the eardrum. Vibration of bones in the middle ear are transferred to fluid waves in the inner ear. Movement of hairs in the cochlea signal the brain to interpret the sound.

Hearing Screening

audi/o = sound, to hear
-gram = record

An audiogram is a graph that shows the results of a hearing test. It shows the frequency, or *pitch*, in hertz (Hz) and the volume in decibels (dB) measured for each ear. People can hear sounds ranging from a volume of about 20 to 20,000 Hz and a pitch of about –10 to 150 dB before experiencing pain. Normal speech ranges from about 50 to 500 Hz and 45 to 65 dB. The speech banana in **Figure 20.27** shows where speech sounds fall on an audiogram. Notice that consonants are generally higher pitched and more softly spoken than most vowels. Hearing loss within the speech banana can affect a child's ability to learn language or an adult's ability to understand what others are saying. Speech therapists help patients produce clear speech and understand words that are heard or read. This growing career area requires a master's degree and clinical fellowship due to the many complexities of speech and hearing conditions.

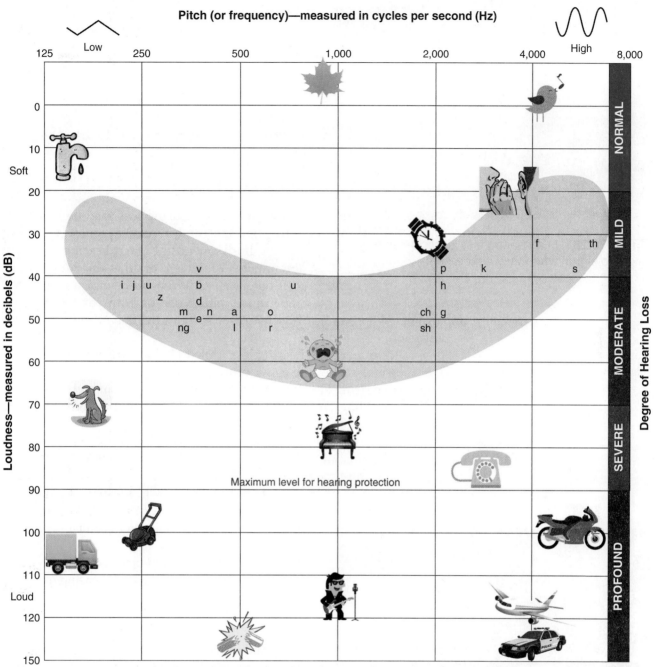

Pitch (or frequency)—measured in cycles per second (Hz)

Figure 20.27   The speech banana in this illustrated audiogram shows the range of hearing required to detect speech sounds. *What sounds would a person with mild hearing loss miss?*

An audiologist may perform a variety of tests for measuring hearing. The method of testing often depends on the patient's ability to participate. For example, auditory brainstem response (ABR) involves attaching electrodes to the head to pick up brain waves in response to hearing. An otoacoustic emission (OAE) test measures the inner ear's echo responses to sound. Behavioral observation audiometry looks for behavioral changes in response to sound.

audi/o = sound, to hear
-metry = process of measuring
ot/o = ear
acous/o = hearing, sound

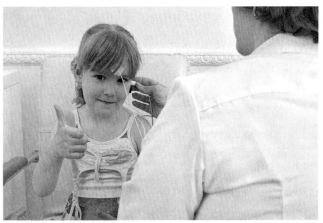

Capifrutta/Shutterstock.com

Figure 20.28 In a hearing test, participants are asked to signal when they hear a tone.

presby/o = old person
acous/o = hearing, sound
-is = pertaining to

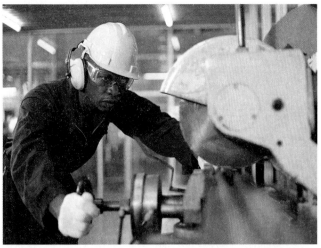

Akarawut/Shutterstock.com

Figure 20.29 Workers in environments with loud, persistent noises must wear protective earplugs or earmuffs. *What type of hearing loss do they help prevent?*

People being tested may be asked to raise their hand when they hear a tone (**Figure 20.28**).

Hearing should be checked at birth because approximately 3 in 1,000 newborns have hearing loss. This limits their ability to collect and process information and communicate with the world around them. Late diagnosis may result in permanent effects on speech, language, and social development.

Hearing Loss

Some types of hearing loss may be inherited. Both dominant and recessive genes can cause hearing impairment. Inherited hearing loss only accounts for 20 percent of all cases. Surprisingly, in 9 out of 10 children born with an inherited impairment, either one or both parents have no impairment. A loss of hearing that results from infection or injury will not be passed on.

Some mild to moderate hearing loss, called *presbycusis* (prehz-bih-KYOO-sihs), is a normal part of the aging process. This condition is different from other types of hearing loss. It particularly relates to sounds in higher frequencies, where an audiogram shows a gradual drop. Older people find it harder to understand high-pitched voices, such as in children. They also may not hear softer speech sounds such as *v*, *p*, and *s*. Background noise can interfere with their hearing. An inability to hear can be frustrating and embarrassing, affecting family, work, and social life.

Noise-induced hearing loss (NIHL) occurs when sounds that are too loud or last too long damage the sensory hair cells in the cochlea. High-frequency sounds cause the most damage. The harmful effects of exposure add up over time, so regular exposure increases your risk for hearing loss. You may have NIHL if you cannot hear yourself speaking, have difficulty understanding sounds around you, noise hurts your ears, or you develop a ringing sound or temporary reduction in hearing after being exposed to loud noise.

Workers who are exposed to noise at 85 dB or higher for extended periods of time are required to wear hearing protection, such as earplugs or earmuffs (**Figure 20.29**). Portable music devices often play at much higher levels than 85 dB. Healthy hearing habits can help prevent NIHL. For example, turn down the sound on TVs and portable devices. Block loud noises with earplugs or earmuffs or move farther away from the noise.

Hearing loss is ranked as mild, moderate, severe, or profound. There are also three specific types of hearing loss.

1. **Conductive hearing loss.** Conductive hearing loss occurs when a sound wave is not carried from the outer ear to the eardrum and into the cochlea. On an audiogram, conductive hearing loss results in loss of sensitivity across the entire range of frequencies and may affect only one ear. A buildup of earwax, or *cerumen*, against the eardrum; a hole in the eardrum; fluid in the middle ear; or the ear bones having a limited ability to vibrate may cause this. If the cause is treated, hearing may be restored.

con- = with, together
duct/o = to lead
-ive = quality of, nature of, pertaining to

2. **Sensorineural hearing loss.** Exposure to loud noises, drug use, or illnesses that damage the cilia may cause sensorineural hearing loss. This type of hearing loss may be hereditary and also includes NIHL. On an audiogram, NIHL creates a characteristic dip in high-pitched sounds around 4 kHz. Sensorineural damage is usually permanent but may be treated with cochlear implants for people who have profound hearing loss. These implants can provide some sound information to support hearing, but the information is different from what others hear.

sensor/i = sensation
neur/o = nerve
-al = pertaining to

3. **Mixed hearing loss.** Mixed hearing loss occurs when a person has both conductive and sensorineural hearing loss.

Hearing aids make sounds louder and can help filter out background noise. Advances in hearing aid technology have made devices smaller and more sensitive to different types of sound. Bluetooth-enabled hearing aids can connect with a smartphone to adjust sounds in different settings. Other technology, such as computers, teletype (TTY), and closed captioning, help people with a hearing impairment communicate with or follow the conversations of people with hearing. People may also use American Sign Language (ASL), a system in which the hands are used to represent letters, numbers, words, and phrases (**Figure 20.30**). This can be like speaking a different language. In healthcare, an interpreter may help a patient who uses ASL communicate with a professional who does not.

Hearing is an important sense for a variety of purposes. It helps people communicate, learn, and understand each other and is important to speech development. It helps alert people to danger and lets people locate a person or scene. Living with a reduced sense of hearing requires adaptation. Members of the deaf community have their own cultural norms, rules of etiquette, and a positive attitude toward being deaf.

20.2-5 **Vision**

Your eyes are *photosensitive*, meaning they can detect light within the visible spectrum (**Figure 20.31**). That light passes through several layers of the eye to reach the photoreceptors. Aging, eye disease, and hereditary conditions can all cause a loss of vision. Ophthalmologists define legal blindness as vision that is less than 20/200. What a person with this diagnosis sees from 20 feet away can be seen by a person with normal vision from 200 feet away. People with a narrow field of vision, or *tunnel vision*, are also considered legally blind. They lack side, or *peripheral*, vision.

phot/o = light

recept/o = receive
ophthalm/o = eye
-logist = specialist in the study of

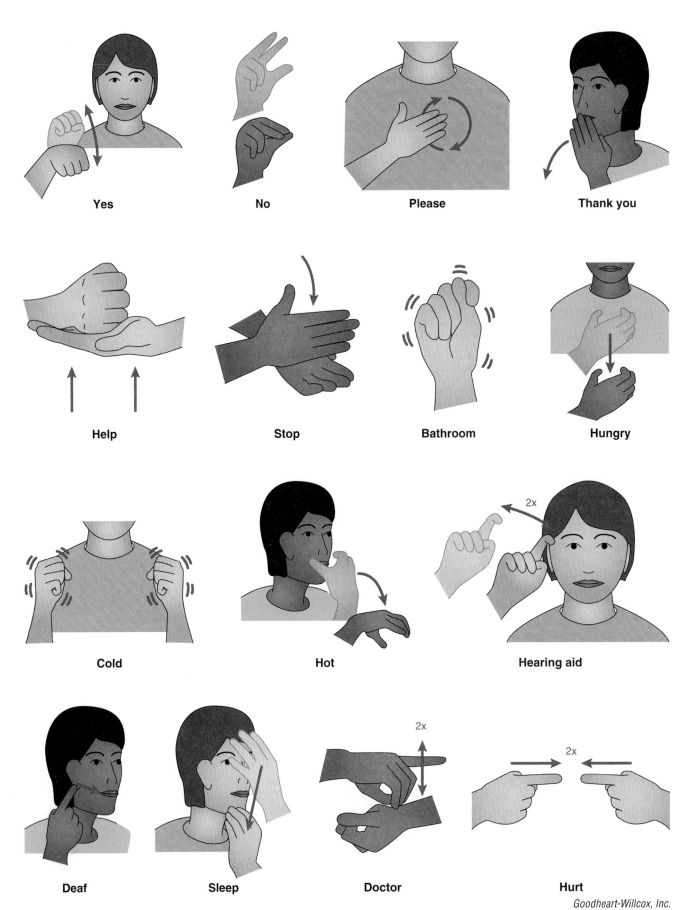

Yes **No** **Please** **Thank you**

Help **Stop** **Bathroom** **Hungry**

Cold **Hot** **Hearing aid**

Deaf **Sleep** **Doctor** **Hurt**

Goodheart-Willcox, Inc.

Figure 20.30 These are common signs in American Sign Language that might be used in a healthcare setting. *Show how you could check if your patient who uses ASL is comfortable.*

The Electromagnetic Spectrum

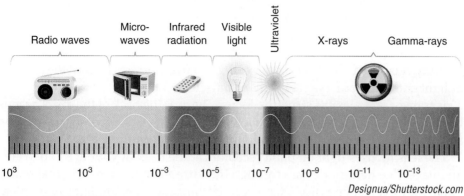

Designua/Shutterstock.com

Figure 20.31 The eyes are photosensitive, meaning they can detect visible light within this spectrum.

A diet that includes vitamin A and omega-3 fatty acids is important for eye health. The structures around your eyes also physically protect them. Your eyelids lubricate and shade your eyeballs. Touching your eyelashes triggers a reflex to close your eye. Tear glands, also known as *lacrimal glands*, produce a fluid to help cleanse your eye (**Figure 20.32**). Excess tears drain away to your nasal cavity through the nasolacrimal duct. That is why your nose runs when you cry.

lacrim/o = tear
-al = pertaining to
nas/o = nose

Parts of the Eye

The white of the eye, or **sclera**, covers your eyeball. Six extraocular muscles attached to the sclera turn your eyes toward the object you want to see. Crossed eyes, or *strabismus*, occurs when the muscles do not keep the eyes focused on the same point. Microsurgery, performed with surgical microscopes and microscopic tools, makes it possible to surgically correct eye muscles and many other eye conditions.

extra- = beyond, more than, outside
ocul/o = eye
-ar = pertaining to
micro- = small
scop/e = to view
-e = instrument
-ic = pertaining to

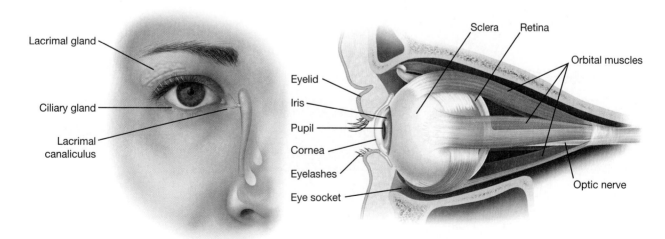

© Body Scientific International

Figure 20.32 The eyes are protected by the structures around them.

aque/o = water

Light enters your eye through the transparent **cornea** at the front of your eye (**Figure 20.33**). Next, light passes through the **aqueous humor**. This clear fluid in the front of your eye maintains pressure and nourishes the cornea and lens. In glaucoma, high pressure in the front of the eye can cause blindness. The light must pass through an opening in the cornea, called the *pupil*, to reach the lens. A circular band of muscles called the *iris* contracts to limit the amount of light entering your eye. Tiny ciliary muscles control the shape of your **lens**. This transparent, flexible structure focuses light at the back of the eye. The lens becomes less flexible and more yellowed with age. A cloudy lens, caused by age or cataracts, will reduce the amount of light entering the eye.

The lens focuses light on photoreceptors at the back of your eye to perceive an image. The light must pass through the **vitreous humor**, a fluid that maintains your eye's shape. Eye shape is important for focusing light that enters your eye. A misshapen eye focuses an image on the wrong area in the eye, resulting in blurry vision (**Figure 20.34**). Nearsightedness, known as *myopia*, results from an eyeball that is too curved or too long. If the eye is too flat or too short, farsightedness, or *hyperopia*, occurs. An astigmatism results when an eye is irregular in shape. Glasses, contact lenses, or refractive surgery can correct vision by changing the focal point.

my/o = muscle
-opia = condition of the eye
hyper- = more than normal, excessive
a- = without
stigmat/o = focus
-ism = condition

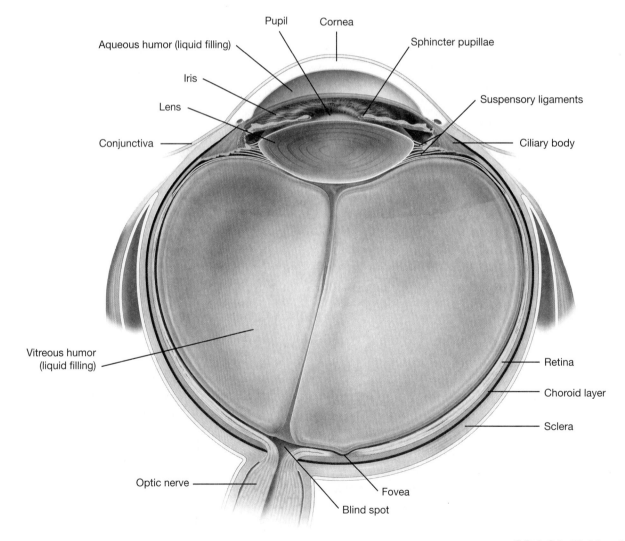

© Body Scientific International

Figure 20.33 The structures of the eye. *Which structure constricts to limit the amount of light that enters the eye?*

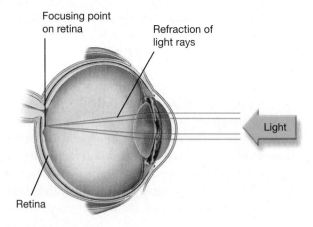

Focusing point
on retina

Refraction of
light rays

Light

Retina

A   Normal vision:
light rays focus on the retina

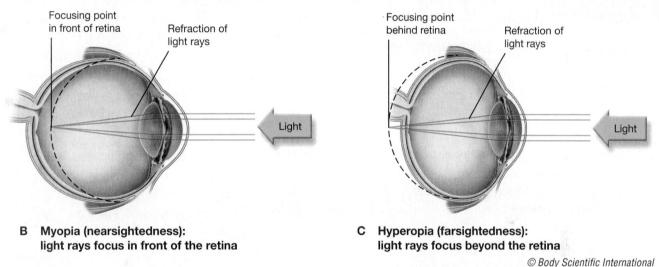

Focusing point
in front of retina

Refraction of
light rays

Light

B   Myopia (nearsightedness):
light rays focus in front of the retina

·Focusing point
behind retina

Refraction of
light rays

Light

C   Hyperopia (farsightedness):
light rays focus beyond the retina

© *Body Scientific International*

Figure 20.34   Common refractive conditions of the eye. *How is vision affected by an eye that is too long from front to back?*

The **choroid**, located at the back of your eye, is a membrane that supplies blood to your eye and controls the light reflected to your retina. "Red eye" occurs in photos when the flash of a camera reflects off the blood-filled retina at the back of your eye. Melanin is a pigment in the choroid that gives your iris its color and absorbs excess light reflection. The less melanin, the lighter your eye color, and the more sensitive you will be to light. The absence of melanin, in the case of albinism, causes low vision in bright light and abnormal development of the retina.

Photoreceptors

Two types of photoreceptors—rods and cones—in your retina interpret light as a visual image. Rods are the most sensitive to light. They are concentrated in an area called the *macula* at the back of the retina. They can pick up images in dim light but do not provide fine detail. A loss of rod function results in night blindness. Macular degeneration, in which the macula is damaged, can make the center of your field of vision look blurry, dark, or distorted. It is the leading cause of blindness in older adults.

phot/o = light
recept/o = receive
-or = one who does
macul/a = spot
-ar = pertaining to

Cones are the photoreceptors that interpret color and take in small details. Cones are most concentrated in the *fovea* at the center of the macula. Red, green, and blue cone receptors each respond to a different range of light wavelengths. Issues with color vision are usually hereditary. The genes for red and green cones are both on the X chromosome, so red-green color blindness affects about 8 percent of males but only 0.5 percent of females. Achromatopsia is a recessive trait for complete color blindness, resulting in black and white vision.

a- = without
chrom/a = color
-opsia = condition of the eye

Each eye gathers information from its own visual field. More than a million axons carry visual information from the eyes to the brain. The blind spot, where the optic nerve leaves your eye, has no room for photoreceptors. The axons join at the optic chiasma. Stem cell research has generated new photoreceptors for the eye, and retinal implants have been developed as new cures for blindness.

Lesson 20.2 Review

 Complete the *Map Your Reading* graphic organizer for the section you just read.

1. Which part of the brain interprets your senses? (20.2-1)
   A. Krause corpuscle
   B. Cerebellum
   C. Brainstem
   D. Primary sensory cortex

2. To access your taste sensory cells, food molecules must (20.2-2)
   A. reach the right area of the tongue
   B. dissolve in saliva
   C. be chewed
   D. be familiar

3. The sense of smell is called (20.2-3)
   A. olfaction
   B. gustation
   C. presbycusis
   D. association

4. Which part of the ear changes sound waves into vibrations? (20.2-4)
   A. Cochlea
   B. Vestibular canal
   C. Tympanic membrane
   D. Ossicles

5. The medical term for nearsightedness is (20.2-5)
   A. hyperopia
   B. astigmatism
   C. myopia
   D. presbyopia

The Endocrine System

Learning Outcomes

After studying this lesson, you will be able to

20.3-1 describe the functions of hormones and the endocrine system, including how hormones work.

20.3-2 explain how the endocrine and nervous systems are connected.

20.3-3 identify the functions of major endocrine glands, including associated diseases and disorders.

20.3-4 analyze factors affecting hormone production.

? **ESSENTIAL QUESTION**
What are the structures, functions, and diseases associated with the endocrine system?

Professional Vocabulary

Essential Terms

endocrine gland   a gland without ducts that produces and releases hormones directly into the bloodstream

hormone   a chemical used to send messages from an endocrine gland to a target organ

negative feedback system   mechanism that reduces a body function in response to a stimulus, such as a hormone

Important Terms

adrenal glands	parathyroid glands	thyroid gland
islets of Langerhans	pituitary gland	

Introduction

Your endocrine system is an important control mechanism for your body. It works closely with your nervous system to stimulate, regulate, and coordinate activities to maintain homeostasis. Maintaining this stable system allows your body to function most efficiently. While your nervous system tends to produce a rapid, short-lived response with electrical stimuli, your endocrine system works much more slowly and over a longer time.

endo- = within
-crine = to secrete

home/o = same
-stasis = stopping, controlling

20.3-1 Understanding Hormones and the Endocrine System

Unlike the glands of your digestive system, **endocrine glands** are ductless. They produce and secrete **hormones** directly into your bloodstream. Hormones are chemical messengers for your body.

metabol/o = change
-ism = condition

They regulate growth and metabolism, maintain fluid and chemical balances, and control sexual processes. Endocrine glands are located in many different areas around your body. **Figure 20.35** lists some of the hormones produced by endocrine glands.

Your hormones are produced in endocrine glands and then travel through the bloodstream to cause specific responses in specific target organs. A hormone must lock onto cell receptors of the target organ to send its chemical instructions into the cell (**Figure 20.36**). This takes much longer than the direct nerve stimulus action of your nervous system.

Blood screening can measure the amount of a hormone, as well as other substances controlled by the endocrine system, that is present in your body. Because your urinary system filters blood, urine tests can also assess hormone levels. Reagent strips change color to indicate the amount of a hormone or other body substance in the urine.

acr/o = extremities
-megaly = enlargement

Under- or overproduction of hormones can cause physical conditions. Because your endocrine system is slow acting, symptoms of an endocrine disorder may take years to develop or become noticeable. Acromegaly (ak-roh-MEHG-uh-lee) is a condition characterized by an oversecretion of growth hormone, usually caused by a tumor of the pituitary gland. It most commonly results in enlarged bones in the hands, feet, and face. The condition may go undiagnosed in adults because they are not screened for growth changes as often as children.

estr/o = female
-gen = origin, formation, producing

Sometimes, people take additional hormones that are not produced by their own body. For instance, people who experience menopause may use hormone replacement therapy to counteract decreasing estrogen levels.

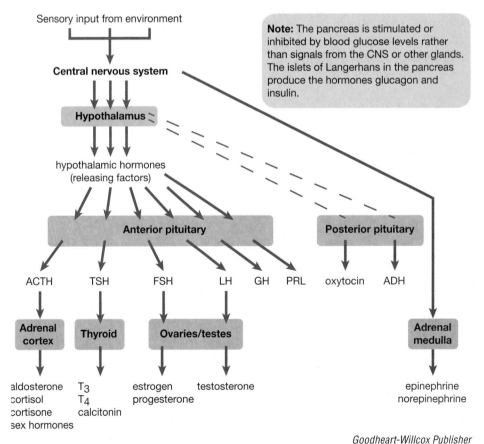

Goodheart-Willcox Publisher

Figure 20.35 Hormones are sent to organs other than the ones in which they originated. *Where are hormones from the anterior pituitary sent?*

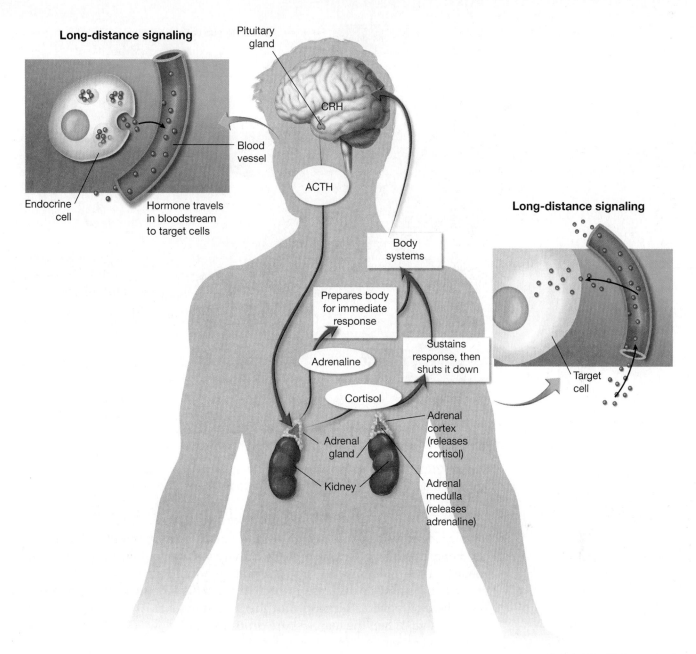

Long-distance signaling

Pituitary gland

CRH

Blood vessel

Endocrine cell

Hormone travels in bloodstream to target cells

ACTH

Long-distance signaling

Body systems

Prepares body for immediate response

Adrenaline

Sustains response, then shuts it down

Cortisol

Target cell

Adrenal cortex (releases cortisol)

Adrenal gland

Kidney

Adrenal medulla (releases adrenaline)

© Body Scientific International

Figure 20.36 Hormones travel through the circulatory system to reach their target organ.

Anabolic steroid abuse is a growing issue among athletes and teens. It is illegal to use these synthetic testosterone hormones without a prescription. They can cause unpleasant physical changes, such as shrunken testicles, development of breast tissue, acne, body hair growth, and baldness. In addition, they can have serious health consequences, such as weight gain, blood clots, high blood pressure, liver damage, and even cancer.

anabol/o = to build up
-ic = pertaining to

Hormones generally work to maintain homeostasis. Blood chemistry, nerve stimulation, or hormones from other glands tell your endocrine glands to release hormones when your system is out of balance. Many hormones, such as insulin and glucagon, are antagonistic pairs that work in opposition to each other. They operate on a **negative feedback system**. This system reverses a condition that is outside of the normal range to restore homeostasis.

home/o = same
-stasis = stopping, controlling

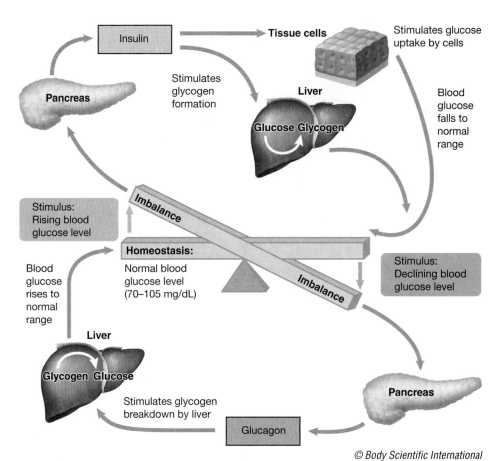

Figure 20.37 Hormones help the body maintain homeostasis in a negative feedback system. *How does insulin contribute to this process?*

© Body Scientific International

In a negative feedback system, when a body activity is out of balance, a hormone is released to encourage the activity to change (**Figure 20.37**). When the activity level is high enough, hormone production ends, or another hormone is triggered to decrease the activity. This is similar to the action of a home heating system. Suppose your thermostat is set at 70°F and is equipped with sensors. When the temperature drops too far below 70°F, the heat comes on. When the temperature rises to a point at or above 70°F, the heat shuts off. Endocrine glands act in a similar way to keep your body systems in balance. Positive feedback systems are less common, but they reinforce a change in the body rather than reversing it.

20.3-2 Connection to the Nervous System

The hypothalamus gland links your nervous system and endocrine system. The hypothalamus is located beneath the thalamus in the center of your brain. In addition to producing oxytocin and antidiuretic hormones, it secretes releasing hormones to encourage or discourage the activity of your pituitary gland.

Your **pituitary gland** is called the *master gland* because it releases hormones that affect the operation of many other glands in your body. A short stalk attaches this small gland to the brain just below the hypothalamus.

Your pituitary gland has two parts: an anterior lobe and a posterior lobe. Hormones produced in the anterior lobe control activities of your thyroid, adrenal, and reproductive glands.

The posterior lobe does not produce its own hormones. Instead, it stores oxytocin and antidiuretic hormones produced by your hypothalamus. Oxytocin acts on the uterus to increase contractions during childbirth. Antidiuretic hormone acts on the kidneys to conserve water in response to low blood volume or low blood pressure. The posterior lobe of the pituitary releases these hormones when stimulated by nerve impulses.

20.3-3 Functions of Endocrine Glands

There are many different glands in your endocrine system (**Figure 20.38**). They are responsible for many body activities. You already learned about the hypothalamus and pituitary glands. Following are some other examples of endocrine glands and their functions.

Thyroid and Parathyroid Glands

Your **thyroid gland** is made up of two lobes that sit like a bowtie on either side of your larynx. This gland controls energy, metabolism, and calcium levels in your blood. It requires iodine to produce its hormones. To get enough iodine in their diets, people use iodized table salt. When the body struggles to make thyroid hormones, a swelling around the neck called a *goiter* may develop.

Four tiny **parathyroid glands** sit on the back of your thyroid. They help balance calcium in your blood by secreting a hormone that triggers the release of calcium from your bones. Calcium is important in many cellular activities. Low levels of calcium in the blood trigger spontaneous nerve impulses and muscle contractions.

Adrenal Glands

Your **adrenal glands** are located just above your kidneys and have two parts that function separately. The adrenal cortex on the outer surface produces a small amount of sex hormones. This becomes important when a person with female anatomy reaches menopause and stops producing sex hormones from the ovaries. The inner part of the adrenal gland, the adrenal medulla, makes two important hormones: epinephrine (ehp-ih-NEHF-rihn) and norepinephrine.

Your sympathetic nervous system triggers the release of epinephrine, or *adrenaline*, and norepinephrine when you are stressed. This produces the "fight-or-flight" response (**Figure 20.39**). Your body prepares itself by increasing your heart and respiration rates, making glucose available for energy, increasing muscle contractions, and slowing other body processes. People have performed superhuman feats of strength in response to stress, such as lifting a car off a person being crushed. After the stress has passed, your parasympathetic nervous system returns your body to its "rest-and-digest" mode. What regulation system is this an example of?

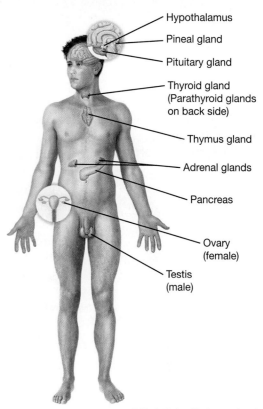

Hypothalamus
Pineal gland
Pituitary gland
Thyroid gland (Parathyroid glands on back side)
Thymus gland
Adrenal glands
Pancreas
Ovary (female)
Testis (male)

© Body Scientific International

Figure 20.38 The major organs and glands of the endocrine system.

thyr/o = an oblong shield
-oid = like
metabol/o = change
-ism = condition
para- = near, beside, abnormal

ad- = to, toward
ren/o = kidney
-al = pertaining to
-ine = substance, chemical

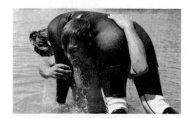

Roy Pedersen/Shutterstock.com

Figure 20.39 The release of adrenaline in stressful or emergency situations can allow people to perform amazing feats, such as rescuing a drowning person.

Ovaries and Testes

Your reproductive system uses hormones to regulate the development of sexual characteristics, production of gametes, and reproductive cycle. In people with female anatomy, the ovaries produce estrogen and progesterone. These hormones prepare the uterus for pregnancy, regulate menstruation, and trigger the development of secondary sexual characteristics such as breast tissue and body fat. During pregnancy, the placenta is a temporary endocrine gland that produces progesterone and human chorionic gonadotropin (hCG). These hormones maintain the pregnancy and tell the breasts when to release milk.

In people with male anatomy, the testes produce testosterone, which is responsible for the development and maintenance of male sexual characteristics. Testosterone supports the development of the testes, increased growth of bones and muscles, enlargement of the larynx, growth of body hair, and increased male sex drive.

estr/o = female
-gen = origin, formation, producing
pro- = before, in front
gest/o = pregnancy, produce
-one = hormone

Pancreas

Your pancreas secretes hormones that are important during digestion. This endocrine and digestive organ sits under your stomach. It secretes enzymes into your digestive system and hormones into your bloodstream. Clusters of cells on your pancreas, called **islets of Langerhans**, make the hormones insulin and glucagon. Insulin is produced when blood sugar levels are high. This hormone helps move sugar into your cells for use and lowers your body's blood sugar level. Glucagon responds to low blood sugar by helping your liver convert glycogen back to glucose. This raises your blood sugar level.

Diabetes mellitus is a chronic illness caused by decreased sensitivity to or secretion of insulin. Type 1 diabetes, or *juvenile diabetes*, begins in childhood and usually requires regular insulin injections. Type 2 diabetes, or *adult-onset diabetes*, used to be seen only in adults, but is becoming more common at all ages for people who are overweight and sedentary. Symptoms, which include excessive thirst, frequent urination, fatigue, and slow healing, may go undiagnosed for many years. Type 2 diabetes has a stronger link to genetic and environmental risk factors than Type 1. Type 2 diabetes has become an epidemic and is even occurring in children due to obesity (**Figure 20.40**).

insul/o = island
-in = substance, chemical
gluc/o = insulin, sugar
glyc/o = glycogen, sugar
-gen = origin, formation, producing

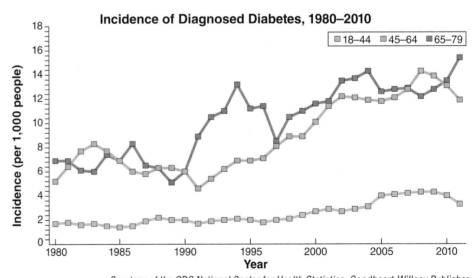

Courtesy of the CDC National Center for Health Statistics, Goodheart-Willcox Publisher

Figure 20.40   The incidence of diabetes diagnosis, grouped by age. *Which age group had the most diagnosed cases of diabetes after 2010?*

Diet and physical activity can help control it. The buildup of sugar in tissues caused by diabetes can slowly damage the blood vessels, kidneys, and nerves. It also slows healing and can lead to nerve disorders such as neuropathy and detachment of the retina. See Figure 20.1 at the beginning of the chapter for more information on this condition.

Several other glands also serve both your endocrine system and another body system. Your thymus is a collection of lymph tissue in the center of your chest. It produces thymosin, which plays an important role in your immune system's production and development of T-cell lymphocytes. The pineal gland in the brain produces melatonin, which makes you sleepy, in response to darkness. Your kidneys produce erythropoietin when blood oxygen is low. This hormone tells your bone marrow to make more red blood cells. Cells in the mucous lining of your stomach and intestines also have endocrine functions. They produce hormones that influence digestive secretions and the movement of substances through your intestines. The liver produces hormones that affect metabolism, mineral levels, and cardiovascular activities. It is also the main source of cholesterol and protein molecules used to produce and carry hormones in the blood.

thym/o = thymus
-in = substance, chemical

erythr/o = red
-poietin = to make

20.3-4 Changes in Hormone Production

There are inherited differences in sensitivity to hormone production. For example, hirsutism is a condition characterized by excessive facial and body hair in people with female anatomy. This condition is caused by an inherited oversensitivity to testosterone. Hormone imbalances increase your risk of obesity, diabetes, heart disease, and other health conditions. Endocrinologists specialize in diagnosing and treating hormone imbalances. Pharmacogenetics focuses on predicting and improving individual metabolic responses to new treatments.

pharmac/o = drugs
genet/o = origin, gene
metabol/o = change
-ic = pertaining to

Lifestyle factors can also affect hormone production. Physiological responses to stress, caffeine consumption, and lack of sleep can cause the release of adrenalin and cortisol. Smoking and alcohol consumption affect the production of reproductive hormones. Some chemicals in plastics and cleaning products have been identified as endocrine disruptors that affect hormone levels. Diet and physical activity also impact hormone production and release. Eating a healthy diet, getting regular physical activity, avoiding stress, and maintaining a regular sleep schedule support endocrine health.

As the body ages, a decrease in hormones may affect sleep patterns, bone density, digestion, urinary function, and regulation of other body activities. The bodies of older people break down hormones more slowly than those of younger people. With age, the body also becomes less able to handle stress.

Lesson 20.3 Review

 Complete the *Map Your Reading* graphic organizer for the section you just read.

1. Unlike other glands, endocrine glands (20.3-1)
   A. secrete substances
   B. are ductless
   C. have specialized cells
   D. produce substances

2. Which gland triggers the activity of the pituitary gland? (20.3-2)
   A. Hypothalamus   C. Adrenal gland
   B. Thyroid gland   D. None of these.

3. Which hormones trigger the "fight-or-flight response"? Choose all that apply. (20.3-3)
   A. Insulin   C. Norepinephrine
   B. Epinephrine   D. Glucagon

4. Which condition is characterized by an oversensitivity to testosterone in people with female anatomy? (20.3-4)
   A. Hirsutism   C. Diabetes mellitus
   B. Gynecomastia   D. Goiter

Chapter 20 Review and Assessment

Chapter Summary

20.1-1 The nervous system and endocrine system are the body's two main pathways for communication and maintaining homeostasis.

20.1-2 Neurons connect the nervous system. Their basic structures include a cell body, an axon, terminal branches and dendrites, and a myelin sheath.

20.1-3 The central nervous system includes the brain and spinal cord. The forebrain includes the frontal, parietal, temporal, and occipital lobes of each hemisphere. The midbrain includes the thalamus, hypothalamus, and pineal gland. The hindbrain includes the cerebellum and brainstem. Sensory, or *afferent*, neurons gather information from the body. Motor, or *efferent*, neurons signal a response.

20.1-4 The CNS is protected by the meninges, the blood-brain barrier, bones, and cerebrospinal fluid. Despite these protections, congenital conditions, diseases, and injuries can affect the CNS.

20.1-5 The glymphatic system transports and cleans fluids and waste in the brain.

20.1-6 The peripheral nervous system includes the nerves that extend out to the rest of the body. Nerves are named for their location and function. There are 12 pairs of cranial nerves and 31 pairs of spinal nerves.

20.2-1 The senses use special sensory receptors to gather information. Different receptors in the skin sense pain, pressure, vibration, stretch, and temperature.

20.2-2 When food molecules are dissolved in saliva, taste buds in the mouth enable your sense of gustation, or taste.

20.2-3 The sense of smell is called olfaction. Scent molecules dissolve in mucus at the back of your nasal passage and trigger chemoreceptors in the olfactory cilia.

20.2-4 The structures in your ear allow you to hear by converting sound waves to electrical impulses. Different types of hearing loss develop for different reasons.

20.2-5 The anatomy of your eyes enables you to detect light for the sense of vision. Changes in the anatomy of your eye can affect vision.

20.3-1 Hormones travel through the bloodstream to a target organ on which they act. This is a slower system than nerve signals to the brain. Hormones have unique functions in regulating body growth, development, and many system functions. Many operate in antagonistic pairs on a negative feedback system to keep the body in homeostasis.

20.3-2 The hypothalamus and pituitary glands link the nervous system to the endocrine system and control the release of hormones.

20.3-3 The endocrine system's major glands include the hypothalamus, pineal gland, pituitary gland, thyroid and parathyroid glands, adrenal glands, pancreas, thymus, ovaries, and testes.

20.3-4 Factors such as hereditary conditions, lifestyle choices, and age can affect hormone production.

Maximize Your Professional Vocabulary

1. **Term Connections.** Make term cards for the word parts that follow. Play *Term Connections* using the following directions:
   - Shuffle together two sets of term cards for every three players joining the game. Pass out seven cards to each player and place the remainder in the center as a "draw pile." Turn over the first card from the draw pile and place it term-side up to begin playing.
   - The player to the left of the dealer goes first. Players will attempt to get rid of their cards by discarding a term card that matches or coordinates with the card that is showing on the discard pile.
   - A discard may "coordinate" with your term card if it has the same meaning, relates to the same part of the body, or rhymes with it. Stretch your brain to come up with creative connections!
   - If the card is challenged by the entire group, then it must be placed back in the player's hand, and a penalty card must be drawn.

- If a player is unable to find a coordinating card in their hand, the player must also draw a card.
- If play goes all the way around the group without anyone being able to play, then a new card may be turned over from the draw pile and play continues.
- The winner is the first player to get rid of their cards, or the player with the fewest cards left at the end of play time.

Prefixes

bi-	hemi-	sym-
ecto-	para-	
extra-	post-	

Root Words

acous/o	genet/o	papill/o
acr/o	gest/o	pathet/a
alges/i	gluc/o	peripher/o
anabol/o	glyc/o	pharmac/o
aque/o	gust/o	phot/o
arachn/o	hippocamp/o	pi/a
audi/o	homin/o	presby/o
callos/o	insul/o	recept/o
cerebell/o	isch/o	ren/o
cerebr/o	lacrim/o	saphen/o
chrom/a	macul/a	sensor/i
corp/o	mening/o	somat/o
dendr/o	ment/o	stigmat/o
dur/a	metabol/o	tempor/o
encephal/o	myel/o	termin/o
enter/o	neur/o	thalam/o
equin/o	oblong/o	thym/o
estr/o	occipit/o	thyr/o
fid/a	ocul/o	trans/i
fiss/i	olfact/o	traum/a
gangli/o	ophthalm/o	vert/o

Suffixes

-ata	-lysis	-plegia
-derm	-megaly	-poietin
-emic	-metry	-sphere
-esthesia	-one	-ure
-ite	-opia	-y
-ive	-opsia	

Reflect on Your Reading

1. Review the questions you wrote for your chapter sections. Attempt to answer each question, then check your reading for correctness. On your deeper question(s), search for an answer online or share the question with a study group or your class to gain further insight.

Review and Recall

1. Which body system carries messages through electrochemical impulses? (20.1-1)
   A. Endocrine system
   B. Nervous system
   C. Skeletal system
   D. All of these.

2. Which structure protects axons from cross-connections that interrupt brain signals? (20.1-2)
   A. White matter
   B. Myelin
   C. Synapse
   D. Neurotransmitters

3. Nerves that bring sensory information from the body to the brain are (20.1-3)
   A. afferent   C. cerebellar
   B. efferent   D. motor

4. The liquid that cushions and provides nutrients to the brain and spinal column is called (20.1-4)
   A. blood   C. meninges
   B. CSF   D. water

5. Which of the following disrupt the glymphatic system? Choose all that apply. (20.1-5)
   A. Sleep deprivation
   B. Physical activity
   C. Aging
   D. Stroke

6. Major nerves travel along the same pathways as major (20.1-6)
   A. bones   C. organs
   B. blood vessels   D. muscle fibers

7. Which of these senses deep pressure in the hypodermis? (20.2-1)
   A. Ruffini ending
   B. Pacinian corpuscle
   C. Merkel disc
   D. Meissner corpuscle

8. Which of these can reduce your sense of taste? Choose all that apply. (20.2-2)
   A. Extreme heat
   B. Youth
   C. Smoking
   D. Thick mucus

9. When scent chemicals trigger _____ in your olfactory cilia, the messages are passed to your brain. (20.2-3)
   A. chemoreceptors
   B. photoreceptors
   C. ossicles
   D. papillae

10. NIHL is a type of _____ hearing loss. (20.2-4)
    A. conductive
    B. hereditary
    C. uncommon
    D. sensorineural

11. Which structure focuses light at the back of the eye? (20.2-5)
    A. Pupil
    B. Cornea
    C. Lens
    D. Retina

12. Hormones adjust activity levels in the body to maintain homeostasis in a _____ feedback system. (20.3-1)
    A. negative
    B. positive
    C. neutral
    D. homeostatic

13. Which lobe of the pituitary gland does *not* produce hormones? (20.3-2)
    A. Anterior lobe
    B. Posterior lobe
    C. Superior lobe
    D. Inferior lobe

14. Which hormone raises blood sugar levels? (20.3-3)
    A. Insulin
    B. Glucagon
    C. Prolactin
    D. Thymosin

15. Compared to younger people, the bodies of older people break down hormones (20.3-4)
    A. faster
    B. more efficiently
    C. more slowly
    D. more easily

Build Core Skills

1. **Reading.** Reread the sections in this chapter that compare the endocrine and nervous systems. How are these systems alike? How are they different? Find an example from the chapter for each system that supports your answers.

2. **Critical Thinking.** Using your knowledge of brain structures, answer the following questions. What is the value of wearing quality helmets for sports like football, snowboarding, or bicycling? From a medical perspective, what types of brain injuries could using a helmet avoid?

3. **Critical Thinking.** Which type of sensory deficit or loss would have the largest impact on your social life and acceptance by others? Why? Explain your response.

4. **Writing.** Research one of the diseases or disorders in this chapter that is not already discussed in Figure 20.1 or Figure 20.10. Describe its etiology, pathology, diagnosis, treatment, and prevention. Write a three- to five-paragraph essay using the information you found.

5. **Problem Solving.** In the endocrine system, what is the role of the hypothalamus? Identify one hypothalamus-related hormone. What conditions cause the hormone to be produced? On which organ does it act? How is the body affected? What makes the body stop sending this hormone?

6. **Math.** Healthcare workers must read and interpret information presented in graphs and charts. What information can you gather from Figure 20.40? What conclusions can you draw? What questions come to mind when you read this information?

7. **Problem Solving.** Study the increase of diabetes shown in Figure 20.40. What electronic devices became popular in the late 1980s and early 1990s that might have contributed to more sedentary activities? What suggestions would you make as a healthcare provider to help counter this issue?

8. **Critical Thinking.** Although most hormones operate on a negative feedback system, oxytocin uses positive feedback to increase contractions for birth of a baby. Reference Figure 20.36 and then draw or describe the positive feedback model of oxytocin.

Activate Your Learning

1. Create cards for the hormones ACTH, TSH, GH, PRL, Testosterone, Oxytocin, ADH, Epinephrine, and Glucagon. Create cards for organs acted on or affected: Adrenal cortex, Thyroid, Bones, Breast, Testes, Uterus, Kidney, Heart, and Liver. Mix the cards, lay them out facedown, then play "concentration." You can play this game alone or with a partner. Take turns turning over two cards to try to make a match, remembering where they are and returning them if they do not match. Continue until all are matched. The person with the most matched cards wins.

2. Simulate the effect of age or disease on senses or muscle control. Work in pairs, switching roles so each person performs the tasks. Record and share your results with the class. Which activities best simulated the feeling of having each condition? How did that make you feel?

How will this impact your treatment of patients in the future?

- **Vision**—Put petroleum jelly on sunglasses to simulate the loss of transparency and ability to focus the lens due to aging or disease. Then perform simple tasks like reading or tying a shoe while wearing the sunglasses.
- **Speech**—Chew two or more pieces of gum while reading a selection from a book out loud to simulate the potential effects of a stroke on muscles required for speech.
- **Hearing**—Walk through a hallway with cotton balls or earplugs in your ears to simulate hearing loss. Then walk through the same hallway without anything in your ears and pay close attention to any sounds you missed the first time. To increase your focus on hearing, try this blindfolded with a partner silently guiding you.
- **Touch**—Perform simple tasks such as writing your name, using a phone, or buttoning a shirt with your nondominant hand to simulate retraining of the brain following a stroke. You can also complete these activities after wrapping your finger joints with aluminum foil and then covering them with gloves to simulate loss of movement with arthritis.
- **Taste**—Suck on a peppermint or wintergreen candy or chew a fresh piece of mint gum for two to three minutes. Spit the candy or gum out, then put on a blindfold and have your partner offer you water flavored with small amounts of spices or drink mixes. Were you able to distinguish the flavors offered?
- **Pain**—Tape a few kernels of unpopped popcorn to the bottom of your sock at the toes, ball, or heel of the foot. Try walking to simulate the effects of bunions, corns, or arthritis.
- **Mobility**—Place a clean, unsharpened pencil in your mouth with the eraser hanging out. Use the eraser to turn the pages of a magazine and type your name on a keyboard without the use of your hands.

Think and Act Like a Healthcare Worker

1. Richard is an audiologist who works with older adults to check their hearing capabilities. Use the speech banana in Figure 20.27 to help him determine which of the following words use sounds his patients will be likely to lose first: *Keep, Hello, Coffee, Animal, Catch,* and *This.*

Go to the Source

1. Go to the Neuroscientifically Challenged website and use the drop-down menu to access their two-minute neuroscience videos. Choose a video about one of the topics from this chapter that you would like to understand better. View the video once, then review the chapter information or diagrams on the topic. View the video a second time and write a short paragraph about a new piece of information you learned and how it connects to what is in the text.

HOSA Event Prep: Behavioral Health

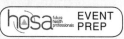

Sara is a 16-year-old who has had increased feelings of sadness and despair over the last six months. Her parents have noticed she has been distant and does not spend time with friends anymore. Last year, she got mostly As and Bs in school and wanted to pursue a career in environmental sciences. Now she gets mostly Cs and got her first D. In her science class, the teacher asked Sara about a missing assignment, and Sara lashed out and ran out of class. She has also had difficulty sleeping. After the science teacher called Sara's mother, Sara's parents decided they needed to seek further help. Their family physician recommended a psychologist.

Think About It

1. What condition is likely affecting Sara?
   A. Dementia
   B. Depression
   C. Obsessive compulsive disorder
   D. Schizophrenia spectrum disorder
2. What type of healthcare professional would likely treat Sara's condition?
   A. Endocrinologist   C. Neurosurgeon
   B. Genetic counselor   D. Psychologist
3. Which of these lifestyle changes might help Sara to manage stress in a healthy way? Choose all that apply.
   A. Regular physical activity
   B. Sleeping more during the day
   C. Using alcohol and illegal drugs
   D. Yelling at people who bother her
4. What area(s) of the brain is (are) most likely involved in producing Sara's emotions?
   A. Brain stem
   B. Broca and Wernicke areas
   C. Occipital lobe
   D. Temporal and frontal lobes

Chapter 21 Body Systems for Maintenance and Continuation

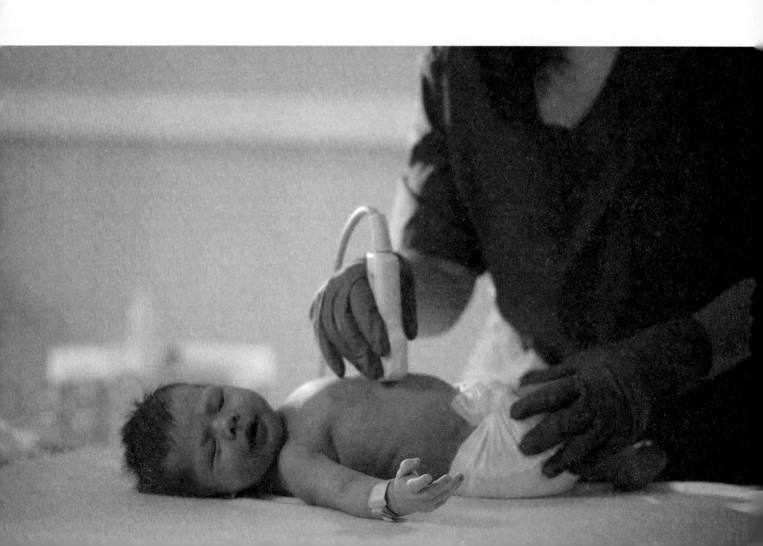

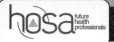
Healthcare focuses on prevention and maintenance. Encouraging regular visits to the doctor can help detect issues early when they are easier to treat. Healthcare professionals have to be good communicators and educators. Teaching patients how to prevent disease or how to manage disease creates a healthier population and decreases hospital admissions and complications from chronic illness. The team event *Health Education* allows students to select a health topic, develop a creative way to teach, provide instruction, showcase their lesson, and evaluate the effectiveness of the lesson.

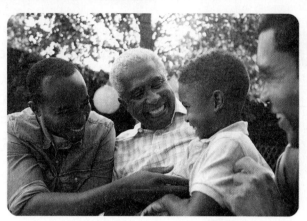

Go to the HOSA website to learn more about the HOSA *Health Education* event. Find out the purpose of the event, what is involved in the event, and what knowledge is demonstrated in the event.

As you prepare for HOSA competitive events, be sure to check the website and talk with your HOSA advisor for the most up-to-date guidelines and procedures. Once you have learned about the *Health Education* event, answer the following questions:

1. How might participating in this event benefit you personally and your future career? Explain.
2. Are you interested in participating in this event? Why or why not?

MBI/Shutterstock.com

Connect with Your Reading

Try a 1-2-3 strategy to gather information from your reading. Use a document or sheet of notebook paper. For each main section of the chapter, pause after you read to write down one main summary point, two points of interest, and three essential facts. This will become an outline of your reading.

Map Your Reading

Make a tablet organizer with two sheets of paper using the example shown here. Stack the sheets, keeping the edges even, but move the top sheet of paper up so its bottom edge is ½ inch to 1 inch above the bottom edge of the sheet below it. Holding both sheets of paper, fold them down so the top edge of the top sheet is ½ inch to 1 inch above the bottom edge of the top sheet. Crease both layers and staple at the folded edge. Write *Systems for Maintenance and Continuation* on the outside flap and list things you know need to happen in the body for humans to continue living and things people can do to keep the body healthy. Label the edges of the flaps below it with the headings *Digestive System*, *Excretory (Urinary) System*, and *Reproductive System*. As you read, add visual cues, definitions of new terms, and notes on the main functions of and careers and diseases related to each system.

Systems for Maintenance and Continuation	
food	reproduction
growth	energy
elimination	nutrients
water	homeostasis

DIGESTIVE SYSTEM
(Urinary System) EXCRETORY SYSTEM
Male and Female REPRODUCTIVE SYSTEM

Goodheart-Willcox Publisher

Chapter opener image: Rattiya Thongdumhyu/Shutterstock.com

The Digestive System

? ESSENTIAL QUESTION

What are the structures, functions, and diseases associated with the digestive system?

Learning Outcomes

After studying this lesson, you will be able to

21.1-1 describe the functions of the digestive system.

21.1-2 explain the process of digestion, including digestive organs and associated diseases and disorders.

Professional Vocabulary

Essential Terms

absorption   the act of taking up a substance into a tissue, such as the movement of nutrients from the small intestines into the bloodstream

defecation   the last stage of digestion in which undigested food and waste from the digestive system are expelled as feces

digestion   the mechanical and chemical breakdown of food into usable nutrients

ingestion   the stage of digestion in which food is taken into the body through the mouth

Important Terms

accessory organs	gallbladder	rectum
alimentary canal	large intestine	salivary glands
anus	liver	small intestines
bile	pancreas	stomach
esophagus	peristalsis	villi

Introduction

At all organizational levels of life, from cells and tissues to complete organisms, growth, repair, regeneration, and new life depend on the processes of your digestive, excretory, and reproductive systems. Your digestive system breaks food down to take in nutrients. Your excretory system removes waste products and helps maintain homeostasis for a healthy environment within your body. The reproductive systems produce, protect, and sustain new life from conception to birth. This provides a means for continuing the species. **Figure 21.1** presents some of the most common disorders of these systems. You will learn about many others as you continue reading.

Common Diseases and Disorders for Body Systems of Maintenance and Continuation

Characteristics	Gastric Ulcer	Hepatitis	Sexually Transmitted Infections (STIs)	Urinary Tract Infection
Etiology	Irritation usually begins with infection by the *H. pylori* bacterium or overuse of pain medications. Stomach acid continues to erode the irritated area until an ulcer appears. Additional risk factors include smoking, drinking alcohol, eating spicy foods, and untreated stress.	Most cases are caused by viruses. Three common types: HAV, HBV, and HCV. Drugs, alcohol, and autoimmune conditions can also cause hepatitis.	A broad group of viral, bacterial, and parasitic infections spread through sexual contact, primarily through body fluids. Pubic lice and scabies are transmitted during close contact. Anyone who is sexually active is at risk. Nearly 20 million cases each year, and one-half are under age 24.	Bacterial infection of any part of the urinary system. Use of catheters increases the risk of UTIs. Females are more prone, due to the shorter urethra and hormone changes in old age.
Pathology	Can occur on the lining of the stomach, small intestine, or esophagus. If left untreated, this can cause perforation, internal bleeding, infection in abdominal cavity, or obstruction of the digestive tract. Symptoms include burning stomach pain, heartburn, belching, fatty food intolerance, and nausea. Vomiting blood, black or tarry stools, trouble breathing, vomiting, and unexplained weight loss are serious.	Inflammation of the liver. Symptoms can include loss of appetite, nausea and vomiting, diarrhea, dark urine, pale stools, stomach pain, and jaundice. Some are mild; others can be serious and lead to cirrhosis or liver cancer.	Infection can cause flu-like symptoms, sores, redness, warts, unusual discharge, odor, itching, pain during intercourse or urination, and pelvic or genital inflammation. If untreated, some infections can lead to organ damage, cancer, infertility, or death. Females often have more serious effects from STIs than males, including infertility.	Infection causes a strong urge to urinate, pelvic pressure, burning pain during urination, and frequently passing small amounts of urine. Urine may appear cloudy, be red with blood, or have a strong odor. May cause pelvic or lower back pain, nausea, or vomiting. Untreated infection can cause kidney damage, narrowing of the urethral opening, and sepsis.
Diagnosis	Breath, stool, or blood tests can identify *H. pylori* in the body. Endoscopy looks for ulcers and can take a biopsy from the stomach lining. A barium swallow makes ulcers more visible during an X-ray series.	Liver function tests, antibody test, ultrasound of the liver and nearby organs, and biopsy.	May have no noticeable symptoms or may be mistaken for flu, urinary tract infection, or yeast infection. A pelvic or physical exam looks for warts, rashes, sores, or discharge. Blood, urine, or vaginal/seminal fluid tests diagnose the type of infection and determine treatment.	Urinalysis, looking for white blood cells, red blood cells, or bacteria. Culture of urine to identify the specific type of bacteria. Imaging of the urinary tract with CT or MRI, sometimes with contrast dye. Cystoscopy to view inside the bladder.

Goodheart-Willcox Publisher

Figure 21.1 Common diseases and disorders of the systems for maintenance and continuation. (continued)

Characteristics	Gastric Ulcer	Hepatitis	Sexually Transmitted Infections (STIs)	Urinary Tract Infection
Treatment	A combination of antibiotics kill the *H. pylori* bacteria. Stomach acid blockers promote healing. Cytoprotective agents protect the stomach and intestine lining. Antacids neutralize stomach acid to relieve symptoms. Acute bleeding may require surgery.	HAV infection generally needs rest and hydration. Antiviral medications are available for acute and chronic HBV and HCV infections. People who develop cirrhosis or liver cancer may need a liver transplant. Corticosteroids may be used for autoimmune hepatitis.	All STIs are treatable, and many are curable. Tests can determine the best treatment. Bacterial STIs are usually treated with antibiotics, and antiviral medications control viral STIs. Both the patient and sexual partner(s) should be treated to prevent reinfection.	Antibiotics and pain medications. IV antibiotics or vaginal estrogen therapy may be required for some cases.
Prevention	Protect yourself from bacterial infections by washing your hands and cooking foods properly. Use pain medications at the lowest dose possible and avoid drinking alcohol with medications. Use antacid or acid blockers to reduce stomach acids that aggravate the stomach lining.	Vaccination is available for HAV and HBV.	Abstinence from vaginal, oral, and anal sex is the only 100% effective way to prevent STIs. Reducing the number of sexual partners and using condoms lessens the risk for many STIs. There is a vaccine for HPV.	Drink plenty of water. Always wipe from front to back after using the toilet. Avoid scented sprays, powders, and douches that may irritate the urethra.

21.1-1 Understanding the Digestive System

nutri/o = nourish
-ent = pertaining to
ex- = out, away from
pel/o = to drive

The digestive system performs several essential functions for the body. It breaks down and extracts nutrients from food. These nutrients are needed for energy, growth, and processes that maintain your body. After the nutrients are absorbed, remaining waste is expelled.

How do you describe a digestive condition to your doctor? With so many different organs involved, one challenge of working with the digestive system is determining which organ is the cause. There are also many interactions between the digestive system and the endocrine, nervous, and circulatory systems. A gastroenterologist uses a wide variety of tests and may consult with other specialists to resolve digestive issues.

gastr/o = stomach
enter/o = intestine
-logist = specialist in the study of

macro- = large

micro- = small

The food services department also plays an important role in maintaining the health of patients, including digestive health. Patients need a balance of nutrients. Macronutrients include carbohydrates, proteins and fats. These are needed in larger amounts for energy and nutrition. Smaller amounts of micronutrients are needed to support chemical reactions in the body.

These include many different vitamins and minerals. Dietitians plan and prepare therapeutic diets to meet patients' unique dietary or nutritional needs. Food service managers oversee the portion sizes, meal requirements, and food presentation. Feeding assistants encourage and support residents in eating a well-balanced diet.

nutri/o = nourish
-ent = pertaining to

These careers may be found in large hospitals, as well as smaller long-term care facilities. Staff typically work regular hours, from early morning to evening, and have limited contact with patients. Dietary workers need knowledge of nutrients, digestion, and dietary principles to protect the health of their patients. They all play a role in analyzing information and investigating solutions so digestive disorders do not deprive the body of the nutrients it needs.

21.1-2 **The Process of Digestion**

The process of breaking down food for use by your body occurs in four stages: ingestion, digestion, absorption, and defecation (**Figure 21.2**). During **ingestion**, food is taken into your **alimentary canal** at the mouth. This long, hollow tube, made up of digestive organs, runs from your mouth to your anus. Digestion takes place in your alimentary canal.

in- = in, not
aliment/o = nourishment
-ary = pertaining to

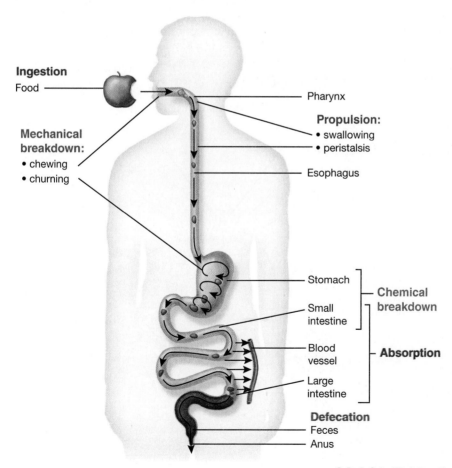

© Body Scientific International

Figure 21.2 The process of digestion. *What is the name of the tube where digestion takes place?*

Mouth and Teeth

in- = in, not
cis/o = to cut
-or = one who does

bi- = two
cusp/o = point
-id = having a particular quality

dent/o = teeth
-in = substance, chemical

gingiv/o = gums
-itis = inflammation

peri- = around
odont/o = tooth
-itis = inflammation

Your mouth contains different types of teeth used to chew your food for ingestion (**Figure 21.3**). Your deciduous teeth, or *baby teeth*, emerged first and were temporary. They were pushed out by permanent teeth that came in behind them. Your incisors have a thin, flat edge for cutting into soft and crispy foods. Your canines and bicuspids are pointed for piercing and tearing through foods, such as meat on a bone. Your molars are shaped for crushing and grinding food into small pieces.

A hard layer of enamel over a softer layer of dentin covers each tooth (**Figure 21.4**). The pulp in the center of your tooth carries its nerves and blood supply to the root. You should brush your teeth regularly to remove plaque and bacteria that build up at the gum line and cause gingivitis. Fluoride and sealants to protect tooth enamel have reduced the rate of dental cavities, or *caries*. Still, caries remain the most common condition found by dentists. Older adults and people with low income are more likely to experience gum disease, or *periodontitis*, the leading cause of tooth loss. Why do you think they are most at risk?

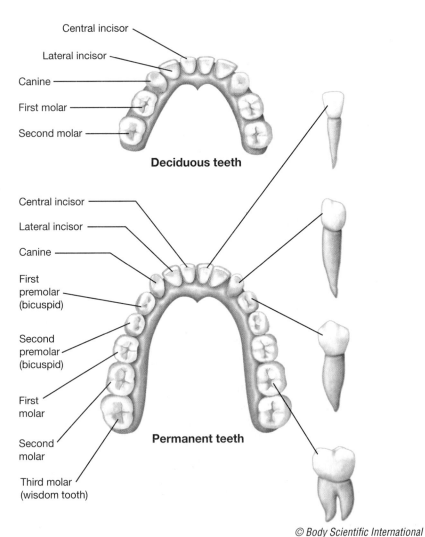

Central incisor
Lateral incisor
Canine
First molar
Second molar

Deciduous teeth

Central incisor
Lateral incisor
Canine
First premolar (bicuspid)
Second premolar (bicuspid)
First molar
Second molar
Third molar (wisdom tooth)

Permanent teeth

© Body Scientific International

Figure 21.3 Different types of teeth help break down food for ingestion. *What is the role of each type of tooth?*

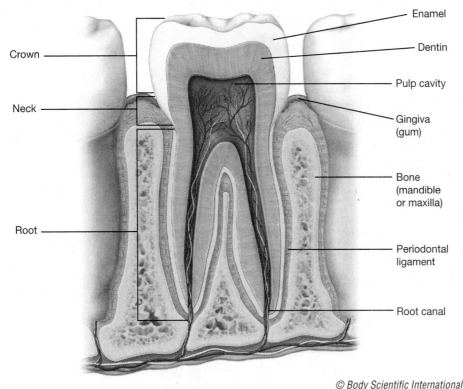

Crown

Neck

Root

Enamel

Dentin

Pulp cavity

Gingiva (gum)

Bone (mandible or maxilla)

Periodontal ligament

Root canal

© Body Scientific International

Figure 21.4 Each tooth consists of several layers. *What part of the tooth do you clean when you brush your teeth?*

The **digestion** stage uses a combination of chemical and mechanical activities to break down food into usable molecules of nutrients. Chemical digestion uses enzymes and acid produced by your body to break apart the chemical bonds in food molecules. **Accessory organs** attached to your alimentary canal produce many of the chemicals used for digestion (**Figure 21.5**). These accessory organs include your salivary glands, pancreas, and liver. **Salivary glands** in your mouth secrete saliva, which contains an enzyme that begins the chemical digestion of starches into sugar. Your tongue and teeth begin mechanical digestion. Their grinding and mixing expose more surface area of each food particle for digestive juices to break down. The resulting soft mass of food and saliva is called a *bolus*. Each organ of your digestive system works on this food bolus. They add chemicals and use smooth muscle to move and mix the bolus to release its nutrients and energy for your body. This smooth muscle in your digestive system is often called visceral muscle because it is found in the walls of most hollow organs, allowing them to squeeze out their contents.

nutri/o = nourish
-ent = pertaining to

viscer/o = internal organ
-al = pertaining to

Pharynx, Esophagus, and Stomach

Swallowing pushes the bolus from your mouth down your throat, or *pharynx* (FA-rinks). Involuntary waves of smooth muscle contractions called **peristalsis** squeeze the bolus along your **esophagus** (eh-SAH-fuh-guhs), the tube from your mouth to your stomach. In the muscular pouch of your **stomach**, the bolus is churned together with hydrochloric acid to break down carbohydrates and proteins. The lining of your stomach produces mucus for protection against the strong acid. Round sphincter muscles at the top and bottom of your stomach hold the food and acid mixture, called *chyme* (kIm), until it is time for the food to move to your intestines.

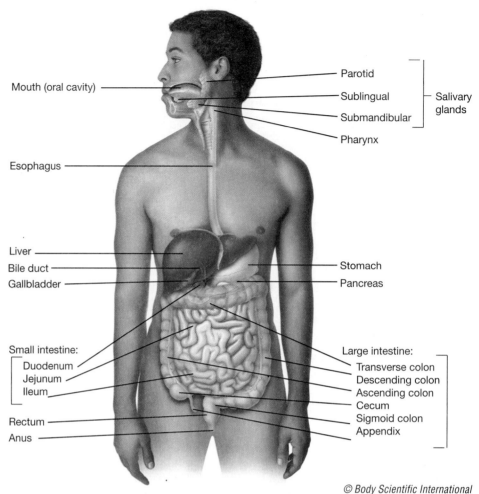

Mouth (oral cavity)

Parotid
Sublingual
Submandibular — Salivary glands
Pharynx

Esophagus

Liver
Bile duct
Gallbladder

Stomach
Pancreas

Small intestine:
Duodenum
Jejunum
Ileum

Large intestine:
Transverse colon
Descending colon
Ascending colon
Cecum
Sigmoid colon
Appendix

Rectum
Anus

© Body Scientific International

Figure 21.5 Food passes through the organs of the alimentary canal as it goes through the digestion process. *How are accessory organs different from those of the alimentary canal? Can you identify which organs in this diagram are accessory organs and which are included in the alimentary canal?*

Heartburn is the pain you feel when acid escapes through the lower esophageal sphincter. This is a symptom of gastroesophageal reflux disease, or *GERD*.

Pancreas

After several hours of digestion in your stomach, food is released into your *duodenum* (doo-AH-deh-nuhm). This first section of your small intestines receives digestive enzymes from your liver and pancreas. Your **pancreas** produces more enzymes to digest carbohydrates, fats, and proteins. Pancreatitis sometimes occurs when the duct to the duodenum is blocked, causing digestive enzymes to inflame and damage the pancreas.

Your pancreas also has an endocrine function. Islets of Langerhans cells within this organ make the hormones insulin and glucagon (GLEW-kuh-gahn) to maintain proper levels of sugar in your blood. High blood sugar, or *hyperglycemia*, can damage nerves, blood vessels, tissues, and organs over time. Diabetes, a disease that can cause hyperglycemia, is an epidemic in the US. There are nearly 35 million cases, and the number is growing. In this condition, the body stops producing or responding to insulin, causing sugar to build up in body tissues.

gastr/o = stomach
esophag/o = esophagus
-eal = pertaining to

pancreat/o = pancreas
-itis = inflammation

gluc/o = insulin, sugar

hyper- = more than normal, excessive
glyc/o = glycogen, sugar
-emia = abnormal blood condition

Metabolic syndrome is a related condition. It is characterized by abdominal obesity (waist size greater than 35 inches for females or 40 inches for males), insulin resistance, hyperlipidemia, and hypertension. The same hereditary and lifestyle factors for diabetes apply, including poor dietary habits and obesity. The incidence of metabolic syndrome is approximately 25 percent of the population. It leads to type 2 diabetes and chronic hypertension if uncontrolled. Treatment and prevention include a commitment to a healthy lifestyle, including physical activity and a plant-based diet.

metabol/o = change
-ic = pertaining to
hyper- = more than normal, excessive
lip/o = fat
-emia = abnormal blood condition

Liver and Gallbladder

The **liver** is your body's largest internal organ, weighing about 3 pounds. It is located in the upper right quadrant of your abdomen, above your stomach. It receives blood from your intestines, spleen, and heart. Your liver breaks down and removes toxic substances, drugs, bacteria, and dead red blood cells from your body. Hemoglobin from dead red blood cells provides the pigment bilirubin, which your liver uses to make **bile**. Bile helps mix fat with digestive enzymes so it breaks down in the intestines.

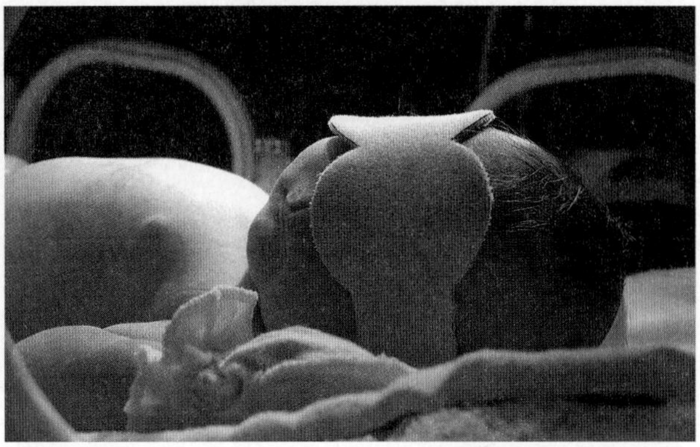

A poorly functioning liver that allows excess bilirubin to build up in the blood causes *jaundice*, a yellow color in the skin and eyes. This is a common condition at birth when the liver is immature (**Figure 21.6**). Phototherapy uses a full-spectrum light to break down bilirubin in the skin.

Cindy Minear/Shutterstock.com

Figure 21.6 Jaundice produces a yellow color in the skin and eyes. When jaundice occurs in infants, they are treated with phototherapy.

tox/i = poison
phot/o = light
hepat/o = liver
-itis = inflammation

Hepatitis is a common cause of liver failure. There are many types of hepatitis, each with different causes and symptoms. Hepatitis A commonly spreads through contaminated food; hepatitis B, through blood and body fluids; and hepatitis C, by contaminated needles. Childhood immunizations have reduced the incidence of hepatitis A by 90 percent and hepatitis B by 80 percent. The liver is involved in so many body processes that you cannot live without it. Luckily, it can regenerate damaged sections.

re = back, again
generat/o = producing
chole/o = gall, bile
ster/o = solid
-ol = alcohol
lith/o = stone
-tomy = to cut into, surgical incision
lapar/o = wall, abdomen
scop/e = to view

Bile from your liver can be stored in a small sac called the **gallbladder** until it is needed. Signals from your stomach trigger the release of bile from your liver and gallbladder into your duodenum. Sometimes gallstones, which are formed from cholesterol and pigments in the bile, block this flow. A cholelithotomy procedure removes the stones with laparoscopic surgery. Several small cuts are made in the abdomen to insert a light, camera, and surgical tools to remove the stones. This technique also allows a surgeon to remove the gallbladder with a shorter recovery and less pain than traditional surgery, which involves larger incisions.

Small Intestines

Absorption, or taking in nutrients, occurs through **villi** in the lining of your small intestines (**Figure 21.7**). These finger-like projections increase the inside surface area of the intestines. Nutrients touch the villi during peristalsis and are absorbed through the thin walls of your intestines. Capillaries and lacteals covering the outside surface of your intestines take the nutrients into the circulatory and lymphatic systems. Celiac disease damages the small intestines, destroying villi and resulting in poor nutrient absorption.

absorpt/o = swallow up
-ion = action, process, condition

celi/o = abdomen
-ac = pertaining to

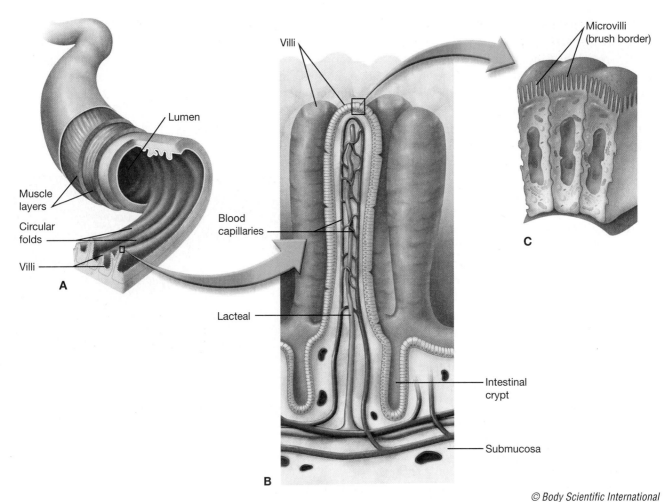

Figure 21.7   The villi in the small intestine absorb nutrients. *What disease destroys the villi?*

nutri/o = nourish
-ent = pertaining to

de- = lack of, away from
tox/i = poison

The 20 to 30 feet of your **small intestines** are divided into three sections, each designed to absorb different nutrients. Your duodenum absorbs iron. The middle section of your small intestines, the *jejunum* (jih-JOO-nuhm), absorbs carbohydrates, proteins, fats, vitamins, and minerals. The *ileum*, the last section of your small intestines, absorbs remaining vitamin B$_{12}$ and bile salts. A portal vein carries the nutrient-rich blood from your small intestines to the liver to be detoxified.

Large Intestines, Rectum, and Anus

Undigested food waste that remains after nutrient absorption is called a bowel movement, or *feces*. Liquid feces continue down your alimentary canal through your colon, or **large intestine**. This tube is about 5 feet long. The *cecum* (SEE-kuhm) is the first section of the large intestine, separating it from your small intestines. Water is absorbed from the feces as feces move through the different sections of the large intestine. The bowel movement travels up the *ascending colon* on the right, across the abdomen in the *transverse colon*, and down the *descending colon* on the left. By the time it reaches the S-shaped *sigmoid colon*, the feces are semisolid. The muscular walls of your sigmoid colon push the feces into your **rectum** for storage. Due to the position of the sigmoid colon and rectum, patients lie on their left side for rectal procedures.

The last step in the process of digestion, called **defecation**, occurs when feces are pushed out of your alimentary canal through the **anus**. If the feces have moved

trans- = across
-verse = to turn

through the colon too quickly, diarrhea may result. When the feces spend too long in the colon, too much water is absorbed from them. This results in constipation, with a firm bowel movement that is difficult to expel. This is more common with slowed digestion and lack of movement in old age. Hemorrhoids, or *piles*, are inflamed veins in the anal canal. They are aggravated by constipation and may cause rectal bleeding. This bright red blood is not a sign of colon cancer.

Colonoscopy is a form of screening for colon cancer that is recommended for people 45 years of age and older. When cancer blocks the intestines, a colostomy must be performed. This surgical procedure brings the intestine to the surface of the abdomen. It creates an opening, or *stoma*, where a bag is attached to collect feces (**Figure 21.8**). A healthy diet that is high in fiber and offers a variety of nutrients can help prevent or improve hemorrhoids, cancer, and many other digestive disorders.

dia- = through, complete
-rrhea = flow, discharge

hem/o = blood
-rrhoid = flow

colon/o = large intestine
-scopy = process of viewing, examination

col/o = large intestine
-stomy = to create an opening

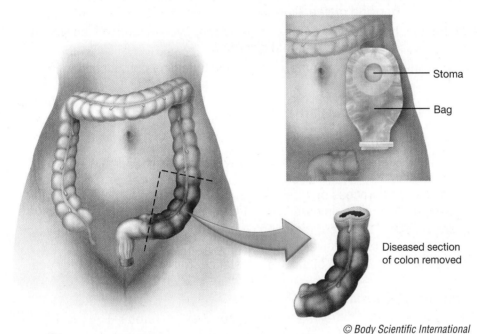

© *Body Scientific International*

Figure 21.8 When part of the colon is damaged, a colostomy must be performed to allow waste to leave the body.

Lesson 21.1 Review

 Complete the *Map Your Reading* graphic organizer for the section you just read.

1. Which of the following is *not* a role of the digestive system? (21.1-1)
   A. Absorb nutrients
   B. Break down food
   C. Extract nutrients
   D. Filter waste from the blood

2. Which of these are part of the alimentary canal? Choose all that apply. (21.1-1)
   A. cecum
   B. duodenum
   C. oral cavity
   D. pancreas

3. The teeth grinding and mixing food is an example of (21.1-2)
   A. chemical digestion
   B. absorption
   C. mechanical digestion
   D. defecation

4. Bile from the liver is stored in the (21.1-2)
   A. pancreas
   B. duodenum
   C. gallbladder
   D. rectum

The Excretory (Urinary) System

ESSENTIAL QUESTION

What are the structures, functions, and diseases associated with the excretory (urinary) system?

Learning Outcomes

After studying this lesson, you will be able to

21.2-1 differentiate between the roles of the excretory and urinary systems in removing metabolic waste.

21.2-2 analyze how the organs of the urinary system function, as well as associated diseases and disorders.

21.2-3 identify the role of the kidneys in maintaining homeostasis.

Professional Vocabulary

Essential Terms

excretion removal from the body of metabolic waste products created by cell activity

filtration the process of separating substances, such as solid from liquid, large from small, or impure from pure

reabsorption the act of returning a substance to the part of the body from which it was previously filtered out

secretion the release of a liquid substance from blood, cells, or tissues

Important Terms

bladder	nephron	ureter
kidneys	renal cortex	urethra

Introduction

Waste produced by your body can provide clues about how your body is working and whether its systems are in balance. Water, vitamins, minerals, hormones, and other substances must be retained in the proper proportions for your body to work efficiently and maintain health.

 Healthcare Professions: Drug Screening

Studying excretions can tell you a great deal about the body. As a human resources manager, Juanita uses this information to make employment decisions at her healthcare facility. All her employees undergo a urine test for drug screening as a condition of employment. Juanita knows it is not legal or ethical to test for other conditions, such as pregnancy or genetic diseases, during an employment screening.

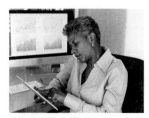

Alfredo Lopez/Shutterstock.com

She is careful to protect the private results of these tests in her records. Juanita's role in healthcare is to ensure patients have the best possible caregivers.

21.2-1 The Excretory System and Waste Removal

Excretion is the removal of waste products created by cell activity. In their study of the excretory system, some sources discuss organs such as sweat glands of the skin. The sweat glands remove excess water and mineral waste and help get rid of the heat produced during physical activity. Other sources might also discuss the lungs, which expel carbon monoxide and water produced by the cells. This lesson, however, will focus on the excretory role of the urinary system.

ex- = out, away from
cret/o = to separate
-ion = action, process, condition

Although the digestive system removes waste, it is not typically included as part of your excretory system. Digestive wastes are the remains of food intake that are not useful in cell metabolism. They are not the metabolic wastes produced by cellular work. Your liver is important for breaking down metabolic waste, but is usually considered a digestive organ.

metabol/o = change
-ism = condition

As your body functions, your cells create nitrogenous waste, carbon dioxide, and excess water that build up in your blood. If allowed to build up too much, this waste becomes toxic to your body. **Figure 21.9** shows the organs of the excretory system.

tox/i = poison
-ic = pertaining to

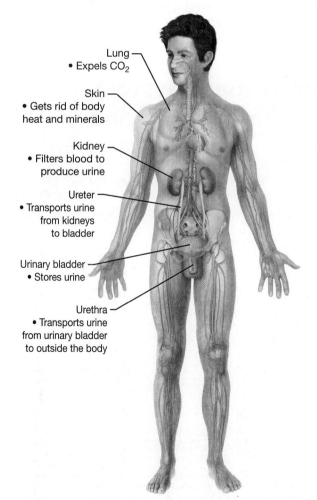

Lung
• Expels CO_2

Skin
• Gets rid of body heat and minerals

Kidney
• Filters blood to produce urine

Ureter
• Transports urine from kidneys to bladder

Urinary bladder
• Stores urine

Urethra
• Transports urine from urinary bladder to outside the body

© Body Scientific International

Figure 21.9 The organs of the excretory system. *Which excretory organs are not part of the urinary system?*

Your kidneys, ureters, bladder, and urethra are involved in filtering waste from your blood. If your kidneys fail, your body will be slowly poisoned to death without intervention.

A hemodialysis machine must be used when the kidneys no longer function properly to filter waste and balance water, vitamins, minerals, and hormones in the blood (**Figure 21.10**). Dialysis technicians monitor patients at a dialysis center during these lifesaving treatments. The technicians test the patient's blood, monitor vital signs, and care for the dialysis equipment. They may see the same patients on a regular basis and can observe changes in patients before and after treatment. This is very different from laboratory technicians who work in a lab setting and test labeled samples. Both careers provide valuable information and support patient health in different ways.

A healthy urinary system excretes about 10 cups of light-yellow urine per day. Urine exiting the body can provide a lot of information. For instance, dark-colored urine can indicate dehydration, while cloudy urine may signal a urinary tract infection (UTI) (**Figure 21.11**). Urine tests can determine diabetes, pregnancy, drug use, kidney disease, and a variety of other conditions in a patient.

hem/o = blood
-dialysis = to separate

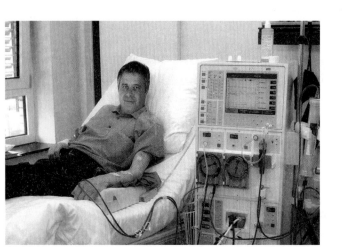

gopixa/Shutterstock.com

Figure 21.10 Dialysis uses equipment to filter waste from the blood when the kidneys no longer can.

21.2-2 The Urinary System and Blood Filtration

Many people confuse the roles of the digestive and urinary systems. The digestive system collects nutrients from food and the circulatory system delivers them from the liver to your cells. Undigested food is removed as feces, but your digestive system does not form urine. As your cells use the nutrients, they create waste. Your liver changes those waste products into urea.

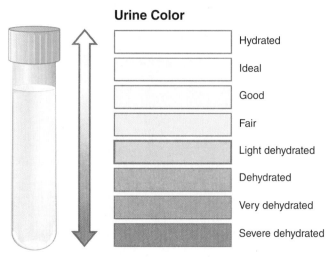

Designua/Shutterstock.com

Figure 21.11 The color of urine can tell you about a person's hydration level and health.

Blood carries that waste to your **kidneys**, which are located just below your liver in your lower back. Your kidneys filter, concentrate, and remove waste from your blood to form urine. Your urinary system does not directly filter the products of your digestive system.

Kidneys and Filtration

About 45 gallons of blood flow through your renal arteries to your kidneys each day (**Figure 21.12**). Blood flow to your kidneys is essential for filtration. When blood flow or blood pressure to your kidneys decreases, this reduces their ability to filter and remove waste. Heart disease, high blood pressure, and diabetes are common conditions that make the kidneys less efficient. Older adults have more risk of kidney failure because they are more likely to have one of these related conditions.

ren/o = kidney
-al = pertaining to

Although people can live for weeks without food, they can only live a few days without water. Dehydration also reduces blood flow to your kidneys and causes electrolyte imbalances that can result in death. Experts recommend drinking eight glasses of water per day to avoid dehydration and keep blood flowing through your kidneys.

de- = lack of, away from
hydr/o = water
-ation = action of, process of

There are three steps to urine formation in your kidneys (**Figure 21.13**):

1. **Filtration. Filtration** is the process of separating the substances in your blood. This occurs in the capillary beds that lie in the **renal cortex** of your kidneys. This dark red, blood-rich, outer portion of each kidney contains millions of *glomeruli* (glah-MER-yuh-lI). Each glomerulus is a ball of capillaries surrounded by a Bowman's capsule that collects water, sugar, salts, urea, and other waste from your blood. Blood cells and protein stay in your blood vessels unless the blood vessels are damaged and allow them to leak out. The waste-filled yellowish liquid that is collected flows through a *collecting tubule*. The glomerulus and tubules form a **nephron** (NEH-fran). More than one million nephrons filter your blood in each kidney.

glomer/o = ball
-ule = small
-us = structure

tub/o = pipe
nephr/o = kidney

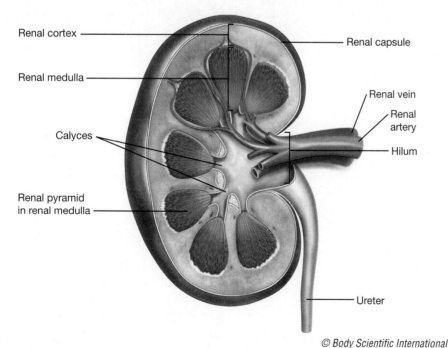

Renal cortex

Renal medulla

Calyces

Renal pyramid
in renal medulla

Renal capsule

Renal vein

Renal
artery

Hilum

Ureter

© Body Scientific International

Figure 21.12 The structure of the kidney. *Where are the kidneys located in the body?*

re- = back, again
absorpt/o = swallow up
-ion = action, process, condition
cret/o = to separate

ren/o = kidney
-al = pertaining to
medull/o = middle
tub/o = pipe
-ule = small

2. **Reabsorption.** Capillaries wrap around the nephron loop of the collecting tubule. Here, **reabsorption** returns some water, sugar, and salts to balance them in your blood for use by your body.

3. **Secretion. Secretion** is the phase in which remaining toxins, drugs, ions, and metabolic waste are pulled back into your collecting tubule to form urine. This occurs in the nephron loop at the same time as reabsorption. After waste products are balanced and excess waste is secreted, your renal vein returns blood to your circulatory system to collect more toxins from your body.

Your *renal medulla* contains pyramid-shaped groups of collecting tubules. These tubules empty into ducts that merge to form *calyces* (KAY-luh-seez), which collect the urine. Calyces connect to form the *renal pelvis* at the center of your kidney.

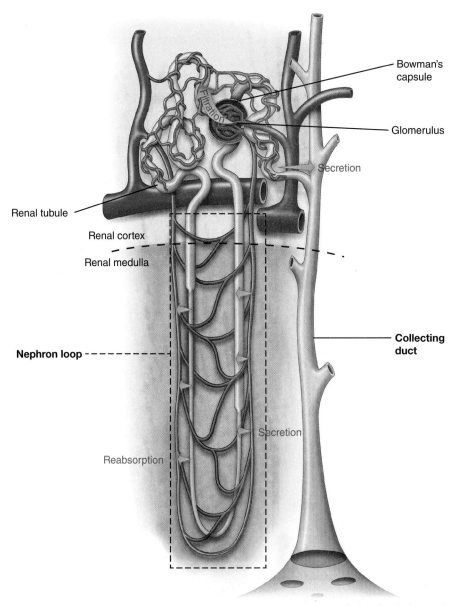

© Body Scientific International

Figure 21.13 Each nephron performs the steps of urine formation. *Where are nephrons located?*

Ureters, Bladder, and Urethra

A **ureter** exits each kidney at its *hilum*, a depression on the medial side of the kidney. This long, thin ureter carries urine from your kidney to your bladder.

Sometimes a kidney stone blocks urine flow. This painful collection of crystals can occur anywhere in the urinary tract. The ureter is a common site because it is a narrow tube. A procedure called lithotripsy uses shock waves to break apart kidney stones without surgery. The tiny pieces flow out with the urine during urination.

lith/o = stone
-tripsy = to crush

When urine reaches your **bladder**, it is stored there temporarily. Your bladder, like your stomach and rectum, is a muscular sac. It has folds called *rugae* (ROO-gee) that allow it to expand without causing damage. Sphincter muscles keep your bladder's exit point closed until it is "time to go." When your brain tells the sphincter muscles to relax, urine flows down your **urethra** to be eliminated. Remember that you have two ureters (two 'e's) to drain your two kidneys and only one urethra (one 'e') to drain your one bladder.

In females, the urethra is only about 1½ inches long, making people with female anatomy more prone to UTIs. This is because bacteria can more easily travel the short distance up to the bladder. The urethra is longer in males, making them less prone to UTIs. People with male anatomy are more likely to have urethritis, which is an inflammation of the urethra. In males, the urethra also serves as a passageway for the reproductive system. This puts males at risk for a variety of sexually transmitted infections (STIs) that can affect the urethra. Painful urination may be a symptom of urethritis or an STI.

urethr/o = urethra
-itis = inflammation

Urination is an issue for many people. *Nocturnal enuresis* is the medical term for bedwetting while sleeping, which sometimes still happens after children are toilet trained. *Urinary incontinence* is the inability to control when you urinate. People who are pregnant may have urinary accidents because of the pressure the developing baby places on the bladder. Older people who have gone through vaginal childbirth may continue to have stress incontinence when they sneeze or laugh.

noct- = night
en- = within, in
ur/e = urine
-sis = condition

in- = in, not
continent/o = holding together

The inability to completely empty the bladder, called *urinary retention*, is most common in males with an enlarged prostate. The prostate gland surrounds the urethra like a donut. *Benign prostatic hyperplasia (BPH)* causes an increase in the number of cells in the prostate. This enlargement squeezes the urethra and may restrict the flow of urine through the urethra. Sometimes, a tube called a *catheter* may be inserted through the urethra to help drain the bladder. *Nocturia* is the need to get up at night to urinate. Frequent urination may indicate urinary retention or diabetes. Most urinary conditions are treatable, and symptoms should be reported to your doctor.

re- = back, again
ten/o = to hold
-tion = action, process, condition
hyper- = more than normal, excessive
-plasia = development, formation
noct- = night
-uria = urine condition

21.2-3 The Kidneys' Role in Maintaining Homeostasis

The kidneys balance your body's fluids and minerals. During the production of urine, your kidneys sense the amounts of different substances in your blood. Healthy kidneys either return or excrete different substances to maintain a proper proportion of each substance in the blood.

Your kidneys influence blood pressure. When you do not have enough fluid in your body and your blood pressure drops, your kidneys produce *renin*. This enzyme helps raise the blood pressure in your kidneys to improve their filtering. Renin signals the *adrenal cortex*, an endocrine gland sitting on top of each kidney.

ren/o = kidney
-in = substance, chemical
ad- = to, toward
-al = pertaining to

-one = hormone
anti- = against
di- = complete, two
uret/o = ureter, urine, urination
-ic = pertaining to

acid/o = acid, low pH
-osis = condition

erythr/o = red
-poietin = to make
calc/i = calcium
tri- = three
-ol = alcohol

The adrenal cortex produces *aldosterone,* a hormone that tells your body to keep sodium and excrete potassium ions. As a result, an *antidiuretic hormone (ADH)* from your brain increases thirst. This cycle increases water retention and raises blood pressure. Medications that interrupt this renin, aldosterone, and ADH production cycle help control high blood pressure.

The kidneys also influence your body's pH level. Your body closely regulates its acid-base balance, keeping blood pH between 7.35 and 7.45. Both your kidneys and your lungs affect pH by reducing the number of free hydrogen ions in your body. Your lungs achieve this by expelling carbon dioxide (CO_2) and water (H_2O). Your kidneys influence pH by reabsorbing bicarbonate (HCO_3) into the blood and excreting hydrogen ions in urine. Without this tight regulation on pH, serious conditions such as acidosis can result in death.

In addition, your kidneys produce and react to hormones and enzymes that control other body functions. When your kidneys sense a low number of red blood cells, they make *erythropoietin* (ih-rihth-roh-POY-eht-ihn), a hormone that tells your bone marrow to make more red blood cells. This process helps prevent conditions such as anemia. Your kidneys also make *calcitriol,* a form of vitamin D_3. Calcitriol tells your intestines to absorb calcium from food and tells your kidneys to retain calcium in the blood. This process increases during breastfeeding because of the greater demand for calcium to produce milk.

The close relationship between the urinary, endocrine, and cardiovascular systems makes it difficult to change one excretory function without affecting other body processes. This means a patient may need to consult two or more specialists for any given condition. A patient advocate performs a support role in this type of complicated medical situation. The advocate helps the patient navigate the healthcare system and can assist in understanding a doctor's diagnosis, arranging appointments, and filing insurance claims. Advocacy is a growing support services career area that brings together many areas of knowledge.

Lesson 21.2 Review

 Complete the *Map Your Reading* graphic organizer for the section you just read.

1. The removal of waste products created by cell activity is called (21.2-1)
   A. secretion
   B. defecation
   C. filtration
   D. excretion

2. Where in the urinary system does filtration occur? (21.2-2)
   A. Bladder
   B. Renal cortex
   C. Renal medulla
   D. Ureter

3. The need to get up at night to urinate is called (21.2-2)
   A. nocturnal enuresis
   B. urinary retention
   C. nocturia
   D. BPH

4. Which hormone do the kidneys produce in response to low numbers of red blood cells? (21.2-3)
   A. Calcitriol
   B. ADH
   C. Aldosterone
   D. Erythropoietin

The Reproductive Systems

Learning Outcomes

After studying this lesson, you will be able to

21.3-1 identify male reproductive organs and their functions.

21.3-2 identify female reproductive organs and their functions.

21.3-3 analyze the impact of sexually transmitted infections (STIs) on the reproductive systems.

21.3-4 describe cellular reproduction and the biomedical therapies used to prevent and treat genetic disorders.

21.3-5 describe how hormones influence the reproductive systems and facilitate reproduction.

21.3-6 summarize the process of reproduction, including prenatal development, and childbirth.

ESSENTIAL QUESTION

What are the structures, functions, and diseases associated with the reproductive systems?

Professional Vocabulary

Essential Terms

gametes reproductive cells that have half the normal number of chromosomes and unite during fertilization; sperm in males and ova in females

gonads reproductive glands that produce gametes and reproductive hormones; testes in males and ovaries in females

gene a unit of heredity within DNA that determines traits and instructs the cell to make molecules that regulate body processes

meiosis the sexual process of cellular reproduction that produces four new haploid cells, each with a unique combination of 23 chromosomes

mitosis the asexual process of cellular reproduction that creates two identical copies of a cell, each with a full set of 46 chromosomes

Important Terms

amniotic sac	fetus	placenta
blastocyst	gene therapy	scrotum
cervix	genetic disorders	semen
chromosome	genetic testing	sperm
cloning	heredity	testes
embryo	morula	uterus
epididymis	ova	vagina
fallopian tube	ovaries	vas deferens
fertilization	penis	zygote

Introduction

While your digestive and excretory systems maintain good health, only your reproductive system can generate new life to continue the species. The reproductive systems include all the organs required to produce sperm, eggs, and sex hormones, as well as organs connected to fertilization, pregnancy, and the development of new life.

Reproduction is a complex process controlled by hormones. Many jobs have emerged from people's ability to control reproductive options. Marriage and family counselors often help couples through the emotions and decisions related to reproduction and sexual relationships. Genetic counselors identify testing options and discuss congenital diseases and the risks of disease inheritance. Clinical fertility coordinators help patients experiencing infertility follow the complicated schedule of appointments and activities for in vitro fertilization. People in these careers enjoy a stable daytime schedule, medical office environment, and growing demand for their skills.

con- = with, together
genit/o = birth, bring forth
-al = pertaining to

in- = in, not
fertiliz/o = to bear, make fruitful

21.3-1 The Male Reproductive Organs

The role of the male reproductive system is to produce and deliver sperm to the female for reproduction (**Figure 21.14**). Sometimes call *testicles*, two oval **testes** are the male reproductive glands, or **gonads**. They produce **sperm**.

gonad/o = gonads, ovaries, testes

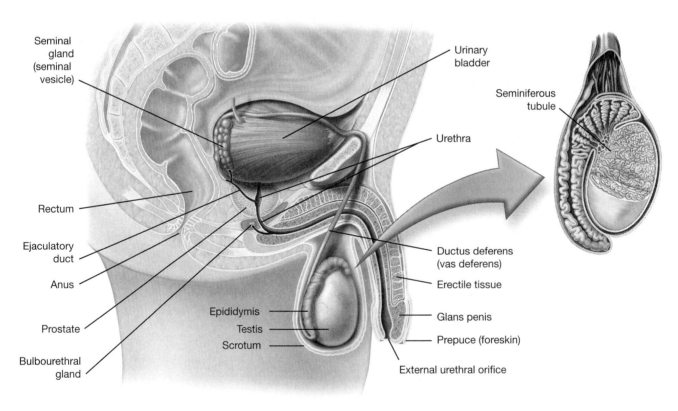

© Body Scientific International

Figure 21.14   The male reproductive system. *What are the male gonads and gametes?*

These tadpole-shaped male **gametes** are the male's reproductive cells. They carry 23 chromosomes, half of the genetic information needed to create a new cell. People with male anatomy are not born with sperm, but they produce millions of them each day. Sperm form in long, thin *seminiferous tubules* of the testes.

Sperm production begins at puberty and continues into old age, although the number of sperm produced declines with age. The sperm mature in the **epididymis** at the top of each testis and are stored until they are ready for release. The **scrotum** is a sac that holds the testes on the outside of the body. Muscles in the scrotum tighten in cold temperatures and loosen when warm to maintain a constant environment ideal for sperm production. Sperm leave the testis through the **vas deferens**, which is sometimes called the *ductus deferens*. Connective tissue called the *spermatic cord* wraps around this tube and supports each testis in the scrotum.

The vas deferens picks up secretions from the testes, seminal vesicles, prostate, and *bulbourethral* (or Cowper) glands. This thick, milky-white fluid called **semen** supports millions of sperm on their way to the uterus in the female body. The seminal vesicles provide nourishment for the sperm. The prostate and bulbourethral glands produce fluid to neutralize acidity in the urethra and vagina that would harm the sperm.

The **penis** is made up of vascular erectile tissue, not muscle. Stimulation increases blood flow, filling the tissue to make the penis erect. The nerve impulses that cause an erection also stimulate the bulbourethral glands to secrete lubricating mucus. During sexual intercourse, about 40 million to 150 million sperm are released into the female's vagina. These small, active cells live for 48 to 72 hours. During this time, they try to swim to reach the egg in the fallopian tube and break through the surface of the egg to fertilize it (**Figure 21.15**). After ejaculation delivers the sperm and semen, blood flow in the erectile tissue returns to normal, and the penis goes back to its normal size. An erection is not under voluntary control.

The head of the penis, or *glans*, is covered by the foreskin, or *prepuce*. Once development separates this skin fold from the glans, it must be retracted for regular cleaning and then returned to its position. The prepuce is sometimes cut away in a procedure called circumcision. This can help to prevent infection.

semin/i = scatter seed, semen
fer/o = bear, carry
-ous = pertaining to

tub/o = pipe
-ule = small

epi- = upon
didym/o = testis
-is = pertaining to

vas/o = vessel
de- = lack of, away from
fer/o = bear, carry
-ent = pertaining to

bulb/o = bulb
urethr/o = urethra
-al = pertaining to
semin/i = scatter seed, semen
-al = pertaining to

erect/o = straight, to set up
-ion = action, process, condition

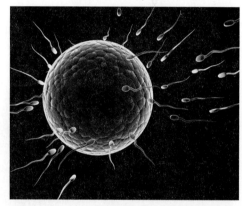

Nejron Photo/Shutterstock.com

Figure 21.15 Sperm attempting to penetrate an egg.

circum- = around
cis/o = to cut
-ion = action, process, condition

21.3-2 The Female Reproductive Organs

The purpose of the female reproductive system is to house, nourish, and protect the egg and fetus during development. Female anatomy plays a larger role in the continuation of the species than male anatomy because the fetus grows in the uterus for nine months.

The major organs of the female reproductive system are found in the lower abdomen (**Figure 21.16**). The **ovaries** are the female gonads. Ovaries store immature **ova** (eggs), which are the female gametes, waiting to be released for development. People with female anatomy are born with their life's supply of about a million immature ova.

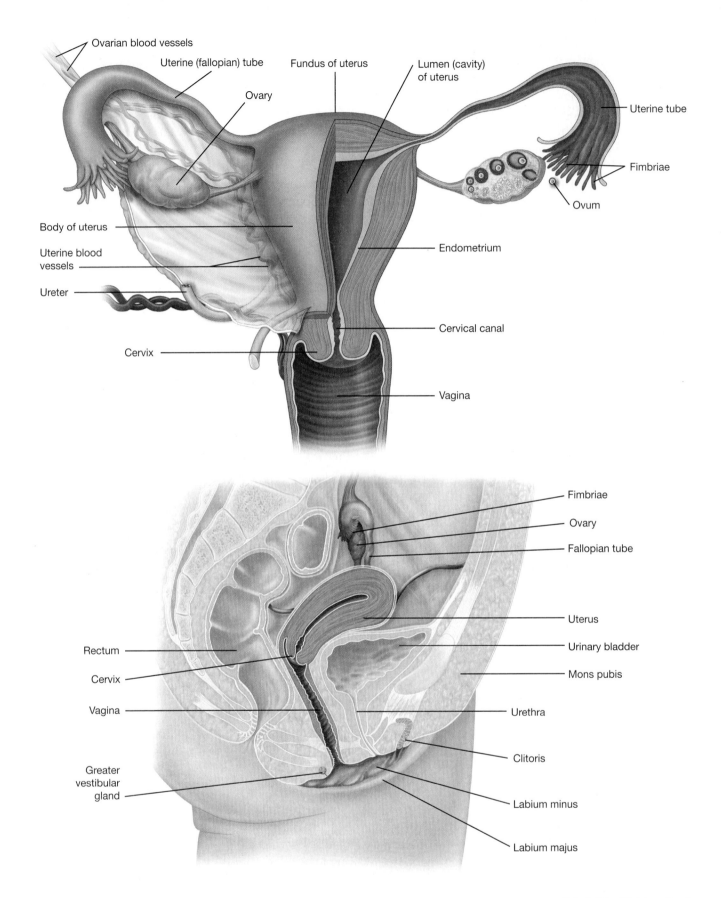

Figure 21.16 The female reproductive system. *What are the female gonads and gametes?*

© *Body Scientific International*

Beginning at puberty, around 10 to 13 years of age, one ovum matures each month. This continues into a female's 40s, when hormone production gradually slows. The older a female is, the greater the risk of having a child with a congenital condition. The risk of pregnancy complications, such as gestational diabetes or preeclampsia, is also greater after 40 years of age. *Menopause*, the end of fertility and monthly menstruation, usually begins around 50 years of age.

When an ovum matures, finger-like *fimbriae* sweep the ovum into the **fallopian tube** for fertilization. This tube carries the ovum on to the **uterus**. This hollow, muscular organ is the shape of an upside-down pear. Each month, the uterine lining develops a thick layer, called the *endometrium*, in preparation for a developing embryo to implant. If an embryo does not attach to the endometrium, the ovum and lining of the uterus are shed during monthly *menstruation*, and they will redevelop during the next monthly hormone cycle.

The uterus houses and protects the growing fetus during pregnancy. The top of the uterus is called the *fundus*. The **cervix** is the narrower neck at the bottom of the uterus. It connects to the **vagina**, a muscular tube leading out of the body. Sperm and menstrual flow can pass through the closed cervix between the vagina and uterus. During birth, the cervix dilates to 10 centimeters so the baby can pass down the birth canal.

From the outside, the vaginal opening is enclosed and protected. A thin mucous membrane called the *hymen* may partly cover the opening of the vagina. The *labia* are folds of skin that cover the vagina, urethra, and clitoris. The clitoris is the sensitive female erectile organ. When the clitoris is stimulated, Bartholin glands—located beside the vaginal opening—produce mucus to lubricate the vagina.

puber/o = grown up
-ty = quality, state
ov/i = egg
-um =structure

gestat/o = pregnancy
pre- = before, in front of
eclamps/o = sudden development
-ia = abnormal condition

men/o = menses, month
-pause = cessation
fertiliz/o = to bear, make fruitful
-ation = action of, process of
endo- = within
metr/o = uterus
-ium = structure

cervic/o = neck

dis- = apart
lat/o = wide

labi/o = lip

21.3-3 Sexually Transmitted Infections (STIs)

Sexually transmitted infections (STIs) are the most common cause of disease within the reproductive system. According to the CDC, there are approximately 20 million new cases of STIs in the US each year. Milky-colored discharge or sores on the penis or labia are signs of possible STIs. Unfortunately, many people have no symptoms, and sores inside the vagina or urethra cannot be seen easily. Condoms provide a barrier that can help reduce the spread of STIs, but sexual abstinence is the only sure way to prevent infection.

The most common STIs are human papillomavirus (HPV), chlamydia, and gonorrhea. Some types of HPV lead to genital warts, cervical cancer, and throat cancer. There may be no symptoms until HPV causes the bumps of genital warts. A vaccination can protect against this virus.

Chlamydia is easily cured with antibiotics, but it can severely damage the female reproductive system before it is even discovered. Those who have symptoms may experience burning during urination and discharge. Males may also have swelling and pain in the testes. Gonorrhea has similar symptoms to chlamydia, but the discharge is typically yellow, white, or green, and females may have more vaginal discharge or bleeding between menstrual periods. If you suspect you have an STI, see your physician immediately to avoid long-term consequences.

abs- = away from
ten/o = to hold
-ense = pertaining to
papill/o = nipple-like
gon/o = seed
-rrhea = flow, discharge

21.3-4 Genetics, Heredity, and Biomedicine

Your cell nuclei contain 23 pairs of **chromosomes**. Each chromosome carries a different chunk of your DNA within its **genes**. These genes provide the instructions for cells to produce molecules, such as protein. Genes also control inherited characteristics. In paired chromosomes, there are two *alleles*, or versions of the gene, for each characteristic. Some alleles are dominant and always express their trait. Others are recessive and may only show if both alleles are recessive.

a- = without

Most human cells divide through **mitosis.** This asexual reproduction creates two identical cells with 46 chromosomes each (**Figure 21.17**).

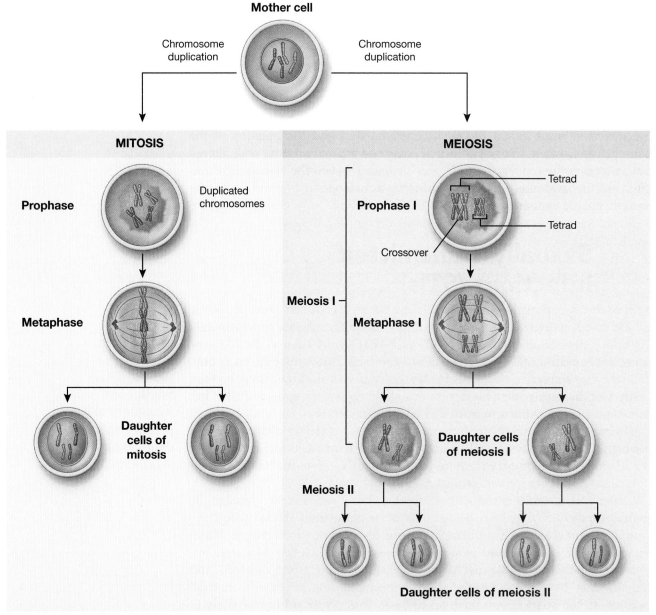

© Body Scientific International

Figure 21.17 Daughter cells of mitosis have 46 chromosomes identical to the mother cell. *How many chromosomes are in each daughter cell of meiosis II?*

Sperm and ova divide through **meiosis** (mI-OH-sihs). This sexual reproduction makes four genetically unique cells. During meiosis, a cell copies all its chromosomes and then divides the chromosomal material between two daughter cells. Each of these daughter cells divides again to produce four daughter cells, each with a unique combination of 23 chromosomes. The ovum and sperm join during **fertilization**. The genetically unique cell that results is called a **zygote**. It has 46 chromosomes, half from each parent. In this manner, the male and female reproductive systems introduce new gene combinations into the population through offspring.

fertiliz/o = to bear, make fruitful
-ation = action of, process of

Heredity describes the process of passing on genetic characteristics from one generation to the next. You may think of eye or hair color when discussing inheritance, but genetic conditions such as Down syndrome and hemophilia are also passed on this way. Some traits are easily traced from parents to children, while others may skip generations. A genetic counselor helps families understand the likelihood of genetic disorders passing on to their children and the occurrence of other congenital conditions. *Congenital conditions* are present from birth, but they are not always genetic, hereditary, or transmissible. Genetic counselors can also help people understand what biomedical therapies are available.

con- = with, together
genit/o = birth, bring forth
-al = pertaining to

Genetic Testing

Better understanding of the human genome has advanced the way scientists approach genetic causes of certain diseases and conditions. Researchers have identified several thousand **genetic disorders**—diseases or conditions that result from damaged, incorrectly located, or abnormal genes. Researchers believe that as many as 1 in 10 adults have some kind of genetic anomaly. Genetic disorders are thought to cause one-half of all miscarriages and nearly one-third of all infant deaths.

Genetic testing uses DNA to identify many serious diseases and conditions. These tests take a small number of cells from a person's body to analyze genetic makeup. Embryonic, fetal, and newborn genetic testing can identify more than 60 different diseases or disorders that impact survival, quality of life, or the need for treatment. This includes conditions such as trisomy 18, Tay-Sachs disease, phenylketonuria, and sickle-cell disease. Adults can be tested for hundreds of conditions, such as Huntington disease, some cancers, or Alzheimer's disease.

Knowledge that you may pass on a genetic disorder can be useful when making decisions about whether to have children. It is common for reproductive clinics to screen for about 170 different genetic conditions before selecting embryos for implanting. Tests that confirm a diagnosis can also help with planning treatment or preparing for health changes and end of life.

Gene Therapy

Gene therapy uses genetic engineering to treat or prevent genetic diseases, adding a correct version of the mutated gene but leaving the faulty gene in the genome. *Gene editing* is a type of gene therapy that revises or replaces the faulty portion of a gene so the mutation is no longer in the genome. With the discovery of CRISPR (clustered regularly interspaced short palindromic repeats), CRISPR-Cas (CRISPR-associated protein), and other tools for gene editing, gene therapy has become more efficient, reliable, and precise. The CRISPR-Cas technology has the potential to cure genetic diseases and cancers with just one treatment.

This process is not yet perfected and has risks that need to be evaluated. It can accidentally create unintended changes such as toxic proteins, mosaic embryos with only partial editing, or other mutations that scientists do not yet understand. While it is not fully ready for use in humans, it is an excellent tool for editing cells outside the body and creating disease-related cell models for research.

As of 2020, the FDA allows gene therapy research targeted at treating cells of the body, such as bone or blood cells. This is called *somatic cell gene therapy*. The FDA does not allow *germline cell gene therapy*, which alters egg or sperm cells, because of the unknown long-term side effects on future generations. The state of California also prohibited the sale of CRISPR kits for modifying human DNA. How do you feel about limitations on genetic engineering, which has so much potential for curing disease?

somat/o = body
-ic = pertaining to

Stem Cells

Another promising area of biotechnology is the use of stem cells as the basis for medical treatments (**Figure 21.18**). *Stem cells* are cells that can develop into other types of cells in the body. All the organs and tissues in your body develop from stem cells. Stem cells can also reproduce themselves in the body to repair damaged tissues.

Scientists distinguish between stem cells taken from embryos and those taken from adults. Embryonic stem cells are obtained from embryos in the blastocyst stage of development. Embryonic stem cells have great potential for use in regenerative therapy because they can reproduce many times and are *unspecialized*. This means they can develop into any kind of cell or tissue in the body, from blood to skin to heart cells. Because of their ability to take many forms, embryonic stem cells are called *pluripotent*.

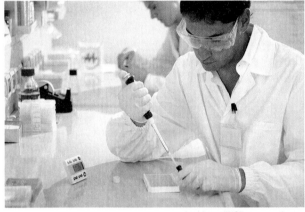

tefanolunardi/Shutterstock.com

Figure 21.18 Stem cell research is done in the hopes of developing new, more effective medical treatments. *What specific types of treatment could stem cells be used for?*

pluri- = more

multi- = many

Somatic stem cells, taken from adults, most easily make cells of their own type. For example, blood stem cells develop into red blood cells, various types of white blood cells, or other immune system cells. In 2007, however, scientists developed *induced pluripotent stem cells* (iPSCs). These are altered adult stem cells that have the flexibility of embryonic stem cells. These *multipotent* cells can develop into more than one type of cell but are more limited than pluripotent cells. Multipotent cells can also be collected from umbilical cord blood at the time of birth.

Scientists hope to use the capabilities of stem cells to develop cellular-level treatments for a variety of diseases and conditions, such as diabetes, heart disease, or degenerative nerve conditions. Stem cells may also restore tissues, as in bone marrow transplants, or generate new tissues for transplant, such as skin. The main hurdle for these treatments is overcoming political, religious, and ethical sentiments that limit their use in research and treatment.

de- = lack of, away from
generat/o = producing
-ive = quality of, nature of, pertaining to

Cloning

The process of **cloning** copies genetic material for use in biomedical research and therapeutic treatments. *Gene cloning* produces copies of DNA segments. *Therapeutic cloning* produces identical embryonic stem cells.

Reproductive cloning creates exact genetic copies of a human or an animal. This process typically involves transferring the nucleus of a somatic cell into an ovum after removing its nucleus. Reproductive cloning became news in 1997, when Scottish scientists announced they had produced a cloned sheep, which they named Dolly (**Figure 21.19**). This marked the first time an animal as complex as a mammal had been cloned from adult somatic stem cells.

The announcement of Dolly prompted questions about whether human cloning was possible or ethical. These questions have become more critical considering the high failure rate and shortened life span of cloned animals. In cloning experiments conducted since Dolly's birth, only about one or two out of a hundred attempts are successful. In addition, nearly one-third of the animals that are born suffer from rare but serious conditions.

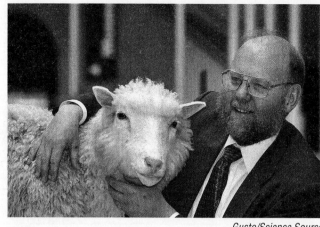

Gusto/Science Source

Figure 21.19 Dolly the sheep is widely known as the first successful attempt at cloning a mammal.

The possibility of putting a human life at such risk is considered immoral and unethical by many people. Both the American Medical Association and the American Association for the Advancement of Science have urged a ban on human reproductive cloning. More than 45 countries have formally banned reproductive cloning of humans. The US Congress has debated such legislation but has not yet passed a federal law controlling this practice in the US. Regulation of cloning has been left to individual states. State laws differ in terms of what types of cloning are allowed, for what purposes, and how long the embryos are allowed to live.

21.3-5 **Reproductive Hormones**

Hormones from the pituitary gland and the gonads regulate many important processes of the reproductive systems. These processes include puberty, the menstrual cycle, pregnancy, childbirth, and menopause.

Puberty and the Menstrual Cycle

Both the male and female reproductive systems produce and respond to hormones that trigger puberty and the development of secondary sexual characteristics. The pituitary gland in the brain produces luteinizing hormone (LH) and follicle-stimulating hormone (FSH). These hormones tell the male's testes to make sperm and *testosterone*. Testosterone is responsible for the development of a deep voice, facial hair, and muscle bulk at puberty. In the female, LH and FSH stimulate the ovaries to produce *estrogen* and *progesterone*, which regulate the menstrual cycle each month. Estrogen is responsible for the development of breasts, the growth of pubic hair, and an increase in body fat during puberty. Progesterone prepares the uterine lining for an egg to implant.

In people with female anatomy, a monthly hormone cycle matures an ovum and prepares the uterus for possible pregnancy (**Figure 21.20**). The first menstrual cycle is called *menarche*. The first day of the cycle is marked by the first day of menstruation, and hormone levels are low.

puber/o = grown up
-ty = quality, state

test/o = testis
sterol/o = steroid
-one = hormone
estr/o = female
-gen = origin, formation, producing
pro- = before, in front of
gest/o = pregnancy, produce
sterol/o = steroid
-one = hormone

men/o = menses, month
-arche = beginning

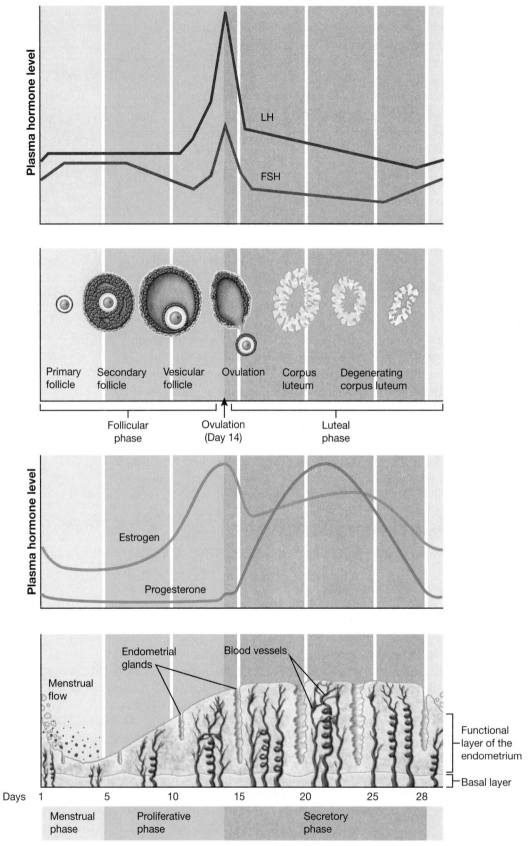

© Body Scientific International

Figure 21.20 Hormonal and structural changes during the female hormone cycle. The events of one complete female cycle, lasting 28 days, are shown. The time scale, shown horizontally at the bottom, applies to all four panels of the figure.

During menstruation, the endometrium is shed from the uterus. From days 6 to 12, estrogen helps rebuild the endometrium in the uterus, while FSH tells the ovaries to mature an ovum follicle. Around day 14, LH and FSH levels increase to trigger ovulation. After the ovum is released, LH and FSH levels decrease until the next cycle. Progesterone from the ovaries continues to build the endometrium through day 28 of the cycle. If an egg is not fertilized or hormone levels are not high enough to support a pregnancy, the endometrium begins to break down, and the cycle starts again. If an egg is fertilized, a different hormone process begins.

endo- = within
metr/o = uterus
-ium = structure

ov/i = egg
-ule = small
-ation = action of, process of

Pregnancy and Childbirth

Hormones also control the processes of pregnancy. Progesterone from the ovaries and human chorionic gonadotropin (kor-ee-AH-nihk goh-nad-oh-TROH-pihn), or *hCG*, from the placenta maintain the placenta during pregnancy. Toward the end of pregnancy, *relaxin* and *prostaglandin* help soften the ligaments in the pelvis and relax and open the cervix in preparation for birth. *Oxytocin* starts the contractions of the uterus that will push the baby out (**Figure 21.21**). *Endorphins* trigger a natural high at the end of labor that helps with pain management. The uterus also secretes *prolactin* at the end of pregnancy to stimulate milk production in the mammary glands. Increased production of all these hormones can affect emotions. After birth, the sudden drop in hormone levels may cause postpartum depression.

gonad/o = gonads, ovaries, testes
-tropin = nourishing, stimulation

ox/y = oxygen
toc/o = labor, birth
-in = substance, chemical
pro- = before, in front of
lact/o = milk
mamm/o = breast
-ary = pertaining to
post- = after
-partum = birth, labor

Hormonal changes continue after birth. When a baby nurses, more oxytocin is released to help shrink the uterus and release milk from the breasts. Nursing maintains hormone levels and may delay the release of ova for several months after birth.

Hormonal birth control methods, such as "the pill," take advantage of the role of hormones in controlling these processes. These methods artificially regulate hormone levels to trick the body into believing it is pregnant, so no eggs are released. Unfortunately, many other side effects come with pregnancy hormones, such as fluid retention and high blood pressure. If you are pregnant or using hormonal birth control, regular consultation with a doctor is important to monitor these effects.

Aging and Reproductive Hormones

Around 50 years of age, menopause begins. Estrogen levels drop, ovulation gradually ends, and people with female anatomy lose their reproductive abilities. Hormonal changes in females during menopause can cause thinning of the uterus, reduced vaginal secretions, hot flashes, night sweats, irritability, fatigue, depression, weight gain, insomnia, and forgetfulness. More hormonal changes occur around 80 years of age, causing a relaxation of ligaments, general loss of muscle tone, and drooping of the breasts. People with male anatomy may experience enlargement of the prostate gland, and a loss of muscle tone and relaxation of ligaments due to a reduction in hormone levels as they age, but they continue to produce sperm.

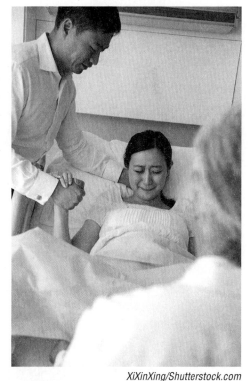

XiXinXing/Shutterstock.com

Figure 21.21 The hormone oxytocin triggers contractions that will begin labor. *What hormone helps with pain management after labor?*

21.3-6 Reproduction, Prenatal Development, and Childbirth

During the reproductive process, a fertilized egg develops into a new baby. This process takes 10 lunar months, which is 280 days or about 9 calendar months. Much growth and development happens during this period, especially in the first few months.

Fertilization and Implantation

ec- = out, outside
top/o = place
-ic = pertaining to

Prenatal development begins with the germinal period, when the sperm fertilizes the ovum in one of the fallopian tubes. The resulting zygote divides quickly to produce a **morula** (MOR-yoo-luh) (**Figure 21.22**). This solid ball of 16 cells travels down the fallopian tube to the uterus to implant. If the morula accidentally implants inside the fallopian tube, the result is an ectopic pregnancy. This is becoming more common due to the increased use of fertility treatments.

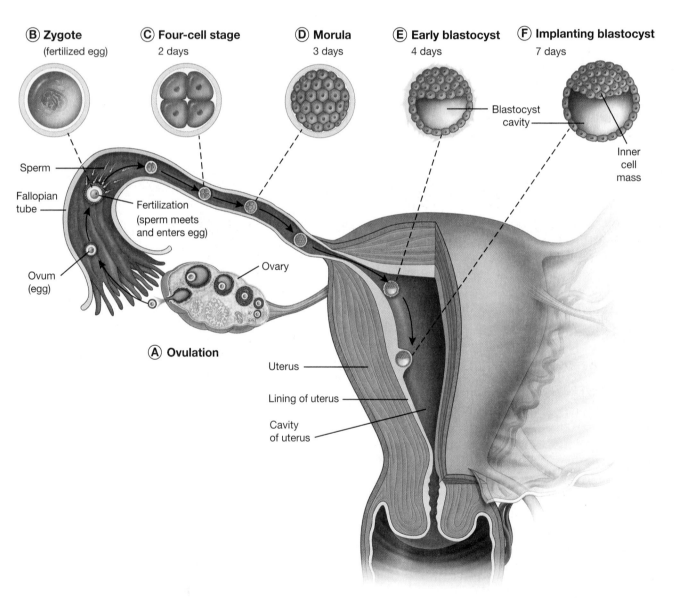

© Body Scientific International

Figure 21.22 Embryonic development begins in the fallopian tube.

An ectopic pregnancy cannot develop normally, and the person who is pregnant may die from internal bleeding if it is not removed.

When the morula reaches the uterus, it attaches to the endometrium. As it grows, the morula becomes a hollow **blastocyst**, developing a fluid sac in its center. The inner cells of the blastocyst become the **embryo** at day seven, eventually developing into a baby. The outer cells release enzymes and hormones that help the embryo implant and form the placenta and **amniotic sac**. This fluid-filled sac protects the developing embryo. At this point, a pregnancy test can detect hCG, but tests are most accurate about three to four weeks after conception.

blast/o = embryonic
-cyst = fluid-filled sac

amni/o = fetal membrane
-tic = pertaining to

Prenatal Development

The embryonic stage begins after the embryo attaches to the uterus. The embryo is unrecognizable in this early stage of development. During the embryonic stage, blood vessels develop between the embryo and the uterus, forming the **placenta**. The embryo's blood and the pregnant person's blood must cross the placental membrane; they never meet directly. This helps prevent the spread of some illnesses to the baby during pregnancy. By the fifth week, the heart is beating.

The fetal stage begins around the ninth week, when all the major internal organs and external features are present. At this point, the developing baby is called a **fetus** and is more than a half-inch long (**Figure 21.23**). The pregnant person has probably missed a second menstrual cycle and may be aware of the pregnancy, although it may not show for several months.

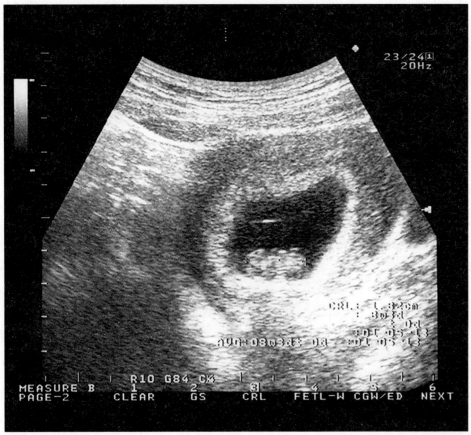

sittipong/Shutterstock.com

Figure 21.23 Sonogram of a fetus at three months.

tri- = three
mens/o = month
terat/o = malformed fetus, monster
-gen = origin, formation, producing

kary/o = nucleus
-type = group, model

de- = lack of, away from
gen/o = origin
-er = one who does
-ate = pertaining to, composed of, process
obstetr/o = midwifery
-ian = relating to, one who does
gynec/o = woman, female
-logist = specialist in the study of

This first *trimester,* or period of three months, is a risky time for the developing fetus. Exposing the developing fetus to harmful teratogens such as drugs and alcohol during this critical development period can have devastating results. However, all the body systems are forming when a person is least aware of their pregnancy. **Figure 21.24** shows the critical periods of development for various structures. A healthy diet that contains all the vitamins, minerals, and nutrients for growth is also essential, although pregnancy often causes nausea or morning sickness in this first trimester.

At this stage, the only way to distinguish between a male and female fetus is by karyotype. This is a visual examination and pairing of the 46 chromosomes. It will show two XX chromosomes in females and an X and Y in males. Male and female gonads develop from the same structures in the embryo. When testosterone is present, the male gonads develop into the vas deferens, seminal vesicles, prostate, scrotum, and penis of a male, while the female gonads degenerate. Without testosterone, the gonads develop into the uterus, fallopian tubes, vagina, labia, and clitoris of a female, while the male gonads degenerate. External genitalia can be seen after 8 to 12 weeks of gestation.

At 12 weeks, the fetus is about 2 inches long and can make small movements. The fetal heartbeat can be detected during regular visits to the obstetrician/gynecologist (OB/GYN). During these visits, the doctor will take urine samples from the pregnant person to check for signs of infection, gestational diabetes, or other conditions that may affect the pregnancy.

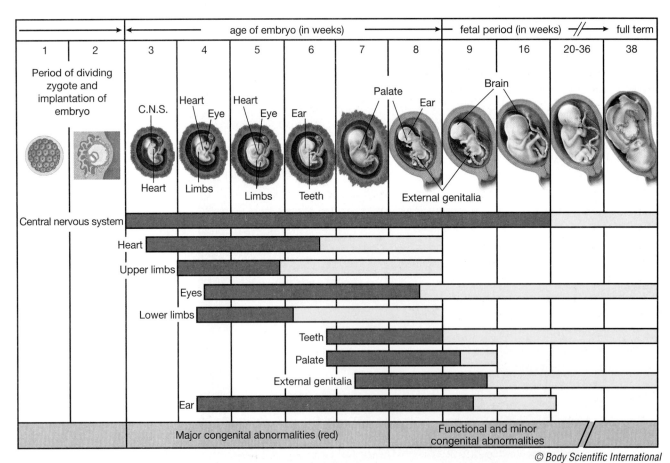

© Body Scientific International

Figure 21.24 This chart shows the timing for development of different parts of the body. It also shows the periods during which major abnormalities (red) and less serious abnormalities (yellow) can occur.

The doctor will also measure the size of the uterus as an estimate of fetal growth. The length from the pubic bone to the fundus (the top of the uterus) will increase by about 1 centimeter each week.

The second trimester, from the sixteenth week until the end of the seventh month, is usually described as the easiest stage of pregnancy. Feelings of morning sickness usually go away. The baby can be felt kicking and moving in the womb. An ultrasound at 20 weeks confirms that the fetus and placenta are growing properly. Because sonography uses sound waves instead of radiation, it is very safe during pregnancy.

son/o = sound
-graphy = process of recording

The third trimester is a period of rapid growth. The fetus grows from about 2 pounds at 28 weeks to 4 pounds at 32 weeks. One-half of a baby's weight is added during the last month of gestation, which explains why premature infants, or *preemies*, are so small. A preemie often remains in the neonatal intensive care unit (NICU) until the full-term due date. Delivery between 38 and 42 weeks is considered full-term. The average baby is 20 inches long and weighs 7.5 pounds at this point.

gestat/o = pregnancy
-ion = action, process, condition
neo- = new
nat/o = birth
-al = pertaining to

Childbirth

Birth is a three-stage process (**Figure 21.25**). It begins with the thinning and *dilation* of the cervix to open the birth canal. Strong contractions of the uterus stretch the cervix opening to 10 centimeters in diameter. The active phase of stage one lasts several hours and can be painful. An anesthesiologist or nurse anesthetist can help control the pain of labor with medications. A birthing coach, doula, or midwife uses breathing, imagery, water baths, and changes in position to help the pregnant person manage pain.

dis- = apart
lat/o = wide
-ion = action of, process of

The second stage is the birth of the baby, or *expulsion*. This happens much faster than the dilation stage. The baby should come out headfirst and face-down. Any other presentation can slow delivery and may cause complications for the baby or person giving birth. If the baby is in breech position, with its bottom or feet down, the doctor may try to turn the baby for an easier delivery. If a vaginal delivery is not safe, the doctor may perform a Cesarean section, or C-section. This is a surgery that cuts through the abdomen and uterus to remove the baby.

ex- = out, away from
pel/o = to drive

At birth, the healthcare providers clear mucus from the baby's nose, mouth, and throat. The baby's lungs inflate with their first breath and all of their systems begin functioning on their own. Crying is normal—it helps to clear fluid from the lungs. The umbilical cord connecting the baby to the placenta is clamped and cut. The newborn's skin may be covered in fine hair, called *lanugo*. The waxy *vernix* that protected their skin from the amniotic fluid is wiped away and the baby is wrapped or placed in an incubator to prevent heat loss. An *APGAR* test is done at 1 minute and 5 minutes after birth. This acronym is a rating of 0 to 2 for their activity level, pulse, grimace reflex, appearance, and respirations. Babies with a score below 7 may need special medical care. Then, the baby will be measured, given vitamin K for blood clotting, treated with antibiotic eye drops, have footprints taken, and be given an identification bracelet.

The final stage of birth is delivery of the placenta. The placenta, commonly called the *afterbirth*, should not detach from the uterus until after the baby is born, but it does need to come out. Some cultures have rituals related to the placenta, so it is important to discuss this before birth. Some people may wish to bury it, eat a portion of it, or save the blood.

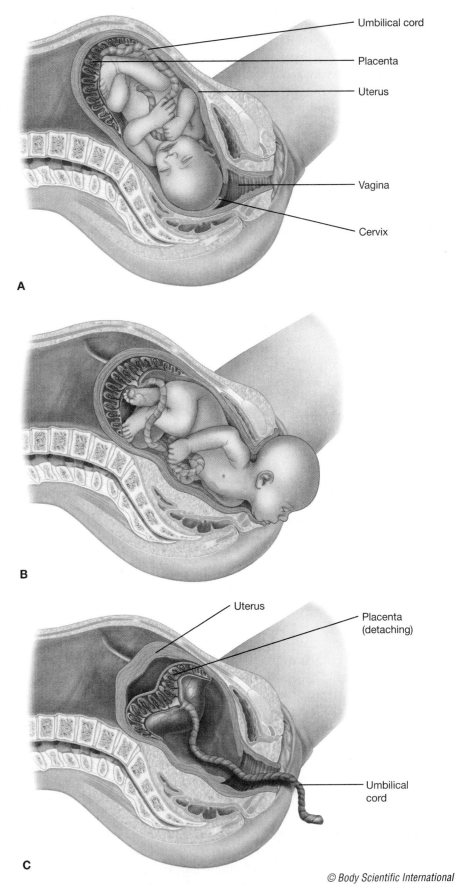

Umbilical cord

Placenta

Uterus

Vagina

Cervix

A

B

Uterus

Placenta (detaching)

Umbilical cord

C

© *Body Scientific International*

Figure 21.25 The stages of labor—dilation (A), expulsion (B), and delivery of the placenta (C). *How wide is the cervix when it is fully dilated?*

After delivery, oxytocin will begin shrinking the uterus and start the flow of breast milk to nourish the baby. Most people spend only a day in the hospital for the birth of a child. During this time, the pediatrician will examine the baby's skin, head, neck, heart, lungs, abdomen, and genitals. The baby may receive initial vaccinations and screening tests. When the parent and child are released, a patient transport technician assists in seeing them out of the hospital safely. A nurse may call new parents after they return home. Regular checkups with the pediatrician follow the healthy development of the new baby.

Lesson 21.3 Review

 Complete the *Map Your Reading* graphic organizer for the section you just read.

1. Where in the male reproductive system do sperm form? (21.3-1)
   A. Penis
   B. Vas deferens
   C. Testes
   D. Epididymis

2. The neck between the uterus and vagina is called the (21.3-2)
   A. uterus
   B. cervix
   C. fundus
   D. fimbria

3. STIs may cause which of the following? Choose all that apply. (21.3-3)
   A. Damage to the reproductive system
   B. No symptoms
   C. Milky-colored discharge
   D. Sores on the penis or labia

4. Sperm and ova divide through (21.3-4)
   A. mitosis
   B. fertilization
   C. meiosis
   D. duplication

5. Which hormone starts contractions in the uterus during childbirth? (21.3-5)
   A. Relaxin
   B. Endorphins
   C. hCG
   D. Oxytocin

6. In an ectopic pregnancy, a morula implants in the (21.3-6)
   A. endometrium
   B. ovary
   C. fallopian tube
   D. vagina

Chapter 21 Review and Assessment

Chapter Summary

21.1-1 The digestive system breaks down and takes nutrients from food and removes waste.

21.1-2 Digestion is a four-step process of ingestion, digestion, absorption of nutrients, and defecation of waste. Food travels through the alimentary canal in this order: mouth, esophagus, stomach, small intestine, large intestine, rectum, and anus. Mechanical processes and chemicals from accessory organs break down food into usable nutrients.

21.2-1 The excretory system, which includes the urinary organs, removes metabolic waste, excess water, urea, and electrolytes from the body as urine.

21.2-2 Kidneys contain millions of nephrons that filter waste from the blood to make urine and return water, protein, sugar, and minerals to the blood. Urine flows from the nephron's collecting tubule to the calyx and then the renal pelvis. From the kidney, it flows down the ureter to the bladder, then out the urethra.

21.2-3 The kidneys help maintain homeostasis in the body by making and responding to a variety of hormones and enzymes. The kidneys influence blood pressure, blood pH, red blood cell production, and calcium levels.

21.3-1 The male testes produce millions of sperm from puberty until death. They mature in the epididymis and are released through the vas deferens.

21.3-2 The female reproductive system houses, nourishes, and protects the ovum and fetus during development. Ova travel from the ovaries to the fallopian tubes, then into the uterus. If they are not fertilized, they will flow out the vagina during menstruation.

21.3-3 Sexually transmitted infections (STIs) can harm the reproductive systems. Sexual abstinence is the most effective way to prevent STIs.

21.3-4 Meiosis produces new gene combinations in offspring. Chromosomes control heredity of dominant and recessive traits. Biomedical therapies can help people prevent and treat diseases. Genetic testing can be used for diagnosis, treatment, genetic counseling, or lifestyle changes. Gene therapy treats genetic diseases. Stem cells can repair damaged tissues. Reproductive cloning creates exact copies of an animal or human cell to research treatments for disease.

21.3-5 The reproductive systems produce new life through a complex process controlled by hormones.

21.3-6 Fertilization occurs in the fallopian tubes. The cells multiply, going from zygote, to morula, to embryo in a week, and fetus at nine weeks. Full term birth occurs between 38 and 42 weeks. Birth is a three-stage process. Dilation and thinning of the cervix open the birth canal. Contractions of the uterus push the baby out. The placenta is delivered last.

Maximize Your Professional Vocabulary

1. **Term Races.** Make flash cards for each word part below. Sit with a partner in a location where you can see a clock with a second hand. Hold up a term card for your partner and have them give the definition. If correct, place it on the table. If incorrect, read the definition and place it back in the deck. Go through all of the cards as quickly as possible until all have been correctly answered. Write down the time. Switch roles and repeat the process. Add your scores and compare with other teams to see who has the fastest time. Repeat the game to see which team makes the most improvement on their time.

2. **Diagram Terms.** Draw or trace a diagram of the digestive, urinary, or reproductive system. Use the medical root words in the list shown below to label the organs associated with the system you chose.

Prefixes

abs-	en-	neo-
di-	in-	noct-
ec-	multi-	pluri-

Root Words

absorpt/o	generat/o	nutri/o
acid/o	genit/o	obstetr/o
aliment/o	gestat/o	odont/o
amni/o	gingiv/o	ov/i
blast/o	glomer/o	pancreat/o
bulb/o	gon/o	pel/o
calc/o	gonad/o	puber/o
celi/o	gynec/o	semin/i
chole/o	hepat/o	son/o
cis/o	kary/o	ster/o
col/o	labi/o	sterol/o
colon/o	lact/o	ten/o
continent/o	lapar/o	terat/o
cret/o	lat/o	test/o
dent/o	lip/o	toc/o
didym/o	lith/o	top/o
eclamps/o	men/o	tub/o
erect/o	mens/o	ur/o
esaphag/o	metr/o	uret/o
fer/o	nat/o	urethr/o
fertiliz/o	nephr/o	uter/o

Suffixes

-arche	-ol	-tropin
-cyst	-partum	-type
-dialysis	-pause	-uria
-ence	-rrhea	-verse
-ent	-rrhoid	
-graphy	-tripsy	

Reflect on Your Reading

1. Review the 1-2-3 notes created as you read the chapter. Using the chapter theme of "Maintenance and Continuation," write a short summary that ties together all these main ideas. How are they related?

Review and Recall

1. Which are functions of the digestive system? Choose all that apply. (21.1-1)
   A. Taking in nutrients
   B. Removing waste
   C. Transporting blood
   D. Transmitting impulses
2. Which part of the small intestines absorbs iron? (21.1-2)
   A. Jejunum
   B. Duodenum
   C. Ileum
   D. All of these.
3. How does constipation occur? (21.1-2)
   A. Feces retain too much water
   B. Feces spend too long in the colon
   C. Feces spend too long in the small intestine
   D. The circulatory system removes too many nutrients
4. Which process can help remove waste from the blood if the kidneys fail? (21.2-1)
   A. Catheter
   B. Hemodialysis
   C. Defecation
   D. Lithotripsy
5. The process by which water, sugar, and salts are returned to the blood is called (21.2-2)
   A. filtration
   B. secretion
   C. reabsorption
   D. absorption
6. How do the kidneys influence blood pH? Choose all that apply. (21.2-3)
   A. Expelling carbon dioxide
   B. Excreting hydrogen ions in urine
   C. Reabsorbing bicarbonate into the blood
   D. Expelling water

7. Which glands help form semen? Choose all that apply. (21.3-1)
   A. Seminal vesicles
   B. Bulbourethral gland
   C. Urethra
   D. Prostate gland

8. The female erectile organ is the (21.3-2)
   A. fallopian tube
   B. ovary
   C. clitoris
   D. vagina

9. What is the most common STI? (21.3-3)
   A. Chlamydia
   B. Gonorrhea
   C. Genital herpes
   D. HPV

10. Which of these treats genetic diseases by editing genes? (21.3-4)
    A. Stem cell therapy
    B. Genetic testing
    C. Gene therapy
    D. All of these.

11. Which hormones regulate the menstrual cycle? Choose all that apply. (21.3-5)
    A. Estrogen
    B. Progesterone
    C. Testosterone
    D. Prolactin

12. Delivery of the placenta happens in which stage of childbirth? (21.3-6)
    A. First stage
    B. Second stage
    C. Third stage
    D. None of these.

Build Core Skills

1. **Writing.** Write a letter of complaint from a sandwich to the digestive system about your travel through the system. Where did you go (which organs), and how were you "treated" there?

2. **Critical Thinking.** Use a Venn diagram to compare meiosis and mitosis. How are they similar? How are they different?

3. **Problem Solving.** For each of the following physical conditions, research the related body system(s), signs or symptoms, and the

healthcare professional(s) the patient or client would have to consult.
   - benign prostatic hyperplasia
   - yeast infection
   - diabetes
   - jaundice
   - UTI
   - kidney failure

4. **Critical Thinking.** Compare the organs of the male and female reproductive systems. What do they have in common?

5. **Problem Solving.** The chapter mentions several medical procedures related to body systems for maintenance and support. For each of the following procedures, write the medical description and then explain it in simpler terminology. Which specific organs are involved in each of these procedures?
   - colonoscopy
   - colostomy
   - dialysis
   - catheterization
   - vaginal childbirth
   - Cesarian section

6. **Math.** Demonstrate the exponential spread of sexually transmitted infections (STIs). Keep a list of every person you touch for one day. Compare your list with the lists of everyone else in your class. Highlight the names of anyone on your list who is also on someone else's list. Choose one name on the list and count how many other people had that name on their list. Then count all the other names on the lists that contain this one name. If this one person had an STI, and these were sexual interactions, how many people would have been exposed?

7. **Writing.** Read the Cloning Fact Sheet on the National Human Genome Research Institute website with an open mind. Your teacher will assign you to either the "affirmative" or "negative" side of a debate team. Based on the information in the fact sheet, prepare a four-minute persuasive speech for your constructive opening argument.

8. **Problem Solving.** In Figure 21.19, Dolly the sheep is shown as a healthy cloned mammal. Why is this misleading?

9. **Critical Thinking.** Where does most of the digestive process occur? Explain your answer.

10. **Critical Thinking.** Explain how the kidneys support homeostasis in the body.

Activate Your Learning

1. Demonstrate the importance of mechanical digestion by comparing the effect of water on a teaspoon of sugar granules versus on a solid sugar cube. Place a teaspoon of sugar and a sugar cube in the bottom of separate cups and add water. Note what happens. Then stir each mixture. Which dissolves fastest: the loose sugar granules or the sugar cube? Use your observations to explain how chewing and mixing are important to digestion.

2. Investigate the alimentary canal. How long is it? Use different-colored yarns and tie them together, then find a comparison for the total length: mouth—8 cm, pharynx—10 cm, esophagus—25 cm, stomach—20 cm, small intestine—700 cm, large intestine—150 cm, rectum—12 cm. Now attach tags for the accessory organs and their digestive juices. Where should they attach? Finally, identify a digestive disorder and where the problem would occur on this "model."

3. Simulate filtration in the kidney. Use a large pan of sand and gravel mix to represent the blood content delivered to the kidney for filtration. Use a sifter to represent the kidney's filter and a cup for the desired amount of sugar, salt, and water in the blood. Filters allow only specific sizes of material to pass through. What would the gravel in the sifter represent? What does the cup represent? Where does the overflow from the cup go? Explain how this process results in homeostasis. How do hormones play a role in this process?

Think and Act Like a Healthcare Worker

1. You are a dentist. Your patient's gums are bleeding, several teeth have caries, and one needs a root canal. The patient asks you to pull the teeth so they no longer hurt. How can you explain the importance of repairing the teeth to support digestive health?

2. You are helping your patient use the toilet. There is very little urine and the color is very dark. Why does this information need to be reported to the nurse? How might you encourage this patient to drink more fluids?

3. Shawna believes she is pregnant. As her primary care physician, what tests could you use to determine if she is pregnant? If she is pregnant, what additional risks and tests would you discuss with her about pregnancy, prenatal, and postnatal care?

Go to the Source

1. Visit NIH's National Institute of Diabetes and Digestive and Kidney Diseases website. Explore the "Health Information" tab. Select one of the diseases listed. Create a poster letting others know about the condition, its causes, treatment (if any), and prevention (if known).

2. Visit the National Kidney Foundation website. Go to "Kidneys and Your Health" to complete the assessment. After answering the eight questions, read the information provided. What is something new you learned about kidney health and kidney disease?

3. Visit the CDC's website and use the search tool to find the page about contraception. Compare two methods listed, such as fertility awareness and oral contraceptives. How do these methods work? When are they used? What are their typical failure rates? Do you think one method is better than the other? Why?

HOSA Event Prep: Health Education

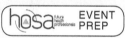

Marietta is a child-life specialist. She uses education and therapeutic play to help children and families cope with change and stress. Her goal is to minimize trauma and increase understanding of their medical situation, diagnosis or treatment.

Her patient, Chase, is a five-year-old male who was recently admitted to the local children's hospital for a possible appendicitis. His doctor ordered labs and a CAT (computed axial tomography) scan to help diagnose his appendicitis. Marietta was called to help prepare Chase for the test and procedures. She used play therapy to show what the CAT scan would be like. Knowing that preschoolers are very concrete and literal thinkers, she kept explanations simple. Chase quickly laughed, saying, "I thought there would be a cat scanning my stomach." She also helped talk him through the IV and lab draw. This helped Chase and his parents feel more comfortable with his hospital stay.

Think About It

1. Explain how the role of a child-life specialist can help prepare young patients for tests and procedures.

2. How would you educate preschoolers about "what it's like to go to the doctor for a checkup"? Give three examples.

3. Does the role of a child-life specialist interest you? Why or why not?

Health Science Careers by Personality Type

John Holland Personality Type	Characteristic	Health Science Career Examples
Realistic doer	Likes mechanical hands-on activities	• Central supply worker • Electrocardiograph technician • Surgeon
Investigative thinker	Is an analytical problem solver	• Medical laboratory technician • Nurse practitioner • Psychologist
Social helper	Is cooperative and people-oriented	• Certified nursing assistant • Health science educator • Physical therapist
Enterprising persuader	Is a competitive leader	• Pharmaceutical sales representative • Healthcare administrator • Dean of nursing at a college or university
Conventional organizer	Pays attention to detail	• Dental assistant • Medical coding specialist • Operating room nurse
Artistic creator	Likes creative activities	• Medical photographer • Music therapist • Community health nurse

Bones of the Human Body

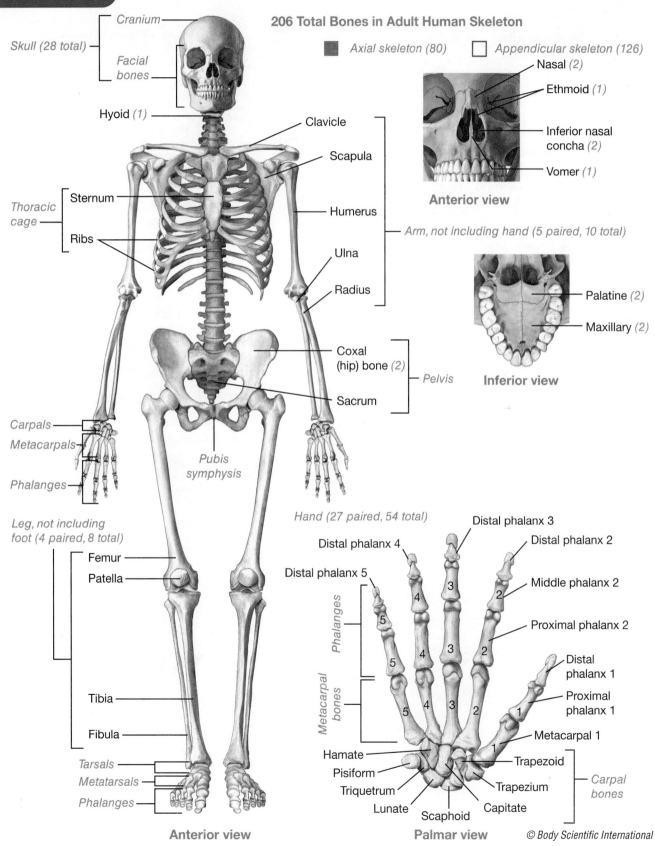

206 Total Bones in Adult Human Skeleton

■ Axial skeleton (80)   □ Appendicular skeleton (126)

Skull (28 total)
Cranium
Facial bones
Hyoid (1)

Nasal (2)
Ethmoid (1)
Inferior nasal concha (2)
Vomer (1)

Anterior view

Clavicle
Scapula

Thoracic cage
Sternum
Ribs

Humerus

Arm, not including hand (5 paired, 10 total)

Ulna
Radius

Palatine (2)
Maxillary (2)

Inferior view

Coxal (hip) bone (2)
Sacrum
Pelvis

Carpals
Metacarpals
Phalanges

Pubis symphysis

Hand (27 paired, 54 total)

Leg, not including foot (4 paired, 8 total)
Femur
Patella

Distal phalanx 3
Distal phalanx 4
Distal phalanx 5
Distal phalanx 2
Middle phalanx 2
Proximal phalanx 2

Phalanges

Distal phalanx 1
Proximal phalanx 1

Tibia
Fibula

Metacarpal bones

Metacarpal 1

Tarsals
Metatarsals
Phalanges

Hamate
Pisiform
Triquetrum
Lunate
Scaphoid
Capitate

Trapezoid
Trapezium
Carpal bones

Anterior view

Palmar view

© Body Scientific International

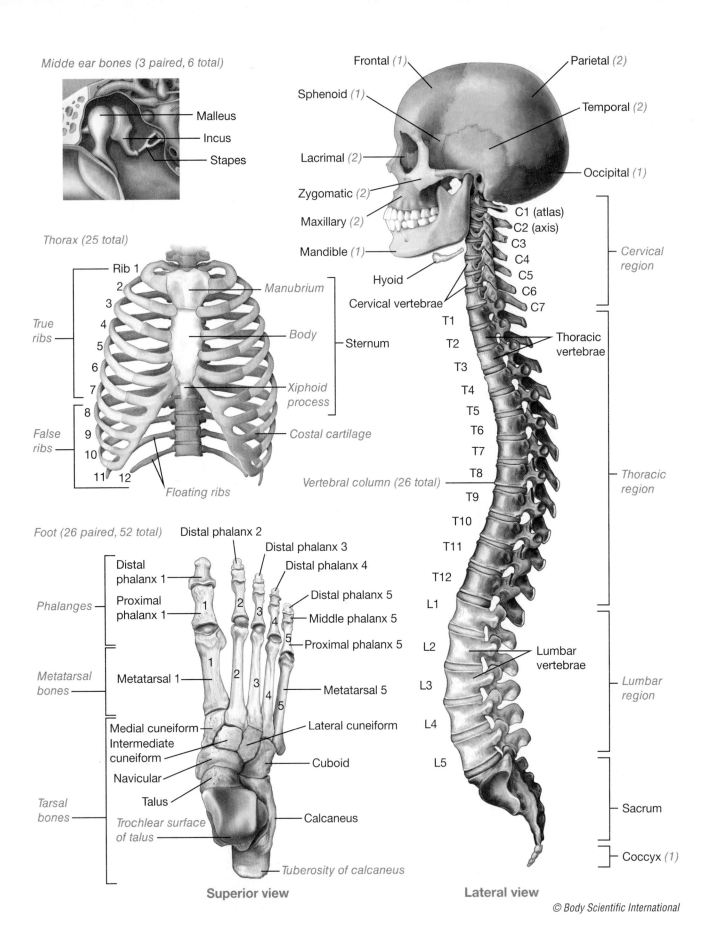

Midde ear bones (3 paired, 6 total)

- Malleus
- Incus
- Stapes

Frontal *(1)*

Parietal *(2)*

Sphenoid *(1)*

Temporal *(2)*

Lacrimal *(2)*

Occipital *(1)*

Zygomatic *(2)*

Maxillary *(2)*

Mandible *(1)*

Hyoid

Cervical vertebrae

C1 (atlas)
C2 (axis)
C3
C4
C5
C6
C7

Cervical region

Thorax (25 total)

Rib 1
2
3
4
5
6
7

Manubrium

Body

Sternum

Xiphoid process

Costal cartilage

True ribs

False ribs

8
9
10
11 12

Floating ribs

T1
T2
T3
T4
T5
T6
T7
T8
T9
T10
T11
T12

Thoracic vertebrae

Vertebral column (26 total)

Thoracic region

Foot (26 paired, 52 total)

Distal phalanx 2

Distal phalanx 3

Distal phalanx 4

Distal phalanx 1

Proximal phalanx 1

Distal phalanx 5

Middle phalanx 5

Proximal phalanx 5

Metatarsal 1

Metatarsal 5

Medial cuneiform

Lateral cuneiform

Intermediate cuneiform

Cuboid

Navicular

Talus

Calcaneus

Trochlear surface of talus

Tuberosity of calcaneus

Phalanges

Metatarsal bones

Tarsal bones

L1
L2
L3
L4
L5

Lumbar vertebrae

Lumbar region

Sacrum

Coccyx *(1)*

Superior view

Lateral view

© *Body Scientific International*

Glossary

24-hour clock: a method of telling time that assigns a number to each hour of the day; also known as *military time.*

3D printing: process of creating three-dimensional solid objects from a digital file.

A

abandonment: the act of leaving a patient dependent on your care.

abbreviation: a shortened way to write or say medical words and phrases.

abdominal cavity: the part of the abdominopelvic cavity that houses the digestive organs.

abdominal quadrants: one of the four regions used to divide the abdomen into sections.

abdominal region: one of nine equal areas of the abdomen that are named and used as reference points.

abdominopelvic cavity: the part of the ventral cavity that lies below the diaphragm muscle; includes the abdominal cavity for the digestive organs and the pelvic cavity that houses the reproductive organs, bladder, and rectum.

abduction: an action that moves a limb laterally away from the side of the body.

absolute risk: ratio of the number of people who have a medical event to those who could have the event because of a medical condition.

absorption: the act of taking up a substance into a tissue, such as the movement of nutrients from the small intestines into the bloodstream.

abuse: an act that inflicts physical or emotional harm.

accessory organs: organs attached to the alimentary canal, including the salivary glands, pancreas, and liver.

accreditation: official recognition from a professional association that an educational program meets minimum educational standards for an occupation.

acronym: an abbreviation in which each letter stands for a word.

active listening: the process of paying attention to and concentrating on understanding what a speaker is saying.

acute care: healthcare for severe illness or injury.

addendum: a note that is added to correct an error, explains the new or corrected information, and gives a reason for the change.

adduction: an action that returns a limb to the side of the body.

adenoids: lymphatic tissues located behind the nose that help protect against infection.

adrenal glands: glands that are located just above the kidneys and contain two parts: the adrenal cortex and the adrenal medulla.

advance directive: a legal document prepared by patients before a health crisis occurs to guide healthcare decisions in situations when patients cannot speak for themselves.

adverse childhood events (ACEs): challenges such as violence, abuse, neglect, and household dysfunction that can create toxic stress and lead to poor physical health.

advocate: to promote or support.

Age Discrimination in Employment Act (ADEA): a federal law that extends civil rights protection to workers 40 years of age and older.

algorithms: sets of rules that computers follow to process and analyze information.

alimentary canal: a long, hollow tube that is made up of digestive organs and runs from the mouth to the anus.

alternative, complementary, or integrative therapies: healthcare practices and treatments that minimize or avoid the use of surgery and drugs.

alternative medicine: entire systems and healthcare practices that have developed independent of Western medicine.

alveoli: tiny, hollow air sacs clustered like bunches of grapes at the ends of the bronchioles, which exchange gas with the surrounding capillaries.

ambulatory care: nonemergency or outpatient services provided at walk-in clinics.

Americans with Disabilities Act (ADA): a federal law that extends civil rights protection to workers with physical or mental disabilities.

amniotic sac: fluid-filled sac that protects the developing embryo in the uterus.

anatomy: the physical structures or parts of the body.

anterior: a directional term that refers to the front side of the body.

antibodies: proteins produced by leukocytes that bind with and disable antigens.

antigen: a foreign substance that causes the body to make antibodies.

antioxidant: a substance that promotes health by reducing cell deterioration and may contribute to disease prevention.

anus: the opening where feces are pushed from the alimentary canal out of the body.

anxiety: a feeling of nervousness, uneasiness, or dread.

aphasia: the loss of ability to understand or express speech.

apical pulse: a pulse measurement taken by listening over the apex (lower tip) of the heart using a stethoscope.

apothecary system: a system of measurement used by early pharmacists, or *apothecaries,* that is sometimes still used for herbal medicines.

appendicular skeleton: the bones of the arms and legs, including the shoulder and hip bones where they are attached.

appendix: structure in the intestines that contains lymphoid tissue that can destroy bacteria.

aptitude: natural inclination.

aqueous humor: a clear fluid in the front of the eye that maintains pressure and nourishes the cornea and lens.

artery: a blood vessel that moves blood from the heart out to the body tissues.

artificial intelligence (AI): technology in which computer systems are taught to do various tasks; also called machine learning.

aseptic techniques: practices used by healthcare professionals to keep an environment free of pathogens and prevent the spread of infections.

aspiration: the inhalation of a liquid into the lungs.

assault: any words or actions that lead an individual to fear that another person intends to cause harm.

assay: analysis done to determine the presence and amount of a substance or the potency of a drug.

assertive communication: a communication style characterized by confidence and consideration for others.

assess: to evaluate.

assessment: evaluation.

assignment of benefits: the process in which adult patients sign a claim form, granting permission to release their medical information to the insurance company; the person carrying the insurance also signs the form, allowing payments to be made directly to the medical office.

atom: the smallest organizational unit of the body.

atrium: a chamber at the top of the heart that receives blood from the veins.

audiologist: a professional who diagnoses hearing and balance conditions and plans treatment.

audiometer: a machine that makes sounds at different frequencies to test hearing.

auditory learners: people who use sounds, rhythm, and music to store and recall information.

auscultation: the use of a stethoscope to listen to sounds made by a patient's internal organs to make a diagnosis.

authenticate: to give legal authority to.

automated analyzer: a piece of equipment that can automatically sort and prepare samples for analysis.

automated external defibrillator (AED): a device that delivers an electric shock to the heart to restore its normal rhythm.

axial skeleton: the skull, spine, and rib cage bones, which rotate around an imaginary center line of the body.

axon: a long, tail-like projection on a neuron, which takes information from the cell body out to the muscles.

B

Background Information Disclosure (BID) form: an application that collects a prospective employee's past history.

bacteria: one-celled microorganisms that are so small they can only be seen under a microscope.

ball-and-socket joints: joints that consist of the rounded head of a bone that fits into the cup-shaped cavity of another bone.

barcode scanners: a device that captures a printed series of numbered black bars and spaces, translates them into numbers and letters, and sends the data to a computer to access information about a patient or product.

bar graph: a chart that shows comparisons between categories of data.

barred: prevented.

base rates: measures that help researchers see the significance of a change that is given in percentages.

battery: the act of touching a person without consent.

behavioral health: involves the daily habits, choices, and actions that affect mental and physical wellness..

benefits: advantages or profits.

bias: a systematic error producing a research finding that deviates from a valid finding.

bile: substance that helps mix fat with digestive enzymes so that it breaks down in the intestines.

bioassays: analysis done to determine the potency of a substance by measuring its effect on living tissues.

biobanking: the collection and storage of human tissue samples and related data for research purposes.

bioethics: the study of ethical practices in medical research and use of advanced technology to treat patients.

biohazard: a biological agent, infectious organism, or insecure laboratory procedure that constitutes a danger to humans or the environment.

Biohazard Prevention Act: a government act that empowers the EPA to investigate workplaces' storage and disposal methods for medical waste.

bioinformatics: a scientific discipline that combines the tools and techniques of mathematics, computer science, and biology to understand the biological significance of data.

bioinformatics scientists: researchers who use their computer skills to organize the expanding overload of data created by improved DNA sequencing technologies.

biomedical engineers: workers who apply a combined knowledge of biology and engineering to the design and development of products such as artificial organs, prostheses, and machines for diagnosing medical conditions.

bioreactors: apparatuses in which a biological process is carried out.

biorepositories: libraries of biological information that may be accessed for medical research.

biotechnology: the manipulation of living organisms to produce useful products.

Biotechnology Research and Development: the career pathway that involves bioscience research and the development of treatments and devices.

biotechnology research laboratories: research facilities that develop new products or treatments and are located on college campuses, in hospitals, and in private biotechnology companies.

bladder: a hollow, muscular organ that stores urine.

blastocyst: a fluid-filled cavity that develops in a morula.

Bloodborne Pathogens Standard: prescribes safeguards to protect workers at risk of being exposed to blood and other potentially infectious materials.

blood pressure: the force of blood pushing against the inside of the blood vessel (artery) walls.

body alignment: a position of the body in which the spine is not crooked or twisted.

body cavity: a hollow space within the body that is lined by a membrane and contains body organs.

body language: nonverbal communication that occurs through conscious or unconscious gestures and movements.

body mass index (BMI): a method of relating weight to height; used to define normal weight, overweight, and obesity.

body mechanics: correct position of the body to help a person avoid injury during a physical task.

body plane: a flat surface seen by cutting away part of the body through surgery or medical imaging; serves as a point of reference when discussing anatomy.

body region: an area of the body with a specific name, which is used as a reference point when discussing location on the body.

body system: a group of organs working together to perform a vital function in the body.

brainstem: area of the brain that controls the smooth muscles of the heart and lungs; also known as the *vital functions center*.

breach: access, use, or disclosure of protected health information that compromises the security or privacy of that information.

bronchi: tubes that branch out from the trachea into the right and left lungs.

bronchioles: tubes that branch out from the bronchi and travel down to the air sacs in the lungs.

business letters: formal letters written to people outside one's healthcare facility.

business-to-business selling: exchanging goods between businesses rather than between businesses and individuals.

C

calories: the units used to measure energy gained from food.

cancer: uncontrolled cell growth.

capillary bed: a network of very fine, thin-walled blood vessels (capillaries) located in body tissues.

carbohydrates: nutrients that are broken down into glucose, the body's first source of energy.

cardiac muscle: an involuntary, striated muscle tissue located in the walls of the heart.

cardiopulmonary resuscitation (CPR): a procedure that keeps the brain and other vital organs supplied with oxygen until advanced medical care arrives.

cardiovascular: related to the heart and blood vessels.

cardiovascular technologists: healthcare workers who assist physicians in diagnosing heart and blood vessel disorders.

career and technical student organizations (CTSOs): membership groups for advancing career skills in career and technical education pathways.

career assessments: tools such as questionnaires and surveys that you can use to find careers that will match your individual needs.

career clusters: groups of similar occupations and industries that share a core set of basic knowledge and skills for all workers.

career ladder: a sequence of job positions progressing from entry-level to higher levels of responsibility and authority based on education, experience, and performance.

career pathways: smaller groups of specialized occupations within a career cluster that require more specific sets of knowledge, skills, and training.

career portfolio: a written record of career planning and preparation.

caregiver laws: laws that protect children, older adults, and people with disabilities from misconduct by those who provide direct care, supervision, and protection.

cartilage: firm, whitish, flexible connective tissue found in various body parts, including where two bones meet to form a joint.

case managers: workers who develop a care plan along with clients and their families and supervise the care being provided.

caudal: a directional term used to talk about a point closer to the tailbone.

cell: a small group of organelles that fulfill a specific purpose and are held together by a membrane.

cell body: part of a neuron that contains the nucleus.

cell membrane: a semipermeable outer covering of a cell with holes that act as its doors and windows.

Celsius scale: a method of measuring temperature that is used in most healthcare facilities around the world (including many US facilities); also called the *Centigrade scale*.

Centers for Disease Control and Prevention (CDC): a division of the HHS that focuses on disease outbreaks and prevention in the United States.

Centers for Medicare & Medicaid Services (CMS): a division of the HHS that provides health insurance for 100 million people under the Medicare program for older adults and the Medicaid program for those with low incomes.

central nervous system (CNS): the brain and spinal cord.

central services: hospital department responsible for receiving, storing, cleaning, disinfecting, sterilizing, and distributing medical and surgical supplies and equipment.

centrifuges: machines with rapidly rotating containers used to separate fluids.

cerebellum: the second-largest area of the brain, which coordinates incoming and outgoing messages to produce smooth skeletal movements.

cerebral cortex: the outer surface of the cerebrum, which has many bumps and grooves.

cerebrum: the largest part of the brain, which is formed by the four lobes of the cerebral cortex.

certified nursing assistant (CNA): a healthcare worker who completes a nursing assisting class and passes a certification test; works under the supervision of a nurse.

cervix: the narrow neck at the bottom of the uterus that connects to the vagina.

chain of infection: the elements required for an infection to spread from one source to another.

charting: the process of recording observations and information about patients.

choroid: a membrane that supplies blood to the eye and controls the light reflected to the retina.

chromosome: a structure that contains genes, which carry chunks of DNA.

chronic: refers to a disease or condition that is long-lasting and potentially lifelong.

cilia: tiny hairs in the mucous membranes that filter out dirt and foreign material, sweeping it toward the throat.

circle graph: a chart that shows the relationship of parts of a data set to the whole; also known as *pie chart*.

circumduction: a motion that makes circles rather than twisting.

cisterna chyli: large vessel near your midline that collects lymph in the abdomen.

civil law: the branch of law that establishes rules for business relationships between people or between individuals and businesses.

Civil Rights Act: a federal law that bans employment discrimination based on a person's race, color, religion, sex, or national origin.

claim: a request for the insurance company to pay for the cost of care using pooled funds.

claims process: the procedure for submitting costs for medical services so payment can be collected or denial can be determined.

clean technique: the practice of disinfecting any object or surface that has come into contact with pathogens.

clear writing: written work that avoids wordiness and uses simple language to explain ideas that may be complex.

clients: people who receive treatment in privately owned offices and treatment facilities, as well as in their own homes.

clinical data: the clinical information found in various forms in a patient chart.

clinical engineers: workers who use medical technology to improve healthcare delivery.

clinical laboratories: facilities that examine materials taken from the human body to discover information related to diagnosis, prognosis, prevention, or treatment of disease.

Clinical Laboratory Improvement Act (CLIA): a government act that regulates how a laboratory test should be performed and how the test results should be interpreted and reported.

clinical training: hands-on work with patients that students do under the supervision of a licensed healthcare provider.

clinical trial: research conducted with patients to evaluate a new medical treatment, drug, or device.

cloning: a process that copies genetic material for use in biomedical research and therapeutic treatments.

cochlea: a fluid-filled chamber of the inner ear that is used for hearing.

code of ethics: a set of guiding principles that tell professionals how they are expected to act.

Coding and Revenue Cycle: health informatics job family that processes patient financial and health information for payment purposes.

cognitive development: the process of gaining thinking, reasoning, and learning abilities.

cognitive impairments: conditions that occur when a patient's ability to think is affected by pain or medication, when the patient is confused or disoriented, or when the patient has dementia.

coinsurance: an individual's share of healthcare costs compared to the insurance company's share.

collaborate: to work together; to consult with each other.

collagen: a protein fiber that connects, supports, and gives strength to body tissues such as the skin, muscle tendons, and bone ligaments.

combining vowel: a letter used to connect root words together when the next root or suffix does not begin with a vowel.

commode hat: a measuring device for urine that is placed under the toilet seat before the patient urinates.

Common Rule: a set of regulations adopted in common by a number of federal agencies to ensure the safety of testing on human subjects.

communication: the act of sharing a message, thought, or idea so it is accurately received and understood.

communication barrier: anything that blocks or interferes with the exchange of information.

communication style: a person's preferred method for exchanging information, which includes words, tone of voice, and nonverbal signals.

community health education outreach programs: programs that serve populations less likely to use preventive health services.

compact bone: the hard, dense, outer layer of bone tissue made to withstand stress.

compassion: sympathy for the distress of others accompanied by a desire to help.

competitive events: HOSA program that recognizes competencies developed by members through health science education and training.

complementary and alternative medicine (CAM): healthcare practices, products, and supplements that are not a part of Western medicine.

complementary medicine: practices used along with mainstream medicine to promote wellness, prevent disease, manage symptoms, and reduce stress.

compliance: adherence and observation of guidelines.

Compliance and Risk Assessment: health informatics job family that manages patient information to satisfy legal storage and security requirements.

computerized patient records: early versions of EHRs that contain patient information for a single organization.

concentration: a term that describes how much of a drug is in a specific volume of liquid.

condylar joints: joints that can bend, straighten, and move side to side.

confidential: private.

conscious: being aware of surroundings or different attitudes.

consistency: the way a liquid flows.

Consolidated Omnibus Budget Reconciliation Act (COBRA): an act that allows employees leaving their job to continue their insurance for up to three years if they pay for it themselves.

consultants: people who provide professional advice.

contamination: the unwanted presence of harmful substances or microorganisms.

continuous compression resuscitation (CCR): a type of CPR that involves using only chest compressions.

contract: a legally binding agreement between two or more people or agencies.

contraindicated: a term that means a patient has a particular condition that makes normal care tasks uncomfortable or dangerous.

conversion factor: a numerical value that represents how much ingredients must be adjusted for a revised recipe; new yield ÷ old yield = conversion factor.

copayment: an out-of-pocket fee paid by a person with health insurance at the time a covered service, such as an office visit or a prescription, is received.

cornea: a transparent tissue through which light enters the eye.

Cornell style notes: a two-column style of notes good for merging notes from multiple sources and reviewing information.

correspondence: written communication.

cover message: a short letter sent with a résumé to introduce the job applicant and give the reasons for applying to a particular job.

cranial: a directional term used to talk about a point closer to the head.

cranial cavity: the part of the dorsal cavity that contains the brain.

cranial nerves: twelve pairs of nerves that provide connections from the brain to the head and neck.

credentials: documents proving a person's qualifications for a particular occupation.

criminal law: the branch of law that aims to protect individuals and society by defining certain actions as crimes, or offenses against society.

cultural competence: the ability to interact effectively with people of different cultures.

cultural differences: variations among people that arise from nationality, ethnicity, race, and family backgrounds; affect beliefs, practices, behavior, and expectations.

cultural diversity: differences in age, gender, sex, physical and intellectual abilities, sexual orientation, nationality, or ethnicity that influence what people believe, think, and do.

customer objections: concerns, doubts, or other reasons a customer gives for not making a purchase.

cytoplasm: semifluid structure contained within the walls of a cell in which chemical reactions take place.

D

data: facts about a specific topic, which are used for reference or analysis.

deductible: the minimum amount a patient must pay out-of-pocket before the insurance company will pay for healthcare.

deep: farther below the surface.

defamation: a term that means damaging someone's good name or reputation.

defecation: the last stage of digestion in which undigested food and waste from the digestive system are expelled as feces.

dehydration: a condition caused by too little fluid in the body tissues.

de-identified information: health documents from which specified personal data has been removed.

delegate: to direct another healthcare worker to perform a care task that is within that worker's training and experience and within the scope of practice of the licensed provider giving the direction.

delegation: process of assigning tasks to team members.

dementia: a condition characterized by memory loss and the decline of other thinking skills.

dendrites: branches of a neuron that collect stimuli and transport them to the cell body.

Department of Health and Human Services (HHS): a government agency with 12 divisions that oversee many programs focused on improving the health of people in the United States.

depression: a long-lasting and overwhelming feeling of sadness.

dermis: the middle layer of the skin, which contains most of the skin's structures.

diagnostic: pertaining to the identification of a disease or syndrome.

Diagnostic Services: the career pathway that involves creating a picture of a patient's health status over time.

diaphysis: the long shaft of bone between the two epiphyses.

dictation: a verbal recording describing a patient's symptoms and the treatment given.

dietetic technician: a worker who plans and produces meals based on established guidelines, teaches principles of food and nutrition, and helps clients make healthy food choices.

dietitians: food and nutrition experts who advise patients on what foods to eat to improve their health condition.

differential diagnosis: a determination made by a doctor that distinguishes a disease or condition from others that have similar symptoms.

digestion: the mechanical and chemical breakdown of food into usable nutrients.

Digital Imaging Communications in Medicine (DICOM): a standard for handling, storing, printing, and transmitting information that enhances the distribution and viewing of medical images.

dilemma: a situation requiring you to make a difficult choice between two or more conflicting options.

dilution ratio: the amount of solvent compared to the amount of solute in a solution.

discretion: the ability to know when to keep sensitive information private.

discrimination: unfair treatment of individuals on the basis of their membership in a specific group (i.e., age, race, color, nationality, citizenship, religion, sex, disability, veteran status, or genetic information).

distal: a directional term that refers to a part that is farther away from the attachment site on the body; can also be used to describe internal organs.

DNA (deoxyribonucleic acid): material present in a cell that contains complete plans for items the cell builds; carries cell's genetic information.

do-not-resuscitate (DNR): an order that states a patient should not be revived with chest compressions or cardiac drugs if the patient stops breathing or the heart stops beating.

dorsal: a directional term used to describe surfaces that are located on the back of the body.

dorsal cavity: the cavity in the back of the body that is protected by the bones of the skull and vertebrae.

dosage: the total quantity of medicine to be administered.

dose: the portion of medicine to be administered at one time.

E

edema: a condition caused by too much fluid in the body tissues.

electrical shock: a physical reaction to electricity passing through the body.

electronic balances: measuring instruments that display the weight of a substance digitally and are used to weigh chemicals in labs.

electronic health record (EHR): a medical document that contains information from all the clinicians involved in a patient's care; can be created and accessed by the patient and by providers across more than one healthcare organization.

electronic medical record (EMR): an earlier version of the EHR that allowed physicians' offices and outpatient clinics to convert their paper records to electronic formats.

embryo: the developing human from the time of implantation to the end of the eighth week after conception.

emergency medical services (EMS): a system that provides rapid response care for those experiencing sudden illness and injury.

emerging diseases: diseases that suddenly increase or threaten to increase.

empathy: the ability to recognize and identify with another person's feelings and thoughts.

employability skills: tasks related to choosing a career, acquiring and keeping a job, changing jobs, and advancing in a career.

employment at will: the basic principle that employment is an equal agreement between employer and employee that either one can end whenever they want.

endocrine gland: glands without ducts that produce and release hormones directly into the bloodstream.

endoplasmic reticulum: the organelle that moves ribosomes in and out of the nucleus as they are assembled; can be rough (covered with ribosomes from the nucleus for building proteins) or smooth (builds and stores fats and carbohydrates and detoxifies harmful substances).

environment: the factor of a system that involves the setting in which the system operates; can be internal or external.

environmental barriers: distractions in the surrounding area that cause a person's attention to wander.

environmental engineers: workers who ensure the health of the public, such as by monitoring safe drinking water and air quality.

environmental services: hospital department responsible for housekeeping, laundry, and facility maintenance.

epidemic: a disease that spreads over a large area.

epidemiologists: scientists who study the spread of diseases.

epidermis: the thin, outer layer of the skin.

epididymis: the structure where sperm mature.

epiglottis: a flap of cartilage that helps direct food and air down the correct tubes.

epiphysis: the knob at the end of a long bone, which is made up of mostly spongy bone.

eponym: a term named after a person.

e-prescribing: electronic generation, transmission, and filling of a medical prescription.

Equal Employment Opportunity Commission (EEOC): a principle that describes employment as a mutual agreement between employer and employee that either party can end whenever they wish.

Equal Pay Act: a federal law that requires employers to pay men and women equally for performing the same job under the same conditions.

ergonomics: the study of designing and arranging a workplace to increase productivity and safety.

erythrocytes: red blood cells that transport oxygen and carbon dioxide to and from body tissues.

esophagus: the digestive tube that runs from the throat to the stomach.

ethical: fitting with someone's personal morals or professional rules of conduct.

ethics committee: a committee that meets to discuss unusual or controversial cases and advises professionals on ethical dilemmas.

ethnocentrism: the evaluation of other cultures using your own culture as the superior model.

etiquette: a code of polite behavior among members of a profession or group.

eugenics: a movement that attempts to promote desirable genetic characteristics.

evidence-based practices: methods of diagnosis and treatment based on the best available current research, clinical expertise, and a patient's needs and preferences.

exclusive provider organization (EPO): insurance plan that charges an access fee for a network of healthcare providers at reduced rates; premiums are usually lower than those of an HMO, but the choice of covered providers is more limited.

excretion: removal from the body of metabolic waste products created by cell activity.

explanation of benefits (EOB): a detailed account of each claim processed by an insurance plan; sent to the patient as notification of claim payment or denial.

exposure control plan: a detailed set of standards that explains how specimens, contaminated equipment, contaminated work surfaces, and contaminated waste materials can be handled safely.

expressed: a term that means the terms are spelled out in detail.

extension: an action that moves a dorsal surface toward a dorsal surface and increases the angle of the ventral surfaces of a joint.

external respiration: process in which capillaries surrounding your alveoli absorb oxygen from the air in your lungs and release carbon dioxide from your blood.

F

face sheet: dashboard in a patient's chart showing contact information, insurance information, and medical history.

Fahrenheit scale: a method of measuring temperature that is sometimes used in US healthcare facilities.

Fair Labor Standards Act (FLSA): a federal law that adopted an eight-hour workday, 40-hour work week, time-and-a-half overtime pay, and restricted employment of minors.

fallopian tubes: tubes that carry the ovum to the uterus.

false imprisonment: the act of holding people against their will or limiting their movement without the right to do so.

Family and Medical Leave Act (FMLA): a federal law that grants workers the right to 12 weeks off work in a 12-month period to give birth to a child, care for a newborn or newly adopted child, care for a family member with a serious illness, or recover from a personal illness or injury.

family history: a record that includes major illnesses and surgeries of a patient's close relatives, including parents, grandparents, aunts and uncles, and siblings.

fascicles: bundles of structures, such as nerve or muscle fibers.

fats: nutrients that provide triglycerides and help the body build insulation, pad vital organs, transport fat-soluble vitamins, make hormones, and store energy.

Federal Insurance Contributions Act (FICA): a government act that established a tax to fund Social Security.

Federal Needlestick Safety and Prevention Act: a government act that requires healthcare facilities to use needles specially engineered for safer injections and blood draws.

federal withholding tax: a tax on personal income.

feedback: the response of an audience to a message.

feedback loop: the factor of a system that involves responses to the functions that are used to keep the system going.

fellowship: highly specialized program or subspecialty, such as endocrinology or pediatric cardiology, that requires even more training than other fi elds.

fermentors: a machine that maintains optimal conditions for the growth of microorganisms and is used to produce drugs or enzymes for use in the biotechnology industry.

fertilization: a process that occurs when the chromosomes of the ovum and sperm unite to produce a zygote.

fetus: a developing human from eight weeks after conception to birth.

filtration: the process of separating substances, such as solid from liquid, large from small, or impure from pure.

fire triangle: the three elements needed for a fire to occur: oxygen, heat, and fuel.

first aid: emergency treatment given before regular medical services can be obtained.

fitness trainers: workers who are trained in specific exercise methods and teach classes.

flat bones: thin bones that are effective as a protective shell.

flexion: an action that moves a ventral surface toward a ventral surface, decreasing the angle of the joint.

fluid balance: a state in which the amount of fluid taken into the body equals the amount of fluid that leaves the body.

fontanel: the soft spot on an infant's head where the bones have not grown together yet.

food insecurity: the lack of consistent access to enough healthy food to support physical health.

foramen: an opening or hole, especially in a bone.

forensic DNA analysts: people who work in a crime lab to extract and match DNA from samples that are used as evidence to solve crimes.

Fowler's: an inclined position in which the patient's body is elevated at 45 degrees.

fraud: a deceitful practice.

frontal lobes: lobes of the brain that are located at the forehead and are responsible for voluntary muscle control, thinking, memory, language, judgment, creativity, and personality.

frontal plane: the body plane that divides the body (or organ) into its front and back sections; also called the coronal plane.

fulcrum: the point at which something pivots; the pin of a goniometer.

functional nursing: a care model in which each nurse is responsible for completing a set of assigned tasks for every patient or resident.

fungi: parasitic microbes that live in soil and on plants.

G

gallbladder: the organ that stores bile and delivers it to the duodenum when needed.

gametes: reproductive cells that have half the normal number of chromosomes and unite during fertilization; sperm in males and ova in females.

ganglion: a swelling located between two neurons.

gene: a unit of heredity within DNA that determines traits and instructs the cell to make molecules that regulate body processes.

generic: a medication that is chemically identical to a brand-name product and meets the same standards for quality and performance, but is usually less expensive.

gene therapy: insertion of a new gene to replace an abnormal or defective gene.

genetic counselors: people who meet with clients to gather medical information and help them understand genetic disorders.

genetic discrimination: the use of genetic information by employers and insurance companies to deny employment or insurance coverage or treat individuals differently because of a genetic condition.

genetic disorders: a disease or condition that results from damaged, incorrectly located, or abnormal genes.

genetic engineering: the deliberate manipulation of genetic materials to eliminate harmful traits or to ensure the presence of desirable traits.

Genetic Information Nondiscrimination Act (GINA): a federal law that protects employees from discrimination based on genetic information.

geneticists: medical scientists who study genes, heredity, and the variation of organisms.

genetic testing: the examination of a person's cells to analyze genes and identify possible genetic disorders.

genomic medicine: personalized medical care that uses a patient's unique combination of genes and chromosomes to prevent illness and maintain health.

gliding joint: a joint in which bones slide over each other.

Golgi apparatus: an organelle made up of layers of membrane in the cytoplasm; inspects, sorts, and packages proteins for use within or removal from the cell.

gonads: reproductive glands that produce gametes and reproductive hormones; testes in males and ovaries in females.

goniometer: an instrument for measuring angles.

good laboratory practices (GLPs): regulations that describe how laboratories must operate.

good manufacturing processes (GMPs): regulations that describe how manufacturers must operate.

graduated cylinder: a tall container used for measuring the volume of liquids.

gross pay: the total amount of money earned in a pay period.

grounding: the act of carrying current safely away from an electrical circuit to prevent shocks from occurring in the event of a problem with the circuit.

H

hair follicle: tube in which hair grows from the root up to the epidermis.

hand hygiene: procedure that includes regular handwashing using plain or antibacterial soap and the use of alcohol-based gels.

harassment: unwelcome, offensive, and repeated language or actions, based on age, race, color, nationality, citizenship, religion, sex, disability, veteran status, or genetic information, that affect an employee's job performance or advancement opportunities or create an uncomfortable working environment.

harms: damages or injuries.

Hazard Communication Standard (HCS) : requires employers to provide information and training for employees about handling potential health hazards in the workplace.

health and safety specialists: workers who focus on making sure the workplace is safe for all employees by ensuring safety regulations are followed.

health and wellness managers: workers who develop and coordinate programs to improve employee wellness.

healthcare-associated infections (HAIs): an infection that is not present when a patient is admitted to a hospital or healthcare facility but develops 48 hours or more after admission.

health disparities: unexpected differences in health outcomes for groups of people due to unequal positions in society.

Health Informatics Services: the career pathway that involves methods, devices, and resources used to acquire, store, retrieve, and work with healthcare and biomedical information.

Health Information Technology for Economic and Clinical Health (HITECH) Act: a law that made significant changes to the HIPAA privacy and security regulations and seeks to increase nationwide use of electronic health records.

Health Insurance Portability and Accountability Act (HIPAA): a federal law that makes it easier to obtain healthcare coverage and protects personal health information.

health literacy: a person's ability to obtain and understand health-related information and make informed decisions using that information.

health maintenance organizations (HMOs): insurance organizations that employ doctors, pharmacists, dentists, laboratories, and hospitals in an integrated and patient-focused network to cover all aspects of medical care for insured individuals.

hemoglobin: a protein that helps red blood cells carry oxygen and gives them their red color.

heredity: the passing of traits (such as eye color, height, and some diseases) from parent or ancestor to offspring through chromosomes.

hierarchy: a term that describes the levels of authority within an organization.

high-deductible health plan (HDHP): insurance plan with a lower monthly premium but higher deductible.

high Fowler's: an inclined position in which the patient's body is elevated at 90 degrees.

hinge joints: joints that only bend and straighten or open and close with no side-to-side movement.

holistic care: therapies that treat the patient as a whole person after assessing the individual's physical, social, mental, and spiritual well-being.

holistic health: provides care for the whole person with a balance between the body, mind, spirit, and emotions; acknowledging that a change in one aspect affects the others.

home healthcare: healthcare provided for those who are weak, older, or have disabilities and live at home; care is provided by nurses, home health aides, clergy, and professionals who provide rehabilitation services.

homeostasis: a state of balance between interdependent elements.

hormone: a chemical used to send messages from an endocrine gland to a target organ.

HOSA—Future Health Professionals: a career and technical student organization for future health professionals.

hospice care: healthcare available for clients who have been diagnosed with a terminal disease and generally have fewer than six months to live.

hospitals: typically a large facility that offers a wide range of services from inpatient care, surgery, and critical care to physical therapy, radiology, and laboratory services.

Human Genome Project: an international scientific research project with the goal of determining the sequence of chemical base pairs that make up human DNA.

human resources: term that describes workers who specialize in maximizing workers' effectiveness and productivity.

human testing: controlled experiments performed on human beings in order to evaluate the safety and effectiveness of medical treatments.

hypertension: a condition in which blood pressure is too high.

hypodermis: the innermost layer of the skin, which stores fat.

hypotension: a condition in which blood pressure is too low.

hypothalamus: the brain's center for emotions and instincts, which controls pleasure, pain, sleep, hunger, and thirst.

hypothesis: a theory or proposed explanation that serves as the starting point for further investigation.

I

Immigration Reform and Control Act: an act that set employment restrictions regarding immigration and people illegally in the United States.

immune response: the lymphatic system makes antibodies to protect against foreign substances in the body.

implied: a term that means an agreement is assumed based on the actions of both parties.

incident report: a form used to record the details of an unusual event, such as an accident or injury.

incompetence: a lack of qualifications or ability to perform job tasks.

industrial engineers: workers who identify the most efficient ways to use space, time, workers, and other resources.

infectious: able to spread.

infectious agent: a pathogen that can cause infection.

inferior: a directional term that means lower down on the body.

inflammation: immune response in which swelling attracts white blood cells to trap and break down the pathogens.

Informatics and Data Analytics: health informatics job family that studies electronic data to further medical research and education.

Information Technology Infrastructure: health informatics job family that focuses on computer science.

informed consent: a patient's choice to accept or reject a procedure after receiving information about available options and possible consequences.

infrastructure: the internal systems a facility needs to operate, such as power supplies; electrical, plumbing, and heating and cooling systems; water; waste management; and phones and computer systems.

infusion: injection of drugs or another solution directly into a vein.

ingestion: the stage of digestion in which food is taken into the body through the mouth.

ingredient cost: a numerical value representing the total cost of one ingredient in a recipe.

initiative: ability to decide independently what to do and when to do it.

innervate: to provide an area with a nerve connection to the brain.

input: the factor of a system that includes the population being served and why they need or want service through this system; also includes the resources the system needs to function, such as workers, equipment, and financial resources.

inspection: visual examination used to assess parts of the body by looking for abnormal color, shape, size, or texture.

insurance: a purchased contract for shared financial protection against an unexpected loss.

intake and output (I&O): measurements of all the fluids that enter and leave the body.

integrity: adherence to ethical principles and professional standards.

integumentary: related to the skin.

intellectual wellness: involves keeping your brain active through stimulating and creative activities that expand your knowledge and skills.

interdisciplinary healthcare team: a group of professionals from different health science training backgrounds working in coordination toward a common goal for the patient.

intern: a term that describes a student doctor completing rotations through various specialties in the first year of residency.

internal respiration: process in which carbon dioxide in your cells is exchanged for oxygen from your blood.

International Classification of Diseases Clinical Modifications (ICD-CM): a system published by the Department of Health and Human Services that contains the coding system for diagnoses based on information from the World Health Organization.

International Units (IU): a system of measurement that describes the effect or potency of manufactured drugs and vitamins.

internship: practical work or training experience that allows students to apply what they have learned in class.

interoperability: the ability of different health information systems to securely access, exchange, and use electronic health information within and across different healthcare organizations.

interview etiquette: accepted appearance and behavior for the interview process.

invasion of privacy: intrusion on a person's privacy; applies to personal information as well as a person's body.

invasive procedure: a test or treatment that requires incisions to the skin or the insertion of instruments or other materials into the body.

in vitro: taking place in a test tube.

involuntary: not under conscious control.

involuntary seclusion: the practice of isolating a person and preventing the person from interacting with others.

irregular bones: bones that are a complex shape and contain mostly spongy bone with a covering of compact bone.

islets of Langerhans: clusters of cells located on the pancreas that make the hormones insulin and glucagon.

isolation: confinement to a private room to prevent the spread of infection.

K

kidneys: organs that filter, concentrate, and remove waste from the blood to form urine.

kinesthetic learners: people who use their body, hands, and sense of touch to learn.

L

lab information system (LIS): a computer system that manages data about patients, lab test requests, and lab test results.

laboratory documentation: written records of observable, measurable, and reproducible findings obtained through examination, testing, research studies, and experiments.

lacteals: specialized lymphatic vessels that pick up digested fats and fat-soluble vitamins in the villi of the small intestine.

large intestine: tube that carries feces from the small intestine to the rectum; water is absorbed from feces in the different sections; also called the *colon*.

larynx: a space near the pharynx that aids in voice production; also known as the *voice box*.

lateral: a directional term that refers to a point toward the side of the body.

learning style: an individual's preferred way of gaining or processing new information.

legal: related to laws made by the government.

legal disability: a condition that results in a person being unable to enter a contract, such as being under the age of consent, being ruled mentally incompetent, or having an altered mental state due to drugs or semiconsciousness.

lens: a transparent, flexible structure that focuses light at the back of the eye.

letter of resignation: a written document that formally states an employee's decision to leave a job.

leukocytes: white blood cells that are involved in fighting infection.

liable: legally responsible.

licensed practical nurse (LPN): a healthcare worker who completes a one-year technical training program and can perform basic nursing tasks such as giving injections, monitoring catheters, and dressing wounds; also called a *licensed vocational nurse (LVN)*.

ligament: a tough, fibrous tissue that connects bones to other bones and holds organs in place.

limbic system: horseshoe-shaped set of structures that includes the cingulate gyrus, hippocampus, and amygdala.

line graph: a chart that shows the changes in data over time.

liver: the organ that breaks down and removes toxic substances, drugs, bacteria, and dead red blood cells from the body.

living will: a patient's written document giving instructions about which procedures may or may not be used to sustain or prolong life, such as feeding tubes or ventilation.

localized: affecting only a small area of the body.

long bones: bones that are longer than they are wide and have a hollow diaphysis.

long-term care facilities: healthcare facilities that provide skilled nursing care and rehabilitation services for residents who will live in the facility for many months or years.

lymph: blood plasma that remains between cells after delivering its oxygen, nutrients, and hormones.

lymphatic: related to or containing the watery fluid (lymph) collected from body tissues.

lymphatic vessels: structures that transport lymph throughout the body.

lymph nodes: small capsules where lymphocytes collect to remove dead cells, destroy pathogens, and create antibodies against infection.

lymphocyte: a type of white blood cell that determines how the body responds to foreign substances.

lysosomes: organelles that use digestive enzymes to destroy used, dead, and foreign materials that are left behind after energy is used up.

M

maladaptive behaviors: nonproductive ways of dealing with emotional challenges.

malpractice: term for actions that violate a professional's scope of practice or standard of care and result in injury to a patient that could reasonably have been expected.

mammogram: X-ray that tests for breast cancer.

managed care: a system that limits access to and use of healthcare to keep costs down.

mandatory reporting: the legal requirement for certain health issues to be reported to authorities.

manufacturing process engineers: workers who design the methods and equipment used to manufacture a product.

marketing: term that describes a field specializing in making others aware of a company's or individual's products and services.

mean: the mathematical average of a set of data.

meaningful use: the use of electronic health records that follows a series of stages with sets of objectives for healthcare providers to meet in each stage.

medial: a directional term that refers to a point closer to the center of the body.

median: term that describes the number found exactly in the middle when a data is listed in numerical order.

Medicaid: a government-provided health insurance program that provides hospital and medical insurance for people with low incomes, children in low-income families, and those who have disabilities and cannot work.

medical coding: the act of assigning numbers to descriptions of a patient's diseases, injuries, and treatments according to established codes.

medical diagnosis: a determination made by a doctor that identifies the cause of a patient's illness.

medical documentation: written reports of observable, measurable, and reproducible findings from examinations, supporting laboratory or diagnostic tests, and assessments of a patient.

medical error: preventable mistake that can occur at any point in the healthcare process and may potentially cause harm to the patient.

medical history: a patient's diseases and surgeries, symptoms, results of examinations and tests, treatments, and other health services.

medical history form: a record of all the diseases and surgeries a patient has had, current symptoms, results of examinations and diagnostic tests, treatments, and other health services.

medical interpreter: an individual who translates between languages for a patient to ensure the patient's needs are being met.

medical terminology: special vocabulary that is used in healthcare and is often formed from Latin and Greek word parts.

Medical Waste Tracking Act: a government act that empowers OSHA to investigate workplaces' storage and disposal methods for medical waste.

Medicare: a government-provided health insurance program designed for people 65 years of age and older.

medication: a substance or mixture of substances proven through research to have a clear value in the prevention, diagnosis, or treatment of diseases.

meiosis: the sexual process of cellular reproduction that produces four new haploid cells, each with a unique combination of 23 chromosomes.

melanin: the brownish-black pigment produced by melanocytes.

memorandums: short, informal messages sent between people within an organization.

meninges: three tough layers of tissue covering the brain and spinal cord, including the dura mater, arachnoid mater, and pia mater.

meniscus: curve at the surface of a liquid caused when it sticks to the walls of a graduated cylinder.

mental health: involves how people think, feel, behave, and cope when faced with life challenges.

metric system: the decimal measurement system based on the meter, liter, and gram as its primary units of length, volume, and weight or mass, respectively.

mHealth: a term that refers to mobile health apps.

micropipette: an instrument designed for the measurement of very small volumes.

midsagittal plane: the body plane that divides the body exactly down the midline.

mind maps: a style of notes that uses visual connections to show how ideas are related.

minimum wage: the lowest hourly earnings that an employer can legally pay a worker.

minimum data set (MDS): a comprehensive evaluation of the functional capabilities of each resident in a long-term care facility.

misappropriation: the unauthorized use of something that belongs to someone else.

misconduct: behavior at work that is unprofessional, unethical, and/or illegal.

mitered corners: neat corner folds used for making beds in hospitals.

mitochondria: organelles that function as power stations for cells.

mitosis: the asexual process of cellular reproduction that creates two identical copies of a cell, each with a full set of 46 chromosomes.

mnemonic device: a learning tool that helps students memorize information.

mode: the number that occurs most frequently in a data set.

mode of transmission: the way in which a pathogen moves from its reservoir to a new host.

molecule: atoms bonded together.

morals: people's beliefs about right and wrong learned from family, friends, traditions, and experiences.

morticians: workers who manage funeral homes and arrange the details of a funeral.

morula: a solid ball of 16 cells that results when a zygote divides.

mucous membranes: thin layers of tissue that line body cavities to provide a natural barrier against pathogens.

multidisciplinary healthcare team: a group of healthcare workers from different healthcare specialties, each providing specific services to the patient.

muscle tone: the normal, partly contracted state of skeletal muscles in the trunk and limbs, which helps maintain the body's balance.

myelin: a fatty layer that protects the axons of some nerves.

N

nail bed: term for the sensitive layer of cells beneath the nail plate at the tips of a person's fingers and toes.

nanotechnology: a field of science that manipulates individual atoms and molecules to create devices that are thousands of times smaller than current technologies allow.

National Health Science Standards: statements developed by the National Consortium for Health Science Education that describe the knowledge and skills workers need to succeed in healthcare careers.

National Institutes of Health (NIH): a division of the HHS that conducts research and provides information toward improving public health through 27 different agencies.

National Labor Relations Act (NLRA): a federal law that gives workers the right to join together, with or without a union, to discuss ways of improving working conditions.

near field communication (NFC): technology that uses an electronic chip in a device or sticker to transmit and exchange information wirelessly using a smartphone.

negative feedback system: mechanism that reduces a body function in response to a stimulus, such as a hormone.

neglect: the failure to provide needed physical or emotional care.

negligence: the failure to do something a person with training should have known enough to do.

nephron: the fundamental excretory unit of each kidney.

net pay: the amount of money received in a pay period after all deductions have been taken out; also known as *take-home pay*.

network: the group of people who work in healthcare that someone might know.

networking: interacting with others to exchange information and develop professional contacts.

neuron: a nerve cell.

neurotransmitter: a chemical used to carry a signal from an axon to a receptor cell to pass along a message.

noninvasive procedure: a test or treatment that does not require incisions to the skin or the insertion of instruments or other materials into the body.

nonprofit organization: business entity that uses any profits to achieve its charitable goals, such as research, education, and low-cost care.

nuclear medicine technologists: healthcare workers who administer radioactive substances as part of the imaging process.

nucleolus: the organelle located at the center of the nucleus, which uses ribosomes to build proteins.

nucleus: the organelle that contains genetic material and controls the cell's activity.

number needed to harm (NNH): the number of patients who must be treated over a specific period to cause harm in an average of one patient who would not otherwise have been harmed.

number needed to treat (NNT): the number of patients who must be treated to prevent the occurrence of the condition under examination.

nursing diagnosis: the description of a client's health condition that a nurse is licensed and competent to treat.

nutrient-dense: foods high in vitamins, minerals, complex carbohydrates, lean proteins, and healthy fats, but low in calories.

nutrients: molecules such as carbohydrates, proteins, fats, vitamins, and minerals used by the body to grow and maintain body processes.

O

obesity: an excessive accumulation of body fat.

objective observations: an indication of a health condition that can be clearly observed; also called a *sign*.

objective writing: written work that draws a conclusion from the facts and makes no assumptions.

occipital lobes: the smallest of the brain's lobes, which are located in the back of the skull and control sight, visual-spatial processes, memory, and storage.

occluder: an implement used to block light to the eye.

Occupational Safety and Health Administration (OSHA): a government agency that creates regulations to prevent work-related injuries, illnesses, and deaths.

off-label: term that describes a type of prescribing in which a doctor uses a medication in a way that is not specified in the product information.

olfactory bulb: the thickened end of the olfactory nerve that sends sensory impulses to the olfactory region of the brain.

on-call: available to answer calls at any time or come in to work on short notice.

open-ended question: a question that requires more than a one- or two-word response.

Operations and Medical Record Administration: health informatics job family that focuses on complete and accurate patient medical records.

ophthalmologist: an eye specialist.

ophthalmoscope: a tool used to examine the eyes.

opioids: a class of drugs often used to manage pain.

optometrist: a professional who performs vision testing and prescribes routine vision corrections.

oral health: the health of the teeth, gums, tongue, and mouth.

organ: a distinct body structure made of different tissues working together for the same purpose.

organelle: a part of a cell that has a specific task.

organizational chart: a diagram that shows how departments in an organization relate to one another.

ossicles: bones that transfer vibrations from the middle ear to the inner ear, including the malleus, incus, and stapes.

ossification: the process of taking calcium from any ingested food and drink and depositing it into cartilage to form bone.

osteoblasts: specialized bone-forming cells that begin the mineralization process.

osteoclast: a cell that breaks down bone during physical activity so it can be remodeled into new bone cells.

otolaryngologist: an ear specialist.

otoscope: a tool used to the examine the ears.

outline notes: a style of notes that follows the headings in a section.

output: the factor of a system that refers to the results produced by the system's functioning.

outsource: to contract out jobs to workers in a different country.

ova: the female gametes, also known as *eggs*.

ovaries: the female gonads.

overtime: payment at one and a half times the regular wage for each hour an employee works beyond 40 hours in a week.

P

pacemakers: devices used to regulate heartbeats.

pain scale: a tool used to help patients describe and identify their pain.

palpation: a medical examination that uses touch to detect growths, changes in the size of organs, or tissue reactions to pressure.

pancreas: the organ that produces enzymes to digest carbohydrates, fats, and proteins.

papillae: tiny bumps on the tongue that house taste buds.

paramedics: workers who respond to emergencies to restore a safe environment and treat patients before they reach a healthcare facility.

parasite: an organism that lives on or inside a host that provides its food.

parathyroid glands: four tiny glands that are located on the back of the thyroid and secrete a hormone that triggers the release of calcium from bones.

parietal lobes: lobes of the brain that are located behind the frontal lobes and integrate sensory information from the skin, internal organs, muscles, and joints.

patent: licenses that give researchers or inventors the sole right to produce and sell a product for a set time.

pathogen: a disease-causing microorganism.

patient interview: a structured communication between a patient and a healthcare worker for the purpose of collecting subjective data such as a medical history.

Patient Protection and Affordable Care Act (ACA): a law that sets minimum standards for insurance products and reduces barriers to gaining insurance coverage; prohibited insurance companies from denying coverage for preexisting conditions and mandated preventive-care coverage at no charge.

patient registration form: a record that includes contact and insurance information for the patient.

patients: people who receive treatment in hospitals and clinics.

Patient Self-Determination Act (PSDA): an act that protects healthcare consumers' rights to make their own decisions; requires many healthcare institutions to provide information about decision-making rights and ask patients if they have advance directives.

pelvic cavity: the part of the abdominopelvic cavity that houses the reproductive organs, bladder, and rectum.

penis: the male reproductive organ, which delivers sperm to the female reproductive tract.

percentiles: measures used to indicate how close to the average a person's height and weight fall.

percussion: a medical examination that includes tapping various body parts and using resulting sounds to assess the condition of internal organs.

percussion hammer: a tool used to check a patient's reflexes.

peripheral devices: pieces of equipment used to gather information and upload it to computer systems.

peripheral nervous system (PNS): the sensory and motor nerves that go out to the body's extremities.

peristalsis: muscle contractions.

personal and professional development: steps taken to improve personal, educational, and career-related performance.

personal bias: an unfair preference for, or dislike of, something or someone.

personal data page: a document that contains personal data and can be used to complete job applications; contains contact information, education, work experience, skills, and references.

personal health record (PHR): an electronic application through which patients can maintain and manage their health information from multiple providers in a private, secure, and confidential environment.

personal hygiene: grooming habits such as bathing, brushing your teeth, and washing your hands.

personal identifying information: information used to connect a patient to the correct record.

personal leadership style: an individual approach to giving directions, implementing plans, and motivating people.

personal protective equipment (PPE): equipment such as gloves, masks, gowns, respirators, and eyewear worn to protect skin, clothing, and the respiratory tract from infectious agents.

personal traits: an individual's unique combination of qualities and characteristics.

pesticides: substances or devices that repel, kill, or prevent the growth of insects, rodents, fungi, weeds, or other pests and plants.

pharmaceutical company: an organization that develops, tests, and markets new medications.

pharynx: the passageway between the nasal cavity and mouth and the esophagus; also known as the *throat*.

phlebotomist: a medical assistant who helps draw blood and receives specimens for testing.

physical wellness: involves balancing diet, physical activity, sleep, and other activities to keep your body healthy.

physician assistant (PA): healthcare worker who practices medicine under the supervision of a physician; can diagnose, treat, and prescribe medication for patients.

Physician's Current Procedural Terminology (CPT): a system created by the American Medical Association that contains the codes used to report procedures and services to public and private insurance companies.

physiology: the functions or inner workings of the body.

pictograph: a chart that presents data using images.

pigment: color.

pituitary gland: gland that releases hormones that affect the operation of many other glands in the body; also called the *master gland*.

pivot joint: a joint that allows movement around a single axis.

placebo: a harmless substance that contains no medication.

placenta: an organ that grows in the uterus to meet the nutritional needs of the embryo and fetus.

plasma: a yellowish liquid containing mostly water; carries nutrients, hormones, and waste for other body systems.

pleurae: membranes that line the surfaces of the lungs.

plexus: an interwoven combination of spinal nerve roots through which messages pass.

plural: a term that means more than one in number.

point-of-care testing: medical diagnostic testing that is performed outside of a laboratory, closer to where a patient is receiving care.

point-of-service (POS): insurance plans that have smaller deductibles and copays than a PPO, but require a referral from a patient's primary care provider before seeing a specialist, like an HMO does.

population health: the physical, mental, and social well-being of groups of people and health differences between groups.

portal of entry: a natural body opening or break in the skin that provides a way for pathogens to enter the body.

portal of exit: a natural body opening or break in the skin that provides a way for pathogens to leave the body.

portion: the amount of food in one serving.

posterior: a directional term that refers to the back side of the body.

postgraduate: education and training completed after receiving a bachelor's degree.

postsecondary education: education past high school that can be obtained at community colleges, vocational or technical colleges, public and private colleges and universities, institutes of technology, and career colleges.

posture: an important part of body mechanics that describes the position of a person's body while performing a task.

power of attorney (POA): the appointment of a person to make healthcare decisions for someone in the event that the patient is unable to make their own choices.

precise writing: written work that uses concrete rather than figurative language and is as specific as possible to avoid confusion.

precision medicine: using population data to customize medical care to an individual's genetic, biological, and lifestyle differences.

preferred provider organization (PPO): insurance organization in which insurers contract with private physicians and hospitals to provide treatment and care at a reduced cost in return for an increased number of patients.

prefix: letters in front of a root word that change the meaning of the word.

prejudice: a strong feeling or belief about a person or subject that is not based on reason or actual experience.

premiums: the monthly fees individuals pay into a shared money pool to receive insurance coverage.

preventive care: practices that help detect or prevent the start of serious diseases.

primary care provider (PCP): a patient's main doctor who provides primary care.

primary care teams: groups of healthcare providers, including the primary care physician along with physician assistants and nurse practitioners, who see the patient in the clinic setting; may also include nutritionists, pharmacists, social workers, or others.

primary motor cortex: an area of the frontal lobe that directs muscle movement through efferent neurons to muscles in the body.

primary nursing: a care model in which one RN, LPN, or LVN is assigned several patients or residents and is responsible for planning and carrying out all aspects of care for as long as the patients are in the care unit.

primary research articles: scientific papers that provide the original data and conclusions of researchers who conducted experiments.

primary sensory cortex: an area of the parietal lobe dedicated to gathering and interpreting information from afferent neurons regarding the five senses of the body.

primary source: a document that describes research in which the authors directly participated.

privileged communication: any private conversations between a healthcare professional and a patient, which cannot be disclosed in court.

probability: the likelihood of something happening.

problem-oriented medical record (POMR): a record that organizes medical information according to the patient's problem.

professional distance: term used to describe the act of showing a caring attitude toward patients without trying to become friends.

professional organization: an association formed to unite and inform people who work in the same occupation.

prone: lying facedown.

proportion: two ratios or fractions that are equal.

proposals: documents that propose or suggest something.

proprietary: privately owned and managed.

prostatectomy: surgical removal of the prostate gland.

prosthetics: artificial body parts.

protected health information (PHI): all individually identifiable personal information obtained through healthcare.

protein: nutrient that provides amino acids to help the body repair and make new cells.

protocol: the appropriate conduct, etiquette, or procedures for communication.

proximal: a directional term that indicates that the part being discussed is closer to the point of attachment to the body; can also be used to describe internal organs.

public health: a branch of medicine focused on protecting and improving health of people and their communities.

public health laboratory professionals: highly educated specialists who have knowledge of one or more scientific disciplines.

public relations: term that describes a field specializing in communication between an organization and the public.

Pull, Aim, Squeeze, Sweep (PASS): an acronym for remembering the steps to use a fire extinguisher.

pulmonary loop: the flow of blood from the heart to the lungs and back to pick up oxygen and drop off carbon dioxide.

pupil: the opening through which light rays enter the eye.

Q

quality assurance specialists: workers who make sure manufacturing processes follow required guidelines and procedures.

quality control technicians: workers who inspect every step in the manufacturing process to ensure quality requirements are met.

quality improvement (QI): a systematic approach to analyzing practices and improving efficiency or success.

quantitative data: information that can be measured.

quick response (QR) codes: a two-dimensional barcode that provides easy access to information through a smartphone; also known as *quick read code*.

R

radial pulse: a pulse measurement taken by placing two or three fingers over the radial artery on the inside of the wrist.

radiation therapist: a healthcare worker who uses CT or other imaging techniques to pinpoint a tumor's location and consults a treatment plan to position the patient for radiation treatment.

radio frequency identification (RFID): a data-collection technology that uses electronic tags for storing data.

radiographers: healthcare professionals who create medical images or treat diseases by passing radiation, such as X-rays or gamma rays, through an object.

range of motion (ROM): the full extent of movement for a joint.

rapport: an empathetic understanding between people.

reabsorption: the act of returning a substance to the part of the body from which it was previously filtered out.

receptor: a nerve cell that receives stimuli.

recipe cost: a numerical value representing the total cost of all ingredients in a recipe.

recommendation reports: documents that provide a way to meet a need in the workplace.

rectal temperature: a body temperature taken by placing the thermometer in the rectum.

rectum: a short segment with a lower end that comprises the anal canal.

recurrence: the return of something after a period of time, such as the return of cancer.

references: people who are willing to discuss someone's skills and job qualifications with potential employers.

regenerative medicine: a form of medical care that creates living tissue to replace tissue or organ functions lost due to age, disease, injury, or birth disorder.

regimens: plans for medical treatment.

registered nurse (RN): a healthcare worker with either an associate's degree in nursing (ADN) or a bachelor's of science in nursing (BSN).

Rehabilitation Act: a federal law that prohibits discrimination on the basis of disability in programs conducted by federal agencies, in programs receiving federal financial assistance, in federal employment, and in the employment practices of federal contractors.

relative risk: ratio of the chance of a disease developing among people who are exposed to a specific factor compared with those who are not exposed.

renal cortex: dark red, blood-rich, outer portion of each kidney contains millions of glomeruli.

Rescue, Alarm, Contain, Extinguish/Evacuate (RACE): an acronym used to remember the steps to take in response to a fire emergency.

reservoir: a place where the pathogen can live, such as the human body, animals, food, or fomites.

residents: (1) individuals living in long-term care facilities; (2) medical school graduates who are completing the last portion of their medical training before becoming licensed physicians.

respiration: one breath in (inhalation) and one breath out (exhalation); the movement of oxygen from air to the cells.

respiratory: related to the act of, or organs involved in, breathing.

respiratory hygiene: practices that seek to protect people from airborne infectious particles; also called *cough etiquette*.

résumé: a short, one-page document that contains your accomplishments and experiences and explains how these relate to a job in which you are interested.

review articles: scientific papers that give an overview of a specific topic by summarizing the data and conclusions from several different studies.

ribosomes: organelles that build proteins for the cell; may be free in the cytoplasm or attached to rough endoplasmic reticulum.

right lymphatic duct: lymphatic vessel that collects fluid from your head and the right side of your upper body.

risk assessments: methods used to calculate and describe a person's chance of becoming ill or dying of a specified condition.

root: the part of a hair where growth begins, which is embedded at the bottom of a hair follicle.

root word: the foundation of a term, giving the term its main meaning.

rotation: the action of turning on an axis.

S

saddle joint: a joint in which one bone forms a shape like a saddle and the other bone fits inside.

Safety Data Sheet (SDS): an OSHA-required document that explains the risks of a chemical product.

safety precaution: information about the safe operation of a piece of equipment, which is usually found in the instruction manual or on equipment labels.

sagittal plane: the body plane that divides the body, organ, or appendage into right and left sections.

sales presentation: a prearranged meeting in which a salesperson presents detailed information and often a demonstration of a product.

sales representatives: workers who contact and meet potential customers to sell a company's products.

salivary glands: glands in the mouth that secrete saliva.

sanitation: procedures and practices that maintain cleanliness and preserve public health.

SBAR system: a method that helps healthcare workers communicate with each other more clearly using a standardized communication format for reporting changes in a patient's status; stands for *Situation, Background, Assessment,* and *Recommendation.*

scientific communication: a type of technical communication used by scientists and nonscientists to provide information and promote understanding.

sclera: the tough, fibrous outer layer of the eye; also known as the *white of the eye.*

scope of practice: tasks an employee is legally allowed to perform based on their training and certification.

screening tools: procedures that assess the risk for many health conditions.

scrotum: a sac that holds the testes on the outside of the body.

sebaceous gland: a small gland in the skin that provides an oily secretion that coats the hair and skin with a softening, waterproof film.

secondary care teams: groups of healthcare providers who deliver specialized services to hospital patients.

secondary source: a document that summarizes the results of several studies.

secretion: the release of a liquid substance from blood, cells, or tissues.

select agents: highly dangerous and strictly controlled substances that can potentially be used to develop biological or chemical weapons.

self-advocate: to speak up for yourself.

semen: a thick, milky white fluid that supports sperm on their way to the uterus.

semi-Fowler's: an inclined position in which the patient's body is elevated at 30 degrees.

sensory impairments: conditions such as hearing loss, vision loss, or speech difficulties that may create communication barriers.

service-learning: an educational experience that integrates academic achievement with community service.

sesamoid bones: small, flat, sesame seed-shaped bones embedded within tendons or joint capsules to withstand friction.

sexual harassment: unwelcome sexual advances; requests for sexual favors; and other verbal, nonverbal, or physical conduct of a sexual nature.

sharps: needles, scalpels, or other sharp-edged objects found in healthcare settings that can puncture the skin.

shift report: a statement that tells oncoming staff the information necessary for a smooth continuation of patient care.

short bones: bones that are as long as they are wide; are made of spongy bone covered by a layer of compact bone.

sign: evidence of a health condition that can be seen or measured.

simulate: to imitate an action.

sinus cavities: air-filled spaces around the nose that contain mucous membranes that help defend against infection.

skeletal muscle: voluntary, striated muscle that connects to bones and is responsible for movement.

sleep deficit: a lack of sufficient sleep.

small intestines: tube that carries digested food from the stomach to the large intestine; nutrient absorption happens in different sections of the small intestines.

smooth muscle: involuntary muscle tissue located in the body's visceral organs and blood vessels; also known as *visceral muscle.*

social determinants of health (SDOH): nonmedical factors related to where a person is born and lives that influence their health status.

social media: a group of online communication tools that allow people to share information and resources via the internet.

Social Security: a government program that provides retirement income, disability, and survivors' benefits.

social wellness: involves building positive relationships and interacting in a meaningful way with those around you.

socioeconomics: the combined force of social class and income.

soft skills: employability skills related to communication, attitude, teamwork, and problem solving that are difficult to teach but critical to workplace success.

solute: a chemical in a solution.

solutions: uniform mixtures of two or more substances, which may be solids, liquids, gases, or a combination of these.

solvent: a liquid that is used to dissolve a chemical in a solution.

sonographers: healthcare professionals who create medical images or treat diseases using high-frequency sound waves.

sperm: male gametes.

sphygmomanometer: a medical instrument that measures blood pressure; may be aneroid or digital.

spinal cavity: the part of the dorsal cavity that contains the spinal cord.

spinal nerve: thirty-one pairs of nerves that connect the spinal cord to the rest of the body.

spleen: a lymphatic organ located just below the diaphragm that makes lymphocytes, filters the blood, and removes old red blood cells.

spongy bone: the lighter, less dense inner layer of bone tissue that contains red bone marrow.

stamina: endurance.

standard anatomical position: the agreed-upon reference for body position when studying anatomy; standing erect, facing frontward, with the arms at the sides and palms facing forward.

standard of care: the level of service a healthcare professional is expected to provide to a patient based on that professional's position and the patient's condition.

standard operating procedures (SOPs): established methods that describe the exact steps to be followed when completing a laboratory task.

standard precautions: steps that a healthcare worker takes with all patients to prevent the spread of infection.

statistics: term for the science that includes the collection, organization, and interpretation of numerical data.

stem cells: cells that can duplicate themselves many times and develop into many different types of cells.

stents: tubular supports used to keep arteries, blood vessels, canals, or ducts open to aid healing or prevent an obstruction.

stereotype: the assumption that everyone in a particular group is the same.

sterile technique: the practice of using sterilization to prevent the introduction of pathogens during invasive procedures.

stethoscope: a medical instrument that amplifies sounds within the body.

stomach: a reservoir in which food is broken down before it enters the small intestine.

stress: physical, mental, or emotional pressure caused by change.

striated: arranged in a striped pattern.

subcutaneous fat: fat below the skin that provides padding to absorb shock, holds in body heat, and stores energy.

subjective observations: an indication of a health condition that is experienced by the patient; also called a *symptom.*

sudoriferous gland: gland in the dermis that secretes sweat.

suffix: letters after a root word that identify the part of speech, if it is singular or plural, or add to the meaning of the word.

superficial: a directional term that refers to the outside surface of the body.

superior: a directional term that means above or higher up on the body.

supine: lying face up with the arms out to the sides and palms facing up.

Support Services: the career pathway that focuses on creating a therapeutic environment for providing patient care.

susceptible host: anyone who can contract a disease.

sutured: term that describes the way cranial bones grow together to form a strong and immovable joint.

symptom: an indication of a disease or disorder experienced by the patient, such as pain.

synapse: a tiny gap between an axon and a receptor cell.

system: an organized structure composed of many parts that work together and depend on each other to carry out a set of functions.

systemic: affecting the entire body.

systemic loop: the flow of blood from the heart to the body systems and back to drop off nutrients and pick up waste.

T

table: a chart that arranges data in rows or columns.

tact: the ability to communicate difficult or embarrassing information without giving offense.

tare weight: the weight of an empty container.

target audience: a specific group of people for whom a technical document is written.

taste bud: a sensory cell that converts flavors into electrical signals.

team nursing: a care model in which an RN functions as a team leader for a group of nursing staff members; together the group divides the nursing care tasks.

technical reading: a skill used to comprehend science, business, or technology publications.

technical service representatives: workers who help solve technical problems that customers encounter.

technical skills: practical tasks performed in a specific healthcare discipline or department.

technical training: education lasting two years or less and leading to an industry certificate, a technical diploma, or an associate's degree.

technical writing: a type of writing used in the workplace to inform or persuade a specific audience.

teleconferencing: the use of telephones to hold meetings that allows healthcare professionals to interact and collaborate over long distances.

telehealth: the use of electronic information and telecommunications technologies to support long-distance clinical healthcare, health-related education, public health, and health administration.

telemedicine: the segment of telehealth that involves the remote diagnosis and treatment of patients using telecommunications technology.

telephone triage: a system for assessing patient needs to determine if patients require emergency treatment, an appointment with a doctor, or self-care at home.

telesurgery: surgery performed by robotic equipment that is monitored and controlled from a remote site.

temporal artery thermometers: devices for measuring body temperature at the temporal artery in the forehead.

temporal lobes: lobes of the brain that lie near the ears and control hearing, balance, emotions, speech planning, and memory associations.

tendon: a tough, fibrous tissue that connects muscles to bones.

terminal branches: branches located at the end of an axon, which connect to other cells.

terminal cleaning: procedure for cleaning and disinfecting a patient hospital room in preparation for a newly admitted patient.

tertiary source: a document compiled from primary and secondary sources that gives an overview of a specific topic.

testes: the male sex organs.

thalamus: area of the brain that acts as a relay station for sorting, interpreting, and directing sensory signals to the appropriate area of the cerebral cortex.

therapeutic: treatment given to maintain or restore health.

therapeutic diet: a special food plan ordered by a physician to help treat a disease.

Therapeutic Services: the career pathway that focuses on changing a patient's health status over time through direct care.

third-party payers: an insurance company that pays the healthcare service provider for services rendered to a patient.

thoracic cavity: the part of the ventral cavity that lies above the diaphragm muscle; includes the pericardial cavity and two pleural cavities.

thoracic duct: lymphatic vessel that collects fluid from your cisterna chyli, lower body, left arm, and chest.

thrombocytes: cell fragments that help form blood clots to repair injured blood vessels.

throughput: the factor of a system that refers to how the system processes or uses the inputs.

thymus: a butterfly-shaped organ in the chest that helps program lymphocytes to respond to infection.

thyroid gland: the largest endocrine gland in the body, which controls energy, metabolism, and calcium levels in the blood.

tier: one of two or more rows, levels, or ranks arranged one above another.

tissue: a group of cells of the same type working together for the same purpose.

tonsils: lymphatic tissues located near the back of the throat that help protect against infection.

tort: an action that harms another person's body or property or takes away freedom of action in some way.

total lung capacity: the amount of air the lungs can hold during the deepest possible breath.

trachea: the tube that leads from the larynx to the lungs; also known as the *windpipe*.

transcriptionist: a health information technician who types medical record information from a physician's recorded dictation.

transmission-based precautions: special steps used in addition to standard precautions, chosen based on how the patient's infection is spread.

transport technicians: healthcare workers who take patients to and from diagnostic imaging appointments and maintain transportation devices.

transverse plane: the body plane that divides the body into top and bottom sections.

trauma-informed: understanding the influence of stressful events on health and behavior.

tympanic membrane: thin membrane that divides the outer and middle ear and changes sound waves into vibrations; also known as the *eardrum*.

U

unconscious: being unaware of surroundings or different attitudes.

union: organization that brings together workers from the same company or region to bargain collectively.

unit cost: the price of one measurable unit of a food item, such as 1 pound, 1 ounce, or 1 piece.

United States Department of Agriculture (USDA): a government agency that regulates the agriculture industry and researches and recommends diets for maintaining and improving general health.

ureter: a tube that leads from the kidney to the bladder.

urethra: a thin tube that leads from the bladder to outside of the body.

urinals: measuring devices for urine that are used by males confined to a bed.

urinalysis: the examination of urine's physical, chemical, and microscopic properties.

US customary units: the main system of weights and measures used in the United States based on the yard, pound, and gallon as units of length, weight, and liquid volume respectively; also known as *household measurements*.

US Department of Veterans Affairs (VA): a government agency that provides healthcare benefits, programs, and facilities to support the unique needs of those who have served in the military.

US Food and Drug Administration (FDA): a government agency that regulates products in the food and drug industries and develops Nutrition Facts labels to help consumers make informed food choices.

US Public Health Service (USPHS): a government agency that supports public health during manmade and natural disasters.

uterus: a hollow, muscular organ that receives and nourishes a fertilized egg.

UV-C disinfection: a device that emits UV-C rays to disinfect areas.

V

vaccinations: substances that stimulate your immune system to build protection against a particular disease; also called *immunizations*.

vacuole: an organelle that allows larger enzymes and waste molecule packages to pass through the cell membrane.

vagina: a muscular tube that leads from the uterus and cervix out of the body.

values: beliefs that express which principles are most important to a person.

valves: parts of a vein that prevent backflow as blood moves against gravity toward the heart.

vas deferens: a duct through which sperm leave a testicle; also called the *ductus deferens*.

vein: a blood vessel that moves blood from body tissues toward the heart.

ventral: a directional term used to describe surfaces that move closer together when you bend a joint.

ventral cavity: the cavity in the front of the body that is surrounded by the ribs and pelvic bones.

ventricle: a chamber at the bottom of the heart that pumps blood out to the rest of the body.

vestibular canals: chamber in the ear that senses movement of fluid.

villi: finger-like projections in the intestines that increase their surface area.

virtual reality: technology that shuts out all parts of a person's environment and provides an entire simulation.

virus: a very small pathogen that invades and reproduces inside other cells.

visual learners: people who prefer to learn through pictures and have a good understanding of direction, spacing, and location.

vital signs: the key measurements that provide information about a person's health; include temperature, pulse, respiration, and blood pressure.

vitreous humor: a clear fluid that maintains the eye's shape.

voluntary: under conscious control.

W

waived tests: simple tests with little risk of error.

Western medicine: the most common form of medical care in the United States; uses medication and surgery to treat the signs and symptoms of illness.

worker's compensation: government healthcare program in which plans cover injuries that happen while people are working on a job.

work ethic: a belief in the benefits of working hard, demonstrating initiative, and being personally accountable for the work you do.

workplace violence: acts of verbal abuse, threats, physical assault, or homicide that occur at work.

work styles: different methods that individuals might prefer to complete a job task.

World Health Organization (WHO): an agency of the United Nations that is concerned with international public health.

wrongful discharge: dismissal from a job without cause.

Y

yield: the number of portions a recipe will produce.

Z

zygote: the genetically unique cell that results from fertilization and contains 46 chromosomes.

Index

appointment scheduling, 137–138
aptitudes, 236
aqueous humor, 792
ARC (American Red Cross), 218, 340, 342, 540
arrhythmia, 732
arteries, 718, 725
arthritis, 674
artificial intelligence (AI), 18–19, 564
ASD (autism spectrum disorder), 288
aseptic practices, 52, 68–73
ASL (American Sign Language), 545, 789–790
aspiration, 222
assault and battery, 615
assays, 234, 237, 241
assertive communication style, 370, 374–375
Association of Surgical Technologists, 358
asthma, 743
astigmatism, 792
atherosclerosis, 730–731
athletic trainers, 700
atoms, 649
atria of heart, 729–730
atrioventricular (AV) node, 731
attrition bias, 519
audiology, 190–191
audiometer, 196
auditory brainstem response (ABR), 787
auditory learners, 94
auscultation, 405
autism spectrum disorder (ASD), 288
autoclaves, 71–72
automated analyzer, 453
automated external defibrillator (AED), 340
autonomic nervous system, 774
autonomy, 579
AV (atrioventricular) node, 731
axial skeleton, 685, 694–695
axons, 762

B

Background Information Disclosure (BID) form, 350
back pain, 44
Back to Sleep® campaign, 13
bacteria, 53, 55–56
balance and position, 785
ball-and-socket joints, 696
barcode technology, 454
bar graph, 512–513
basal cell carcinoma, 678
basal ganglia, 764, 767–769
base rates, 527
basophils, 736

BATHE technique, 288–289
B-cells, 737
bedmaking, 220–221
behavioral health
    maladaptive and risky behaviors, 290–293
    mental and behavioral development, 286–289
    mental health conditions, 289–290, 560–561
behavioral observation audiometry, 787–788
beneficence, 579
bias, 509, 519
BID (Background Information Disclosure) form, 350
bile, 815
bioassays, 241
biobanking, 594
bioethics, 593–594. *See also* ethical issues
Biohazard Prevention Act, 625
biohazards
    protections from, 624–625
    signs warning of, 67
    types of, 247–248
bioinformatics, 245, 447, 464
biomechanical technology, 19–20
biomedical engineers, 243
biomedicine, 830–833
bioreactors, 242
biorepositories, 464
biosafety guidelines, 248–249
biotechnology research and development
    advances in, 236–237, 570–571
    biosafety guidelines, 248–249
    career choices, 239–245
    clinical laboratories, 238
    description of, 101–102
    HOSA connections, 258–259
    laboratory safety protocols, 249–250
    laboratory tasks, 250–256
    overview, 234–235, 248
    personal traits for, 235–236
    regulation of research in, 565–568
    research funding for, 568
    sales and technical support skills, 256–258
    technology applications, 457–463
bioterrorism, 80–81
bipolar disorder, 768
blastocyst, 837
blood, 721–724
bloodborne pathogen exposure, 68
Bloodborne Pathogens Standard, 623, 625
blood-brain barrier, 771
blood filtration, 820–823
blood pressure, 333–336, 732–733
blood vessels, 725–727, 730–731

BLS (Bureau of Labor Statistics), 44
BMI (body mass index), 509, 514–516
body alignment, 192–194
body language, 403–404, 416
body mass index (BMI), 509, 514–516
body mechanics, 34, 45
body organization
    abdominal regions and quadrants, 660–661
    anatomical position, 657
    atoms and molecules, 649
    cavities, 661–663
    cells and organelles, 649–652
    directions, 657–659
    organs and systems, 653–655
    planes, 663–664
    regions and sections, 660
    tissues and membranes, 652
body systems
    cardiovascular system, 718–733
    digestive system, 808–817
    endocrine system, 795–801
    excretory (urinary) system, 818–824
    integumentary system, 672–684
    lymphatic system, 734–741
    muscular system, 699–710
    nervous system, 758–780
    reproductive systems, 825–841
    respiratory system, 742–751
    skeletal system, 685–698
    special senses, 781–794
bones
    central nervous system protected by, 771–772
    development of, 688–691
    markings on, 692–694
    ossicles, in ear, 785
    parts of, 687–688
    types of, 691–692
boundaries, 278–279
bradypnea, 749
brain
    blood-brain barrier, 771
    dementia, 759
    development of, 761–764
    forebrain, 764–769
    hindbrain, 770
    imaging of, 188–189
    midbrain, 769
    spinal cord, 770
    traumatic brain injury, 759
brainstem, 770
breach, 428, 433
breach of contract, 609
brittle bone disease, 688
bronchi, 746–747
Bureau of Labor Statistics (BLS), 44
business letters, 391
business operations, 208–211
business-to-business selling, 247, 256

C

call screening, 380–381
CAM (complementary and alternative medicine), 23, 296, 303–305
cancellations of appointments, 139
cancer, 678, 735, 739
capillary bed, 718, 726
CAPTA (Child Abuse Prevention and Treatment Act), 617
carbohydrates, 268–269
cardiac muscle, 699, 701
cardiographic technicians, 188
cardiologists, 721
cardiopulmonary resuscitation (CPR), 340
cardiovascular system
    blood, 721–724
    blood vessels, 725–727
    cardiac cycle and vital signs, 731–733
    diseases and disorders, 719–721
    heart, 728–730
    overview, 719
career and technical student organizations (CTSOs), 115
career assessments, 111
career ladders
    clinical laboratory, 185
    dental office, 106–107
    medical imaging, 185
    medical research, 241
    nursing, 106–107, 158
    occupational therapy, 153
    overview, 99
    physical therapy, 153
career portfolios, 108, 114–115, 348, 358–359
career preparation
    career clusters and pathways, 100–104
    career selection, 109–113
    job titles and credentials, 105
    national health science standards, 108–109
    student organizations and, 115
career skills in healthcare
    biotechnology research and development, 247–259
    changing jobs, 359–361
    conflict resolution, 319–321
    cultural competence, 415–421
    decision-making, 582
    diagnostic services, 192–199
    employability skills, 344–345, 353–354
    health informatics services, 132–139
    healthy relationships, 278–279, 301–303
    leadership, 322–325
    reading and writing, 383–401

    speaking and listening, 370–382
    stress management, 277–278
    succeeding at work, 353–354
    support services, 219–227
    teamwork, 312–321
    therapeutic services, 163–171
    time management, 299–301
    universal technical skills, 325–342
caregiver background form, 350
caregiver laws, 614
carpal tunnel syndrome, 706
Carson, Benjamin, 9
case managers, 217. 316
cataracts, 759, 792
cavities, in body organization, 656, 661–663
CBER (Center for Biologics Evaluation and Research) of FDA, 597
CCR (continuous compression resuscitation), 342
CDC (Centers for Disease Control and Prevention). *See* Centers for Disease Control and Prevention (CDC)
cell body, 762
cell membrane, 651–652
cells, 648–652
Celsius scale of temperature, 497–499
Center for Biologics Evaluation and Research (CBER, FDA), 597
Centers for Disease Control and Prevention (CDC)
    clinical laboratories, 238
    hand hygiene, 12
    healthcare environment, 69
    infant and children's measurements, 517–519
    infectious diseases, 53
    laboratory quality improvement, 626
    multidrug-resistant organisms (MDROs), 56
    overview, 539
    reporting health and safety incidents, 624
    safety, 34, 44
    standard precautions, 58
    vaccinations, 283, 591
Centers for Medicare and Medicaid Services (CMS), 431, 434, 539
central nervous system
    blood-brain barrier, 771
    bones protecting, 771–772
    brain development, 761–764
    cerebrospinal fluid (CSF), 772–773
    description of, 758
    forebrain, 764–769
    hindbrain, 770
    meninges, 770–771
    midbrain, 769
    spinal cord, 770

central services, 206, 212
cerebellum, 770
cerebral cortex, 764
cerebrospinal fluid (CSF), 772–773
cerebrovascular accident (CVA), 719, 764
cerebrum, 758, 764
Certification Board for Sterile Processing and Distribution, 212
certified nursing assistant (CNA), 158
CERT (Community Emergency Response Team) skills, 33
cervix, 828–829
CEUs (continuing education units), 358
chain of infection, 52, 56–58
CHAMPVA, 551
charts and graphs, 512–514
Child Abuse Prevention and Treatment Act (CAPTA), 617
childbirth, 835, 839–841
child protective services (CPS), 617
Children's Health Insurance Program (CHIP), 550
children's measurements, 517–519
chlamydia, 829
choroid, 793
chronic illness, 16
chronic obstructive pulmonary disease (COPD), 747
chronological filing, 136
cilia, 744
circle graph, 512, 514
circular muscles, 707
circulatory system. *See* cardiovascular system
cisterna chyli vessel, 740
civil law, 606–607
Civil Rights Act of 1964, 607, 631–632
claims process, 480, 482–486
CLIA (Clinical Laboratory Improvement Act) practices, 625–626
clinical data, 438
clinical engineers, 213
clinical laboratories
    career ladder, 185
    careers in, 181–184
    certifications, 238
Clinical Laboratory Improvement Act (CLIA) practices, 625–626
clinical laboratory technicians, 184
clinical nursing, 145
clinical simulators, 454
clinical training, 146, 153
clinical trials, 234, 240
cloning, 832–833
clusters and pathways for careers, 99–104
CMS (Centers for Medicare and Medicaid Services), 431, 434, 539
CNA (certified nursing assistant), 158

glands of endocrine system, 799–801
glial cells, 773
gliding joints, 697
gloving, sterile, 169–170
GLPs (good laboratory practices), 240
glymphatic system, 773
GMPs (good manufacturing processes), 241–242
goal setting, 298–299
Golgi apparatus, 651–652
gonads, 825–826
goniometer, 480, 494–495
gonorrhea, 829
good laboratory practices (GLPs), 240
good manufacturing processes (GMPs), 241–242
Good Samaritan laws, 340
Government Accounting Office, 598
government agencies, 538–540
graduated cylinder, 506
granulocytes, 736
graphic design, 246
graphing vital signs, 336–339
greenstick fracture, 697–698
grief management, 294–295
gross pay, 356
ground-fault circuit interrupter (GFCI), 80
gustation (taste), 783

H

hair follicles, 680–681
HAIs (healthcare-associated infections), 56
hand hygiene, 12, 60–62
harassment, 44, 627, 632
harm *versus* benefit, 525–527
Hazard Communication Standard (HCS), 623–625
hazardous chemicals, 40–41
HCS (Hazard Communication Standard), 623–625
HDHP (high-deductible health plan), 553
Healing the Children, 358
health and safety incident reporting, 623–624
health and safety specialists, 244
health and wellness managers and coaches, 215
healthcare
    accessibility and affordability, 24–25, 589–590
    clusters and pathways, 100–104
    delivery systems, 536–546
    disparities in, 284, 558–559
    economic systems, 547–553
    evolution of, 4–31
    facility environment, 212–213
    management of, 209–210

mandates for, 591–592
    privacy in, 621–622
healthcare-associated infections (HAIs), 56
health disparities, 284, 558–559
health educators, 130
health informatics services, 120–143
    careers in, 124–127
    description of, 101–102
    education and training, 128–129
    filing, 136–137
    HOSA connections, 139
    patient interaction, 129–131
    patient records, 132–136
    personal traits, 123–124
    scheduling, 137–139
    technology, 127–128
health information exchange (HIE), 431
health information technology (HIT), 431
Health Information Technology for Economic and Clinical Health (HITECH) Act of 2009, 431–434, 622
Health Insurance Exchange Marketplace, 550, 560
Health Insurance Portability and Accountability Act (HIPAA)
    description of, 619
    Privacy Rule of, 318, 431, 435, 621–622
    regulatory and paperwork additions, 553
health literacy, 409, 412–413, 559
health maintenance, 264–309
    complementary and alternative medicine (CAM), 303–305
    food nutrition, 268–273
    grief management, 294–295
    holistic health, 296–297
    intellectual wellness, 297–301
    mental and behavioral health, 286–293
    oral health, 283
    personal hygiene, 281
    physical activity, 274
    physical wellness, 267–268
    public health, 284–285
    relationships, 278–279
    screenings and examinations, 281–282
    sleep habits, 275–276
    social wellness, 301–303
    stress management, 277–278
    suicide, 293
    support, 293–294
    vaccinations, 283
    weight management, 275
health maintenance organizations (HMOs), 26, 551–552

Health Resources and Services Administration (HRSA), 539
health savings account (HSA), 553
hearing
    careers in, 189–190
    hearing loss, 788–789
    parts of ear, 785–786
    screenings for, 195–196, 786–788
heart, 728–730
heart and brain imaging, 188–189
heart murmur, 730
height and weight measurement, 326–328, 514–516
hemodialysis, 820
hemoglobin, 721
hepatitis, 809–810, 815
hepatitis B vaccines, 16
heredity, 831. *See also* genetics; reproductive system
HHS. *See* US Department of Health and Human Services (HHS)
HIE (health information exchange), 431
hierarchy, 542–543
high-deductible health plan (HDHP), 553
highlighting reading material, 91
Hill-Burton Act, 606
hindbrain, 770
hinge joints, 697
HIPAA (Health Insurance Portability and Accountability Act). *See* Health Insurance Portability and Accountability Act (HIPAA)
Hippocrates (ancient Greece), 12
Hippocratic Oath for Physicians, 579–580
hiring and discharge laws, 628–629
HIT (health information technology), 431
HITECH (Health Information Technology for Economic and Clinical Health) Act of 2009, 431–434, 622
HMOs (health maintenance organizations), 26, 551–552
holistic care, 6, 11–12, 296–297
Holland, John, 112, 322
Holter monitor procedures, 188
home health aides, 160
home healthcare, 541
homeostasis, 758, 760, 797
hormones
    endocrine system, 795–798, 801
    reproductive system, 833–835
HOSA—Future Health Professionals, 5, 89, 108, 110, 115, 121, 139, 145, 171, 177, 199, 205, 226–227, 233, 258–259, 265, 311, 369, 427, 471, 535, 577, 605, 641, 671, 717, 757, 807

PET (positron emission tomography) scans, 184
pharmaceutical companies, 542
pharmacogenetics, 801
pharmacogenomics, 570
pharynx, 745–746, 813–814
PHI (protected health information), 133, 432, 622
phlebotomists, 182, 184, 720
photoreceptors, 793–794
PHRs (personal health records), 428, 430, 435–436
physical activity, 274
physical examinations, 197–198, 406–407
physical therapist assistant, 700
physical therapists, 700
physical therapy, 153
physical wellness, 266–268
physician assistants (PAs), 27, 157–158
physician-assisted suicide, 581
physicians, 89, 156
Physician's Current Procedural Terminology (CPT, AMA), 481
Physician's Pledge, 579–580
physiology, 648–649. *See also* anatomy and physiology
pictograph, 512
pigment, 678
pineal gland, 801
pituitary gland, 798–799
pivot joints, 697
placebos, 240
placenta, 837, 839
Plan-Do-Check-Act (PDCA) model, 556
planes of body, 656, 663–664
plasma, 721–722
platelets (thrombocytes), 721–722
pleurae membranes, 748
plexus of spinal nerve roots, 778
plural medical terms, 645
pneumonia, 747
POA (power of attorney) for healthcare documents, 621
point-of-care testing, 182, 238, 451
point-of-service (POS) plans, 551–552
POMR (problem-oriented medical record) method of organization, 440
population health, 284
portfolios, career, 348, 358–359
portion, 497, 500
position and balance, 785
positioning patients, 193–194
positron emission tomography (PET) scans, 184
POS (point-of-service) plans, 551–552
posterior, 657–658
postgraduate education, 146, 154
postsecondary education, 101–105

post-traumatic stress disorder (PTSD), 769
power of attorney (POA) for healthcare documents, 621
PPE (personal protective equipment), 52, 60–64
PPOs (preferred provider organizations), 26, 551–552
precision medicine, 554, 570–571
pre-exposure prophylaxis (PrEP), 738
preferred provider organizations (PPOs), 26, 551–552
prefixes, 642, 644
pregnancy, 835
prejudice, 415, 421
premiums, insurance, 549
prenatal development, 837–839
PrEP (pre-exposure prophylaxis), 738
presbycusis (hearing loss), 788
prescriptions, filling, 169
preventive care, 280–281
preview of reading material, 91
primary care provider (PCP), 552
primary care teams, 315
primary motor cortex of brain, 765–766
primary nursing model, 316
primary sensory cortex, 781–782
primary source document, 447, 460–461
privacy
    healthcare and, 621–622
    notices of, 135
    patients and, 615–616
privileged communication, 616–618
probability, 521–522
problem-oriented medical record (POMR) method of organization, 440
problem solving, 301
professional development, 344, 357–358
professional distance, 303
professional organizations, 344, 357–358
professional standards, 354–355
prone, 657
pronunciation of medical terminology, 646–647
proportions, 475
proposals, 397–398
proprietary systems, 430
prospective payment system, 551
protected health information (PHI), 133, 432, 622
protein, 268, 270
protocols, 372, 377
proximal, 658
PSDA (Patient Self-Determination Act) of 1990, 620
psychosocial development stages (Erikson), 287
PTSD (post-traumatic stress disorder), 769

puberty, 833–835
publication bias, 520
public health, 280, 284–285
public health laboratory professionals, 183
public relations, 210–211
pull, aim, squeeze, sweep (PASS fire extinguishers), 74, 78
pulmonary loop, 718, 728
pulse, 330–331, 732
pulse oximeters, 332, 732

Q

quadriplegia, 772
quality and regulation careers, 244–245
quality assurance specialists, 244
quality control technicians, 244
quality improvement (QI) in feedback loop, 554–556
quantitative data, 527
quick response (QR) codes, 454

R

race. *See* diversity; health disparities
RACE (rescue, alarm, contain, extinguish/evacuate) in fire emergencies, 74, 76–77
radial pulse, 331
radiation exposure, 42
radiation therapist, 186–187
radio frequency identification (RFID) tracking technology, 455–456
radiology, 178, 186–187
Radium Girls, The (Moore), 31
range-of-motion (ROM) exercises, 163, 166–168
rapport, 419
rate, respiratory, 748–751
RDs (registered dietitians), 214
reabsorption, 818
reading strategies, 90–91
receptors, 781–782
recipes, standardized, 500–504
recommendation reports, 397–398
recreational therapy, 152, 701
rectal temperature, 329
rectum, 816–817
red blood cells, 721–722
reflexes, 774
regenerative medicine, 14, 16–17
regimens, drug, 464
regions and sections of body, 660
registered dietitians (RDs), 214
Registered Health Information Technician (RHIT) certification, 357
registered nurse (RN), 158–160. *See also* nursing

visual learners, 94
vital signs
blood pressure, 333–336
cardiac cycle, 731–733
graphing, 336–339
height and weight, 326–328
oxygen saturation, 332–333
pain assessment, 336
pulse, 330–331
respiration, 332
temperature, 328–330
vitamin C, 673
vitamins and minerals, 268, 270
vitreous humor, 792
vocabulary, studying, 95–96
vocal biomarkers, 19
voice technologies, 19
volume
measurement of, 251–253
respiratory system, 748–751
voluntary movement, 699, 704
volunteering opportunities, 227
VRE (vancomycin-resistant
Enterococcus), 56

W

wages, hours, and minimum age laws,
629–631
waived tests, 238, 254
Weed, Lawrence, 439
weight
charting, 514–516
managing, 275
measuring, 326–328
wellness promotion, 213–215
Western medicine, 6, 11
wheelchair transport, 48, 225–226
white blood cells, 721–722
WHO (World Health Organization).
See World Health Organization
(WHO)
whole medical systems, 23
WMA (World Medical Association), 580
Wolff's Law, 693
word parts, 643–644
work. *See* employment in healthcare
worker's compensation plans, 551
work ethic, 584

workplace harassment, 44
workplace violence, 42–44
work styles, 320
World Health Organization (WHO)
description of, 539
diagnosis coding system, 481
genetic engineering, 597
growth charts, 519
infectious diseases, 53, 569
World Medical Association (WMA), 580

X

X-rays, 184

Y

yield, 497, 500, 502

Z

zygotes, 831